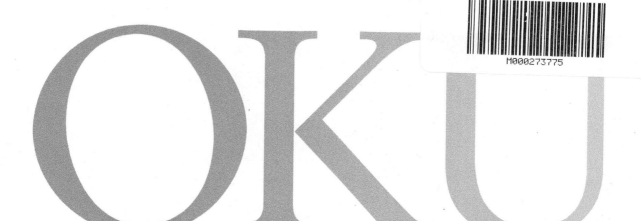

OKU 5

Orthopaedic Knowledge Update

Sports Medicine

M000273775

AAOS
AMERICAN ACADEMY OF ORTHOPAEDIC SURGEONS

OKU

5

Orthopaedic
Knowledge
Update

Sports Medicine

EDITOR

Mark D. Miller, MD
Head, Division of Sports Medicine
S. Ward Casscells Professor
Department of Orthopaedic Surgery
University of Virginia
Charlottesville, Virginia

Developed by the American Orthopaedic Society for Sports Medicine

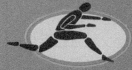
The American Orthopaedic
Society for Sports Medicine

AAOS
AMERICAN ACADEMY OF
ORTHOPAEDIC SURGEONS

AAOS
AMERICAN ACADEMY OF ORTHOPAEDIC SURGEONS

Board of Directors, 2015-2016

David D. Teuscher, MD
President

Gerald R. Williams Jr, MD
First Vice-President

William J. Maloney, MD
Second Vice-President

Frederick M. Azar, MD
Treasurer

Frederick M. Azar, MD
Past-President

Lisa K. Cannada, MD

Howard R. Epps, MD

Daniel C. Farber, MD

Daniel K. Guy, MD

Lawrence S. Halperin, MD

David A. Halsey, MD

David J. Mansfield, MD

Raj D. Rao, MD

Brian G. Smith, MD

Ken Sowards, MBA

Jennifer M. Weiss, MD

Karen L. Hackett, FACHE, CAE (*ex officio*)

Staff

Ellen C. Moore, *Chief Education Officer*

Hans Koelsch, PhD, *Director, Department of Publications*

Lisa Claxton Moore, *Senior Manager, Book Program*

Steven Kellert, *Senior Editor*

Courtney Dunker, *Editorial Production Manager*

Abram Fassler, *Publishing Systems Manager*

Suzanne O'Reilly, *Graphic Designer*

Susan Morritz Baim, *Production Coordinator*

Karen Danca, *Permissions Coordinator*

Charlie Baldwin, *Digital and Print Production Specialist*

Hollie Muir, *Digital and Print Production Specialist*

Emily Nickel, *Page Production Assistant*

Rachel Winokur, *Editorial Coordinator*

Genevieve Charet, *Editorial Coordinator*

Sylvia Orellana, *Publications Assistant*

The material presented in *Orthopaedic Knowledge Update: Sports Medicine 5* has been made available by the American Academy of Orthopaedic Surgeons for educational purposes only. This material is not intended to present the only, or necessarily best, methods or procedures for the medical situations discussed, but rather is intended to represent an approach, view, statement, or opinion of the author(s) or producer(s), which may be helpful to others who face similar situations. Some drugs or medical devices demonstrated in Academy courses or described in Academy print or electronic publications have not been cleared by the Food and Drug Administration (FDA) or have been cleared for specific uses only. The FDA has stated that it is the responsibility of the physician to determine the FDA clearance status of each drug or device he or she wishes to use in clinical practice. Furthermore, any statements about commercial products are solely the opinion(s) of the author(s) and do not represent an Academy endorsement or evaluation of these products. These statements may not be used in advertising or for any commercial purpose.

All rights reserved. No part of this publication may be reproduced, stored in a retrieval system, or transmitted, in any form, or by any means, electronic, mechanical, photocopying, recording, or otherwise, without prior written permission from the publisher.

Published 2016 by the
American Academy of Orthopaedic Surgeons
9400 West Higgins Road
Rosemont, IL 60018

Copyright 2016
by the American Academy of Orthopaedic Surgeons

Library of Congress Control Number:
2015945902

ISBN 978-1-62552-328-0
Printed in the USA

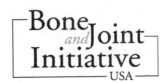

Acknowledgments

Editorial Board, Orthopaedic Knowledge Update: Sports Medicine 5

Mark D. Miller, MD
Head, Division of Sports Medicine
S. Ward Casscells Professor
Department of Orthopaedic Surgery
University of Virginia
Charlottesville, Virginia

Stephen F. Brockmeier, MD
Associate Professor
Department of Orthopaedics
University of Virginia
Charlottesville, Virginia

Cree M. Gaskin, MD
Associate Professor, Vice Chair, Associate Chief
*   Medical Information Officer*
Department of Radiology and Medical Imaging,
*   Orthopaedic Surgery*
University of Virginia Health System
Charlottesville, Virginia

F. Winston Gwathmey, MD
Assistant Professor of Orthopaedic Surgery
Department of Orthopaedic Surgery
University of Virginia Health System
Charlottesville, Virginia

James J. Irrgang, PhD, PT, ATC, FAPTA
Professor and Director of Clinical Research
Department of Orthopedic Surgery
University of Pittsburgh
Pittsburg, Pennsylvania

David R. McAllister, MD
Professor and Chief, Sports Medicine
Department of Orthopaedic Surgery
David Geffen School of Medicine at UCLA
Los Angeles, California

Matthew D. Milewski, MD
Assistant Professor of Orthopaedic Surgery and
*   Sports Medicine*
Elite Sports Medicine
Connecticut Children's Medical Center
Farmington, Connecticut

Sourav K. Poddar, MD
Associate Professor and Director, Primary Care
*   Sports Medicine*
Department of Family Medicine/Orthopedics
University of Colorado
Denver, Colorado

Francis H. Shen, MD
Warren G. Stamp Endowed Professor
Division Head, Spine Surgery
Department of Orthopaedic Surgery
University of Virginia Health Systems
Charlottesville, Virginia

Stephen R. Thompson, MD, Med, FRCSC
Associate Professor of Sports Medicine
Eastern Maine Medical Center
The University of Maine
Bangor, Maine

Kevin E. Wilk, PT, DPT, FAPTA
Clinical Director
Physical Therapy
Champion Sports Medicine
Birmingham, Alabama

AOSSM Board of Directors, 2015

Annunziato Amendola, MD
President-Elect

Charles A. Bush-Joseph, MD
Vice President

Rick D. Wilkerson, DO
Secretary

Andrew J. Cosgarea, MD
Treasurer

Robert A. Arciero, MD
Past President

Jo A. Hannafin, MD, PhD
Past President

Joseph H. Guettler, MD
Member at Large

C. Benjamin Ma, MD
Member at Large

Rick W. Wright, MD
Member at Large

Christopher C. Kaeding, MD
Ex-Officio

Bruce Reider, MD
Executive Editor, Medical Publishing
*   Board of Trustees*

Irv Bomberger
Executive Director

Explore the full portfolio of AAOS educational programs and publications across the orthopaedic spectrum for every stage of an orthopaedic surgeon's career, at www.aaos.org. The AAOS, in partnership with Jones & Bartlett Learning, also offers a comprehensive collection of educational and training resources for emergency medical providers, from first responders to critical care transport paramedics. Learn more at www.aaos.org/ems.

Contributors

Eduard Alentorn-Geli, MD, MSc, PhD, FEBOT
Orthopaedic Sport Medicine Fellow
Division of Sports Medicine
Department of Orthopaedic Surgery
Duke University Medical Center
Durham, North Carolina

David W. Altchek, MD
Attending Orthopaedic Surgeon
Department of Sports Medicine & Shoulder
    Surgery
Hospital for Special Surgery
New York, New York

George S. Athwal, MD, FRCSC
Orthopaedic Surgeon
Hand and Upper Limb Centre
St. Joseph's Health Care
London, Ontario, Canada

Christopher M. Bader, PhD, LP, CC-AASP
Counseling and Sports Psychologist
Intercollegiate Athletics
University of Colorado Boulder
Boulder, Colorado

Champ L. Baker, III, MD
Staff Physician
Department of Orthopaedic Surgery
Hughston Clinic
Columbus, Georgia

Champ L. Baker, Jr, MD
Staff Physician
Department of Orthopaedic Surgery
Hughston Clinic
Columbus, Georgia

Brenden J. Balcik, MD
Sports Medicine Fellow
Department of Family and Community
    Medicine
University of Arizona
Tucson, Arizona

F. Alan Barber, MD, FACS
Fellowship Director
Plano Orthopedic Sports Medicine and Spine
Plano, Texas

James T. Beckmann, MD, MS
Fellow
Department of Orthopaedics
Stanford University
Palo Alto, California

Sagir Girish Bera, DO, MPH, MS
Physician
Sports Medicine – Family Physician
University of Arizona
Tucson, Arizona

Johnathan A. Bernard, MD, MPH
Fellow
Department of Sports Medicine
Hospital for Special Surgery
New York, New York

Jacqueline R. Berning, PhD, RD, CSSD
Professor and Chair
University of Colorado, Colorado Springs
Health Science Department
Colorado Springs, Colorado

Ljiljana Bogunovic, MD
Sports Medicine Fellow
Department of Orthopaedic Surgery
Rush University Medical Center
Chicago, Illinois

Stephen F. Brockmeier, MD
Associate Professor
Department of Orthopaedics
University of Virginia
Charlottesville, Virginia

Robert H. Brophy, MD
Associate Professor, Sports Medicine
Department of Orthopaedic Surgery
Washington University School of Medicine
St. Louis, Missouri

Christopher A. Burks, MD
Bienville Orthopaedic Specialists
Pascagoula, Mississippi

Charles A. Bush-Joseph, MD
Professor of Orthopaedic Surgery
Department of Orthopaedic Surgery
Rush Medical Center
Chicago, Illinois

J.W. Thomas Byrd, MD
Nashville Sports Medicine Foundation
Clinical Professor, Department of Orthopaedic
*   Surgery and Rehabilitation*
Vanderbilt University School of Medicine
Nashville, Tennessee

A. Bobby Chhabra, MD
Professor and Chair
Department of Orthopaedic Surgery
University of Virginia
Charlottesville, Virginia

Brian J. Chilelli, MD
Orthopaedic Surgeon
Cadence Physician Group Orthopaedics,
*   Sports Medicine*
Northwestern Medicine, West Region
Warrenville, Illinois

Terese L. Chmielewski, PT, PhD, SCS
Associate Professor
Department of Physical Therapy
University of Florida
Gainesville, Florida

J.H. James Choi, MD
Orthopaedic Sports Medicine Fellow
Division of Sports Medicine
Department of Orthopaedic Surgery
Duke University
Durham, North Carolina

Melissa A. Christino, MD
Orthopedic Sports Medicine Fellow
Division of Sports Medicine
Boston Children's Hospital
Boston, Massachusetts

Thomas O. Clanton, MD
Director, Foot and Ankle Sports Medicine
The Steadman Clinic
Vail, Colorado

Nathan Coleman, MD
Sports Medicine Fellow
Department of Orthopaedic Surgery
Hospital for Special Surgery
New York, New York

Evan J. Conte, MD
Sports Medicine Fellow
University of Virginia
Department of Orthopaedics
Charlottesville, Virginia

Andrew J. Cosgarea, MD
Professor, Department of Orthopaedic Surgery
Director, Division of Sports Medicine
Johns Hopkins University
Baltimore, Maryland

Aristides I. Cruz, Jr, MD
Clinical Assistant Professor
Warren Alpert Medical School of Brown
*   University*
Hasbro Children's Hospital
Division of Pediatric Orthopedics
Providence, Rhode Island

George J. Davies, MD, DPT, MED, PT, SCS,
**   ATC, LAT, CSAS, PES, FAPTA**
Professor, Physical Therapy Program
Armstrong State University
Savannah, Georgia

Thomas M. DeBerardino, MD
Associate Professor
Department of Orthopaedic Surgery
University of Connecticut Health Center
Farmington, Connecticut

Ryan M. Degen, MD, MSc, FRCSC
Orthopedic Sports Medicine Fellow
Department of Orthopedics, Sports Medicine
*   and Shoulder Service*
Hospital for Special Surgery
New York, New York

Joshua S. Dines, MD
Associate Attending Orthopedic Surgeon
Department of Orthopaedic Surgery
Hospital for Special Surgery
New York, New York

Laurie D. Donaldson, MD
Team Physician, USA Hockey National Team
*   Development Program*
Department of Orthopaedic Surgery
University of Michigan
Ann Arbor, Michigan

Jonathan A. Drezner, MD
Professor
Department of Family Medicine
University of Washington
Seattle, Washington

Guillaume D. Dumont, MD
Assistant Professor
Department of Orthopaedic Surgery and Sports
    Medicine
University of South Carolina School of
    Medicine
Columbia, South Carolina

Warren R. Dunn, MD, MPH
Associate Professor
Department of Orthopedics and Rehabilitation
University of Wisconsin
Madison, Wisconsin

Alexander E. Ebinger, MD
Assistant Professor
Department of Emergency Medicine
University of Colorado Hospital
Aurora, Colorado

Eric W. Edmonds, MD
Director of Orthopaedic Research
Rady Children's Hospital San Diego
University of California San Diego
San Diego, California

Youssef El Bitar, MD
Orthopaedic Sports Medicine Fellow
Department of Orthopaedics and Rehabilitation
University of Iowa Hospitals and Clinics
Iowa City, Iowa

John J. Elias, PhD
Senior Research Scientist
Department of Orthopaedic Surgery
Akron General Medical Center
Akron, Ohio

Todd S. Ellenbecker, DPT, MS, SCS, OCS,
    CSCS
Clinic Director
Physiotherapy Associates
Scottsdale Sports Clinic
Scottsdale, Arizona

Keelan Enseki, MS, PT, OCS, SCS, ATC, CSCS
Orthopaedic Physical Therapy Program
    Director
Center for Rehab Services – Center for Sports
    Medicine
University of Pittsburgh Medical Center
Pittsburgh, Pennsylvania

Rafael F. Escamilla, PhD, PT, CSCS, FACSM
California State University, Sacramento
Department of Physical Therapy
Sacramento, California

Michael S. Ferrell, MD
Orthopedic Surgeon
Bridger Orthopedic and Sports Medicine
Bozeman, Montana

Ted J. Ganley, MD
Director of Sports Medicine
Division of Orthopaedics
The Children's Hospital of Philadelphia
Philadelphia, Pennsylvania

Penny Lauren Goldberg, PT, DPT, ATC
Physical Therapist
Sports Physical Therapy
Request Physical Therapy
Gainesville, Florida

Petar Golijanin, BS
Research Coordinator
Sports Medicine Service
Massachusetts General Hospital
Boston, Massachusetts

Andreas H. Gomoll, MD
Associate Professor of Orthopedic Surgery
Harvard Medical School
Cartilage Repair Center
Department of Orthopedic Surgery
Brigham and Women's Hospital
Boston, Massachusetts

Marci A. Goolsby, MD
Assistant Attending Physician
Primary Care Sports Medicine Service
Hospital for Special Surgery
New York, New York

Joshua A. Greenspoon, BSc
Research Scholar
Steadman Philippon Research Institute
Vail, Colorado

Imran Hafeez, MD
Sports Medicine Specialist
Elite Sports Medicine
Connecticut Children's Medical Center
Hartford, Connecticut

Kimberly G. Harmon, MD
Professor
Department of Family Medicine
Department of Orthopaedics and Sports
*   Medicine*
University of Washington
Seattle, Washington

Hamid Hassanzadeh, MD
Assistant Professor
Department of Orthopaedic Surgery
University of Virginia
Charlottesville, Virginia

John P. Haverstock, MD, FRCSC
Clinical Fellow
Roth McFarlane Hand and Upper Limb Center
St. Joseph's Health Care
London, Ontario, Canada

Benton E. Heyworth, MD
Orthopaedic Surgeon, Clinical Instructor in
*   Orthopaedic Surgery*
Department of Orthopaedic Surgery
Boston Children's Hospital
Boston, Massachusetts

Todd R. Hooks, PT, ATC, OCS, SCS,
   NREMT-1, CSCS, CMTPT, FAAOMPT
Assistant Athletic Trainer/Physical Therapist
New Orleans Pelicans
Metairie, Louisiana

Jeffrey A. Housner, MD, MBA
Team Physician
Department of Orthopaedic Surgery
University of Michigan Athletic Department
Ann Arbor, Michigan

Jeffrey Taylor Jobe, MD
Clinical Volunteer
Department of Orthopedic Surgery
University of Virginia Health Systems
Charlottesville, Virginia

Nicholas S. Johnson, MD
Research Fellow
The Steadman Clinic
Vail, Colorado

Debi Jones, PT, DPT, SCS, OCS, CSCS
Staff Physical Therapist
Department of Rehabilitation
University of Florida Health
Gainesville, Florida

Jeremy B. Kent, MD, CAQSM
Assistant Professor, Team Physician
University of Virginia Athletics
Department of Family Medicine
University of Virginia Health Systems
Charlottesville, Virginia

A. Jay Khanna, MD, MBA
Professor
Department of Orthopaedic Surgery
Johns Hopkins University
Bethesda, Maryland

W. Benjamin Kibler, MD
Medical Director
Shoulder Center of Kentucky
Lexington Clinic
Lexington, Kentucky

David Kohlrieser, DPT, PT, OCS, SCS, CSCS
Physical Therapist
OSU Sports Medicine
The Ohio State University Wexner Medical
*   Center*
Columbus, Ohio

Regina Kostyun, MSEd, ATC
Concussion Program Coordinator
Elite Sports Medicine
Elite Sports Medicine
Connecticut Children's Medical Center
Farmington, Connecticut

Christopher M. Larson, MD
Program Director
FV/MOSMI Sports Medicine Fellowship
Program
Twin Cities Orthopedics
Edina, Minnesota

Matthew S. Leiszler, MD
Football Team Physician
University Health Services
University of Notre Dame
Notre Dame, Indiana

John M. MacKnight, MD, FACSM
Medical Director and Team Physician
Department of Internal Medicine and Primary
Care Sports Medicine
University of Virginia
Charlottesville, Virginia

RobRoy L. Martin, PhD, PT
Professor
Department of Physical Therapy
Duquesne University
Pittsburgh, Pennsylvania

Richard Charles Mather III, MD
Surgeon, Assistant Professor
Duke Sports Medicine
Duke University
Durham, North Carolina

Stephanie W. Mayer, MD
Fellow
Orthopaedic Surgery
Hospital for Special Surgery
New York, New York

Lucas S. McDonald, MD, MPH,&TM
Fellow
Sports Medicine and Shoulder Surgery
Hospital for Special Surgery
New York, New York

William R. Miele, MD
Assistant in Orthopaedic Surgery
Department of Orthopaedic Surgery
The Johns Hopkins Hospital
Baltimore, Maryland

Matthew D. Milewski, MD
Assistant Professor of Orthopaedic Surgery and
Sports Medicine
Elite Sports Medicine
Connecticut Children's Medical Center
Farmington, Connecticut

Peter J. Millett, MD, MSc
Orthopaedic Surgeon
Director of Shoulder Service
The Steadman Clinic
Vail, Colorado

Claude T. Moorman III, MD
Orthopaedic Surgeon
Division of Sports Medicine
Department of Orthopaedic Surgery
Duke University
Durham, North Carolina

Nicholas C. Nacey, MD
Assistant Professor
Radiology and Medical Imaging
University of Virginia
Charlottesville, Virginia

Brian J. Neuman, MD
Assistant Professor of Orthopaedic Surgery
Department of Orthopaedic Surgery
Johns Hopkins University
Baltimore, Maryland

Kelly L. Neville, MS
Department of Biology
University of Colorado, Colorado Springs
Colorado Springs, Colorado

Shane J. Nho, MD, MS
Assistant Professor
Department of Orthopaedic Surgery
Rush University Medical Center
Chicago, Illinois

Carl W. Nissen, MD
Physician
Elite Sports Medicine
Connecticut Children's Medical Center
Farmington, Connecticut

Meredith C. Northam, MD
Assistant Professor
Department of Musculoskeletal Radiology
University of North Carolina
Chapel Hill, North Carolina

Brett D. Owens, MD
Orthopaedic Surgeon
John A. Feagin, Jr. Sports Medicine Fellowship
Keller Army Hospital
West Point, New York

Mark V. Paterno, PT, PhD, MBA, SCS, ATC
Associate Professor
Division of Sports Medicine, Division of
*   Occupational Therapy, and Physical Therapy*
Cincinnati Children's Hospital Medical Center
Cincinnati, Ohio

Jeanne C. Patzkowski, MD
Orthopaedic Surgery Fellow
John A. Feagin Jr. Sports Medicine Fellowship
Keller Army Community Hospital
West Point, New York

Stephen E. Paul, MD
Associate Professor
Department of Sports Medicine
University of Arizona
Tucson, Arizona

Andrew D. Pearle, MD
Orthopedic Surgeon
Shoulder and Sports Medicine Service
Hospital for Special Surgery
New York, New York

Maximilian Petri, MD
Orthopaedic Surgeon, Research Fellow
The Steadman Clinic
Steadman Philippon Research Institute
Vail, Colorado

Jennifer L. Pierce, MD
Musculoskeletal Radiologist
Department of Radiology
University of Virginia
Charlottesville, Virginia

Matthew T. Provencher, MD
Chief
Sports Medicine Service
Massachusetts General Hospital
Boston, Massachusetts

Jeremy L. Riehm, DO
Sports Medicine Fellow
Family Medicine Practice
University of Virginia
Charlottesville, Virginia

Scott A. Rodeo, MD
Professor, Orthopaedic Surgery
Sports Medicine and Shoulder Service
The Hospital for Special Surgery
New York, New York

David M. Rowley, MD
Orthopedic Sports Medicine Fellow
Department of Orthopedics
Fairview/MOSMI
Minneapolis, Minnesota

Marc R. Safran, MD
Professor
Department of Orthopaedics
Stanford University
Palo Alto, California

Kari Sears, MD
Sports Medicine Fellow
Primary Care Sports Medicine
South Bend-Notre Dame Sports Medicine
*   Fellowship*
South Bend, Indiana

Kevin G. Shea, MD
Surgeon
Department of Sports Medicine
St. Luke's Health System
Boise, Idaho

Anuj Singla, MD
Instructor, Spine Surgery
Department of Orthopedics
University of Virginia
Charlottesville, Virginia

David I. Smith, DO
Fellow
Primary Care Sports Medicine
St. Joseph Regional Medical Center
Mishawaka, Indiana

Marissa M. Smith, MD
Fellow Physician
Primary Care Sports Medicine
Hospital for Special Surgery
New York, New York

Matthew V. Smith, MD
Assistant Professor, Sports Medicine
Department of Orthopedics
Washington University in St. Louis
St. Louis, Missouri

Siobhan Statuta, MD, CAQSM
Director, Primary Care Sports Medicine
Fellowship
Department of Family Medicine
University of Virginia
Charlottesville, Virginia

James Derek Stensby, MD
Instructor
Department of Musculoskeletal Radiology
Mallinckrodt Institute of Radiology
St. Louis, Missouri

Sophia Strike, MD
Physician
Department of Orthopaedic Surgery
Johns Hopkins Hospital
Baltimore, Maryland

Joseph J. Stuart, MD
Orthopaedic Sports Medicine Fellow
Division of Sports Medicine
Department of Orthopaedic Surgery
Duke University
Durham, North Carolina

Miho J. Tanaka, MD
Assistant Professor, Department of
Orthopaedics
Director, Women's Sports Medicine Program
Johns Hopkins University
Baltimore, Maryland

Jeffery A. Taylor-Haas, PT, DPT, OCS, CSCS
Coordinator – OT/PT
Division of Occupational Therapy and Physical
Therapy
Cincinnati Children's Hospital Medical Center
Cincinnati, Ohio

Ekaterina Y. Urch, MD
Department of Orthopaedic Surgery
Hospital for Special Surgery
New York, New York

Bryan G. Vopat, MD
Fellow
Sports Medicine Service
Massachusetts General Hospital
Boston, Massachusetts

Norman E. Waldrop III, MD
Orthopaedic Surgeon
Department of Orthopaedics
Andrews Sports Medicine & Orthopaedic
Center
Birmingham, Alabama

Andrew Watson, MD, MS
Team Physician
Department of Orthopedics and Rehabilitation
University of Wisconsin
Madison, Wisconsin

Scott R. Whitlow, MD
Foot and Ankle Fellow
The Steadman Clinic
Vail, Colorado

Kevin E. Wilk, PT, DPT, FAPTA
Clinical Director
Physical Therapy
Champion Sports Medicine
Birmingham, Alabama

Trevor Wilkes, MD
Orthopedic Surgeon
Orthopedics-Sports Medicine Center
Lexington Clinic
Lexington, Kentucky

Brian R. Wolf, MD, MS
Ralph and Marcia Congdon Professor
Department of Orthopaedics and Rehabilitation
University of Iowa
Iowa City, Iowa

Jeffrey E. Wong, MD
Fellow
Sports Medicine Service
Massachusetts General Hospital
Boston, Massachusetts

Justin Shu Yang, MD
Orthopedic Sports Fellow
Department of Orthopedics
University of Connecticut Health Center
Farmington, Connecticut

Ashley Young, PT, DPT, CSCS
Outpatient Orthopedics
Center for Rehab Services – Center for Sports
  Medicine
University of Pittsburgh Medical Center
Pittsburg, Pennsylvania

Tracy L. Zaslow, MD, FAAP, CAQSM
Physician, Medical Director
Department of Orthopedics
Children's Hospital Los Angeles
Los Angeles, California

Giorgio Zeppieri, Jr, PT, SCS, CSCS
Physical Therapist
Orthopaedic and Sports Medicine Institute
University of Florida Health
Gainesville, Florida

©2016 American Academy of Orthopaedic Surgeons

Preface

I have always been a fan of the American Academy of Orthopaedic Surgeons (AAOS) Orthopaedic Knowledge Update (OKU) series. As a resident when the first OKU was published, I literally read the cover off the edition in the department library and have referred to subsequent editions ever since.

Two years ago, Jo Ann Hannafin, then President of the American Orthopaedic Society for Sports Medicine (AOSSM), asked me to edit *OKU Sports Medicine 5*. As is often the case with time-consuming requests from respected leaders, I agreed, knowing that time invested would lead to value for both authors and readers. As an academic project designed to be a useful resource for practitioners, the OKU series ultimately benefits our patients in clinics and operating rooms. So... 2 years and 57 chapters later, it is with great pride that I introduce the fifth edition of Orthopaedic Knowledge Update--Sports Medicine.

The fifth edition is not a rehash of *OKU Sports Medicine 4*. Much of the credit goes to the 10 section editors, Drs. Brockmeier, Gwathmey, McAllister, Irrgang, Wilk, Shen, Thompson, Poddar, Milewski, and Gaskin. They played a key role in deciding on chapter topics, many of which are new, and selecting authors. They also did an outstanding job encouraging the contributors and editing their work. In addition, new figures were found or created specifically for this edition, adding a rich and informative context to the written descriptions of medical processes and terminology. Video is also included for some of the chapters.

Finally, I want to give a shout-out to Lisa Claxton Moore and the other members of the AAOS publications department who worked on this project. As one of many invested in the future of sound practice in orthopaedic sports medicine, I am honored to be part of the team that put together this book. Thank you.

Mark D. Miller, MD
Editor

Table of Contents

Video Abstracts

Chapter 15 Cruciate Ligament Injuries

Video 15.1 Kim SJ, Kim SG, Kim SH, Lee DY, Jo IK: Video Excerpt. Arthroscopic Double-Bundle ACL Reconstruction Using Quadriceps Tendon Autograft. Rosemont, IL, American Academy of Orthopaedic Surgeons, 2010. (10 min)

This video demonstrates an arthroscopic reconstruction of the ACL using a quadriceps tendon autograft on a 30-year-old man. Examination reveals grade 2 instability during the anterior drawer test, a grade 3 Lachman test, and jumping during the pivot shift test. The graft is harvested with a rectangular bone plug and is split sagittally at a 3:2 ratio with regard to the anteromedial and posterolateral bundles. The graft is whip stitched at the ends. Portals include a high anterolateral, a low anteromedial, and an accessory anteromedial. Tunnels are reamed, and the graft is passed. The bundles are passed alternately to prevent jamming. Sutures are tensioned while the knee is cycled, and all ends are fixed with absorbable interference screws. All tests are negative and do not indicate instability, and rehabilitation is discussed.

Video 15.2 Bach Jr BR: Video Excerpt. Revision Single Bundle ACL Reconstruction Using BPTB Autograft pt 1. River Forest, IL, 2010. (21 min)

This video demonstrates the first part of a two-part video showing a revision single bundle ACL reconstruction using a transfibular endoscopic technique with a bone-tendon-bone autograft for a 19-year-old woman who is an athlete. An examination under anesthesia reveals a grade two pivot shift, and the importance of checking for medial- or lateral-side instability is discussed. The graft is harvested through an incision along the medial edge of the patellar tendon. The tibial bone plug is cut first, and the soft tissue is left attached to the infrapatellar fat pad for stability while cutting the patellar plug. Diagnostic arthroscopy is carried out through a standard infralateral portal through the wound incision, which allows for better visualization. A medial portal is made adjacent to the patellar tendon at the level of the patella. The remnants of the ACL are removed with arthroscopic scissors, and a posterior notchplasty is performed with a spherical burr. An accessory inframedial portal is made with a spinal needle, which aids in distalization of the insertion on the tibial entrance site, as well as allowing for a more oblique orientation with the tibial tunnel. An aiming device is inserted through the transpatellar portal.

Video 15.3 Bach Jr BR: Video Excerpt. Revision Single Bundle ACL Reconstruction Using BPTB Autograft pt 2. River Forest, IL, 2010. (18 min)

This video demonstrates the second part of a two-part video showing a revision single bundle ACL reconstruction using a transfibular endoscopic technique with a bone-tendon-bone autograft for a 19-year-old woman who is an athlete. The orientation of the guide pin is checked in flexion and extension. The femoral tunnel is drilled with a cannulated reamer, and the removed bone is saved for grafting, and the tibial tunnel is cleared with a shaver. The graft is delivered into the femoral tunnel intra-articularly, and the knee is hyperflexed while placing the interference screw. Improvements in Lachman and pivot shift tests are demonstrated. The tibial plug is rotated 180° and secured with an interference screw with the knee in extension. The screw is placed on the cortical edge of the anterior aspect of the bone plug. Pivot shift and translation are tested for, bupivacaine is used intra-articularly and in the surgical wound, and rehabilitation and physical therapy are discussed.

Video 15.4 Johnson DH: Video Excerpt. Pitfalls in ACL Reconstruction. Rosemont, IL, American Academy of Orthopaedic Surgeons, 2010. (12 min)

This video demonstrates various pitfalls that can occur with ACL reconstruction. One is that a tendon stripper may get caught on a band branching off the tendon, which kinks the main tendon and causes it to be cut short. The next pitfall is patellar fracture resulting from an "overrun" horizontal cut when harvesting a bone-to-bone graft. Overzealous use of an osteotome on the patella is also demonstrated and discussed. Improperly positioned tunnels and solutions for fixing them are discussed extensively. Insufficiently large or broken bone plugs are also discussed.

Video 15.5 Miller MD, Hart J, Kurkis G: Anatomic ACL Reconstruction--All Comers. Charlottesville, VA, 2013. (20 min)

In this video, techniques are presented for achieving anatomic anterior cruciate ligament (ACL) reconstructions in a variety of clinical scenarios. The introduction demonstrates a primary single-bundle anatomic ACL reconstruction using a hamstring autograft. Subsequent sections focus on adaptations to this technique for primary single-bundle anatomic ACL reconstruction with a bone-patellar tendon graft, revision ACL reconstruction, and femoral physeal reconstruction. All of the techniques that are shown focus on restoring the native ACL in its anatomic footprint.

Video 15.6 Shino K: Video Excerpt. Anatomical Rectangular Tunnel ACL Reconstruction Using BTB Graft. Osaka, Japan, 2010. (16 min)

Three benefits of this procedure are outlined: that it uses the double bundle concept with a single bone-to-bone graft, that it maximizes the graft-tunnel contact area, and that notch anatomy is preserved. Fiber arrangement is demonstrated with a diagram, and the rectangular profile of the graft is overlaid. The graft is harvested and bone plugs shaped. Portals are made: anteromedial, anterolateral, and the far anteromedial. The ACL stump is excised, and attachment points are made. The tibial and femoral tunnel rectangular profiles are demonstrated. The femoral interference screw is introduced with an outside-in technique, then the graft is passed through the tibial and then femoral tunnels. Both ends are fixed, and notch or PCL impingement is not present. Rehabilitation is discussed.

Video 15.7 Fulkerson JP: Video Excerpt. ACL Reconstruction Using a Free-Tendon Quadriceps Autograft. Farmington, CT, 2010. (20 min)

This video demonstrates ACL reconstruction using a free-tendon quadriceps autograft.

Video 15.8 Howell SM: Video Excerpt. Technique for Harvesting Hamstring Tendons for ACL Reconstruction. Sacramento, CA, 2010. (8 min)

This video demonstrates a technique for harvesting hamstring tendons for ACL reconstruction for a 28-year-old man who plays soccer. The incision is made and a right angle clamp is placed over the gracilis, and its tendon and that of the semitendinosus are identified. Both are retracted with a Penrose drain, stripped with a blunt open-ended tendon stripper, and remaining muscle is removed. The tendons are combined, doubled over, and the ends have sutures placed. The choice of allograft versus autograft is discussed. The graft is sized and submerged in a saline bath while still inside an 8-mm sizing sleeve to prevent drying out of the graft.

Video 15.9 Shelbourne KD: Video Excerpt. Tips for Harvesting BTB Autograft. Indianapolis, IN, 2010. (13 min)

This video demonstrates tips for the contralateral harvesting of a bone-to-bone autograft for ACL reconstruction. The patella and patellar tendon are marked, and an incision is made along the medial border of this tendon. An incision is made into the paratenon to expose the tendon, and flaps are maintained for closure. A 10-mm graft is taken from the central third of the tendon from proximal to distal. Centimeter-deep bone plugs are cut first medially, then laterally for each end. Holes are drilled in bone plug ends and sutures passed, and a sizing guide is used to ensure the graft passes through an 11-mm hole. The soft tissues of the graft are injected with bupivacaine and epinephrine. Bone graft is packed into the patellar and tibial defects, and the paratenon is closed over both. Rehabilitation is discussed and includes high-repetition low-weight exercises; then flexion and extension are checked, a subcutaneous drain is placed, and closure is performed.

Video 15.10 Looney CG, Sterett WI: Video Excerpt. ACL Reconstruction Using Achilles Allograft and Interference Screws. Franklin, TN, 2010. (7 min)

This video demonstrates the preparation and placement of an Achilles allograft for ACL reconstruction. The graft soaks in a solution of kanamycin and sterile saline, and is prepared on a graft preparation table. The bone plug is sculpted; and the graft is cut to size, marked, and the ends are whip stitched. Arthroscopy portal locations are demonstrated, and a notchplasty is performed. The tibial and femoral tunnels are drilled, and the graft is inserted and fixed at both ends with bone interference screws over guidewires. Flexion and extension are tested, and rehabilitation is discussed.

Video 15.11 Howell SM, Andres O: Video Excerpt. Anatomic Single Bundle ACL Reconstruction without Roof and PCL Impingement - Tibialis Allograft. Sacramento, CA, 2010. (20 min)

This video demonstrates a single-bundle ACL reconstruction with a tibialis allograft and the important steps to avoid roof and PCL impingement. Portals are made at the joint line at the medial edge of the patellar tendon and at the approximate midline of the patellar tendon. A 65° guide is used to gauge the space between the lateral femoral condyle and the PCL; this space is too narrow, so a wallplasty is performed. The femoral tunnel drill point should be halfway between the apex and the bottom of the intercondylar notch. The sagittal trajectory is aimed to avoid roof impingement, and the coronal trajectory is aimed to avoid PCL impingement. The tunnels are reamed and the graft passed. The knee is cycled 15 to 20 times, and the tibial end is fixed in full extension. The desirable triangular space between the PCL and the graft is demonstrated.

Chapter 16 Collateral Ligament Injuries

Video 16.1 Gordon D, Pinczewski L: Medial Collateral Ligament - MCL - Acute Meniscotibial Repair. Sydney, Australia, 2012. (9 min)

Grade 3 medial collateral ligament (MCL) injuries involve tearing of both the superficial and deep components of the MCL. These structures may be torn from either the femur or the tibia. Tibial-sided (meniscotibial) injuries require surgery to close the knee capsule and stop synovial fluid extrusion, which prevents adequate healing of the MCL. In this video, the surgical technique for repair of acute meniscotibial MCL injuries, including diagnosis, operating theater set-up, surgical steps, and rehabilitation, is shown and described.

Video 16.2 Miller MD, Werner BC, Higgins S: Posterolateral Corner Primary Repair and Reconstruction. Case Based. Charlottesville, VA, 2014 (18 min)

This video uses three case examples to demonstrate surgical techniques for repair and reconstruction of the posterolateral corner of the knee. The first case presented is a primary repair backed up by a free soft-tissue graft. The second case is a reconstruction of the posterolateral corner. The final case is a reconstruction of an isolated lateral collateral ligament (LCL) injury using a strip of biceps tendon. The posterolateral corner of the knee is often misunderstood, and this video simplifies repair and reconstruction techniques.

Chapter 18 Articular Cartilage of the Knee

Video 18.1 Chalmers P, Yanke A, Sherman S, Karas V, Cole BJ: Combined Cartilage Restoration and Distal Realignment for Patellar and Trochlear Chondral Lesions. Chicago, IL, 2012. (24 min)

Chondral lesions of the patellofemoral joint are relatively common and pose a treatment challenge to the orthopaedic surgeon because of the complex three-dimensional topography and high-contact stresses. Anterior knee pain, either at or surrounding the patella, is the most common symptom in patients with patellofemoral cartilage defects; however, posterior knee pain may also suggest a trochlear defect. Given the wide differential diagnosis for anterior knee pain, the patient history and physical examination should focus on osseous, cartilaginous, and tendinous structures from the hip to the ankle. MRI and CT should be considered to better visualize the state of the underlying cartilage and to quantify the patellar alignment and tilt. Treatment options for patellofemoral cartilage defects include realignment procedures such as anteromedialization of the tibial tubercle, or cartilage restoration procedures such as autologous chondrocyte implantation, microfracture, and osteochondral allograft transplantation. Although reasonable results have been reported with distal realignment and cartilage restoration used in isolation, better outcomes are seen when these types of procedures are combined.

Chapter 20 Meniscal Injuries

Video 20.1 Shelton WR: Video Excerpt. All-Inside Meniscus Repair - FAST-FIX. Jackson, MS, 2011. (12 min)

This video demonstrates meniscal repair using the FAST-FIX system. FAST-FIX is introduced with its blue sheath and the first grommet is deployed automatically, and sutures are made from the periphery to the middle. A slip knot is tied and tightened with a ringed tightener, and excess suture is trimmed with an arthroscopic scissors. The most difficult suture to make is above the tear, and this is demonstrated. The importance of vertically oriented sutures is emphasized. A bucket-handle tear repair is demonstrated.

Video 20.2 Lawhorn KW: Video Excerpt. All-Inside Meniscus Repair - MaxFire MarXmen. Fairfax, VA, 2011. (8 min)

This video demonstrates meniscal repair with the MaxFire MarXmen system. Setup includes a leg holder, and the lateral and medial portal placements are demonstrated. A tourniquet is not used, and bupivacaine or lidocaine with epinephrine is injected into the portal sites. A posterior horn tear of the medial meniscus is repaired with a horizontal mattress suture. Suture tensioning is demonstrated with the inner and outer loops. Anchors are spaced 1 cm apart to ensure a soft-tissue bridge to enhance fixation. Vertical mattress repair of a posterior horn tear of the medial meniscus is also demonstrated, and again suture tensioning is demonstrated. A probe is used to assess repair, and suture ends are trimmed.

©2016 American Academy of Orthopaedic Surgeons

Video 20.3 Vyas D, Harner CD: Video Excerpt. Posterior Horn Medial Meniscus Root Repair. Blawnox, PA, 2011. (14 min)

This video demonstrates a posterior horn medial meniscus root repair for a 45-year-old man. The tear is demonstrated on MRI, and the difficulty of making this diagnosis is discussed. Patient positioning and portals are demonstrated. A diagnostic arthroscopy is performed, along with a reverse notchplasty to improve visualization. The first suture, a monofilament, is pierced into the root with a suture shuttle; and then a braided suture is looped through the monofilament and passed. The tear is reduced. A tibial tunnel is drilled. The braided ends are passed through the tunnel, and the ends are fixed on the tibia with a 6.5-mm cancellous screw with a washer. Suture ends are trimmed.

Video 20.4 Sgaglione NA, Chen E: Video Excerpt. All-Arthroscopic Meniscus Repair With Biological Augmentation. Rosemont, IL, American Academy of Orthopaedic Surgeons, 2011. (28 min)

This video is a cadaver demonstration of an all-arthroscopic repair of both a posterior and an anterior horn tear of the medial meniscus. The importance of evaluating a tear for stability and vascularity is discussed, as are spacing and number of sutures. A portal skid is used to introduce needles and sutures, and is also used as a retractor. The index vertical mattress suture is placed with a curved, proprietary device, and then platelet-rich fibrin matrix is inserted in the tear. Two more sutures are made in the posterior horn of the medial meniscus, and a final suture is placed in the anterior junction. Repair of an anterior horn of the medial meniscus is demonstrated on a different cadaver specimen. Two sutures are placed with a clot of platelet-rich fibrin matrix, and an outside-in technique is demonstrated. The suture ends are retrieved through a cut-down incision, and the sutures are tied down against the capsule. Stability is checked with a probe, and closure performed.

Video 20.5 Shaffer BS: Video Excerpt. Lateral Meniscus Transplantation. Rosemont, IL, American Academy of Orthopaedic Surgeons, 2011. (6 min)

This video demonstrates a lateral meniscus transplantation in a 31-year-old woman who plays soccer with a 2-year history of lateral right knee pain. The patient has normal gait and alignment, but the primary positive findings are joint line tenderness and mild valgus deformity. Graft size is determined from measuring an AP radiograph and MRI. A diagnostic arthroscopy is performed, and the meniscus is resected. Then, the tourniquet is inflated and an anterolateral incision is made in line with the lateral arthroscopic portal. A posterolateral incision is also made in preparation for the meniscal repair. The graft is prepared and the bone block checked in a trough gauge. Colinear placement is discussed, as is the need to possibly make an incision in the patellar tendon to achieve this. A shallow gouge is used to create a preliminary trough, and then a deep gouge the size of the bone block is used. This is checked with a template. The graft is inserted through the posterior corner, and its sutures are retrieved through the posterolateral incision. The graft is seated and then secured with an inside-out technique using vertical mattress sutures.

Video 20.6 Cole BJ: Video Excerpt. Lateral Meniscus Transplantation - Bridge-in-Slot. Rosemont, IL, American Academy of Orthopaedic Surgeons, 2011. (15 min)

This video demonstrates a lateral meniscus transplantation using the bridge-in-slot technique for a 14-year-old girl. The graft is prepared with only two cuts needed to shape the bone block, and soft tissue posterior to the posterior horn is cut away to improve visibility during placement. The graft width is confirmed in an 8-mm slot gauge, and the meniscus is marked posterior to the expected site of the popliteal hiatus. A diagnostic arthroscopy is performed with a standard two-portal setup, and a standard meniscectomy is performed. A trans-patellar tendon approach is used for the arthrotomy to establish anterior-posterior direction. A reference slot is made, checked with a depth gauge, converted to a rectangular channel with a three-sided box cutter, and rasped. A lateral-side incision is made while taking care to avoid the common peroneal nerve. A nitinol pin pulls the graft in through the arthrotomy from the lateral-side incision, and the graft is seated. The bone bridge is fixed anteriorly with a screw, and the meniscus is fixed with vertical mattress sutures. The meniscus is assessed for balance, and the sutures tied down with the knee in extension.

Video 20.7 Carter TR: Video Excerpt. Medial Meniscus Transplantation - Double Bone Plug. Pheonix, AZ, 2011. (11 min)

This video is a demonstration of a medial meniscus transplantation with a double bone plug graft. The difference between medial and lateral meniscal repair is illustrated. A diagnostic arthroscopy ensures that the patient is a candidate for transplant before the allograft packaging is opened. Tissue is removed at the medial notch to improve visualization, and the meniscus remnant is debrided until bleeding to ensure healing. The graft is shown and the dimensions of the bone plugs are marked, cut, and their size checked. Holes are drilled through the plugs and sutures passed. A 7-mm sizer is brought through the notch to ensure that the drill guide and guide pin will fit. Drilling is similar to that used in PCL repair, and the tibial tunnel is drilled over a guide pin. A looped wire is brought up through the tunnel and will be used to pass the posterior plug sutures. The needles for the anterior reduction sutures are passed using an inside-out technique. The graft is pulled into the joint with all reduction sutures engaged. The graft pops into place posteriorly as with a bucket-handle tear repair. Bone plug sutures are secured anteriorly, and a polyethylene button is used in this case. The meniscus is repaired as it is with a bucket-handle tear repair. The anterior horn and plug are secured last, as these are more amenable to adjustment. Typically, eight sutures are needed. The anterior bone plug has a guide pin placed and then a socket drilled for press-fit fixation. The repair is shown again at 5 months.

Video 20.8 Richmond JC: Video Excerpt. Medial Meniscus Transplantation During ACL Repair. Boston, MA, 2011. (11 min)

This video demonstrates a medial meniscal transplant in an active young adult woman prior to ACL reconstruction. Piecrusting is performed to stretch the tight medial collateral ligament to improve visualization of the medial meniscal remnant. Residual meniscal tissue is débrided, and a mini notchplasty is performed on the medial femoral condyle to allow passage of the graft. The allograft is prepared and bone plugs are harvested from the bone block with a coring reamer. Sutures are passed through the bone and the soft tissue. If an ACL is being reconstructed with the transplantation, the ACL tunnels would be fashioned at this time. A counterincision is made at the posteromedial corner to retrieve the graft sutures. The tibial tunnel is reamed, and suture retrievers are passed. The meniscus graft is passed up through the tibial tunnel, and the sutures retrieved. The bone block and meniscus are seated, and the meniscus is captured with classic inside-out technique. The ACL graft is passed into place and fixed. This is considered a salvage procedure, and the

©2016 American Academy of Orthopaedic Surgeons

patient is asked to commit to no running or cutting sports for a year; though it is encouraged to permanently give up these activities for the preservation of the joint.

Chapter 22 Ankle and Foot Injuries and Other Disorders

Video 22.1 Ferkel RD, Stuart KD: Video Excerpt. Autologous Chrondrocyte Implantation. Van Nuys, CA , 2011. (13 min)

The program begins with a review of published studies on ACI. Patient indications are reviewed, and a two-stage procedure is summarized. Cultivation of biopsy tissue is discussed and one patient case is demonstrated beginning with imaging studies (x-ray, CT, and MRI). Preoperative planning is discussed using x-ray imaging. The initial incision is made at the medial malleolus and the surgical site is dissected for complete visualization of the talar dome. The osteotomy is completed using an oscillating saw and osteotome. The osteochondral lesion is identified and removed.

Video 22.2 Glazebrook M: Video Excerpt. Conventional Treatment - Débridement Abrasion Microfracture Drilling. Halifax, Nova Scotia, 2011. (4 min)

Anatomical structures are outlined on the patient's skin, and the ankle joint is infused with saline. Portals are made and tissue débridement to improve visualization of the ankle joint space is completed. Loose bodies are identified using a probe and then removed. Cartilage defects are identified. Using a Kirschner wire, subchondral bone penetration commences. Alternative methods for bone penetration and gaining access to more difficult lesions are discussed. After the surgeon makes the necessary holes in the bone, blood and fat can be seen extruding from the holes. This sets the stage for fibrocartilangeous scar formation. Postoperative protocols are discussed.

Video 22.3 Hangody L: Video Excerpt. OATS Procedure. Budapest, Hungary, 2011. (10 min)

Radiographic imaging demonstrates osteoarthritis dissecans in the ankle joint. Patient positioning, application of tourniquet, and anatomic landmarks are discussed. A longitudinal incision is made for access to the surgical site, and anatomical structures are protected. A medial malleolar osteotomy begins the procedure. The defect is visualized. The affected tissue at the site is removed and graft sizing is discussed. Two grafts, 8.5 mm and 6.5 mm, are harvested at the knee using an arthroscopic approach. Tips and pearls regarding graft harvesting are discussed. Optimal positioning for graft placement is determined, and the two grafts are tapped into the defect. Tips, including the need for congruency, are discussed. The larger graft is placed first. Discussion on managing larger defects with more than two grafts is discussed. When the grafts are in place, screws are used to place the medial malleolus into correct position and the site is closed. Postoperative management and rehabilitation are discussed, and a follow-up radiograph demonstrates the repair.

Video 22.4 Coetzee JC: Video Excerpt. Anterior Ankle Impingement. Edina, MN, 2011. (7 min)

This video demonstrates arthroscopic débridement of soft tissue and bone spurs to relieve impingement of the ankle joint. Surface anatomic landmarks and arthroscopic portals are demonstrated, along with patient positioning to distract the ankle. Soft-tissue and bone spur removal on the distal tibia causing impingement are demonstrated. Use of fluoroscopy to determine the amount of débridement and correct contour of the ankle is shown. Identification of additional pathology is discussed.

Video 22.5 Wiegerinck JI, de Leeuw PAJ, van Dijk CN: Video Excerpt. Posterior Ankle Arthroscopy - Impingement Os Trigonum FHL Tenosynovitis. Amsterdam, Netherlands, 2011. (8 min)

The program begins with a demonstration of patient positioning and portal placement. The nick and spread method is used to create posterolateral and posteromedial portals. Soft-tissue shaving is demonstrated to improve visualization and to create operating space in the joint capsule. Removal of the os trigonum is demonstrated in the first of three cases. A loose body forceps or rongeur is used to remove the os trigonum when débridement is completed. The second case involves management for chronic flexor hallucis longus (FHL) tenosynovitis. Nonsurgical treatments failed in this patient. The FHL is viewed and wear is seen. The FHL is decompressed using a basket forceps. After complete release there is unimpaired motion of the FHL. The final case involves posteromedial ankle pain. A cyst on the talus is seen on MRI. Edema is also present. Anatomic landmarks are seen and then a shaver is use to improve visualization of the joint space. A curette is used to unroof the cyst and then complete débridement is accomplished. Decompression of the lesion is seen. Postoperative care is discussed.

Video 22.6 Wiegerinck JI, de Leeuw PAJ, van Dijk CN: Video Excerpt. Haglund Deformity, Achilles Problems. Amsterdam, Netherlands, 2011. (3 min)

This video demonstrates an endoscopic technique for a calcaneoplasty. The patient is in a prone position with a bolster, and posteromedial and posterolateral portals are made adjacent to the Achilles tendon and superior to the palpable superior border of the calcaneus. The large posterior calcaneal prominence is demonstrated radiographically, and arthroscopy begins with the scope in the lateral portal. A burr is introduced through the medial portal, and bone is removed gradually without compromising the Achilles insertion. The arthroscope is then changed to the medial portal, and the burr to the lateral portal to complete the procedure. Postoperative radiographs and arthroscopic views are shown. Rehabilitation protocol is discussed, as are the benefits of an arthroscopic versus an open procedure.

Chapter 25 Hip Rehabilitation
Video 25.1 Enseki K: Video. Manual Perturbation, Prone and Quadruped. Pittsburgh, PA, 2015. (0:28 min)

This activity emphasizes dynamic hip and pelvic control in a non–weight-bearing position. The patient assumes the prone position. The clinician applies randomly directed forces to the free end of the lower extremity forcing the patient to utilize various hip muscles to maintain stability of the limb. This activity emphasizes dynamic hip and pelvic control in a partial weight-bearing position. The patient assumes the quadruped position. The clinician applies randomly directed forces to the pelvis, forcing the patient to utilize various muscles to maintain stability.

Chapter 26 Current Rehabilitation Concepts Following Anterior Cruciate Ligament Reconstruction
Video 26.1 Goldberg P: Video. Perturbation Training for Neuromuscular Control and Dynamic Stability. Gainesville, FL, 2015. (0:13 min)

Rollerboards or wobble boards create an unstable support surface in perturbation training to challenge knee stability and enhance proprioception and neuromuscular control.

©2016 American Academy of Orthopaedic Surgeons

Video 26.2 Goldberg P: Video. Anticipatory Strategies to Enhance Neuromuscular Control and Proprioception. Gainesville, FL, 2015. (0:16 min)

Anticipatory balance strategies can be trained by placing an object, such as a cone, outside of the patient's base of support for reaching tasks. The uninvolved lower extremity may also be used to reach outside of the base of support.

Video 26.3 Goldberg P: Video. Reactive Strategies to Enhance Neuromuscular Control and Proprioception. Gainesville, FL, 2015. (0:17 min)

Postural perturbations can also be applied with a ball thrown to the patient by another individual or a device such as a "Rebounder." The patient maintains a balanced position on a stable or unstable surface while catching the ball.

Chapter 32 The Cervical Spine

Video 32.1 Faldini C, Gasbarrini A, Chehrassan M, Miscione MT, Acri F, D'Amato M, Boriani L, Boriani S, Giannini S: Video. Anterior Interbody Fusion in Cervical Disc Herniation. Bologna, Italy, 2012. (18 min)

Combined anterior interbody fusion and cervical diskectomy is a surgical technique to treat a variety of cervical spine disorders, such as nerve root or spinal cord compression. This technique permits the surgeon to decompress the spinal cord and nerve roots and perform interbody fusion to provide segmental alignment in lordosis and solid arthrodesis with minimal surgical risk. The aim of this video is to show the anterior cervical diskectomy and interbody fusion of a 55-year-old patient who was suffering from cervical pain associated with intractable radiculopathy of the left C6 root for 6 months. We took an anterior approach to the cervical spine and made a longitudinal skin incision on the medial border of the sternocleidomastoideus (SCM) muscle. We gently incised the platisma muscle and isolated the medial border of the SCM muscle. Then we isolated and partially retracted the homoyoid muscle and separated the longus colli to expose the C5-C6 space. The diskectomy was performed; the posterior osteophyte was removed, along with the posterior longitudinal ligament to expose the dural sac. With the arthroscope, it was possible to visualize and remove the posterior longitudinal ligament and expose the dura. A 6-mm anatomic cage was placed into the intervertebral space to achieve the correct height of the intervertebral space and correct the physiologic lordosis. Finally, the incised fascia and muscles were reattached. Postoperative care consisted of having the patient wear a soft collar for 4 weeks and then undergo physiotherapy. Two-year clinical and radiographic follow-up demonstrated solid anterior interbody fusion of the C5-C6 space.

Chapter 49 Patellofemoral Instability and Other Common Knee Issues in the Skeletally Immature Athlete

Video 49.1 Ellis HB, Jr, Wilson PL: Video. A Surgical Technique for Medial Patellofemoral Ligament Reconstruction in the Skeletally Immature. Dallas, TX, 2014. (14 min)

A surgical technique to treat skeletally immature patients with patellar instability and open physes is described. With recent evidence supporting anatomic origin of the medial patellofemoral ligament (MPFL) distal to the physis, a safe surgical technique to reconstruct the MPFL with a physeal-sparing technique is presented. Thirty-five consecutive patients with open physes have undergone MPFL reconstruction with four revisions and no physeal injury.

Upper Extremity

SECTION EDITOR

Stephen F. Brockmeier, MD

Chapter 1

Shoulder Instability

Jeanne C. Patzkowski, MD   Brett D. Owens, MD

Abstract

Glenohumeral instability is common in young athletes. Most instability events are traumatic anterior subluxations. Both traumatic anterior dislocation and subluxation events result in Bankart lesions in young athletes. Early surgical repair is recommended to optimize outcome and minimize risk of bone and soft-tissue damage. Many in-season athletes can return to play (depending on their sport and position) but two-thirds will experience recurrent events. Attention to glenoid and humeral bone loss is increasing along with renewed interest in bone augmentation procedures. Posterior instability comprises approximately 10% of events and usually is a subluxation. Posterior labral tears are often seen, as well as loose posterior capsules, and arthroscopic repair is the mainstay of treatment with excellent results. Multidirectional instability continues to be a common area of study, with good reported outcomes with physical therapy and surgical stabilization in select patients.

Keywords: shoulder; instability; repair

Introduction

Glenohumeral instability is endemic in young athletes. Instability comprises 23% of all shoulder injuries (including contusions and strains) among National Collegiate Athletic Association athletes.[1] Given this high incidence, instability should be actively ruled out in a young athlete with shoulder problems. Although solely epidemiologic studies of instability are rare, one study has confirmed that most instability events are anterior, and only 10% are posterior events.[2] Posterior instability is an area of increased awareness and study. Approximately 85% of traumatic anterior events are subluxation or incomplete instability events not requiring manual reduction. This is important because these injuries sometimes present with a variable history and examination and can be difficult to diagnose.

Anterior Instability

Pathophysiology

Acute anterior or anteroinferior instability is the most common injury pattern in shoulder instability. The glenohumeral joint moves through a large range of motion, but translation of the humeral head on the glenoid is limited by multiple static and dynamic restraints. Static restraints include the glenoid labrum, which deepens the otherwise shallow glenoid, joint capsule, and glenohumeral ligaments. The anterior band of the inferior glenohumeral ligament (IGHL) is the primary restraint to anterior translation with the arm in abduction and external rotation (ABER). The middle glenohumeral ligament prevents anterior translation in mid ABER, whereas the superior glenohumeral ligament and rotator interval resist anterior and inferior translation with the arm at the side.

The Bankart lesion, a separation of the anteroinferior labrum and IGHL from the glenoid, is found in up to 90% of anterior shoulder dislocations. Humeral avulsion of the glenohumeral ligament (Figure 1) is identified in up to 10% of shoulder instability cases.[3] In the setting of a bony Bankart lesion, variations such as glenolabral articular disruptions and anterior labroligamentous periosteal sleeve avulsion lesions as well as acute glenoid rim fractures can be present. Hill-Sachs lesions, or impression fractures of the posterosuperior humeral head, are common following acute dislocations. In severe cases, the labrum can be injured at multiple locations. Careful

Dr. Owens or an immediate family member serves as a paid consultant to Mitek and the Musculoskeletal Transplant Foundation, and serves as a board member, owner, officer, or committee member of the American Orthopaedic Society for Sports Medicine. Neither Dr. Patzkowski nor any immediate family member has received anything of value from or has stock or stock options held in a commercial company or institution related directly or indirectly to the subject of this chapter.

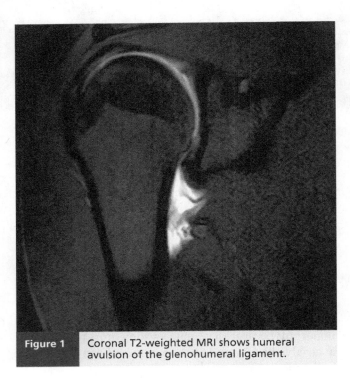

Figure 1 Coronal T2-weighted MRI shows humeral avulsion of the glenohumeral ligament.

inspection of postinjury imaging studies and recognition of all intra-articular pathology at the time of surgery is important to ensure that all instability components are addressed.

The pathoanatomy of first-time traumatic subluxation events is similar to acute dislocations. A prospective study of high-risk individuals identified 27 patients who sustained a primary traumatic subluxation event.[4] MRI identified Bankart lesions in 26 patients and Hill-Sachs lesions in 25. Fourteen patients underwent surgery, 13 of whom had Bankart lesions. Subluxation events represent a wide spectrum of injury from microinstability to the spontaneous reduction of a dislocation event.

Known risk factors for anterior instability include a history of shoulder instability and participation in contact or collision sports. In high-risk athletic and military populations, those with prior instability in any direction have a fivefold increase in the risk for the development of subsequent instability.[5] Identifying modifiable risk factors can help mitigate these troublesome outcomes. A recent prospective study of 714 young athletes without prior instability found that only positive apprehension and relocation signs on physical examination, increased glenoid index (a tall, thin glenoid), and increased coracohumeral distance were predictive of future shoulder instability;[6] modifiable risk factors such as strength, range of motion, and signs of hyperlaxity were not. Increased age at the time of dislocation and the presence of a bony Bankart

lesion can be associated with a positive prognosis for future shoulder stability.[7]

Presentation

For the patient who presents with an acute dislocation, the joint should be reduced as soon as possible. This can be performed on the field or sidelines by a physician or certified athletic trainer or in the emergency department. With a delayed reduction, muscle spasm can prevent successful reduction and may require the use of intravenous sedation or intra-articular local anesthesia. Postreduction radiographs, including axillary lateral views, should be obtained to confirm concentric reduction and evaluate for bony injury. Standard radiographs can be supplemented with a West Point or Stryker notch view to evaluate for glenoid bone loss or Hill-Sachs lesions, respectively.

A thorough physical examination, to include neurovascular status and rotator cuff testing, is essential. Assessment of scapulothoracic kinetics can elicit weakness patterns amenable to physical therapy. Ligamentous laxity should also be assessed (typically with Beighton criteria) because this can have a substantial effect on surgical treatment outcome. Physical examination findings in the patient with anterior shoulder instability can include positive results for the apprehension and relocation tests in the ABER position. The load-and-shift test helps assess laxity in all directions, and the results should be compared with the contralateral side. The Gagey sign, or passive abduction with the arm in a neutral position, can indicate injury to the IGHL if more than 105° of abduction is noted or if substantial asymmetry to the uninjured extremity is seen. The Gagey test can also be used to delineate the presence of inferior capsular laxity most commonly associated with hyperlaxity/multidirectional instability.

Advanced imaging is often obtained following shoulder reduction or in cases of recurrent instability. Magnetic resonance arthrography (MRA) is performed with intra-articular gadolinium to delineate soft-tissue detail. The diagnostic accuracy of MRA has recently been questioned. In a prospective study of 18 patients with traumatic anterior instability undergoing arthroscopic surgery, MRA had only moderate agreement ($\kappa = 0.47$) with arthroscopic findings for Bankart lesions and did not identify two labral lesions that required fixation at the time of surgery.[8] MRA had poor results for identifying superior labrum anterior to posterior tears and glenohumeral ligament lesions. Given the additional time and cost associated with MRA, the authors recommended against routine use of MRA. The ABER view has been used for improved visualization of the inferior labrum (Figure 2), but this is anecdotal. Including the

© 2016 American Academy of Orthopaedic Surgeons

ABER sequence has not been shown to improve accuracy; instead, the experience level of the radiologist and consensus agreement were found to be more important. The ABER view has a high rate of motion artifact, and 12% of patients with instability could not tolerate the ABER position for imaging.[9] MRI has known limitations regarding bony detail, and CT is indicated in cases of suspected bone loss. In a prospective, blinded study comparing MRA and CT arthrography with arthroscopic findings, CT arthrography had superior results overall, with excellent identification of labral and bony pathology.[10] MRA outperformed CT in identifying glenohumeral ligament tears, but the studies were equivalent in identifying humeral avulsion of the glenohumeral ligament lesions. CT can be an acceptable alternative to MRA for instability evaluation in the shoulder, but its lower cost and decreased time are balanced by the risks of exposure to ionizing radiation.

Natural History

Multiple studies have demonstrated a high rate of recurrent dislocation in young, active patients, particularly in contact and collision athletes. Recurrent instability rates can be as high as 94%. Recurrence rates decrease substantially with each decade after age 20 years, and older patients are more likely to sustain a concomitant rotator cuff tear or greater tuberosity fracture after shoulder dislocation.[11]

Treatment

Treatment of the patient with a first-time dislocation remains controversial. For patients who choose nonsurgical treatment, the shoulder is immobilized until pain resolves and early motion is initiated. Physical therapy focuses on regaining motion, strengthening the rotator cuff and periscapular muscles, and proprioceptive training. Initial immobilization in external versus internal rotation may better reduce the torn labrum to the anteroinferior glenoid. Although initial clinical results were promising, follow-up studies could not reproduce the original results and meta-analysis showed no benefit in rates of recurrence or validated outcomes with external rotation bracing. Compliance was reported as problematic with the external rotation brace.[12]

The goal of surgical management is to restore stability by repairing the injured labrum or glenohumeral ligaments, and if needed, plication of the redundant capsule. Arthroscopic Bankart repair (Figure 3) has become common because it allows excellent visualization of the entire joint and is minimally invasive; it is now the treatment of choice among new surgeons in the United States.[13] Determining which patients need surgery after a

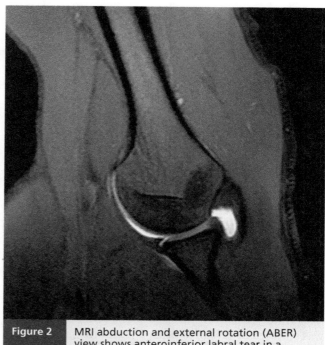

Figure 2 MRI abduction and external rotation (ABER) view shows anteroinferior labral tear in a patient experiencing recurrent subluxations who did not demonstrate pathology in other imaging sequences. This correlated with arthroscopic findings at time of repair.

first-time dislocation and how soon remains in question. In a double-blind, randomized clinical trial evaluating arthroscopic Bankart repair versus sham surgery, patients with a first-time dislocation had decreased recurrence of instability and improved outcome scores after repair.[14] Surgery resulted in lower costs and higher patient satisfaction, but overall outcomes were related to shoulder stability, not necessarily the surgery itself. Patients in the repair group also had a higher rate of return to contact sports. Similarly, a systematic review of only level I and II studies demonstrated decreased recurrence of instability following arthroscopic Bankart repair when compared with physical therapy and sham surgery, both together and in isolation.[15] The patients in the repair group were noted to have one-fifth the rate of recurrent instability and improved Western Ontario Shoulder Instability Index (WOSI) scores. The patients were 22 to 25 years old and primarily male, representing the highest risk cohort of shoulder instability patients.

Technologic advances have increased the orthopaedic surgeon's ability to manage shoulder instability arthroscopically. High rates of patient satisfaction and improved outcome scores have been reported in the short term and mid term, with low rates of recurrent instability and disability.[16] Radiographic evidence of dislocation arthropathy can present with longer term follow-up and

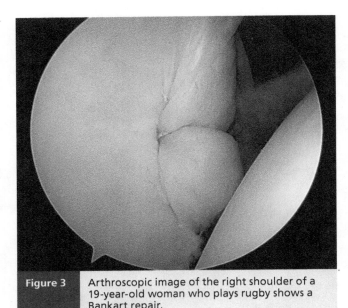

Figure 3 Arthroscopic image of the right shoulder of a 19-year-old woman who plays rugby shows a Bankart repair.

was reported in 41% of patients 8 years after arthroscopic Bankart repair.[17] The presence of radiographic arthritis did not correlate with outcome scores.

Open Bankart repair has historically provided good results for shoulder stability. The procedure requires transection, or splitting, of the subscapularis tendon, and mild losses in forward elevation and external rotation can occur, typically between 8° and 10°. In a series of 49 patients, including 31 elite rugby players, 16% had recurrence of instability during the 26-year follow-up period after open Bankart repair.[18] Of these patients, 65% had radiographic evidence of arthritis at final follow-up, most of which was considered mild, and 80% reported being pain free. Ninety-four percent of patients resumed athletic activity, 75% of those at their original level of competition.

The treatment of contact or collision athletes remains controversial, and some reports suggested higher rates of recurrent instability in these patients following arthroscopic management. In a recent randomized clinical trial comparing open versus arthroscopic Bankart repair, an increased rate of recurrence was noted after arthroscopic repair (23% versus 11% in open repair).[19] The highest rate of recurrence was noted in males younger than 25 years with Hill-Sachs lesions. The arthroscopic group comprised more contact athletes and bone loss was not evaluated; both factors have been shown to influence recurrence. In a trial of isolated Bankart lesions randomized to arthroscopic versus open repair, improved Disability of the Arm, Shoulder and Hand (DASH) scores were noted in the arthroscopic group, with no substantial difference in recurrence noted.[20] A differential loss

to follow-up between groups was noted, and more than 50% of patients had no more than two suture anchors placed during the repair in both groups. A systematic review of more recent meta-analyses demonstrated no difference in recurrence between the two techniques, but noted that the analyses performed before 2007 favored open surgery in recurrence rates, whereas those published after 2007 showed no difference.[21] Similarly, the latest Cochrane database review stated that evidence was insufficient to claim superiority of one technique over another in recurrence, need for subsequent surgery, and shoulder function.[22]

Many athletes want to return to sport following a traumatic anterior shoulder instability event during his or her athletic season. In a prospective study of 45 intercollegiate contact athletes, 73% returned to sport after accelerated rehabilitation.[23] Sixty-seven percent finished the season, but 64% had recurrent instability during the season. No difference in recurrence was reported between those who sustained an initial dislocation versus subluxation event, but those with subluxations had a higher overall rate of return to sport and did so more quickly. WOSI and Simple Shoulder Test (SST) scores at the time of injury were predictive of ability to return to play, and WOSI, SST, and American Shoulder and Elbow Surgeons (ASES) scores could predict the time needed to return to play. None of the outcome scores were predictive of recurrence.

Recurrent shoulder instability increases the risk that existing intra-articular pathology will worsen, including bony attrition of the anteroinferior glenoid, enlargement or engagement of a Hill-Sachs lesion, and soft-tissue compromise. Over the long term, osteoarthritis of the glenohumeral joint can develop in these patients. With excellent outcomes reported after surgical management of instability, it must be questioned whether continuing sports participation or rehabilitation only in the setting of recurrent instability is wise for future shoulder function. A systematic review compared arthroscopic management of instability performed after the initial instability event or in a delayed fashion after multiple recurrences and reported no substantial differences in postoperative recurrence, range of motion, or complications.[24] Outcome measures varied across studies, precluding in-depth analysis. The lowest rates of recurrence were noted with suture anchor fixation over older implants. In the short term, delaying surgical management did not appear to have adverse effects.

Recurrence

Recurrent instability after surgical repair is a challenging problem. Some studies demonstrated recurrence rates ranging between 4% and 19% for arthroscopic repair, most of which occurred during the first year after surgery.[16] Independent risk factors included age at time of surgery, glenoid bone loss greater than 25%, an engaging Hill-Sachs lesion, male sex, competitive sports participation, fewer than three suture anchors, ligamentous laxity, and the presence of an anterior labroligamentous periosteal sleeve avulsion lesion.[16,25]

Revision open Bankart repair has demonstrated reliable results after failed arthroscopic repair. Improved outcome scores, pain, and return to almost preinjury activity levels have been shown with low rates of recurrence. Patients with substantial bone loss are still at risk for recurrent instability following open Bankart repair.[26] In appropriately selected patients, revision arthroscopic stabilization can be a reasonable option. Recurrence rates ranging from 6% to 10% have been demonstrated with revision arthroscopic Bankart repair in patients without substantial glenoid or humeral head bone loss, without hyperlaxity, and in those willing to comply with postoperative restrictions and therapy.[27,28] Revision arthroscopic surgery including bony augmentation can be considered after an open index procedure, but patient selection is critical. Low recurrence rates and high patient satisfaction can be achieved with meticulous attention to detail and surgical technique. Patients should be cautioned that pain may persist and osteoarthritis can still progress.[29] Studies of revision arthroscopic Bankart repair demonstrated the importance of good surgical technique. In a study of 56 patients with recurrent postoperative instability, more than one-half had suture anchors placed above the equator during the index procedure.[27]

Instability With Bone Loss

Bone loss should be suspected in patients with unsuccessful instability repair, multiple subluxations and/or dislocations, or instability with minimal provocation (such as activities of daily living or during sleep). Attritional bone loss can be noted on the anteroinferior glenoid, resulting in an inverted pear glenoid or as a large Hill-Sachs lesion. Glenoid and humeral head bone loss typically do not occur in isolation, and the interaction of the two is important in determining the risk of continued instability. The humeral head defect can fall into, or engage with, the area of the glenoid bone defect. In the glenoid track concept, glenoid bone loss narrows the track available for the humeral head to articulate. If a concomitant Hill-Sachs lesion is wide or occurs in a medial enough location, the humeral head can slip off track, resulting in an anterior dislocation[30] (Figure 4).

Suspicion of bone loss warrants advanced imaging to quantify the defect for preoperative planning. Glenoid bone loss of greater than 20% to 25% is the generally

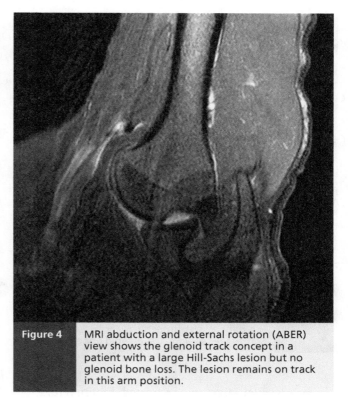

Figure 4 MRI abduction and external rotation (ABER) view shows the glenoid track concept in a patient with a large Hill-Sachs lesion but no glenoid bone loss. The lesion remains on track in this arm position.

accepted threshold for choosing a bony restoration procedure because this is an independent risk factor for postoperative recurrence.[16,25] Multiple techniques have been described to measure glenoid bone loss, but no gold standard currently exists. CT, particularly three-dimensional (3D) CT, appears to be the most reliable means of calculating glenoid bone loss when compared with plain radiography and MRI. All imaging modalities underestimated the degree of bone loss to some extent, but 3D CT demonstrated the least inconsistency.[31] 3D CT has also demonstrated high specificity and positive predictive values for the detection of Hill-Sachs lesions, with an overall accuracy of 80%. Shallower lesions and lesions without subchondral bone damage are not as easily appreciated.[32]

Glenoid augmentation procedures include open or arthroscopic coracoid transfer, iliac crest autograft, distal clavicle autograft, and various allograft techniques. The open coracoid transfer, or Latarjet procedure (Figure 5), has demonstrated excellent long-term results with low rates of recurrence and high patient satisfaction.[33] The procedure is technically challenging, and a recent systematic review of level IV case series found a 30% complication rate with an average follow-up of 6.8 years.[34] Recurrent instability was found in 8.7% of patients, most within the first year after surgery, and was associated with suboptimal graft placement. Most complications were related to coracoid fracture, nonunion, or lysis. Low rates

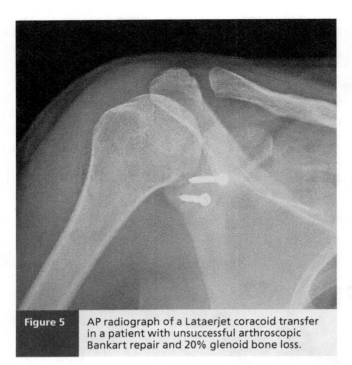

Figure 5 AP radiograph of a Lataerjet coracoid transfer in a patient with unsuccessful arthroscopic Bankart repair and 20% glenoid bone loss.

of neurovascular injury were reported. External rotation was reduced by an average of 13°. An all-arthroscopic technique has been described with rates of recurrence approaching those of the open procedure, but is associated with a steep learning curve.[35] Iliac crest and allograft glenoid augmentation have also demonstrated reliable long-term results,[36] and the most recent systematic review available found no evidence to support one technique over another.[37]

Management of a large Hill-Sachs lesion may also be necessary to restore shoulder stability. In cases of substantial glenoid bone loss and a large Hill-Sachs lesion, treatment of the glenoid bone loss may be all that is needed to stabilize a joint. In cases with minimal glenoid bone loss, the Hill-Sachs lesion can be addressed using multiple techniques. Remplissage involves suturing the infraspinatus tendon into the humeral head defect using either an arthroscopic or open approach. In a study of recurrent anterior shoulder instability with glenoid bone loss less than 25% and an engaging Hill-Sachs lesion, patients who underwent combined primary arthroscopic remplissage and Bankart repair were compared with control patients undergoing Bankart repair only.[38] All patients demonstrated healing of the tendon to bone at the remplissage site at 2 years on MRI; no recurrent instability was reported in patients undergoing the combined procedure. In those undergoing Bankart repair only, instability recurrence was 20%. Eighty percent of patients treated using remplissage returned to sport at their previous level and showed substantial improvements in University of California Los Angeles (UCLA), Rowe, and Constant scores. Similar results were reported in a series of 47 patients who underwent remplissage with Bankart repair.[39] Only one patient experienced recurrence of instability, and 68% returned to sports participation at their previous level. External rotation was reduced by an average of 8° and abduction by an average of 9°.

Other procedures can be used to treat a Hill-Sachs lesion, including osteochondral allograft, rotational (Weber) osteotomy, and arthroplasty. Allograft reconstruction may be indicated in young patients with very large defects, whereas arthroplasty is reserved for large defects in elderly patients. Currently, no absolute guidelines exist to indicate these procedures. A recent systematic review demonstrated high rates of serious complications with Weber osteotomy, allograft reconstruction, and arthroplasty.[40] The lowest rate of recurrent instability was found with allograft reconstruction, but complications such as osteonecrosis and collapse were seen in up to 74% of patients. Arthroscopic remplissage remains a viable option, with low rates of recurrence and the highest safety profile.

Posterior Instability

Epidemiology

Posterior shoulder dislocation is much less common than anterior dislocation, comprising approximately 5% of all shoulder dislocations, with a prevalence of 1.1/100,000 per year.[41] A slight male predominance exists, and frank posterior dislocations are more commonly associated with seizure activity and electrocution than are anterior dislocations. Almost two-thirds of posterior dislocations are the result of trauma such as motor vehicle collisions or falls, and 31% are related to seizure activity.[41] Up to 50% of posterior dislocations can be missed in the emergency department setting; obtaining an axillary lateral radiograph is critical for correct diagnosis. In athletes, posterior instability can be more subtle, with primarily subluxation events in the at-risk position of forward flexion, adduction, and internal rotation.[2] Football linebackers are at particularly increased risk. Posterior instability in athletes can primarily manifest as pain, particularly during the bench press, push-ups, or other upper extremity weight-bearing activities. Recent reports suggest that combined instability pathology may be more common than previously thought in certain populations. Of 231 consecutive military patients undergoing surgery for shoulder instability, only 57% had isolated anterior pathologic changes.[42] Twenty-four percent had isolated posterior pathology, and 19% of patients had combined anterior and posterior findings. MRI was only 68% accurate for predicting intra-articular lesions.

Pathophysiology

Multiple lesions are associated with posterior instability. Kim et al[43] described multiple lesions on the posterior labrum in the setting of posterior instability, most commonly, an incomplete stripping of the posteroinferior labrum without displacement. A prospective cohort of 200 shoulders with isolated posterior instability found a patulous posterior capsule in 69% and posterior labral tears in 64%.[44] Of note, patients with labral tears had lower preoperative ASES scores, with no differences noted postoperatively. Other lesions include damage to the rotator interval, reverse Hill-Sachs lesions, bony deficiency of the posterior glenoid, injury to the posterior capsule or posterior band of the IGHL, and glenoid retroversion. In a prospective series of military cadets, increased glenoid retroversion at baseline was predictive for the development of posterior shoulder instability, with every 1° increase in retroversion increasing the risk of posterior instability by 17%.[45]

Presentation

Patients presenting with an acute posterior dislocation typically hold the arm in an adducted, internally rotated position. Full radiographic work-up that includes an axillary lateral view is critical to determine the presence of an acute dislocation. A high index of suspicion should be maintained in patients presenting to the emergency department after sustaining a seizure or electrocution event. These patients are also at higher risk for bilateral dislocations. Patients presenting with chronic posterior dislocations can have profound lack of external rotation with a mechanical block. Radiographic evaluation can demonstrate large reverse Hill-Sachs lesions or humeral head erosion. Chronic dislocations typically require an open reduction. Arthroplasty may be required in chronic cases with excessive bone loss.

Patients with posterior shoulder subluxation may present primarily with pain. Symptoms are typically noted in the position of forward flexion, adduction, and internal rotation, and may be exacerbated by push-ups, bench press, and other activities that place a posteriorly directed load on the shoulder. Physical examination should include a posterior load-and-shift test, jerk test, and posterior apprehension sign, along with testing for anterior and inferior instability because these conditions frequently coexist. A sulcus sign that persists in external rotation can indicate rotator interval incompetence. MRI with or without intra-articular contrast can be used to evaluate the status of the posterior labrum, capsule, and other intra-articular structures, whereas CT scanning can help determine humeral head bone loss, glenoid bone loss, and glenoid retroversion.

Treatment

Nonsurgical management is the first-line treatment of posterior shoulder instability. Physical therapy focuses on periscapular and rotator cuff strengthening, particularly of the infraspinatus. In a prospective series of 112 patients with posterior dislocations, recurrent instability did not develop after a formalized physical therapy regimen in 82% of shoulders. Persistent deficits in shoulder motion and function were seen in all patients at 2-year follow-up, irrespective of recurrence. Recurrent instability was independently predicted by age younger than 40 years, dislocation resulting from seizure, and a large reverse Hill-Sachs lesion. Hyperlaxity was not predictive of dislocation recurrence.[41]

Surgery is indicated for patients with recurrent instability, pain, or functional limitations following appropriate therapy. Although both arthroscopic and open techniques are described to treat the various lesions that can contribute to posterior instability, most surgeons currently prefer arthroscopic management (Figure 6). In a prospective cohort of 200 patients undergoing surgical stabilization for isolated posterior instability, Bradley et al[44] reported good results with arthroscopic capsular plication and/or labral repair; 94% of patients were satisfied with the result and would undergo surgery again, and 90% returned to sports (64% at their previous level of competition). Similar results were noted in contact/collision athletes. Six percent of patients had failing ASES scores in pain and function, and 7% were noted to have continued instability. All failures were identified within the first 7 months after surgery. Of those patients in whom treatment failed, 62.5% had signs of multidirectional instability (MDI) at the time of revision. In the remaining patients in whom treatment failed, poor tissue quality was noted, typically a result of prior thermal capsulorrhaphy or early aggressive rehabilitation outside the established protocol.

Open procedures to address posterior instability include open capsular shift and bone block augmentation. A retrospective series of 44 patients with posterior instability undergoing open capsulorrhaphy reported 84% overall satisfaction with a 74% rate of return to sport.[46] Recurrent instability developed in 19% of patients, but in patients without signs of MDI at the time of surgery, the recurrence rate was only 13%. Anterior instability developed subsequently in an additional 13% of patients, highlighting the risk of overaggressive posterior constraint. Chondral injury and age older than 38 years at the time of surgery were associated with worse outcomes.

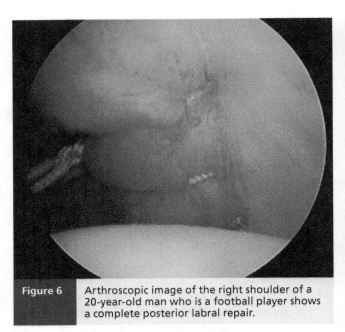

Figure 6 | Arthroscopic image of the right shoulder of a 20-year-old man who is a football player shows a complete posterior labral repair.

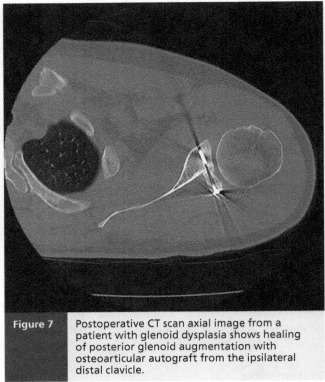

Figure 7 | Postoperative CT scan axial image from a patient with glenoid dysplasia shows healing of posterior glenoid augmentation with osteoarticular autograft from the ipsilateral distal clavicle.

Instability With Bone Loss

Bone loss is a rare but challenging problem in the setting of posterior shoulder instability. Although posterior glenoid bone loss has been studied less than its anterior counterpart, both arthroscopic and open posterior bone block augmentation techniques have been described for this rare condition (Figure 7). A biomechanical cadaver study demonstrated that the bone block can overconstrain posterior translation while not treating inferior translation in the setting of an incompetent posterior band of the IGHL.[47] Precise positioning of the bone block is critical to achieve the preferred mechanical effect.

An all-arthroscopic technique using autograft iliac crest for recurrent posttraumatic posterior shoulder instability has been described in 18 patients.[48] Graft union was reported in all cases; however, complete lysis of the graft requiring revision proceeded to develop in one patient. Sixteen patients reported satisfaction with the procedure, but a complication rate of 36%, steep learning curve, and worse outcomes in patients with glenoid dysplasia were noted.

Long-term follow-up after open bone block procedures may not be as promising. Of 11 patients followed for 18 years, 8 had residual instability, 2 of whom eventually required arthrodesis.[49] All patients had evidence of radiographic osteoarthritis at long-term follow-up, and clinical outcomes diminished over time. The worst outcomes were found in patients with hyperlaxity or MDI, and this procedure should be avoided in these populations.

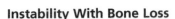

Multidirectional Instability

Pathophysiology

MDI is poorly defined, but most authors agree that it encompasses a shoulder joint with excessive translation in two or more directions. Patients may or may not have a structural lesion such as a labral tear. Although many cases are atraumatic, traumatic onset does not rule out the diagnosis. Patients with multidirectional laxity (asymptomatic) can sustain a traumatic injury, and the treatment needs to incorporate an understanding of the physiologic laxity for a particular patient, with the need for capsular tightening to augment a labral repair or capsulorrhaphy. Multiple underlying etiologies exist with the common theme of a patulous inferior capsule, increased glenohumeral joint volume, and IGHL laxity.

Treatment

The natural history of MDI is poorly documented, and various definitions of the disease have made interpretation of the literature difficult. Classically, MDI was considered a self-limited condition that partially resolves with increasing age, resulting in its universal treatment with physical therapy alone. Multiple protocols exist but share a common theme of rotator cuff and periscapular muscle strengthening as well as proprioceptive training.

However, athletic patients may not be willing to modify their activities and symptoms may continue even with aggressive rehabilitation.

In the largest longitudinal study to date, 64 patients with MDI were followed for a minimum of 8 years.[50] All patients underwent formal physical therapy with a home exercise program. At 2 years, 20 patients had undergone surgery, and of those who had not, only one-half reported good or excellent outcomes for pain and stability. Of those who improved with therapy, substantial gains were noted by 3 months. At 8-year follow-up, one additional patient had undergone surgery, seven had given up sports completely, and an additional nine admitted to substantial lifestyle and occupational changes to accommodate their shoulders. The need for surgery was associated with unilateral involvement, more severe laxity, and difficulty performing activities of daily living. All patients who underwent surgery had persisted with formal physical therapy for at least 6 months. At long-term follow-up, only 30% of all patients reported good or excellent Rowe scores. This population was younger and more active than those of previous reports, but the diminishing subjective outcomes and need to modify lifestyles evident at longer term follow-up were concerning.

A recent prospective cohort compared patients with MDI who underwent physical therapy only, physical therapy after open capsular shift, and normal control subjects without history or physical findings of instability.[51] Subjects underwent kinematic and electromyographic testing during humeral elevation. In the physical therapy–only group, the strengthening program did not restore the muscular activity or duration parameters of the normal shoulder, and at the 2- and 4-year points, the values tested were similar to those obtained before therapy began. In contrast, the subjects who underwent capsular shift and postoperative therapy had values similar to those of the control group that persisted throughout follow-up. Surgery combined with therapy could restore the stability and muscular control of the shoulder, whereas therapy alone was less reliable.

Both open capsular shift and arthroscopic capsular plication have been described for the treatment of MDI, with the main goals of decreasing capsular volume and tightening the IGHLs.[52] In a systematic review of available level IV studies, similar outcomes were reported for recurrent instability, return to sport, loss of external rotation, and complications between the two techniques. The arthroscopic technique demonstrated a small increase in rate of recurrence and improved rate of return to sport, but these results did not reach significance. The systematic review was limited by variability in the definition of MDI used in the literature and inconsistent reporting of athletic activity. In the studies that stratified results by sport played, overhead athletes, elite athletes, and swimmers had the lowest rates of returning to sport at their previous level. Overall, both open and arthroscopic techniques can be considered safe, effective options for the management of MDI unresponsive to nonsurgical measures.

Summary

Shoulder instability is a common problem in a young, athletic population. Traumatic anterior instability comprises most instability events and can be treated using arthroscopic or open techniques. Preoperative evaluation for bone loss is important because unrecognized bone loss is a substantial risk factor for recurrence and poor outcomes. Further research is needed to determine the most accurate, reliable way to quantify bone loss, determine which patients are at highest risk of recurrence, and identify the best procedure to restore stability. Posterior shoulder instability may be more common in athletes and excellent outcomes can be achieved with arthroscopic repair. MDI is treated with formal physical therapy, but some patients have persistent muscular deficits and unsatisfactory outcomes. Selected patients will benefit from arthroscopic or open repair of the capsule and injured structures.

Key Study Points

- Traumatic anterior instability comprises the majority of shoulder instability cases, with subluxation events more common than dislocations.
- Most traumatic anterior subluxations and dislocations in young athletes result in a Bankart lesion, but physicians should be cautious of the HAGL, which occurs in up to 10% of patients.
- Preoperative risk stratification – including advanced imaging for bone loss assessment—is critical to a successful outcome when selecting a surgical stabilization approach in patients with anterior instability.
- Posterior instability may present with pain alone, and most cases have good outcomes with arthroscopic repair/plication.

Annotated References

1. Owens BD, Agel J, Mountcastle SB, Cameron KL, Nelson BJ: Incidence of glenohumeral instability in collegiate athletics. *Am J Sports Med* 2009;37(9):1750-1754.

This retrospective analysis of the National Collegiate Athletic Association injury database over a 15-year period reported the incidence of shoulder instability events was 0.12 per 1,000 athlete exposures. Males and football players sustained the most injuries, with more instability events noted during competitions than practices.

2. Owens BD, Duffey ML, Nelson BJ, DeBerardino TM, Taylor DC, Mountcastle SB: The incidence and characteristics of shoulder instability at the United States Military Academy. *Am J Sports Med* 2007;35(7):1168-1173.

3. Bui-Mansfield LT, Banks KP, Taylor DC: Humeral avulsion of the glenohumeral ligaments: The HAGL lesion. *Am J Sports Med* 2007;35(11):1960-1966.

4. Owens BD, Nelson BJ, Duffey ML, et al: Pathoanatomy of first-time, traumatic, anterior glenohumeral subluxation events. *J Bone Joint Surg Am* 2010;92(7):1605-1611.

   This prospective cohort reported on 27 patients who sustained a primary, traumatic anterior subluxation event. MRI and surgical findings demonstrated high rates of Bankart and Hill-Sachs lesions. Four of thirteen had recurrence of instability with nonsurgical management. Level of evidence: II.

5. Cameron KL, Mountcastle SB, Nelson BJ, et al: History of shoulder instability and subsequent injury during four years of follow-up: A survival analysis. *J Bone Joint Surg Am* 2013;95(5):439-445.

   This prospective cohort studied 714 high-risk subjects. Subsequent instability was 5.6 times more likely to develop in patients with prior instability in any direction than those without a history of instability. Level of evidence: I.

6. Owens BD, Campbell SE, Cameron KL: Risk factors for anterior glenohumeral instability. *Am J Sports Med* 2014;42(11):2591-2596.

   This prospective cohort studied 714 high-risk young athletes. The risk of shoulder instability was associated with positive apprehension and relocation signs on physical examination, increased glenoid index, and increased coracohumeral distance. Modifiable risk factors and hyperlaxity were not predictive of instability. Level of evidence: II.

7. Salomonsson B, von Heine A, Dahlborn M, et al: Bony Bankart is a positive predictive factor after primary shoulder dislocation. *Knee Surg Sports Traumatol Arthrosc* 2010;18(10):1425-1431.

   In 39 patients treated nonsurgically after a first-time anterior dislocation, the only prognostic factors for a stable shoulder at 8 years after injury were age older than 30 years at time of injury and the presence of a bony Bankart lesion on MRI.

8. van der Veen HC, Collins JP, Rijk PC: Value of magnetic resonance arthrography in post-traumatic anterior shoulder instability prior to arthroscopy: A prospective evaluation of MRA versus arthroscopy. *Arch Orthop Trauma Surg* 2012;132(3):371-375.

   This prospective, blinded evaluation of 18 patients with posttraumatic anterior instability compared MRA findings with arthroscopy. Moderate agreement was seen for Bankart lesions; otherwise, poor agreement was seen for other intra-articular pathology.

9. van Grinsven S, Hagenmaier F, van Loon CJ, van Gorp MJ, van Kints MJ, van Kampen A: Does the experience level of the radiologist, assessment in consensus, or the addition of the abduction and external rotation view improve the diagnostic reproducibility and accuracy of MRA of the shoulder? *Clin Radiol* 2014;69(11):1157-1164.

   In this blinded prospective evaluation of 58 patients with shoulder instability undergoing arthroscopy, radiologists evaluated MRAs and ABER views. The ABER view did not improve accuracy or reproducibility, but the experience level of the radiologist and consensus agreements did. Many patients were unable to tolerate the ABER position.

10. Acid S, Le Corroller T, Aswad R, Pauly V, Champsaur P: Preoperative imaging of anterior shoulder instability: Diagnostic effectiveness of MDCT arthrography and comparison with MR arthrography and arthroscopy. *AJR Am J Roentgenol* 2012;198(3):661-667.

    This prospective evaluation of 40 patients compared multidetector row CT and MRA with arthroscopy. Multidetector row CT identified labral and bony pathology and was recommended as the preoperative imaging study of choice. MRA had superior results for identifying lesions of the glenohumeral ligaments.

11. Robinson CM, Shur N, Sharpe T, Ray A, Murray IR: Injuries associated with traumatic anterior glenohumeral dislocations. *J Bone Joint Surg Am* 2012;94(1):18-26.

    This prospective analysis reported on 3,633 consecutive patients with a traumatic anterior shoulder dislocation at an average age of 47.6 years. Neurologic deficits were found in 13.5% following reduction, and 33.4% had either a rotator cuff tear or greater tuberosity fracture. The likelihood of neurologic deficit was increased in patients with a rotator cuff tear or greater tuberosity fracture. Level of evidence: II.

12. Liu A, Xue X, Chen Y, Bi F, Yan S: The external rotation immobilisation does not reduce recurrence rates or improve quality of life after primary anterior shoulder dislocation: A systematic review and meta-analysis. *Injury* 2014;45(12):1842-1847.

    This meta-analysis of seven rotator cuff tears compared external and internal bracing after acute glenohumeral dislocation. No difference was found in rates of recurrence or outcome scores. Worse compliance was reported in the external rotation group.

13. Owens BD, Harrast JJ, Hurwitz SR, Thompson TL, Wolf JM: Surgical trends in Bankart repair: An analysis of data from the American Board of Orthopaedic Surgery certification examination. *Am J Sports Med* 2011;39(9):1865-1869.

© 2016 American Academy of Orthopaedic Surgeons

This retrospective analysis of the American Board of Orthopaedic Surgeons database from 2003 to 2008 reported that prior to 2005, 71% of Bankart repairs were performed arthroscopically, versus 88% after 2006.

14. Robinson CM, Jenkins PJ, White TO, Ker A, Will E: Primary arthroscopic stabilization for a first-time anterior dislocation of the shoulder. A randomized, double-blind trial. *J Bone Joint Surg Am* 2008;90(4):708-721.

15. Chahal J, Marks PH, Macdonald PB, et al: Anatomic Bankart repair compared with nonoperative treatment and/or arthroscopic lavage for first-time traumatic shoulder dislocation. *Arthroscopy* 2012;28(4):565-575.

    This systematic review of level I and II studies compared arthroscopic Bankart repair with physical therapy or sham surgery. Patients who underwent Bankart repair had substantially decreased recurrence and improved WOSI scores. Level of evidence: II.

16. Ahmed I, Ashton F, Robinson CM: Arthroscopic Bankart repair and capsular shift for recurrent anterior shoulder instability: Functional outcomes and identification of risk factors for recurrence. *J Bone Joint Surg Am* 2012;94(14):1308-1315.

    In this study, 302 patients were treated with arthroscopic Bankart repair. Recurrent instability was noted in 13.2%. Improved WOSI and DASH scores were noted at 2 years, but scores were decreased in patients with recurrence. Three independent risk factors for recurrence were age, glenoid bone loss greater than 25%, and an engaging Hill-Sachs lesion. Level of evidence: I.

17. Elmlund AO, Ejerhed L, Sernert N, Rostgård LC, Kartus J: Dislocation arthropathy and drill hole appearance in a mid- to long-term follow-up study after arthroscopic Bankart repair. *Knee Surg Sports Traumatol Arthrosc* 2012;20(11):2156-2162.

    In this study, 41% of patients demonstrated radiographic signs of osteoarthritis 8 years after arthroscopic Bankart repair for shoulder dislocation. Outcome scores did not correlate with radiographic findings. Level of evidence: III.

18. Fabre T, Abi-Chahla ML, Billaud A, Geneste M, Durandeau A: Long-term results with Bankart procedure: A 26-year follow-up study of 50 cases. *J Shoulder Elbow Surg* 2010;19(2):318-323.

    This 26-year follow-up reviewed 50 shoulders that underwent open Bankart repair after shoulder dislocation. Most patients were elite rugby players. At final follow-up, 16% had recurrent instability, 65% showed signed of arthritis, 94% returned to sports, and 80% were pain free. Level of evidence: IV.

19. Mohtadi NG, Chan DS, Hollinshead RM, et al: A randomized clinical trial comparing open and arthroscopic stabilization for recurrent traumatic anterior shoulder instability: Two-year follow-up with disease-specific quality-of-life outcomes. *J Bone Joint Surg Am* 2014;96(5):353-360.

    Higher recurrence of instability was noted in patients in the arthroscopic Bankart group, particularly in young

males with Hill-Sachs lesions. The arthroscopic group had more contact athletes, and no quantification of bone loss was performed. Level of evidence: I.

20. Archetti Netto N, Tamaoki MJ, Lenza M, et al: Treatment of Bankart lesions in traumatic anterior instability of the shoulder: A randomized controlled trial comparing arthroscopy and open techniques. *Arthroscopy* 2012;28(7):900-908.

    Improved DASH scores were noted in the arthroscopy group, but no substantial differences were noted in Rose or UCLA scores, range of motion, or recurrent instability. Level of evidence: II.

21. Chalmers PN, Mascarenhas R, Leroux T, et al: Do arthroscopic and open stabilization techniques restore equivalent stability to the shoulder in the setting of anterior glenohumeral instability? A systematic review of overlapping meta-analyses. *Arthroscopy* 2015;31(2):355-363.

    Overall, no difference was noted in recurrence rates noted. Studies published before 2007 favored open surgery in recurrence rates, whereas those published after 2007 demonstrated no difference. Level of evidence: IV.

22. Pulavarti RS, Symes TH, Rangan A: Surgical interventions for anterior shoulder instability in adults. *Cochrane Database Syst Rev* 2009;4:CD005077.

    Insufficient evidence exists from available randomized clinical trials to favor one technique over another.

23. Dickens JF, Owens BD, Cameron KL, et al: Return to play and recurrent instability after in-season anterior shoulder instability: A prospective multicenter study. *Am J Sports Med* 2014;42(12):2842-2850.

    Forty-five intercollegiate athletes with in-season shoulder instability were followed after accelerated rehabilitation and return to play; 73% returned to contact sports, but 64% had recurrent instability during the season. Level of evidence: II.

24. Grumet RC, Bach BR Jr, Provencher MT: Arthroscopic stabilization for first-time versus recurrent shoulder instability. *Arthroscopy* 2010;26(2):239-248.

    This systematic review compared arthroscopic Bankart repair immediately after first dislocation versus after multiple recurrences. No difference was noted in postoperative recurrence of instability, range of motion, or complications. Level of evidence: II.

25. Randelli P, Ragone V, Carminati S, Cabitza P: Risk factors for recurrence after Bankart repair a systematic review. *Knee Surg Sports Traumatol Arthrosc* 2012;20(11):2129-2138.

    Factors associated with recurrent instability after arthroscopic Bankart repair included age younger than 20 years, male sex, competitive sports participation, fewer than three suture anchors, glenoid bone loss, large Hill-Sachs lesions, ligamentous laxity, and anterior labroligamentous periosteal sleeve avulsion lesions. Level of evidence: II.

26. Cho NS, Yi JW, Lee BG, Rhee YG: Revision open Bankart surgery after arthroscopic repair for traumatic anterior shoulder instability. *Am J Sports Med* 2009;37(11):2158-2164.

Of 26 shoulders that underwent revision open Bankart repair after failed arthroscopic procedures, 88% had good or excellent results, with improved pain and stability scores. Three additional dislocations occurred in patients with engaging Hill-Sachs lesions and hyperlaxity. Level of evidence: IV.

27. Bartl C, Schumann K, Paul J, Vogt S, Imhoff AB: Arthroscopic capsulolabral revision repair for recurrent anterior shoulder instability. *Am J Sports Med* 2011;39(3):511-518.

Fifty-six patients underwent revision arthroscopic surgery following unsuccessful open or arthroscopic anterior stabilization. Rose, Constant, and SST scores substantially improved with 86% good or excellent results, with 11% recurrence. Level of evidence: IV.

28. Arce G, Arcuri F, Ferro D, Pereira E: Is selective arthroscopic revision beneficial for treating recurrent anterior shoulder instability? *Clin Orthop Relat Res* 2012;470(4):965-971.

In this retrospective analysis, 16 patients underwent revision arthroscopic Bankart repair. Strict exclusion criteria included substantial glenoid or humeral head bone loss, hyperlaxity, and participation in contact sports. UCLA, Constant, and Rowe scores improved substantially, and three recurrences were reported at mean 31-month follow-up. Level of evidence: IV.

29. Boileau P, Richou J, Lisai A, Chuinard C, Bicknell RT: The role of arthroscopy in revision of failed open anterior stabilization of the shoulder. *Arthroscopy* 2009;25(10):1075-1084.

Twenty-two patients with unsuccessful open anterior stabilization procedures underwent arthroscopic revision. Good or excellent results obtained in 85%, and one case of recurrent dislocation was reported. Osteoarthritis progressed by one stage in three patients. Level of evidence: IV.

30. Trivedi S, Pomerantz ML, Gross D, Golijanan P, Provencher MT: Shoulder instability in the setting of bipolar (glenoid and humeral head) bone loss: The glenoid track concept. *Clin Orthop Relat Res* 2014;472(8):2352-2362.

This systematic review reports on the biomechanical and cadaver data related to the glenoid track concept. Restoration of the glenoid track should be a primary goal of instability surgery.

31. Rerko MA, Pan X, Donaldson C, Jones GL, Bishop JY: Comparison of various imaging techniques to quantify glenoid bone loss in shoulder instability. *J Shoulder Elbow Surg* 2013;22(4):528-534.

This cadaver study reviewed three sizes of glenoid bone defects created and then imaged using 3D CT, CT, MRI, and plain radiography. Although 3D CT was the most accurate and reliable, all imaging modalities underestimated bone loss to some extent. Level of evidence: III.

32. Ozaki R, Nakagawa S, Mizuno N, Mae T, Yoneda M: Hill-sachs lesions in shoulders with traumatic anterior instability: Evaluation using computed tomography with 3-dimensional reconstruction. *Am J Sports Med* 2014;42(11):2597-2605.

3D CT performed in 135 patients with traumatic anterior shoulder instability undergoing arthroscopic Bankart repair identified 80% of Hill-Sachs lesions with a sensitivity of 76%, a specificity of 100%, a positive predictive value of 100%, and a negative predictive value of 46%. 3D CT was less accurate in shallow lesions and those without subchondral bone damage. Level of evidence: II.

33. Hovelius L, Sandström B, Olofsson A, Svensson O, Rahme H: The effect of capsular repair, bone block healing, and position on the results of the Bristow-Latarjet procedure (study III): Long-term follow-up in 319 shoulders. *J Shoulder Elbow Surg* 2012;21(5):647-660.

In three series of patients undergoing open Latarjet procedure with between 5 and 23 years of follow-up, 1% of patients required revision surgery for recurrence and 96% reported satisfaction with the procedure. Recurrence was associated with graft placement that was too medial.

34. Griesser MJ, Harris JD, McCoy BW, et al: Complications and re-operations after Bristow-Latarjet shoulder stabilization: A systematic review. *J Shoulder Elbow Surg* 2013;22(2):286-292.

This systematic review of open and arthroscopic Latarjet procedures reported an overall complication rate of 30%, most of which related to healing or fracture of the coracoid. Recurrent instability was noted in 8.7%, 73% of those within the first year following surgery. The mean loss of external rotation was 13°. Level of evidence: IV.

35. Dumont GD, Fogerty S, Rosso C, Lafosse L: The arthroscopic latarjet procedure for anterior shoulder instability: 5-year minimum follow-up. *Am J Sports Med* 2014;42(11):2560-2566.

This retrospective case series reported on 62 patients who underwent an arthroscopic Latarjet procedure with a minimum 5-year follow-up. Recurrent instability was seen in 1.6%, and high WOSI scores were reported in all domains. Level of evidence: IV.

36. Sayegh ET, Mascarenhas R, Chalmers PN, Cole BJ, Verma NN, Romeo AA: Allograft reconstruction for glenoid bone loss in glenohumeral instability: A systematic review. *Arthroscopy* 2014;30(12):1642-1649.

This systematic review evaluated multiple allograft techniques for anterior glenoid reconstruction. At an average 44-month follow-up, 93% of patients were satisfied with the outcome, despite 10% with residual pain. High Rowe scores and recurrent instability in 7.1% were reported; 100% graft incorporation was noted. Level of evidence: IV.

37. Beran MC, Donaldson CT, Bishop JY: Treatment of chronic glenoid defects in the setting of recurrent anterior shoulder instability: A systematic review. *J Shoulder Elbow Surg* 2010;19(5):769-780.

    A systematic review of the current evidence demonstrated no data to support one glenoid bone restoration technique over another. Level of evidence: IV.

38. Franceschi F, Papalia R, Rizzello G, et al: Remplissage repair—new frontiers in the prevention of recurrent shoulder instability: A 2-year follow-up comparative study. *Am J Sports Med* 2012;40(11):2462-2469.

    This retrospective cohort of patients with Bankart and engaging Hill-Sachs lesions was treated with remplissage and Bankart repair or Bankart repair alone. Patients in the remplissage group had substantially decreased recurrence. All had improved outcome scores, returned to sports, and had minimal motion loss. All remplissage tendons were fully healed at 2 years on MRI. Level of evidence: III.

39. Boileau P, O'Shea K, Vargas P, Pinedo M, Old J, Zumstein M: Anatomical and functional results after arthroscopic Hill-Sachs remplissage. *J Bone Joint Surg Am* 2012;94(7):618-626.

    A retrospective analysis evaluated 47 patients undergoing arthroscopic remplissage with Bankart repair for recurrent instability. Recurrence was reported in one patient; 68% returned to previous level of sport. The average motion loss in ABER was 8° to 9°. Level of evidence: IV.

40. Longo UG, Loppini M, Rizzello G, et al: Remplissage, humeral osteochondral grafts, weber osteotomy, and shoulder arthroplasty for the management of humeral bone defects in shoulder instability: Systematic review and quantitative synthesis of the literature. *Arthroscopy* 2014;30(12):1650-1666.

    This systematic review evaluated all four techniques to treat humeral head defects. Overall, remplissage was an effective, safe technique. High rates of substantial complications were reported with other techniques. Level of evidence: IV.

41. Robinson CM, Seah M, Akhtar MA: The epidemiology, risk of recurrence, and functional outcome after an acute traumatic posterior dislocation of the shoulder. *J Bone Joint Surg Am* 2011;93(17):1605-1613.

    This prospective cohort of 120 patients with isolated posterior dislocations reviewed epidemiology, associated injuries, and functional outcomes. The risk of recurrence was independently predicted by young age, large reverse Hill-Sachs lesions, and seizure as an etiology of dislocation. Level of evidence: II.

42. Song DJ, Cook JB, Krul KP, et al: High frequency of posterior and combined shoulder instability in young active patients. *J Shoulder Elbow Surg* 2015;24(2):186-190.

    In this retrospective analysis, 231 patients underwent surgical stabilization for shoulder instability. Isolated anterior labral tears were found in 57% of patients, with isolated posterior tears in 24% and combined labral injuries in 19%. Level of evidence: III.

43. Kim SH, Ha KI, Park JH, et al: Arthroscopic posterior labral repair and capsular shift for traumatic unidirectional recurrent posterior subluxation of the shoulder. *J Bone Joint Surg Am* 2003;85-A(8):1479-1487.

44. Bradley JP, McClincy MP, Arner JW, Tejwani SG: Arthroscopic capsulolabral reconstruction for posterior instability of the shoulder: A prospective study of 200 shoulders. *Am J Sports Med* 2013;41(9):2005-2014.

    This prospective case series evaluated 200 shoulders with unidirectional posterior shoulder instability treated with arthroscopic capsulolabral reconstruction. At 36-month follow-up, patients demonstrated improved outcomes related to stability, pain, and function. Level of evidence: II.

45. Owens BD, Campbell SE, Cameron KL: Risk factors for posterior shoulder instability in young athletes. *Am J Sports Med* 2013;41(11):2645-2649.

    This prospective cohort study of high-risk, young athletes in whom posterior shoulder instability develops reported that the most substantial risk factor for subsequent posterior instability was increased glenoid retroversion. A 17% increase in risk of acute posterior instability with every 1° increase in retroversion was demonstrated. Level of evidence: II.

46. Wolf BR, Strickland S, Williams RJ, Allen AA, Altchek DW, Warren RF: Open posterior stabilization for recurrent posterior glenohumeral instability. *J Shoulder Elbow Surg* 2005;14(2):157-164.

47. Wellmann M, Bobrowitsch E, Khan N, et al: Biomechanical effectiveness of an arthroscopic posterior bankart repair versus an open bone block procedure for posterior shoulder instability. *Am J Sports Med* 2011;39(4):796-803.

    This cadaver biomechanical study evaluated eight matched pairs of shoulders with a simulated posterior Bankart lesion and laceration of the posterior band of the IGHL. Pathologic translation in all directions was returned to the intact state using an arthroscopic posterior Bankart repair, whereas the joint was overconstrained to posterior translation and inferior instability was not addressed with the bone block procedure.

48. Schwartz DG, Goebel S, Piper K, Kordasiewicz B, Boyle S, Lafosse L: Arthroscopic posterior bone block augmentation in posterior shoulder instability. *J Shoulder Elbow Surg* 2013;22(8):1092-1101.

    This retrospective case series reviewed 19 arthroscopic posterior bone block procedures for patients with recurrent posterior instability and bone loss. Level of evidence: IV.

49. Meuffels DE, Schuit H, van Biezen FC, Reijman M, Verhaar JA: The posterior bone block procedure in posterior shoulder instability: A long-term follow-up study. *J Bone Joint Surg Br* 2010;92(5):651-655.

    In this prospective case series of 11 patients who underwent posterior bone block procedure with 18-year follow-up, patients with traumatic etiology of instability had the best results versus hyperlaxity or MDI. More than one-half of patients had residual instability, and diminishing outcomes were noted over time. Level of evidence: IV.

50. Misamore GW, Sallay PI, Didelot W: A longitudinal study of patients with multidirectional instability of the shoulder with seven- to ten-year follow-up. *J Shoulder Elbow Surg* 2005;14(5):466-470.

51. Nyiri P, Illyés A, Kiss R, Kiss J: Intermediate biomechanical analysis of the effect of physiotherapy only compared with capsular shift and physiotherapy in multidirectional shoulder instability. *J Shoulder Elbow Surg* 2010;19(6):802-813.

A cohort of patients with MDI who underwent physical therapy alone was compared with those who underwent physiotherapy after an open capsular shift. At 2 and 4 years after therapy, the combined surgical/therapy group had kinematic and electromyographic values similar to those of control patients. Therapy alone was unable to restore normal joint kinematics and prevent instability. Level of evidence: II.

52. Jacobson ME, Riggenbach M, Wooldridge AN, Bishop JY: Open capsular shift and arthroscopic capsular plication for treatment of multidirectional instability. *Arthroscopy* 2012;28(7):1010-1017.

This systematic review compared open and arthroscopic surgical management of MDI. No substantial differences were reported; both appear to be safe, effective techniques. Overhead athletes and swimmers were least likely to return to prior level of sport. Level of evidence: IV.

Chapter 2

Disorders of the Acromioclavicular Joint, Sternoclavicular Joint, and Clavicle

Brian R. Wolf, MD, MS   Youssef El Bitar, MD

Abstract

Acromioclavicular (AC) joint separations and clavicle fractures are common injuries involving the shoulder girdle; injuries to the sternoclavicular (SC) joint are less common. Management of AC joint separations depends on the injury type; management of type III is the most controversial. Clavicle fracture management depends on the fracture location along the clavicle shaft. Neer type II lateral third fractures and complex unstable middle shaft fractures require surgical intervention. SC joint injuries are mostly treated nonsurgically, except in cases of instability and pain. An understanding of the mechanism of injury for these shoulder injuries is important, along with knowledge about the most commonly used classification systems for each injury, management options based on classification, postoperative rehabilitation, outcomes reported in the literature, and possible complications.

Keywords: acromioclavicular joint separation; clavicle fracture; sternoclavicular joint dislocation

Introduction

Shoulder injuries can result in various pathologies including subluxations, dislocations, and fractures. Acromioclavicular (AC) joint injuries are common in young athletes, ranging from a simple sprain to frank dislocation. Managing the AC joint separation is usually nonsurgical in type I and II injuries, and type IV to VI injuries are treated surgically. The management of type III AC joint separation is controversial, with proponents for both nonsurgical and surgical treatment. Clavicle fractures are common injuries in adults, affecting patients who are both young and elderly. These fractures are divided into lateral third, middle third, and medial third clavicle fractures. Although most clavicle fractures are treated nonsurgically, some require surgical intervention, mainly unstable type II lateral third fractures and complicated, substantially shortened middle third fractures. The sternoclavicular (SC) joint is injured less often than the AC joint or the clavicle because the surrounding ligaments are strong. The most common type of management of SC joint injury is nonsurgical. Closed reduction is required in type 3 SC joint dislocation whether anterior or posterior. Occasionally, open reduction and internal stabilization is required for unstable, symptomatic dislocations.

AC Joint Injuries

Injuries to the AC joint comprise 9% of shoulder injuries and are often caused by direct trauma to the shoulder or a fall on an outstretched hand.[1] Younger, physically active athletes are at particularly increased risk,[2] especially

Dr. Wolf or an immediate family member serves as a paid consultant to CONMED Linvatec; has received research or institutional support from the Orthopaedic Research and Education Foundation; has received nonincome support (such as equipment or services), commercially derived honoraria, or other non–research-related funding (such as paid travel) from Arthrex; and serves as a board member, owner, officer, or committee member of the American Academy of Orthopaedic Surgeons, the American Orthopaedic Society for Sports Medicine, and the Mid-America Orthopaedic Association. Neither Dr. El Bitar nor any immediate family member has received anything of value from or has stock or stock options held in a commercial company or institution related directly or indirectly to the subject of this chapter.

those involved in contact and extreme sports, as well as high-risk activities such as skiing and cycling. The extent of injury to the AC and coracoclavicular (CC) ligaments as well as the amount and direction of clavicle displacement often determine the severity of AC joint separation. Debate continues regarding the best management of such injuries, especially type III AC joint separation. Several factors play a role in decision making on the management of these common injuries including age of patient, type of injury, time from injury, activity level, and to some extent, aesthetic appearance. Treatment involves nonsurgical and surgical measures, including acute repairs with or without augmentation or late reconstruction. Overall, the outcomes are favorable with most treatment options.

Mechanism of Injury

Injuries to the AC joint are usually the result of a direct blow to the superior and lateral aspects of the shoulder with the arm in an adducted position, resulting in the displacement of the acromion inferiorly and medially relative to the clavicle. The first ligament injured is the AC ligament. With increasing severity of injury, the CC ligaments are injured next, followed by the deltotrapezial fascia.[3] Another less common mechanism of injury is a fall on an outstretched hand, resulting in the proximal humerus being pushed into the acromion with a superiorly directed force.[3]

Classification

In 1963, AC joint injuries were initially classified in 1963 into types I, II, and III.[4] The classification was later expanded by Rockwood in 1984 to include types IV, V, and VI,[5] relying on comparative films of the contralateral shoulder to determine each type (**Figure 1**). A type I injury involves AC ligament sprain without injury to the CC ligaments, and no AC joint widening or clavicular displacement. Type II injuries consist of complete rupture of the AC ligament, CC ligament sprain, widening of the AC joint, and increase of the CC distance by more than zero to less than 25% compared to the contralateral shoulder. In type III injuries, the AC and CC ligaments are disrupted, the AC joint is widened, and the CC distance is increased 25% to 100% compared to the contralateral shoulder. A type IV AC joint separation is diagnosed when the distal clavicle is displaced posteriorly into the trapezius muscle. Type V injury is similar to type III, except the CC distance is increased by more than 100% compared to the contralateral shoulder because of disruption of the deltotrapezial fascia and tenting of the overlying skin can result. Type VI injury is rare and involves inferior displacement of the clavicle into the subcoracoid space (Table 1).

Management

Type I and Type II AC Joint Injuries

Nonsurgical management has been the first-line treatment of type I and type II AC joint separations, using an arm sling for immobilization and pain control. Additionally, several other therapeutic modalities are used including rest, oral analgesics, NSAIDs, icing, and activity modification. Some studies advocate the use of intra-articular long-acting anesthetic injections into the AC joint in highly competitive athletes to allow faster return to play in the acute setting. The arm sling is usually used for approximately 1 week in type I injuries, and for 2 to 3 weeks in type II AC joint separations. When the pain subsides, the arm sling is discontinued and physical therapy is initiated with active and passive shoulder range-of-motion (ROM) exercises. Strengthening exercises are started after full ROM is obtained. Patients should refrain from returning to contact sports or heavy lifting for approximately 2 to 3 months, until restoration of full, painless shoulder ROM.

Currently, no evidence supports early surgical management for type I or type II AC joint separations. However, patients are at risk for recurrent or persistent shoulder symptoms after type I and type II injuries. Injury can occur to the AC joint articular cartilage or articular disk that can result in shoulder complaints subsequent to the injury. Retrospective studies have reported persistent symptoms in up to 40% to 50% of patients at 1, 6, and 10 years after injury.[6-8] Despite the relatively high percentage of persistent symptomatic patients, nonsurgical treatment is still the standard of care in type I and type II AC joint injuries. In one study, 27% of patients underwent surgical intervention at a mean of 26 months after injury.[7] Distal clavicle resection, either arthroscopic or open, could provide a potential solution in patients whose nonsurgical treatment failed secondary to the development of osteoarthritis in the AC joint.[9]

Type III AC Joint Injuries

The initial management of type III AC joint separations is still controversial in the literature and in clinical practice. Several studies have advocated nonsurgical treatment with good to excellent outcomes at final follow-up;[10] other studies have reported persistent pain and symptoms.[11] A 2011 study recommended surgical management for type III AC joint separation in young, active patients in the acute setting.[12] Therefore, no consensus has been reached regarding the best treatment option for type III AC joint injuries. These injuries should be treated on a case-by-case basis, depending on the age and activity level of the patient. A 2007 study reported the results of a survey of 664 members and residency directors from the American Orthopaedic Society for Sports Medicine:

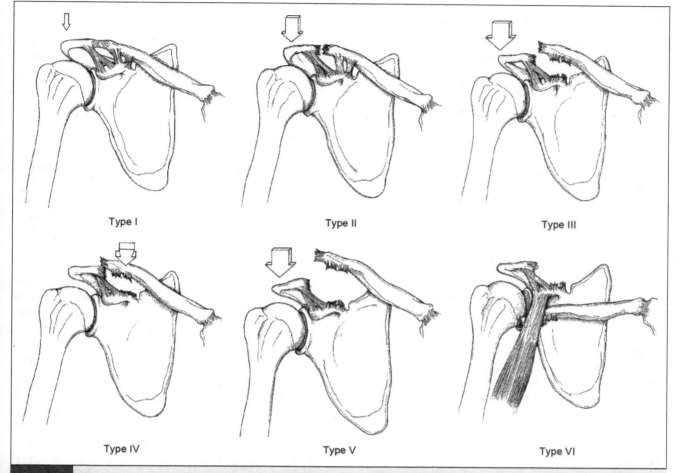

Type I

Type II

Type III

Type IV

Type V

Type VI

Figure 1   Illustration demonstrates the six types of acromioclavicular joint separation. (Reproduced from Nuber GW, Bowen MK: Acromioclavicular joint injuries and distal clavicle fractures. *J Am Acad Orthop Surg* 1997;5[1]:11-18.)

Table 1

Classification of AC Joint Separation

Type	AC Ligaments	CC Ligaments	Deltotrapezial Fascia	Increase in Radiographic CC Distance	AC Radiographic Appearance	AC Joint Reducible
I	Sprained	Intact	Intact	Normal (1.1 to 1.3 cm)	Normal	NA
II	Disrupted	Sprained	Intact	<25%	Widened	Yes
III	Disrupted	Disrupted	Disrupted	25% to 100%[a]	Widened	Yes
IV	Disrupted	Disrupted	Disrupted	Increased	Posterior clavicle displacement	No
V	Disrupted	Disrupted	Disrupted	100% to 300%[a]	NA	No
VI	Disrupted	Intact	Disrupted	Decreased	NA	No

AC = acromioclavicular, CC = coracoclavicular, NA = not applicable.

[a]. Displacement is compared with that of the contralateral shoulder (described by Rockwood) and not determined according to clavicular diameter.

86.3% preferred nonsurgical treatment of uncomplicated type III AC joint injuries.[13]

Several studies have compared results of nonsurgical and surgical management to treat type III AC joint separations using randomized trials, cohort studies, and retrospective designs. Support for both initial nonsurgical treatment[14,15] and early surgery[16] was found. A 2011 meta-analysis of six nonrandomized studies compared nonsurgical and surgical management of type III AC joint injuries in 380 patients.[17] No difference was found between the groups in pain, strength, throwing ability, or incidence of AC joint osteoarthritis. Patients in the surgical group had substantially greater duration of sick leave with better cosmetic appearance.[17]

If surgery is preferred or deemed necessary, early surgical repair of type III AC joint injuries with or without augmentation seems to result in better patient satisfaction and clinical outcomes compared with delayed reconstruction.[18] A 2014 systematic review compared early and delayed surgical intervention in complete AC joint dislocation involving mostly type III injuries.[19] Overall, superior functional outcomes were found in the early surgical group ($P < 0.05$) compared with delayed surgery. Partial dislocations or redislocations were found in 26% of cases in the early treatment group compared with 38.1% of cases in the delayed group ($P < 0.05$).

Type IV, V, and VI AC Joint Injuries and Surgical Management

Surgical management is usually indicated for type IV and V AC joint separations given the high likelihood of shoulder pain and dysfunction and substantial deformity of the shoulder. Type VI injuries are extremely rare and are treated surgically. Surgery for type IV and type V injuries is usually recommended in the acute or subacute setting, but can be performed on a delayed basis if nonsurgical treatment fails or if the patient presents for treatment late. A recent retrospective study looked at conservative treatment of type V AC joint separations in active-duty service members.[20] After exclusions, 21 underwent conservative treatment initially, whereas 8 underwent acute repair. In the conservative group, 11 patients (61%) returned to full duty without surgery at an average of 97.8 days, whereas in the acute surgical group, 6 patients (75%) returned to full duty at an average of 169.3 days. Type IV and type V injuries are relatively less common, with most published data involving small case series, case reports, or as part of larger series involving type III injuries. Several key elements of surgical intervention are critical for successful outcomes in treating those high-grade injuries. Anatomic reduction of the dislocated clavicle to correct posterior, superior, or anterior translation is important

for successful outcomes. Repairing and/or reconstructing the CC ligaments are important for maintaining anatomic reduction. Supplementing the CC ligament repair and/or reconstruction with synthetic material or plate fixation can provide adequate stability for CC ligament healing. Repairing or imbricating the damaged deltotrapezial fascia are integral parts of surgical management to optimize outcomes.

Numerous surgical techniques are described in the literature for the surgical management of AC joint injuries. No consensus exists on technique or timing of surgery. For type III injuries, options for primary fixation without reconstruction are available. The objective is to reduce the AC joint and directly repair the CC ligaments or allow them to scar or heal together. Reduction of the AC joint promotes healing of the damaged CC ligament tissue. AC joint reduction can be maintained using various techniques. A hook plate is a clavicular plate that includes a lateral extension that goes under the acromion, reducing the AC joint. Other methods focus on direct fixation between the clavicle and the coracoid and include a screw through the clavicle into the coracoid, heavy sutures around or through the coracoid and clavicle, or button suture constructs around/through the coracoid and clavicle (Figure 2). A 2014 study compared arthroscopically assisted reduction of acute AC joint separation using the double-button suture technique compared with the hook plate technique.[21] Both techniques had good to excellent results, with comparable outcome scores and complication rates. A 2013 study followed 23 patients who underwent arthroscopically assisted acute CC ligament reduction using two double-button sutures (one for each CC ligament).[22] There were 3 type III, 3 type IV, and 17 type V AC joint injuries, and patients were followed for an average of 58 months; 96% of patients were very satisfied or satisfied at final follow-up, with a significant improvement in the visual analog scale and Constant scores, even with eight radiographic failures.

Ligament reconstruction is another method for surgical management and is commonly used for acute surgical management of grade IV and V injuries, as well as for delayed treatment (longer than 6 weeks) after type III injury. Reconstruction is performed to reconstruct or replace soft-tissue stabilizers of the AC joint using hamstring autograft or allograft, tibialis anterior allograft, or coracoacromial ligament transfer (the Weaver-Dunn procedure). The ligament reconstruction techniques provide options for managing both acute and chronic AC joint injuries. In 2010, free tendon anatomic reconstruction of the CC ligaments became widely accepted for surgical management of AC joint.[23] Anatomic reconstruction uses a free tendon graft and nonabsorbable sutures that wrap

© 2016 American Academy of Orthopaedic Surgeons

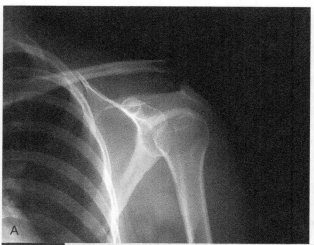
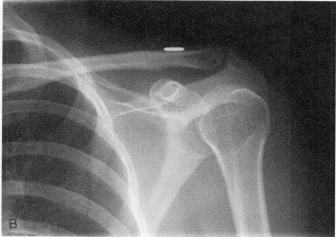

Figure 2 **A,** Preoperative AP radiograph of the left shoulder of a 26-year-old woman who is an athlete demonstrates a type V acromioclavicular (AC) joint separation. **B,** AP radiograph obtained 2 weeks following acute repair using a double-endobutton suture technique, demonstrates adequate reduction of the AC joint separation.

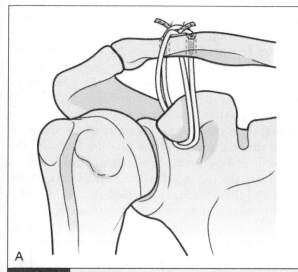
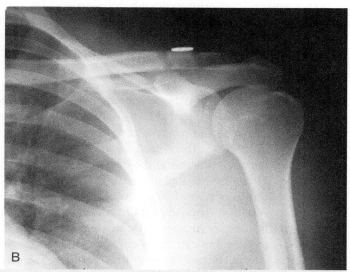

Figure 3 **A,** Illustration demonstrates the double-loop coracoclavicular ligament reconstruction technique for chronic unstable acromioclavicular (AC) joint separation. **B,** Postoperative AP radiograph of the left shoulder of a 49-year-old man with type III AC joint separation whose nonsurgical treatment was unsuccessful shows adequate reduction of the AC joint.

around the base of the coracoid and are passed through the clavicle using small bone tunnels. Several variations of this technique have been reported.[23-25] A small distal clavicle resection is occasionally performed with AC joint reconstruction if the distal clavicle has become deformed and cannot be reduced. The decision to routinely perform a distal clavicle resection with reconstruction is controversial. A 2010 study reported on 17 cases managed using anatomic ligament reconstruction, 14 of which were successful with excellent improvement in American Shoulder and Elbow Surgeon and Constant scores.[23] A 2014 study reported on seven patients who underwent reconstruction

using a doubled loop of tendon graft with zero failures at short-term follow-up[24] (Figure 3).

Postoperative Rehabilitation

Following surgery, the shoulder is usually immobilized in a sling or supportive brace for 6 to 8 weeks. Elbow, wrist, and hand exercises are encouraged as long as the shoulder is kept stable. Passive supine shoulder flexion and abduction up to 90° in the plane of the scapula can be considered safe early in the rehabilitation phase. However, motion can also be delayed until 6 to 8 weeks with minimal risk of stiffness. Gradual progression of shoulder ROM exercises are usually started 6 to 8 weeks after surgery and slowly progressed until 12 to 14 weeks. Strengthening exercises for the shoulder muscles can be started when the patient achieves painless shoulder ROM at approximately 12 weeks postoperatively, taking care to avoid downward force on the arm and shoulder. Return to work without restrictions usually occurs at 16 to 24 weeks following surgery, with full-contact athletic activities resumed at approximately 6 months postoperatively, after the patient has achieved similar shoulder strength and ROM compared with the unaffected shoulder. Full recovery can take 9 to 12 months.[3,22,25]

Complications

Both nonsurgical and surgical management of AC joint separations can result in complications. Complications associated with nonsurgical management include persistent pain, crepitus, and swelling at the AC joint; late arthrosis; and persistent instability. Osteolysis of the distal clavicle also has been reported. Postoperative complications depend on the type of surgical technique used. Implant failure and migration, resulting in vascular injuries, have been reported. Hence, Kirschner wires and pins are not advised. Aseptic foreign body reaction and erosion of the coracoid or clavicle have been reported with the use of synthetic suture loops. Early or late fractures of the clavicle or coracoid process have been reported as well, especially with surgical techniques that involve tunnels through the coracoid and/or clavicle. Painful hardware related to the hook plate or CC screw usually requires a second procedure for implant removal. Loss of AC joint reduction, persistent pain, and instability can potentially complicate surgical outcomes. Neurologic injuries are rare, but can involve nerve root injuries secondary to traction during surgery, direct injury to the suprascapular nerve resulting from aggressive dissection during reconstruction, or injury to the brachial plexus with techniques that pass grafts or suture loops under the coracoid process.[6]

Clavicle Fractures

Fractures of the clavicle comprise 2% to 5% of all fractures in adults and 35% to 44% of all fractures in the shoulder, with an incidence of 50 to 64 per 100,000 persons annually.[26-28] The risk for clavicle fracture is increased in men age 30 years or younger and all patients older than 70 years. Middle third fractures are the most common types of injuries, comprising approximately 69% to 81% of all clavicle fractures. Lateral third fractures account for approximately 17% to 28% of all clavicle fractures, and medial third fractures comprise the remaining 2% to

3%.[26-28] Nonsurgical management has been the preferred initial mode of treatment for most clavicle fractures. However, according to more recent literature, nonunion can be a substantial cause of morbidity, with some publications reporting unfavorable patient-based outcomes. Therefore, treatment of clavicle fractures should be tailored to each patient and the type of fracture, amount of displacement and comminution, age and level of activity of the patient, and to some extent, the esthetic appearance of the shoulder, should be considered.

Mechanism of Injury and Classification

The most common mechanism of injury in clavicle fractures is a direct blow to the shoulder, whether following a fall or because of direct trauma. Less commonly, a fall on an outstretched hand can result in clavicle fracture; this mechanism was initially thought to be the most common cause of these fractures. These injuries are rarely open, despite being caused by high-energy trauma.[26,27]

Clavicle fractures were initially described in 1967 based on their anatomic location and in descending order of incidence.[28] Type I fractures involve the middle third of the clavicle; type II and type III fractures involve the lateral and medial thirds, respectively. In 1968 (Neer classification)[29] and 1996 (Craig classification),[30] type II (lateral third) clavicle fractures were subclassified into three types, depending on the integrity of the CC ligaments and the relationship of the fracture line with the CC ligaments and AC joint. Type I lateral third fractures occur lateral to the CC ligaments and are usually stable. Type II lateral third fractures are medial to the CC ligaments, are usually unstable, and require surgical management. Type II was further subclassified into type IIA, in which the fracture is medial to the intact conoid and trapezoid ligaments, and type IIB, in which the fracture is lateral to the torn conoid ligament but medial to the intact trapezoid ligament. Type III lateral third fractures are intra-articular fractures through the AC joint with intact CC ligaments. These fractures are usually stable, but can result in the development of AC joint arthritis. Type IV fractures are rare and involve disruption of the clavicular periosteal sleeve in pediatric patients, in whom the epiphysis and physis remain with the AC joint and the displacement occurs at the junction of the metaphysis and physis. In type V fractures, a small, inferior cortical bone fragment remains attached to the CC ligaments, with the proximal and distal fragments of the clavicle fracture not connected to the coracoid process (Figure 4). These fractures are rare and generally require surgical intervention for reduction and stabilization.

The Edinburgh classification was proposed in 1998, with clavicular fractures divided by anatomic location

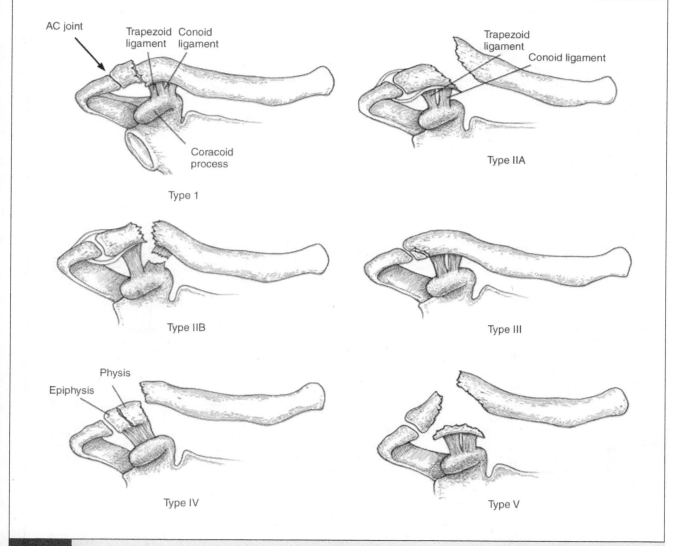

Figure 4 Illustration demonstrates the Neer classification for distal clavicle fractures. AC = acromioclavicular. (Reproduced from Banerjee R, Waterman B, Padalecki J, Robertson W: Management of distal clavicle fractures. *J Am Acad Orthop Surg* 2011;19[7]:392-401.)

into type I (medial third), type II (middle third), and type III (lateral third).[31] Further subclassification of each type was based on fracture magnitude and displacement. Subgroup A indicates displacement less than 100% and subgroup B indicates displacement more than 100%. Articular involvement determined further subdivision of types I and III. Subgroup 1 indicates no articular involvement and subgroup 2 indicates intra-articular extension of the fracture. Type II fractures are also subdivided: subgroup 1 indicates simple or wedge-type fractures and subgroup 2 indicates comminuted or segmented fractures (**Figure 5**). A 2011 study compared the previous classification systems and reported that the Craig classification

best predicted nonunion or delayed union of lateral third clavicle fractures, and the Robinson classification had the best prognostic potential for middle third clavicle fractures.[32]

Management and Complications
Medial Third Clavicle Fractures
The treatment of medial third clavicle fractures is usually nonsurgical, with satisfactory outcomes and low nonunion rates of 4% to 8%.[31] These fractures are uncommon and are usually nondisplaced. The SC joint is rarely involved in such injuries. Treatment consists of an arm sling for comfort, with shoulder immobilization for

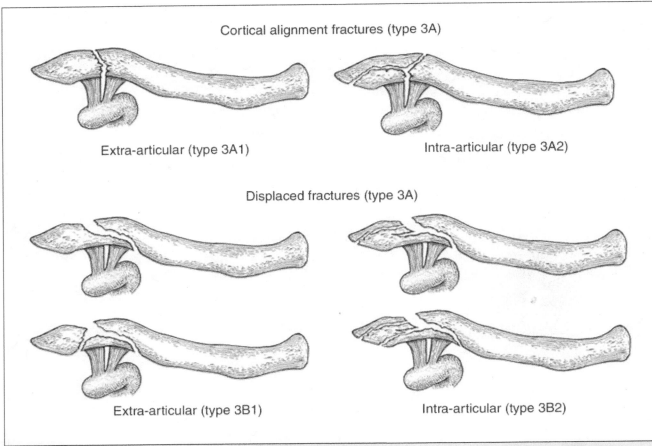

Cortical alignment fractures (type 3A)

Extra-articular (type 3A1)

Intra-articular (type 3A2)

Displaced fractures (type 3A)

Extra-articular (type 3B1)

Intra-articular (type 3B2)

Figure 5 Illustration demonstrates the Robinson classification for distal clavicle fractures. (Reproduced from Banerjee R, Waterman B, Padalecki J, Robertson W: Management of distal clavicle fractures. *J Am Acad Orthop Surg* 2011;19[7]:392-401.)

2 to 6 weeks. Shoulder ROM is started as soon as the pain subsides or becomes tolerable. Ice can help decrease the swelling, with oral medications for pain control. Use of NSAIDs is controversial, with some studies not recommending them because of the possibility of delayed fracture healing. Contact sports should be avoided for at least 2 to 3 months to allow complete fracture healing and shoulder rehabilitation.[27]

Surgical management of medial third clavicle fractures is usually reserved for fractures associated with injury to the mediastinal structures secondary to fracture displacement. These fractures should be reduced fairly emergently, with an attempt at closed reduction. Open reduction and internal fixation (ORIF) is sometimes necessary to maintain reduction of an unstable fracture. Several techniques have been used for ORIF of displaced medial third clavicle fractures including wire fixation, plate-and-screw constructs, or interosseous sutures. Because this type of clavicle fracture is rare, few case reports or small series exist on this subject, with favorable outcomes.[33]

Middle Third Clavicle Fractures

Middle third clavicle fractures comprise most clavicle fractures and have been treated nonsurgically with reported successful outcomes. A nonunion rate less than 1% has been reported for nonsurgical management, less than rates reported for surgical management.[29] High patient satisfaction has also been reported following nonsurgical treatment. However, the more recent literature has provided more information about clavicle fracture management, with many studies reporting less favorable outcomes following nonsurgical management with high nonunion rates.[34-37] A 2005 meta-analysis compared surgical and nonsurgical treatment of middle third clavicle fractures in 2,144 cases with a mean follow-up of 61 months.[34] Nonsurgical management was performed in 1,145 (53.4%) cases, with a nonunion rate of 5.9%, as opposed to a nonunion rate of 2.2% in 999 surgically treated cases. When examining displaced fractures separately, 159 cases were treated nonsurgically, resulting in a nonunion rate of 15.1%, as opposed to 2.1% for 612 surgically treated cases. A 2012 meta-analysis compared surgical and nonsurgical management of middle third clavicle fractures.[36] The nonunion rate was substantially higher in the nonsurgical group, with both groups achieving comparable Constant shoulder and Disabilities of the Arm, Shoulder and Hand scores at final follow-up.

Two multicenter randomized clinical trials compared the clinical outcomes of surgical and nonsurgical management of displaced middle third clavicle fractures.[35,37] The Constant and Disability of the Arm, Shoulder and Hand scores as well as patient satisfaction were substantially superior in patients in the surgical group.[35,37] The risk of nonunion and malunion was significantly higher in patients in the nonsurgical group, and patients in the surgical group had higher risk of wound infection and implant irritation requiring removal.[35,37] The mean time to union in a 2007 study was substantially shorter in the surgical group (16.4 weeks) compared with the nonsurgical group (28.4 weeks, $P = 0.001$).[35] Surgical treatment of middle third clavicle fractures is usually reserved for patients between age 16 and 60 years, with no infection or skin compromise at the surgical site, and who are medically fit and have an active lifestyle. In general, the indications for surgical management of middle third clavicle fractures include fracture displacement with shortening of more than 2 cm, skin tenting with an impending or open fracture, neurovascular compromise, floating shoulder, and obvious clinical deformity.[38]

ORIF of middle third clavicle fractures is usually performed with a plate-and-screw construct or with intramedullary pinning. The plate-and-screw fixation technique provides rigid fixation, allowing early mobilization. However, implant prominence and irritation usually results in a second surgical procedure for implant removal. Other complications such as infection, implant failure with nonunion, subsequent fracture following implant removal, hypertrophic scarring, and adhesive capsulitis of the shoulder have been reported. Intramedullary pin fixation has become more common because of better cosmetic appearance following surgery. However, some intramedullary pins lack a locking mechanism, resulting in no rotational control at the fracture site. Those pins require routine removal, with complications such as implant migration or breakage, skin breakdown and infection, and temporary brachial plexus palsy reported.[27]

Lateral Third Clavicle Fractures

Most lateral third clavicle fractures are nondisplaced or minimally displaced extra-articular fractures; therefore, treatment has been typically nonsurgical. The nonsurgical management modalities are similar to those used for middle third and medial third clavicle fractures.[31]

Surgical management of distal clavicle fractures depends on several factors including fracture stability (which relies on the status of the CC ligaments), fracture displacement, and patient age. Displacement of the clavicle occurs in Neer type II or Edinburgh type 3B fractures, with nonunion rates up to 28% for nonsurgical treatment.[29,39] Older age has also been associated with an increased risk of nonunion.[39] Intra-articular extension of the fracture can increase the risk of AC joint arthrosis, requiring distal clavicle resection when symptomatic.

Several surgical techniques have been described in the treatment of lateral third clavicle fractures, which are more technically challenging than middle third fractures. Wire fixation has been abandoned because of reported cases of pin migration. CC screw fixation has resulted in mostly favorable outcomes, with only small cohorts reported.[40] Hook plate, standard plating, and locking plate fixation have also been successful despite the reported rare incidence of complications such as nonunion, stiffness, fracture around the plate, and progression of AC joint arthritis.[41] Last, some unstable lateral third clavicle fractures can be repaired using reconstruction techniques also used for high-grade AC joint separations and include CC ligament reconstruction and suture augmentation. Hybrid plating of the clavicle and CC ligament reconstruction is also an option for unstable lateral fractures. Hook plates and CC screws require removal at a later stage secondary to decreased ROM and discomfort and are associated with a risk of screw breakage and hook plate damage to the AC joint. In addition, use of CC screws or traditional plate-and-screw constructs is occasionally not possible when the distal fragment is small, although the number of plates designed for the lateral clavicle has increased. CC ligament suture or ligament reconstruction techniques have resulted in generally acceptable functional results with high union rates.[42]

Postoperative Rehabilitation

Postoperative rehabilitation for lateral third clavicle fractures generally follows that used following surgical management of grade III through VI AC joint dislocations, with shoulder immobilization for 6 weeks. Generally, rehabilitation is slower and more conservative for lateral third fractures compared with medial or middle third fractures. Following surgical management of medial or middle third clavicle fractures, an arm sling is used for pain control and comfort, with shoulder ROM started as soon as postoperative day 1. Overhead lifting is withheld until approximately 6 weeks after surgery. Resolution of pain is successful enough following ORIF using plate-and-screw constructs that patients sometimes need to be prevented from overdoing shoulder exercises and activities to protect the construct. When intramedullary pinning is performed in middle third clavicle fractures and some concern exists regarding rotational stability of the fixation, forward flexion and abduction exercises for the shoulder should be restricted to 90° for the first 4 weeks. Shoulder muscle strengthening can be started as soon as 2 weeks postoperatively as long as fracture reduction is maintained and confirmed on shoulder radiographs. Some athletes return to noncontact athletic activities as soon as 2 to 3 weeks and to contact sports in 6 to 8 weeks following surgical management of middle third clavicle fractures.

SC Joint Injuries

SC joint injuries comprise 3% of all injuries involving the shoulder girdle and are uncommon because of the high energy required to disrupt the SC ligaments. Although rare, these injuries sometimes result in damage to adjacent structures such as the trachea, esophagus, lungs, and great vessels. The management of such injuries depends on the direction of subluxation or dislocation. Acute anterior SC joint strain or subluxation in any direction is usually treated nonsurgically as long as the joint is reduced. Acute anterior or posterior dislocations are treated in the acute setting with closed reduction, especially when mediastinal structures are at risk, with ORIF reserved for certain unstable cases. Chronic pain and instability of the SC joint can be managed by ligament reconstruction as well as medial clavicle resection, either open or arthroscopic. The risk of major complications is associated with open surgical intervention because of the proximity of major vital structures to the SC joint.[43,44]

Mechanism of Injury and Classification

SC joint dislocation usually requires a large force because of the strong support provided by the surrounding ligaments. Athletic injuries and motor vehicle accidents comprise more than 80% of injuries to the SC joint. Anterior dislocation, the most common form of SC joint dislocation, usually results from an indirect force to the shoulder, with forces transmitted through the clavicle to the SC joint. Posterior SC joint dislocation can result from both indirect and direct forces, with direct anteromedial force usually resulting in the clavicle being pushed posteriorly into the mediastinum. The medial clavicle epiphysis does not fuse with the shaft until age 23 to 25 years.[43] Therefore, the injury to the SC joint can, in some instances, result in a fracture through the medial physis, with the clavicle shaft subluxating or dislocating anteriorly or posteriorly, leaving the epiphysis attached to the sternum.[45]

Classification of SC joint instability can be based on the direction of clavicle subluxation/dislocation (anterior or posterior), cause of injury (traumatic or atraumatic), injury severity (sprain, subluxation, or dislocation), and the onset of injury (acute or chronic). SC joint injuries have been classified into three types based on the extent of SC joint ligament injuries.[28] Type 1 involves SC ligament and capsule sprain, with no subluxation or dislocation. Type 2 involves disruption of the SC ligaments and capsule, with subluxation of the medial clavicle anteriorly or posteriorly. Type 3 involves rupture of all supporting ligaments to the SC joint, with complete anterior or posterior dislocation of the medial clavicle.[28]

Management and Complications

Type 1 and Type 2 SC Joint Injuries

The management of type 1 SC joint injury is typically nonsurgical. The shoulder is immobilized in an arm sling for approximately 1 week for pain control. Ice application and oral NSAIDs can help decrease pain and control inflammation. After the pain subsides, generally a few days following the injury, the arm sling can be discarded and the patient can resume normal daily activities, with gradual integration into competitive sports.[43,44] With type 2 injuries, the medial clavicle is typically subluxated anteriorly. The subluxation can be reduced in a closed manner by pushing the shoulder posteriorly and medially. Generally, a longer period is spent in an arm sling with or without a figure-of-8 clavicle brace, typically 4 to 6 weeks, until the SC ligaments are healed. At 4 to 6 weeks, the shoulder is mobilized, with ROM and strengthening exercises started for rehabilitation.[43,44]

Type 3 SC Joint Injuries

The management of type 3 SC joint dislocations depends on the direction of clavicle dislocation. Anterior dislocations are more common than posterior dislocations. Acute anterior dislocations are usually treated with closed reduction under anesthesia or sedation. The patient is placed supine on the table, with a pad between both scapulae. Direct posterior pressure is applied to the medial clavicle until reduction is obtained. When reduction is successful and stable, figure-of-8 sling immobilization is applied for 6 weeks to allow soft tissues to heal. However, unlike posterior dislocations, anterior dislocations are usually unstable because of the loss of the stabilizing effect of the torn SC ligaments, and could require acute or delayed open surgical reduction with stabilization.[43,44]

Acute posterior dislocation can be associated with concomitant injuries to vital surrounding structures that could require urgent management by a cardiothoracic surgeon. In stable patients, closed reduction under

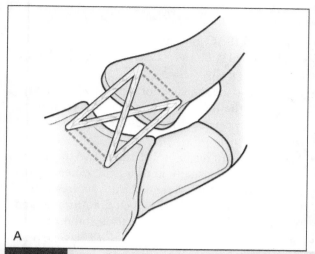
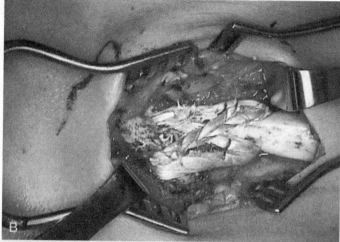

Figure 6 **A,** Illustration demonstrates the "Roman numeral X" reconstruction technique for SC joint separation. **B,** Intraoperative photograph demonstrates the finished reconstruction.

anesthesia is the first-line treatment, preferably with a cardiothoracic surgeon available in case of mediastinal injury. The patient is placed supine on the table, with a pad between both scapulae and the affected shoulder positioned at the edge of the table. In a slender patient, the clavicle can be manually grasped and pulled anteriorly into position. Shoulder and arm extension can assist in the reduction. Alternatively, traction is applied to the affected extremity, with countertraction applied to the chest using a large sheet. Traction is then increased with the upper extremity moved into extension. This can help lever a posteriorly dislocated clavicle into a reduced position. Last, traction can be applied to a fully adducted arm, in addition to posteriorly directed pressure to the shoulder to lever the clavicle anteriorly. If those two techniques fail, a clamp can be used under sterile conditions to hold the medial aspect of the clavicle and pull it anteriorly while extending the abducted upper extremity. When reduction is obtained, it is usually stable, and the patient requires shoulder immobilization in a figure-of-8 brace for 4 to 6 weeks to allow soft-tissue healing.[43,44] Reduction can be confirmed using an O-arm in the operating room or CT postoperatively.

Open reduction and internal stabilization is indicated for acute anterior or posterior dislocations that have failed closed reduction or are unstable, posterior dislocations in patients with an open physis,[45] and in cases of chronic anterior or posterior subluxations/dislocations that have become symptomatic. Internal stabilization can be performed by various means, including suture fixation and ligament reconstruction. Wire-and-pin fixation has been abandoned because of fatal complications, and suture fixation has yielded suboptimal biomechanical results.

Currently, ligament reconstruction is the most widely used technique for SC joint stabilization.[43,44]

In 2004, a biomechanical study compared three different types of ligament reconstruction techniques of the SC joint ligaments.[46] The figure-of-8 technique had substantially higher mechanical strength in both the anterior and posterior directions compared with the subclavian tendon technique and the intramedullary tendon technique. However, all three techniques were found to be biomechanically inferior to the native SC joint ligaments. Most clinical studies published on ligament reconstruction of the SC joint are case reports or case series with generally favorable outcomes. A 2014 study reported on the reconstruction of chronic anterior SC joint instability using autograft (palmaris longus tendon or gracilis tendon).[47] Twenty-seven patients were followed for a median of 54 months (minimum, 2 years), with significant improvement in Western Ontario Shoulder Instability scores. Two patients underwent successful revision surgery for recurrent instability. A 2013 case series reported on six patients undergoing SC joint reconstruction using a modified extra-articular "Roman numeral X" reconstruction using hamstring tendon autograft for anterior instability[48] (Figure 6). All patients had substantial improvement in their functional scores and visual analog scale scores at a mean follow-up of 40 months. All patients returned to preinjury activity level including sports, with one patient requiring revision surgery 4 years later for SC joint arthrosis.

Posttraumatic arthritis of the SC joint can become symptomatic in patients treated nonsurgically or surgically following an SC joint injury. When nonsurgical treatment fails, medial clavicle resection, either open or arthroscopic, can be performed to alleviate pain and improve outcomes.[49,50] To avoid recurrent instability, it is recommended to avoid resecting more than 1.5 cm of the medial clavicle. The arthroscopic technique is advantageous because it is minimally invasive, with faster rehabilitation possible. However, this procedure is still associated with the risk for damage to vital nearby structures such as carotid arteries, subclavian veins, and the trachea.[49]

Postoperative Rehabilitation

The postoperative care of patients undergoing open reduction and internal stabilization of unstable SC joints is the same for anterior or posterior dislocations. The surgical upper extremity is immobilized in an arm sling for 6 to 8 weeks to allow soft-tissue healing, and only pendulum exercises are allowed during this period. Active shoulder ROM is started at 6 to 8 weeks postoperatively, with the arm maintained at 90° or less. The patient can be weaned from the arm sling over a period of 1 to 2 weeks. Full, active ROM and strengthening exercises are initiated at 12 weeks, with return to manual labor or athletic activities allowed at 5 to 6 months.[44,45,48]

Summary

Managing AC joint separations, clavicle fractures, and SC joint dislocations depends on several factors, including patient age, level of activity, level of pain, presence of instability or deformity, and potential complications in performing surgical intervention. Applying these guidelines provides the orthopaedic surgeon with an appropriate plan to treat any of the injuries discussed in this chapter.

Key Study Points

- Type I and II AC joint injuries are treated nonsurgically; type IV, V, and VI AC joint separations are treated surgically.
- Nonsurgical management of type III AC joint separation is the most common first-line treatment, followed by surgical intervention if nonsurgical treatment fails.
- Management of medial third and lateral third clavicle fractures is usually nonsurgical, except in the case of Neer type II lateral third fractures (Edinburgh type 3B fractures), which are unstable and require open reduction and internal stabilization.
- Surgical management of middle third clavicle fractures yields improved results, with fewer cases of nonunion and malunion and improved patient satisfaction compared with nonsurgical management.
- Anterior SC joint dislocations are usually unstable, even after closed reduction, often requiring surgical intervention.
- Posterior SC joint dislocations can result in injury to vital surrounding structures, with surgical intervention being associated with substantial complications.

Annotated References

1. Mazzocca AD, Arciero RA, Bicos J: Evaluation and treatment of acromioclavicular joint injuries. *Am J Sports Med* 2007;35(2):316-329.

2. Kaplan LD, Flanigan DC, Norwig J, Jost P, Bradley J: Prevalence and variance of shoulder injuries in elite collegiate football players. *Am J Sports Med* 2005;33(8):1142-1146.

3. Johansen JA, Grutter PW, McFarland EG, Petersen SA: Acromioclavicular joint injuries: Indications for treatment and treatment options. *J Shoulder Elbow Surg* 2011;20(2, Suppl)S70-S82.

   The study reviews the pathoanatomy, biomechanics, classification, presentation, and evaluation of AC joint injuries, with analysis of the literature involving both surgical and nonsurgical management.

4. Tossy JD, Mead NC, Sigmond HM: Acromioclavicular separations: Useful and practical classification for treatment. *Clin Orthop Relat Res* 1963;28(28):111-119.

5. Rockwood CA: Injuries to the acromioclavicular joint, in Rockwood CA, Green DP, eds: *Fractures in Adults*, ed 2. Philadelphia, JB Lippincott, 1984, pp 860-910, 974-982, vol 1.

© 2016 American Academy of Orthopaedic Surgeons

6. Mikek M: Long-term shoulder function after type I and II acromioclavicular joint disruption. *Am J Sports Med* 2008;36(11):2147-2150.

7. Mouhsine E, Garofalo R, Crevoisier X, Farron A: Grade I and II acromioclavicular dislocations: Results of conservative treatment. *J Shoulder Elbow Surg* 2003;12(6):599-602.

8. Shaw MB, McInerney JJ, Dias JJ, Evans PA: Acromioclavicular joint sprains: The post-injury recovery interval. *Injury* 2003;34(6):438-442.

9. Nuber GW, Bowen MK: Arthroscopic treatment of acromioclavicular joint injuries and results. *Clin Sports Med* 2003;22(2):301-317.

10. Calvo E, López-Franco M, Arribas IM: Clinical and radiologic outcomes of surgical and conservative treatment of type III acromioclavicular joint injury. *J Shoulder Elbow Surg* 2006;15(3):300-305.

11. Schlegel TF, Burks RT, Marcus RL, Dunn HK: A prospective evaluation of untreated acute grade III acromioclavicular separations. *Am J Sports Med* 2001;29(6):699-703.

12. Lizaur A, Sanz-Reig J, Gonzalez-Parreño S: Long-term results of the surgical treatment of type III acromioclavicular dislocations: An update of a previous report. *J Bone Joint Surg Br* 2011;93(8):1088-1092.

    This study followed 38 patients for a mean of 24.2 years following surgical management of type III AC joint separation, with satisfactory results and complete resolution of pain in 35 patients, and comparable outcome scores in both the surgical and contralateral shoulders. Level of evidence: IV.

13. Nissen CW, Chatterjee A: Type III acromioclavicular separation: Results of a recent survey on its management. *Am J Orthop (Belle Mead NJ)* 2007;36(2):89-93.

14. Bannister GC, Wallace WA, Stableforth PG, Hutson MA: The management of acute acromioclavicular dislocation. A randomised prospective controlled trial. *J Bone Joint Surg Br* 1989;71(5):848-850.

15. Taft TN, Wilson FC, Oglesby JW: Dislocation of the acromioclavicular joint. An end-result study. *J Bone Joint Surg Am* 1987;69(7):1045-1051.

16. Gstettner C, Tauber M, Hitzl W, Resch H: Rockwood type III acromioclavicular dislocation: Surgical versus conservative treatment. *J Shoulder Elbow Surg* 2008;17(2):220-225.

17. Smith TO, Chester R, Pearse EO, Hing CB: Operative versus non-operative management following Rockwood grade III acromioclavicular separation: A meta-analysis of the current evidence base. *J Orthop Traumatol* 2011;12(1):19-27.

    This meta-analysis reported on surgical versus nonsurgical management of type III AC joint separation, with surgical management resulting in better cosmetic appearance but increased sick leave. No difference was reported in strength, pain, throwing ability, or incidence of AC joint osteoarthritis.

18. Rolf O, Hann von Weyhern A, Ewers A, Boehm TD, Gohlke F: Acromioclavicular dislocation Rockwood III-V: Results of early versus delayed surgical treatment. *Arch Orthop Trauma Surg* 2008;128(10):1153-1157.

19. Song T, Yan X, Ye T: Comparison of the outcome of early and delayed surgical treatment of complete acromioclavicular joint dislocation. *Knee Surg Sports Traumatol Arthrosc* 2014; Aug 14 [Epub ahead of print].

    This review compared outcomes of early and delayed surgical management of AC joint separations, with early surgery resulting in better functional outcomes and fewer resubluxations/redislocations. Overall complication rates were comparable. Level of evidence: IV.

20. Krul KP, Cook JB, Ku J, Cage JM, Bottoni CR, Tokish JM: Successful conservative therapy in Rockwood type V acromioclavicular dislocations. *Orthop J Sports Med* 2015;3(3, suppl 1).

    In a retrospective study, the authors assessed conservative treatment of type V AC joint separations in active-duty service members. In the conservative group, 11 patients (61%) returned to full duty without surgery at an average of 97.8 days, whereas in the acute surgical group, 6 patients (75%) returned to full duty at an average of 169.3 days. Level of evidence: IV.

21. Jensen G, Katthagen JC, Alvarado LE, Lill H, Voigt C: Has the arthroscopically assisted reduction of acute AC joint separations with the double tight-rope technique advantages over the clavicular hook plate fixation? *Knee Surg Sports Traumatol Arthrosc* 2014;22(2):422-430.

    This study compared 26 arthroscopically assisted AC joint repairs with 30 hook plate fixation procedures for acute AC joint separation. Both techniques resulted in comparable clinical and radiographic outcomes as well as comparable complication rates. Level of evidence: IV.

22. Venjakob AJ, Salzmann GM, Gabel F, et al: Arthroscopically assisted 2-bundle anatomic reduction of acute acromioclavicular joint separations: 58-month findings. *Am J Sports Med* 2013;41(3):615-621.

    This study reported outcomes following arthroscopically assisted AC joint reduction in 23 patients at a mean follow-up of 58 months. Outcome scores showed substantial improvement: 96% of patients were very satisfied or satisfied at final follow-up. Level of evidence: IV.

23. Carofino BC, Mazzocca AD: The anatomic coracoclavicular ligament reconstruction: Surgical technique and indications. *J Shoulder Elbow Surg* 2010;19(Suppl 2):37-46.

    The authors reported their technique for CC ligament reconstruction in the treatment of AC joint separation in 17 patients. Outcome scores were substantially improved. Three failures were reported, two of which required revision surgery. Level of evidence: IV.

24. Westermann RW, Martin W, Wolf BR: Double-loop Anatomic Acromioclavicular Reconstruction: Surgical Technique and Early Results. *Tech Shoulder Elbow Surg* 2014;15:71-74.

   The authors reported their technique for AC joint reconstruction using semitendinosis tendon for AC joint separations. Seven patients were included with good results at final follow-up, no complications, and no loss of reduction. Level of evidence: IV.

25. Yoo JC, Ahn JH, Yoon JR, Yang JH: Clinical results of single-tunnel coracoclavicular ligament reconstruction using autogenous semitendinosus tendon. *Am J Sports Med* 2010;38(5):950-957.

   The study reported clinical results following CC ligament reconstruction for AC joint separation. All 21 patients had good to excellent results at final follow-up; 17 patients maintained reduction. Level of evidence: IV.

26. Postacchini F, Gumina S, De Santis P, Albo F: Epidemiology of clavicle fractures. *J Shoulder Elbow Surg* 2002;11(5):452-456.

27. van der Meijden OA, Gaskill TR, Millett PJ: Treatment of clavicle fractures: Current concepts review. *J Shoulder Elbow Surg* 2012;21(3):423-429.

   This review article describes the classification, surgical indications, and techniques for treatment of clavicle fractures.

28. Allman FL Jr: Fractures and ligamentous injuries of the clavicle and its articulation. *J Bone Joint Surg Am* 1967;49(4):774-784.

29. Neer CS II: Fractures of the distal third of the clavicle. *Clin Orthop Relat Res* 1968;58(58):43-50.

30. Craig EV: Fractures of the clavicle, in Rockwood CA, Green DP, Bucholz RW, Heckman JD, eds: *Fractures in Adults*, ed 4. Philadelphia, PA, Lippincott-Raven, 1996, pp 1109-1193.

31. Robinson CM: Fractures of the clavicle in the adult. Epidemiology and classification. *J Bone Joint Surg Br* 1998;80(3):476-484.

32. O'Neill BJ, Hirpara KM, O'Briain D, McGarr C, Kaar TK: Clavicle fractures: A comparison of five classification systems and their relationship to treatment outcomes. *Int Orthop* 2011;35(6):909-914.

   This article compared five classification systems for clavicle fractures. The Craig classification showed the greatest prognostic value for lateral third fractures and the Robinson classification showed the greatest prognostic value for middle third fractures. Nonunion was more common in lateral third fractures.

33. Hanby CK, Pasque CB, Sullivan JA: Medial clavicle physis fracture with posterior displacement and vascular compromise: The value of three-dimensional computed tomography and duplex ultrasound. *Orthopedics* 2003;26(1):81-84.

34. Zlowodzki M, Zelle BA, Cole PA, Jeray K, McKee MD; Evidence-Based Orthopaedic Trauma Working Group: Treatment of acute midshaft clavicle fractures: systematic review of 2144 fractures: on behalf of the Evidence-Based Orthopaedic Trauma Working Group. *J Orthop Trauma* 2005;19(7):504-507.

35. Canadian Orthopaedic Trauma Society: Nonoperative treatment compared with plate fixation of displaced midshaft clavicular fractures. A multicenter, randomized clinical trial. *J Bone Joint Surg Am* 2007;89(1):1-10.

36. McKee RC, Whelan DB, Schemitsch EH, McKee MD: Operative versus nonoperative care of displaced midshaft clavicular fractures: A meta-analysis of randomized clinical trials. *J Bone Joint Surg Am* 2012;94(8):675-684.

   This meta-analysis examined surgical and nonsurgical management of middle third clavicle fractures in 412 patients. Nonunion rates and symptomatic malunion rates were higher in nonsurgical cases.

37. Robinson CM, Goudie EB, Murray IR, et al: Open reduction and plate fixation versus nonoperative treatment for displaced midshaft clavicular fractures: A multicenter, randomized, controlled trial. *J Bone Joint Surg Am* 2013;95(17):1576-1584.

   This randomized, controlled trial compared ORIF and nonsurgical treatment of displaced middle third clavicle fractures: 105 patients were treated nonsurgically, 95 were treated with ORIF. Better functional outcomes and reduced nonunion rates were found in the surgical group. Level of evidence: I.

38. Altamimi SA, McKee MD; Canadian Orthopaedic Trauma Society: Nonoperative treatment compared with plate fixation of displaced midshaft clavicular fractures. Surgical technique. *J Bone Joint Surg Am* 2008;90(Suppl 2 Pt 1):1-8.

39. Robinson CM, Court-Brown CM, McQueen MM, Wakefield AE: Estimating the risk of nonunion following nonoperative treatment of a clavicular fracture. *J Bone Joint Surg Am* 2004;86-A(7):1359-1365.

40. Yamaguchi H, Arakawa H, Kobayashi M: Results of the Bosworth method for unstable fractures of the distal clavicle. *Int Orthop* 1998;22(6):366-368.

41. Good DW, Lui DF, Leonard M, Morris S, McElwain JP: Clavicle hook plate fixation for displaced lateral-third clavicle fractures (Neer type II): A functional outcome study. *J Shoulder Elbow Surg* 2012;21(8):1045-1048.

   The study examined functional outcomes following ORIF for displaced lateral third clavicle fractures: 36 patients were included with a mean time to union of 3 months and 95% union rates. However, 92% of plates required later removal. Level of evidence: IV.

42. Levy O: Simple, minimally invasive surgical technique for treatment of type 2 fractures of the distal clavicle. *J Shoulder Elbow Surg* 2003;12(1):24-28.

43. Groh GI, Wirth MA: Management of traumatic sternoclavicular joint injuries. *J Am Acad Orthop Surg* 2011;19(1):1-7.

    This review discusses injuries to the SC joint, describing anatomy, mechanisms of injury, classification on SC joint injuries, imaging, and management options including nonsurgical, closed reduction, or open reduction and internal stabilization.

44. Martetschläger F, Warth RJ, Millett PJ: Instability and degenerative arthritis of the sternoclavicular joint: A current concepts review. *Am J Sports Med* 2014;42(4):999-1007.

    This review examines instability and degenerative arthritis of the SC joint. Diagnostic modalities and classification as well as management options and complications are described.

45. Van Hofwegen C, Wolf B: Suture repair of posterior sternoclavicular physeal fractures: A report of two cases. *Iowa Orthop J* 2008;28:49-52.

46. Spencer EE Jr, Kuhn JE: Biomechanical analysis of reconstructions for sternoclavicular joint instability. *J Bone Joint Surg Am* 2004;86-A(1):98-105.

47. Bak K, Fogh K: Reconstruction of the chronic anterior unstable sternoclavicular joint using a tendon autograft: Medium-term to long-term follow-up results. *J Shoulder Elbow Surg* 2014;23(2):245-250.

    The study reported mid-term to long-term results of SC joint reconstruction in 27 patients followed for a minimum of 2 years, with substantial improvement in outcome scores. Two failures were treated successfully with revision surgery. Level of evidence: IV.

48. Guan JJ, Wolf BR: Reconstruction for anterior sternoclavicular joint dislocation and instability. *J Shoulder Elbow Surg* 2013;22(6):775-781.

    This article reported the results of surgical management of anterior SC joint dislocation and instability. Six patients were followed for a mean of 40 months; all patients showed improved functional scores and all had no or minimal pain. Level of evidence: IV.

49. Tytherleigh-Strong G, Griffith D: Arthroscopic excision of the sternoclavicular joint for the treatment of sternoclavicular osteoarthritis. *Arthroscopy* 2013;29(9):1487-1491.

    This article reported the results of arthroscopic excision of the SC joint for treatment of osteoarthritis. Of 10 patients, all had no or minimal pain at final follow-up, and 9 had good to excellent results. Level of evidence: IV.

50. Rockwood CA Jr, Groh GI, Wirth MA, Grassi FA: Resection arthroplasty of the sternoclavicular joint. *J Bone Joint Surg Am* 1997;79(3):387-393.

Chapter 3

Rotator Cuff Disease

Evan J. Conte, MD   Stephen F. Brockmeier, MD

Abstract

Disease of the rotator cuff is common and increases in prevalence with age in the general population. Rotator cuff disease can present as an acute injury or insidiously with shoulder pain and weakness. Physical examination and imaging studies can help guide treatment. Surgical and nonsurgical treatment can be effective in correctly chosen patient groups. The sequelae of untreated long-standing larger tears of the rotator cuff can cause joint destruction and profound disability.

Keywords: rotator cuff; impingement syndrome; rotator cuff tear; rotator cuff repair; reverse total shoulder arthroplasty

Introduction

Rotator cuff disease is one of the most commonly treated upper extremity ailments, and management strategies continue to evolve. Modern understanding of this entity can be traced to 1934 when rotator cuff function, pathology, and proposed treatment were first described. During the next 80 years, abundant basic science and clinical investigations have expanded knowledge of the natural history of rotator cuff disease and helped refine treatment options. Although rotator cuff pathology can present in younger patients after trauma or in overhead athletes, it

Dr. Brockmeier or an immediate family member serves as a paid consultant to Biomet and MicroAire Surgical Instruments; has received research or institutional support from Arthrex, Biomet, Tornier; and serves as a board member, owner, officer, or committee member of the American Orthopaedic Society for Sports Medicine and the MidAtlantic Shoulder and Elbow Society. Neither Dr. Conte nor any immediate family member has received anything of value from or has stock or stock options held in a commercial company or institution related directly or indirectly to the subject of this chapter.

is predominantly prevalent in middle-aged and elderly patients.[1] Treatment ranges from nonsurgical modalities focusing on rest and phased rehabilitation to arthroscopic or open tendon repair to salvage options including reverse total shoulder arthroplasty.

Natural History and Societal Effect

Numerous studies have reported an age-associated increase in the prevalence of rotator cuff tears beginning in patients approximately 50 years old and increasing with each decade of life (Figure 1). Rotator cuff abnormalities are prevalent in both symptomatic and asymptomatic patients, and bilateral rotator cuff tears are common in patients with unilateral symptoms. The prevalence of tears has been reported to range from 13% for patients in their 50s to 50% for patients 80 years or older.[2,3] The factors that cause an asymptomatic tear to become symptomatic have not been completely elucidated, but natural history data collected in recent studies have linked symptom emergence to progression from a partial- to a full-thickness tear, an increase in size of a full-thickness tear, development of muscle atrophy, fatty infiltration of the muscle, or new biceps pathology.[4,5] The societal burden of rotator cuff disease can be substantial when lost days of work are factored in, and a 2013 study reported that a rotator cuff repair procedure could result in a cost savings of up to $78,000 when compared with nonsurgical management, depending on the age of the patient.[1]

Biomechanics, Anatomy, and Genetics

The rotator cuff has a dual function for the shoulder: it helps initiate and assist with active shoulder motion and it provides dynamic stability to the glenohumeral joint during this motion. Given the short arc length of the glenoid, the humeral head requires not only substantial stabilization from soft-tissue structures including the glenohumeral ligaments, but also the force-couple moment provided by contraction of the four rotator cuff muscles during motion. The supraspinatus and infraspinatus tendons, which comprise the posterosuperior rotator cuff,

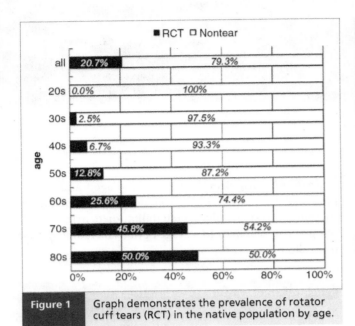

Figure 1 Graph demonstrates the prevalence of rotator cuff tears (RCT) in the native population by age.

Table 1

Classification of Rotator Cuff Muscle Degeneration

Grade	Description
0	No fatty streaks
1	Some fatty streaks
2	More muscle than fat
3	As much muscle as fat
4	Less muscle than fat

are confluent centrally and insert on the greater tuberosity of the humeral head. Studies have shown that most tears occur in the anterior portion of the supraspinatus tendon and are more likely to be larger and associated with fatty muscle degeneration.[6,7] Additionally, the common types of tear geometry have resulted in the "cable-crescent" concept: a thickened, horseshoe-shaped region that comprises the anteriormost 8 to 12 mm of the supraspinatus, termed the rotator "cable," which is critical for the structural and functional integrity of the superior cuff. The relatively stress-shielded center section is called the "crescent." Biomechanical test results have shown that tears involving the cable result in increased tear gap distance and strain when compared with those in the crescent area[8]

The etiology of rotator cuff disease involves both intrinsic and extrinsic factors. Most early studies focused on mechanical phenomena secondary to external impingement against the undersurface of a prominent anterior or lateral acromion, eventually resulting in the development of a tear. New studies investigating genetic influence have suggested that rotator cuff disease is not a purely mechanical problem, but is most attributable to intrinsic degenerative tendinopathic changes. These are thought to involve changes in both the molecular composition of the tendon substance as well as its vascularity, which allows for the gradual development of tendinosis and eventual structural failure and tearing. As with other degenerative tendinopathies, certain individuals may be more at risk. One study has shown a familial hereditary pattern of rotator cuff disease;[9] another has identified five genes found more commonly in patients with substantial disease.[10]

Classification

Rotator cuff tears can be described and classified based on several factors, including size, location, number of tendon units involved, tear geometry, level of tendon retraction, and muscle atrophy and fatty infiltration. Tears were first classified based on size in 1984;[11] a subsequent classification combined coronal and sagittal variables as well as tear thickness.[12] The quality of the injured myotendinous unit is also important. Atrophy of the muscle belly diameter as well as the degree of fatty infiltration, as classified in 1994 (Table 1), can help indicate tendon quality during repair.[13] Most recently, a new classification was presented to assist with surgeon-to-surgeon communication as well as provide prognostic and treatment considerations. This new geometric classification describes rotator cuff tears as viewed directly via the lateral arthroscopic portal.[14] The patterns include crescent-shaped, L-shaped, reverse L-shaped, U-shaped, or massive contracted-type tears that require more advanced techniques such as interval slides and marginal convergence to repair successfully (Figure 2).

Physical Examination

Initial evaluation of a patient with symptoms of rotator cuff disease starts with a comprehensive history and physical examination. The examination should be broad, including the cervical spine, scapula, shoulder girdle, and neurologic testing of the extremity, followed by a systematic shoulder examination with specific tests for the rotator cuff and common concomitant pathology. Visual inspection of the shoulder can reveal rotator cuff musculature atrophy as well as signs of rotator cuff dysfunction and anterosuperior escape. Assessment of passive range of motion is important to rule out adhesive capsulitis, which would ideally be treated before attempting surgical repair. It is important to assess for other pathology that could be the cause of concurrent symptoms and potentially

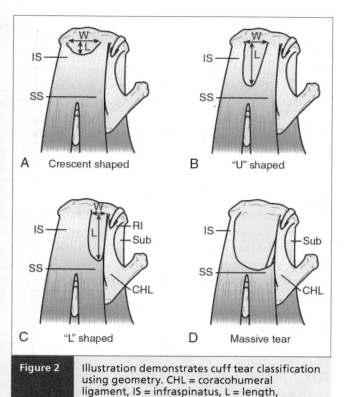

A Crescent shaped

B "U" shaped

C "L" shaped

D Massive tear

Figure 2 Illustration demonstrates cuff tear classification using geometry. CHL = coracohumeral ligament, IS = infraspinatus, L = length, RI = rotator interval, Sub = subscapularis, SS = supraspinatus, W = width.

treated during rotator cuff repair such as biceps tendon disease, acromioclavicular joint arthrosis, or impingement syndrome.

The muscles of the rotator cuff should be tested individually. The Jobe test, or empty can test, isolates the supraspinatus and is performed with the arm at 90° of abduction, 30° of flexion in the scapular plane, and with the forearm pronated. The infraspinatus can be tested by assessing external rotation strength with the arm in adduction and the elbow at 90° of flexion. The subscapularis can be assessed by using the lift-off and belly-press tests. Other tests commonly used are the external rotation lag sign and the hornblower sign, both of which assess for failure of the infraspinatus and teres minor, and the drop arm test for the superior rotator cuff. No single test for rotator cuff disease has proved to be of greater diagnostic value. Rather, a 2014 study validated a combination of positive tests that greatly increases the specificity of a rotator cuff disease diagnosis.[15]

Diagnostic Imaging

A series of plain radiographs of the shoulder, including a Grashey AP view, lateral outlet view/scapular Y view, and an axillary lateral view should be the first diagnostic studies obtained. The presence of superior migration of the humeral head with a diminished acromiohumeral interval, glenohumeral joint space narrowing that suggests osteoarthritis, acromioclavicular joint arthrosis, and features of rotator cuff arthropathy with morphologic changes of the humeral head, glenoid, and acromial arch are all detectable findings on plain film radiographs.

MRI has proved incredibly useful in diagnosing rotator cuff disease. Not only does MRI provide the surgeon with a qualitative diagnosis, it also can help determine the condition of the muscle, the size and location of the tear, the amount of tendon retraction, and perhaps most importantly, the presence of other pathology that should be managed during surgery to provide the best possible outcome. A new method to assess the quality of the musculature on MRI is the tangent sign (Figure 3), which is the failure of the supraspinatus to intersect the line from the superior border of the coracoid process to the superior border of the scapular spine. This method is quick and has been shown to predict the reparability of rotator cuff tears.[16]

The use of ultrasonography has steadily increased in recent years, and it can be as accurate as MRI in diagnosing rotator cuff tears. Ultrasonography has also been recently shown to accurately assess the degree of degeneration of muscle in chronic rotator cuff tears.[17] It is less expensive than MRI, and may best be used not as an initial diagnostic agent but to assess repair integrity in postoperative patients.

Nonsurgical Treatment

Nonsurgical management of rotator cuff pathology typically consists of 6 to 12 weeks of rest, symptom management, and physical therapy with a home exercise regimen that focuses on passive and active range of motion and strengthening the scapular stabilizing muscles and rotator cuff musculature. NSAIDs and the occasional subacromial injection can also be considered in the painful shoulder but could affect the potential for postoperative healing. Bursal injection can be performed using an anterior, lateral, or posterior approach; the anterior and lateral approaches demonstrated increased accuracy in one recent study.[18]

Efforts have increasingly focused on determining which patients can be most predictably treated nonsurgically, and those who are more likely to be recalcitrant to nonsurgical efforts and require intervention. The Multicenter Orthopaedic Outcomes Network shoulder group studied a group of 452 patients with asymptomatic full-thickness rotator cuff tears initially treated nonsurgically with a physical therapy protocol. At 2-year follow-up, 75% of

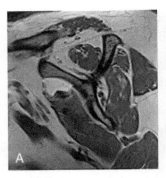
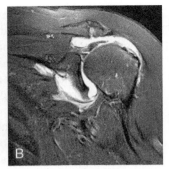
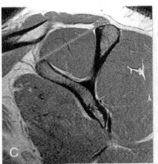
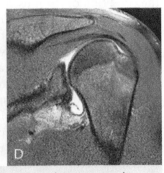

Figure 3 Magnetic resonance image demonstrate the tangent sign. **A,** Medial sagittal T1-weighted image depicts supraspinatus muscle atrophy and fatty infiltration just below the tangent line of the scapula (red line). **B,** Coronal T2-weighted image depicts a corresponding large, retracted posterosuperior rotator cuff tear. **C,** Medial sagittal T1-weighted image depicts a healthy supraspinatus muscle occupying the entire suprascapular fossa and without fatty infiltration (red line). **D,** Coronal T2-weighted image depicts a corresponding normal supraspinatus myotendinous unit.

patients did not go on to surgery, and most therapeutic failures occurred in the first 12 weeks.[19]

Large, well-designed studies comparing surgical and nonsurgical treatment of rotator cuff tears have only recently been published. A Norwegian group compared physical therapy with immediate repair in a single-center randomized controlled study.[20] Small and medium (<3 cm) tears were confirmed on MRI. Overall, patients in the surgical group had slightly better Constant and American Shoulder and Elbow Surgeons scores, but the data, although significant, were likely not clinically important. Of note, one-third of the nonsurgically treated patients had poor outcomes with an associated increase in tear size greater than 5 mm.

Surgical Considerations

The rate of arthroscopic rotator cuff repair has increased dramatically since its development, with a concurrent decrease in open rotator cuff repairs. A shift toward outpatient treatment of rotator cuff tears has also occurred.[21] Numerous studies have demonstrated equivalent outcomes when comparing open and arthroscopic techniques. The arthroscopic technique has become more mechanically similar to the open technique, with the development of a medial- and lateral-row suture bridge construct commonly referred to as a transosseous-equivalent repair. This type of arthroscopic repair has shown excellent outcomes with maintenance of functional outcomes scores and strength at 5 years.[22] A typical approach to arthroscopic rotator cuff repair has been illustrated (Figures 4 and 5).

Despite these advances, primary repair can still fail, especially in the setting of large and massive, retracted tears. Thus, the ability to augment or biologically enhance a repair has received substantial attention. Biologic augmentation with products in the family of platelet-rich plasma (PRP), platelet-rich fibrin matrix (PRFM), or platelet-leukocyte membrane has been studied extensively. The preparation, method of delivery, and incorporation into repairs has not been standardized and continues to make evaluation of these new products challenging. Several recent randomized controlled studies have provided new data that could help to discern the potential benefit of biologic augmentation of rotator cuff repairs. Longer follow-up and an assessment of patient subgroups (such as age, sex, and tear size and location) could help find specific indications for use of PRP/PRFM in repairs. Several large, blinded, randomized studies have shown no substantial difference in outcomes.[23,24] Additionally, a systematic review of all level I or II studies on PRP for rotator cuff repair augmentation did not identify any benefit greater than the minimum clinically important difference.[25]

The incorporation of either synthetic or natural graft material can also be used to augment repairs. Xenografts, dermal or collagen grafts, and synthetic mesh-type grafts have been studied. A few short-term outcomes studies have shown promise, but further longer term review is lacking.[26,27]

Although most studies show that rotator cuff repairs have successful, enduring clinical outcomes that can result in the assumption of tendon-to-bone healing, evidence increasingly shows that the integrity of many repairs may not be what is expected. Actual tendon-to-bone healing may not always be necessary to achieve a successful clinical outcome, especially in the short term. Both MRI and ultrasonography have been used to quantify the structural success after rotator cuff repair. A systemic review identified an overall re-tear rate of 20.4%.[28] Another study reported a re-tear rate for medium to massive tears of 12% to 22%, with no difference in patient outcome versus

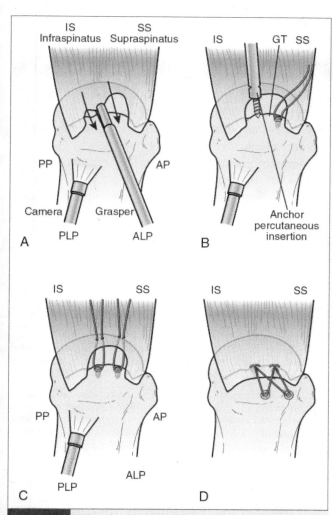

1: Upper extremity

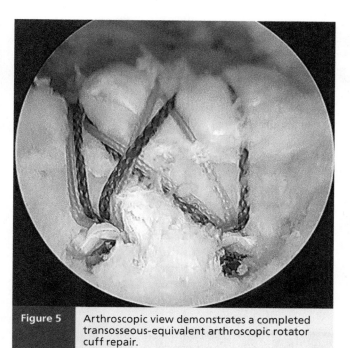

Figure 5 Arthroscopic view demonstrates a completed transosseous-equivalent arthroscopic rotator cuff repair.

Figure 4 Illustration demonstrates a typical approach to arthroscopic transosseous-equivalent rotator cuff repair. **A,** The cuff tissue is viewed from the lateral portal for débridement of bursal adhesions. The tear pattern is determined and the tissue mobility is assessed using a nontraumatic grasper. **B,** The greater tuberosity (GT) is débrided of soft tissue to allow punctate bleeding. Medial-row anchors are placed just lateral to the articular margin percutaneously to allow a more favorable insertion angle. **C,** The sutures are passed through the rotator cuff tendon lateral to the myotendinous junction and tied to reduce the tendon to the medial row anchors. **D,** The suture limbs are brought to lateral row knotless anchors to complete the repair. ALP = anterolateral portal, AP = anterior portal, IS = infraspinatus, PLP = posterolateral portal, PP = posterior portal, SS = supraspinatus.

Postoperative Concerns

Traditional postoperative rehabilitation regimens have emphasized an immobilization period of 6 weeks, with gradual passive range of motion followed by active-assisted range of motion starting in the early postoperative period. The rationale for early motion has been to limit the development of tissue adhesions; extended immobilization encourages tissue healing in a low-stress environment followed by subsequent return of range of motion. The optimum time to start passive range of motion has been debated considerably. A prospective randomized study showed no difference in outcome and final range of motion with early versus late initiation of motion for small- or medium-size tears (≤3 cm).[31] This finding was supported by a recent meta-analysis, which concluded that small- or medium-size tears have a lower risk of re-tear when motion is started within 1 week. However, it also reported that massive tears (>5 cm) have a greater risk of re-tear when motion is started early, suggesting that patient-specific postoperative protocols can be beneficial.[32]

Tendon Transfers

Younger patients with massive, irreparable tears represent a particularly difficult subset to treat. Although elderly, low-demand patients can often be treated effectively with reverse total shoulder arthroplasty, this is not yet an accepted option in the middle-aged patient with a massive

the intact repairs.[29] Although tendon-to-bone healing may not result from all repairs, outcomes remain favorable. A meta-analysis of seven level I or II studies suggests that the integrity of the repair does not correspond with outcome but it does correspond with strength.[30]

tear that has become irreparable. Direct transfers of the latissimus dorsi musculotendinous unit for irreparable posterosuperior tears has been used by many authors as a salvage option for irreparable tears in patients younger than 60 years. The transferred tendon has been postulated to function as a tissue augment, an external rotator of the shoulder joint, a humeral head depressor, and to act in concert with the intact subscapularis (which is a prerequisite for consideration of a latissimus dorsi transfer) to restore the rotator cuff force couple and assist the deltoid in elevation and abduction. A successful latissimus dorsi transfer can improve patient subjective outcomes, decrease pain, and improve strength and range of motion, but not as well as that of a reparable tear.[33] Poorer results can be expected in patients with concomitant deficiencies of the subscapularis and teres minor.[34] In the setting of a tendon transfer, it is important to counsel patients not to expect an undeliverable outcome.

Reverse Total Shoulder Arthroplasty

In patients with irreparable massive tears with a low shoulder functional demand and in the setting of rotator cuff tear arthropathy, reverse total shoulder arthroplasty is a proven, effective treatment. The function of the procedure is to alter the joint mechanics, thus providing a mechanical advantage to the deltoid muscle by medializing the center of rotation and translating the humeral side inferiorly, allowing the deltoid to function without the assistance of the rotator cuff musculature while replacing the worn articular surfaces. Concerns related to longevity should be considered in patients younger than 60 years because long-term implant survivorship is not yet clear. The outcomes for reverse total shoulder arthroplasty in patients with rotator cuff disease have been favorable.[35] Patient selection is paramount because studies including patients younger than 65 years can have less favorable long-term outcomes.[36]

Summary

Rotator cuff disease increases in prevalence with age, with many patients having both symptomatic and asymptomatic tears. Tears typically occur in reliable patterns, and for chronic tears in older patients, most can initially be treated nonsurgically with a high success rate. Repair is now commonly performed arthroscopically, with equivalent outcomes to open surgery despite a less-than-ideal rate of definitive healing, especially in larger tears. Physical therapy tailored to patient- and tear-specific factors should be started in the postoperative period. Salvage operations including tendon transfers and

reverse total shoulder arthroplasty have favorable outcomes and should be considered on a case-by-case basis.

Key Study Points

- Rotator cuff disease is common and the incidence increases with age in patients older than 50 years.
- History and physical examination followed by MRI confirmation help guide treatment.
- Many chronic small rotator cuff tears can be treated successfully nonsurgically.
- Both arthroscopic and open repair techniques can yield good results.
- Postoperative therapy protocols are best when individualized based on tear size.

Annotated References

1. Mather RC III, Koenig L, Acevedo D, et al: The societal and economic value of rotator cuff repair. *J Bone Joint Surg Am* 2013;95(22):1993-2000.

   This study examined the effect of rotator cuff disease on earnings, missed workdays, and disability payments using a Markov decision model to determine the economic effect of the disease on society. Societal cost savings were estimated at approximately $3.44 billion per year due to rotator cuff repairs.

2. Yamamoto A, Takagishi K, Osawa T, et al: Prevalence and risk factors of a rotator cuff tear in the general population. *J Shoulder Elbow Surg* 2010;19(1):116-120.

   This study used ultrasonography to determine the prevalence of rotator cuff tears in a mountain village in Japan for patients of all ages. Rotator cuff tears are rare in young patients but increase steadily for each decade in life after age 50 years.

3. Yamaguchi K, Ditsios K, Middleton WD, Hildebolt CF, Galatz LM, Teefey SA: The demographic and morphological features of rotator cuff disease. A comparison of asymptomatic and symptomatic shoulders. *J Bone Joint Surg Am* 2006;88(8):1699-1704.

   This article investigated the correlation between symptoms and cuff tear size progression. Larger tears were more likely to be symptomatic and be accompanied by a contralateral cuff tear.

4. Moosmayer S, Tariq R, Stiris M, Smith H-J: The natural history of asymptomatic rotator cuff tears: A three-year follow-up of fifty cases. *J Bone Joint Surg Am* 2013;95(14):1249-1255.

   This study followed patients with asymptomatic cuff tears using ultrasonography to determine the natural history of the disease and which factors were associated with symptom generation. Increase in tear size and decrease of muscle quality were associated with development of symptoms. Level of evidence: II.

5. Mall NA, Kim HM, Keener JD, et al: Symptomatic progression of asymptomatic rotator cuff tears: A prospective study of clinical and sonographic variables. *J Bone Joint Surg Am* 2010;92(16):2623-2633.

   This research study followed asymptomatic patients using ultrasonography to determine that symptoms begin with increases in tear size or progression from partial- to full-thickness tears. Level of evidence: III.

6. Kim HM, Dahiya N, Teefey SA, Keener JD, Galatz LM, Yamaguchi K: Relationship of tear size and location to fatty degeneration of the rotator cuff. *J Bone Joint Surg Am* 2010;92(4):829-839.

   This article determined that fatty degeneration of the rotator cuff musculature is associated with both location and tear size. The loss of the fibers of the anterior supraspinatus tendon can result in development of fatty degeneration of the muscle.

7. Namdari S, Donegan RP, Dahiya N, Galatz LM, Yamaguchi K, Keener JD: Characteristics of small to medium-sized rotator cuff tears with and without disruption of the anterior supraspinatus tendon. *J Shoulder Elbow Surg* 2014;23(1):20-27.

   This article examined the results of rotator cuff tear repairs that involved the anterior supraspinatus tendon and those that did not. Anterior tears involving the rotator cuff cable were larger and more likely to have associated muscle degeneration but had no influence on structural results after surgery. Level of evidence: III.

8. Mesiha MM, Derwin KA, Sibole SC, Erdemir A, McCarron JA: The biomechanical relevance of anterior rotator cuff cable tears in a cadaveric shoulder model. *J Bone Joint Surg Am* 2013;95(20):1817-1824.

   This biomechanical cadaver study showed that tears involving the anterior 8 to 12 mm of the supraspinatus tendon, in which the rotator cuff cable is present, develop larger gaps when subject to loading that tears in the posterior supraspinatus, the crescent area. This supports the importance of the rotator cuff cable in load bearing versus the more stress-shielded crescent area.

9. Motta GdaR, Amaral MV, Rezende E, et al: Evidence of genetic variations associated with rotator cuff disease. *J Shoulder Elbow Surg* 2014;23(2):227-235.

   The authors investigated the link between 23 single-nucleotide polymorphisms within six genes and their association with degenerative processes in the development of rotator cuff disease. These genes correlated with the presence of rotator cuff disease as well as female sex and Caucasian race. Level of evidence: III.

10. Tashjian RZ, Farnham JM, Albright FS, Teerlink CC, Cannon-Albright LA: Evidence for an inherited predisposition contributing to the risk for rotator cuff disease. *J Bone Joint Surg Am* 2009;91(5):1136-1142.

    This study used genealogic data from a population in Utah to determine the presence of excess familial clustering for rotator cuff disease. The findings strongly supported a heritable predisposition to rotator cuff disease. Level of evidence: III.

11. DeOrio JK, Cofield RH: Results of a second attempt at surgical repair of a failed initial rotator-cuff repair. *J Bone Joint Surg Am* 1984;66(4):563-567.

12. Patte D: Classification of rotator cuff lesions. *Clin Orthop Relat Res* 1990;254:81-86.

13. Goutallier D, Postel JM, Bernageau J, Lavau L, Voisin MC: Fatty muscle degeneration in cuff ruptures. Pre- and postoperative evaluation by CT scan. *Clin Orthop Relat Res* 1994;304:78-83.

14. Davidson J, Burkhart SS: The geometric classification of rotator cuff tears: A system linking tear pattern to treatment and prognosis. *Arthroscopy* 2010;26(3):417-424.

    The authors proposed a new classification for rotator cuff tears based on geometry of the cuff tear that was linked to prognosis and treatment technique.

15. Somerville LE, Willits K, Johnson AM, et al: Clinical assessment of physical examination maneuvers for rotator cuff lesions. *Am J Sports Med* 2014;42(8):1911-1919.

    This study investigated the sensitivity and specificity of various physical examination tests for rotator cuff disease when correlated with surgical evidence of tear. No test in isolation provides enough data for diagnosis but rather that a combination of tests improves the ability to diagnose rotator cuff disease. Level of evidence: I.

16. Kissenberth MJ, Rulewicz GJ, Hamilton SC, Bruch HE, Hawkins RJ: A positive tangent sign predicts the repairability of rotator cuff tears. *J Shoulder Elbow Surg* 2014;23(7):1023-1027.

    The authors proposed the tangent sign, a novel, quick method to determine muscle quality in the setting of rotator cuff tears. This method was shown to be predictive of reparability of cuff tears. Level of evidence: II.

17. Wall LB, Teefey SA, Middleton WD, et al: Diagnostic performance and reliability of ultrasonography for fatty degeneration of the rotator cuff muscles. *J Bone Joint Surg Am* 2012;94(12):e83.

    This study compared the diagnostic performance and observer reliability of ultrasonography in grading fatty degeneration of the rotator cuff musculature when compared with MRI. The group found that ultrasonography and MRI were comparable. Level of evidence: II.

18. Maman E, Harris C, White L, Tomlinson G, Shashank M, Boynton E; EranMaman: Outcome of nonoperative treatment of symptomatic rotator cuff tears monitored by magnetic resonance imaging. *J Bone Joint Surg Am* 2009;91(8):1898-1906.

This retrospective study investigated the natural history of patients with rotator cuff disease using nonsurgical methods with MRI at 6 months or longer. After age 60 years, fatty infiltration or the presence of a full-thickness tear were associated with tear progression. Level of evidence: IV.

19. Kuhn JE, Dunn WR, Sanders R, et al; MOON Shoulder Group: Effectiveness of physical therapy in treating atraumatic full-thickness rotator cuff tears: A multicenter prospective cohort study. *J Shoulder Elbow Surg* 2013;22(10):1371-1379.

    This prospective multicenter study examined the effectiveness of physical therapy as a treatment modality for atraumatic full-thickness rotator cuff tears in a cohort of 452 patients. All patients began physical therapy and were subsequently allowed to choose surgery or further physical therapy. Fewer than 25% of patients elected to undergo surgery, and most commonly did so between 6 and 12 weeks.

20. Moosmayer S, Lund G, Seljom US, et al: Tendon repair compared with physiotherapy in the treatment of rotator cuff tears: A randomized controlled study in 103 cases with a five-year follow-up. *J Bone Joint Surg Am* 2014;96(18):1504-1514.

    This randomized controlled study compared surgical and nonsurgical treatment of rotator cuff tears less than 3 cm in size: 24% of patients in the nonsurgical group underwent secondary tendon repair with inferior results compared with those treated with primary repair. Overall, the differences in outcomes between the groups were small, and the clinical significance may be minor. Level of evidence: I.

21. Iyengar JJ, Samagh SP, Schairer W, Singh G, Valone FH III, Feeley BT: Current trends in rotator cuff repair: Surgical technique, setting, and cost. *Arthroscopy* 2014;30(3):284-288.

    This study reported on current trends in rotator cuff repair using a Florida database. A rapid increase in arthroscopic repair, decrease in open repair, and increase in the number of cases performed in outpatient centers were reported.

22. Gulotta LV, Nho SJ, Dodson CC, Adler RS, Altchek DW, MacGillivray JD; HSS Arthroscopic Rotator Cuff Registry: Prospective evaluation of arthroscopic rotator cuff repairs at 5 years: Part I—functional outcomes and radiographic healing rates. *J Shoulder Elbow Surg* 2011;20(6):934-940.

    This prospective cohort study of 193 patients who underwent all-arthroscopic rotator cuff repair was followed for 5 years. The midrange results were good, with lasting functional improvements. The healing rate, determined using ultrasonography, continued to increase over time. Level of evidence: II.

23. Weber SC, Kauffman JI, Parise C, Weber SJ, Katz SD: Platelet-rich fibrin matrix in the management of arthroscopic repair of the rotator cuff: A prospective, randomized, double-blinded study. *Am J Sports Med* 2013;41(2):263-270.

This investigation of the use of PRFM in rotator cuff repair showed no substantial difference in outcome or structural integrity. Level of evidence: I.

24. Castricini R, Longo UG, De Benedetto M, et al: Platelet-rich plasma augmentation for arthroscopic rotator cuff repair: A randomized controlled trial. *Am J Sports Med* 2011;39(2):258-265.

    The authors performed a randomized controlled trial to determine if PRP augmentation improved rotator cuff repair of small- or medium-size tears. No improvement was detected. Level of evidence: I.

25. Warth RJ, Dornan GJ, James EW, Horan MP, Millett PJ: Clinical and structural outcomes after arthroscopic repair of full-thickness rotator cuff tears with and without platelet-rich product supplementation: A meta-analysis and meta-regression. *Arthroscopy* 2015;31(2):306-320.

    This meta-analysis of level I and II studies of PRP augmentation of rotator cuff repairs found no substantial difference in overall gain in outcome score or re-tear rates. However, evidence supported decreased re-tear rates for tears greater than 3 cm, which received PRP augmentation during repair. Level of evidence: II.

26. Ciampi P, Scotti C, Nonis A, et al: The benefit of synthetic versus biological patch augmentation in the repair of posterosuperior massive rotator cuff tears: A 3-year follow-up study. *Am J Sports Med* 2014;42(5):1169-1175.

    The authors investigated mechanical augmentation of rotator cuff repair with two patch types versus a control group. Polypropylene patches were found to improve outcomes at 36 months. Level of evidence: III.

27. Gupta AK, Hug K, Boggess B, Gavigan M, Toth AP: Massive or 2-tendon rotator cuff tears in active patients with minimal glenohumeral arthritis: Clinical and radiographic outcomes of reconstruction using dermal tissue matrix xenograft. *Am J Sports Med* 2013;41(4):872-879.

    This study determined that reconstruction of irreparable two-tendon rotator cuff tears with dermal xenograft could improve outcomes at 2 years. Level of evidence: IV.

28. Slabaugh MA, Nho SJ, Grumet RC, et al: Does the literature confirm superior clinical results in radiographically healed rotator cuffs after rotator cuff repair? *Arthroscopy* 2010;26(3):393-403.

    This systematic review assessed the literature to determine a correlation between cuff healing and outcome. The overall re-tear rate was 20.4% and the study suggested that intact cuff repairs can improve some outcome scores. Level of evidence: IV

29. Kim KC, Shin HD, Lee WY: Repair integrity and functional outcomes after arthroscopic suture-bridge rotator cuff repair. *J Bone Joint Surg Am* 2012;94(8):e48.

    This study used ultrasonography or MRI to assess healing rates of rotator cuff repairs. The authors found an increased rate of re-tear for larger tears but found no correlation between integrity of the repair and clinical outcome. Level of evidence: IV.

30. Russell RD, Knight JR, Mulligan E, Khazzam MS: Structural integrity after rotator cuff repair does not correlate with patient function and pain: A meta-analysis. *J Bone Joint Surg Am* 2014;96(4):265-271.

   This meta-analysis of level I or II studies found a 21.7% overall rate of re-tear, no difference in tear size between intact and failed repairs, and no correlation between intact repairs and re-torn repairs on clinical outcomes. Level of evidence: II.

31. Keener JD, Galatz LM, Stobbs-Cucchi G, Patton R, Yamaguchi K: Rehabilitation following arthroscopic rotator cuff repair: A prospective randomized trial of immobilization compared with early motion. *J Bone Joint Surg Am* 2014;96(1):11-19.

   This level I study of patients undergoing arthroscopic repair of small or medium-sized tears randomized to early or delayed postoperative range of motion groups found no clinical advantage to early passive motion versus immobilization. Level of evidence: I.

32. Kluczynski MA, Nayyar S, Marzo JM, Bisson LJ: Early versus delayed passive range of motion after rotator cuff repair: A systematic review and meta-analysis. *Am J Sports Med* 2015;43(8):2057-2063.

   This study analyzed the literature to determine re-tear rates when postoperative passive motion is started within 1 week or delayed 3 to 6 weeks. Grouped level I studies found no difference in re-tear rates. However, re-tear rates were higher for massive tears when early motion was initiated and higher for smaller tears when early motion was delayed, suggesting that rehabilitation programs should be patient-specific based on tear size.

33. Namdari S, Voleti P, Baldwin K, Glaser D, Huffman GR: Latissimus dorsi tendon transfer for irreparable rotator cuff tears: A systematic review. *J Bone Joint Surg Am* 2012;94(10):891-898.

   This systematic review of available literature confirmed that latissimus dorsi tendon transfers for irreparable rotator cuff tears improve shoulder function, strength, motion, and pain relief. Level of evidence: IV.

34. Gerber C, Rahm SA, Catanzaro S, Farshad M, Moor BK: Latissimus dorsi tendon transfer for treatment of irreparable posterosuperior rotator cuff tears: Long-term results at a minimum follow-up of ten years. *J Bone Joint Surg Am* 2013;95(21):1920-1926.

   A long-term study of 57 shoulders followed for at least 10 years confirmed that latissimus dorsi transfers are successful and provide lasting improvement to patients with irreparable rotator cuff tears. Level of evidence: IV.

35. Wall B, Nové-Josserand L, O'Connor DP, Edwards TB, Walch G: Reverse total shoulder arthroplasty: A review of results according to etiology. *J Bone Joint Surg Am* 2007;89(7):1476-1485.

   This study stratified the outcomes of reverse total shoulder arthroplasty by indication, finding that patients with rotator cuff arthropathy had better clinical results that patients undergoing the procedure for posttraumatic arthritis or in revision cases. Level of evidence: II.

36. Ek ET, Neukom L, Catanzaro S, Gerber C: Reverse total shoulder arthroplasty for massive irreparable rotator cuff tears in patients younger than 65 years old: Results after five to fifteen years. *J Shoulder Elbow Surg* 2013;22(9):1199-1208.

   The authors studied the outcome of reverse total shoulder arthroplasty for patients younger than 65 years. Substantial, lasting improvement was found in overall function up to 10 years from surgery. Level of evidence: IV.

Chapter 4

Superior Labrum and Biceps Pathology

Bryan G. Vopat, MD   Jeffrey E. Wong, MD   Petar Golijanin, BS   Matthew T. Provencher, MD

1: Upper Extremity

Abstract

Superior labrum anterior to posterior (SLAP) tears and pathology involving the long head of the biceps (LHB) tendon are both common issues that can result in shoulder pain, dysfunction, and activity limitation. However, it can be difficult to identify SLAP and LHB pathologies as the sole culprit because they are commonly seen with other injuries. The treatment of both issues remains controversial and a subject of continued research. SLAP repairs have had more beneficial results in patients younger than 40 years and when not associated with a rotator cuff repair. Ideal treatment of LHB tendon pathology is still evolving; patient desire and surgeon preference will help decide if repair, tenotomy, or tenodesis is best, depending on the type of SLAP tear, age, and demographics. The literature has not clearly demonstrated a superior surgical option. However, when tenodesis or tenotomy is indicated, tenodesis should be performed in those with higher levels of physical activity, patients concerned with cosmesis, and workers' compensation cases. Several types of tenodesis procedures can be performed, but the literature has not yet identified optimal treatment. Future research is needed to help identify the best treatment options for patients.

Keywords: biceps tendinopathy; SLAP; biceps tenodesis; biceps tenotomy; biceps tendinitis

Introduction

Superior labrum tears were first described in 1985[1]; they were subsequently classified in 1990.[2] These detachment injuries, or superior labrum anterior to posterior (SLAP) tears, also can possibly involve the long head of the biceps (LHB) tendon. The LHB tendon has been identified as an important pain generator in the shoulder; however, it can be difficult to isolate the LHB involvement because it commonly occurs with other disorders. Currently, this pathology can be treated with either a tenodesis or tenotomy.

Anatomy

The glenoid labrum is composed of fibrocartilaginous tissue. The suprascapular artery, the circumflex scapular branch of the subscapular artery, and the posterior humeral circumflex artery provide the labrum's vascular supply. These vessels arborize within the peripheral aspect of the labrum. The inner portion of the labrum is avascular, and the superior labrum is less vascular compared with the inferior and posterior labrum.[3]

The superior labrum is usually triangular but can have a meniscoid shape. It commonly attaches medial to the articular margin of the glenoid rim. This medial attachment at the supraglenoid tubercle creates a subsynovial recess; 40% to 60% of the LHB tendon originates from the supraglenoid tubercle, and the remaining fibers insert directly into the superior labrum. The LHB can have an entirely posterior, posterior-dominant, or equally

Dr. Vopat or an immediate family member serves as a paid consultant to DePuy. Dr. Provencher or an immediate family member has received royalties from Arthrex; serves as a paid consultant to Arthrex and the Joint Restoration Foundation; and serves as a board member, owner, officer, or committee member of the American Academy of Orthopaedic Surgeons, the American Orthopaedic Society for Sports Medicine, American Shoulder and Elbow Surgeons, the Arthroscopy Association of North America, the International Society of Arthroscopy, Knee Surgery, and Orthopaedic Sports Medicine, the San Diego Shoulder Institute, and the Society of Military Orthopaedic Surgeons. Neither of the following authors nor any immediate family member has received anything of value from or has stock or stock options held in a commercial company or institution related directly or indirectly to the subject of this chapter: Dr. Wong and Mr. Golijanin.

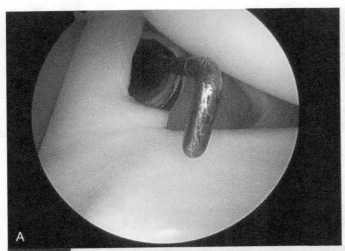
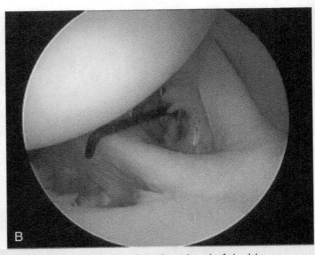

Figure 1   **A,** Arthroscopic view via the posterior portal demonstrates normal attachment of the long head of the biceps tendon with the patient in the decubitus position. **B,** Arthroscopic view demonstrates a cordlike middle glenohumeral ligament, a normal variant, which can be identified with the probe inserted via the anterior portal. This structure should not be repaired.

anterior-posterior attachment at the superior labrum. In most cases, the LHB has a posterior-dominant or entirely posterior labral insertion.[4] The LHB anchor has some inherent physiologic motion, and overconstraint from repair can contribute to stiffness.

Anatomic variants in the superior labrum must also be recognized. Variants include a sublabral foramen or absence of the superior labrum, often seen together with a cordlike middle glenohumeral ligament (MGHL). The following labral anatomic variants were identified: 3.3% had a sublabral foramen, 8.6% had a sublabral foramen with cordlike MGHL, also called a Buford complex (Figure 1), and 1.5% had an absent anterosuperior labrum.[5] Surgical repair of these anatomic variants can result in loss of external rotation.

The LHB passes intra-articularly over the humeral head before exiting the glenohumeral joint in the bicipital groove.[3] The LHB pulley, especially the coracohumeral ligament and superior fibers of the subscapularis, stabilize the extra-articular LHB as it enters the bicipital groove. A subscapularis tear should be highly suspected in the setting of LHB instability, and vice versa. The subscapularis tendon, supraspinatus tendon, coracohumeral ligament, and superior glenohumeral ligament comprise the soft-tissue sling.[6] The LHB tendon is innervated by thinly myelinated sensory neurons. Most of this innervation occurs at the LHB origin; therefore, pathology in this region can generate pain.[7] Blood is supplied to the LHB tendon from the thoracoacromial and brachial arteries via the osteotendinous and musculotendinous junctions, respectively.[8] A hypovascular zone found near the tendon origin at the superior glenoid attachment corresponds to where it commonly tears at the LHB pulley near the proximal groove.[3,8]

Pathophysiology

SLAP tears can be caused by forceful traction to the arm, direct compression loads, and repetitive overhead throwing. Certain anatomic and biomechanical factors can predispose the overhead athlete to SLAP tears. Increased external rotation of the shoulder in the late cocking phase increases torsional force at the LHB root, resulting in a peel-back injury to the posterosuperior labrum (Figure 2). Injuries can also result from repetitive contact of the posterosuperior labrum with the undersurface of the rotator cuff in the late cocking phase.[9] Studies have shown that SLAP tears are seen more frequently in the late cocking position. It has been proposed that the essential lesion is posterior capsular contracture.[10] Because of this, throwing athletes have increased shoulder external rotation and decreased internal rotation in abduction, which causes posterosuperior migration of the humeral head in the late cocking phase, which can result in a peel-back SLAP tear. Increased external rotation results in greater torsional loads across the superior labrum from the more posteriorly oriented LHB tendon. The labrum and LHB tendon displace medially over the glenoid rim, creating a SLAP tear (Figure 3). The proximal LHB tendon has been recognized as a source of substantial pain;[11] this can be difficult to diagnose because it is known to occur with other pathologies including SLAP lesions, rotator cuff disorders, impingement, bursitis, and other acromioclavicular joint disorders.

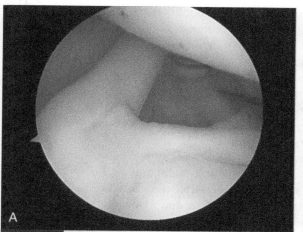
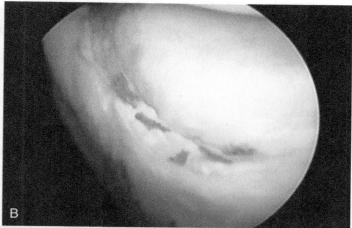

Figure 2 Arthroscopic views obtained via the posterior portal with the patient in the lateral decubitus position. **A,** View shows the biceps attachment to the labrum. **B,** View shows the peel-back sign of the labrum with abduction and external rotation.

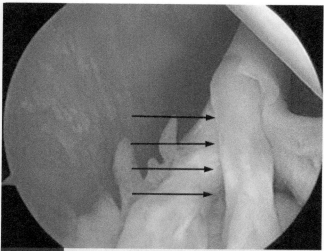

Figure 3 Arthroscopic view obtained via the posterior portal with the patient in the lateral decubitus position demonstrates a type III superior labrum anterior to posterior tear. Note the biceps displaced medially over the glenoid rim as a bucket-handle tear of the long head of the biceps tendon (arrows).

Pathology of the LHB tendon can include tendinitis, tears, subluxation, entrapment, delamination, and dislocations out of the bicipital groove.[12] Because of the relatively anterior position of the bicipital groove along the humeral head along with humeral retroversion, the tendon is exposed to medial instability, which can increase degeneration.[13] The different variations of the bicipital groove can also increase the risk of LHB tendon pathology. However, isolated LHB tendon pathology can still occur in isolation but is frequently associated with other shoulder pathologies, especially rotator cuff pathology.

When seen in isolation, primary LHB tendinitis usually occurs in younger patients who participate in overhead activities such as volleyball and baseball.[14] With LHB tendon instability, the patient describes a clicking or snapping with overhead motions. In addition, a subscapularis tear is associated with LHB medial instability and a supraspinatus tear is associated with posterolateral instability.[15]

Classification

Snyder's original classification system of SLAP tears is the most widely used and recognized[2] (**Figure 4**). Type I lesions consist of fraying of the superior labrum with localized degeneration (**Figure 5, A**). The superior labrum and LHB anchor remain intact. Type II lesions are the most common and are characterized by detachment of the superior labrum and/or LHB anchor from the glenoid (**Figure 5, B**). These lesions demonstrate abnormal mobility of the labrum and LHB anchor. Type III lesions are characterized by a bucket-handle tear of the superior labrum with an intact LHB anchor (**Figure 5, C**). Type IV lesions have a bucket-handle tear of the superior labrum that extends into the LHB anchor (**Figure 5, D**). The original classification system has been expanded to include type V, a SLAP tear combined with a Bankart lesion; type VI, a SLAP tear combined with an unstable flap tear of the labrum; and type VII, a SLAP tear that continues to the MGHL origin.[16]

Physical Examination

The clinical diagnosis and physical examination of a SLAP tear or symptomatic LHB tendinopathy is often challenging because the findings are similar to other

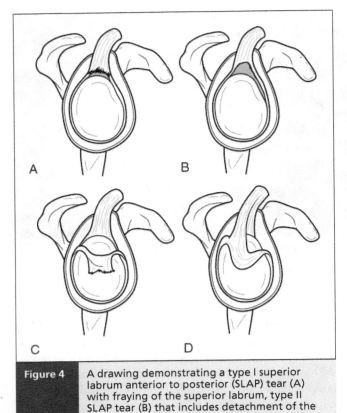

Figure 4 A drawing demonstrating a type I superior labrum anterior to posterior (SLAP) tear (A) with fraying of the superior labrum, type II SLAP tear (B) that includes detachment of the superior labrum, type III SLAP tear (C) consisting of a bucket handle-tear of the superior labrum, and a type IV SLAP tear (D) demonstrating a bucket-handle tear that extends into the bicep.

pathologies within the glenohumeral joint.[17] No single physical examination finding is completely accurate for diagnosing a SLAP tear. It is important to inspect for shoulder asymmetry and atrophy of the rotator cuff muscles. Isolated atrophy of the infraspinatus can indicate the presence of a spinoglenoid cyst, which is often associated with a superior labral tear. Range of motion and rotator cuff strength must be assessed and both are usually preserved. LHB-specific tests (such as the Speed and Yergason tests) can re-create shoulder pain in patients with SLAP tears. Apprehension, relocation, and load-and-shift tests can be performed to assess for shoulder stability. However, overt instability in the setting of an isolated SLAP tear is rare. Glenohumeral internal rotation deficit should be assessed in overhead athletes; extreme deficits greater than 25° to 30° can predispose patients to internal impingement and SLAP tears.[9] The O'Brien active compression test is the most commonly used maneuver to evaluate for a possible SLAP tear.[18] Clinical examination alone is unreliable in diagnosing SLAP tears when

multiple physical examination tests have been compared with intraoperative findings.[19,20]

A deformity of the LHB tendon such as a Popeye sign indicates tendon rupture. The most common physical examination for LHB disorder is tenderness caused by palpating the tendon within the bicipital groove.[17] An examiner can test for synovitis that is localized in the bicipital groove by palpating the tendon medial to the pectoralis major insertion during internal rotation with resistance.[21] For a more accurate diagnosis, the examiner should test the contralateral side and compare it with the affected side. Multiple tests have been established to identify LHB tendinitis and associated pathologies but none have a reported positive predictable value. Both the Yergason and Speed tests are specific but not sensitive in detecting LHB tendinitis, rupture, and SLAP lesions.[22] A painful click or tenderness to palpation at full abduction and external rotation indicates medial LHB instability. If the tendon is dislocated, it can be rolled under the examiner's fingers.[21] Different types of injections can be used for further treatment and diagnosis. Most commonly, a subacromial cortisone injection is given first to differentiate pain caused by impingement from LHB tendinitis. If the pain persists, a cortisone injection into the bicipital groove can be given to diagnose and treat LHB tendinitis.

Imaging

For all cases, typical plain radiographic views (scapular Y, AP, and axillary lateral) should be obtained to assess the joint for abnormalities. MRI is used to assess the bicipital groove, LHB tendon, fluid, and bony osteophytes and can help identify concomitant pathologies. However, studies have demonstrated poor correlation between MRI and arthroscopic findings regarding LHB pathology and poor to moderate sensitivity for inflammation, partial-thickness tears, and ruptures.[23] Magnetic resonance arthrography (MRA) is more specific and sensitive for LHB pathology and SLAP tears (Figure 6) than MRI.[24] MRA in patients with no pathology shows the tendon surrounded by contrast fluid and it resembles a kidney bean. Both MRI and MRA are needed in the sagittal oblique and axial planes because LHB subluxation and dislocation are associated with partial- and full-thickness subscapularis tendon tears[25] (Figure 7).

Ultrasonography is accurate and cost-effective in the diagnosis of LHB dislocation, subluxation, and rupture. However, it is not as accurate in diagnosing partial-thickness tendon tears.[26] The exact role of ultrasonography for the diagnosis of tendon inflammation has not been fully defined.

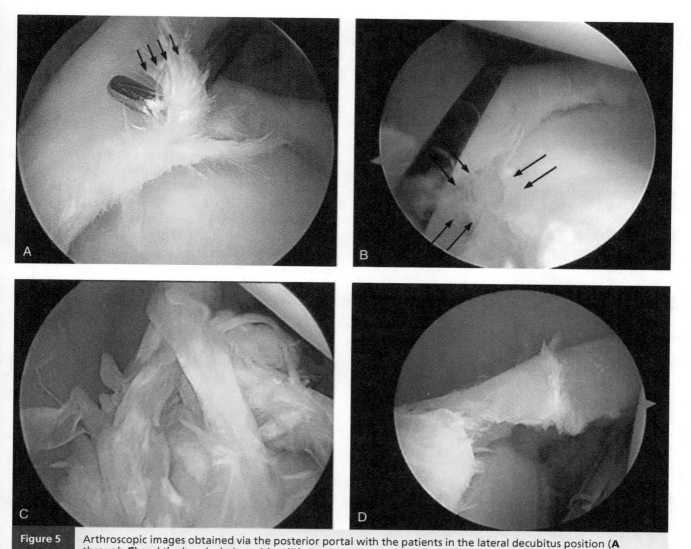

Figure 5 Arthroscopic images obtained via the posterior portal with the patients in the lateral decubitus position (**A** through **C**) and the beach chair position (**D**). **A,** View shows a type I superior labrum anterior to posterior (SLAP) lesion, with fraying of the superior labrum and localized degeneration (arrows). **B,** View shows a type II SLAP lesion with the superior labrum and biceps anchor detached from the glenoid (arrows). **C,** View shows a type III SLAP lesion with a bucket-handle tear of the superior labrum and an intact biceps anchor. **D,** View shows a type IV SLAP tear of more than 50% diameter of the long head of the biceps tendon; the tear extends up the biceps tendon.

Nonsurgical Treatment

Nonsurgical treatment of SLAP tears consists of rehabilitation focused on improving posterior capsular flexibility and strengthening of the rotator cuff muscles and scapular stabilizers. Intra-articular steroid injections can help in the diagnosis and treatment of patients with a possible SLAP tear. In the only study reporting on the nonsurgical treatment of SLAP tears,[27] the authors found that functional scores, quality-of-life scores, and pain scores all improved substantially in 19 patients at an average follow-up of 3.1 years; 71% of athletes returned to preparticipation levels, but only 66% of overhead athletes returned to sport at the

same level. The nonsurgical protocol consisted of NSAIDs and a physical therapy protocol focused on scapular stabilization and posterior capsular stretching.

The initial step for the treatment of LHB tendon pathology is nonsurgical and should encompass physical therapy to correct scapulothoracic dyskinesia. Because the LHB is continuous with the synovium of the glenohumeral joint, cortisone injections can also be used for initial treatment in the subacromial space or the glenohumeral joint. Some authors have recommended a diagnostic and potentially therapeutic corticosteroid injection in the tendon sheath at the groove; however, this can increase the risk of LHB rupture if injected within the tendon itself. The authors of a 2011 study reported an 86.7% accuracy of injection in the sheath using ultrasonography versus 26.7% without, and another 40.0% was injected into the tendon itself; therefore, ultrasonographic guidance was recommended.[28]

Surgical Treatment

Surgical treatment for SLAP tears should be considered in patients with persistent symptoms whose nonsurgical

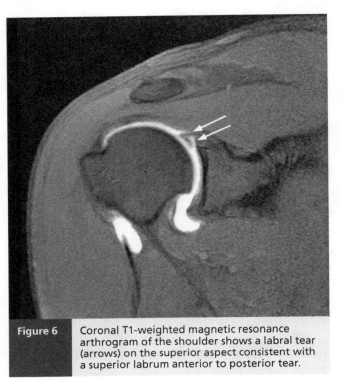

| Figure 6 | Coronal T1-weighted magnetic resonance arthrogram of the shoulder shows a labral tear (arrows) on the superior aspect consistent with a superior labrum anterior to posterior tear. |

treatment was unsuccessful for approximately 3 months. High-level athletes with a SLAP tear are usually allowed to compete and finish the season. Earlier intervention can be offered to those patients with evidence of suprascapular nerve compression from a spinoglenoid cyst.

Arthroscopic surgery can be performed in the lateral decubitus or beach chair position. Type I tears are usually débrided. Type II lesions should be repaired when the history and examination suggest a SLAP tear and the arthroscopic examination confirms findings of a type II tear (Figure 8). The gold standard for the diagnosis of SLAP tears on arthroscopic examination uses the Snyder criteria. This includes separation of the chondrolabral junction, erythema at the LHB anchor junction, and a minimum 5 mm of labral excursion.[2] Degenerative type II tears associated with other lesions in older patients do not require repair but can be better addressed with débridement, tenodesis, or tenotomy. Type III tears are treated with either repair of the bucket handle or, depending on size and tissue quality, a resection of the unstable labral fragment and repair of the MGHL if it is attached to the torn fragment. Treatment of type IV tears depends on the patient age and the extent of LHB tendon involvement. If less than 30% of the tendon is involved, these tears are usually treated with débridement. Tears of more than 30% of the LHB tendon are usually treated with LHB tenodesis. Although some studies have suggested superior labral ring repair, what to do with the remaining potentially unstable superior labrum after tenodesis remains controversial.[29]

Bioabsorbable tacks are no longer used because of concerns about synovitis and cartilage damage caused by the degradation and release of loose bodies.[30] SLAP repair

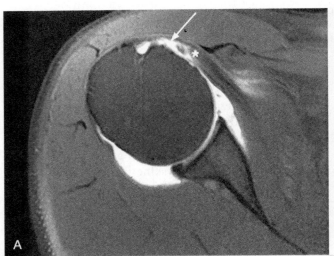
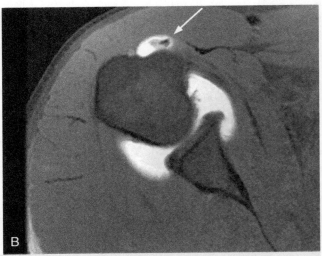

| Figure 7 | Axial T2-weighted magnetic resonance arthrograms demonstrate an empty bicipital groove. The biceps tendon can be seen medial to the groove (arrows), indicating a subscapularis tear (asterisk in **A**). |

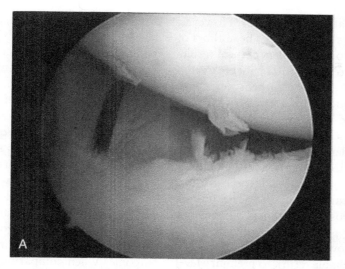

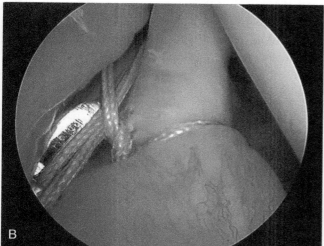

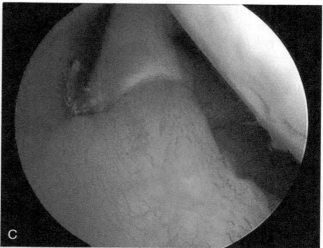

Figure 8 Arthroscopic views demonstrate a type II superior labrum anterior to posterior (SLAP) tear with posterior extension via the posterior portal, with the patient in the lateral decubitus position. **A,** Probe inserted via the anterior portal. **B,** The sutures are passed via the anterosuperior portal around the tear. **C,** The repaired SLAP tear.

failure is not limited to the use of bioabsorable tacks. A reoperation rate of 6.3%, with a 4.3% rate of revision SLAP repair, has been reported.[31] Revision surgery and failure after index SLAP repair correlated with the use of absorbable poly-L–D-lactic acid suture anchors. Paralabral ganglion cysts associated with SLAP tears can successfully be treated arthroscopically.[32] The authors of a 2014 study examined patients who underwent open subpectoral tenodesis for a failed repair of type II SLAP tears in a military population.[33] An 81% return to sport and active duty was reported. LHB tenodesis is a predictable, safe, and effective treatment of failed arthroscopic SLAP repairs.

Concomitant repair of rotator cuff tears and SLAP tears have shown good clinical outcomes with high patient satisfaction. In patients 50 years and older with a degenerative SLAP tear, a combined LHB tenotomy or tenodesis and rotator cuff repair have shown superior outcomes compared with rotator cuff and SLAP repair combined.[34]

Data suggest that the rate of SLAP repairs is increasing. A statewide database study in New York reported a 464% increase in the number of SLAP repairs from 2002 to 2010.[35] The authors of a 2012 study found that the percentage of SLAP repairs reported by American Board of Orthopaedic Surgery candidates was three times the incidence reported in the current literature.[36] A substantial increase in the number of SLAP repairs was also noted in a database study.[37] The authors noted that this trend is slightly worrisome given the relatively high number of SLAP repairs performed.

Most studies have reported on the outcomes of patients treated for type II SLAP tears. Pain relief and return of function can be expected after SLAP repair. However, return to sports is often less predictable. The authors of one study reported 97% good to excellent clinical results and an 84% rate of return to sport in 102 patients treated with suture anchors for SLAP repair.[38] Other studies have reported 90% to 94% good to excellent results, with return to preinjury athletic levels ranging from 75% to 91%. Long-term outcomes after isolated SLAP repair were found to be independent of patient age, with 88% reporting good or excellent results at 5-year follow-up.[39-41] The authors of a 2010 study also reported favorable results independent of patient vocation or sport.[42] The authors of a 2014 study reported prospective clinical outcomes of arthroscopic treatment of type II SLAP tears in young, active patients.[43] The study showed substantial improvement in shoulder outcomes. A reliable return to preinjury level of activity was less predictable: a 37% failure rate and a 28% revision rate were reported. In addition, an increased relative risk of failure was reported for patients older than 36 years. It has been reported that 37% of patients had an unsatisfactory result and 9% to 55% were unable to return to prior activity levels.[44] Given these findings, the reported outcomes after primary SLAP repair have some inconsistencies.

The optimal surgical treatment of LHB tendon pathology remains controversial. No definitive consensus exists regarding LHB tenodesis compared with an LHB tenotomy.[45] An increased incidence of cosmetic deformity (Popeye deformity) in LHB tenotomies was found when compared with LHB tenodesis (43% versus 8%).[46] For postoperative bicipital pain, similar results were found in the tenodesis group compared with the tenotomy group (24% versus 9%).

Current indications proposed for LHB tenodesis include degenerative SLAP tears, high-grade SLAP tears, failed SLAP repairs, those patients who are reasonably active, patients concerned with cosmesis, and workers' compensation cases.[45] Relative indications for tenodesis include a tear of 25% or more of the tendon, longitudinal tears that decrease gliding in the bicipital groove, subluxation of the LHB tendon, an hourglass (hypertrophy) LHB,[47] disruption of the sling, or if a concomitant subscapularis tear is present.[21] However, the surgeon must also consider the characteristics of the patient, such as age and activity level. as well when deciding to perform tenodesis. Other proposed relative indications include a symptomatic type II tear in a patient older than 50 years, failed SLAP repair, a type IV SLAP tear, and LHB tendinitis pain for which conservative management has failed.[13]

Among LHB tenodesis procedures, no technique is clearly superior. Tenodesis techniques include arthroscopic, mini-open, and open procedures; proximal versus distal fixation; and multiple types of fixation constructs. The authors of a 2015 study found degenerative changes in the proximal intra-articular and middle intragroove portions in all 36 cases and up to the distal extra-articular portion in 29 (80.6%).[47] Therefore, subpectoral tenodesis was optimal for these patients. However, no clinical outcome studies have demonstrated any tenodesis technique as superior to other techniques. It was demonstrated in a 2013 study that the open subpectoral approach placed the tenodesis tunnel 2.2 cm distal to the arthroscopic suprapectoral approach.[48] However, both of these techniques placed the tenodesis tunnel distal to the bicipital groove, which may allay concerns about the bicipital groove as a source of pain after this procedure. According to a 2014 study, there were no significant differences in clinical outcomes when comparing arthroscopic suprapectoral and open subpectoral LHB tenodesis with a minimum 2-year follow-up.[49] No difference was found regarding failure of fixation type when comparing unicortical and interference screw fixation for subpectoral tenodesis.[49,50] Substantially less displacement was found during cyclic loading for the interference screw compared with the unicortical button.[50] However, arthroscopic suprapectoral and open subpectoral LHB tenodesis techniques using an interference screw implant in a cadaver model were compared; arthroscopic tenodesis overtensioned the LHB and has a substantially decreased ultimate load to failure compared with the open technique[51] (Figure 9). In the future, studies should define when a tenodesis is indicated, along with the position and type of fixation used when performing an LHB tenodesis.

Summary

The treatment of SLAP tears and LHB pathologies remains controversial. The clinical diagnosis and physical examination of a SLAP tear or symptomatic LHB tendinopathy is often challenging because the findings are similar to the other pathologies within the glenohumeral joint. No single physical examination finding is completely accurate for the diagnosis of a SLAP tear. MRA helps diagnose LHB pathology and SLAP tears because it is more specific and more sensitive than MRI. SLAP repairs have had more beneficial results in patients younger than 40 years and if they are not associated with a rotator cuff repair. The ideal treatment of LHB pathology is also still evolving. Both tenotomy and LHB tenodesis are acceptable treatment options, but the literature has not clearly demonstrated which surgery is superior. Several types of tenodesis surgeries can be performed and the literature has not identified which is optimal. Future research is needed to help identify the best treatment options.

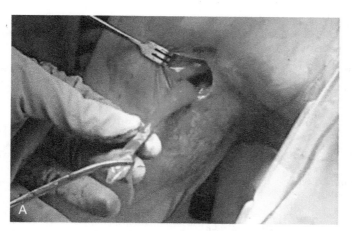

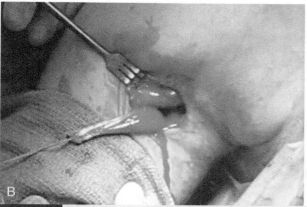

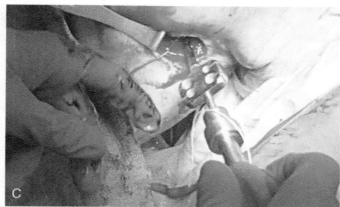

Figure 9 Photographs of the open subpectoral biceps tenodesis. **A,** The tendon pulled out of the skin. **B,** The tendon is stitched 2 cm proximal to the musculotendinous junction with No. 2 suture. **C,** Completed tenodesis.

Key Study Points

- SLAP repairs have proved more beneficial than tenodesis in patients younger than 40 years and may be even more successful if not associated with rotator cuff repair.

- No clear advantage has been reported when comparing LHB tenodesis and tenotomy. An increase of Popeye deformities is seen with tenotomies. However, current indications proposed for LHB tenodesis include patients with high levels of physical activity, patients concerned with cosmesis, and workers' compensation cases.

- Different tenodesis techniques include proximal arthroscopic fixation, in which the tendon remains in the bicipital groove, or the tendon can be fixed distally so it is removed from the groove. The location of tenodesis has shown substantial differences in clinical outcomes when comparing arthroscopic suprapectoral and open subpectoral LHB tenodesis.

Annotated References

1. Andrews JR, Carson WG Jr, McLeod WD: Glenoid labrum tears related to the long head of the biceps. *Am J Sports Med* 1985;13(5):337-341.

2. Snyder SJ, Karzel RP, Del Pizzo W, Ferkel RD, Friedman MJ: SLAP lesions of the shoulder. *Arthroscopy* 1990;6(4):274-279.

3. Cooper DE, Arnoczky SP, O'Brien SJ, Warren RF, DiCarlo E, Allen AA: Anatomy, histology, and vascularity of the glenoid labrum. An anatomical study. *J Bone Joint Surg Am* 1992;74(1):46-52.

4. Tuoheti Y, Itoi E, Minagawa H, et al: Attachment types of the long head of the biceps tendon to the glenoid labrum and their relationships with the glenohumeral ligaments. *Arthroscopy* 2005;21(10):1242-1249.

5. Rao AG, Kim TK, Chronopoulos E, McFarland EG: Anatomical variants in the anterosuperior aspect of the glenoid labrum: A statistical analysis of seventy-three cases. *J Bone Joint Surg Am* 2003;85-A(4):653-659.

1: Upper Extremity

6. Werner A, Mueller T, Boehm D, Gohlke F: The stabilizing sling for the long head of the biceps tendon in the rotator cuff interval: A histoanatomic study. *Am J Sports Med* 2000;28(1):28-31.

7. Alpantaki K, McLaughlin D, Karagogeos D, Hadjipavlou A, Kontakis G: Sympathetic and sensory neural elements in the tendon of the long head of the biceps. *J Bone Joint Surg Am* 2005;87(7):1580-1583.

8. Cheng NM, Pan WR, Vally F, Le Roux CM, Richardson MD: The arterial supply of the long head of biceps tendon: Anatomical study with implications for tendon rupture. *Clin Anat* 2010;23(6):683-692.

   This cadaver study found that the region of hypovascularity zone for the LHB tendon (via injection with either a radiopaque lead oxide/milk mixture or India ink) was 1.2 to 3.0 cm from the tendon origin, extending from midway through the glenohumeral joint to the proximal intertubercular groove. Although this was found to be a vital reason for tendon rupture, mechanical factors also play an important role. Level of evidence: IV.

9. Keener JD, Brophy RH: Superior labral tears of the shoulder: Pathogenesis, evaluation, and treatment. *J Am Acad Orthop Surg* 2009;17(10):627-637.

   This review discussed the advances in surgical techniques for secure SLAP injuries repair. This is supported by recent outcomes demonstrating good functional results and an acceptable rate of return to athletic activities. Level of evidence: V.

10. Burkhart SS, Morgan CD, Kibler WB: The disabled throwing shoulder: Spectrum of pathology. Part I: Pathoanatomy and biomechanics. *Arthroscopy* 2003;19(4):404-420.

11. Hitchcock HH, Bechtol CO: Painful shoulder: Observations on the role of the tendon of the long head of the biceps brachii in its causation. *J Bone Joint Surg Am* 1948;30-A(2):263-273.

12. Szabó I, Boileau P, Walch G: The proximal biceps as a pain generator and results of tenotomy. *Sports Med Arthrosc* 2008;16(3):180-186.

13. Ahrens PM, Boileau P: The long head of biceps and associated tendinopathy. *J Bone Joint Surg Br* 2007;89(8):1001-1009.

14. Patton WC, McCluskey GM III: Biceps tendinitis and subluxation. *Clin Sports Med* 2001;20(3):505-529.

15. Lafosse L, Reiland Y, Baier GP, Toussaint B, Jost B: Anterior and posterior instability of the long head of the biceps tendon in rotator cuff tears: A new classification based on arthroscopic observations. *Arthroscopy* 2007;23(1):73-80.

16. Maffet MW, Gartsman GM, Moseley B: Superior labrum-biceps tendon complex lesions of the shoulder. *Am J Sports Med* 1995;23(1):93-98.

17. Nho SJ, Strauss EJ, Lenart BA, et al: Long head of the biceps tendinopathy: Diagnosis and management. *J Am Acad Orthop Surg* 2010;18(11):645-656.

    This review article described arthroscopic and open biceps tenodesis techniques; both show promising results. Level of evidence: V.

18. O'Brien SJ, Pagnanwi MJ, Fealy S, McGlynn SR, Wilson JB: The active compression test: A new and effective test for diagnosing labral tears and acromioclavicular joint abnormality. *Am J Sports Med* 1998;26(5):610-613.

19. Parentis MA, Glousman RE, Mohr KS, Yocum LA: An evaluation of the provocative tests for superior labral anterior posterior lesions. *Am J Sports Med* 2006;34(2):265-268.

20. Cook C, Beaty S, Kissenberth MJ, Siffri P, Pill SG, Hawkins RJ: Diagnostic accuracy of five orthopedic clinical tests for diagnosis of superior labrum anterior posterior (SLAP) lesions. *J Shoulder Elbow Surg* 2012;21(1):13-22.

    This study analyzed five clinical tests for SLAP lesion diagnosis. The Biceps Load II test demonstrated efficacy for diagnosing SLAP-only lesions. The results had a positive predictive value of 26 (95% confidence interval [CI]: 18-31), negative predictive value of 93 (95% CI: 84-97), positive likelihood ratio of 1.7 (95% CI: 1.1-2.6), and negative likelihood ratio of 0.39 (95% CI: 0.14-0.91). No other tests demonstrated diagnostic utility for SLAP lesion diagnosis, including those with concomitant diagnoses. Level of evidence: III.

21. Sethi N, Wright R, Yamaguchi K: Disorders of the long head of the biceps tendon. *J Shoulder Elbow Surg* 1999;8(6):644-654.

22. Holtby R, Razmjou H: Accuracy of the Speed's and Yergason's tests in detecting biceps pathology and SLAP lesions: Comparison with arthroscopic findings. *Arthroscopy* 2004;20(3):231-236.

23. Mohtadi NG, Vellet AD, Clark ML, et al: A prospective, double-blind comparison of magnetic resonance imaging and arthroscopy in the evaluation of patients presenting with shoulder pain. *J Shoulder Elbow Surg* 2004;13(3):258-265.

24. Pfirrmann CW, Zanetti M, Weishaupt D, Gerber C, Hodler J: Subscapularis tendon tears: Detection and grading at MR arthrography. *Radiology* 1999;213(3):709-714.

25. Gambill ML, Mologne TS, Provencher MT: Dislocation of the long head of the biceps tendon with intact subscapularis and supraspinatus tendons. *J Shoulder Elbow Surg* 2006;15(6):e20-e22.

26. Wall LB, Teefey SA, Middleton WD, et al: Diagnostic performance and reliability of ultrasonography for fatty degeneration of the rotator cuff muscles. *J Bone Joint Surg Am* 2012;94(12):e83.

    This study analyzed diagnostic performance and reliability of ultrasonography for fatty degeneration of the rotator cuff muscles by comparing it with MRI. Ultrasonography can be used as the primary diagnostic modality. The agreement between MRI and ultrasonography was substantial for the supraspinatus and infraspinatus (κ = 0.78 and 0.71, respectively) and moderate for the teres minor (κ = 0.47). Level of evidence: II.

27. Edwards SL, Lee JA, Bell JE, et al: Nonoperative treatment of superior labrum anterior posterior tears: Improvements in pain, function, and quality of life. *Am J Sports Med* 2010;38(7):1456-1461.

The outcomes of nonsurgical treatment of SLAP tears in 39 patients were analyzed. Nonsurgical treatment can be trialed in patients with an isolated superior labral tear. Overall, mean American Shoulder and Elbow Surgeon scores increased from 58.5 to 84.7, Simple Shoulder Test scores increased from 8.3 to 11.0, and visual analog scale pain scores decreased from 4.5 to 2.1. In overhead athletes and in those patients where pain relief and functional improvement is not achieved, surgical treatment should be considered. Level of evidence: IV.

28. Hashiuchi T, Sakurai G, Morimoto M, Komei T, Takakura Y, Tanaka Y: Accuracy of the biceps tendon sheath injection: Ultrasound-guided or unguided injection? A randomized controlled trial. *J Shoulder Elbow Surg* 2011;20(7):1069-1073.

This study analyzed the accuracy of ultrasonographically guided or unguided biceps tendon sheath injection in 30 patients. Injection into the LHB tendon sheath is more accurate under ultrasonographic guidance. Level of evidence: II.

29. Chalmers PN, Trombley R, Cip J, et al: Postoperative restoration of upper extremity motion and neuromuscular control during the overhand pitch: Evaluation of tenodesis and repair for superior labral anterior-posterior tears. *Am J Sports Med* 2014;42(12):2825-2836.

This study evaluated shoulder motion in overhand pitchers after biceps tenodesis and SLAP repair in 18 patients. SLAP repair and biceps tenodesis can restore physiologic neuromuscular control, but pitchers who undergo SLAP repair may have altered thoracic motion when compared with control patients. Level of evidence: IV.

30. Sassmannshausen G, Sukay M, Mair SD: Broken or dislodged poly-L-lactic acid bioabsorbable tacks in patients after SLAP lesion surgery. *Arthroscopy* 2006;22(6):615-619.

31. Park MJ, Hsu JE, Harper C, Sennett BJ, Huffman GR: Poly-L/D-lactic acid anchors are associated with reoperation and failure of SLAP repairs. *Arthroscopy* 2011;27(10):1335-1340.

32. Abboud JA, Silverberg D, Glaser DL, Ramsey ML, Williams GR: Arthroscopy effectively treats ganglion cysts of the shoulder. *Clin Orthop Relat Res* 2006;444(444):129-133.

33. McCormick F, Nwachukwu BU, Solomon D, et al: The efficacy of biceps tenodesis in the treatment of failed superior labral anterior posterior repairs. *Am J Sports Med* 2014;42(4):820-825.

This study prospectively evaluated revision biceps tenodesis after failed arthroscopic repair for type II SLAP tear. Most patients obtained good to excellent outcomes using validated measures with a substantial improvement in range of motion. Level of evidence: IV.

34. Franceschi F, Longo UG, Ruzzini L, Rizzello G, Maffulli N, Denaro V: No advantages in repairing a type II superior labrum anterior and posterior (SLAP) lesion when associated with rotator cuff repair in patients over age 50: A randomized controlled trial. *Am J Sports Med* 2008;36(2):247-253.

35. Onyekwelu I, Khatib O, Zuckerman JD, Rokito AS, Kwon YW: The rising incidence of arthroscopic superior labrum anterior and posterior (SLAP) repairs. *J Shoulder Elbow Surg* 2012;21(6):728-731.

The study analyzed the increase of arthroscopic SLAP repairs in New York state from 2002 to 2010. Substantial increases in the number of arthroscopic SLAP repairs (464%) and in the age of patients treated with arthroscopic SLAP repairs were noted. Level of evidence: V.

36. Weber SC, Martin DF, Seiler JG III, Harrast JJ: Superior labrum anterior and posterior lesions of the shoulder: Incidence rates, complications, and outcomes as reported by American Board of Orthopedic Surgery. Part II: candidates. *Am J Sports Med* 2012;40(7):1538-1543.

A database of cases was examined for board certification on the demographics of SLAP lesion repair. A concerning number of repairs was noted in middle-aged (9.4% of all shoulder cases, increased to 10.1% in 2008) and elderly patients and emphasized the importance of educating orthopaedic surgeons to appropriately recognize and treat symptomatic SLAP lesions to reduce the rate of SLAP repairs. Level of evidence: III.

37. Zhang AL, Kreulen C, Ngo SS, Hame SL, Wang JC, Gamradt SC: Demographic trends in arthroscopic SLAP repair in the United States. *Am J Sports Med* 2012;40(5):1144-1147.

Demographic trends in arthroscopic SLAP repairs were examined. From 2004 to 2009, the findings show substantially more arthroscopic SLAP repairs were performed each year, with the highest incidence rates in the 20- to 29-year-olds (29.1 per 10,000) and 40- to 49-year-olds (27.8 per 10,000) and in men. Level of evidence: V.

38. Morgan CD, Burkhart SS, Palmeri M, Gillespie M: Type II SLAP lesions: Three subtypes and their relationships to superior instability and rotator cuff tears. *Arthroscopy* 1998;14(6):553-565.

39. Schrøder CP, Skare O, Gjengedal E, Uppheim G, Reikerås O, Brox JI: Long-term results after SLAP repair: A 5-year follow-up study of 107 patients with comparison of patients aged over and under 40 years. *Arthroscopy* 2012;28(11):1601-1607 .

40. Ide J, Maeda S, Takagi K: Sports activity after arthroscopic superior labral repair using suture anchors in overhead-throwing athletes. *Am J Sports Med* 2005;33(4):507-514.

41. Kim SH, Ha KI, Kim SH, Choi HJ: Results of arthroscopic treatment of superior labral lesions. *J Bone Joint Surg Am* 2002;84-A(6):981-985.

42. Friel NA, Karas V, Slabaugh MA, Cole BJ: Outcomes of type II superior labrum, anterior to posterior (SLAP) repair: Prospective evaluation at a minimum two-year follow-up. *J Shoulder Elbow Surg* 2010;19(6):859-867.

    The outcomes of SLAP II lesion repairs via bioabsorbable sutures were examined. At an average 3.4-year follow-up, this type of suture anchor provided a significant improvement in functional capacity and pain relief (mean American Shoulder and Elbow Surgeon scores improved from 59.49 to 83.37; mean Simple Shoulder Test scores improved from 7.28 to 10.20; visual analog scale 3.98-1.52). Level of evidence: IV.

43. Provencher MT, McCormick F, Dewing C, McIntire S, Solomon D: A prospective analysis of 179 type 2 superior labrum anterior and posterior repairs: Outcomes and factors associated with success and failure. *Am J Sports Med* 2013;41(4):880-886.

    This prospective analysis of SLAP II repairs in 179 patients examined factors associated with success and failure and found a 37% rate of returning to previous athletic activity and a 28% rate of failure. Patients aged 36 years and older have higher risk of failure. Level of evidence: III.

44. Katz LM, Hsu S, Miller SL, et al: Poor outcomes after SLAP repair: Descriptive analysis and prognosis. *Arthroscopy* 2009;25(8):849-855.

    This study examined failed SLAP repairs in 39 patients (40 shoulders). After revision, 32% of patients still had suboptimal results. Conservative treatment resulted in poor outcomes (71% of patients; mean patient age, 43 years) after failed repair. Level of evidence: V.

45. Hsu AR, Ghodadra NS, Provencher MT, Lewis PB, Bach BR: Biceps tenotomy versus tenodesis: A review of clinical outcomes and biomechanical results. *J Shoulder Elbow Surg* 2011;20(2):326-332.

    This review compared biceps tenotomy and tenodesis for biceps tendon rupture from 1966 to 2010. Higher cosmetic deformity and lower load to tendon failure were found in patients who underwent tenotomy (40%). Level of evidence: V.

46. Slenker NR, Lawson K, Ciccotti MG, Dodson CC, Cohen SB: Biceps tenotomy versus tenodesis: Clinical outcomes. *Arthroscopy* 2012;28(4):576-582.

    This systematic review analyzed clinical outcomes of biceps tenodesis versus tenotomy and found that tenotomies result in cosmetic deformities (43%) more often than tenodesis. No consensus was reported regarding the use of tenotomy versus tenodesis for the treatment of LHB lesions. Level of evidence: V.

47. Moon SC, Cho NS, Rhee YG: Analysis of "hidden lesions" of the extra-articular biceps after subpectoral biceps tenodesis: The subpectoral portion as the optimal tenodesis site. *Am J Sports Med* 2015;43(1):63-68.

    This study examined the optimal tenodesis site by analyzing the extension and delamination of extra-articular lesions in the retrieved biceps after subpectoral biceps tenodesis in 36 patients. Lesions were observed beyond the bicipital groove, extending to the distal extra-articular portion (80%). The subpectoral portion may be the optimal tenodesis site. Level of evidence: IV.

48. Johannsen AM, Macalena JA, Carson EW, Tompkins M: Anatomic and radiographic comparison of arthroscopic suprapectoral and open subpectoral biceps tenodesis sites. *Am J Sports Med* 2013;41(12):2919-2924.

    The authors conducted anatomic and radiographic evaluation of arthroscopic and open subpectoral biceps tenodesis. In 20 specimens, the open subpectoral approach placed the tunnel 2.2 cm distal to the arthroscopic suprapectoral approach. Thus, patients undergoing the arthroscopic suprapectoral approach may still have postoperative bicipital groove pain. Level of evidence: V.

49. Buchholz A, Martetschläger F, Siebenlist S, et al: Biomechanical comparison of intramedullary cortical button fixation and interference screw technique for subpectoral biceps tenodesis. *Arthroscopy* 2013;29(5):845-853.

    This study analyzed intramedullary cortical button fixation and interference screw technique for subpectoral biceps tenodesis. Intramedullary cortical button fixation showed no failures during cyclic testing; however, a 30% failure rate was reported for screw fixation. Cortical button fixation provides an alternative technique for subpectoral biceps tenodesis with comparable and, during cyclic loading, even superior biomechanical properties to interference screw fixation. Level of evidence: V.

50. DeAngelis JP, Chen A, Wexler M, et al: Biomechanical characterization of unicortical button fixation: A novel technique for proximal subpectoral biceps tenodesis. *Knee Surg Sports Traumatol Arthrosc* 2013. [Epub ahead of print]

    This study analyzed mechanical properties of unicortical metal buttons and interference screws in proximal biceps tenodesis in six pairs of fresh-frozen shoulders. The ultimate load to failure and stiffness for both methods were the same. A unicortical button provides a reliable alternative method of fixation with a potentially lower risk of postoperative humeral fracture and a construct that permits early mobilization following biceps tenodesis. Level of evidence: IV.

51. Werner BC, Evans CL, Holzgrefe RE, et al: Arthroscopic suprapectoral and open subpectoral biceps tenodesis: A comparison of minimum 2-year clinical outcomes. *Am J Sports Med* 2014;42(11):2583-2590.

    This cohort study compared open subpectoral (32 patients) and arthroscopic suprapectoral (50 patients) biceps tenodesis at a minimum 2-year follow-up. Both groups had excellent clinical and standardized outcomes; no clinical differences were seen in clinical or standardized outcomes. Level of evidence: III.

© 2016 American Academy of Orthopaedic Surgeons

Chapter 5

Adhesive Capsulitis, Cartilage Lesions, Nerve Compression Disorders, and Snapping Scapula

Maximilian Petri, MD   Joshua A. Greenspoon, BSc   Peter J. Millett, MD, MSc

Abstract

The most common shoulder pathologies in sports medicine are rotator cuff tears, instability of the glenohumeral and acromioclavicular joints, and tears of the long head of the biceps tendon. However, other disorders such as stiffness, focal chondral lesions, neural compression, and pathologies of the scapulothoracic joint can cause pain and loss of function for patients. It is important to be cognizant of the current concepts for treatment of adhesive capsulitis, cartilage lesions, nerve compression disorders, and snapping scapula syndrome for optimal outcomes.

Keywords: adhesive capsulitis; cartilage lesions; nerve compression disorders; suprascapular nerve entrapment; snapping scapula

Dr. Petri or an immediate family member has received nonincome support (such as equipment or services), commercially derived honoraria, or other non–research-related funding (such as paid travel) from Arthrex. Dr. Millett or an immediate family member has received royalties from Arthrex; serves as a paid consultant to Arthrex and MYOS; has stock or stock options held in Game Ready and VuMedi; and has received research or institutional support from Arthrex, Össur, Siemens, and Smith & Nephew. Neither Mr. Greenspoon nor any immediate family member has received anything of value from or has stock or stock options held in a commercial company or institution related directly or indirectly to the subject of this chapter.

Introduction

Glenohumeral instability, rotator cuff tears, pathologies of the long head of the biceps tendon, and instability of the acromioclavicular joint represent most shoulder disorders. Although disorders such as adhesive capsulitis, chondral defects, suprascapular nerve entrapment, and snapping scapula syndrome are less common, they can cause substantial disability in patients. Comprehensive knowledge of these pathologies is necessary to establish the proper diagnosis. Open and arthroscopic surgical treatments can be used to manage these disorders. Clinical outcomes studies have primarily been conducted as case series (level IV evidence); comparative studies are challenging because each entity is relatively rare. However, good to excellent results can be achieved with appropriate patient selection and surgical technique.

Adhesive Capsulitis

Adhesive capsulitis, commonly known as frozen shoulder, is characterized by spontaneous onset of pain and progressive restriction of shoulder movement. A cascade of inflammation involving abnormal tissue repair and fibrosis modulated by abnormal production of growth factors and cytokines is pathogenetic.[1,2]

Adhesive capsulitis can be idiopathic in origin (primary) or occur secondary to systemic diseases such as diabetes mellitus[3] or hypothyroidism. Additional secondary causes include previous trauma or surgery.[4] Breast cancer treatment with surgery and radiotherapy has also been linked to the development of adhesive capsulitis.[5] The condition is generally self-limiting; however, it often has a prolonged course, taking more than 2 years to resolve.[4]

The diagnosis for primary adhesive capsulitis is usually established by sudden onset of pain without history of major trauma, infection, or surgery of the affected shoulder, combined with a global limitation of both active and passive range of motion. Similar findings apply for secondary adhesive capsulitis, but with a history of previous trauma or surgery or medical disease. Differential diagnoses include calcific tendinitis, glenohumeral and acromioclavicular osteoarthritis, rotator cuff tendinopathy or tear, and lesions of the long head of the biceps tendon. Imaging modalities such as radiography, MRI, and ultrasonography should support the clinical diagnosis.[6]

Nonsurgical Treatment

Nonsurgical management should be recommended to patients initially; reported success rates range from 70% to 90%.[7] Adhesive capsulitis is commonly treated with physical therapy and exercise in primary cases. A recent randomized controlled trial found that group exercise classes for physical therapy achieved substantially higher Constant and Oxford Shoulder scores than both individual physical therapy sessions with a therapist and home exercises completed by the patient alone.[8]

NSAIDs and corticosteroid injections have proved to be useful adjuncts to therapy.[9] Calcitonin has also been suggested as an adjunct therapy. Patients should attempt nonsurgical management for at least 6 months before considering surgical intervention.[4,10]

Electrotherapy, Extracorporeal Shock Wave Therapy, and Suprascapular Nerve Stimulation

Electrotherapy aims to reduce pain and improve function by means of an increase of electrical, sound, light, and thermal energy into the body. Two recent Cochrane reviews[9,11] found no evidence regarding the addition of pulsed electromagnetic field therapy and other electrotherapeutic modalities to the standard regimens of manual therapy and exercise, corticosteroid injection, or NSAIDs. However, low-level laser therapy combined with exercise appeared to be more effective than exercise alone for pain and function.[11] In a recent randomized clinical trial of 36 patients, extracorporeal shock wave therapy was shown to substantially improve pain and range of motion.[12]

Given that the suprascapular nerve accounts for 70% of shoulder capsule sensitivity,[4,10] pulsed radiofrequency stimulation of the suprascapular nerve guided by ultrasonography represents a new therapeutic approach. This suprascapular nerve stimulation combined with physical therapy provided better and faster pain relief and improved passive range of motion compared with physical therapy alone.[13]

Distension Arthrography

Arthrographic joint distension with corticosteroids and saline improves patients' pain, satisfaction, and active range of motion.[9,14] Improvements in range of motion and pain relief were reported in 172 patients who underwent treatment with distension arthrography using radiopaque contrast material and lidocaine.[15] This approach provides both a therapeutic and diagnostic intervention in depicting rotator cuff tears by extrusion of the contrast agent. A recent randomized controlled clinical trial found no difference in outcomes between ultrasonographically guided posterolateral capsular distension and fluoroscopically guided anterior capsular distension.[16]

Differences between corticosteroid and hyaluronate injections in patients with adhesive capsulitis were investigated in a randomized clinical trial.[6] Both groups demonstrated improvements in clinical outcomes scores and range of motion, however no significant differences were found between the two groups.

Nonsurgical treatment of adhesive capsulitis commonly consists of manual therapy and exercise, often with the addition of NSAIDs. Corticosteroid injections and distension arthrography can effectively improve patient pain, satisfaction, and range of motion, but is associated with the inherent risks of invasive procedures such as bleeding, infection, and nerve damage. Laser therapy, extracorporeal shockwave therapy, and pulsed radiofrequency stimulation of the suprascapular nerve can be considered if standard nonsurgical treatments fail.

Surgical Treatment

If nonsurgical management fails to relieve symptoms, surgical treatment can improve range of motion and alleviate pain. For surgical intervention, regional anesthesia with an interscalene nerve catheter is particularly important postoperatively. This allows aggressive physical therapy with aggressive range-of-motion and stretching exercises.[4]

Manipulation under anesthesia (MUA) is often combined with local anesthetic and corticosteroid injections, and good results have been reported.[5] However, because MUA does not allow a controlled release of adherent tissues, this procedure is associated with the risk of humeral fractures and labral and rotator cuff tears.[4]

Various surgical techniques have been suggested for the treatment of adhesive capsulitis, particularly the extent of capsular release.[17,18] No benefit has been proved with combined anterior, inferior, and posterior capsular releases compared with anterior capsular release alone.[17,18] The contractures of the coracohumeral ligament and rotator interval must be treated. Most shoulder specialists advocate for selective capsular release, starting anteriorly and with the rotator interval. If the shoulder is still tight, posterior and inferior releases are performed. Extra-articular releases also can be performed, particularly in secondary adhesive capsulitis.

© 2016 American Academy of Orthopaedic Surgeons

The authors of a 2014 study compared arthroscopic capsular release and subacromial decompression with subacromial decompression combined with MUA and selective arthroscopic capsular release and reported that all surgical treatments substantially improved glenohumeral range of motion.[19] No substantial difference was found between the techniques.

Arthroscopic capsular releases between patients with and without diabetes at 2-year follow-up were prospectively compared.[3] Both groups had substantial improvements in modified Constant scores; however, the clinical results in diabetic patients were substantially inferior. Similarly, nonsurgical treatment and MUA yielded fewer good results in diabetic patients.

Currently, the literature lacks studies detailing long-term outcomes on the treatment of adhesive capsulitis. In a cohort of 10 patients with refractory adhesive capsulitis, arthroscopic treatment substantially improved range of motion at a minimum 6-year follow-up.[4]

Cartilage Lesions

Chondral lesions of the shoulder can result from trauma, instability, osteonecrosis, osteochondritis dissecans, osteoarthritis, or iatrogenically.[20,21] Focal cartilage lesions should be suspected in patients with previous shoulder trauma or surgery, dislocations, mechanical symptoms such as clicking or catching, pain, interrupted sleep, weakness, or loss of range of motion.[22]

Cartilage lesions are graded according to the International Cartilage Repair Society, or Outerbridge classification, with grade IV a full-thickness lesion.[21,22] Full-thickness chondral lesions are encountered in 5% to 29% of patients undergoing arthroscopy.[21,22] Differentiating between focal chondral lesions and generalized glenohumeral osteoarthritis is important because treatment varies between the two.

Nonsurgical Treatment

Nonsurgical treatment options include activity modification, physical therapy, NSAIDs, steroid joint injections, and viscosupplementation (such as hyaluronic acid). These options can mitigate symptoms; however, nonsurgical treatment cannot fill cartilage defects or alter the progression of osteoarthritis.[21] Also, if loose bodies are associated with the defect, surgical treatment is recommended to mitigate the effects of third-body wear.

Surgical Treatment
Palliative Treatment

For older patients with lower physical demands, palliative treatment consisting of débridement and chondroplasty can provide symptomatic pain relief. However, these procedures do not restore cartilage.[23-26]

Reparative Treatment

Microfracture has been performed in the shoulder with good success. The hyaline cartilage of the humerus is 1.2 to 1.3 mm thick at the center, thinning to 1.0 mm in the periphery.[22] Thin cartilage can limit the use of microfracture in the shoulder. Interest has recently increased in the outcomes of microfracture for treating focal glenohumeral cartilage defects.[21] Improvements in pain and mean American Shoulder and Elbow Surgeons scores have been noted,[27,28] along with substantial improvement in mean Constant scores[29] (Figure 1). The best results were seen in humeral lesions, and even bipolar lesions improved.[27]

Restorative Treatment

Restorative treatment attempts to re-create the damaged or absent cartilage. The two treatment options for restorative treatment are osteochondral grafting and autologous chondrocyte implantation. Both procedures require open surgery and can potentially result in donor site morbidity. Patient selection is important for success: the ideal patient is young, active, and has isolated cartilage defects.[30] As with microfracture, these procedures have been investigated in the knee with good results, but the shoulder is much less studied. Osteochondral grafts obtained from the knee can help treat both bone and cartilage defects. Good clinical results with osteochondral grafts in the shoulder have been demonstrated; however, a significant incidence of donor site morbidity was reported. [31] Autologous chondrocyte implantation eliminates the risk of donor site morbidity. One case report of this technique performed in the shoulder of a young baseball player was published.[32] Recently, use of a CT-matched medial tibial plateau surface has been suggested for osteoarticular allograft reconstruction of the glenoid.[33]

Nerve Compression Disorders/Suprascapular Nerve Entrapment

Suprascapular Nerve Entrapment

Patients with suprascapular nerve entrapment usually present with vague posterolateral shoulder pain and may report rapid onset of muscle fatigue with overhead activities. Atrophy of the infraspinatus and/or supraspinatus muscles with weakness in external rotation and/or abduction may be noted, depending on the location of the lesion. However, patients can also be asymptomatic. Differential diagnoses of peripheral nerve injury of the shoulder include central neurologic disorders such as cervical spinal

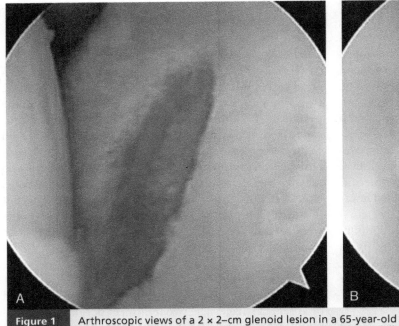
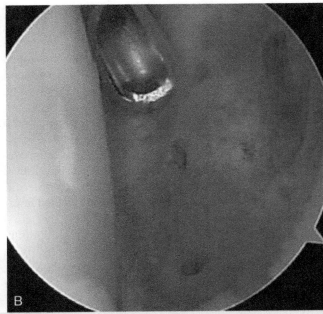

Figure 1 Arthroscopic views of a 2 × 2–cm glenoid lesion in a 65-year-old man before (**A**) and after (**B**) microfracture. (Reproduced with permission from van der Meijden OA, Gaskill TR, Millett PJ: Glenohumeral joint preservation: A review of management options for young, active patients with osteoarthritis. *Adv Orthop* 2012;2012:160923. doi: 10.1155/2012/160923. Epub Mar 27, 2012.)

disk protrusion, cervical spine instability, and spinal cord contusion, as well as transient brachial plexopathy.

Suprascapular nerve entrapment can occur at several locations. If the nerve is compressed proximally at the transverse scapular ligament, both the supraspinatus and infraspinatus are involved. If the nerve is compressed distally by the spinoglenoid ligament or a structural lesion at the spinoglenoid notch such as a paralabral cyst, only the infraspinatus is involved[34] (Figure 2).

Most diagnoses can be made using physical examination alone. For appropriate diagnosis and localization of the lesion, electromyography and nerve conduction velocity can be helpful. However, sensitivity and specificity of these tests are not 100% and their results must be correlated with clinical findings.[34,35] Three-dimensional soft-tissue imaging using MRI can help measure the degree of atrophy of the infraspinatus and/or supraspinatus muscles, and more importantly, help determine whether a compressive lesion such as a ganglion cyst exists. MRI also provides information about other concomitant shoulder pathologies, such as superior labrum anterior to posterior tears, which are often associated with spinoglenoid notch cysts.[34]

Suprascapular nerve entrapment can also have idiopathic causes. Four cases of complete fatty infiltration of intact supraspinatus and infraspinatus muscles caused by suprascapular neuropathy without any traction or compression mechanisms have been reported.[36] Immediate improvement in pain and subjective shoulder values were reported following arthroscopic suprascapular nerve decompression.

The shape and size of the suprascapular notch are among the most important risk factors for suprascapular nerve entrapment. A five-part classification of entrapment according to morphologic features and anatomic variations has been suggested.[37] A narrow, deep suprascapular notch (type I) with sharp bony margins could be predispose a patient to suprascapular nerve injury by repeated microtrauma resulting from "kinking" the nerve.

Nonsurgical Treatment

Acute injuries to the suprascapular nerve can be treated with rest and pain control, followed by physical therapy with progressive range-of-motion and strengthening exercises as tolerated. Overhead athletes should be followed for 6 to 12 months with recommended activity restriction and periscapular therapy. Periodic electromyographic/nerve conduction velocity studies should be performed to monitor electrophysiologic nerve recovery.[34]

Surgical Treatment

Nerve decompression is usually performed arthroscopically. The surgical technique was described in detail in 2006.[34] After standard diagnostic arthroscopy, the arthroscope is briefly placed in an anterolateral portal, and accessory anterior and posterior portals are established.

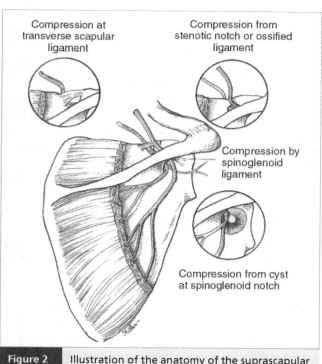

Figure 2 Illustration of the anatomy of the suprascapular nerve as it passes through the suprascapular and spinoglenoid notches. Common compression mechanisms are depicted at each site. (Reproduced with permission from Millett PJ, Barton RS, Pacheco IH, Gobezie R: Suprascapular nerve entrapment: Technique for arthroscopic release. *Tech Shoulder Elbow Surg* 2006;7[2]:88-94.)

The coracoid process is visualized with dissection carried medially along the posterior aspect of the coracoid process. The supraspinatus muscle belly is posteriorly retracted to visualize the coracohumeral and coracoclavicular ligaments. The suprascapular notch is identified at the medial base of the coracoid. The suprascapular artery is cauterized with the radiofrequency ablation device, and the ligament is released using handheld arthroscopic tissue punches. The nerve is probed to ensure full decompression (Figure 3). Good to excellent outcomes can be expected following arthroscopic decompression, with decreased pain and improved function for releases at both the spinoglenoid notch and the suprascapular notch.[34,38]

Snapping Scapula

Snapping scapula syndrome is uncommon and likely underdiagnosed. It can produce substantial pain and disability; however, the precise origin remains unknown. Potential factors causing snapping scapula syndrome include bony changes at the superomedial scapular angle, dysbalance of the periscapular muscles, and scapulothoracic bursitis.[39,40] Patients often present with decreased athletic performance and increased pain with overhead activities. Crepitus also can be reported.[41] Plain radiographs and CT scans provide detailed information about osseous abnormalities; MRI characterizes bursal and other soft-tissue pathologies.[41]

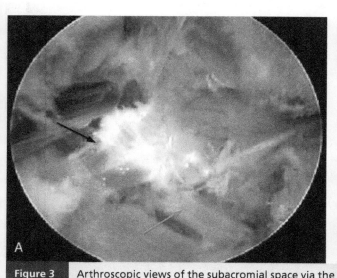
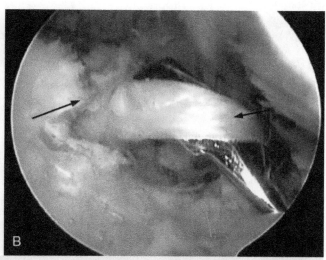

Figure 3 Arthroscopic views of the subacromial space via the posterolateral portal. **A,** Suprascapular nerve (red arrow) is under the transverse scapular ligament (arrow). **B,** Elevator is in the anterolateral portal, exposing the nerve (short arrow) after releasing the transverse scapular ligament (long arrow) at the notch (red arrow). (Reproduced with permission from Millett PJ, Barton RS, Pacheco IH, Gobezie R: Suprascapular nerve entrapment: Technique for arthroscopic release. *Tech Shoulder Elbow Surg* 2006;7[2]:88-94.)

1: Upper extremity

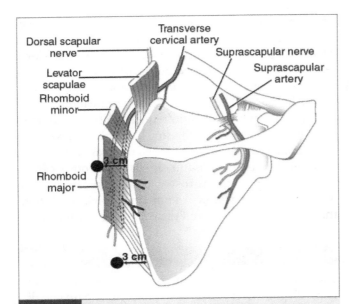

Figure 4 Illustration of the right posterior shoulder demonstrates the gross location of neurovascular structures important in scapulothoracic articulation. Black dots indicate typical portal locations, noting the distance from the medial scapular border. (Reproduced with permission from Millett PJ, Gaskill TR, Horan MP, van der Meijden OA: Technique and outcomes of arthroscopic scapulothoracic bursectomy and partial scapulectomy. *Arthroscopy* 2012;28[12]:1776-1783.)

Nonsurgical Treatment

Nonsurgical management remains the first treatment option;[41,42] surgery is recommended after 6 months of nonsurgical treatment with no improvement. Strengthening weak periscapular muscle groups combined with simultaneous stretching of contracted muscles and training of antagonistic muscle groups can yield good clinical results.[39,41] In addition, physical therapy, injections with local anesthetics and/or steroids, and NSAIDs can be useful. Nonsurgical treatment will likely fail if scapulothoracic masses such as osteochondromas of the rib or scapula are present.[41]

Surgical Treatment

Scapulothoracic bursectomy with or without partial scapulectomy is currently the most effective primary method of treatment in patients whose nonsurgical therapy is unsuccessful. This procedure can be performed open,[42] arthroscopically,[39,40,43-46] or using a combined approach.[47] Detailed knowledge of neurovascular anatomy of the periscapular region is crucial. The main branches of the spinal accessory nerve are at risk if portals are placed above the scapular spine. The dorsal scapular nerve and accompanying dorsal scapular artery run 1 to 2 cm medial to the medial border of the scapula, deep to the major and minor rhomboid muscles. Therefore, portals or incisions should be placed 2 to 3 cm from the medial scapular border[41,45] (Figure 4). The amount of resection of the superomedial angle is still debated, ranging from 1 to 7 cm[48,49] (Figure 5).

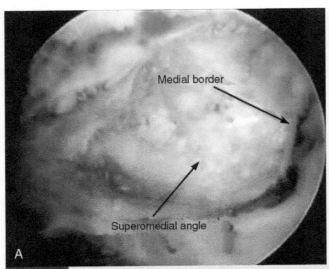

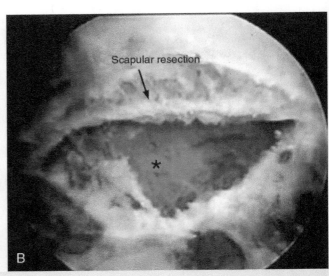

Figure 5 Arthroscopic views of a left scapula viewed from the inferomedial portal demonstrate the superomedial scapular border. **A,** Before resection. **B,** Completed resection of the superomedial border. Note the absence of the hooked superomedial border of the scapula; the supraspinatus musculature (*) also can be visualized. (Reproduced with permission from Millett PJ, Gaskill TR, Horan MP, van der Meijden OA: Technique and outcomes of arthroscopic scapulothoracic bursectomy and partial scapulectomy. *Arthroscopy* 2012;28[12]:1776-1783.)

Table 1

Results of Surgical Treatment of Snapping Scapula Syndrome

Authors and Year	Treatment	No. of Patients	Results
Nicholson and Duckworth[42] 2002	Open	17 (all with bursectomy, 4 also with bony scapular resection)	ASES score, VAS, and simple shoulder test all substantially improved after 2.5 years
Lien et al[47] 2008	Combined	12	ASES score, VAS, and simple shoulder test all substantially improved after 3.1 years
Harper et al[39] 1999	Arthroscopy	7	Successful outcome in 6 patients (86%)
Pavlik et al[46] 2003	Arthroscopy	10	Mean VAS postoperatively 2.6 of 10; UCLA score: 4 excellent, 5 good, 1 fair
Pearse et al[44] 2006	Arthroscopy	13	Nine improved with mean Constant score of 87 of 100; four unchanged or worse, with mean Constant score of 55 of 100
Millett et al[45] 2012	Arthroscopy	23 (2 with bursectomy only, 21 with bursectomy + scapuloplasty)	ASES, SANE and QuickDASH scores all substantially improved at mean 2.5 years follow-up
Merolla et al[43] 2014	Arthroscopy	10	Substantial improvement for WORC and Constant score after 2 years ($P < 0.01$)

ASES = American Shoulder and Elbow Surgeons score, quickDASH = quick Disabilities of the Arm, Shoulder and Hand, SANE = single assessment numeric evaluation, UCLA = University of California – Los Angeles score, VAS = visual analog scale, WORC = Western Ontario Rotator Cuff index.

A recent review identified 81 articles dealing with snapping scapula syndrome, including 9 level IV outcomes studies.[50] The results of the relevant studies after surgical therapy are summarized in Table 1. The largest series reported on 23 shoulders and found substantial pain and functional improvement following arthroscopic bursectomy and scapuloplasty.[45]

Although most patients improve after surgical treatment, some patients continue to experience shoulder disability. Further studies are needed to investigate the modifiable factors associated with poor outcomes after surgical and nonsurgical management for snapping scapula syndrome.

Summary

Glenohumeral stiffness, focal chondral lesions, neural compression, and pathologies of the scapulothoracic joint are relatively uncommon. However, these disorders can be debilitating for the patient and require specific treatment. A sound awareness and working knowledge of these pathologies is necessary to arrive at the appropriate diagnosis. If nonsurgical treatment fails, open and arthroscopic surgical techniques can be used to treat these disorders. A thorough understanding of the local anatomy including neurovascular structures is crucial for success with surgical treatment. Good to excellent results can be achieved with appropriate patient selection and surgical technique.

Key Study Points

- It is important to include adhesive capsulitis, focal chondral defects, suprascapular nerve compression, and snapping scapula syndrome in the differential diagnosis of shoulder pathologies.
- Nonsurgical treatment has a success rate of 70% to 90% in patients with adhesive capsulitis.
- Microfracture yields good clinical results for glenohumeral focal chondral lesions.
- Arthroscopic suprascapular nerve decompression yields good results when nonsurgical treatment fails.
- Arthroscopic scapulothoracic bursectomy with partial scapulectomy is currently the most effective treatment in patients whose nonsurgical therapy for snapping scapula syndrome is unsuccessful.

Annotated References

1. Bunker TD, Reilly J, Baird KS, Hamblen DL: Expression of growth factors, cytokines and matrix metalloproteinases in frozen shoulder. *J Bone Joint Surg Br* 2000;82(5):768-773.

2. Mullett H, Byrne D, Colville J: Adhesive capsulitis: Human fibroblast response to shoulder joint aspirate from patients with stage II disease. *J Shoulder Elbow Surg* 2007;16(3):290-294.

3. Mehta SS, Singh HP, Pandey R: Comparative outcome of arthroscopic release for frozen shoulder in patients with and without diabetes. *Bone Joint J* 2014;96-B(10):1355-1358.

   Patients with diabetes had substantially worse results than nondiabetic patients after arthroscopic release for frozen shoulder. Level of evidence: III.

4. Fernandes MR: Arthroscopic treatment of refractory adhesive capsulitis of the shoulder. *Rev Col Bras Cir* 2014;41(1):30-35.

   Arthroscopic treatment is effective in refractory adhesive capsulitis of the shoulder resistant to nonsurgical treatment. Level of evidence: IV.

5. Leonidou A, Woods DA: A preliminary study of manipulation under anaesthesia for secondary frozen shoulder following breast cancer treatment. *Ann R Coll Surg Engl* 2014;96(2):111-115.

   MUA, corticosteroid injection and subsequent physiotherapy showed good results in a series of patients with adhesive capsulitis secondary to breast cancer treatment. Level of evidence: III.

6. Lim TK, Koh KH, Shon MS, Lee SW, Park YE, Yoo JC: Intra-articular injection of hyaluronate versus corticosteroid in adhesive capsulitis. *Orthopedics* 2014;37(10):e860-e865.

   Treatment for idiopathic adhesive capsulitis using intra-articular injection of hyaluronate or corticosteroid for idiopathic adhesive capsulitis both showed substantial improvement in clinical scores and range of motion without substantial differences between groups. Level of evidence: I.

7. Levine WN, Kashyap CP, Bak SF, Ahmad CS, Blaine TA, Bigliani LU: Nonoperative management of idiopathic adhesive capsulitis. *J Shoulder Elbow Surg* 2007;16(5):569-573.

8. Russell S, Jariwala A, Conlon R, Selfe J, Richards J, Walton M: A blinded, randomized, controlled trial assessing conservative management strategies for frozen shoulder. *J Shoulder Elbow Surg* 2014;23(4):500-507.

   Hospital-based exercise classes result in rapid recovery from a frozen shoulder with a minimum number of hospital visits and were more effective than individual physical therapy or a home exercise program. Level of evidence: I.

9. Page MJ, Green S, Kramer S, et al: Manual therapy and exercise for adhesive capsulitis (frozen shoulder). *Cochrane Database Syst Rev* 2014;8:CD011275.

   Oral NSAIDs, glucocorticoid injections, and arthrographic joint distension with glucocorticoid and saline are effective treatment options for adhesive capsulitis. The role of manual therapy, exercise, and electrotherapy as adjuncts is still debated. Level of evidence: I.

10. Tasto JP, Elias DW: Adhesive capsulitis. *Sports Med Arthrosc* 2007;15(4):216-221.

11. Page MJ, Green S, Kramer S, Johnston RV, McBain B, Buchbinder R: Electrotherapy modalities for adhesive capsulitis (frozen shoulder). *Cochrane Database Syst Rev* 2014;10:CD011324.

    Only low to moderate evidence exists that shows low-level laser therapy and pulsed electromagnetic field therapy to be effective adjuncts in the treatment of adhesive capsulitis. Level of evidence: I.

12. Vahdatpour B, Taheri P, Zade AZ, Moradian S: Efficacy of extracorporeal shockwave therapy in frozen shoulder. *Int J Prev Med* 2014;5(7):875-881.

    Extracorporeal shockwave therapy showed quicker return to daily activities and quality-of-life improvement compared with sham shockwave in the treatment of frozen shoulders. Level of evidence: I.

13. Wu YT, Ho CW, Chen YL, Li TY, Lee KC, Chen LC: Ultrasound-guided pulsed radiofrequency stimulation of the suprascapular nerve for adhesive capsulitis: A prospective, randomized, controlled trial. *Anesth Analg* 2014;119(3):686-692.

    Ultrasonographically guided pulsed radiofrequency stimulation of the suprascapular nerve combined with physical

© 2016 American Academy of Orthopaedic Surgeons

therapy provided better and faster relief from pain, reduced disability, and improved passive range of motion compared with physical therapy alone in patients with adhesive capsulitis. Level of evidence: I.

14. Buchbinder R, Green S, Youd JM, Johnston RV, Cumpston M: Arthrographic distension for adhesive capsulitis (frozen shoulder). *Cochrane Database Syst Rev* 2008;1:CD007005.

15. Waters D, Collins J: Distension arthrogram improves pain and range of movement in adhesive capsulitis of the shoulder. *Int J Surg* 2013;11(8):672.

    The distension arthrogram can provide good improvement in range of motion and pain for patients with adhesive capsulitis at 3 months, providing both therapeutic and diagnostic intervention. Level of evidence: IV.

16. Bae JH, Park YS, Chang HJ, et al: Randomized controlled trial for efficacy of capsular distension for adhesive capsulitis: Fluoroscopy-guided anterior versus ultrasonography-guided posterolateral approach. *Ann Rehabil Med* 2014;38(3):360-368.

    Ultrasonographically guided capsular distension using a posterolateral approach has similar effects on patients with adhesive capsulitis compared with a fluoroscopically guided anterior approach. Level of evidence: I.

17. Chen J, Chen S, Li Y, Hua Y, Li H: Is the extended release of the inferior glenohumeral ligament necessary for frozen shoulder? *Arthroscopy* 2010;26(4):529-535.

    An additional posterior capsular release did not improve patient function or range of motion over an anterior capsular release alone in patients with frozen shoulder. Level of evidence: I.

18. Snow M, Boutros I, Funk L: Posterior arthroscopic capsular release in frozen shoulder. *Arthroscopy* 2009;25(1):19-23.

    Arthroscopic capsular release for primary and secondary frozen shoulder results in an overall rapid substantial clinical improvement. An additional posterior release did not substantially affect the overall outcome. Level of evidence: III.

19. Walther M, Blanke F, Von Wehren L, Majewski M: Frozen shoulder—comparison of different surgical treatment options. *Acta Orthop Belg* 2014;80(2):172-177.

    Arthroscopic capsular release, alone or with subacromial decompression, showed better results postoperatively compared with subacromial decompression combined with MUA. Level of evidence: III.

20. McCarty LP III, Cole BJ: Nonarthroplasty treatment of glenohumeral cartilage lesions. *Arthroscopy* 2005;21(9):1131-1142.

21. van der Meijden OA, Gaskill TR, Millett PJ: Glenohumeral joint preservation: A review of management options for young, active patients with osteoarthritis. *Adv Orthop* 2012;2012:160923.

    Arthroplasty may not be a practical treatment option in young, active patients with osteoarthritis of the shoulder. Arthroscopic joint débridement with a capsular release, humeral osteoplasty, and transcapsular axillary nerve decompression seems promising when humeral osteophytes are present.

22. Elser F, Braun S, Dewing CB, Millett PJ: Glenohumeral joint preservation: Current options for managing articular cartilage lesions in young, active patients. *Arthroscopy* 2010;26(5):685-696.

    Substantial controversy persists regarding the repair of glenohumeral cartilage lesions in young, active patients. Applicable techniques include microfracture, osteoarticular transplantation, autologous chondrocyte implantation, bulk allograft reconstruction, and biologic resurfacing.

23. de Beer JF, Bhatia DN, van Rooyen KS, Du Toit DF: Arthroscopic debridement and biological resurfacing of the glenoid in glenohumeral arthritis. *Knee Surg Sports Traumatol Arthrosc* 2010;18(12):1767-1773.

    Arthroscopic débridement and biologic resurfacing of the glenoid is a minimally invasive therapeutic option for glenohumeral osteoarthritis that can provide pain relief and improved function and patient satisfaction in the intermediate term. Level of evidence: IV.

24. Kerr BJ, McCarty EC: Outcome of arthroscopic débridement is worse for patients with glenohumeral arthritis of both sides of the joint. *Clin Orthop Relat Res* 2008;466(3):634-638.

25. Richards DP, Burkhart SS: Arthroscopic debridement and capsular release for glenohumeral osteoarthritis. *Arthroscopy* 2007;23(9):1019-1022.

26. Van Thiel GS, Sheehan S, Frank RM, et al: Retrospective analysis of arthroscopic management of glenohumeral degenerative disease. *Arthroscopy* 2010;26(11):1451-1455.

    Arthroscopic débridement for glenohumeral osteoarthritis can potentially help avoid arthroplasty and increase function with decreased pain. Grade 4 bipolar disease, joint space less than 2 mm, and large osteophytes are substantial risk factors for failure. Level of evidence: IV.

27. Millett PJ, Huffard BH, Horan MP, Hawkins RJ, Steadman JR: Outcomes of full-thickness articular cartilage injuries of the shoulder treated with microfracture. *Arthroscopy* 2009;25(8):856-863.

    Microfracture for full-thickness cartilage lesions of the shoulder showed the greatest improvement for smaller lesions of the humerus; the worst results were in patients with bipolar lesions, with a total failure rate of 19%. Level of evidence: IV.

28. Frank RM, Van Thiel GS, Slabaugh MA, Romeo AA, Cole BJ, Verma NN: Clinical outcomes after microfracture of the glenohumeral joint. *Am J Sports Med* 2010;38(4):772-781.

    Microfracture of the glenohumeral joint resulted in substantial improvements in pain relief and shoulder function in patients with isolated, full-thickness chondral injuries at a mean follow-up of 28 months. Level of evidence: IV.

29. Snow M, Funk L: Microfracture of chondral lesions of the glenohumeral joint. *Int J Shoulder Surg* 2008;2(4):72-76.

30. Cole BJ, Yanke A, Provencher MT: Nonarthroplasty alternatives for the treatment of glenohumeral arthritis. *J Shoulder Elbow Surg* 2007;16(Suppl 5):S231-S240.

31. Scheibel M, Bartl C, Magosch P, Lichtenberg S, Habermeyer P: Osteochondral autologous transplantation for the treatment of full-thickness articular cartilage defects of the shoulder. *J Bone Joint Surg Br* 2004;86(7):991-997.

32. Romeo AA, Cole BJ, Mazzocca AD, Fox JA, Freeman KB, Joy E: Autologous chondrocyte repair of an articular defect in the humeral head. *Arthroscopy* 2002;18(8):925-929.

33. Rios D, Jansson KS, Martetschläger F, Boykin RE, Millett PJ, Wijdicks CA: Normal curvature of glenoid surface can be restored when performing an inlay osteochondral allograft: An anatomic computed tomographic comparison. *Knee Surg Sports Traumatol Arthrosc* 2014;22(2):442-447.

The radius of curvature of the glenoid and the medial tibial plateau surface have a statistically similar relationship as measured using three-dimensional CT. This can allow the medial tibial plateau to be used as a donor for osteoarticular allograft reconstruction of the glenoid.

34. Millett PJ, Barton RS, Pacheco ICH, Gobezie R: Suprascapular nerve entrapment: Technique for arthroscopic release. *Tech Shoulder Elbow Surg* 2006;7(2).

35. Post M: Diagnosis and treatment of suprascapular nerve entrapment. *Clin Orthop Relat Res* 1999;368:92-100.

36. LeClere LE, Shi LL, Lin A, Yannopoulos P, Higgins LD, Warner JJ: Complete Fatty infiltration of intact rotator cuffs caused by suprascapular neuropathy. *Arthroscopy* 2014;30(5):639-644.

Suprascapular neuropathy with complete neurogenic fatty infiltration can also occur in the absence of traction or compression mechanisms. Arthroscopic suprascapular nerve decompression resulted in immediate improvement in pain and subjective shoulder values in all four patients. Level of evidence: IV.

37. Polguj M, Sibiński M, Grzegorzewski A, Grzelak P, Majos A, Topol M: Variation in morphology of suprascapular notch as a factor of suprascapular nerve entrapment. *Int Orthop* 2013;37(11):2185-2192.

Knowledge of the anatomic variations of the suprascapular notch is important for both endoscopic and open procedures of the suprascapular region.

38. Oizumi N, Suenaga N, Minami A: Snapping scapula caused by abnormal angulation of the superior angle of the scapula. *J Shoulder Elbow Surg* 2004;13(1):115-118.

39. Harper GD, McIlroy S, Bayley JI, Calvert PT: Arthroscopic partial resection of the scapula for snapping scapula: A new technique. *J Shoulder Elbow Surg* 1999;8(1):53-57.

40. Millett PJ, Pacheco IH, Gobezie R, Warner JJ: Management of recalcitrant scapulothoracic bursitis: Endoscopic scapulothoracic bursectomy and scapuloplasty. *Tech Shoulder Elbow Surg* 2006;7:200-205.

41. Gaskill T, Millett PJ: Snapping scapula syndrome: Diagnosis and management. *J Am Acad Orthop Surg* 2013;21(4):214-224.

Nonsurgical therapy is the initial treatment of choice for snapping scapula syndrome. If nonsurgical treatment fails, open and endoscopic techniques have been used with satisfactory results. Familiarity with the neuroanatomic structures surrounding the scapula is critical to avoid iatrogenic complications.

42. Nicholson GP, Duckworth MA: Scapulothoracic bursectomy for snapping scapula syndrome. *J Shoulder Elbow Surg* 2002;11(1):80-85.

43. Merolla G, Cerciello S, Paladini P, Porcellini G: Scapulothoracic arthroscopy for symptomatic snapping scapula: A prospective cohort study with two-year mean follow-up. *Musculoskelet Surg* 2014 March 2013. Epub ahead of print.

Arthroscopic decompression showed substantial clinical improvements in 10 patients with snapping scapula syndrome at 2-year follow-up. Level of evidence: IV.

44. Pearse EO, Bruguera J, Massoud SN, Sforza G, Copeland SA, Levy O: Arthroscopic management of the painful snapping scapula. *Arthroscopy* 2006;22(7):755-761.

45. Millett PJ, Gaskill TR, Horan MP, van der Meijden OA: Technique and outcomes of arthroscopic scapulothoracic bursectomy and partial scapulectomy. *Arthroscopy* 2012;28(12):1776-1783.

Although substantial pain and functional improvement can be expected following arthroscopic bursectomy and scapuloplasty in patients with snapping scapula syndrome, the mean postoperative American Shoulder and Elbow Surgeons and Single Assessment Numeric Evaluation scores remain lower than expected. Level of evidence: IV.

46. Pavlik A, Ang K, Coghlan J, Bell S: Arthroscopic treatment of painful snapping of the scapula by using a new superior portal. *Arthroscopy* 2003;19(6):608-612.

47. Lien SB, Shen PH, Lee CH, Lin LC: The effect of endoscopic bursectomy with mini-open partial scapulectomy on snapping scapula syndrome. *J Surg Res* 2008;150(2):236-242.

48. Lehtinen JT, Tetreault P, Warner JJ: Arthroscopic management of painful and stiff scapulothoracic articulation. *Arthroscopy* 2003;19(4):E28.

49. Oizumi N, Suenaga N, Funakoshi T, Yamaguchi H, Minami A: Recovery of sensory disturbance after arthroscopic

decompression of the suprascapular nerve. *J Shoulder Elbow Surg* 2012;21(6):759-764.

The sensory disturbance at the posterolateral aspect of the shoulder can be a diagnostic criterion for suprascapular nerve palsy. Arthroscopic release of the suprascapular nerve is useful to treat nerve entrapment at the suprascapular notch. Level of evidence: IV.

50. Warth RJ, Spiegl UJ, Millett PJ: Scapulothoracic bursitis and snapping scapula syndrome: A critical review of current evidence. *Am J Sports Med* 2015;43(1):236-245.

Snapping scapula syndrome is a likely underdiagnosed condition and can produce substantial shoulder dysfunction. Scapulothoracic bursectomy with or without partial scapulectomy is currently the most effective primary method of treatment in patients whose nonsurgical therapy is unsuccessful.

Chapter 6

Elbow Arthroscopy and the Thrower's Elbow

Ekaterina Y. Urch, MD   Lucas S. McDonald, MD, MPH&TM   Joshua S. Dines, MD   David W. Altchek, MD

Abstract

The throwing athlete is at increased risk for various elbow injuries due to the substantial repetitive forces exerted on the joint during the throwing motion. The management of these injuries requires a resolute understanding of the underlying biomechanics involved in this complex motion. Surgical intervention is often required to attain acceptable clinical outcomes and to allow the athlete to return to his or her sport. Along with the various open surgical techniques available, elbow arthroscopy has quickly come to the forefront of surgical treatment in these athletes.

Keywords: elbow arthroscopy; thrower's elbow; valgus extension overload; lateral epicondylitis; posteromedial impingement; ulnar collateral ligament

Introduction

Elbow arthroscopy is a modern surgical technique popularized in 1985; the first study on the topic described visualization of the elbow joint through anterolateral, anteromedial, and posterolateral portals with the patient supine.[1] Historically, elbow arthroscopy was associated with inconsistent outcomes and an unacceptably high complication rate. Since the initial outcome studies, improved instrumentation, advanced surgical technique, and better understanding of arthroscopic elbow anatomy have made arthroscopy a safe, effective treatment for elbow pathology.

Indications and Contraindications

The advantages of elbow arthroscopy include decreased surgical morbidity and improved joint visualization, making the technique an excellent option for numerous elbow conditions. However, the small size and compartmentalization of the joint, along with the proximity of portals to neurovascular structures, makes the procedure technically challenging. The treating surgeon must not only be familiar with the anatomy and surgical technique, but also must be proficient in identifying patients most likely to benefit from the procedure. Classically, the indications for elbow arthroscopy include the removal of loose bodies, olecranon osteophyte excision, synovectomy, capsular release, and the evaluation and treatment of osteochondritis dissecans (OCD) lesions.[2] More recently, indications have expanded to include treatment of septic arthritis, lateral epicondylitis, intra-articular fracture management, and plica excision.[3,4]

Arthroscopy is contraindicated in patients with distorted soft tissue or osseous anatomy, precluding safe portal placement. Such situations include ankylosed joints, history of prior elbow trauma or surgical intervention, soft-tissue pedicle flaps, skin grafts, burns, and the presence of heterotopic ossification.[4,5] Additionally, soft-tissue infection at the portal sites is an absolute contraindication. Because of the increased risk of ulnar nerve injury, elbow arthroscopy is relatively contraindicated in patients with prior ulnar nerve transposition. If arthroscopy is performed in these patients, it is critical to visualize the ulnar nerve before establishing the medial portal.[5]

Dr. Dines or an immediate family member has received royalties from Biomet; is a member of a speakers' bureau or has made paid presentations on behalf of Arthrex; and serves as a paid consultant to Arthrex and CONMED Linvatec. None of the following authors or any immediate family member has received anything of value from or has stock or stock options held in a commercial company or institution related directly or indirectly to the subject of this chapter: Dr. Altchek, Dr. McDonald, and Dr. Urch.

I: Upper extremity

Patient Positioning

Patient positioning is based primarily on surgeon preference. Advantages and disadvantages of the various methods have been described. Classically, elbow arthroscopy was performed supine with the surgical arm draped across the chest over a bolster.[5]

The modern concept of arm suspension from the supine position, keeping the arm in 90° of shoulder abduction and 90° of elbow flexion, was introduced in 1985.[1] The advantages of the supine position include simplified airway access, familiar orientation, and ease of conversion to an open procedure. Disadvantages include elbow instability during the procedure and difficult access to the posterior compartment.[5]

To address these concerns, the modified supine position was developed, suspending the arm over the chest with the elbow in 90° of flexion while the forearm, wrist, and hand are secured in a commercially available mechanical holder (Figure 1). This position facilitates easy arm adjustment, providing access to both the anterior and posterior compartments of the elbow. Furthermore, this arm position decreases the risk of injury to the anterior neurovascular structures by allowing them to drop away from the anterior capsule.[2]

Other options include the lateral decubitus and the prone positions. In the lateral decubitus position, the patient is positioned laterally on a beanbag with the surgical arm flexed to 90° and suspended over a well-padded post. Joint distraction is provided by a weight attached to the hand. The advantages of the lateral position include improved arm stability, posterior elbow access, and relatively easy airway management. The disadvantages include orientation challenges from reversed anatomic landmarks and difficult access to the anterior compartment. In the prone position, the arm is suspended off the table in an arm holder with the arm in 90° of shoulder abduction and the elbow in 90° of flexion in a similar position to the lateral decubitus position. The advantages of the prone position include natural traction, easy access to the posterior compartment, and a theoretically increased space between vascular structures and the anterior capsule. The disadvantages include the necessity for general anesthesia, difficult airway access, reversed anatomy, and poor access to the anterior compartment.

Irrespective of the position used, it is crucial to assess the elbow for access to each compartment and to portal sites before starting the procedure. Pressure on the antecubital fossa should be avoided to decrease the risk of injury to anterior neurovascular structures. A tourniquet is placed as proximal on the arm as possible and can be insufflated as needed.

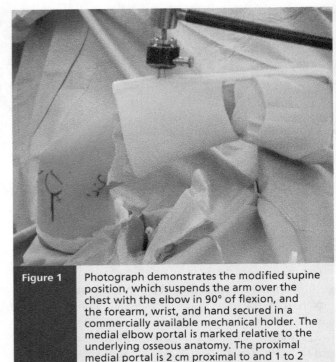

Figure 1 Photograph demonstrates the modified supine position, which suspends the arm over the chest with the elbow in 90° of flexion, and the forearm, wrist, and hand secured in a commercially available mechanical holder. The medial elbow portal is marked relative to the underlying osseous anatomy. The proximal medial portal is 2 cm proximal to and 1 to 2 cm anterior to the medial epicondyle. The transtriceps portal is visible posteriorly.

Portal Placement

Prior to portal creation, the elbow joint is insufflated with 30 mL of saline through the lateral soft spot located in the center of a triangle created by the radial head, the lateral epicondyle, and the tip of the olecranon. This distends the capsule, moving the neurovascular structures further away from the joint and facilitating easier access to the space. Anatomic landmarks are marked, including the medial and lateral epicondyles, ulnar nerve, radial head, and olecranon.

Although many different methods and locations are used for portal placement, the authors of this chapter prefer to first create the proximal lateral portal, located 1 to 2 cm proximal to the lateral epicondyle and 1 cm anterior to the humerus (Figure 2). The radial and posterior antebrachial cutaneous nerves are at greatest risk during creation of this portal; therefore, only the skin is incised sharply, and a trocar is used to enter the ulnohumeral joint.[5] This portal is primarily used as a viewing portal. To access the anterior compartment, a proximal medial portal can be established 2 cm proximal and 1 to 2 cm anterior to the medial epicondyle (Figure 1); it is important to stay anterior to the medial intermuscular septum, minimizing the risk of ulnar nerve injury. An additional working anteromedial portal can be established 2 cm anterior and 2 cm distal to the medial humeral epicondyle.

This portal is near the medial antebrachial cutaneous nerve and should be localized first under direct visualization with a spinal needle.

Diagnostic arthroscopy of the anterior elbow is performed while viewing through the proximal lateral portal. Trochlear and coronoid fossa articular cartilage lesions, coronoid process osseous spurs, synovitis, and loose bodies can be identified. The anterior radiocapitellar joint is evaluated for osteochondral lesions and any concomitant pathology of the radial head. If débridement is performed in this area, extreme caution must be used because of the proximity of the radial nerve to the anterolateral joint capsule. If ulnar collateral ligament (UCL) insufficiency is suspected, an arthroscopic valgus stress test is performed. A standard 3.4-mm hook probe is inserted through the proximal medial portal to help measure gapping, and based on a 1996 cadaver study, a gap of only 1 or 2 mm suggests a complete anterior bundle UCL injury. Large increases in gapping suggest injury to the posterior bundle as well[6] (Figure 3).

For visualization of the posterior compartment, the posterolateral portal is created 1 cm posterior to the lateral epicondyle at the level of the olecranon tip (Figure 2). To access the posterior compartment, a midlateral portal can be created through the lateral soft spot or a transtriceps portal (the portal preferred by the authors of this chapter) can be created in the midline of the triceps just proximal to the tip of the olecranon (Figure 2). The posterior compartment is evaluated for olecranon osteophytes, posterior recess loose bodies, capitellar OCD, and chondral injuries.

Complications

Elbow arthroscopy has historically been associated with complication rates as high as 20%.[7-9]

The most common complication is neurovascular injury resulting from surgeon inexperience, poor technique, and lack of knowledge of elbow anatomy. Compression

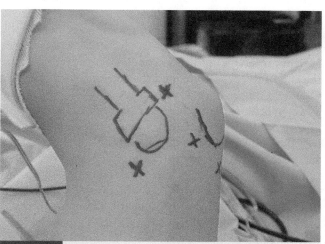

Figure 2 Photograph demonstrates the lateral elbow portals marked relative to the underlying osseous anatomy. The proximal lateral portal is 1 to 2 cm proximal to the lateral epicondyle and 1 cm anterior to the humerus. The posterolateral portal is 1 cm posterior to the lateral epicondyle at the level of the olecranon tip. The transtriceps portal is marked posteriorly in the midline of the triceps tendon just proximal to the tip of the olecranon.

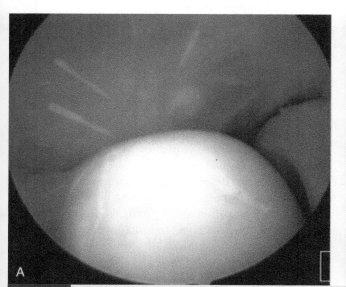

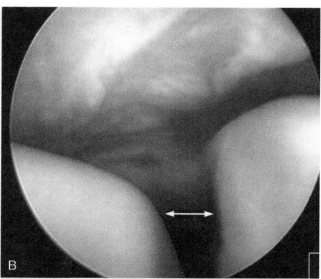

Figure 3 **A,** Arthroscopic view depicts the valgus stress test of an elbow without an ulnar collateral ligament (UCL) injury, demonstrating no medial-side ulnohumeral joint opening. **B,** Arthroscopic view depicts the valgus stress test on an elbow with a UCL injury, demonstrating 3 mm of ulnohumeral joint opening (arrow).

1: Upper Extremity

from cannulas, fluid extravasation into surrounding soft tissues, local anesthesia, and laceration with the scalpel or cannula are the most commonly cited insults.[4] Most of these injuries are transient, resolving without residual deficit. Improved surgeon training, better understanding of elbow anatomy, and surgical technique standardization have all increased the safety of elbow arthroscopy. A recent study demonstrated that most complications, including wound healing and infection, are now those ubiquitous to arthroscopy of other joints.[10] Specifically, an increased risk of postoperative infection was noted in patients receiving an intra-articular steroid injection at the end of the procedure, and the authors of this chapter do not recommend this treatment.

Currently, nerve injuries are exceedingly rare, with reported transient nerve injury rates ranging from 1.7% to 2.0%.[10,11] Despite the advent of more complex arthroscopic procedures including complete synovectomy, radial head resection, osteocapsular arthroplasty, and medial epicondylectomy, no substantial association has been found between complication rate and surgical complexity.[10] Other known complications include articular cartilage injury, synovial fistula formation, instrument breakage, and tissue injury secondary to use of a tourniquet.

Specific Procedures

Loose Bodies

Loose bodies are osteochondral or chondral fragments caused by either traumatic insult to the elbow or underlying pathology such as OCD. Loose body removal from the elbow joint is the most commonly performed arthroscopic therapeutic intervention.[2] The surgeon should perform a thorough diagnostic arthroscopy, assessing all compartments for loose bodies, chondral injury, and any other pathology. Loose bodies are most commonly located in the posterior recess. Prior to completion of the procedure, an intraoperative arthroscopic valgus stress test to assess UCL insufficiency is recommended.

OCD Lesions

OCD is most often seen in young athletes ranging between 11 and 21 years of age.[5] It classically affects the capitellum and is caused by repetitive microtrauma to the vulnerable epiphysis, which has a tenuous blood supply.[2] Repetitive loading of the lateral compartment of the elbow results in subchondral bone degeneration causing cartilage fragmentation. Management of OCD depends on the integrity and stability of the overlying cartilage, as well as the size and location of the lesion. Indications for arthroscopic débridement include failure of nonsurgical

treatment, the presence of loose bodies, and mechanical symptoms. OCD lesions are most commonly seen at the posteroinferior aspect of the capitellum, an area best visualized via the posterolateral portal with the elbow flexed more than 90°. Use of a 70° arthroscope can assist with visualization. The midlateral portal is used for cartilage flap débridement, loose body removal, and percutaneous drilling.

Lateral Epicondylitis

Lateral epicondylitis affects between 1% to 3% of the population and is an angiofibroblastic hyperplasia of the extensor carpi radialis tendon (ECRB), a noninflammatory, dysvascular degenerative process caused by repetitive microtrauma.[12,13] Up to 90% of cases are self-limiting, resolving within 1 to 2 years.[14] Patients whose nonsurgical therapy fails are candidates for surgical treatment. Classically, the procedure is performed through a small incision, focusing on débridement of the degenerative tendon; repair of the tendon to the lateral epicondyle should be considered. After the advent of elbow arthroscopy, some surgeons advocated arthroscopic treatment to include débridement of both the tendon and the anterolateral capsule. The advantages include the ability to visualize the entire joint and to treat concomitant pathology, including synovial plicae, which can mimic lateral epicondylitis.[15,16] Arthroscopic release is performed using a medial visualization portal and a lateral working portal. The medial portal is placed proximally enough to ensure visualization of the entire ECRB insertion. The lateral portal is placed directly through the site of the damaged ECRB tendon (the Nirschl lesion), 2 cm anterior to the intermuscular septum. The joint is entered just proximal to the articular margin of the capitellum.[12] The capsule is débrided first, followed by débridement of the ECRB tendon until healthy tissue is visualized. The lateral epicondyle is decorticated with a shaver, working anterior to the equator of the radial head to avoid injury to the lateral collateral ligament complex. The ECRB tendon can be plicated to the overlying extensor carpi radialis longus tendon or secured to the anterior aspect of the lateral epicondyle using a suture anchor.[12]

Arthroscopic débridement of lateral epicondylitis demonstrates substantial improvement in symptoms with good overall outcomes.[12,17,18] Furthermore, it has been suggested that arthroscopic treatment provides substantial improvement in functional outcomes when compared with the open method.[17] The same study found no difference in complication or failure rates between open and arthroscopic treatment.[17] Careful patient selection remains paramount: manual laborers and patients with workers' compensation claims are associated with a substantially

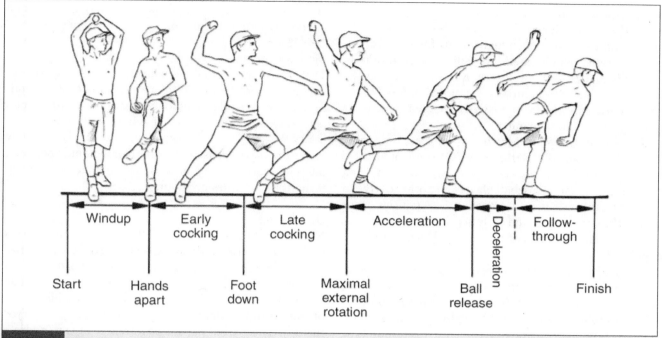

| Figure 4 | Illustration depicts the throwing motion divided into six distinct stages: windup, early arm cocking, late cocking, acceleration, deceleration, and follow-through. (Reproduced from Limpisvasti O, ElAttrache NS, Jobe FW: Understanding shoulder and elbow injuries in baseball. *J Am Acad Orthop Surg* 2007;15[3]:139-147.) |

increased risk of poor functional outcomes following arthroscopic treatment.[18]

Thrower's Elbow

Biomechanics of Throwing

The overhead throw involves coordination of the upper extremity, trunk, and lower extremity in one fluid motion. Elbow static and dynamic stabilizers play a critical role throughout this motion. Static stabilizers of the elbow include the anterior joint capsule, the UCL complex, and the radial collateral ligament complex. Dynamic stabilizers include the flexor pronator mass made of the pronator teres, the flexor carpi radialis, the palmaris, the flexor digitorum superficialis, and the flexor carpi ulnaris. To better understand the biomechanics of overhead throwing, the motion is divided into six distinct stages: windup, early arm cocking, late cocking, acceleration, deceleration, and follow-through[19,20] (Figure 4).

During wind-up, the elbow is flexed with the forearm in pronation. The arm is moved overhead and into adduction. In early cocking, elbow flexion and pronation are maintained while the shoulder is abducted and externally rotated. The leading lower extremity is advanced forward. In late cocking, elbow flexion is increased to between 90° and 120°. The forearm is pronated with maximum shoulder abduction and external rotation. At this stage,

a valgus force as high as 64 Nm is generated in the elbow by the forward rotation of the upper trunk and pelvis with associated external rotation of the shoulder.[19] Concomitantly, up to 500 Nm of compression can be placed on the lateral radiocapitellar joint.[20] As the arm is driven forward into acceleration, the elbow is rapidly extended as the humerus adducts and internally rotates. The trunk and upper extremity shift forward. During this time, the elbow accelerates at up to 600,000° per second.[20] A countering varus torque generated through the elbow opposes the valgus torque created by shoulder external rotation and rapid acceleration. The UCL has been found to supply almost 50% of the force required to oppose the valgus force when the elbow is in 90° of flexion.[19]

Such high loads exceed the ultimate tensile strength of the UCL and over time result in attritional changes. The deceleration phase is initiated at ball release. Deceleration occurs at a rate of 500,000° per second over a span of approximately 50 ms.[19] During this stage, maximum elbow extension velocity can reach 2,700° per second.[19] The shoulder reaches maximum internal rotation, the elbow is extended to roughly 20°, and the flexor-pronator muscles contract to prevent posteromedial impingement of the olecranon.[19,20] The arm moves into the follow-through stage, marking the end of the throwing motion.

Valgus Extension Overload

Most throwing injuries of the elbow occur during the acceleration stage in which high valgus forces are countered by rapid elbow extension. This motion results in three distinct pathologic forces: a tensile force on the medial stabilizing structures, a compression force at the radiocapitellar joint, and a medially directed shear force in the posterior compartment.[19]

These forces cause a spectrum of injuries comprising the valgus extension overload (VEO) syndrome. This injury pattern is the most common diagnosis requiring surgical treatment in baseball players and other overhead throwing athletes.[2] Because most of these injuries occur during the late cocking and early acceleration stages, it is not surprising that 85% of overhead athletes with VEO experience symptoms during the acceleration phase of throwing.[21] Athletes usually present with chronic medial elbow pain and concomitant changes in performance, including decreased pitch speed and stamina. Some report elbow clicking or locking. Key physical examination maneuvers include the moving valgus stress test and the milking maneuver. Evaluation for ulnar neuritis or subluxation is critical for future surgical planning.

Pathophysiology of VEO

The large valgus force exerted on the elbow in overhead throwing, created by humeral torque and trunk rotation, is countered by rapid elbow extension. As repetitive, near-failure tensile stresses are exerted on the UCL, the ligament is subjected to microtrauma and subsequent attenuation of the anterior bundle. The anterior bundle of the UCL is the most important static stabilizer of the medial elbow and damage to this structure results in valgus instability. Even subtle UCL laxity results in stretch of other medial structures, including the ulnar nerve and the flexor-pronator mass causing ulnar neuritis and flexor mass tendinitis or tears. In skeletally immature athletes, medial epicondyle apophysitis can occur. Similarly, as a result of UCL incompetency, osseous constraints of the posteromedial elbow become key stabilizers during throwing. The repetitive shear stresses from continued throwing cause posterior compartment impingement. Valgus laxity secondary to UCL stretching further exacerbates the condition by altering the contact area between the medial humeral crista and the olecranon.[22] The abnormal ulnohumeral congruency results in increased contact pressures causing posteromedial impingement. With chronic impingement, athletes become susceptible to synovitis, olecranon tip osteophyte formation, olecranon stress fractures, loose bodies, and chondral lesions of the posteromedial trochlea. Finally, because of the high compression forces exerted on the lateral radiocapitellar joint, athletes are at risk for chondromalacia, loose bodies, and lateral osteophyte formation.

Management

The management of elbow injuries in throwing athletes begins with prevention. Youth pitchers are most susceptible to this injury. Athletes logging more than 100 games per year are 3.5 times more likely to sustain an elbow injury.[23] Other factors known to increase the risk of elbow injury are playing baseball more than 8 months per year, pitching more than 80 pitches per game, and throwing faster than 85 miles per hour.[24]

UCL Injuries

Nonsurgical management is indicated in young athletes with acute injuries and athletes with partial UCL injuries (grade I or II sprains).[20,25] These patients are placed on active rest for 6 to 12 weeks. Nonsurgical modalities include physical therapy emphasizing elbow and shoulder range of motion and strengthening, NSAIDs, bracing, and cryotherapy. The goal of nonsurgical treatment is to address any issues with pitching mechanics, shoulder kinematics, shoulder motion deficits, as well as core strengthening.[26] After painless range of motion is established, the patient is progressed to an isometric program followed by an isotonic upper arm and forearm-based strengthening program with close attention given to flexor-pronator mass training.[20] An integrated gradual throwing program is initiated after pain has resolved and all kinetic chain deficits have been treated. Approximately 40% of patients return to sports participation at or above their preinjury level of play after an appropriate rehabilitation protocol.[27] A 2010 study reported successful nonsurgical treatment of professional football quarterbacks with UCL injuries.[28] Most cases were contact injuries, suggesting an acute, traumatic UCL rupture. The study concluded that these types of injuries could be amenable to nonsurgical management. However, this does not apply to chronic UCL injury seen more often in baseball pitchers. The use of platelet-rich plasma (PRP) can be considered as an augment to healing, with one study reporting an 88% rate of return to preinjury play in athletes treated with PRP.[29] Although scattered reports appear promising, data on the efficacy of PRP remain limited.[20,25] Steroids are not recommended because of the risk of tendon rupture.

Athletes whose nonsurgical treatment was unsuccessful or those preferring to quickly return to their preinjury level of play are candidates for surgical treatment. Some studies have suggested the value of diagnostic elbow arthroscopy to evaluate for articular cartilage lesions and loose bodies, as well as for osteophyte débridement and capsular release.[5,19] Additionally, an intraoperative arthroscopic valgus stress test can confirm UCL insufficiency. However, with a thorough clinical history, accurate physical examination, and corresponding imaging, diagnostic arthroscopy is rarely needed and is recommended only if presentation suggests intra-articular pathology.

Direct repair of the UCL is indicated in the few patients with acute avulsion injuries, with good outcomes reported in young, nonprofessional athletes.[30] The surgical management of choice for a chronically injured, attenuated UCL is reconstruction using an ipsilateral palmaris tendon autograft. Alternative graft options include the gracilis tendon or contralateral palmaris tendon.

In 1974, UCL reconstruction of the elbow, commonly referred to as Tommy John surgery, was popularized. This "3-ply technique" used two convergent bone tunnels in the ulna and two divergent bone tunnels in the humerus. Autograft tendon was passed through the tunnels and sutured to itself for tensioning. Concerns over graft fixation and appropriate tensioning prompted several modifications, including the Jobe modification (a muscle-splitting approach without ulnar nerve transposition), the American Sports Medicine Institute modification (a posterior approach between the two heads of the flexor carpi ulnaris, flexor-pronator elevation without takedown, and ulnar nerve transposition), the docking technique (a muscle-splitting approach, reconstruction performed via converging tunnels distally and a Y-shaped humeral tunnel with graft docking in a single proximal tunnel), the hybrid technique (humeral fixation with suture anchors), and the Tommy John DANE TJ modification.[19]

The DANE TJ method uses a muscle-splitting approach through the posterior one third of the common flexor mass, within the anterior fibers of the flexor carpi ulnaris. The procedure reconstructs the deep central fibers of the UCL. After the remnant of the ligament is taken down, the ulnar side of the graft is fixed by placing an interference screw into a single drill hole at the UCL insertion. On the humeral side, the docking technique is used, with the limbs of the graft secured within a single 15-mm bone tunnel made using a 4-mm burr. The graft is secured with two suture limbs that are passed through two divergent drill holes and tied over the top of the epicondyle.

The Authors' Preferred Technique

Preoperatively, the patient is evaluated for the presence of an ipsilateral palmaris tendon; if absent, gracilis tendon autograft is used. If present, the palmaris tendon graft is harvested first through a 1-cm transverse incision just proximal to the volar wrist crease, where the tendon is easily identified and isolated. Using blunt dissection, the

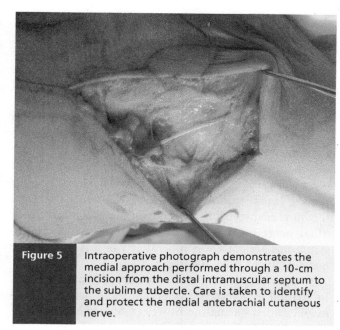

Figure 5 Intraoperative photograph demonstrates the medial approach performed through a 10-cm incision from the distal intramuscular septum to the sublime tubercle. Care is taken to identify and protect the medial antebrachial cutaneous nerve.

tendon is delivered out of the incision using two mosquito clamps. A locked Krakow stitch is run along the tendon using No. 1 nonabsorbable, braided suture and the tendon is cut distal to the suture before harvesting with a closed tendon stripper. The wound is irrigated and closed with interrupted nylon sutures.

Under tourniquet for visualization, the medial elbow is approached through a 10-cm incision from the distal third of the intramuscular septum to 2 cm distal to the sublime tubercle, protecting the medial antebrachial cutaneous nerve (Figure 5). The flexor pronator mass is split through the posterior third of the muscle belly, taking care to identify the ulnar nerve by palpation and remaining anterior to it. The native UCL is identified and the anterior bundle is split, longitudinally exposing the joint. Two bone tunnels are made in the ulna 4 to 5 mm distal to the sublime tubercle. A 3-mm burr is used create the tunnels, one anterior and one posterior to the tubercle. The tunnels are connected with small curved curet, maintaining a 2-cm osseous bridge. For humeral fixation, a 4-mm burr is used to create a longitudinal tunnel along the axis of the medial epicondyle. Care is taken to avoid violating the posterior cortex. On the upper border of the epicondyle, at the proximal end of the tunnel, two small anterior exit points are made using a 1.5-mm drill or a small burr. These points are positioned anterior to the intramuscular septum 0.5 to 1.0 cm apart. The native UCL is repaired using a 2-0 absorbable, synthetic suture.

For graft passing and fixation, the forearm is maintained in supination with a mild varus stress applied to the elbow. The graft is passed from anterior to posterior through the ulnar tunnel. The previously placed traction sutures are passed into the humeral tunnel and out through one of the two exit holes. This limb is held taught while the elbow is moved from flexion to extension to confirm isometry. Optimal graft length is determined using the exit hole as a reference point. This point is marked on the graft, and a second locked Krakow stitch is placed into the free end of the graft just proximal to the mark before trimming excess graft. The second limb of the graft is passed up into the humeral tunnel and through the empty exit hole, completely docking the graft (Figure 6). The sutures are tied over the osseous bridge on the humerus, securing the graft in place. Subcutaneous ulnar nerve transposition is performed only if clinical symptoms are present preoperatively or it is found to be unstable at the time of surgery.

Outcomes following UCL reconstruction are favorable. In 2010, a large case series evaluated clinical outcomes in 743 athletes using the American Sports Medicine Institute modification[31] and found that 83% of athletes returned to the same level of competition after surgery or higher, with an average time of 11.6 months from surgery to competition. Other studies have found excellent functional outcomes in 90% of patients following the docking technique with a trend to greater rates of return to play when compared with the Jobe modification.[32,33] The DANE TJ modification has also been shown to have excellent outcomes, with 86% of athletes returning to preinjury level of play.[34]

The most common complication following UCL reconstruction is ulnar nerve neurapraxia, which usually resolves over the course of several months.[25] Rates of ulnar nerve neurapraxia can be as high as 16%, although these results are associated with older surgical techniques in which transposition of the ulnar nerve was regularly performed.[31] Outcomes studies involving the docking and DANE TJ methods have shown a substantial decline in postoperative neurapraxia secondary to limited handling of the nerve. Other reported complications are rare and include iatrogenic fractures, wound complications, and stiffness.[25]

Flexor-Pronator Mass Injuries

The flexor-pronator muscles are key dynamic stabilizers in the elbow, countering the high valgus load during the throwing motion. During the acceleration phase of the throwing motion, these muscles contract repetitively to stabilize the elbow. Similarly, the muscles contract eccentrically to protect the elbow from posteromedial impingement in the deceleration phase as the elbow moves into extension. Acute rupture, although rare in overhead athletes, can occur during such forceful movements. In

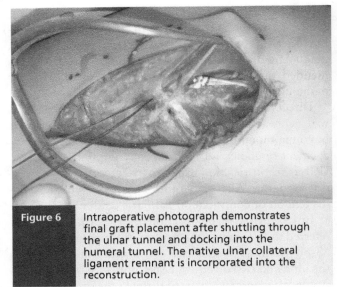

Figure 6 Intraoperative photograph demonstrates final graft placement after shuttling through the ulnar tunnel and docking into the humeral tunnel. The native ulnar collateral ligament remnant is incorporated into the reconstruction.

most cases, acute rupture is preceded by prodromal symptoms manifesting as the final stage of a chronic pathologic process. More commonly, flexor-pronator injuries occur on a spectrum ranging from mild overuse and chronic tendinitis to partial tears. These injuries are often associated with UCL attenuation, exposing the muscles to increased stress.[35] Similarly, age is a substantial risk factor for combined UCL and flexor-pronator injuries.[35] Nonsurgical treatment of these injuries is the mainstay of management. Treatment with active rest, ice, NSAIDs, and physical therapy with gradual return to throwing is almost always curative.

Surgical management, consisting of débridement and repair, is indicated in patients whose nonsurgical treatment has failed. This commonly presents as recurrence of weakness and/or pain with throwing. In such cases, a missed underlying pathology such as a UCL injury may be the cause.[20] A high level of suspicion and careful reevaluation of the athlete and imaging are critical.

Radiocapitellar Joint Overload

Radiocapitellar joint overload is a phenomenon caused by the tremendous compression forces exerted on the joint during the overhead throw. Although the underlying pathophysiology is thought to be the combination of repetitive compressive trauma, ischemia, and genetic predisposition, the distinct cause remains unclear.[20] The injury most commonly presents with loss of elbow extension, swelling, joint effusion, and lateral elbow pain with both palpation and valgus stress. Radiocapitellar joint overload can manifest in various injury patterns, including marginal osteophytes, chondromalacia, or OCD of the capitellum. A trial of nonsurgical treatment is indicated

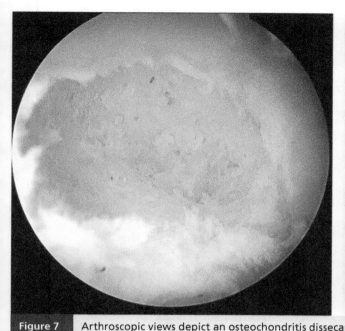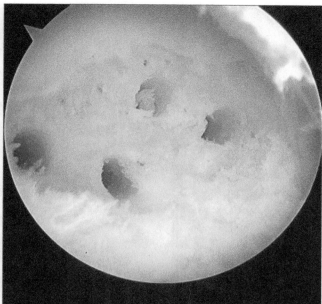

Figure 7 Arthroscopic views depict an osteochondritis dissecans (OCD) lesion of the elbow before (**A**) and after (**B**) microfracture.

for patients in whom early (stage I) OCD lesions have been diagnosed. Young patients with open capitellar growth plates, localized flattening or radiolucency without subchondral bone involvement, and good elbow function are prime candidates for nonsurgical care.[36]

Patients whose nonsurgical treatment has failed and those with advanced (stage II and III) OCD lesions are indicated for surgery. Stage II lesion are unstable, partially detached fragments of cartilage with lateral buttress involvement.[3] Treatment consists of arthroscopic débridement using the lateral and posterolateral portals. Although fracture fixation of acute grade II lesions has been described, healing rates are unpredictable.[37] Alternatively, fragment excision and arthroscopic or mini-open microfracture can be performed for lesions smaller than 7 mm in diameter[5,36] (Figure 7). Mosaicplasty can be performed for defects greater than 7 mm, with good early outcomes.[5,38,39] In these cases, graft can be harvested from the far lateral or medial edges of the lateral femoral condyle.

Stage III lesions are unstable, fully detached cartilage fragments that present as intra-articular loose bodies. These injuries are treated in a manner similar to stage II lesions; microfracture is indicated for smaller lesions and grafting can be considered for larger lesions. Reports demonstrate good early outcomes with improved range of motion and a high rate of return to sport in properly selected adolescent athletes. Overall, approximately 85% of patients return to their preinjury level of play.[36,40] Outcomes in younger patients with open radial physes and those with large lesions are less consistent.[40] In skeletally immature athletes, radial head enlargement can develop and may predispose these patients to early osteoarthritis. Similarly, patients with large lesions can also be at increased risk for early arthritis and are thus less likely to report good long-term outcomes.[40] It is imperative for treating physicians to educate patients about these risks to manage long-term goals and expectations.

Posteromedial Impingement

Commonly, symptomatic posteromedial impingement in overhead athletes is treated surgically. Nonsurgical management is reserved for overhead athletes with radiographic signs of impingement and who remain asymptomatic. Similarly, symptomatic individuals who modify their sports activity, either by changing positions or reducing the intensity or frequency of play, can defer to nonsurgical management, including rest and physical therapy with dynamic stabilizing and strengthening exercises.

Rehabilitation for competitive athletes with symptomatic posterior medial osteophytes or intra-articular loose bodies is usually unsuccessful and surgery is indicated. As described previously, posteromedial impingement is frequently secondary to underlying UCL insufficiency. Treatment of impingement without appropriately treating the UCL injury results in poor functional outcomes. Therefore, arthroscopic management of posteromedial impingement is preferred because it allows surgeons to evaluate the integrity of the UCL using the arthroscopic valgus stress test and performing reconstruction if necessary. The posterolateral and posterior portals provide visualization

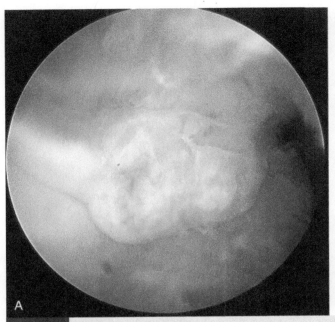
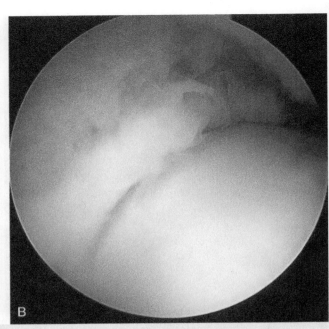

Figure 8   Arthroscopic views of posteromedial olecranon osteophytes obtained from the posterolateral portal before (**A**) and after (**B**) resection of the osteophytes to the level of native bone, avoiding excessive resection and instability.

of the posterior recess and the entire olecranon. Resection of the posteromedial olecranon osteophytes is performed with the arthroscope in the posterolateral portal and the shaver in the transtriceps portal (Figure 2). A small, curved osteotome can also be used. Resection should be limited to the osteophyte itself without débridement of native bone because excessive olecranon resection is associated with valgus elbow instability in the setting of concomitant chronic UCL insufficiency[41] (Figure 8). Multiple studies have demonstrated the role of the proximal olecranon in elbow stability. Studies vary based on the specific type of resection; however, a 1986 study demonstrated that resection of the proximal 25% of the olecranon reduces constraint by 30% in extension and 50% in 90° of flexion.[42] A 2003 study found only 3 mm of posteromedial resection caused changes in valgus angulation.[43] An intraoperative arthroscopic valgus stress test must be performed to avoid missing any underlying UCL injury. The posteromedial gutter must be débrided with caution to avoid iatrogenic injury to the ulnar nerve. In patients with preoperative ulnar neuritis, a concomitant ulnar nerve transposition is indicated.

Some throwing athletes demonstrate more advanced arthritic changes associated with posteromedial impingement. Treatment can be challenging because of contractures and the proximity of neurovascular structures to the anterior elbow. Osseous spur removal and capsular release can assist with motion and pain relief. A 2013 study described a stepwise approach to prevent nerve injury during capsulectomy and débridement of the elbow, including the use of blunt retractors to sweep neurovascular structures out of the working field.[44] Additionally, supine positioning using an arm holder limits pressure on the antecubital fossa, allowing critical neurovascular structures to fall away from the surgical field.

Olecranon Stress Fractures

Olecranon stress fractures result from repetitive microtrauma and excessive tensile stress from the triceps tendon and posterior impingement of the olecranon. The injury presents as posteromedial olecranon pain during and after throwing and has a prevalence of 5.4% in baseball-related elbow injuries.[45] The same study found that 70% to 90% of these injuries occur concomitantly with a UCL injury. First-line treatment consists of rest, immobilization, and limiting full extension to allow the bone to heal.

Surgical treatment is performed in patients with persistent pain after prolonged rest and in competitive throwers with complete fractures. The basic principles of fracture fixation apply, and compression through the fracture is the primary goal. Open reduction and internal fixation using a cannulated screw has high success rates in returning athletes to their previous level of preinjury play or higher[46] (Figure 9). The most common complication following surgery is painful hardware, with 33% of patients requiring additional surgery for removal.[46] Fracture nonunion, although rare, can be seen in young patients with undiagnosed chronic elbow pain or in those

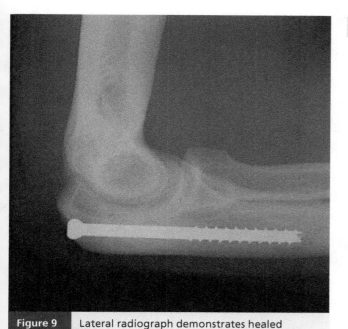

Figure 9 Lateral radiograph demonstrates healed olecranon stress fracture following fixation with a partially threaded, cannulated screw.

treated nonsurgically. In such cases, surgical fixation with a cannulated screw has been shown to be an excellent treatment option.[47]

Summary

Elbow injuries are a prominent phenomenon among overhead athletes. As athletes become competitive at younger ages, the incidence of these types of injuries will continue to grow. Consequently, research needs to be directed toward improving on and developing new treatment methods for the various pathologies associated with competitive throwing. Currently, arthroscopic management is a viable treatment option for many of these injuries, providing promising functional outcomes and minimal morbidity. As surgical techniques evolve and surgeons become familiarized with the arthroscopic method, the applications of elbow arthroscopy will continue to expand.

Key Study Points

- Elbow arthroscopy, although technically challenging, is an important tool in an elbow surgeon's armamentarium.
- Knowledge of throwing biomechanics is crucial for understanding injuries seen in overhead athletes.
- Injury to the UCL must be considered in an overhead athlete with elbow pain.

Annotated References

1. Andrews JR, Carson WG: Arthroscopy of the elbow. *Arthroscopy* 1985;1(2):97-107.

2. Dodson CC, Nho SJ, Williams RJ III, Altchek DW: Elbow arthroscopy. *J Am Acad Orthop Surg* 2008;16(10):574-585.

3. Ahmad CS, ElAttrache NS: Treatment of capitellar osteochondritis dissecans. *Tech Shoulder Elbow Surg* 2006;7:169-174.

4. Bennett JM: Elbow arthroscopy: The basics. *J Hand Surg Am* 2013;38(1):164-167.

    This article focuses on the basic surgical setup and technique for elbow arthroscopy. The author discusses current indications and contraindications for the procedure, as well as common complications.

5. Byram IR, Kim HM, Levine WN, Ahmad CS: Elbow arthroscopic surgery update for sports medicine conditions. *Am J Sports Med* 2013;41(9):2191-2202.

    This article provides an update on the current indications, modern techniques, and outcomes following elbow arthroscopy. The authors describe the most common surgical techniques to treat the most common pathologies within the elbow joint. The importance of appropriate indications and proper technique are highlighted.

6. Field LD, Altchek DW: Evaluation of the arthroscopic valgus instability test of the elbow. *Am J Sports Med* 1996;24(2):177-181.

7. Baker CL Jr, Jones GL: Arthroscopy of the elbow. *Am J Sports Med* 1999;27(2):251-264.

8. Kelly EW, Morrey BF, O'Driscoll SW: Complications of elbow arthroscopy. *J Bone Joint Surg Am* 2001;83-A(1):25-34.

9. Savoie FH III, Field LD: Complications of elbow arthroscopy, in Savoie FH, Field LD, eds: *AANA Advanced Arthroscopy: The Wrist and Elbow.* Philadelphia, Saunders/Elsevier, 2010, pp 146-150.

    The textbook covers basic and complex elbow pathologies that can be treated using arthroscopy. A thorough review of arthroscopic indications, surgical techniques, outcomes, and complications are reviewed. The future of elbow arthroscopy is also discussed.

10. Nelson GN, Wu T, Galatz LM, Yamaguchi K, Keener JD: Elbow arthroscopy: Early complications and associated risk factors. *J Shoulder Elbow Surg* 2014;23(2):273-278.

    This case series of 417 elbow arthroscopies evaluated early complications following the procedure and reviewed associated risk factors. The study found an overall complication rate of 14%. Most complications were minor and transient in nature. Major complications, the most common of which was deep infection, occurred in 5% of cases. Level of evidence: IV.

11. Marti D, Spross C, Jost B: The first 100 elbow arthroscopies of one surgeon: Analysis of complications. *J Shoulder Elbow Surg* 2013;22(4):567-573.

    This case series of 100 consecutive elbow arthroscopies analyzed complications seen following elbow arthroscopy. The overall complication rate was 5%, with no major complications occurring. No association was seen between complications and the complexity of the procedure or the surgeon's learning curve. Level of evidence: IV.

12. Savoie FH III, VanSice W, O'Brien MJ: Arthroscopic tennis elbow release. *J Shoulder Elbow Surg* 2010;19(2, Suppl)31-36.

    This review details surgical technique for treating lateral epicondylitis using elbow arthroscopy. The results of recent studies evaluating functional outcomes are discussed. The authors conclude that arthroscopic release of lateral epicondylitis is an excellent option for patients whose nonsurgical treatment has failed.

13. Nirschl RP, Ashman ES: Elbow tendinopathy: Tennis elbow. *Clin Sports Med* 2003;22(4):813-836.

14. Coonrad RW, Hooper WR: Tennis elbow: Its course, natural history, conservative and surgical management. *J Bone Joint Surg Am* 1973;55(6):1177-1182.

15. Kim DH, Gambardella RA, Elattrache NS, Yocum LA, Jobe FW: Arthroscopic treatment of posterolateral elbow impingement from lateral synovial plicae in throwing athletes and golfers. *Am J Sports Med* 2006;34(3):438-444.

16. Lattermann C, Romeo AA, Anbari A, et al: Arthroscopic debridement of the extensor carpi radialis brevis for recalcitrant lateral epicondylitis. *J Shoulder Elbow Surg* 2010;19(5):651-656.

    This retrospective review of 36 patients with lateral epicondylitis treated with surgery assessed the outcome of arthroscopic release of the ECRB with a mean follow-up of 3.5 years. The results showed substantial improvement in postoperative pain and a mean return to full activity of 7 weeks. No major complications were identified. Level of evidence: III.

17. Solheim E, Hegna J, Øyen J: Arthroscopic versus open tennis elbow release: 3- to 6-year results of a case-control series of 305 elbows. *Arthroscopy* 2013;29(5):854-859.

    This case-control study compared the outcome of arthroscopic and open treatment of lateral epicondylitis in 80 patients at a minimum follow-up of 3 years. Patients were evaluated using the QuickDASH scale. Substantially better scores were reported in the arthroscopic group. Level of evidence: III.

18. Grewal R, MacDermid JC, Shah P, King GJ: Functional outcome of arthroscopic extensor carpi radialis brevis tendon release in chronic lateral epicondylitis. *J Hand Surg Am* 2009;34(5):849-857.

    This case series of 36 patients with chronic lateral epicondylitis treated with athroscopic release reported on postoperative functional outcomes. Thirty patients improved with surgery; most reported good to excellent results. Workers' compensation and heavy labor were associated with substantially worse outcomes. Level of evidence: IV.

19. Jones KJ, Osbahr DC, Schrumpf MA, Dines JS, Altchek DW: Ulnar collateral ligament reconstruction in throwing athletes: A review of current concepts. AAOS exhibit selection. *J Bone Joint Surg Am* 2012;94(8):e49.

    This review article details the anatomy and functional biomechanics of the UCL. Work-up and management of the throwing athlete with UCL injury is described, and a thorough review of surgical techniques and clinical outcomes was conducted.

20. Patel RM, Lynch TS, Amin NH, Calabrese G, Gryzlo SM, Schickendantz MS: The thrower's elbow. *Orthop Clin North Am* 2014;45(3):355-376.

    This comprehensive overview includes the functional anatomy of the elbow, the biomechanics of throwing, and the various pathologies incurred with repetitive throwing in overhead athletes. Clinical presentation, work-up, and management of the most common injuries are covered in detail.

21. Callaway GH, Field LD, Deng XH, et al: Biomechanical evaluation of the medial collateral ligament of the elbow. *J Bone Joint Surg Am* 1997;79(8):1223-1231.

22. Osbahr DC, Dines JS, Breazeale NM, Deng XH, Altchek DW: Ulnohumeral chondral and ligamentous overload: Biomechanical correlation for posteromedial chondromalacia of the elbow in throwing athletes. *Am J Sports Med* 2010;38(12):2535-2541.

    This cadaver study evaluated the pathologic biomechanics of an elbow with valgus laxity in six specimens subjected to static valgus load. Contact forces and contact area shift across the posteromedial elbow were measured before and after sectioning of the anterior bundle of the UCL. The results show abnormal contact across the posteromedial elbow secondary to valgus laxity.

23. Fleisig GS, Andrews JR, Cutter GR, et al: Risk of serious injury for young baseball pitchers: A 10-year prospective study. *Am J Sports Med* 2011;39(2):253-257.

    This cohort followed 481 youth pitchers over 10 years to quantify the cumulative incidence of throwing injuries. The overall incidence of injury was found to be 5%. A substantial increase in risk of injury was seen in athletes pitching more than 100 innings per year. Level of evidence: III.

24. Olsen SJ II, Fleisig GS, Dun S, Loftice J, Andrews JR: Risk factors for shoulder and elbow injuries in adolescent baseball pitchers. *Am J Sports Med* 2006;34(6):905-912.

© 2016 American Academy of Orthopaedic Surgeons

25. Bruce JR, Andrews JR: Ulnar collateral ligament injuries in the throwing athlete. *J Am Acad Orthop Surg* 2014;22(5):315-325.

This review provides a comprehensive overview of UCL injuries in overhead athletes and the treatments used for these injuries.

26. Wilk KE, Macrina LC, Cain EL, Dugas JR, Andrews JR: Rehabilitation of the overhead athlete's elbow. *Sports Health* 2012;4(5):404-414.

This review article discusses the basic principles behind rehabilitation following elbow injury. The authors review the various phases of a standard rehabilitation protocol and describe specific nonsurgical and postoperative rehabilitation guidelines for common elbow injuries and procedures.

27. Rettig AC, Sherrill C, Snead DS, Mendler JC, Mieling P: Nonoperative treatment of ulnar collateral ligament injuries in throwing athletes. *Am J Sports Med* 2001;29(1):15-17.

28. Dodson CC, Slenker N, Cohen SB, Ciccotti MG, DeLuca P: Ulnar collateral ligament injuries of the elbow in professional football quarterbacks. *J Shoulder Elbow Surg* 2010;19(8):1276-1280.

The article reviewed 10 cases of UCL elbow injury in NFL quarterbacks, describing the type and mechanism of injury, player demographics, method of treatment, and return to play. In nine athletes, nonsurgical management resulted in successful return to play at an average of 26.4 days. Level of evidence: IV.

29. Podesta L, Crow SA, Volkmer D, Bert T, Yocum LA: Treatment of partial ulnar collateral ligament tears in the elbow with platelet-rich plasma. *Am J Sports Med* 2013;41(7):1689-1694.

This case series reported on the functional outcomes of 34 overhead athletes with partial-thickness UCL tears treated with PRP. At an average follow-up of 70 weeks, 88% of athletes had returned to their previous level of play at an average time of 12 weeks. The authors concluded that PRP is an effective treatment option for partial UCL tears. Level of evidence: IV.

30. Savoie FH III, Trenhaile SW, Roberts J, Field LD, Ramsey JR: Primary repair of ulnar collateral ligament injuries of the elbow in young athletes: A case series of injuries to the proximal and distal ends of the ligament. *Am J Sports Med* 2008;36(6):1066-1072.

31. Cain EL Jr, Andrews JR, Dugas JR, et al: Outcome of ulnar collateral ligament reconstruction of the elbow in 1281 athletes: Results in 743 athletes with minimum 2-year follow-up. *Am J Sports Med* 2010;38(12):2426-2434.

This case series evaluated the functional outcomes of 743 athletes treated with surgical UCL reconstruction using a modified Jobe technique. At a minimum follow-up of 2 years, results demonstrated an 83% rate of return to previous level of competition less than 1 year after surgery. Level of evidence: IV.

32. Bowers AL, Dines JS, Dines DM, Altchek DW: Elbow medial ulnar collateral ligament reconstruction: Clinical relevance and the docking technique. *J Shoulder Elbow Surg* 2010;19(Suppl 2):110-117.

This case series documented the treatment course of 21 overhead athletes with UCL insufficiency. A modified version of the docking technique for UCL reconstruction was used to treat the injury. At follow-up, 90% of athletes had excellent results. No complications occurred. Level of evidence: IV.

33. Watson JN, McQueen P, Hutchinson MR: A systematic review of ulnar collateral ligament reconstruction techniques. *Am J Sports Med* 2014;42(10):2510-2516.

This systematic review of 21 studies reported on outcomes following various UCL reconstruction techniques. The overall complication rate was 18.6%; the most common complication was ulnar nerve neurapraxia. The overall rate of return to play was 78.9%. Level of evidence: IV.

34. Dines JS, ElAttrache NS, Conway JE, Smith W, Ahmad CS: Clinical outcomes of the DANE TJ technique to treat ulnar collateral ligament insufficiency of the elbow. *Am J Sports Med* 2007;35(12):2039-2044.

35. Osbahr DC, Swaminathan SS, Allen AA, Dines JS, Coleman SH, Altchek DW: Combined flexor-pronator mass and ulnar collateral ligament injuries in the elbows of older baseball players. *Am J Sports Med* 2010;38(4):733-739.

This case series of 187 baseball players undergoing UCL reconstruction evaluated the athletes for concomitant flexor-pronator mass injury, with 8 players undergoing flexor-pronator débridement. Athletes older than 30 years were substantially more likely to sustain combined UCL and flexor-pronator mass injuries. Level of evidence: IV.

36. Jones KJ, Wiesel BB, Sankar WN, Ganley TJ: Arthroscopic management of osteochondritis dissecans of the capitellum: Mid-term results in adolescent athletes. *J Pediatr Orthop* 2010;30(1):8-13.

This case series of 25 adolescent athletes undergoing arthroscopic treatment of capitellar OCD evaluated functional outcomes. Patients were treated with arthroscopic débridement, drilling, and/or bone grafting. At a mean follow-up of 4 years, patients were found to have substantially improved range of motion and a high rate of return to sports. Level of evidence: IV.

37. Takahara M, Mura N, Sasaki J, Harada M, Ogino T: Classification, treatment, and outcome of osteochondritis dissecans of the humeral capitellum. *J Bone Joint Surg Am* 2007;89(6):1205-1214.

38. Iwasaki N, Kato H, Ishikawa J, Masuko T, Funakoshi T, Minami A: Autologous osteochondral mosaicplasty for osteochondritis dissecans of the elbow in teenage athletes. *J Bone Joint Surg Am* 2009;91(10):2359-2366.

This study reported on the functional outcomes of 19 adolescent competitive athletes undergoing mosaicplasty for elbow OCD. At a mean follow-up of 45 months, 18 athletes had excellent or good clinical results, and all but 2 returned to their previous level of play. Level of evidence: IV.

39. Yamamoto Y, Ishibashi Y, Tsuda E, Sato H, Toh S: Osteochondral autograft transplantation for osteochondritis dissecans of the elbow in juvenile baseball players: Minimum 2-year follow-up. *Am J Sports Med* 2006;34(5):714-720.

40. Miyake J, Masatomi T: Arthroscopic debridement of the humeral capitellum for osteochondritis dissecans: Radiographic and clinical outcomes. *J Hand Surg Am* 2011;36(8):1333-1338.

    This retrospective review reported on outcomes of arthroscopic débridement of the capitellum in 106 adolescent patients diagnosed with OCD. At an average follow-up of 13 months, 84% of patients were pain free and 85% had returned to their previous level of play. Large lesions or an open proximal radial physis at the time of surgery were associated with poor outcomes. Level of evidence: III.

41. Kamineni S, ElAttrache NS, O'driscoll SW, et al: Medial collateral ligament strain with partial posteromedial olecranon resection. A biomechanical study. *J Bone Joint Surg Am* 2004;86-A(11):2424-2430.

42. An KN, Morrey BF, Chao EY: The effect of partial removal of proximal ulna on elbow constraint. *Clin Orthop Relat Res* 1986;209:270-279.

43. Kamineni S, Hirahara H, Pomianowski S, et al: Partial posteromedial olecranon resection: A kinematic study. *J Bone Joint Surg Am* 2003;85-A(6):1005-1011.

44. Blonna D, Wolf JM, Fitzsimmons JS, O'Driscoll SW: Prevention of nerve injury during arthroscopic capsulectomy of the elbow utilizing a safety-driven strategy. *J Bone Joint Surg Am* 2013;95(15):1373-1381.

    This retrospective review reports on the incidence of nerve injury in a series of 502 arthroscopic elbow contracture releases. Twenty-five patients (5%) had nerve palsies associated with prolonged tourniquet time, ulnar nerve transposition, or retractor use. All deficits had resolved at 2-year follow-up. Level of evidence: III.

45. Furushima K, Itoh Y, Iwabu S, Yamamoto Y, Koga R, Shimizu M: Classification of olecranon stress fractures in baseball players. *Am J Sports Med* 2014;42(6):1343-1351.

    This case series of 200 baseball players diagnosed with olecranon stress fractures evaluated the orientation of the fractures using various imaging modalities. A novel classification system was presented for these fractures based on the origin and direction of the fracture plane. Level of evidence: IV.

46. Paci JM, Dugas JR, Guy JA, et al: Cannulated screw fixation of refractory olecranon stress fractures with and without associated injuries allows a return to baseball. *Am J Sports Med* 2013;41(2):306-312.

    This case series reported functional outcomes in 18 patients treated with open reduction and internal fixation for an olecranon stress fracture. All 18 fractures went on to union, and 94% of athletes returned to their previous level of play. At an average follow-up of 6.2 years, six patients had undergone removal of hardware, two of which for infection. Level of evidence: IV.

47. Rettig AC, Wurth TR, Mieling P: Nonunion of olecranon stress fractures in adolescent baseball pitchers: A case series of 5 athletes. *Am J Sports Med* 2006;34(4):653-656.

© 2016 American Academy of Orthopaedic Surgeons

Chapter 7

Acute/Traumatic Elbow Injuries

John P. Haverstock, MD, FRCSC   George S. Athwal, MD, FRCSC

Abstract

Fractures and dislocations around the elbow range from simple isolated injuries to complex injuries of multiple bony and ligamentous stabilizers. Orthopaedic surgeons and sports medicine physicians may encounter several patterns of elbow injuries. Thorough knowledge of classic studies and recent evidence for the diagnosis and treatment of radial head fractures, simple elbow dislocations, complex elbow instability, triceps and biceps injuries is necessary for optimal outcomes.

Keywords: elbow trauma; acute elbow injury; elbow dislocation; radial head fracture; terrible triad; PLRI; posterolateral rotatory instability; coronoid fracture; posteromedial rotatory instability; complex elbow instability; triceps rupture; biceps rupture

Introduction

The elbow is a complex assembly of joints that requires prompt diagnosis and treatment after acute injury to maximize outcomes and avoid instability, stiffness, and pain. Physical examination in combination with radiographs, and frequently advanced imaging, is required for adequate assessment of complex fractures or soft-tissue injury patterns.

Most physical examination special tests are more effective after initial inflammation and pain have settled; however, the elbow extension test can be used to help rule

Dr. Athwal or an immediate family member has the potential to receive royalties from Imascap; serves as a paid consultant to DePuy, Smith & Nephew, and Tornier; and has received research or institutional support from DePuy, Exactech, Smith & Nephew, Tornier, and Zimmer. Neither Dr. Haverstock nor any immediate family member has received anything of value from or has stock or stock options held in a commercial company or institution related directly or indirectly to the subject of this chapter.

out fracture in the acute setting. It is a sensitive screening tool (96.8%) to identify patients who would benefit from further radiographic assessment. The elbow extension test is performed by asking the seated patient with exposed and supinated forearms to flex his or her shoulders to 90° and fully extend and lock both elbows. In a study of patients who were unable to perform the elbow extension test, almost 50% had sustained a fracture.[1] The negative predictive value for fracture in adults and children able to extend the elbow was 98.4% and 95.8%, respectively.

The elbow is a commonly injured joint in the upper extremity. At the 2012 Summer Olympics Games more than one-half of elbow injuries occurred in judo and weightlifting; elbow injuries in throwing athletes were less common.[2] Surveillance of National Football League injuries over a 10-year period revealed that the elbow was commonly injured (58% of 859 upper extremity injuries); 75% of elbow injuries occurred in offensive and defensive lineman, and most were ligament and instability problems.[3]

Elbow stability depends on the bony and soft-tissue stabilizers, which must be assessed with every elbow injury. Primary stabilizers include the ulnohumeral joint, the lateral ulnar collateral ligament (LUCL) and the anterior bundle of the medial collateral ligament (MCL). Secondary stabilizers include the radial head, the common extensor origin, and the common flexor origin, which become increasingly important after injury to the primary stabilizers.[4]

Radial Head Fractures

Radial head fractures, the most common fracture around the elbow, were classified by Mason in 1954 and modified further in 1997.[5] Type 1 fractures are displaced less than 2 mm without a mechanical block to forearm rotation and can be effectively treated nonsurgically. Type 2 fractures are displaced greater than 2 mm, may block forearm motion, and are not substantially comminuted. The treatment of type 2 fractures is controversial; however, most authors agree that with the best available evidence and without a block to rotation, this group can be effectively treated nonsurgically. In patients with a block to forearm rotation that can be attributed to the fracture, surgical intervention is indicated. Type 3 fractures are severely comminuted and typically require surgical intervention to restore elbow and forearm function. In type 3 fractures associated with instability, radial head excision is contraindicated. Although type 3 fractures are highly comminuted and typically indicated for arthroplasty, in the younger, active athletic population an attempt at open reduction and internal fixation should be considered.

Injuries commonly associated with radial head fractures include ligamentous injuries, and chondral injuries to the capitellum. When complete loss of cortical contact of at least one fragment from a radial head fracture occurs, one study reported that 91% of these fractures were associated with complex elbow instability patterns.[6] In a series of 50 surgically treated Mason type 2 and 3 fractures, 10 had sustained chondral injury.[7] Chondral injury to the capitellum was most common in higher-grade radial head fractures.

Treatment of radial head fractures depends on the character of the fracture, blocks to pronation and supination, and associated injuries (elbow dislocation, MCL, and Essex-Lopresti injuries). Controversy exists regarding the best method of treating type 2 fractures, and a large prospective trial is underway.[8] Stable, displaced partial articular fractures and those with minimal comminution and displacement can be treated nonsurgically as long as range of motion recovers and no associated elbow or forearm stability exists.[9,10]

The nonsurgical treatment of minimally displaced radial head fractures without a block to rotation includes a brief period of immobilization preceding range of motion and active therapy. A prospective randomized controlled trial of 180 patients with simple radial head fractures reported that immobilization for 2 days with a sling followed by active mobilization had superior results in motion, strength, and functional outcomes compared with immediate mobilization and immobilization for 8 days.[11] In addition, a fragment displaced more than 4 mm or angulated more than 30° impaired outcome.

Radial head fractures with more than three fragments are often not amenable to open reduction and internal fixation because of small fragment size, comminution, and osteopenia;[12] however, in the younger, active population, an initial attempt at fixation is appropriate. To maximize elbow stability, radial head arthroplasty is an option, which is especially important for complex instability patterns.[13] The early results of metallic smooth stem and bipolar radial head implants have been good, with minimal posttraumatic arthritis and high rates of good to excellent patient-rated outcomes at follow-up.[14]

Simple Elbow Dislocations

Simple elbow dislocations include those without fracture, in which the medial and lateral ligament complexes are ruptured or avulsed. Elbow dislocations most often occur in adolescent males participating in football, wrestling, and basketball; or in females participating in gymnastics and skating.[15] A review of video footage of 62 elbow dislocations showed that the typical injury occurs with the arm in near-full extension with a valgus force, which suggests MCL rupture is common, although numerous mechanisms are described.[16]

Treatment of simple elbow dislocation includes closed reduction beginning with stabilization of the humerus, traction, correction of varus/valgus angulation, and flexion. Alternatively, the physician can use one hand to grasp the patient's wrist to apply traction and use his or her other hand to grasp the distal humerus, while using the thumb to push the olecranon anteriorly to obtain reduction. An examination for stability should be documented to guide rehabilitation by gradually extending the elbow from flexion with the forearm in pronation, neutral, and supination, noting the angle where subluxation begins. Radiographs obtained before and after reduction should be scrutinized for radial head fractures, coronoid fractures, intra-articular fragments, or a nonconcentric reduction. These occult findings can result in substantial instability, stiffness, or pain if missed.

Therapy for elbow dislocations with a concentrically reduced joint must begin within 7 to 10 days. Overhead motion protocols have been shown to decrease the "drop sign," a radiographic finding of ulnohumeral subluxation that is worsened by gravity and extra forearm weight (larger arms and elbow hinge braces).[17] Isometric exercises and protective splinting with forearm rotation (pronation for lateral collateral ligament [LCL] insufficiency and supination for MCL insufficiency) can facilitate protected range of motion. Therapy using this protocol allows healing in the reduced position and decreases the incidence of recurrent instability.[18] Elbows with both MCL and LCL injuries should undergo rehabilitation with active motion, neutral pronation/supination of the forearm, and with the humerus oriented vertically or horizontally to minimize forces that promote rotational subluxation[19] (Figure 1).

A review of 110 patients at a mean follow-up of 88 months following simple elbow dislocation revealed that although outcomes are generally good with appropriate treatment, 62% have residual pain, 56% report subjective stiffness, and 8% have subjective instability.[20] Additionally, a reduced elbow flexion-extension arc predicted poorer overall satisfaction, with reduced flexion influencing patient outcome more than reduced extension.

In elbows that remain unstable after successful reduction attempts or become unstable subacutely, surgical treatment should be considered. In a series of 15 patients with persistent instability following simple elbow dislocation, 12 were treated with LUCL repair alone and 3 required the addition of hinged external fixation.[21] Of those treated with LUCL repair alone, 5 experienced resubluxation: 1 required later external fixation and 4 were treated with physical therapy alone, all of whom eventually achieved a concentric and stable reduction.

Patients in whom persistent posterolateral rotatory instability (PLRI) develops have several treatment options. If PLRI is identified subacutely within 6 weeks from injury, an attempt at nonsurgical management is reasonable with splinting at 90° in full pronation. Extension range of motion can be blocked to 45° to 50°, and increased 10° per week. In patients whose nonsurgical management is unsuccessful or who present delayed with symptomatic instability, surgical intervention to repair or reconstruct the LUCL is indicated.

Posterolateral Rotatory Instability

Originally described in 1991, PLRI occurs following injury to the LUCL, allowing rotatory subluxation of the ulnohumeral joint and dislocation of the radiohumeral joint with a combination of extension, valgus, and supination.[22]

The diagnosis of PLRI can be difficult because symptoms of painful locking or snapping and apprehension are hard to elicit. The lateral pivot-shift test is best performed with the patient lying supine with the arm overhead, maximal external rotation at the shoulder, and with the examiner grasping the wrist and forearm to provide a valgus and supination force in full extension. A positive test result presents as subluxation in extension, and as the elbow is flexed, it pops or slides in to reduction at 30° to 40°. Although poorly tolerated by patients who are awake, the test is reproducible at various levels of training with full muscle relaxation.[23] The posterolateral drawer test, chair sign, and the inability to do a push-up with the forearms in supination are also useful special tests. Terminal forearm supination (hypersupination) by the examiner while palpating the radiocapitellar joint can reveal subtle instability in patients both awake and under anesthesia.

PLRI can be treated in the acute setting as described for simple elbow dislocations, with rehabilitation performed with the arm in pronation. For those patients with ongoing symptoms or instability, repair or reconstruction of the LUCL with tissue plication or tendon graft is recommended[24] (Figure 2).

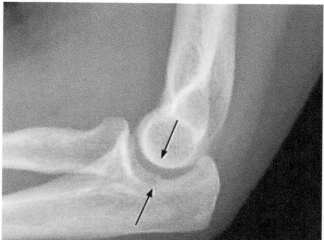

Figure 1 Lateral radiograph of the ulnohumeral joint demonstrates the drop sign, which indicates a noncongruent reduction. This finding usually occurs because of periarticular muscle pain-related atony and hemarthrosis. If only axial distraction (no medial or lateral translation of the joint) exists, the elbow can be treated with isometric exercises and overhead rehabilitation can be considered. The patient should be followed with weekly radiographs to ensure improvement. (Reproduced with permission from Pipicelli JG, Chinchalkar SJ, Grewal R, King GJ: Therapeutic implications of the radiographic "drop sign" following elbow dislocation. J Hand Ther 2012;25[3]:346-353, quiz 354. http://dx.doi.org/10.1016/j.jht.2012.03.003.)

In a study of 19 patients with acute PLRI treated by LCL repair using nonabsorbable, braided suture or a suture anchor,[25] Mayo Elbow Performance Score was 86.9 of 100, with 12 excellent results, 5 good results, and 1 fair result. Reported complications included heterotopic ossification in five and knot irritation in one. In a study of a technique describing the use of tensionable suture anchors to fine-tune the tension of collateral ligament repair, good outcomes in two patients were reported.[26]

When treating chronic PLRI, the best results are obtained with ligament reconstruction with tendon graft.[27] However, LUCL reconstruction can also fail. A 2014 study reported that revision of failed LUCL reconstruction is challenging and that the outcomes are guarded: one half of patients at follow-up had persistent instability and poorer elbow scores.[28]

Complex Elbow Instability

Complex elbow dislocations include those with associated fractures and are typically classified into three broad groups: radial head fracture-dislocations (including terrible triad injuries), varus posteromedial rotatory instability ([PMRI] with anteromedial coronoid fractures) and

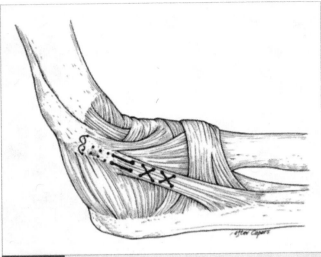

Figure 2 Illustration depicts the lateral collateral ligament complex, including the primary stabilizer, the lateral ulnar collateral ligament, running from the geometric center of the capitellum to the crista supinatorus. Suture marks indicate a transosseous repair or a suture anchor proximally, which can be used to repair acute injuries. (Reproduced from Mehta, JA, Bain GI: Posterolateral rotatory instability of the elbow. *J Am Acad Orthop Surg* 2004;12[6]:405-415.)

fracture-dislocations of the proximal radius and ulna (including transolecranon and Monteggia-type injuries). Outcomes following treatment of complex elbow instability are guarded and poor general health, lack of cooperation, obesity, delayed surgery, and high-energy trauma are all poor prognostic factors.[29]

Terrible Triad

A terrible triad injury is named for the historically poor results seen after an elbow dislocation combined with radial head and coronoid fractures. A more complete understanding of the primary and secondary stabilizers of the elbow and treatments that allow early range of motion following surgical stabilization has substantially improved outcomes. Biomechanical and clinical research has resulted in the development of successful surgical treatment protocols that also have improved patient outcomes.

Diagnosis is often clear using plain radiographs, although subtle avulsions of the coronoid can be difficult to detect and spontaneous reduction of the elbow dislocation is possible. On radiographs, these areas should be assessed carefully, as well as the shape of the posterolateral capitellum, where an Osborne-Coterill lesion can indicate elbow instability, as would a Hill-Sachs lesion on the humeral

head.[30] It is recommended that all patients with radiographic findings of a possible coronoid fracture should undergo advanced imaging using CT to fully characterize the fractures and instability pattern.

Strict indications for the successful nonsurgical treatment of terrible triad injuries have enabled good results. Nonsurgical treatment is only advised in patients with a concentric joint reduction, a radial head fracture without block to rotation, a smaller coronoid fracture (Regan-Morrey type 1 or 2), and a stable arc of motion to a minimum extension of 30° to 45°, allowing active range of motion within 10 days.[31,32]

Surgical treatment should be considered for most patients with terrible triad injuries. A stepwise approach to fixation results in good results with minimization of complications.[33] Typically, a posterior skin incision with full-thickness fasciocutaneous flaps is advised for versatility and to avoid injury to the superficial cutaneous nerves; however, a direct lateral skin incision is also acceptable.

If the radial head fracture is not reconstructable, the coronoid fracture can usually be accessed via the lateral approach following radial neck osteotomy in preparation for radial head arthroplasty. Otherwise, a medial approach can be suitable for exposure, depending on the fracture configuration. Irrespective, repair of a type 2 or 3 coronoid fracture should be performed to stabilize the elbow to varus loading, which is encountered with shoulder abduction during daily activities.[34]

Coronoid fracture fixation is accomplished with sutures, screws, or plates, depending on the size, approach, and comminution of the fragment. During the surgical approach, the coronoid fragment will appear larger than measured on preoperative CT scan; cartilage is a mean 3 mm thick at the coronoid tip, with greater ulnar height and length associated with thicker cartilage.[35] For smaller or comminuted fractures unlikely to be repaired with screw fixation, the authors of this chapter use an anterior cruciate ligament drill guide to create two tunnels from the dorsal ulna and secure the capsule and fragments with a nonabsorbable suture. Larger fragments should be fixed with screws in a dorsal to volar trajectory. The biomechanical strength of two different screw trajectories was assessed in coronoid fixation and the posterior to anterior screw was found to be stronger, stiffer, and technically easier to use.[36]

In the younger, athletic population, after the coronoid is secured, all radial head fractures should be fixed. However, if stable fixation cannot be obtained, radial head arthroplasty is indicated to provide elbow stability.[12] Because the radial head is a primary stabilizer to PLRI, especially in the context of a coronoid fracture, the orthopaedic surgeon should not hesitate to proceed with arthroplasty to restore stability. A review of 24 patients treated for terrible triad injuries compared the results for those who underwent radial head open reduction and internal fixation with arthroplasty.[37] Good results were noted for the entire group, and patients in the radial head arthroplasty group scored higher in the Disabilities of the Arm, Shoulder and Hand assessment. Although these outcomes may not translate to the younger athletic population, they stress the importance of a radial head stabilized using either fixation or arthroplasty.

Varus PMRI

Anteromedial coronoid facet fractures are associated with varus PMRI.[38] This fracture pattern is described in O'Driscoll's comprehensive coronoid facture classification,[39] which is based on the anatomic location of the main fragments: the tip, the anteromedial facet, and the basal coronoid, often as noted on CT. Anteromedial facet fractures are further subclassified based on tip and sublime tubercle involvement.

A biomechanical study reported that PMRI increases with the size of the anteromedial coronoid fracture.[40] The instability associated with small O'Driscoll subtype 1 anteromedial coronoid facet fractures can be improved using LUCL repair alone, whereas larger fractures require bony fixation in addition to LCL repair to achieve stability.

Exposure of an anteromedial coronoid fracture is possible via the approach through the floor of the ulnar nerve, flexor carpi ulnaris splitting, or Hotchkiss over-the-top approaches, although access to the proximal ulna for plate application is limited in the over-the top approach.[41]

Type 2 anteromedial coronoid fractures were assessed and a treatment algorithm created based on the fragment size and the stability to varus and pronation stress testing under fluoroscopy. Selective fixation of the anteromedial coronoid, LUCL repair, or a combination of both were indicated for increasingly unstable patterns.[42]

Distal Triceps Injuries

Distal triceps tendon injuries are less common than distal biceps tendon ruptures, and diagnosis is often missed acutely because of edema and pain. Patients report weakness and pain, but may have some active elbow extension because of an intact lateral triceps expansion. On clinical examination, patients will have difficulty with extension against gravity and a palpable defect in the extensor mechanism may be present. Standard radiography should be performed because avulsion of an associated olecranon traction spur with the distal triceps tendon can be seen on the lateral view as a sign of proximal tendon retraction. Ultrasonography or MRI

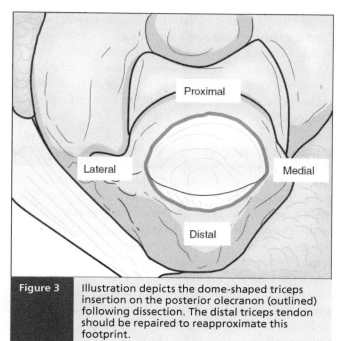

Figure 3 Illustration depicts the dome-shaped triceps insertion on the posterior olecranon (outlined) following dissection. The distal triceps tendon should be repaired to reapproximate this footprint.

are useful to confirm and characterize the rupture location in cases that are unclear or to assess for other pathology.

An anatomic cadaver study was performed to quantify tendon insertion characteristics.[43] The triceps tendon insertion is a confluence of the long, lateral, and medial heads on the posterior surface of the olecranon in a dome shape. At the insertion site on the olecranon, the medial head is deep to both the long and lateral heads. The mean triceps insertion footprint was 20.9 mm wide and 13.4 mm long (**Figure 3**).

Partial triceps tendon ruptures of the medial head insertion have been reported. Following an appropriate trial of nonsurgical management for patients with persistent pain and dysfunction, surgery can be suggested. Surgery is typically performed open; however, an arthroscopic repair technique has been described that uses suture anchors. Surgical repair for partial triceps tendon injuries has been reported as successful at eliminating pain and improving strength.[44]

Complete distal triceps tendon avulsions are debilitating and result in pain and weakness. Presently, in the younger athletic population, primary repair allows for early rehabilitation and predictably good outcomes. Primary open repair with transosseous tunnels or suture anchors have both been described. In addition triceps repair, the lateral triceps expansion, if disrupted, should be repaired because it constitutes a substantial portion of the total tendon width.[43] To re-create the full depth of the triceps tendon insertion, a double-row repair has been described using Keith needles and nonabsorbable, braided sutures with anchors for the superficial layer.[45] Repair is most successful when performed within the first 3 weeks; all patients in a 2003 series regained 4/5 manual strength, but a mean of 10° of terminal extension was lost.[46]

Distal Biceps Injuries

Distal biceps tendon avulsion injuries are common and occur most frequently in the dominant extremity of middle-aged men. Typically, the mechanism of injury is a sudden eccentric muscle contraction that occurs while lifting heavy loads. The underlying pathophysiology is most likely related to degenerative changes to the tendon at its insertion on the bicipital tuberosity. Vascular, inflammatory, and mechanical factors are thought to be associated with biceps avulsion injuries.

Patients will often hear an audible snap or pop at the time of injury and report pain and weakness to resisted elbow supination and flexion. Physical examination usually identifies an elevated muscle belly, an abnormal hook test result, and loss of the normal rise and fall of the biceps muscle with forearm rotation. Recently, a study suggested that three physical examination special tests to diagnose complete distal biceps tendon ruptures can expedite diagnosis and avoid the need for MRI or ultrasonography. Positive hook test results, passive forearm pronation, and biceps crease interval test together had 100% sensitivity and specificity for a complete distal biceps rupture. If test results were negative or equivocal, MRI was performed to detect partial injuries.[47]

Partial rupture of the distal biceps tendon can also produce pain and weakness and often results in a delay in diagnosis. The direct radial tuberosity compression test, in which the examiner compresses 2.5 cm distal to the radiocapitellar joint to elicit pain with passive pronation and supination of the forearm,[48] was performed in patients with a presumed partial rupture. MRI can assist with the diagnosis by visualizing the biceps insertion. The flexed, abducted, supinated view is a method of patient positioning in the MRI unit, with the shoulder fully abducted so the arm is beside the head, the elbow flexed to 90°, and the forearm fully supinated. These images along the long axis of the tendon from the musculotendinous junction to the insertion ease interpretation and reduce errors due to volume averaging.[49]

Nonsurgical management can be considered in patients with acute distal biceps tendon injuries. Good results have been reported with nonsurgical management and historic reports suggested a 40% loss of supination and 30% loss of flexion strength.[50] In a more recent, larger study of 18 patients treated nonsurgically at a median of 38 months, supination strength recovered to 63% and flexion strength to 93% compared with the uninjured side.[51]

In the only prospective randomized controlled trial, the outcomes and complications of single- versus double-incision distal biceps tendon repair were compared.[52] At 2-year follow-up, no clinically substantial differences were reported in the Disabilities of the Arm, Shoulder and Hand score, the Patient-Rated Elbow Evaluation score, the American Shoulder and Elbow Surgeon elbow score, or elbow range of motion. Additionally, no differences were found in supination, pronation, or extension strength; however, the double-incision repair group had substantially greater flexion strength at follow-up. Furthermore, the complication rate was significantly higher in the single-incision group. Most complications were transient neurapraxias of the lateral antebrachial cutaneous nerve.

Excellent clinical outcomes and advances in fixation techniques have enabled a resurgence of single-incision technique; however, some concern exists that supination strength may not be fully reestablished. Single-incision repairs place the insertion of the distal biceps tendon more anteriorly and midline than the native insertion.[53] The radial tuberosity is oriented at a mean of 56° ulnar to the midsagittal plane of the radius (range, 43° to 67°). One study showed that the anatomic insertion on the radial tuberosity could not be re-created using an anterior incision, and that this may be responsible for supination weakness.[54] A recent systematic review of repair techniques for distal biceps tendon ruptures found that bone tunnel (20.4%) and cortical button (0) methods had substantially lower complication rates compared with suture anchors (26.4%) and intraosseous screws (44.8%)[55,56] (Figure 4).

Irrespective of the approach or type of fixation used, surgeons should be confident in their knowledge of the anatomy and the best exposure to minimize injury to the lateral antebrachial cutaneous nerve of the forearm, the posterior interosseous nerve, and the recurrent branch of the radial artery. Repairs are easiest in the first 2 weeks following avulsion before scarring of the tendon track has occurred. In subacute and chronic cases, a primary repair should still be attempted even if up to 90° to 100° of elbow flexion is required to reduce the tendon to the tuberosity. Repairs in extreme flexion eventually lengthen and still yield good results.[57] In chronic cases in which primary repair is not possible, autologous or allograft distal biceps tendon reconstruction is an option that yields satisfactory outcomes.

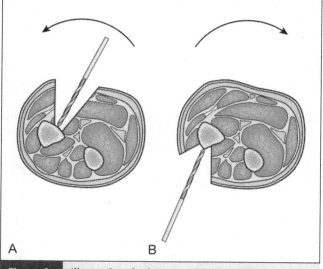

| Figure 4 | Illustration depicts an axial schematic of the forearm at the level of the radial tuberosity. **A,** Drill placement from an anterior approach with the forearm in full supination. The results indicate a limited ability to repair the tendon to its anatomic footprint. **B,** Drill trajectory for the double-incision with the forearm in pronation, re-creating the anatomic insertion of the biceps brachii tendon. |

Summary

Acute elbow injuries require a thorough physical examination and often advanced imaging to determine the full extent of injury and instability patterns. Examination under anesthetia and intraoperatively helps to determine the plan of sequential repair of primary and secondary stabilizers and dictates postoperative rehabilitation. Achieving a concentric reduction and allowing early range of motion is critical to maximizing outcomes of acute elbow injuries.

Key Study Points

- Primary stabilizers of the elbow include the ulnohumeral joint, LUCL, and the anterior bundle of the MCL. Secondary stabilizers include the radial head, the common flexor and extensor origins, and the joint capsule. These structures should be assessed with every elbow injury.
- Simple elbow dislocations benefit greatly from an early rehabilitation protocol started within 7 to 10 days and routine imaging to ensure concentric reduction.
- PLRI of the elbow can be difficult to diagnose, and patients presenting with locking or snapping should be assessed for subtle instability findings.

Key Study Points (continued)

- Complex elbow fractures and instability cases should be assessed with CT to fully delineate the bony injury and plan fixation strategies.
- Varus PMRI typically requires fixation of the anteromedial coronoid facet, and/or repair of the LUCL to regain stability.

Annotated References

1. Appelboam A, Reuben AD, Benger JR, et al: Elbow extension test to rule out elbow fracture: Multicentre, prospective validation and observational study of diagnostic accuracy in adults and children. *BMJ* 2008;337:a2428.

   This multicenter prospective development and validation of a study was performed to rule out elbow fracture in both children and adults as they present to the emergency department. Level of evidence: I.

2. Bethapudi S, Robinson P, Engebretsen L, Budgett R, Vanhegan IS, O'Connor P: Elbow injuries at the London 2012 Summer Olympic Games: Demographics and pictorial imaging review. *AJR Am J Roentgenol* 2013;201(3):535-549.

   This review analyzed elbow injuries sustained during the 2012 London Summer Olympic Games. Level of evidence: III.

3. Carlisle JC, Goldfarb CA, Mall N, Powell JW, Matava MJ: Upper extremity injuries in the National Football League: Part II: elbow, forearm, and wrist injuries. *Am J Sports Med* 2008;36(10):1945-1952.

4. O'Driscoll SW, Jupiter JB, King GJ, Hotchkiss RN, Morrey BF: The unstable elbow. *Instr Course Lect* 2001;50:89-102.

5. Hotchkiss RN: Displaced fractures of the radial head: Internal fixation or excision? *J Am Acad Orthop Surg* 1997;5(1):1-10.

6. Rineer CA, Guitton TG, Ring D: Radial head fractures: Loss of cortical contact is associated with concomitant fracture or dislocation. *J Shoulder Elbow Surg* 2010;19(1):21-25.

   This retrospective review of a large series of radial head fractures was performed to determine the clinical significance of loss of cortical contact in Mason type 2 injuries. Level of evidence: IV.

7. Nalbantoglu U, Gereli A, Kocaoglu B, Aktas S, Turkmen M: Capitellar cartilage injuries concomitant with radial head fractures. *J Hand Surg Am* 2008;33(9):1602-1607.

8. Bruinsma W, Kodde I, de Muinck Keizer RJ, et al: A randomized controlled trial of nonoperative treatment versus open reduction and internal fixation for stable, displaced,

partial articular fractures of the radial head: The RAMBO trial. *BMC Musculoskelet Disord* 2014;15(1):147.

This study describes the RAMBO trial to determine optimal treatment of Mason type 2 radial head fractures; the results of this trial are pending.

9. Lindenhovius AL, Felsch Q, Ring D, Kloen P: The long-term outcome of open reduction and internal fixation of stable displaced isolated partial articular fractures of the radial head. *J Trauma* 2009;67(1):143-146.

This study reported on long-term follow-up of surgically treated Mason type 2 radial head fractures in 16 patients. Level of evidence: IV.

10. Furey MJ, Sheps DM, White NJ, Hildebrand KA: A retrospective cohort study of displaced segmental radial head fractures: Is 2 mm of articular displacement an indication for surgery? *J Shoulder Elbow Surg* 2013;22(5):636-641.

This retrospective cohort study reported on whether successful nonsurgical treatment of radial head fractures is influenced by displacement greater or less than 2 mm. No evidence was found to support 2 mm of fracture displacement as an indication for surgery. Level of evidence: II.

11. Paschos NK, Mitsionis GI, Vasiliadis HS, Georgoulis AD: Comparison of early mobilization protocols in radial head fractures. *J Orthop Trauma* 2013;27(3):134-139.

This prospective, randomized controlled study compared two early motion protocols with 1 week of cast immobilization after radial head fracture. Level of evidence: I.

12. Ring D, Quintero J, Jupiter JB: Open reduction and internal fixation of fractures of the radial head. *J Bone Joint Surg Am* 2002;84-A(10):1811-1815.

13. Ring D, King G: Radial head arthroplasty with a modular metal spacer to treat acute traumatic elbow instability. Surgical technique. *J Bone Joint Surg Am* 2008;90(Suppl 2 Pt 1):63-73.

14. Zunkiewicz MR, Clemente JS, Miller MC, Baratz ME, Wysocki RW, Cohen MS: Radial head replacement with a bipolar system: A minimum 2-year follow-up. *J Shoulder Elbow Surg* 2012;21(1):98-104.

The short-term clinical and radiographic results of 29 patients with a bipolar radial head prosthesis were reported. Level of evidence: IV.

15. Stoneback JW, Owens BD, Sykes J, Athwal GS, Pointer L, Wolf JM: Incidence of elbow dislocations in the United States population. *J Bone Joint Surg Am* 2012;94(3):240-245.

The epidemiology of simple elbow dislocations was recorded by the National Electronic Injury Surveillance System database. Level of evidence: II.

16. Schreiber JJ, Warren RF, Hotchkiss RN, Daluiski A: An online video investigation into the mechanism of elbow dislocation. *J Hand Surg Am* 2013;38(3):488-494.

This video analysis reviewed arm position and deforming forces during elbow dislocations from YouTube.com and noted that most elbow extensions occur with the elbow in relative extension. Level of evidence: IV.

17. Lee AT, Schrumpf MA, Choi D, et al: The influence of gravity on the unstable elbow. *J Shoulder Elbow Surg* 2013;22(1):81-87.

This biomechanical assessment of seated, overhead, and hinged-brace elbow rehabilitaiton protocols reported on the optimal protocol for unstable elbows.

18. Pipicelli JG, Chinchalkar SJ, Grewal R, King GJ: Therapeutic implications of the radiographic "drop sign" following elbow dislocation. *J Hand Ther* 2012;25(3):346-353, quiz 354.

A description of the ulnohumeral drop sign and a therapeutic program to aid in a congruent joint reduction is based on ligament injury pattern.

19. Alolabi B, Gray A, Ferreira LM, Johnson JA, Athwal GS, King GJ: Rehabilitation of the medial- and lateral collateral ligament-deficient elbow: An in vitro biomechanical study. *J Hand Ther* 2012;25(4):363-373.

This biomechanical study used cadaver elbows in an elbow motion simulator to describe safe positions for the rehabilitation of complex elbow injuries.

20. Anakwe RE, Middleton SD, Jenkins PJ, McQueen MM, Court-Brown CM: Patient-reported outcomes after simple dislocation of the elbow. *J Bone Joint Surg Am* 2011;93(13):1220-1226.

A trauma center review of 110 patients with simple elbow dislocations described outcome and patient satisfaction. Level of evidence: IV.

21. Duckworth AD, Ring D, Kulijdian A, McKee MD: Unstable elbow dislocations. *J Shoulder Elbow Surg* 2008;17(2):281-286.

22. O'Driscoll SW, Bell DF, Morrey BF: Posterolateral rotatory instability of the elbow. *J Bone Joint Surg Am* 1991;73(3):440-446.

23. Lattanza LL, Chu T, Ty JM, et al: Interclinician and intraclinician variability in the mechanics of the pivot shift test for posterolateral rotatory instability (PLRI) of the elbow. *J Shoulder Elbow Surg* 2010;19(8):1150-1156.

Biomechanical testing was performed to determine the influence of training level on the performance of the lateral pivot shift test.

24. Mehta JA, Bain GI: Posterolateral rotatory instability of the elbow. *J Am Acad Orthop Surg* 2004;12(6):405-415.

25. Kim BS, Park KH, Song HS, Park SY: Ligamentous repair of acute lateral collateral ligament rupture of the elbow. *J Shoulder Elbow Surg* 2013;22(11):1469-1473.

Clinical outcomes of lateral ligament repair for 19 patients with acute PLRI were reported. Level of evidence: IV.

26. Lee YC, Eng K, Keogh A, McLean JM, Bain GI: Repair of the acutely unstable elbow: Use of tensionable anchors. *Tech Hand Up Extrem Surg* 2012;16(4):225-229.

A technique for the use of tensionable suture anchors for the repair of collateral ligaments is described.

27. Sanchez-Sotelo J, Morrey BF, O'Driscoll SW: Ligamentous repair and reconstruction for posterolateral rotatory instability of the elbow. *J Bone Joint Surg Br* 2005;87(1):54-61.

28. Baghdadi YM, Morrey BF, O'Driscoll SW, Steinmann SP, Sanchez-Sotelo J: Revision allograft reconstruction of the lateral collateral ligament complex in elbows with previous failed reconstruction and persistent posterolateral rotatory instability. *Clin Orthop Relat Res* 2014;472(7):2061-2067.

A case series documented the outcomes of elbows treated with revision allograft reconstruction of the LCL for persistent PLRI after failure of index surgery. Level of evidence: IV.

29. Giannicola G, Polimanti D, Bullitta G, Scacchi M: Negative prognostic factors in complex elbow instability: A prospective study on 76 patients. *J Orthop Traumatol* 2013;14(Suppl 1):S38.

A cohort of 78 patients with complex elbow instability was reviewed to determine negative prognostic factors. Level of evidence: III.

30. Jeon IH, Micic ID, Yamamoto N, Morrey BF: Osborne-cotterill lesion: An osseous defect of the capitellum associated with instability of the elbow. *AJR Am J Roentgenol* 2008;191(3):727-729.

31. Guitton TG, Ring D: Nonsurgically treated terrible triad injuries of the elbow: Report of four cases. *J Hand Surg Am* 2010;35(3):464-467.

Case series reported on four patients with terrible triad injuries treated nonsurgically. Level of evidence: IV.

32. Chan K, MacDermid JC, Faber KJ, King GJ, Athwal GS: Can we treat select terrible triad injuries nonoperatively? *Clin Orthop Relat Res* 2014;472(7):2092-2099.

Specific indications for nonsurgical treatment of terrible triad injuries and the results of treatment were reported for 12 patients. Level of evidence: IV.

33. Pugh DM, Wild LM, Schemitsch EH, King GJ, McKee MD: Standard surgical protocol to treat elbow dislocations with radial head and coronoid fractures. *J Bone Joint Surg Am* 2004;86-A(6):1122-1130.

34. Hartzler RU, Llusa-Perez M, Steinmann SP, Morrey BF, Sanchez-Sotelo J: Transverse coronoid fracture: When does it have to be fixed? *Clin Orthop Relat Res* 2014;472(7):2068-2074.

This biomechanical cadaver study assessed the effect of a 50% coronoid fracture and fixation on elbow stability with and without an intact radial head.

35. Rafehi S, Lalone E, Johnson M, King GJ, Athwal GS: An anatomic study of coronoid cartilage thickness with special reference to fractures. *J Shoulder Elbow Surg* 2012;21(7):961-968.

A CT study was performed to determine the thickness of cartilage on the coronoid tip.

36. Moon JG, Zobitz ME, An KN, O'Driscoll SW: Optimal screw orientation for fixation of coronoid fractures. *J Orthop Trauma* 2009;23(4):277-280.

This biomechanical study assessed optimal screw orientation for the fixation of coronoid fractures.

37. Leigh WB, Ball CM: Radial head reconstruction versus replacement in the treatment of terrible triad injuries of the elbow. *J Shoulder Elbow Surg* 2012;21(10):1336-1341.

The results following surgical repair of terrible triad injuries were reviewed in 23 patients. Level of evidence: III.

38. Doornberg JN, Ring DC: Fracture of the anteromedial facet of the coronoid process. *J Bone Joint Surg Am* 2006;88(10):2216-2224.

39. O'Driscoll SW, Jupiter JB, Cohen MS, Ring D, McKee MD: Difficult elbow fractures: Pearls and pitfalls. *Instr Course Lect* 2003;52:113-134.

40. Pollock JW, Brownhill J, Ferreira L, McDonald CP, Johnson J, King G: The effect of anteromedial facet fractures of the coronoid and lateral collateral ligament injury on elbow stability and kinematics. *J Bone Joint Surg Am* 2009;91(6):1448-1458.

A biomechanical study assessed the effect of various sizes of anteromedial coronoid facet fracture and the influence of LCL repair on elbow stability.

41. Huh J, Krueger CA, Medvecky MJ, Hsu JR; Skeletal Trauma Research Consortium: Medial elbow exposure for coronoid fractures: FCU-split versus over-the-top. *J Orthop Trauma* 2013;27(12):730-734.

A cadaver dissection compared the exposure obtained by the flexor carpi ulnaris–splitting versus the Hotchkiss over-the-top approach.

42. Rhyou IH, Kim KC, Lee JH, Kim SY: Strategic approach to O'Driscoll type 2 anteromedial coronoid facet fracture. *J Shoulder Elbow Surg* 2014;23(7):924-932.

The authors suggested a strategic approach to dealing with fractures of the anteromedial coronoid facet based on the O'Driscoll classification and the degree of lateral soft-tissue injury. Level of evidence: IV.

43. Keener JD, Chafik D, Kim HM, Galatz LM, Yamaguchi K: Insertional anatomy of the triceps brachii tendon. *J Shoulder Elbow Surg* 2010;19(3):399-405.

A cadaver dissection study detailed the triceps tendon anatomy and the lateral triceps expansion.

44. Athwal GS, McGill RJ, Rispoli DM: Isolated avulsion of the medial head of the triceps tendon: An anatomic study and arthroscopic repair in 2 cases. *Arthroscopy* 2009;25(9):983-988.

   The authors described the insertion of the triceps tendon and an arthroscopic repair technique for isolated medial head triceps avulsions. Level of evidence: IV.

45. Kokkalis ZT, Mavrogenis AF, Spyridonos S, Papagelopoulos PJ, Weiser RW, Sotereanos DG: Triceps brachii distal tendon reattachment with a double-row technique. *Orthopedics* 2013;36(2):110-116.

   The authors described a technique for a double-row repair of the triceps tendon using Keith needles and suture anchors, and the results for a series of patients were reviewed. Level of evidence: IV.

46. van Riet RP, Morrey BF, Ho E, O'Driscoll SW: Surgical treatment of distal triceps ruptures. *J Bone Joint Surg Am* 2003;85-A(10):1961-1967.

47. Devereaux MW, ElMaraghy AW: Improving the rapid and reliable diagnosis of complete distal biceps tendon rupture: A nuanced approach to the clinical examination. *Am J Sports Med* 2013;41(9):1998-2004.

   The physical examination for distal biceps tendon ruptures and an evidence-based diagnositic algorithm are described. Level of evidence: II.

48. Abboud JA, Ricchetti ET, Tjoumakaris FP, Bartolozzi AR, Hsu JE: The direct radial tuberosity compression test: A sensitive method for diagnosing partial distal biceps tendon ruptures. *Curr Orthop Pract* 2011;22(1):76-80.

   The authors describe and validate the direct radial tuberosity compression test to diagnose partial biceps tendon injuries. Level of evidence: II.

49. Giuffrè BM, Moss MJ: Optimal positioning for MRI of the distal biceps brachii tendon: Flexed abducted supinated view. *AJR Am J Roentgenol* 2004;182(4):944-946.

50. Morrey BF, Askew LJ, An KN, Dobyns JH: Rupture of the distal tendon of the biceps brachii. A biomechanical study. *J Bone Joint Surg Am* 1985;67(3):418-421.

51. Freeman CR, McCormick KR, Mahoney D, Baratz M, Lubahn JD: Nonoperative treatment of distal biceps tendon ruptures compared with a historical control group. *J Bone Joint Surg Am* 2009;91(10):2329-2334.

   The results of surgical and nonsurgical treatment are compared: nonsurgical treatment results in 63% of the supination strength that surgical treatment does; flexion strength is the same. Level of evidence: IV.

52. Grewal R, Athwal GS, MacDermid JC, et al: Single versus double-incision technique for the repair of acute distal biceps tendon ruptures: A randomized clinical trial. *J Bone Joint Surg Am* 2012;94(13):1166-1174.

   This is the only prospective, randomized controlled trial to evaluate the outcomes of distal biceps tendon repair using a single- versus double-incision technique. Level of evidence: I.

53. Schmidt CC, Diaz VA, Weir DM, Latona CR, Miller MC: Repaired distal biceps magnetic resonance imaging anatomy compared with outcome. *J Shoulder Elbow Surg* 2012;21(12):1623-1631.

   A substantial decrease in strength at 60° of supination appears to be an effect of an anterior tendon reattachment location. Level of evidence: III.

54. Hansen G, Smith A, Pollock JW, et al: Anatomic repair of the distal biceps tendon cannot be consistently performed through a classic single-incision suture anchor technique. *J Shoulder Elbow Surg* 2014;23(12):1898-1904.

   This retrospective review of single-incision distal biceps repairs with CT was performed to determine if the anatomic insertion on the radial tuberosity can be re-created. Level of evidence: IV.

55. Watson JN, Moretti VM, Schwindel L, Hutchinson MR: Repair techniques for acute distal biceps tendon ruptures: A systematic review. *J Bone Joint Surg Am* 2014;96(24):2086-2090.

   The authors conducted a systematic review of techniques for distal biceps tendon repair with a focus on complication rate. Level of evidence: IV.

56. Schmidt CC, Jarrett CD, Brown BT: The distal biceps tendon. *J Hand Surg Am* 2013;38(4):811-821, quiz 821.

57. Morrey ME, Abdel MP, Sanchez-Sotelo J, Morrey BF: Primary repair of retracted distal biceps tendon ruptures in extreme flexion. *J Shoulder Elbow Surg* 2014;23(5):679-685.

   This retrospective case-control study examined the outcomes of distal biceps repairs requiring repair in greater than 60° of flexion. Level of evidence: III.

Chapter 8

Chronic/Overuse Elbow Disorders

Champ L. Baker III, MD   Champ L. Baker Jr, MD

Abstract

Overuse disorders of the elbow are common and can be a substantial cause of pain and disability to the athlete. Despite increased understanding of the causes and pathoanatomy of elbow tendinopathy, a lack of consensus remains regarding optimal management. Many different nonsurgical and surgical interventions have been reported with varied outcomes. Irrespective of the methods chosen, nonsurgical treatment typically allows safe return to sport. Surgical intervention is reserved only for the few cases with recalcitrant symptoms.

Keywords: medial epicondylitis; lateral epicondylitis; tendinopathy

Introduction

Elbow tendinopathy is the most common cause of elbow pain. Competitive and recreational athletes, laborers, and office workers engaged in repetitive upper extremity activities are all susceptible to this painful, sometimes disabling condition. It remains a substantial cause of activity restriction, with lost time from sports, recreation, and occupation. Despite increased understanding of the causes and pathoanatomy of elbow tendinopathy, a lack of consensus remains regarding its optimal management. Multiple treatment options have been described, with most patients ultimately responding to nonsurgical care over an extended period. Many different surgical

procedures have been described for those patients with recalcitrant symptoms despite appropriate nonsurgical treatment. Optimal management of elbow tendinopathy requires a thorough understanding of the pathophysiology, clinical evaluation, available treatment options, and reported outcomes.

Medial Epicondylitis

Elbow tendinopathy of the flexor pronator origin arising from the medial epicondyle is commonly referred to as medial epicondylitis. Although lateral epicondylitis is diagnosed up to 7 to 10 times more frequently, medial elbow tendinopathy can cause substantial disability to athletes and those individuals with repetitive occupational requirements.[1,2] Athletes who are particularly susceptible to the development of medial epicondylitis include baseball players, golfers, and those involved in racquet sports such as tennis.[3] Medial epicondylitis primarily affects patients in the fourth or fifth decades of life.

Pathophysiology

The primary etiology appears to be repetitive overuse of or stress to the flexor pronator muscle origin. In the late cocking and early acceleration phases of the overhand throwing motion, high medial tensile forces and lateral compression forces are generated at the elbow. The extreme valgus forces are transmitted medially to the ulnar collateral ligament and the flexor pronator muscle group, which acts as an important secondary and dynamic stabilizer of the elbow. The repetitive stress and loading over time can result in tendon degeneration and tendinopathy in throwers. Similarly, overuse injuries are common in golfers, especially those who have poor technique. A recent electromyographic (EMG) analysis of amateur and professional golfers demonstrated substantially increased activity in the pronator teres in the trailing arm of the amateur golfers during the forward swing phase and a trend toward increased activity of the pronator teres during the acceleration phase compared with the professional golfers.[4] In tennis players, EMG analysis has showed substantially increased activity of the pronator

Dr. Champ L. Baker III or an immediate family member has stock or stock options held in Arthrex. Dr. Champ L. Baker, Jr, or an immediate family member has received royalties from Arthrex; serves as an unpaid consultant to Arthrex and Smith & Nephew; has stock or stock options held in Arthrex; and serves as a board member, owner, officer, or committee member of the American Orthopaedic Society for Sports Medicine.

© 2016 American Academy of Orthopaedic Surgeons

teres and flexor carpi radialis during the acceleration phase of the overhand serve.[5]

Repetitive overuse results in microscopic tears of the flexor pronator origin with subsequent tendinous repair and replacement with immature reparative tissue. Histologically, the tissue is characterized by the absence of inflammatory cells and the presence of fibroblasts, disorganized collagen, and vascular hyperplasia. This tendon degeneration has been termed angiofibroblastic tendinosis.[3,6,7] In medial epicondylitis, the pathologic tendinosis tissue most commonly involves the pronator teres and the flexor carpi radialis. In one study of surgical treatment of 50 elbows, the degenerated tissue was localized at the flexor carpi radialis–pronator teres interval in 56% of cases, the flexor carpi ulnaris in 12%, and diffuse changes were noted in the common flexor origin in the remaining 32%.[3]

Evaluation

Patients with medial elbow tendinopathy tend to report a gradual onset of elbow pain localized to the medial epicondyle and over the flexor pronator muscle mass. Pain is increased with the offending activity such as throwing or playing golf. Physical examination typically reveals tenderness over the flexor pronator origin anterior and distal to the medial epicondyle. Pain on resisted pronation of the forearm has been found to be the most sensitive physical examination finding.[8] Pain can also be reproduced from resisted wrist flexion. Grip strength can be decreased as well. The examination of the athlete with medial elbow pain should also include a complete evaluation of the integrity of the ulnar collateral ligament and assessment for ulnar neuritis, both of which can coexist with medial epicondylitis. Ulnar neuritis has been reported in up to 60% of patients ultimately requiring surgery for medial epicondylitis.[3,8-11]

Plain radiographs are typically normal, although calcifications can sometimes be seen adjacent to the medial epicondyle. Although primarily a clinical diagnosis, advanced imaging can help evaluate for suspected associated conditions. One study evaluated the MRI findings of 13 patients with a clinical diagnosis of medial epicondylitis.[12] Compared with age-matched control patients, the most specific MRI findings for medial epicondylitis are the presence of intermediate to high T2-weighted signal intensity or high T2-weighted signal intensity within the common flexor tendon and the presence of paratendinous soft-tissue edema. Another study found a sensitivity of 95% and specificity of 92% for ultrasonography in the diagnosis of clinical medial epicondylitis.[13] The most common positive ultrasonographic findings in patients with medial epicondylitis were focal hypoechoic regions demonstrating tendinopathy, focal anechoic areas indicating partial common flexor tendon tears, cortical irregularities, and tendon thickening. The use of ultrasonography in the office setting is increasing recently, especially in the treatment of medial and lateral elbow tendinopathy with injections and other procedures.

Treatment

Although the existing literature is replete with reports of widely varied nonsurgical treatment options for lateral epicondylitis, relatively little is dedicated specifically to medial epicondylitis. Reported nonsurgical treatment options include rest, activity modifications, counterforce bracing, physical therapy, oral and topical NSAIDs, and injections with corticosteroids in addition to the more recent use of platelet-rich plasma (PRP) and autologous blood. Although commonly used in clinical practice, a randomized double-blind study comparing an injection of methylprednisolone with an injection of saline in patients with medial epicondylitis found only short-term benefit in pain relief at 6 weeks for patients in the methylprednisolone group. No substantial differences were found regarding pain relief at 3 months or 1 year after injection.[14] One case series investigated the use of dry needling and injections of autologous blood under ultrasonographic guidance in 20 patients with medial elbow tendinopathy.[15] At final follow-up of 10 months, 3 patients were considered to have unsuccessful results and the remaining patients demonstrated substantial decreases in their visual analog scale (VAS) pain scores and modified Nirschl pain scores. Although the use of PRP has been studied in the treatment of lateral epicondylitis, to date, no reports are available on the treatment of medial elbow tendinopathy.

Successful nonsurgical treatment has been reported in 85% to 90% of cases.[8,11] Surgical treatment is reserved for those patients with refractory symptoms even after at least 6 months of nonsurgical care. In contrast to the numerous reports of surgical treatment of lateral elbow tendinopathy, few reports regarding surgical management of medial epicondylitis are published. Although percutaneous and open flexor releases[10] have been described, the current consensus for surgical treatment is open resection of pathologic tendinosis tissue from the flexor pronator origin[3,8,9,11,16] (Figure 1). The success of débridement is substantially influenced by the presence of concurrent ulnar neuritis.[8,10] Overall, 87% good to excellent results were reported in 30 patients treated with flexor pronator origin débridement at a mean follow-up of 7 years; however, the status of the ulnar nerve correlated with the outcome.[8] Good to excellent results were found in 96% of patients with no or associated mild ulnar neuropathy

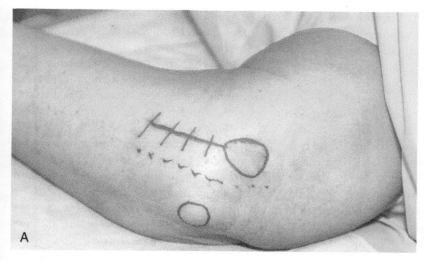

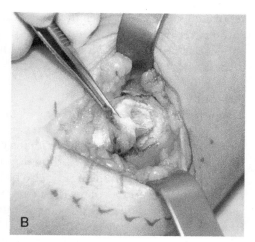

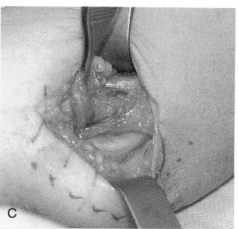

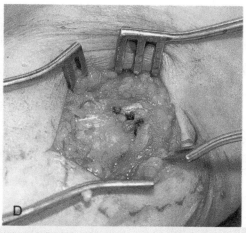

Figure 1 Photographs demonstrate open treatment of medial epicondylitis. **A,** The planned incision is marked, progressing distally from the medial epicondyle. The medial epicondyle, the olecranon, and the position of the ulnar nerve are outlined on the skin. **B,** A portion of the flexor pronator origin is detached from the medial epicondyle and reflected distally. A good cuff of tissue remains proximally for later repair. **C,** The tendinosis tissue is removed from the undersurface of the flexor pronator tendons. The ulnar nerve is identified and either simply decompressed or transposed, based on the presence and severity of preoperative ulnar nerve symptoms. **D,** The flexor pronator mass is securely repaired back to the medial epicondyle with heavy suture. (Reproduced from Baker CL III, Akins J, Baker CL Jr: Open treatment of medial and lateral epicondylitis, in Flatow E, Colvin AC, eds: *Atlas of Essential Orthopaedic Procedures*. Rosemont, IL, American Academy of Orthopaedic Surgeons, 2013, pp 39-42.)

compared with only 40% good to excellent results in those patients with moderate to severe ulnar neuropathy. Currently, no studies have evaluated the results of ulnar nerve decompression versus anterior transposition in patients with associated ulnar neuritis. Most case series detail high rates of pain relief and success with various outcome measures. Overall rate of return to the same level of sport ranges from 69% to 95%.[3,11] A recent case series of 22 elbows treated with open flexor pronator tendinosis resection detailed 93% improvement in mean VAS scores for pain, 94% improvement for pain at rest, and 83% improvement for pain with heavy activity at a mean follow-up of 36 months.[9] The patient's perception of their arm function as measured by the Disability of the Arm, Shoulder and Hand (DASH) scores substantially improved to the levels of the general, healthy population (mean improvement, 51.6 to 8.0), with 90% of patients overall satisfied with their outcome.

Lateral Epicondylitis

Lateral elbow tendinopathy, or tennis elbow, is the most common cause of lateral elbow pain in the adult population. Although it can occur in up to 50% of recreational tennis players, lateral elbow tendinopathy frequently affects other athletes and workers whose occupation requires repetitive wrist extension activities.[17] The dominant arm is most commonly involved with an equal incidence

1: Upper Extremity

in men and women in the general population. Acute onset of symptoms can be seen in young athletes, whereas chronic, recalcitrant symptoms typically occur in older patients. It primarily affects patients in their fourth or fifth decades of life.[18,19]

Pathophysiology

The primary etiology for lateral elbow tendinopathy appears to be repetitive overuse or stress to the wrist extensor origin. The extensor carpi radialis brevis (ECRB) is most commonly affected, although portions of the extensor digitorum communis can also be involved. Several authors have promoted the most commonly accepted theory of the pathogenesis of lateral epicondylitis.[6,7,17] Repetitive overuse results in microscopic tears of the ECRB. Attempted repair and failure of healing results in degenerative changes in the tendon characterized by fibroblasts, disorganized collagen, and vascular hyperplasia with an absence of inflammatory cells. The degenerated angiofibroblastic tendinosis tissue is similar histologically to that found in medial elbow tendinopathy. One study noted increased rates of cellular apoptosis and autophagic cell death in surgical specimens of ECRB tendon with associated collagen deterioration and breakdown.[20] A recent cadaver study demonstrated impingement of the ECRB origin on the lateral edge of the capitellum during extension as a potential anatomic contribution to the development of lateral epicondylitis.[21]

Evaluation

Patients with lateral elbow tendinopathy report lateral elbow pain that can radiate down the forearm. Occasionally, the patient may recall a specific injury to the area, but the history is typically of a gradual, progressive nature. Symptoms include weakness of grip strength affecting work activities, sports performance, and sometimes even activities of daily living. Difficulty picking up objects and shaking hands may be noted. On examination, point tenderness is located at and just anterior and distal to the lateral epicondyle. Pain is reproduced on resisted wrist extension, which can be greater with the elbow extended than with the elbow flexed. The differential diagnosis for lateral elbow pain includes synovial plica, radiocapitellar arthritis, posterolateral rotatory instability, radial tunnel syndrome, osteochondritis dissicans of the capitellum, and cervical radiculopathy.

Plain radiographs are typically normal, although calcifications can sometimes be seen adjacent to the lateral epicondyle. Although primarily a clinical diagnosis, advanced imaging can be useful in patients with symptoms refractory to treatment and those with atypical symptoms or presentation. MRI may demonstrate increased T2-weighted signal and extensor tendon thickening. MRI findings have been shown to correlate well with surgical and histologic findings.[22] However, one study noted that severity of MRI signal changes consistent with tendon degeneration did not correlate positively with patient symptoms.[23] Ultrasonography has been described as a useful diagnostic tool and as an adjunct to treatment of lateral epicondylitis. One study reported on 62 elbows with lateral epicondylitis that underwent ultrasonographic assessment of the common extensor tendon at diagnosis and after 6 months of physical therapy.[24] Pain and functional disability were assessed using a validated tennis elbow questionnaire. The presence of a large intrasubstance tear was found to be predictive of a poor outcome and less likely to respond to noninvasive treatment.

Treatment

In 1936, it was proposed that tennis elbow have only one type of treatment.[25] However, the increasing literature of myriad proposed nonsurgical treatment options with sometimes conflicting results, different outcome measurements, and varied levels of evidence makes direct comparison difficult. A recent systematic review of randomized controlled trials of nonsurgical treatment concluded no conclusive evidence exists of one preferred method of nonsurgical treatment of lateral epicondylitis.[26] An assessment of all nonsurgical treatment options must also consider the favorable natural history of the condition with resolution of approximately 80% of cases within 1 year.[27] In general, nonsurgical treatment options have included benign neglect, rest, activity modification, physical therapy, bracing or splinting, oral and topical medications including NSAIDs, extracorporeal shockwave therapy, and injections of corticosteroid and newer biologic alternatives. Irrespective of the type of nonsurgical care, almost 90% of patients ultimately respond successfully, sometimes after an extended period. Poor overall improvement has been noted in patients whose employment involves manual labor, who have dominant arm involvement, and who have higher levels of baseline pain.[28]

Initial treatment includes active rest and refraining from the repetitive offending activity. Modifications to improper technique, if contributory, must also be made. Physical therapy with stretching in conjunction with modalities including iontophoresis, friction massage, ultrasonography, and electrical stimulation can be instituted, although the efficacy of these modalities remains unproved. The addition of eccentric extensor strengthening has been investigated based on prior success with patellar and Achilles tendinopathy.[29] A recent systematic review evaluating the utility of eccentric extensor strengthening supported its inclusion as part of a multimodal treatment program for improved outcomes in patients with lateral epicondylitis.[30] Forearm counterforce straps and wrist extension splints are two common orthoses prescribed as part of a nonsurgical treatment regimen. Few studies have evaluated the use of orthoses, especially in comparison with other treatment modalities; however, the authors of a 2010 randomized trial compared a counterforce brace with a wrist extension splint and found greater pain relief in the wrist extension splint group after 6 weeks of treatment despite no functional differences between the groups.[31]

Although the pathology of elbow tendinopathy does not support an inflammatory component, both oral and topical NSAIDs are commonly prescribed. In a 2013 Cochrane review, 15 clinical trials were examined to determine the benefits and disadvantages of both oral and topical NSAIDs.[32] Although firm conclusions were not drawn from the available evidence, data suggest that topical NSAIDs are more effective than placebo in providing short-term pain relief in patients with lateral epicondylitis, with a small risk of a transient skin rash. Conflicting evidence regarding the use of oral NSAIDs precluded any recommendations, although gastrointestinal side effects were noted in several studies.[32] The use of other topical agents has been described, including compounding creams and nitric oxide. A prospective, randomized, double-blinded clinical trial compared patients receiving therapy and a glyceryl trinitrate transdermal patch with those receiving therapy and a placebo patch.[33] Patients in the glyceryl trinitrate group demonstrated substantially decreased elbow pain, reduced epicondyle tenderness, and improved wrist extensor strength compared with the placebo group. At 6 months, 81% of the treated patients were asymptomatic with activities of daily living versus 60% of those treated with rehabilitation alone. These results were not maintained in a follow-up study at 5 years after discontinuation of treatment, with no differences seen between groups, although both had improved compared with baseline.[34] Extracorporeal shockwave therapy has been proposed as an effective treatment option, but evidence remains mixed with one systematic review finding that most trials showed no benefit over placebo.[35]

Multiple injection therapies have been described, including the use of glucocorticoids, PRP, autologous blood, autologous tenocytes, sodium hyaluronate, botulinum toxin, polidocanol, and glycosaminoglycan polysulfate.[36] The use of glucocorticoid injections are common in clinical practice despite the lack of inflammation seen in chronic elbow tendinopathy. Randomized studies comparing glucocorticoid injection with naproxen or placebo[37] or with physiotherapy or a wait-and-see approach[27] demonstrated substantial improvements in pain and

function with glucocorticoid injection compared with other treatment arms at short-term evaluation of 4 to 6 weeks. No benefit remained at 12-month follow-up. A recent network meta-analysis of injection therapies in the treatment of lateral epicondylitis found no substantial benefit of glucocorticoid injections versus placebo in outcomes greater than 8 weeks.[36] Potential side effects from steroid injections include subcutaneous fat atrophy and skin depigmentation. In this same network meta-analysis, botulinum toxin was found to have a marginally significant reduction of pain intensity compared with placebo. Several high-level studies have evaluated the use of PRP injections. In one study, an injection of leukocyte-rich PRP was compared with an injection of corticosteroid using a peppering technique in a randomized controlled trial of 100 patients.[38] Outcomes were determined by VAS pain scores and DASH scores. The PRP cohort demonstrated substantial improvements in pain and function at 6 months and at 1 year compared with baseline and the corticosteroid cohort. These results were maintained in a follow-up study at 2 years: PRP-treated patients demonstrated 69% improvement in pain versus 36% improvement in the corticosteroid cohort. Similarly, the PRP cohort maintained substantial differences in improvement in function: almost 68% in the DASH outcome measurement versus only 16% in the corticosteroid group.[39] In a multicenter randomized, controlled trial of 230 patients, a leukocyte-rich PRP injection was compared with a control group of needling without PRP.[40] Substantial differences were not noted until final follow-up at 24 weeks when 84% of the PRP group was determined to have successful treatment compared with 68% of the control group. A 2013 a systematic review of the use of PRP in the treatment of lateral epicondylitis suggests PRP has been shown to be of benefit over corticosteroid treatment,[41] and a network meta-analysis concluded PRP and autologous blood injections were all substantially more efficacious than placebo.[36] Important questions remain regarding the cost-effectiveness of PRP, optimal preparation, and the timing and frequency of intervention, although these early results of biologic enhancement of healing appear promising.

Surgical treatment is recommended in patients with recalcitrant symptoms even after 6 months or more of nonsurgical care. Numerous reports of surgical management have been published with a wide variety of techniques used; the most common currently include percutaneous extensor tendon release,[42,43] open tendinosis resection,[7,16,19,43] and arthroscopic resection.[18] Most studies detail high rates of success with limited follow-up. A paucity of well-designed controlled studies support one technique over another; therefore, the type of procedure

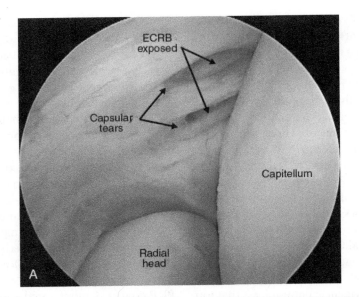

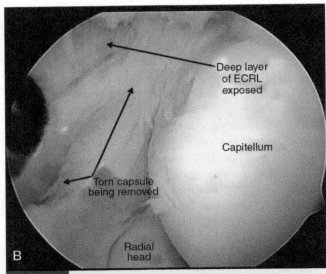

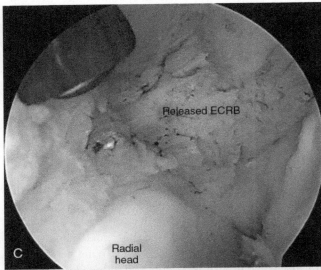

Figure 2 Arthroscopic images of treatment of lateral epicondylitis obtained from the proximal anteromedial portal. **A,** The capitellum, radial head, and capsular tears are visualized. **B,** After capsular débridement, the deep extensor carpi radialis longus is exposed. **C,** The diseased extensor carpi radialis brevis origin is resected off its origin using a radiofrequency probe. (Reproduced from Baker CL Jr: Arthroscopic release for lateral epicondylitis, in Yamaguchi K, King GJW, McKee MD, O'Driscoll SWM, eds: *Advanced Reconstruction: Elbow.* Rosemont, IL, American Academy of Orthopaedic Surgeons, 2007, pp 25-30.)

used should be based on surgeon comfort and experience. Currently, open treatment includes resection of the ECRB tendinosis tissue with or without repair of the extensor tendon origin. One study reported an overall improvement rate of 98% in a cohort of 88 elbows, with 85% of patients returning to full activities including sports.[7] A long-term follow-up study of the Nirschl open tendinosis resection technique reported 84% good to excellent results based on outcome measurements, with 93% of patients available at 10-year follow-up returning to sports.[19] Proponents of arthroscopic resection similarly detail high rates of

success with additional benefits of identifying and treating concurrent intra-articular pathology. Of 30 patients at a mean follow-up of 130 months,[18] none reported pain at rest, with overall high function demonstrated using the Mayo Elbow Performance Index; 23 (77%) reported pain as "much better," 6 (20%) as "better," and 1 (3%) as the same. Twenty-six patients (87%) were satisfied with the procedure and 28 (93%) stated they would undergo the surgery again if necessary. Arthroscopic resection of tendinosis tissue was determined to be an effective treatment of recalcitrant lateral epicondylitis. High rates of early success are maintained at long-term follow-up (Figure 2). A 2006 study compared 23 percutaneous releases, 41 arthroscopic procedures, and 38 open Nirschl procedures, all with a mean follow-up of 48 months.[43] No significant differences were reported among the groups regarding complications, recurrences, failures, VAS pain scores, or preoperative or postoperative Andrews-Carson scores. The rate at which these patients returned to their activities of daily living and work without discomfort could not be measured. Each method is considered a highly effective way to treat recalcitrant ECRB tendinosis.

Summary

Elbow tendinopathy is a common cause of pain and disability resulting from repetitive overuse activities. Nonsurgical treatment is successful in most cases, with surgical intervention reserved for those patients with continued symptoms after 6 months or more of treatment. Many treatment options are available, but currently, no consensus exists regarding optimal management. Additional well-designed comparative studies are needed to better evaluate an ideal treatment algorithm with comparison with the natural history of the condition.

Key Study Points

- Overuse disorders of the elbow are common and can be a substantial cause of pain and disability, resulting in loss of time from work and sport.
- Elbow tendinopathy is not an inflammatory condition but rather tendon degeneration resulting from continued microtrauma and failed attempts at healing.
- Many nonsurgical treatment options are available; rest and activity modification are paramount.
- The current literature provides no definitive recommendations regarding efficacy of nonsurgical interventions.
- Regardless of treatment type, most symptoms improve.

Annotated References

1. Leach RE, Miller JK: Lateral and medial epicondylitis of the elbow. *Clin Sports Med* 1987;6(2):259-272.

2. Ciccotti MC, Schwartz MA, Ciccotti MG: Diagnosis and treatment of medial epicondylitis of the elbow. *Clin Sports Med* 2004;23(4):693-705, xi.

3. Ollivierre CO, Nirschl RP, Pettrone FA: Resection and repair for medial tennis elbow. A prospective analysis. *Am J Sports Med* 1995;23(2):214-221.

4. Farber AJ, Smith JS, Kvitne RS, Mohr KJ, Shin SS: Electromyographic analysis of forearm muscles in professional and amateur golfers. *Am J Sports Med* 2009;37(2):396-401.

   This fine-wire electromyographic study noted differences in pronator teres activity during golf swings between professional and amateur golfers.

5. Morris M, Jobe FW, Perry J, Pink M, Healy BS: Electromyographic analysis of elbow function in tennis players. *Am J Sports Med* 1989;17(2):241-247.

6. Kraushaar BS, Nirschl RP: Tendinosis of the elbow (tennis elbow). Clinical features and findings of histological, immunohistochemical, and electron microscopy studies. *J Bone Joint Surg Am* 1999;81(2):259-278.

7. Nirschl RP, Pettrone FA: Tennis elbow. The surgical treatment of lateral epicondylitis. *J Bone Joint Surg Am* 1979;61-A(6):832-839.

8. Gabel GT, Morrey BF: Operative treatment of medial epicondylitis. Influence of concomitant ulnar neuropathy at the elbow. *J Bone Joint Surg Am* 1995;77(7):1065-1069.

9. Kwon BC, Kwon YS, Bae KJ: The fascial elevation and tendon origin resection technique for the treatment of chronic recalcitrant medial epicondylitis. *Am J Sports Med* 2014;42(7):1731-1737.

   The authors of this case series noted substantial improvements in VAS and DASH scores and improvements in grip strength using their tendinosis resection technique in 22 elbows at a mean 3-year follow-up. Level of evidence: IV.

10. Kurvers H, Verhaar J: The results of operative treatment of medial epicondylitis. *J Bone Joint Surg Am* 1995;77(9):1374-1379.

11. Vangsness CT Jr, Jobe FW: Surgical treatment of medial epicondylitis: Results in 35 elbows. *J Bone Joint Surg Br* 1991;73(3):409-411.

12. Kijowski R, De Smet AA: Magnetic resonance imaging findings in patients with medial epicondylitis. *Skeletal Radiol* 2005;34(4):196-202.

13. Park GY, Lee SM, Lee MY: Diagnostic value of ultrasonography for clinical medial epicondylitis. *Arch Phys Med Rehabil* 2008;89(4):738-742.

14. Stahl S, Kaufman T: The efficacy of an injection of steroids for medial epicondylitis: A prospective study of sixty elbows. *J Bone Joint Surg Am* 1997;79(11):1648-1652.

15. Suresh SP, Ali KE, Jones H, Connell DA: Medial epicondylitis: Is ultrasound guided autologous blood injection an effective treatment? *Br J Sports Med* 2006;40(11):935-939, discussion 939.

16. Schipper ON, Dunn JH, Ochiai DH, Donovan JS, Nirschl RP: Nirschl surgical technique for concomitant lateral and medial elbow tendinosis: A retrospective review of 53 elbows with a mean follow-up of 11.7 years. *Am J Sports Med* 2011;39(5):972-976.

    The authors of this case series reported substantial improvements in Nirschl tennis elbow scores, American Shoulder and Elbow Surgeons scores, and 85% good to excellent results with open combined medial and lateral tendinosis resection at long-term follow-up: 96% of patients returned to sports. Level of evidence: IV.

17. Nirschl RP: Elbow tendinosis/tennis elbow. *Clin Sports Med* 1992;11(4):851-870.

18. Baker CL Jr, Baker CL III: Long-term follow-up of arthroscopic treatment of lateral epicondylitis. *Am J Sports Med* 2008;36(2):254-260.

19. Dunn JH, Kim JJ, Davis L, Nirschl RP: Ten- to 14-year follow-up of the Nirschl surgical technique for lateral epicondylitis. *Am J Sports Med* 2008;36(2):261-266.

20. Chen J, Wang A, Xu J, Zheng M: In chronic lateral epicondylitis, apoptosis and autophagic cell death occur in the extensor carpi radialis brevis tendon. *J Shoulder Elbow Surg* 2010;19(3):355-362.

    Ten lateral epicondylitis surgical specimens were examined histologically. Increasing rates of tenocyte apoptosis and autophagic cell death were noted with associated increasing collagen degradation.

21. Bunata RE, Brown DS, Capelo R: Anatomic factors related to the cause of tennis elbow. *J Bone Joint Surg Am* 2007;89(9):1955-1963.

22. Potter HG, Hannafin JA, Morwessel RM, DiCarlo EF, O'Brien SJ, Altchek DW: Lateral epicondylitis: Correlation of MR imaging, surgical, and histopathologic findings. *Radiology* 1995;196(1):43-46.

23. Walton MJ, Mackie K, Fallon M, et al: The reliability and validity of magnetic resonance imaging in the assessment of chronic lateral epicondylitis. *J Hand Surg Am* 2011;36(3):475-479.

    There was substantial interobserver reliability and intraobserver agreement in the MRI evaluation of 21 elbows with clinical lateral epicondylitis. A negative correlation with tendinosis severity on MRI was seen with patient symptoms as reported by quick DASH and maximum pain levels.

24. Clarke AW, Ahmad M, Curtis M, Connell DA: Lateral elbow tendinopathy: Correlation of ultrasound findings with pain and functional disability. *Am J Sports Med* 2010;38(6):1209-1214.

    In this cohort study, 62 elbows with lateral epicondylitis were evaluated ultrasonographically and with Patient-Rated Tennis Elbow Evaluation (PRTEE) scores. After 6 months of physical therapy, PRTEE scores were again determined. Large intrasubstance tears and lateral collateral ligament tears seen on initial ultrasonography were predictive of a poor outcome with this form of nonsurgical treatment. Level of evidence: II.

25. Cyriax JH: The pathology and treatment of tennis elbow. *J Bone Joint Surg Am* 1936;178:921-940.

26. Sims SE, Miller K, Elfar JC, Hammert WC: Non-surgical treatment of lateral epicondylitis: A systematic review of randomized controlled trials. *Hand (N Y)* 2014;9(4):419-446.

    In a systematic review of 58 randomized, controlled trials evaluating nonsurgical treatment options for lateral epicondylitis, the authors determined no conclusive evidence of one preferred option. Corticosteroid injections can provide short-term pain relief with long-term advantages. Level of evidence: II.

27. Smidt N, van der Windt DA, Assendelft WJ, Devillé WL, Korthals-de Bos IB, Bouter LM: Corticosteroid injections, physiotherapy, or a wait-and-see policy for lateral epicondylitis: A randomised controlled trial. *Lancet* 2002;359(9307):657-662.

28. Haahr JP, Andersen JH: Prognostic factors in lateral epicondylitis: A randomized trial with one-year follow-up in 266 new cases treated with minimal occupational intervention or the usual approach in general practice. *Rheumatology (Oxford)* 2003;42(10):1216-1225.

29. Tyler TF, Thomas GC, Nicholas SJ, McHugh MP: Addition of isolated wrist extensor eccentric exercise to standard treatment for chronic lateral epicondylosis: A prospective randomized trial. *J Shoulder Elbow Surg* 2010;19(6):917-922.

    In a small trial of 21 elbows, patients with lateral epicondylitis were randomized to treatment groups of standard physical therapy and standard physical therapy with the addition of eccentric wrist extensor exercises. Patients in the eccentric exercise group improved substantially in all outcome measures of VAS, DASH, tenderness, and strength compared with control patients.

30. Cullinane FL, Boocock MG, Trevelyan FC: Is eccentric exercise an effective treatment for lateral epicondylitis? A systematic review. *Clin Rehabil* 2014;28(1):3-19.

    In a systematic review of eight randomized trials evaluating eccentric exercise, the authors reported most studies demonstrated improved clinical outcomes with the addition of eccentric exercise compared with those treatment programs without eccentric exercise.

31. Garg R, Adamson GJ, Dawson PA, Shankwiler JA, Pink MM: A prospective randomized study comparing a forearm strap brace versus a wrist splint for the treatment of lateral epicondylitis. *J Shoulder Elbow Surg* 2010;19(4):508-512.

    In a randomized clinical trial of 44 elbows, patients receiving a wrist splint compared with a forearm counterforce brace demonstrated improved pain relief after 6 weeks, although no functional differences were seen between groups based on American Shoulder and Elbow Surgeons or Mayo Elbow Performance scores.

32. Pattanittum P, Turner T, Green S, Buchbinder R: Non-steroidal anti-inflammatory drugs (NSAIDs) for treating lateral elbow pain in adults. *Cochrane Database Syst Rev* 2013;5:CD003686.

   A Cochrane review concluded that topical NSAIDs are more effective than placebo in providing short-term pain relief in patients with lateral epicondylitis, with a small risk of a transient skin rash. Conflicting evidence regarding the use of oral NSAIDs prevented any recommendations, although gastrointestinal side effects were noted in several studies.

33. Paoloni JA, Appleyard RC, Nelson J, Murrell GA: Topical nitric oxide application in the treatment of chronic extensor tendinosis at the elbow: A randomized, double-blinded, placebo-controlled clinical trial. *Am J Sports Med* 2003;31(6):915-920.

34. McCallum SD, Paoloni JA, Murrell GA: Five-year prospective comparison study of topical glyceryl trinitrate treatment of chronic lateral epicondylosis at the elbow. *Br J Sports Med* 2011;45(5):416-420.

   In this prospective follow-up study of a prior report, the authors reported no sustained benefit 5 years after treatment with a topical glyceryl patch compared with those treated with physical therapy alone.

35. Buchbinder R, Green SE, Youd JM, Assendelft WJ, Barnsley L, Smidt N: Systematic review of the efficacy and safety of shock wave therapy for lateral elbow pain. *J Rheumatol* 2006;33(7):1351-1363.

36. Krogh TP, Bartels EM, Ellingsen T, et al: Comparative effectiveness of injection therapies in lateral epicondylitis: A systematic review and network meta-analysis of randomized controlled trials. *Am J Sports Med* 2013;41(6):1435-1446.

   In this systematic review and meta-analysis of injection therapies for lateral epicondylitis, the authors concluded glucocorticoids were no better than placebo beyond 8 weeks, botulinum toxin was marginally better than placebo with risk of extensor paresis, and PRP and autologous blood were substantially better than placebo; however, most studies were associated with risks of bias.

37. Hay EM, Paterson SM, Lewis M, Hosie G, Croft P: Pragmatic randomised controlled trial of local corticosteroid injection and naproxen for treatment of lateral epicondylitis of elbow in primary care. *BMJ* 1999;319(7215):964-968.

38. Peerbooms JC, Sluimer J, Bruijn DJ, Gosens T: Positive effect of an autologous platelet concentrate in lateral epicondylitis in a double-blind randomized controlled trial: Platelet-rich plasma versus corticosteroid injection with a 1-year follow-up. *Am J Sports Med* 2010;38(2):255-262.

   This randomized, controlled trial compared leukocyte-rich PRP and corticosteroid injections. The PRP cohort demonstrated progressive improvement. At 1 year, the PRP cohort demonstrated 73% success in substantial pain reduction versus 49% in the corticosteroid group. Based on DASH scores, the PRP cohort demonstrated substantially more success at 73% versus 51%. Level of evidence: I.

39. Gosens T, Peerbooms JC, van Laar W, den Oudsten BL: Ongoing positive effect of platelet-rich plasma versus corticosteroid injection in lateral epicondylitis: A double-blind randomized controlled trial with 2-year follow-up. *Am J Sports Med* 2011;39(6):1200-1208.

   At 2-year follow-up of a randomized, controlled trial, PRP-treated patients demonstrated 69% improvement in pain versus 36% improvement in the corticosteroid cohort. Similarly, the PRP cohort maintained substantial improvement in function of almost 68% in the DASH outcome versus only 16% in the steroid group. Level of evidence: I.

40. Mishra AK, Skrepnik NV, Edwards SG, et al: Efficacy of platelet-rich plasma for chronic tennis elbow: A double-blind, prospective, multicenter, randomized controlled trial of 230 patients. *Am J Sports Med* 2014;42(2):463-471.

   In a multicenter randomized controlled trial of 230 patients, a leukocyte-rich PRP injection was compared with a control group of needling without PRP. Substantial differences were not noted until final follow-up of 24 weeks when 84% of the PRP group was determined to have successful treatment compared with 68% of the control group. Level of evidence: II.

41. Ahmad Z, Brooks R, Kang SN, et al: The effect of platelet-rich plasma on clinical outcomes in lateral epicondylitis. *Arthroscopy* 2013;29(11):1851-1862.

   In a systematic review of the clinical efficacy of PRP in the treatment of lateral epicondylitis, the authors concluded limited evidence in the use of PRP. Recommendations regarding future studies involving its use were made. Level of evidence: III.

42. Baumgard SH, Schwartz DR: Percutaneous release of the epicondylar muscles for humeral epicondylitis. *Am J Sports Med* 1982;10(4):233-236.

43. Szabo SJ, Savoie FH III, Field LD, Ramsey JR, Hosemann CD: Tendinosis of the extensor carpi radialis brevis: An evaluation of three methods of operative treatment. *J Shoulder Elbow Surg* 2006;15(6):721-727.

1: Upper extremity

Chapter 9

Hand and Wrist Injuries

Jeffrey Taylor Jobe, MD   A. Bobby Chhabra, MD

Abstract

Athletes commonly sustain injuries to the hand and wrist. An understanding of both common and uncommon injuries, diagnostic modalities and treatments of the athletes' hand and wrist, along with the most recent published data and treatment methods, are important to maximize treatment outcomes.

Keywords: hand and wrist injuries; hand fractures; carpal fractures; wrist instability; finger dislocations; return to play; skier's thumb; mallet finger; central slip; flexor pulley rupture; hook of hamate fracture; triangular fibrocartilage complex; scapholunate ligament; Bennett fracture; sagittal band; extensor carpi ulnaris tendinitis; flexor carpi radialis tendinitis; extensor carpi ulnaris instability; jersey finger; intersection syndrome; de Quervain; ganglion; ulnar tunnel syndrome; ulnar artery thrombosis

Introduction

Hand and wrist injuries in the athlete are frequently encountered by orthopaedic surgeons. Although treatment of many of these injuries is effective, management of these injuries can present a challenge to the physician. An understanding of diagnosis and treatment of common hand and wrist injuries in the athlete, along with guidelines for return to play will help the physician provide optimal care for a specific injury.

Dr. Chhabra or an immediate family member has received nonincome support (such as equipment or services), commercially derived honoraria, or other non–research-related funding (such as paid travel) from DePuy/Synthes. Neither Dr. Jobe nor any immediate family member has received anything of value from or has stock or stock options held in a commercial company or institution related directly or indirectly to the subject of this chapter.

Hand Injuries

Not only are the hands used in almost every sport for sport-specific tasks, but they are also instinctively used to protect the body from the initial impact of a fall or contact with another person. Hand injuries are common in athletes and occur in almost every sport played. Neglected injuries can have detrimental consequences; therefore, it is important to quickly and accurately identify and treat hand injuries.[1]

Metacarpal and Phalangeal Fractures

Metacarpal and phalangeal shaft fractures are the most common fractures and are frequently encountered in athletes. Most injuries can be treated nonsurgically in the general population, but athletes require special consideration. When treating hand fractures, "Deformity follows undertreatment, stiffness follows overtreatment, and deformity and stiffness follow poor treatment."[1]

Distal phalanx fractures (tuft fractures) are the most common hand fractures and require only short periods of immobilization (10 to 14 days). The nail bed should be inspected because this is a common associated injury. Substantial nail bed injuries require meticulous repair technique to avoid nail plate abnormalities.

More proximal fractures in the phalanges and metacarpal bones can usually be treated with approximately 3 weeks of immobilization followed by early protected range of motion to prevent stiffness if minimal displacement and no rotational deformity exist. Early edema control, along with motion and elevation, should be incorporated into therapy. Fractures of the metacarpal head are rare intra-articular fractures, most commonly occurring in the index finger. Surgery with Kirschner wires or minifragment plate and screws is required if more than 1 mm of intra-articular step-off exists. These injuries are commonly associated with fight bites, which should be treated with appropriate irrigation and débridement and a course of antibiotics.

Metacarpal neck fractures (boxer's fractures) usually occur in the ring and little fingers, although other metacarpal bones can be involved. Lateral radiographs are necessary to evaluate the amount of angular deformity;

15° of deformity can be tolerated in the index and middle finger metacarpals, 30° to 40° in the ring finger, and 50° to 60° in the little finger. The interossei are the deforming forces that cause dorsal angulation. Traditionally, an ulnar gutter splint has been applied for 2 to 3 weeks, but data from 2007 showed no difference in Disabilities of the Arm, Shoulder and Hand scores with buddy taping alone.[2] Malunion is common after metacarpal neck fractures, but is rarely a functional deficit in the athlete.[2,3] In rare circumstances, open reduction and internal fixation (ORIF), closed reduction and percutaneous pinning (CRPP), or an intramedullary technique can be considered if malunion is not tolerated, such as for a tennis player in whom the metacarpal head prominence in the palm can make gripping a racquet difficult.

For metacarpal shaft fractures, less angular deformity is tolerated than for metacarpal neck fractures: 10° for the index and middle fingers, and 30° for the ring and little fingers. Malrotation is unacceptable because 5° of malrotation results in 1.5 cm of digital overlap. Shortening is acceptable up to 5 mm, but 7° of extensor lag occurs with every 2 mm of shortening. ORIF is commonly performed in athletes with metacarpal shaft fractures if surgical criteria are met, but CRPP can be considered.[4,5]

Metacarpal base fractures are uncommon, usually stable, and minimally displaced. Displaced fractures at the base of the metacarpal can result in arthrosis. Fourth and fifth carpometacarpal (CMC) fracture-dislocations are unstable injuries and require pinning of the CMC joint.

Proximal phalanx shaft fractures result in volar angulation because the proximal fragment is flexed by the interossei, and the distal fragment is extended by the central slip. Middle phalangeal shaft fractures can have volar or dorsal angulation, depending on the location of the fracture. Malrotation is unacceptable, and only 10° of angulation in any plane is tolerable. CRPP can be considered, but ORIF with a plate in the athlete may be a better option. Oblique/spiral fractures can be treated with interfragmentary lag screws if the fracture line is twice the bone diameter.[5]

Phalangeal head fractures can be unicondylar or bicondylar. The collateral ligament attachment provides blood supply. Surgery must be considered with displaced unstable fractures, usually with ORIF with interfragmentary screws.[6]

Athletes can return to play with appropriate protection after the fracture is stable and sport-specific range of motion is obtained. Recent data have shown successful early return to play (less than 1 month) after ORIF for metacarpal and phalangeal fractures with appropriate protection.[7] Contact sports are not allowed without protection (casting or splinting) until 6 to 8 weeks after injury

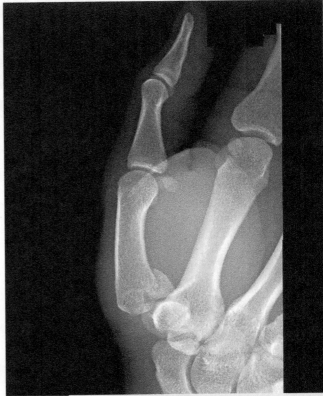

Figure 1 Radiograph shows a Bennett fracture. (Reproduced from Grewal R, Faber KJ, Graham TJ, Rettig LA: Hand and wrist injuries, in Kibler WB, ed: *Orthopaedic Knowledge Update: Sports Medicine*, ed 4. Rosemont, IL, American Academy of Orthopaedic Surgeons, 2009, pp 69-80.)

to ensure adequate healing.

Bennett fractures are intra-articular fractures that involve the base of the thumb and occur when an axial load is applied to the flexed and adducted thumb (Figure 1). The abductor pollicis longus displaces the metacarpal base proximally, and the anterior oblique ligament pulls the Bennett fragment to the base of the second metacarpal. Bennett fractures are surgical injuries and require CRPP or ORIF if the fragment is large enough. Extra-articular thumb metacarpal base fractures can tolerate up to 30° of angulation as a result of CMC joint hypermobility and most cases can be treated nonsurgically, but ORIF or CRPP should be considered in the high-level athlete for earlier rehabilitation and return to play.

Finger Dislocations

Dorsal dislocations of the proximal interphalangeal (PIP) joint are the most common finger dislocation. Simple dislocations are usually reducible with hyperextension of the middle phalanx followed by distal translation. The volar

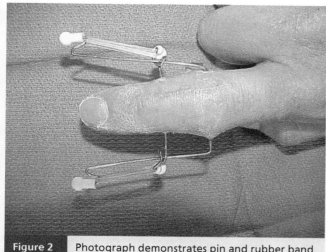

Figure 2 Photograph demonstrates pin and rubber band traction used to treat middle phalanx pilon fractures.

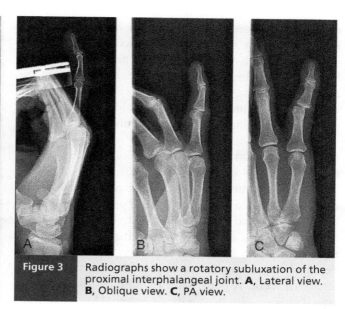

Figure 3 Radiographs show a rotatory subluxation of the proximal interphalangeal joint. **A,** Lateral view. **B,** Oblique view. **C,** PA view.

plate can block reduction. If stable after reduction, buddy taping and range of motion are initiated. If unstable, a dorsal blocking splint is applied. Avulsion fractures of the volar plate should be monitored carefully because a flexion contracture can develop.[8] Early return to play is possible with buddy taping based on comfort and stability after reduction.

Dorsal fracture-dislocations often involve fracture of the volar base of the middle phalanx. The Hastings classification summarizes these injuries and guides treatment, and is based on the size of the middle phalanx articular fragment. For Hastings type I fractures, less than 30% of the articular surface is considered stable. Type II fractures have 30% to 50% articular involvement and are considered tenuous. Type III fractures have more than 50% articular involvement and are considered unstable. If reducible, types I and II can be treated with a dorsal extension block splint, carefully decreasing the amount of flexion by 10° every week. Unstable fractures must be treated surgically using ORIF or hemihamate arthroplasty.[9,10] Chronic fracture-dislocations are treated using volar plate arthroplasty or hemihamate arthroplasty.[11] Pilon fractures of the base of the middle phalanx are treated using longitudinal traction (pin and rubber band traction) and immediate motion.[12] Good results have been obtained using pin and rubber band traction[13] (Figure 2).

Volar PIP dislocations are less common and are associated with a central slip disruption. After reduction, the PIP should be splinted in extension for 6 weeks to prevent a boutonnière deformity and allow healing of the central slip. If the dislocation is still unstable after reduction, pinning for 3 weeks is required.

Rotatory subluxation-dislocations of the PIP also can occur, leaving the central slip intact, but the condyle buttonholes through the central slip and lateral band (Figure 3). These injuries often require surgical intervention for reduction.

Skier's Thumb

Injury to the ulnar collateral ligament of the thumb metacarpophalangeal (MCP) joint is referred to as skier's thumb, or gamekeeper's thumb. A competent ulnar collateral ligament is critical for effective pinch.

It is important to obtain radiographs before stressing the MCP joint to avoid displacing an otherwise nondisplaced fracture. Physical examination is performed with a valgus stress applied to the thumb in both extension (testing the accessory ligament) and 30° flexion (proper ligament). The ulnar side of the joint should be palpated for a Stener lesion (both the proper and accessory ligament are retracted and lie on the adductor aponeurosis). The adductor aponeurosis interposition prevents direct ligament healing without surgery. More than 35° of laxity alone or more than 15° of laxity compared with the contralateral side is considered a positive test result. Stress radiographs are useful for identifying Stener lesions, as are MRIs and ultrasonographs.[14]

Incomplete acute tears and nondisplaced avulsion fractures are treated with a thumb spica cast for 4 weeks, followed by removable protective splinting for 3 more weeks with active range-of-motion exercises. Complete tears require open repair with suture anchors or bone tunnels placed at the site of the avulsion, which most commonly is the proximal phalanx. Although complete minimally retracted tears can heal with nonsurgical treatment, the tear will not heal in the setting of a Stener lesion because of adductor aponeurosis interposition. Strenuous activity is avoided for 3 months, with unrestricted return to sport usually at 2 to 3 months. Recent data have reported good long-term outcomes following repair with two suture anchors in collegiate football players. Skill position players were repaired acutely; lineman were able to complete the season with bracing or casting before undergoing repair.[15]

Extensor Tendon Injuries
Mallet Finger
Mallet finger occurs when the extensor tendon attachment to the distal phalanx becomes incompetent, resulting in inability to extend the distal phalanx. This can be either a soft-tissue or a bony avulsion. Soft-tissue mallets are treated with 6 to 8 weeks of extension. A slight residual extensor lag of approximately 10° should be expected after treatment. A bony mallet should be assessed with lateral radiographs, both without external force and with the joint held in extension to assess if the fracture reduces appropriately. Bony mallet injuries also are treated with 6 weeks of extension splinting. If the distal interphalangeal (DIP) joint is subluxated or the fragment is large and results in substantial articular incongruity, ORIF or dorsal block pinning should be considered (Figure 4). Chronic mallet fingers result in swan neck deformities. Recent data have shown good outcomes with splinting for soft-tissue mallets that were treated within 6 weeks of injury.[16] Previously, splinting at night for 1 month after cessation of full-time splinting has been performed, but recent data reported equivocal outcomes without night splinting.[17]

Central Slip Injury (Acute Boutonnière Deformity)
A boutonnière deformity is the result of a central slip rupture, triangular ligament attenuation, and volar migration of the lateral bands. On examination, the PIP joint is passively placed in extension; if the patient can maintain PIP extension, the triangular ligaments are likely intact and splinting usually provides good outcomes. The Elson test is used to assess a central slip rupture. The PIP is flexed to 90° and blocked while extension of the PIP is attempted and the DIP is assessed. The test result for a central slip injury is positive if the DIP becomes rigid or actively extends to neutral. Radiographs may show an avulsion fracture. A closed acute boutonnière injury is treated with extension splinting of the PIP for 6 weeks followed by 6 weeks of night splinting. Surgery is indicated if closed treatment fails, for open injuries, for large displaced avulsion fractures, or in the setting of an unstable volar PIP dislocation (Figure 5). For large fracture fragments, ORIF can be performed or the fragment can be excised and the tendon repaired with suture anchors.[11]

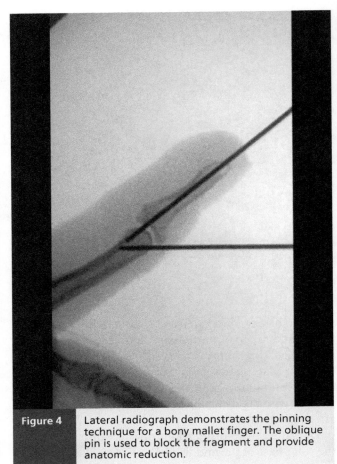

Figure 4 | Lateral radiograph demonstrates the pinning technique for a bony mallet finger. The oblique pin is used to block the fragment and provide anatomic reduction.

Sagittal Band Injury
If an extensor lag of the finger is present, laceration or rupture of the sagittal band should be considered, which results in ulnar subluxation of the extensor tendon. This injury, also known as boxer's knuckle, also can be associated with a capsular injury of the MCP joint. The middle finger is the most commonly affected. On examination, the patient is unable to initiate MCP joint extension, but can maintain extension after passive finger extension. The extensor tendon dislocates to the contralateral side when the MCP joint is flexed and reduces when the joint is extended. The mainstay of treatment of acute injuries in the general population is flexion block splinting of the MCP joint for 8 weeks, but in athletes, surgical repair must be considered, depending on when in the season the injury occurs and the athlete's preferences.[18] Numerous techniques can be used for repair, depending on the local soft-tissue availability and need for reconstruction. Patients with chronic injuries can undergo a trial of splinting, but surgery is required more often than for acute injuries.

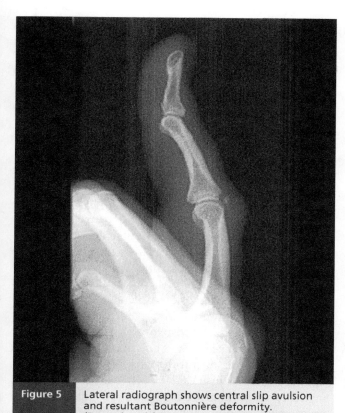

Figure 5   Lateral radiograph shows central slip avulsion and resultant Boutonnière deformity. (Reproduced from Grewal R, Faber KJ, Graham TJ, Rettig LA: Hand and wrist injuries, in Kibler WB, ed: *Orthopaedic Knowledge Update: Sports Medicine*, ed 4. Rosemont, IL, American Academy of Orthopaedic Surgeons, 2009, pp 69-80.)

Flexor Tendon Injuries

Jersey Finger

Jersey finger is the result of a flexor digitorum profundus avulsion from its insertion on the distal phalanx. The ring finger is most commonly involved. Physical examination reveals inability to flex the DIP. Ultrasonography can help assess the level of tendon retraction in a timely fashion, although MRI also has good results if performed soon enough postinjury. The Leddy classification is based on the level of retraction. In type I injuries, the flexor digitorum profundus is retracted to the palm and the vincula (blood supply) is compromised. Primary early repair (within 10 days) is warranted. Type II injuries involve a tendon that is retracted but still in the flexor sheath, at the level of the A2 pulley. Surgical repair is warranted and should be performed in a timely fashion, usually within 4 weeks. Type III injuries include a bone fragment that is caught on the A4 pulley. ORIF is performed on the fragment that involves the tendon insertion. Type IIIA injuries are less common and involve a bone fragment

and tendon retraction to the palm. ORIF is performed, as well as tendon repair, and should be done within 10 days as in type 1 injuries.[19]

Pulley Rupture

Flexor tendon pulley ruptures occur when a sudden extension force is generated on a flexed finger. This is most commonly seen in rock climbers when they slip and frequently affects the ring and middle finger. The patient will have acute pain over the flexor tendon. On examination, bowstringing may be visible if the A2 or A4 pulleys are involved and the patient will have difficulty making a full fist. Dynamic ultrasonography and MRI are useful in diagnosis.

Single-pulley ruptures should be immobilized for 10 to 14 days, followed by therapy for motion and taping or rings to support the pulleys. Multiple ruptured pulleys should be treated surgically. Repair can be performed with extensor retinaculum sutured to the remnant of the pulleys. If no pulley edges remain for suturing, a triple loop repair is performed using tendon autograft (Figure 6). Return to sport is permitted at 6 to 8 weeks with continued pulley protection. Full sports participation begins at 3 months. Taping or pulley ring use should be continued for at least 6 months.[19]

Scaphoid Fractures

Scaphoid fractures are a common problem encountered by orthopaedic hand surgeons. A high index of suspicion is necessary to make the diagnosis because radiographs are often negative at initial presentation. Any history of wrist trauma and tenderness should increase suspicion. On physical examination, tenderness over the anatomic snuffbox prevents the surgeon from ruling out a scaphoid fracture. Resisted pronation also elicits pain on examination. In addition to standard wrist radiographs, a scaphoid view should be obtained, with the wrist in 30° of extension and 20° of ulnar deviation. In the athlete, an MRI is useful if radiographs are inconclusive. This can allow earlier return to play if no fracture is identified. MRI is also used to assess osteonecrosis of the proximal pole of the scaphoid, a common complication of these injuries, and can help assess for a scapholunate ligament injury, another common cause of radial-side wrist pain in the athlete after a fall.

Scaphoid fractures are often a missed injury. Fractures treated less than 28 days from injury result in a 5% nonunion rate. If treatment is delayed longer than 28 days, the nonunion rate increases to 28%. It is imperative that the surgeon educate all trainers and other athletic staff about scaphoid fractures; any suspected injury should be promptly evaluated and treated.

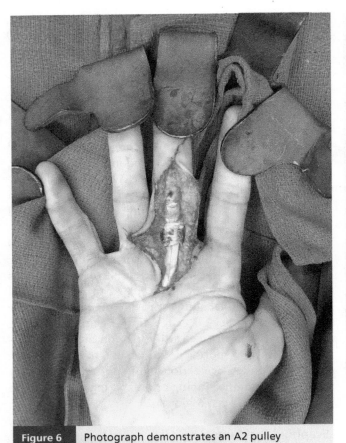

| Figure 6 | Photograph demonstrates an A2 pulley reconstruction with a triple-looped tendon graft. |

Scaphoid fracture treatment depends on the location and displacement of the fracture, as well as the skills required for the sport and/or position. If clinical suspicion is high for fracture, but the radiographs are negative, the athlete should be placed in a short arm thumb spica splint and an MRI should be obtained. Nondisplaced fractures of the scaphoid waist can be treated with thumb spica casting in football lineman with frequent follow-up repeat radiographs, but percutaneous compression screw fixation is strongly considered for more skilled position players such as receivers. Casting generally lasts for at least 3 months or until healing is confirmed on sequential radiographs or a CT scan. Displaced scaphoid waste fractures are treated using ORIF with a compression screw. Proximal pole fractures are treated using ORIF with compression screw fixation in all cases because of the high rate of osteonecrosis and nonunion for these fracture patterns. Other surgical indications include 15° humpback deformity, comminuted fractures, and displacement greater than 1 mm. In general, surgical fixation decreases the time to union, thus allowing a quicker return to sport. Athletes are not allowed to return to

unprotected play until evidence of radiographic union is confirmed. Healing is assessed by tenderness on clinical examination and using radiographs and CT scans. CT is the most reliable imaging study for assessing union.[6] Arthroscopically assisted reduction and fixation has been performed in athletes, but substantial fluoroscopy is also required for this procedure.[20]

Hook of Hamate Fractures

Hook of hamate fractures are often a source of chronic ulnar-side hand pain in baseball players, hockey players, golfers, and those who play racquet sports. Patients present with vague ulnar-side pain in the palm. Tenderness is elicited over the hamate, and ulnar nerve symptoms may be present. The fracture can also cause flexor tendon irritation or rupture. Standard hand radiographs usually will not reveal the fracture, so a carpal tunnel view is necessary. Because diagnosis is difficult, a CT scan should be obtained if a fracture is suspected.

Acute injuries can be treated with 6 weeks in a short arm cast; however, the risk of nonunion is high. Surgical excision of the fragment is the most reliable option for a pain-free outcome in athletes. ORIF has been described, but hardware prominence is a common complication. After fragment excision, range of motion and strengthening can begin immediately. Baseball players are often able to return to play by 6 weeks after surgery. On return to sports, a glove with a donut-shaped pad can be worn for protection until the scar is no longer tender.[21]

Differential Diagnosis of Wrist Pain in the Athlete

Radial Wrist Pain

Intersection Syndrome

Intersection syndrome is acute bursitis at the intersection of the first and second extensor compartment tendons in the forearm. This injury is most commonly seen in rowers and golfers. It presents with tenderness 5 cm proximal to the radial styloid, and must be differentiated from de Quervain tenosynovitis, which is more distal. A characteristic crepitus is located at the site of intersection. Treatment consists of splinting in a thumb spica brace, activity modification, NSAIDs, and sometimes, steroid injections. Surgery is rarely indicated, and is reserved for those in whom nonsurgical treatment has been unsuccessful for at least 3 months. Surgery includes bursal débridement and second extensor compartment release.

de Quervain Tenosynovitis

de Quervain tenosynovitis is an overuse syndrome that involves inflammation of the tenosynovium of the first extensor compartment tendons and is seen in racquet sport athletes and golfers. Symptoms include dorsoradial wrist pain and swelling, with crepitus over the tendons detected with thumb circumduction. Individuals with de Quervain tenosynovitis will have tenderness over the first dorsal compartment and a positive Finklestein test result. Pain is also elicited with resisted thumb MCP extension. Treatment is similar to intersection syndrome, but with a lower threshold level for surgical intervention. At the time of surgical release of the first dorsal compartment, careful inspection for a separate subsheath that contains the extensor pollicis brevis tendon is needed.[22] In 2011, a novel four-point steroid injection technique for recalcitrant cases in high-resistance athletes was described that yielded better outcomes than the standard two-point injection technique.[10]

Volar Wrist Ganglions

Volar wrist ganglions can cause pain on the radial aspect of the wrist, usually emanating from the joint via a tear in the radioscaphocapitate ligament. Pain is caused by compression of the surrounding structures. If the cyst is appreciable on physical examination, it will transilluminate. Usually, no correlation is found with underlying pathology, although other diagnoses, such as a radial artery aneurysm, should be excluded before undertaking surgical excision. The cyst should be excised if painful, although 20% recur. A volar cyst (versus a dorsal cyst) should not be aspirated or injected with steroid because of the proximity of the radial artery and potential for injury to this structure.[23]

Flexor Carpi Radialis Tendinitis

Athletes engaging in forceful, repetitive wrist flexion can develop inflammation of the wrist flexors, especially the flexor carpi radialis. Symptoms include volar radial and/or ulnar wrist and forearm pain, and are elicited with resisted wrist flexion and radial or ulnar deviation. Localized tenderness is present over the involved tendon. Splinting and steroid injections into the tendon sheath are the first line of treatment. Surgical release of the flexor carpi radialis sheath has good results in 80% of cases.[24]

Dorsal Wrist Pain

Dorsal Wrist Ganglions

Approximately 70% of dorsal wrist ganglions emanate from the scapholunate wrist ligament. Pain associated with a dorsal wrist ganglion should increase concern for a scapholunate ligament injury. Ganglions not associated with pain may be observed. They can be aspirated if painful, but have recurrence rates of 20% to 50%. Steroid injection of the cyst has no benefit. Surgical excision is usually successful at relieving symptoms, although up to 20% of ganglions recur. Arthroscopic excision allows direct visualization of the scapholunate ligament as well as the remainder of the wrist joint, and débridement of the capsular stalk at the base of the cyst. Arthroscopic excision has a slightly lower recurrence rate than open excision.[25,26]

Scapholunate Ligament Injuries

Scapholunate ligament injuries also cause dorsal wrist pain. As with scaphoid fractures, scapholunate ligament injuries are often missed on initial presentation and are challenging for the orthopaedic hand surgeon to treat if they present in a delayed fashion. Examination will reveal tenderness at the scapholunate interval, as well as a positive scaphoid shift test result. Wrist radiographs should be obtained and include a clenched fist view to evaluate for widening between the scaphoid and lunate. More than 3 mm of widening (the Terry Thomas sign) suggests a ligament tear. On the lateral view, an increased scapholunate angle may be appreciated (greater than 90°). Dynamic widening of the interval is appreciated when the widening only occurs with the clenched fist view (Figure 7). Static widening can be seen on all views, is usually associated with a chronic injury, and will result in arthritis over time. MRI can be helpful in the diagnosis, although it only has 70% to 81% accuracy.[27] Arthroscopy is the gold standard in diagnosis[28] (Figure 8). Acute tears should undergo surgical treatment acutely when possible, with open reduction of the scaphoid and lunate with dorsal wrist capsulodesis or ligament repair and percutaneous pin fixation. Numerous reconstruction techniques have been described for static chronic injuries more than 6 weeks post-injury. More recent data have shown better radiographic outcomes with ligament reconstruction over wrist capsulodesis for chronic injuries.[29,30]

Ulnar Wrist Pain

Extensor Carpi Ulnaris Tendinitis

Extensor carpi ulnaris (ECU) tendinitis is seen in racquet sport athletes and baseball players. The sixth extensor compartment is a unique fibro-osseous compartment that holds the ECU tendon tight against the ulnar groove. As the forearm is supinated, the sheath prevents ulnar translation of the tendon. Tenderness is elicited directly over the ECU tendon on examination. Radiographs are obtained to rule out fractures of the ulnar styloid and other bony pathologies. MRI sometimes shows splits in the tendon or increased signal intensity in the tendon on T2-weighted images. Nonsurgical management is preferred using NSAIDs, splints, and restricted activity. Steroid injections can help relieve pain. If nonsurgical management fails, the ECU tendon can be débrided. The

I: Upper Extremity

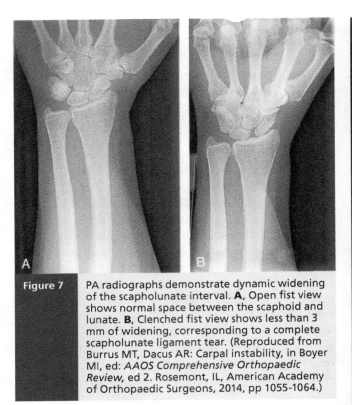

Figure 7 PA radiographs demonstrate dynamic widening of the scapholunate interval. **A,** Open fist view shows normal space between the scaphoid and lunate. **B,** Clenched fist view shows less than 3 mm of widening, corresponding to a complete scapholunate ligament tear. (Reproduced from Burrus MT, Dacus AR: Carpal instability, in Boyer MI, ed: *AAOS Comprehensive Orthopaedic Review*, ed 2. Rosemont, IL, American Academy of Orthopaedic Surgeons, 2014, pp 1055-1064.)

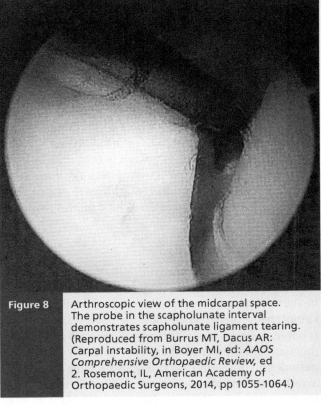

Figure 8 Arthroscopic view of the midcarpal space. The probe in the scapholunate interval demonstrates scapholunate ligament tearing. (Reproduced from Burrus MT, Dacus AR: Carpal instability, in Boyer MI, ed: *AAOS Comprehensive Orthopaedic Review*, ed 2. Rosemont, IL, American Academy of Orthopaedic Surgeons, 2014, pp 1055-1064.)

retinaculum of the sixth extensor compartment must be repaired carefully to prevent instability.

ECU Tendon Subluxation

ECU tendon subluxation is most commonly seen in tennis players, usually resulting from a hypersupination and/or ulnar deviation injury. On examination, the ECU tendon painfully snaps out of the groove with supination and ulnar deviation. The displaced tendon is palpable. Acute treatment is with a long arm cast in pronation and slight radial deviation. Chronic instability requires compartment reconstruction performed with direct repair supplemented using a radial-based sling of retinaculum or a free graft from the retinaculum. The ulnar groove can also be deepened to further stabilize the tendon. This is strongly (almost 50%) associated with triangular fibrocartilage complex (TFCC) tears.[31] Wrist arthroscopy should be considered at the time of surgery if a TFCC tear is suspected.

Ulnar Tunnel Syndrome

Ulnar tunnel syndrome consists of entrapment of the ulnar nerve in the Guyon canal at the wrist. Also known as handlebar palsy in cyclists, it can be associated with carpal tunnel syndrome. Depending on the location of the compression, patients can have motor or sensory symptoms or both. Paresthesias are noted in the ring and little fingers, and the intrinsic muscles are often weak. This condition is often caused by a mass lesion such as an ulnar artery thrombosis or aneurysm, hook of hamate fracture, ganglion (most common) or lipoma, inflammatory arthritis, bone anomalies, or continuous pressure.[32] Nerve conduction velocity studies and electromyography can support the diagnosis, and MRI can be helpful if a mass lesion is suspected. Nonsurgical therapy includes wrist splints and avoidance of aggravating activities. Surgery involves nerve decompression and removal of any masses or lesions. If the patient has concomitant carpal tunnel syndrome, release of the carpal tunnel is sufficient for release of the ulnar tunnel as well.

Ulnar Artery Thrombosis

Ulnar artery thrombosis, also known as hypothenar hammer syndrome, can occur in baseball catchers because of repetitive impact to the ulnar artery while catching. Symptoms include pain, cramping, and sensory disturbance. The Allen test should be performed if diagnosis is suspected, with delayed reperfusion appreciated while occluding the radial artery. Ulnar artery reconstruction with interposition vein grafting is required.[33]

TFCC Injury

The TFCC is the primary stabilizer of the distal radioulnar joint and is composed of a central disk and peripheral disk–carpal ligaments that are more volarly based. TFCC tears can be degenerative or acute.

Injury to the TFCC causes pain or perceived instability that can prevent athletic participation. Peripheral injury has the best likelihood of healing because this portion has the best blood supply. Tenderness over the fovea of the ulna (a positive fovea sign) is evident on examination. Radiographs are obtained to assess ulnar variance and rule out ulnar styloid fractures. MRI helps determine a diagnosis, although studies have shown magnetic resonance arthrography to be more helpful.[34] Wrist arthroscopy confirms the diagnosis (Figure 9). Classification is based on the location of the tear and chronicity. Type 1 tears are traumatic (Table 1); type 2 tears are degenerative. Treatment consists of rest, splinting, NSAIDs, and steroid injections versus arthroscopic surgical débridement or repair.

Ulnar-side peripheral tears should be repaired; central and radial tears can only be débrided.[35] Ulnar tears that are repaired within 3 months regain 80% of motion and strength.[36] The surgeon should be aware that a knot tied in the floor of the ECU sheath can cause ECU tendinitis. If a central tear is débrided, a 2-mm peripheral rim of the TFCC should be preserved after débridement to maintain a stable joint. Partial-thickness tears of the ulnar fovea do well with repair and patients who play racquet sports are often able to return to sport. However, athletes who bear weight through the wrist have less favorable return-to-sport outcomes.[37] If ulnar variance of more than 2 mm exists, resulting in symptomatic ulnocarpal abutment, an ulnar shortening procedure should also be performed. Excellent results have been achieved with ulnar shortening osteotomy because this stabilizes the distal radioulnar joint, reduces the effect of ulnocarpal abutment, and decreases forces on the TFCC.[38]

Summary

Hand and wrist injuries of the athlete provide a substantial challenge to the treating physician because of the sheer number and diversity of injuries seen in this patient population. Furthermore, many injuries are initially missed, presenting the challenge of treating a chronic injury in an athlete. The complexity of the hand and wrist can make diagnosis difficult; thus, it is imperative to have a deep understanding of all types of injuries that can occur in the hand and wrist. With the appropriate knowledge base, orthopaedic hand surgeons can usually confirm the diagnosis of athletic injuries of the hand and wrist and provide the appropriate therapy to allow the athlete to return to his or her sport as quickly and safely as possible.

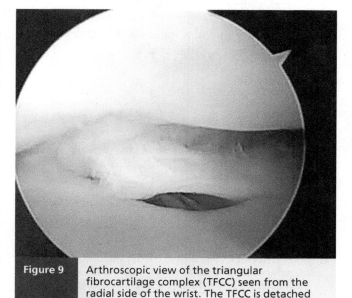

Figure 9 Arthroscopic view of the triangular fibrocartilage complex (TFCC) seen from the radial side of the wrist. The TFCC is detached from the radius.

Table 1

Palmer Classification of Class 1 (Acute) Triangular Fibrocartilage Complex Tears

Type	Location	Characteristics
1A	Central	Traumatic tears of articular disk
1B	Ulnar	Ulnar avulsion
1C	Volar distal	Distal traumatic disruption of the ulnolunate or ulnotriquetral ligaments
1D	Radial	Traumatic avulsion from sigmoid notch of radius

(Reproduced from Goldfarb CA: Wrist arthroscopy, in Boyer MI, ed: *AAOS Comprehensive Orthopaedic Review*, ed 2. Rosemont, IL, American Academy of Orthopaedic Surgeons, 2014, pp 1197-1200.)

Key Study Points

- Metacarpal and phalangeal fractures are at risk of deformity and functional loss if not treated appropriately. The hand/fingers are at high risk of stiffness if immobilized for extended periods of time.

- Direction of finger PIP joint dislocation is important in guiding treatment.

- Acute pain in the snuffbox region in an athlete should be treated aggressively with immobilization for 3 weeks and then reassessment to rule out a scaphoid fracture. Occult scaphoid fractures may not be visible on radiographs until 3 weeks postinjury. For early evaluation and diagnosis, an MRI is beneficial in the diagnosis of an occult scaphoid fracture if return to play is critical for a high-level athlete. Untreated scaphoid fractures can have dire consequences to the patient.

- Advancements in wrist arthroscopy have lowered the recurrence rates of dorsal wrist ganglions.

- Ulnar-side peripheral tears of the TFCC should be repaired as opposed to débrided.

Annotated References

1. Swanson AB: Fractures involving the digits of the hand. *Orthop Clin North Am* 1970;1(2):261-274.

2. van Aaken J, Kämpfen S, Berli M, Fritschy D, Della Santa D, Fusetti C: Outcome of boxer's fractures treated by a soft wrap and buddy taping: A prospective study. *Hand (N Y)* 2007;2(4):212-217.

3. Soong M, Got C, Katarincic J: Ring and little finger metacarpal fractures: Mechanisms, locations, and radiographic parameters. *J Hand Surg Am* 2010;35(8):1256-1259.

   The authors reviewed 101 ring and little finger metacarpal fractures and reported that punching injuries usually cause a neck fracture of the little finger versus a shaft fracture of the ring finger. The isthmus of the ring finger is narrower. Level of evidence: IV.

4. Roth JJ, Auerbach DM: Fixation of hand fractures with bicortical screws. *J Hand Surg Am* 2005;30(1):151-153.

5. Hardy MA: Principles of metacarpal and phalangeal fracture management: A review of rehabilitation concepts. *J Orthop Sports Phys Ther* 2004;34(12):781-799.

6. Rizzo M, Shin AY: Treatment of acute scaphoid fractures in the athlete. *Curr Sports Med Rep* 2006;5(5):242-248.

7. Kodama N, Takemura Y, Ueba H, Imai S, Matsusue Y: Operative treatment of metacarpal and phalangeal fractures in athletes: Early return to play. *J Orthop Sci* 2014;19(5):729-736.

   Of 101 metacarpal or phalangeal shaft fractures, 20 were treated with ORIF so athletes could return for important event. All 20 returned by 1 month and eventually achieved union with excellent range of motion. Level of evidence: III.

8. Arora R, Angermann P, Fritz D, Hennerbichler A, Gabl M, Lutz M: [Dorsolateral dislocation of the proximal interphalangeal joint: Closed reduction and early active motion versus static splinting].[Article in German.] *Handchir Mikrochir Plast Chir* 2007;39(3):225-228.

9. Elfar J, Mann T: Fracture-dislocations of the proximal interphalangeal joint. *J Am Acad Orthop Surg* 2013;21(2):88-98.

   The authors reviewed dorsal, volar, and pilon PIP fracture-dislocations in this review article. Acceptable outcomes were achieving a well-aligned joint and reestablishing motion. Anatomic articular congruity is preferable but not absolutely necessary for good outcomes.

10. Pagonis T, Ditsios K, Toli P, Givissis P, Christodoulou A: Improved corticosteroid treatment of recalcitrant de Quervain tenosynovitis with a novel 4-point injection technique. *Am J Sports Med* 2011;39(2):398-403.

    The authors compared two similar groups of 24 athletes treated with one- to two-point injection technique versus their new four-point technique. Symptom relief was better in the four-point group at 2 and 52 weeks. Level of evidence: II.

11. Williams RM, Kiefhaber TR, Sommerkamp TG, Stern PJ: Treatment of unstable dorsal proximal interphalangeal fracture/dislocations using a hemi-hamate autograft. *J Hand Surg Am* 2003;28(5):856-865.

12. Nilsson JA, Rosberg HE: Treatment of proximal interphalangeal joint fractures by the pins and rubbers traction system: A follow-up. *J Plast Surg Hand Surg* 2014;48(4):259-264.

    Forty-two patients with complex PIP joint fractures were treated with a pins–and–rubber band system. The device was easy to apply and well tolerated. Volar lip fractures had the best outcome. Osteoarthritis and loss of motion are still common. Level of evidence: III.

13. Kiral A, Erken HY, Akmaz I, Yildirim C, Erler K: Pins and rubber band traction for treatment of comminuted intra-articular fractures in the hand. *J Hand Surg Am* 2014;39(4):696-705.

    This retrospective review of 33 patients treated with pins–and–rubber band system at the PIP, DIP, thumb interphalangeal, and thumb MCP joints reported satisfactory results. Level of evidence: IV.

14. Heyman P: Injuries to the ulnar collateral ligament of the thumb metacarpophalangeal joint. *J Am Acad Orthop Surg* 1997;5(4):224-229.

15. Werner BC, Hadeed MM, Lyons ML, Gluck JS, Diduch DR, Chhabra AB: Return to football and long-term clinical outcomes after thumb ulnar collateral ligament suture anchor repair in collegiate athletes. *J Hand Surg Am* 2014;39(10):1992-1998.

    The authors reported on a two-suture anchor technique of ulnar collateral ligament repair performed on 18 collegiate football players. All returned to at least their original level of play. Skilled players returned in 7 weeks, nonskilled returned in 4 weeks. Level of evidence: IV.

16. Altan E, Alp NB, Baser R, Yalçın L: Soft-tissue mallet injuries: A comparison of early and delayed treatment. *J Hand Surg Am* 2014;39(10):1982-1985.

17. Gruber JS, Bot AG, Ring D: A prospective randomized controlled trial comparing night splinting with no splinting after treatment of mallet finger. *Hand (N Y)* 2014;9(2):145-150.

    In this study, 51 patients were enrolled in a prospective trial to either receive night splinting after 6 to 8 weeks of continuous splinting for mallet fingers or no splinting. No difference in extensor lag was reported between the two groups at final outcome. Level of evidence: II.

18. Lin JD, Strauch RJ: Closed soft tissue extensor mechanism injuries (mallet, boutonniere, and sagittal band). *J Hand Surg Am* 2014;39(5):1005-1011.

    The authors summarize mechanism and treatment of closed soft-tissue injuries in zone I, III, and V extensor mechanism injuries. Level of evidence: V.

19. Freilich AM: Evaluation and treatment of jersey finger and pulley injuries in athletes. *Clin Sports Med* 2015;34(1):151-166.

    The author discussed flexor tendon injuries and pulley injuries in the athlete. Level of evidence: V.

20. Geissler WB: Arthroscopic management of scaphoid fractures in athletes. *Hand Clin* 2009;25(3):359-369.

    This article discussed the indications and treatment strategy for arthroscopic management of scaphoid fractures and nonunions in athletes. Level of evidence: V.

21. Bachoura A, Wroblewski A, Jacoby SM, Osterman AL, Culp RW: Hook of hamate fractures in competitive baseball players. *Hand (N Y)* 2013;8(3):302-307.

    The authors presented their experience with hook of hamate fractures in baseball players treated surgically. Ulnar tunnel decompression with hook excision provides good outcomes. Mean return to play was 5.7 weeks. Level of evidence: IV.

22. Stein AH Jr, Ramsey RH, Key JA: Stenosing tendovaginitis at the radial styloid process (DeQuervain's disease). *AMA Arch Surg* 1951;63(2):216-228.

23. Lidder S, Ranawat V, Ahrens P: Surgical excision of wrist ganglia; literature review and nine-year retrospective study of recurrence and patient satisfaction. *Orthop Rev (Pavia)* 2009;1(1):e5.

    The authors followed up 117 patients who underwent volar or dorsal wrist ganglia excision. An overall recurrence of 41.8% was reported; it was concluded that surgery may have better results with a hand specialist. Level of evidence: IV.

24. Sauvé PS, Rhee PC, Shin AY, Lindau T: Examination of the wrist: Radial-sided wrist pain. *J Hand Surg Am* 2014;39(10):2089-2092.

    The authors provided a thorough review of causes of radial-side wrist pain. Level of evidence: V.

25. Fernandes CH, Miranda CD, Dos Santos JB, Faloppa F: A systematic review of complications and recurrence rate of arthroscopic resection of volar wrist ganglion. *Hand Surg* 2014;19(3):475-480.

    Of 232 wrists treated with arthroscopic volar wrist ganglion excision, 14 had recurrence. Recurrence rates in the papers reviewed ranged from 0 to 20%. The procedure was reported as technically difficult, and had higher rates of associated complications than open excision. Level of evidence: III.

26. Kang L, Akelman E, Weiss AP: Arthroscopic versus open dorsal ganglion excision: A prospective, randomized comparison of rates of recurrence and of residual pain. *J Hand Surg Am* 2008;33(4):471-475.

27. Spaans AJ, Minnen Pv, Prins HJ, Korteweg MA, Schuurman AH: The value of 3.0-tesla MRI in diagnosing scapholunate ligament injury. *J Wrist Surg* 2013;2(1):69-72.

    The authors reviewed the sensitivity and specificity of 3.0-T MRI in the diagnosis of TFCC tears by comparing the imaging findings with arthroscopic findings. Level of evidence: II.

28. Schädel-Höpfner M, Iwinska-Zelder J, Braus T, Böhringer G, Klose KJ, Gotzen L: MRI versus arthroscopy in the diagnosis of scapholunate ligament injury. *J Hand Surg Br* 2001;26(1):17-21.

29. Pappou IP, Basel J, Deal DN: Scapholunate ligament injuries: A review of current concepts. *Hand (N Y)* 2013;8(2):146-156.

    The authors reviewed classification of and treatment options for scapholunate injuries, focusing on stages in which reconstruction procedures may work as opposed to salvage procedures. Level of evidence: V.

30. Rohman EM, Agel J, Putnam MD, Adams JE: Scapholunate interosseous ligament injuries: A retrospective review of treatment and outcomes in 82 wrists. *J Hand Surg Am* 2014;39(10):2020-2026.

    The authors reviewed 27 acute and 50 chronic scapholunate tears treated surgically. Chronic injuries had better radiographic outcomes with ligament reconstruction compared with capsulodesis. Acute repair within 6 weeks was preferred. Level of evidence: III.

31. MacLennan AJ, Nemechek NM, Waitayawinyu T, Trumble TE: Diagnosis and anatomic reconstruction of extensor carpi ulnaris subluxation. *J Hand Surg Am* 2008;33(1):59-64.

32. Jayakumar P, Jayaram V, Nairn DS: Compressive neuropathies related to ganglions of the wrist and hand. *Hand Surg* 2014;19(1):113-116.

    The authors discussed the pathoanatomy of wrist and hand ganglions that cause compressive neuropathies. Motor and/or sensory deficits can be encountered and correlate to the location of the ganglion. Level of evidence: V.

33. Dreizin D, Jose J: Hypothenar hammer syndrome. *Am J Orthop (Belle Mead NJ)* 2012;41(8):380-382.

    Hypothenar hammer syndrome was discussed in this study, including the importance of early diagnosis and imaging studies. Definitive evaluation was made with catheter-directed angiography. Management options were also discussed. Level of evidence: V.

34. Berná-Serna JD, Martínez F, Reus M, Alonso J, Doménech G, Campos M: Evaluation of the triangular fibrocartilage in cadaveric wrists by means of arthrography, magnetic resonance (MR) imaging, and MR arthrography. *Acta Radiol* 2007;48(1):96-103.

    The authors examined the value of arthrography, MRI, and magnetic resonance arthrography in diagnosing TFCC tears, and their ability to identify the location of the tear. Level of evidence: II.

35. Estrella EP, Hung LK, Ho PC, Tse WL: Arthroscopic repair of triangular fibrocartilage complex tears. *Arthroscopy* 2007;23(7):729-737.e1.

    The authors reviewed 26 patients who underwent repairs of partial-thickness TFCC fovea tears. Patients were more likely to return to racquet sports and less likely to return to sports that required weight bearing through the hands. Level of evidence: VI.

36. Ruch DS, Papadonikolakis A: Arthroscopically assisted repair of peripheral triangular fibrocartilage complex tears: Factors affecting outcome. *Arthroscopy* 2005;21(9):1126-1130.

37. Wysocki RW, Richard MJ, Crowe MM, Leversedge FJ, Ruch DS: Arthroscopic treatment of peripheral triangular fibrocartilage complex tears with the deep fibers intact. *J Hand Surg Am* 2012;37(3):509-516.

38. Constantine KJ, Tomaino MM, Herndon JH, Sotereanos DG: Comparison of ulnar shortening osteotomy and the wafer resection procedure as treatment for ulnar impaction syndrome. *J Hand Surg Am* 2000;25(1):55-60.

© 2016 American Academy of Orthopaedic Surgeons

Hip and Pelvis

SECTION EDITOR

F. Winston Gwathmey, MD

Chapter 10
Athletic Hip Injuries

Richard Charles Mather III, MD, MBA   Michael S. Ferrell, MD

Abstract

Indications for hip arthroscopy are rapidly expanding and include pathology in the central, peripheral, and peritrochanteric compartments. The anterolateral and anterior portals are the primary portals with several described accessory portals. The most common surgical complications include iatrogenic chondrolabral injury, transient neurapraxia, and the inadequate resection of femoroacetabular impingement. The acetabular labrum is a critical structure and should be repaired or reconstructed whenever possible to preserve its function, especially that of creating negative pressure seal to the femoral head. Hip microinstability is proving to be a source of chronic hip pain and disability with several soft-tissue structures, including the ligamentum teres, playing key roles in maintaining stability. Appropriate capsular management, including capsular repair and plication in indicated cases, is proving to be a key step in preserving or establishing hip stability and optimizing surgical outcomes. Tears of the ligamentum teres are a source of pain in the hip and require a high index of suspicion to make the diagnosis. Débridement of partial-thickness ligamentum teres tears has demonstrated good clinical outcomes. Ligamentum teres reconstruction in instability cases may prove to be a useful adjunct along with capsular plication in certain settings but is still unproved at this point.

Dr. Mather or an immediate family member serves as a paid consultant to KNG Health Consulting, Pivot Medical, Smith & Nephew, and Stryker; has stock or stock options held in for[MD]; and serves as a board member, owner, officer, or committee member of the Arthroscopy Association of North America, the American Academy of Orthopaedic Surgeons, and the North Carolina Orthopaedic Association. Neither Dr. Ferrell nor any immediate family member has received anything of value from or has stock or stock options held in a commercial company or institution related directly or indirectly to the subject of this chapter.

Keywords: hip arthroscopy; labral tears; ligamentum teres; hip instability

Introduction

Hip arthroscopy has been one of the most rapidly developing fields in orthopaedic surgery over the past decade.[1] As improved equipment and evolving techniques have made the procedure safer and relatively easier to perform, indications have continued to expand. Furthermore, as the understanding and appreciation of femoroacetabular impingement (FAI)—the most common indication for hip arthroscopy—have evolved, the diagnosis has become better recognized and surgical outcomes have improved.[2]

The current indications for hip arthroscopy address pathology in the central, peripheral, and peritrochanteric compartments of the hip joint. Central compartment pathology includes labral tears, loose bodies, ligamentum teres (LT) tears, chondral defects, and pincer lesions associated with FAI. Peripheral compartment pathology includes cam lesions associated with FAI, capsular laxity associated with hip instability, loose bodies, and recalcitrant internal snapping hip secondary to chronic iliopsoas bursitis. Peritrochanteric compartment pathology includes recalcitrant trochanteric bursitis, tears of the gluteus medius and minimus, and painful external snapping hip. Successful surgical outcomes in these compartments have expanded the application of endoscopic techniques to other conditions, including proximal hamstring repairs and sciatic nerve decompression in the deep gluteal space.

The portals for hip arthroscopy have evolved to improve access and safety (Figure 1). In general, the central and peripheral compartments can be accessed through two or three portals. The anterolateral portal is typically the first portal established, using anatomic landmarks and fluoroscopy to determine the appropriate trajectory with which to enter the joint. Typically, this portal is 2 cm anterior and 2 cm distal to the greater trochanter and has the objective of entering the joint parallel to the sourcil without violating the labrum. The anterior portal typically is made next, using a spinal needle for localization via an inside-out technique through the anterior triangle,

© 2016 American Academy of Orthopaedic Surgeons

2: Hip and Pelvis

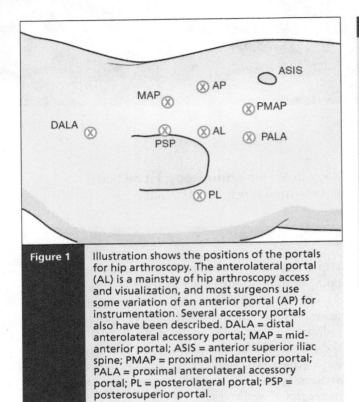

Figure 1 Illustration shows the positions of the portals for hip arthroscopy. The anterolateral portal (AL) is a mainstay of hip arthroscopy access and visualization, and most surgeons use some variation of an anterior portal (AP) for instrumentation. Several accessory portals also have been described. DALA = distal anterolateral accessory portal; MAP = mid-anterior portal; ASIS = anterior superior iliac spine; PMAP = proximal midanterior portal; PALA = proximal anterolateral accessory portal; PL = posterolateral portal; PSP = posterosuperior portal.

Table 1
Complications Associated With Hip Arthroscopy
Iatrogenic chondrolabral injury
Neurapraxia
FAI underresection
Sequela of FAI overresection, including iatrogenic instability and femoral neck fracture
Heterotopic ossification
Deep vein thrombosis
Pulmonary embolism
Osteonecrosis
Abdominal compartment syndrome
FAI = femoroacetabular impingement.

as in other joints. The key landmark is a line parallel to the femur extending distal from the anterior superior iliac spine (ASIS). Remaining lateral to this line will minimize the risk to the femoral neurovascular bundle, and the more lateral the portal is, the farther away it is from the lateral femoral cutaneous nerve. The position of the anterior portal varies and can be placed farther distal and lateral to facilitate anchor placement, particularly for two-portal approaches.

Additional portals include the distal anterolateral portal, which is typically 4 to 5 cm distal to the anterolateral portal. This portal provides a safe trajectory for anchor placement in the acetabulum and provides easy access for cam resection in FAI. The Dienst portal is placed a few centimeters proximal to the anterolateral portal and offers a different trajectory into the central and peripheral compartments. The trochanteric space can be accessed via the same anterolateral portal as well as via a posterolateral portal, which is 2 cm posterior and 2 cm distal to the greater trochanter. A third portal distal to the vastus ridge insertion of the vastus lateralis provides a good viewing angle for gluteus medius and minimus repairs while working through the anterolateral and posterolateral portals.

Hip arthroscopy has a unique set of complications that differ from those of other joints because of the steep learning curve associated with the procedure, the techniques required to access the deep, highly congruent joint through its thick soft-tissue envelope, and the longer surgical times (Table 1). Iatrogenic chondrolabral injury can occur while the surgeon is gaining access to the central compartment; it was the most reported complication in one systematic review.[3] Another common but transient complication following hip arthroscopy is neurapraxialan with incidence approaching 50% in one series.[4] The lateral femoral cutaneous nerve (LFCN) is most commonly involved. It is unclear whether LFCN neurapraxia is related to direct injury from portal placement, traction from the portals and cannulas, swelling associated with arthroscopy, or a combination of causes, but LFCN neurapraxia is now considered by many hip arthroscopists to be a sequela of hip arthroscopy rather than a complication. Permanent injury is less than 5%, however. Pudendal neurapraxia also can occur, even with short traction times, especially in stiff, prearthritic hips. Traction injuries related to the post, which are substantial but avoidable, also include skin and soft-tissue necrosis.

Inadequate resection in FAI surgery, more commonly on the femoral side, is the most common reason for revision hip preservation surgery.[5] Fluoroscopy, hip rotation, and the performance of a T-capsulotomy allow visualization of the cam lesion in its entirety and minimize the risk of an inadequate resection. The most common reason for reoperation following hip arthroscopy is conversion to a total hip arthroplasty (THA).[5] Whether conversion to THA is a complication related to hip arthroscopy or merely a progression of the natural history of FAI remains unclear.

Rare but catastrophic hip arthroscopy complications include femoral neck fracture, abdominal compartment

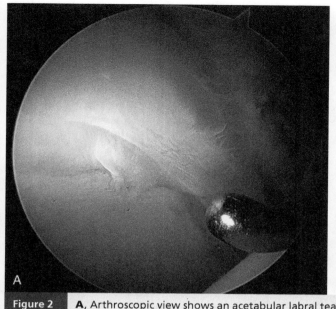
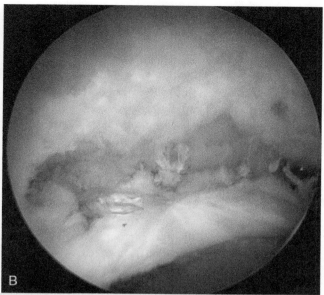

Figure 2 **A,** Arthroscopic view shows an acetabular labral tear, which is a common finding at arthroscopy and typically occurs anteriorly and/or anterolaterally. **B,** Arthroscopic view shows acetabular labral repair, which is essential to restore the multiple functions of the labrum. (Courtesy of F. Winston Gwathmey, MD, Charlottesville, VA.)

syndrome, iatrogenic instability including hip dislocation, thromboembolic disease, and fatal pulmonary embolism.[6-10]

Acetabular Labral Tears

Acetabular labral tears have been shown to be a substantial source of pain and disability and comprise the most common pathologic finding at the time of hip arthroscopy[11] (Figure 2). The acetabular labrum is a triangular fibrocartilaginous ring, which is attached firmly to the acetabular rim and encompasses nearly the entire acetabulum, except for the most inferior aspect, which is bridged by the transverse acetabular ligament. The labrum deepens the acetabulum, increases coverage of the femoral head, and plays a role in shock absorption, joint lubrication, and pressure distribution. Its most critical role may be the creation of a negative pressure seal with the femoral head, which aids in joint stability. Removal of the labrum has been shown to lead to a shift in the femoral contact point toward the acetabular rim, a decrease in intra-articular fluid pressurization, and a loss of lateral restraint to femoral head motion. It also has been shown to increase contact stresses between the articular cartilage of the femoral head and the acetabulum by 92%.[12-14]

The labrum is injured most often in FAI and acetabular dysplasia. Hip trauma leading to a labral tear generally involves a high-energy contact mechanism, which results in a frank dislocation or subluxation. Traumatic hip instability is frequently associated with chondral lesions to

the femoral head and acetabulum analogous to those seen in a shoulder dislocation. Sports that require a great deal of hip torsion can lead to capsule attenuation and laxity secondary to repetitive microtrauma. Attenuation of the capsule leads to microinstability of the joint, in which the femoral head subluxates anteriorly and rides on the anterior superior labrum.[15] Microinstability can also occur outside of sports in patients with collagen disorders such as Ehlers-Danlos syndrome, Marfan syndrome, and Down syndrome. Degenerative labral tears are analogous to degenerative meniscus tears in the knee and are frequently associated with diffuse articular changes in an arthritic joint. Degenerative labral tears are thought to be extremely common in the aging hip and likely occur early in the arthritic process.

Iliopsoas impingement on the anterior hip joint recently has been suggested as an additional mechanism for labral tears. The authors of a 2011 study[16] described an atypical labral tear pattern in a series of patients in which the labral tear occurs on the anterior acetabulum directly beneath where the iliopsoas tendon crosses the hip joint, unlike the common location in FAI and dysplasia, which is more superior on the anterior acetabulum. The presentation was similar to that of FAI, with groin pain in flexion, adduction, and internal rotation. These patients were successfully treated with an iliopsoas lengthening and a labral débridement or repair.

In the pediatric literature, several case series describe labral tears in association with avulsions of the rectus femoris. The reflected head of the rectus femoris is near the anterior labrum and inferior to the ASIS. It is theorized that a traction injury of sufficient energy can tear the labrum in this location.[17]

Several labral tear classification systems exist based on tear morphology, histology, and location. Tear patterns based on morphology have been described.[18] Stable tear patterns include radial, fibrillated, and longitudinal peripheral tear patterns. Radial flap tears occur with an intra-articular free-edge disruption. Radial fibrillated tears are degenerative tears with fibrillated free margins. Longitudinal peripheral tears are stable labral separations from the acetabular margin. Unstable tears include the bucket-handle tear. Two types of labral tears based on histology have been described.[19] Type 1 tears occurred at the junction between the fibrocartilaginous labrum and the articular hyaline cartilage. Type 2 tears occurred in various planes within the substance of the labrum. Labral tear classification based on location is described by the tear position in relation to the acetabulum. Anterior labral tears have been prevalent in most of the studies because of their association with FAI.

The diagnosis of a labral tear often can be made clinically. Patients may report mechanical symptoms, such as clicking and catching, as well as groin pain in positions of hip flexion. It is not uncommon to feel pain laterally or posteriorly with anterior labral tears. Pain with prolonged sitting is another common symptom. Physical examination findings can include pain in the provocative position of flexion, adduction, and internal rotation if the tear is anterior or pain in flexion, abduction, and external rotation if the tear is lateral. Table 2 describes the tests used to detect a labral tear. Imaging includes plain radiographs and magnetic resonance arthrography. The most valuable diagnostic sign is a positive response to an intra-articular joint injection that brings complete pain relief, even for a brief period. This assessment is especially helpful in patients with atypical referred pain locations to confirm the joint as the source of pain.

Treatment options for labral tears include débridement, repair, and reconstruction, with the goal of restoring or preserving the function of the native labrum (Figure 3). Débridement is reserved for tear patterns that are stable and in which the function of the labrum will be maintained. Repair is appropriate for unstable tear patterns, in which excision would render the labrum incompetent. Several studies have shown improved results with repair versus débridement in groups treated with an open surgical hip dislocation as well as an arthroscopic repair. A comparison of labral débridement versus repair in open surgical hip dislocation for FAI showed substantial improvement in clinical outcomes, with 80% excellent results in the labral repair group versus 28% excellent

Table 2	
Tests for Labral Tears During the Physical Examination	
Anterior tears	Flexion, adduction, internal rotation (FADIR) test
	Dynamic internal rotation impingement test
Lateral tears	Flexion, abduction, external rotation (FABER) test
	Dynamic external rotation impingement test
Hip instability	Extension and external rotation test
	External rotation log-roll test
Ligamentum teres tears	Ligamentum teres test

results in the débridement group.[20] In addition, radiographic signs of osteoarthritis were significantly more prevalent in the débridement group at final follow-up. Furthermore, superior clinical outcomes and patient satisfaction were seen with arthroscopic labral repair versus labral débridement, with 67% good or excellent results in the débridement group versus 90% in the repair group.[21] Labral repair and débridement were compared in a randomized controlled trial and significantly greater improvement in the hip outcome score in the repair group was found, although both groups demonstrated improvement from the preoperative state.[22] In addition, 72% of the patients in the repair arm self-rated their hips as normal versus 28% in the débridement arm. Labral reconstruction traditionally has been reserved for revision cases in which the primary labral repair has failed. Reconstruction may be considered in young athletes with an irreparable tear or a hypoplastic labrum that renders the labrum incompetent, especially in a high-demand sport that requires cutting and pivoting at high speed or repetitive rotational maneuvers or for patients at risk of instability. Good outcomes and high patient satisfaction were seen with labral reconstruction using iliotibial band autograft; better results occurred in younger patients with no joint space narrowing less than 2 mm.[23]

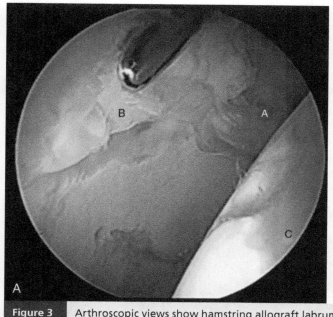
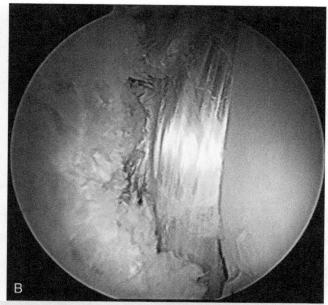

Figure 3 Arthroscopic views show hamstring allograft labrum reconstruction for iatrogenic instability after hip arthroscopy. **A,** Point A shows a normal labrum. Point B shows labral insufficiency. Point C shows an iatrogenic cartilage injury of the femoral head. **B,** Restoration of the suction seal after hamstring allograft labral reconstruction is shown.

Hip Instability

Hip instability has been increasingly recognized as a pathologic entity and a source of chronic pain and disability over the past decade, especially in cases of more subtle atraumatic instability. Unlike those in the shoulder, the major stabilizers in the hip are the static restraints and include both osseous and soft-tissue structures. The osseous components consist of the highly constrained femoral head inside the concentric acetabulum. The degree of acetabular coverage and the femoral and acetabular version are key determinants of stability. It is in the setting of diminished acetabular coverage and alterations in normal version that the hip joint increasingly relies on soft-tissue structures to maintain stability.[24]

The soft-tissue static restraints include the labrum, the capsule, and the ligaments. The labrum is a triangular fibrocartilaginous ring encompassing the acetabulum at all but its most inferior aspect, which is spanned by the transverse acetabular ligament. The labrum deepens the acetabulum, increases the coverage of the femoral head, and enables the joint to have a negative suction seal, which increases stability.[12-14] Three primary ligaments span the joint and blend with the capsule (Table 3). The strongest is the iliofemoral ligament (IFL), which is an inverted Y-shaped ligament that originates just inferior to the anterior inferior iliac spine and attaches distally along the femoral intertrochanteric line. The IFL has been shown to limit hip extension and external rotation.[25] The

pubofemoral ligament (PFL) is inferior to the IFL, originates on the pubis, and blends in with the IFL at its medial attachment, extending along the femoral intertrochanteric line. The PFL has been shown to limit external rotation and abduction. The ischiofemoral ligament (ISL) is located posteriorly, connecting the posterior acetabulum to a portion of the posterior femoral neck. The ISL provides some support to the posterior femoral neck. Because of their helical orientation, the three ligaments twist when they are taut and are thought to provide a "screw home" mechanism to the joint when the hip is in extension. The zona orbicularis is a circumferential structure that forms a collar around the base of the femoral neck and is thought to resist hip distraction. The LT appears to play a secondary role to these soft-tissue restraints, having been shown to restrict the motion of the femoral head.[26,27] Furthermore, isolated tears of the LT have been found in hip dysplasia, in which it may play a more prominent role in stabilization.[28]

Hip instability is thought to have traumatic and atraumatic origins (Table 4). Traumatic origins include high-energy and low-energy mechanisms. High-energy mechanisms can lead to osseous disruptions and an unstable hip joint, as in a posterior acetabular rim fracture. The classic example is the motor vehicle accident in which the knee strikes the dashboard, resulting in a posterior hip dislocation. High-energy mechanisms also can lead to disruptions of the soft tissue, such as labral tears and ligament sprains, resulting in instability in the absence

Table 3

Hip Ligaments and Their Motion Restrictions

Iliofemoral ligament	Extension and ER
Ischiofemoral ligament	Flexion and IR
	Extension and IR
Pubofemoral ligament	Abduction and ER
Ligamentum teres	Flexion and ER
	Extension and IR

ER = external rotation, IR = internal rotation.

Table 4

Risk Factors for Hip Instability

Acetabular dysplasia

Abnormal femoral and acetabular version

Generalized ligamentous laxity

Iatrogenic capsular insufficiency

Sports requiring extreme hip motion

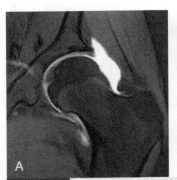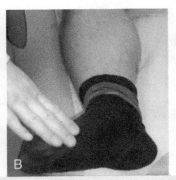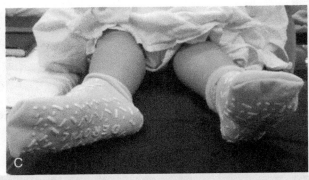

Figure 4 Images depict assessment of the iliofemoral ligament. **A,** Coronal magnetic resonance arthrogram demonstrates a large capsular defect after hip arthroscopy. **B,** Photograph shows the external rotation log-roll test for iliofemoral ligament insufficiency. The examiner externally rotates the leg at the foot. A normal ligament will display spring back. **C,** Photograph shows capsular plication of the left leg with an end point in external rotation, whereas the right leg shows the preoperative iliofemoral ligament instability.

of fracture. Sports with repetitive torsional movements can produce soft-tissue attenuation due to repetitive microtrauma to the capsule and ligaments. A common example is the athlete engaged in a sport requiring extreme amounts of hip motion and rotation, such as gymnastics, ballet, and golf. Atraumatic origins also can be seen in patients with congenital soft-tissue deficiency or laxity, such as the capsular and ligamentous laxity seen in Ehlers-Danlos syndrome, Marfan syndrome, and Down syndrome. The atraumatic mechanism most recently described is a sequela of a large cam-based deformity in FAI. In this case, impingement of the cam lesion inside the acetabulum in flexion levers the femoral head posteriorly, which can cause a posterior contrecoup cartilage lesion, with posterior subluxation and instability.[29]

The concept of atraumatic hip instability has led to the emerging idea of hip microinstability. This type of instability can occur in athletes with mild osseous hip dysplasia superimposed on ligamentous laxity during sports requiring high degrees of hip motion. In the setting of hip dysplasia, the individual is much more reliant on soft-tissue structures to stabilize the hip. The athlete with hip microinstability may report mechanical symptoms

and feelings of instability, especially in hip positions that rely more on soft-tissue restraint like hip extension and external rotation. These patients tend to be highly symptomatic in pain and can have difficulty with tasks as simple as walking. Secondary iliopsoas tendinitis, resulting from strain on the iliopsoas as it attempts to stabilize the anterior hip joint, can develop in these patients.

On examination, these patients may show global signs of generalized ligamentous laxity. The log-roll external rotation test may show a capsular laxity, with diminished spring back during external rotation (Figure 4). The results of this test can be compared with those of the contralateral hip. These patients also may have pain and apprehension during hip extension and external rotation if the primary component of instability is anterior. This pain and apprehension can be improved with a posteriorly directed force to the proximal femur in this position of anterior instability with external rotation and extension, a maneuver comparable to the Jobe relocation test in the shoulder.

Patients with hip microinstability in whom nonsurgical treatment has failed may benefit from a hip arthroscopy to address ligamentous and capsular laxity as well as

© 2016 American Academy of Orthopaedic Surgeons

labral tears. The labrum can be repaired after addressing any associated rim pathology using a mattress suture, which will restore the suction seal. Several procedures have been described to address the capsule in instability, including thermal capsulorrhaphy and capsular plication. Thermal capsulorrhaphy was described in 95 patients having a monopolar radiofrequency probe to reduce capsular redundancy, with resolution of hip instability in 100% of his patients at 12 months and improvement in their modified Harris Hip Scores.[30] To date, no reports have been recorded of chondrolysis secondary to thermal capsulorrhaphy in the hip, as has been described in the shoulder. Capsular plication also has been described by several authors as a method to reduce capsular redundancy. A technique has been described, in which the medial and lateral limbs of the IFL were tied together to reduce capsular laxity.[31] Another technique, in which the capsule is plicated by including it in a labral repair using double-loaded suture anchors at the acetabular rim, has been described.[32] This second technique is thought to restore normal anatomy and appropriately tension the capsule with good short-term results.

The evolution of the concept of capsular laxity as a source of hip instability has led some authors to stress the importance of capsular management and the recognition of risk factors for instability in hip arthroscopy performed to address other pathology. This concept has been reinforced by recent case reports of hip dislocations following hip arthroscopy. The authors of one study reported hip subluxation in a patient with a dysplastic hip 3 months following an arthroscopic labral resection and capsulotomy.[33] A case of a traumatic anterior hip dislocation was reported in a postoperative patient following a fall down stairs that was successfully treated with a revision capsular repair.[34] The authors of another study reported a hip dislocation in the recovery room in a patient who had undergone an arthroscopic capsulotomy for a cam resection and rim trimming; the dislocation was successfully treated with mini-open anterior capsulorrhaphy.[8]

Recently, improved outcomes have been demonstrated in patients undergoing hip arthroscopy with a complete capsular repair versus a matched cohort that underwent a partial repair only.[35] The complete repair group demonstrated superior sport-specific outcomes and had a 0% revision rate compared with a 13% arthroscopic revision rate in the partial repair group. Current recommendations for capsular management involve performing an interportal capsulotomy between the standard anterior and anterolateral portals to address central compartment pathology. This procedure is followed by adding a longitudinal capsulotomy to form a T-capsulotomy down the neck of the femur in the interval between the iliocapsularis and the gluteus minimus. This longitudinal component typically is stopped just proximal to the zona orbicularis to protect the lateral femoral circumflex artery. This exposure typically allows ample visualization of a cam lesion. Hip rotation provides visualization from the medial to lateral synovial folds, which are landmarks for the synovial vessels. Both limbs of the T-capsulotomy are repaired at the completion of the case with several side-to-side stitches. The capsule can be plicated at this stage, if indicated, by resecting a portion of the capsule before repair or by taking bigger bites in the side-to-side closure to tighten the capsule. In general, three or four sutures are used on the longitudinal portion, and two or three sutures are used on the interportal portion. Typically, the patient is placed in a brace for 6 weeks postoperatively to limit extension and external rotation, with a period of protected weight bearing as indicated for other procedures.

The Ligamentum Teres

The LT can be a common source of hip pain and has been found to be torn at arthroscopy in 8% to 51% of cases.[36-38] It is a pyramid-shaped structure, with its broad base at the posteroinferior acetabular fossa and its point attaching to the femoral fovea capitis. It forms some attachment to the transverse acetabular ligament at its base and transitions to a round and ovoid attachment to the femur. It has been shown to contain free nerve endings with both nocioceptive and proprioceptive innervation concentrated primarily in the center of the ligament, confirming its role as a potential pain generator in the hip.[39]

The function and pathologic role of the LT remains controversial. Currently, it is thought to serve as a secondary restraint to hip stability. The first suggestion that the LT might play a role in hip stability surfaced in an early cadaver study demonstrating that sectioning the LT resulted in increasing amounts of hip abduction and adduction.[27] A string model was used to assess LT excursion during hip motions and showed the greatest excursion during hip external rotation and flexion, which occurs in squatting, and during internal rotation and extension, which occurs when crossing one leg under the other.[28] The LT moved into an anterior and inferior position around the femoral head during a squat.[40] This was thought to provide a sling-like effect, analogous to the actions of the conjoint tendon in the coracoid transfer procedure in the shoulder. Further, in a survey of 161 postoperative patients who had undergone a surgical hip dislocation, which includes resection of the LT, it was reported that 35% of patients described popping and locking, and 24% experienced feelings of instability.[41] The LT may play a more important role in stability in dysplastic patients lacking acetabular coverage. These patients may be more reliant on primary soft-tissue restraints such as the labrum, capsule, and ligaments. If one or more of these soft-tissue restraints also is compromised, increased reliance on the LT to maintain a concentric hip joint may occur with certain motions.

Injury to the LT is thought to occur from one of several mechanisms. The LT is at risk with any major hip trauma causing a hip dislocation. It has been torn with lower levels of trauma, however, including a case report of a tear occurring while a patient pushed a shopping cart.[42] LT tears also can occur from repetitive microtrauma in sports requiring extreme amounts of hip motion such as dance, gymnastics, and martial arts. Microtrauma to the LT may be exacerbated in patients with ligamentous laxity or insufficiency, in which the LT is thought to play a larger role in instability. Finally, a degenerative tear can occur due to abrasive wear against osteophytes in osteoarthritis.[43]

The clinical assessment of LT tears traditionally has been difficult. Patients may report an injury during a twisting mechanism, a fall onto a flexed knee, or a hyperadduction mechanism. Patient reports may include pain, mechanical symptoms, and feelings of instability with giving way, especially during squatting and when crossing the affected leg behind the other when standing. Some patients may present with pain as their only symptom. Physical examination findings in patients with LT tears are consistent with findings in other tests for intra-articular pathology. These nonspecific tests include pain with flexion and internal rotation, log rolling in extension, and during the McCarthy test, in which the hip is alternately taken from flexion to extension in internal rotation and then external rotation. A test called the LT test was recently described that may aid in the diagnosis.[44] The LT test is performed by placing the patient supine, flexing in the hip to 70°, abducting it 30°, and rotating it into maximum internal and external rotation. This test was found to have a sensitivity of 90% and a specificity of 85%.

Imaging to identify LT pathology also has proven difficult traditionally. The authors of one study noted that only 2 of 23 LT tears in their series were diagnosed preoperatively.[37] In an attempt to distinguish partial LT tears from normal anatomy, the authors of a 2012 study found similar radiographic findings on 3-T magnetic resonance arthrography between the partial tear and normal anatomy.[45] Their ability to diagnose LT tears ranged from 42% to 67%. Finally, a sensitivity of 34% and a specificity of 50% in identifying pathology in the LT was found, also using 3-T MRI.[46]

Treatment options for LT tears include débridement and reconstruction. A systematic review compared the short-term benefit of the two modalities.[47] The 6-patient reconstruction group was compared with 81 patients in the débridement group. The débridement group showed an increase in modified Harris Hip Scores from poor (60.73; 95% confidence interval [CI], 47.0-74.46) to good (88.4; 95% CI, 85.95-90.82) and showed an improvement in pain and function in the mean nonarthritic hip score from 65.1 (95% CI, 62.94-67.26) to 86.35 (95% CI, 85.66-87.04). Although having very small numbers, the reconstruction group also showed improved subjective and objective outcome scores despite using different graft sources and fixation techniques. The indications for repair versus reconstruction are not yet defined clearly.[47]

Summary

Hip arthroscopy continues to evolve rapidly along with the understanding of pathology in and around the hip joint. The indications for surgery include pathology in the central, peripheral, and peritrochanteric compartments, and the indications are expanding to include pathology in the surrounding soft tissues. The acetabular labrum is a critical structure and should be repaired or reconstructed whenever possible to preserve its function, especially the negative suction seal function. Hip instability has proven to be a source of chronic pain and disability. Soft-tissue structures, including the LT, play a key role in maintaining stability, especially in the setting of abnormal bony morphology. Appropriate capsular management, including capsular repair and plication in indicated cases, is proving to be a key step in preserving or establishing hip stability and optimizing surgical outcomes. Tears of the LT are a source of pain in the hip and require a high index of suspicion to make the diagnosis. The LT test is a new physical examination tool to aid in making the diagnosis. Débridement of partial-thickness tears has demonstrated good clinical outcomes. LT reconstruction in instability cases may prove to be a useful adjunct along with capsular plication in certain settings but is still unproved at this point.

© 2016 American Academy of Orthopaedic Surgeons

Key Study Points

- Acetabular labral tears are the most commonly noted pathology at hip arthroscopy and should be repaired or reconstructed whenever possible to restore the labral function of creating a negative pressure seal to the femoral head.

- Hip microinstability is an increasingly recognized source of pain and instability because of soft-tissue restraint incompetency in the borderline dysplastic hip. The acetabular labrum, the ligamentum teres, and the joint capsule play critical secondary roles to bony restraint.

- Tears of the ligamentum teres can be an important source of pain and disability, which require a high index of suspicion to diagnose but are successfully treated with surgical débridement and reconstruction.

Annotated References

1. Colvin AC, Harrast J, Harner C: Trends in hip arthroscopy. *J Bone Joint Surg Am* 2012;94(4):e23.

   The authors determined that the number of hip arthroscopy cases submitted by American Board of Orthopaedic Surgery Part II candidates during the period from 1999 to 2009 increased 18-fold, with most performed by sports medicine fellowship–trained candidates

2. Bozic KJ, Chan V, Valone FH III, Feeley BT, Vail TP: Trends in hip arthroscopy utilization in the United States. *J Arthroplasty* 2013;28(8, Suppl)140-143.

   The authors determined that the incidence of hip arthroscopy procedures among American Board Of Orthopaedic Surgery Part II candidates increased over 600% from 2006 to 2010, with an overall complication rate of approximately 5%.

3. Harris JD, McCormick FM, Abrams GD, et al: Complications and reoperations during and after hip arthroscopy: A systematic review of 92 studies and more than 6,000 patients. *Arthroscopy* 2013;29(3):589-595.

   The authors reviewed 92 studies, of which 88% are level IV evidence with short-term follow-up at a mean of 2.0 years. The rate of major complications after hip arthroscopy was 0.58% and minor complications was 7.5%. The reoperation rate was 6.3% at a mean of 16 months, with the most common reoperation being conversion to total hip arthroplasty. Level of evidence: IV.

4. Dippmann C, Thorborg K, Kraemer O, Winge S, Hölmich P: Symptoms of nerve dysfunction after hip arthroscopy: An under-reported complication? *Arthroscopy* 2014;30(2):202-207.

   The authors reviewed 52 consecutive hip arthroscopy patients from March to October 2010 and determined that 46% report symptoms of nerve dysfunction during the first postoperative week, which decreased to 28% at 6 weeks and 18% after 1 year. Traction time during surgery was not different in patients with and without symptoms of nerve dysfunction. Level of evidence: IV.

5. Clohisy JC, Nepple JJ, Larson CM, Zaltz I, Millis M; Academic Network of Conservation Hip Outcome Research (ANCHOR) Members: Persistent structural disease is the most common cause of repeat hip preservation surgery. *Clin Orthop Relat Res* 2013;471(12):3788-3794.

   The authors reviewed a prospective, multicenter hip preservation database of 2,386 surgery cases to identify 352 patients, or 15%, who had prior surgery. Inadequately corrected structural disease was the most common reason for secondary surgery. Level of evidence: III.

6. Ayeni OR, Bedi A, Lorich DG, Kelly BT: Femoral neck fracture after arthroscopic management of femoroacetabular impingement: A case report. *J Bone Joint Surg Am* 2011;93(9):e47.

   The authors present a case report of a nondisplaced, subcapital femoral neck fracture after arthroscopic management of femoroacetabular impingement. Level of evidence: IV.

7. Fowler J, Owens BD: Abdominal compartment syndrome after hip arthroscopy. *Arthroscopy* 2010;26(1):128-130.

   Authors present a case report of abdominal compartment syndrome resulting from fluid extravasation following hip arthroscopy for FAI. A distended abdomen was noted at time of drape removal, and a decompressive laparotomy was performed. Level IV evidence.

8. Matsuda DK: Acute iatrogenic dislocation following hip impingement arthroscopic surgery. *Arthroscopy* 2009;25(4):400-404.

   The authors discuss a case report of an iatrogenic hip dislocation after arthroscopic hip surgery for femoroacetabular impingement. Noted in the report is supranormal hip distraction to extract a loose body. A mini-open capsulorrhaphy was required to restore hip stability. Level of evidence: IV.

9. Salvo JP, Troxell CR, Duggan DP: Incidence of venous thromboembolic disease following hip arthroscopy. *Orthopedics* 2010;33(9):664.

   The authors retrospectively reviewed 81 consecutive patients undergoing standard hip arthroscopy and determined a 3.7% incidence of clinically symptomatic venous thromboembolic disease, which was suspected clinically and confirmed with the use of Doppler ultrasonography. No patients developed symptomatic pulmonary emboli.

10. Bushnell BD, Dahners LE: Fatal pulmonary embolism in a polytraumatized patient following hip arthroscopy. *Orthopedics* 2009;32(1):56.

2: Hip and Pelvis

The authors present a case report of a fatal pulmonary embolism after hip arthroscopy performed to removal multiple intra-articular loose bodies following a closed reduction and percutaneous fixation of an acetabular fracture secondary to a gunshot wound.

11. Kelly BT, Weiland DE, Schenker ML, Philippon MJ: Arthroscopic labral repair in the hip: Surgical technique and review of the literature. *Arthroscopy* 2005;21(12):1496-1504.

12. Ferguson SJ, Bryant JT, Ganz R, Ito K: The acetabular labrum seal: A poroelastic finite element model. *Clin Biomech (Bristol, Avon)* 2000;15(6):463-468.

13. Ferguson SJ, Bryant JT, Ganz R, Ito K: The influence of the acetabular labrum on hip joint cartilage consolidation: A poroelastic finite element model. *J Biomech* 2000;33(8):953-960.

14. Ferguson SJ, Bryant JT, Ganz R, Ito K: An in vitro investigation of the acetabular labral seal in hip joint mechanics. *J Biomech* 2003;36(2):171-178.

15. Philippon MJ: Hip arthroscopy in the athlete, in McGinty JB, ed: *Operative arthroscopy*, ed 3. Philadelphia, Lippincott Williams & Wilkins, 2002.

16. Domb BG, Shindle MK, McArthur B, Voos JE, Magennis EM, Kelly BT: Iliopsoas impingement: A newly identified cause of labral pathology in the hip. *HSS J* 2011;7(2):145-150.

The authors identified 25 patients who underwent isolated, primary, unilateral iliopsoas release with either labral débridement or repair of a labral tear. In this series, they identified a distinct pattern of labral pathology that occurs in the direct anterior location thought be secondary to iliopsoas impingement. Level of evidence: IV.

17. Foote CJ, Maizlin ZV, Shrouder J, Grant MM, Bedi A, Ayeni OR: The association between avulsions of the reflected head of the rectus femoris and labral tears: A retrospective study. *J Pediatr Orthop* 2013;33(3):227-231.

The authors reviewed electronic medical records over a 10-year period of patients between the ages of 12 and 18 years and identified 9 patients with avulsion injuries of the rectus femoris muscle during sports activities, with 7 of the 9 demonstrating labral tears on magnetic resonance arthrography. All patients were initially managed nonsurgically, and 2 of the 9 went on to arthroscopy secondary to substantial refractory pain. Level of evidence: IV.

18. Lage LA, Patel JV, Villar RN: The acetabular labral tear: An arthroscopic classification. *Arthroscopy* 1996;12(3):269-272.

19. Seldes RM, Tan V, Hunt J, Katz M, Winiarsky R, Fitzgerald RH Jr: Anatomy, histologic features, and vascularity of the adult acetabular labrum. *Clin Orthop Relat Res* 2001;382:232-240.

20. Espinosa N, Rothenfluh DA, Beck M, Ganz R, Leunig M: Treatment of femoro-acetabular impingement: Preliminary results of labral refixation. *J Bone Joint Surg Am* 2006;88(5):925-935.

21. Larson CM, Giveans MR: Arthroscopic debridement versus refixation of the acetabular labrum associated with femoroacetabular impingement. *Arthroscopy* 2009;25(4):369-376.

The authors compared two groups that underwent arthroscopic labral débridement versus labral repair for pincer-type or combined pincer- and cam-type FAI with a minimum of 1-year follow-up. The labral repair group demonstrated better modified Harris Hip Scores (94.3 versus 88.9) and a greater percentage of good to excellent results compared with the labral débridement group (89.7% versus 66.7%). Level of evidence: IV.

22. Krych AJ, Thompson M, Knutson Z, Scoon J, Coleman SH: Arthroscopic labral repair versus selective labral débridement in female patients with femoroacetabular impingement: A prospective randomized study. *Arthroscopy* 2013;29(1):46-53.

The authors report outcomes of 36 female patients undergoing arthroscopic hip treatment for pincer- or combined-type FAI randomized to either labral repair versus labral débridement between June 2007 and June 2009 with the same rehabilitation protocol postoperatively with average follow-up of 32 months. The labral repair group demonstrated superior improvement in hip functional outcomes with a greater number rating their hip function as normal or nearly normal. Level of evidence: I.

23. Philippon MJ, Briggs KK, Hay CJ, Kuppersmith DA, Dewing CB, Huang MJ: Arthroscopic labral reconstruction in the hip using iliotibial band autograft: Technique and early outcomes. *Arthroscopy* 2010;26(6):750-756.

The authors discuss the technique of labral reconstruction for labral deficiency or advanced labral degeneration using an iliotibial band autograft and outcomes of 95 arthroscopic labral reconstructions with mean follow-up of 18 months. This study showed good outcomes and high patient satisfaction, with better outcomes for those within 1 year from the time of injury. Level of evidence: IV.

24. Shindle MK, Ranawat AS, Kelly BT: Diagnosis and management of traumatic and atraumatic hip instability in the athletic patient. *Clin Sports Med* 2006;25(2):309-326, ix-x.

25. Shu B, Safran MR: Hip instability: Anatomic and clinical considerations of traumatic and atraumatic instability. *Clin Sports Med* 2011;30(2):349-367.

The authors reviewed the anatomy of the hip and how each structure contributes to hip stability. They also reviewed the causes of instability and treatment techniques.

26. Demange MK, Kakuda CMS, Pereira CAM, Sakaki MH, Albuquerque RFM: Influence of the femoral head ligament on hip mechanical function. *Acta Ortop Bras* 2007; 15(4):187-190.

© 2016 American Academy of Orthopaedic Surgeons

27. Martin RL, Palmer I, Martin HD: Ligamentum teres: A functional description and potential clinical relevance. *Knee Surg Sports Traumatol Arthrosc* 2012;20(6):1209-1214.

The authors created a string model to examine ligamentum teres excursion during various hip positions and found the ligamentum teres to have the greatest hip excursion when the hip was externally rotated in flexion and internally rotated in extension. A total of 350 consecutive surgical patients were then retrospectively reviewed to identify 20 patients with complete ligamentum teres rupture. Nine of the 20 subjects were available for follow-up, and 5 of the 9 noted feelings of instability with squatting into external rotation and flexion and crossing one leg behind the other into internal rotation and extension. Level of evidence: IV.

28. Domb BG, Lareau JM, Baydoun H, Botser I, Millis MB, Yen YM: Is intraarticular pathology common in patients with hip dysplasia undergoing periacetabular osteotomy? *Clin Orthop Relat Res* 2014;472(2):674-680.

The authors documented arthroscopic incidence of intra-articular pathology of 16 patients undergoing peri-acetabular osteotomy for hip dysplasia and concomitant hip arthroscopy for mechanical symptoms consistent with labral pathology identified on MRI and found significant intra-articular pathology in all patients, to include pathology of the labrum, chondral surface, ligamentum teres, cam deformity, and psoas tendon.

29. Krych AJ, Thompson M, Larson CM, Byrd JW, Kelly BT: Is posterior hip instability associated with cam and pincer deformity? *Clin Orthop Relat Res* 2012;470(12):3390-3397.

The authors reviewed the records of 22 athletes presenting with a posterior acetabular rim fracture confirming a posterior hip instability episode and identified a potential association between the occurrence of posterior hip instability and structural abnormalities associated with FAI, which may contribute to a mechanism of femoroacetabular-induced posterior subluxation.

30. Philippon MJ: The role of arthroscopic thermal capsulorrhaphy in the hip. *Clin Sports Med* 2001;20(4):817-829.

31. Bayer JL, Sekiya JK: Hip instability and capsular laxity. *Oper Tech Orthop* 2010;20(4):237-241.

The authors describe their surgical technique for treatment of hip instability including evaluation with fluoroscopy and arthroscopy capsular plication.

32. Slikker W, Van Thiel GS, Chahal JC, Nho SJ: Hip instability and arthroscopic techniques for complete capsular closure and capsular plication. *Oper Tech Sports Med* 2012;20:301-309.

The authors describe two different techniques that provide anatomic repair of the capsule and aim to decrease the capsular volume to minimize the risk of iatrogenic hip instability after hip arthroscopy.

33. Benali Y, Katthagen BD: Hip subluxation as a complication of arthroscopic debridement. *Arthroscopy* 2009;25(4):405-407.

The authors reported the case of a 49-year-old woman with moderate hip dysplasia who underwent arthroscopic labral resection with removal of an acetabular exostoses in whom hip instability developed 3 months after surgery. It was concluded that the labrum performed a more stabilizing function in dysplastic joints.

34. Ranawat AS, McClincy M, Sekiya JK: Anterior dislocation of the hip after arthroscopy in a patient with capsular laxity of the hip. A case report. *J Bone Joint Surg Am* 2009;91(1):192-197.

The authors reported on a case of anterior hip dislocation after hip arthroscopy.

35. Frank RM, Lee S, Bush-Joseph CA, Kelly BT, Salata MJ, Nho SJ: Improved outcomes after hip arthroscopic surgery in patients undergoing T-capsulotomy with complete repair versus partial repair for femoroacetabular impingement: A comparative matched-pair analysis. *Am J Sports Med* 2014;42(11):2634-2642.

The authors reported outcomes of 64 patients undergoing hip arthroscopy for FAI that were divided into two treatment groups comparing a partial T-capsulotomy repair versus complete repair with minimum 2-year follow-up. Patients with complete capsular closure demonstrated superior sport-specific outcomes and no revision surgery versus 13% revision rate in the partial repair group.

36. Botser IB, Martin DE, Stout CE, Domb BG: Tears of the ligamentum teres: Prevalence in hip arthroscopy using 2 classification systems. *Am J Sports Med* 2011;39(Suppl):117S-125S.

The authors reviewed 558 primary hip arthroscopies by the senior author between February 2008 and January 2011 and determined that 51% had partial or complete ligamentum teres tears. Patients with tears were older and had worse preoperative functional scores. Magnetic resonance arthrography demonstrated low accuracy and sensitivity in detection of tears. Level of evidence: IV.

37. Byrd JW, Jones KS: Traumatic rupture of the ligamentum teres as a source of hip pain. *Arthroscopy* 2004;20(4):385-391.

38. Villar RN: *Hip Arthroscopy* .Oxford, Butterworth Heineman, 1992.

39. Haversath M, Hanke J, Landgraeber S, et al: The distribution of nociceptive innervation in the painful hip: A histological investigation. *Bone Joint J* 2013;95-B(6):770-776.

The authors performed a histologic investigation of the nociceptive innervation of the acteabular labrum, the ligamentum teres, and capsule of the hip in order to prove pain- and proprioceptive-associated marker expression. The labrum demonstrated pain-associated free nerve ending expression at its base, decreasing in the periphery. The ligamentum teres was concentrated at its center, and the capsule demonstrated almost homogenous marker expression in all investigated areas.

2: Hip and Pelvis

40. Kivlan BR, Richard Clemente F, Martin RL, Martin HD: Function of the ligamentum teres during multi-planar movement of the hip joint. *Knee Surg Sports Traumatol Arthrosc* 2013;21(7):1664-1668.

   The authors dissected the soft tissue of eight cadaver hips except for the ligamentum teres and placed the joints into flexion and abduction to simulate a deep squat position until ligamentous endpoint of the ligamentum teres was achieved. The orientation of the ligamentum teres was described and found to prevent the femoral head from anterior/inferior subluxation because of its sling-like effect in support of the femoral head.

41. Phillips AR, Bartlett G, Norton M, Fern D: Hip stability after ligamentum teres resection during surgical dislocation for cam impingement. *Hip Int* 2012;22(3):329-334.

   Questionnaires completed by 161 patients who had undergone surgical hip dislocation with excision of the ligamentum teres revealed 39% experience pain with exercise, 35% popping and locking, and 24% subjective feelings of giving way. Level of evidence: IV.

42. Yamamoto Y, Villar RN, Papavasileiou A: Supermarket hip: An unusual cause of injury to the hip joint. *Arthroscopy* 2008;24(4):490-493.

43. O'Donnell JM, Pritchard M, Salas AP, Singh PJ: The ligamentum teres—its increasing importance. *J Hip Preserv Surg* 2014;1:3-11.

   The authors reviewed the function, mechanism of injury, clinical assessment, imaging, arthroscopic assessment, treatment, outcomes, reconstruction, and unusual conditions of the ligamentum teres.

44. O'Donnell J, Economopoulos K, Singh P, Bates D, Pritchard M: The ligamentum teres test: A novel and effective test in diagnosing tears of the ligamentum teres. *Am J Sports Med* 2014;42(1):138-143.

   The authors reported results from a new test to detect ligamentum teres tears. The ligamentum teres test is performed by placing the patient supine, flexing the hip to 70°, abducting it 30°, and rotating it into maximum internal and external rotation. A sensitivity of 90% and a specificity of 85% were reported.

45. Blankenbaker DG, De Smet AA, Keene JS, Del Rio AM: Imaging appearance of the normal and partially torn ligamentum teres on hip MR arthrography. *AJR Am J Roentgenol* 2012;199(5):1093-1098.

   The authors reviewed magnetic resonance arthrography images of 116 patients who later underwent hip arthroscopy and reported a high level of difficulty of distinguishing partially torn versus intact ligamentum teres on imaging because of similar findings. Edema and peripheral irregularity were not associated with partial tears.

46. Devitt BM, Philippon MJ, Goljan P, Peixoto LP, Briggs KK, Ho CP: Preoperative diagnosis of pathologic conditions of the ligamentum teres: Is MRI a valuable imaging modality? *Arthroscopy* 2014;30(5):568-574.

   The authors review 3-Tesla MRI in detecting ligamentum teres tears in 142 patients who underwent hip arthroscopy. They reported that MRI demonstrated sensitivity and specificity of 50% and 34%, respectively, in identifying any pathologic process of the ligamentum teres. MRI was reported to have a 91% sensitivity and 67% positive predictive value at detecting a partial ligamentum teres tear. Level of evidence: II.

47. de SA D, Phillips M, Philippon MJ, Letkemann S, Simunovic N, Ayeni OR: Ligamentum teres injuries of the hip: A systematic review examining surgical indications, treatment options, and outcomes. *Arthroscopy* 2014;30(12):1634-1641.

   The authors performed a systematic review of all articles from 1946 to 2013 pertaining to surgical treatment of the ligamentum teres, identifying nine studies meeting eligibility criteria with 89 hips undergoing arthroscopic débridement or reconstruction of a torn ligamentum teres. Débridement demonstrated good outcomes for partial tears, whereas reconstruction may be indicated for full-thickness tears that resulted in instability, failure of previous débridement, or a combination of these conditions.

© 2016 American Academy of Orthopaedic Surgeons

Chapter 11

Femoroacetabular Impingement

Ljiljana Bogunovic, MD   Shane J. Nho, MD, MS

Abstract

Femoroacetabular impingement can lead to pain, limited motion, and decreased function in active adolescents and young adults. The condition arises from an osseous deformity in the proximal femur and/or acetabulum that results in abnormal joint contact force with hip range of motion. Damage to the labrum and articular cartilage develops with time, leading to early joint degeneration and osteoarthritis. In the symptomatic patient, early recognition and characterization of the deformity is critical to the success of surgical intervention.

Keywords: femoroacetabular impingement; FAI; cam deformity; pincer deformity; dysplasia; labral tear

Introduction

Femoroacetabular impingement (FAI) is an increasingly recognized cause of hip pain and dysfunction. FAI has been described as a condition resulting from a structural mismatch between the osseous anatomy of the proximal femur and that of the acetabulum, leading to abnormal loading of the hip joint and subsequent damage to the underlying labrum and articular cartilage.[1] In the non-dysplasic hip, increasing evidence suggests that FAI may lead to the development of early joint degeneration and osteoarthritis.[2,3] Over the past decade, the understanding of the pathomorphology and pathomechanics of FAI has

Dr. Nho or an immediate family member serves as a paid consultant to Össur and Stryker, and has received research or institutional support from AlloSource, Arthrex, Athletico, DJ Global Orthopaedics, ConMed Linvatec Miomed Orthopedics, Smith & Nephew, and Stryker. Neither Dr. Bogunovic nor any immediate family member has received anything of value from or has stock or stock options held in a commercial company or institution related directly or indirectly to the subject of this chapter.

increased significantly, allowing improved recognition, earlier diagnosis, and the development of effective treatment options.

Etiology

Structural deformity can occur secondary to the sequelae of pediatric hip disease such as slipped capital femoral epiphysis, Legg-Calvé-Perthes disease, and hip dysplasia. In most cases of primary FAI, no prior history of disease is present, and the condition is likely caused by a combination of genetic and environmental factors. The prevalence of FAI deformity in asymptomatic adults is estimated at approximately 14%, with 24% in males and 5% in females.[4] Males are three to five times more likely to have cam deformities than are females, and the deformity also is more likely to be bilateral in males.[4-7] A 2.8 relative risk of cam deformity in the siblings of affected individuals suggests additional genetic contributions.[8]

Several studies suggest a link between participation in high-level sports at a young age and the development of symptomatic disease.[9-13] Studies of young athletes demonstrate a lack of cam deformity in skeletally immature individuals but a presence after physeal closure.[9] Several studies have reported an increased prevalence of femoroacetabular deformities in football, soccer, and hockey players compared with the general population.[9,11,14,15] According to the data from the National Football League Scouting Combine, 90% of players showed radiographic evidence of FAI, of whom 31% were symptomatic and 69% were asymptomatic. The greater the α angle the more likely was the athlete to present with symptoms.[16] The repetitive stress that occurs in athletic activities is believed to influence physeal growth and potentially contribute to the development of deformity.

Types of Impingement

The deformity of primary FAI can involve the proximal femur (cam), the acetabulum (pincer), or both (combined). Isolated cam deformity or combined deformity appears to be most common, and each occurs with nearly equal frequency (45%). Isolated pincer deformity is less common, occurring in fewer than 10% of patients with symptomatic FAI.[17,18] Extra-articular impingement, which includes trochanteric-pelvic impingement, ischiofemoral impingement, and anterior inferior iliac spine (AIIS) impingement, is another infrequent, but increasingly recognized, source of symptomatic impingement. A thorough understanding of the pathomorphology and pathomechanics of each individual deformity is critical to the successful surgical management of FAI.

Cam Impingement

Cam deformity is characterized by decreased offset between the femoral head and neck, most commonly occurring at the anterolateral head-neck junction. With attempted hip flexion and internal rotation, the osseous cam lesion impinges on the acetabulum, limiting motion and causing damage at the chondrolabral junction with repetitive impingement. In cam impingement, inclusion of the deformity into the acetabulum results in shear stress and disruption of the chondrolabral junction, causing delamination of the articular cartilage from the underlying subchondral bone.[19] Over time, intrasubstance damage to the labrum occurs, and the chondral injury can progress to a full-thickness defect. The location and severity of the acetabular injury can be predicted by the size of the cam deformity, because a higher ⍺ angle is associated with increased incidence of full-thickness chondral defects.[20] In most patients, decreased offset occurs at the anterolateral head-neck junction, resulting in damage to the anterosuperior acetabulum.[3] In long-standing cam impingement, degenerative changes can progress to involve the weight-bearing spherical portion of the femoral head.

Pincer Impingement

Pincer impingement is characterized by excessive acetabular coverage. The acetabular overcoverage can be global (coxa protrusio and coxa profunda) or focal (cephalad retroversion) or can result from true acetabular retroversion.[21] Pincer impingement leads to intrasubstance damage of the labrum as it is compressed between the femoral neck and the abnormal acetabular rim during extremes of hip range of motion. As in cam impingement, the anterosuperior acetabulum is most commonly affected; less chondral delamination is present with isolated rim impingement, however. Over time, repeated levering of the femoral head against the excessive acetabular rim can result in contrecoup chondral injury to the posteroinferior femoral head and acetabulum.

Extra-articular Impingement

Subspine impingement is a distinct form of pincer impingement, in which the anterior capsule and/or iliocapsularis muscle becomes pinched between the femoral head-neck junction and a prominent AIIS.[22] Pathologic AIIS morphology can be developmental (types I and II) or can arise following pelvic osteotomy or secondary to prior rectus femoris injury or avulsion (type III). Affected patients may report activity-related groin pain, pain during prolonged sitting, limitations in motion, and a grinding sensation during deep flexion and lateral movements. Impingement between the lesser trochanter and the ischium (ischiofemoral impingement) and the great trochanter and the ilium (trochanteric-pelvic impingement) are other potential, although uncommon, sources of extra-articular impingement that can cause pain and restricted hip extension and abduction, respectively. Intra-articular steroid injection typically provides no relief or only partial relief of symptomatic extra-articular impingement.[22] Both open and arthroscopic resection have been shown to improve motion and alleviate pain.[22,23]

Femoral Version

Femoral version can affect the severity of cam and pincer deformities and should be assessed in all patients with symptomatic FAI. The normal adult femur has 10° to 15° of femoral anteversion. In the setting of relative or absolute femoral retroversion, external rotation of the hip is increased, and internal rotation is decreased. When femoral retroversion coexists with a focal cam or pincer lesion, the osseous lesion engages earlier (with less internal rotation) than would be seen in a hip with normal femoral anteversion.[21] The motion restriction in patients with combined FAI and femoral retroversion is typically more severe than in those patients with isolated FAI.

Acetabular Dysplasia

Symptomatic FAI must be differentiated from acetabular dysplasia. In dysplasia, abnormal joint loading occurs secondary to a relative undercoverage of the femoral head by an abnormally deficient acetabulum. Preoperative radiographs are essential to the diagnosis, and common radiographic parameters should be measured to ensure proper diagnosis. Although FAI may coexist with acetabular dysplasia, the surgical treatment for the combined condition varies dramatically from that of an isolated FAI.[24] Correction of dysplasia typically requires an open approach, most commonly performed using the Bernese periacetabular osteotomy.[25]

History

Given the overlap in symptomatology between the lumbar spine, hip, and pelvis, it is common for patients to present in a delayed fashion following previous failed treatment, or with an incorrect diagnosis. A layered approach should be applied to assess not only the mechanics of the hip joint but also the surrounding joints and musculature. A primary hip disorder may be obscured by compensatory injury to the pelvic musculature, lumbar spine, pubic joint, or sacroiliac joint as the patient attempts to maintain a high level of activity in the setting of restricted hip motion.[26] Patients may present with chronic gluteal pain, abductor irritability, trochanteric bursitis, osteitis pubis, or trochanteric bursitis.

The location, duration, and inciting factors of the patient's pain should be elicited. Although most patients with symptomatic impingement (80%) present with pain in the anterior groin or lateral hip, approximately 25% of patients report pain in the lumbar spine, buttock, or even referred pain to the knee.[27] Patients may display the classic "C" sign (**Figure 1**) when describing the location of pain. Most report an insidious onset of symptoms without a specific injury; however, athletes may recall a specific event.[27] Pain is often worse with activity (running, cutting, and pivoting) and is exacerbated in positions of hip flexion, such as prolonged sitting or squatting.

Physical Examination

Gait should be examined in all patients. A mild, intermittent limp is common but can be extremely subtle, occurring in up to 75% of patients.[27] Abductor weakness on the affected side often is seen with a positive Trendelenberg sign. Range of motion should be assessed on supine examination at full extension and at 90° of hip flexion. The contralateral limb should be examined for comparison. Bilateral disease is seen in approximately 75% of patients but is symptomatic in fewer than 25%.[28] Restricted hip motion is a defining feature of symptomatic FAI, and affected individuals often have less than 100° of straight flexion and less than 10° of internal rotation with the hip at 90° of flexion.

Several dynamic tests can be used to assess for the presence of impingement and to compare with the contralateral limb. A positive test should re-create the characteristic pain that the patient experiences. The positive anterior impingement test (**Figure 2**) causes pain in the anterior groin with flexion, adduction, and internal rotation, which is present in most patients (88%) with symptomatic FAI. Although sensitive for hip pathology, the anterior impingement test is not specific for impingement and may be positive in any patient with a labral or chondral injury. The apprehension test (**Figure 3**) is performed with the patient supine at the edge of the examination table. The hip is extended and externally rotated. Patients with

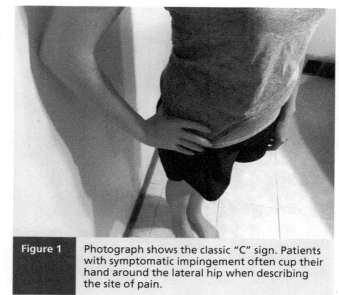

Figure 1 Photograph shows the classic "C" sign. Patients with symptomatic impingement often cup their hand around the lateral hip when describing the site of pain.

a dysplastic or unstable hip may report uneasiness or apprehension during this maneuver. The same maneuver also may re-create pain in patients with symptomatic posterior impingement. The subspine impingement test is performed with the patient in the supine position (**Figure 4**). Maximal anterior groin pain with direct hip flexion beyond 90° is consistent with subspine impingement.

Intra-articular anesthetic injection can be a useful adjunct to diagnosis. The injection can be performed in the office setting via ultrasound or fluoroscopic guidance. Following injection, patients are instructed to perform activities that would typically elicit pain. Substantial or complete relief with injection signifies an intra-articular source of pathology. Little to no pain relief following injection warrants further investigation. Such patients should be assessed for potential extra-articular sources of impingement (subspine impingement) or other pelvic or lumbar pathology.[22]

Imaging

Plain Radiographs

Preoperative imaging is critical to the diagnosis of FAI and in planning for potential surgical intervention. A systematic approach should be implemented and should include the following standard radiographs: standing AP pelvis, false profile, Dunn views, and frog-lateral views.[29] For an accurate standing AP pelvis view, the pelvis should be aligned with neutral rotation and tilt such that the coccyx is centered in the midline, the tip is within 1 to 3 cm of the pubic symphysis, and the obturator foramen is symmetric.[30] The joint space should be assessed for evidence of narrowing, sclerosis, or cystic change indicative

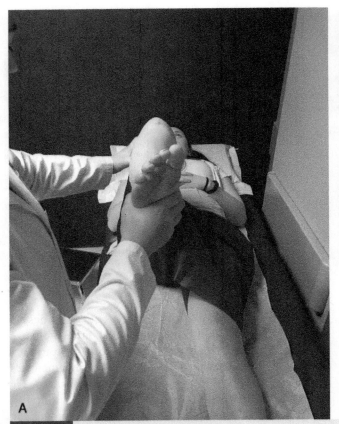
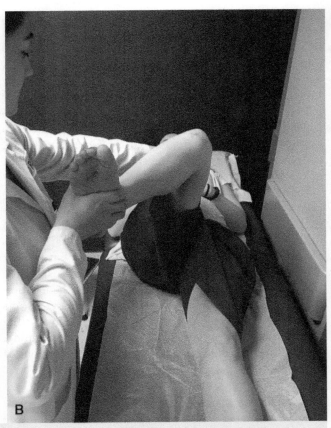

Figure 2   Photographs depict the anterior impingement test. This test is performed with the patient in the supine position. The affected hip is maximally flexed (**A**) and then adducted and internally rotated (**B**). Reproduction of the patient's anterior groin pain during this maneuver indicates clinically significant impingement and/or intra-articular pathology.

of early osteoarthritis. Acetabular depth and coverage should be assessed. Global overcoverage is easily identified when the medial femoral head lies adjacent to the ilioischial line (coxa profunda) or medial to it (coxa protrusio). Excessive anterior overcoverage, also referred to as cephalad retroversion, may be signaled by a crossover sign. In cephalad retroversion, relative retroversion of the anterosuperior acetabulum coexists with normal version of the anteromedial acetabulum. This must be differentiated from true acetabular retroversion, in which anterior overcoverage is associated with a deficient posterior wall, a condition that places the patient at risk for iatrogenic instability with isolated anterior wall decompression. A crossover sign, combined with an ischial spine sign and a posterior wall sign (the posterior wall lies medial to the center of the femoral head), is indicative of true acetabular retroversion[30] (Figure 5). The lateral center edge angle (LCEA) can be used to assess lateral overcoverage. Values greater than 40° indicate pincer morphology.[30] Additional findings concerning for rim impingement include rim fractures, a downsloping sourcil, a Tonnis angle less than

0°, and impingement cysts or a trough along the femoral head-neck junction.

The false profile view provides additional radiographic information regarding acetabular morphology. This image is obtained with the patient rotated at an angle of 65° between the pelvis and x-ray source and profiles the anterior acetabulum. An anterior center edge angle (ACEA) greater than 40° indicates excessive anterior overcoverage.[30] The morphology of the AIIS also can be assessed with this view (Figure 6).

The Dunn and frog-lateral views are used for assessment of the femoral cam morphology. The α angle is drawn to quantify the severity of the asphericity. Values greater than 50° indicate cam deformity (Figure 7). The different radiographic views help identify the loss of head-neck offset at different locations along the proximal femur. Nepple et al[29] used a clock face technique, in which the superior femoral neck is at 12 o'clock, and the anterior neck is at 3 o'clock, to correlate the position of the head-neck junction profiled on plain radiographs to radial oblique CT reformats. The 12 o'clock position is seen

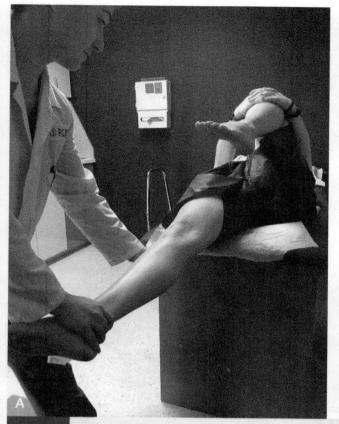
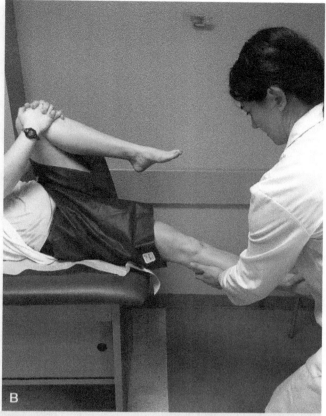

Figure 3 Photographs show the anterior apprehension test, which is performed with the patient supine and positioned at the end of the examination table. **A**, The contralateral hip is held in flexion; **B**, The affected hip is extended and externally rotated. Patients with structural instability may report a sense of instability or apprehension with this maneuver. Pain during this maneuver may signify posterior impingement.

with the AP pelvis view, the 1 o'clock with the 45° Dunn view, the 2 o'clock with the frog-lateral view, and the 3 o'clock with the cross-table lateral view. Given the typical location of cam deformities at the anterolateral head-neck junction (1 o'clock), deformity is identified most readily on the Dunn view, where the hip has abducted 20° and flexed to 45° (45° Dunn) or 90° (90° Dunn).[29,30] The 45° Dunn view has been shown to be more sensitive in detecting the presence and severity of cam deformity than the 90° Dunn view.[31] When compared with the Dunn view, the frog-lateral view has improved specificity for cam morphology.[29] It is crucial that all radiographs be scrutinized for evidence of acetabular dysplasia, which may coexist with FAI or be the primary pathology in a patient presenting with hip pain.

Radiographic findings on the AP pelvis that are concerning for acetabular undercoverage and structural instability include an LCEA less than 20° and a Tonnis angle greater than 10° (Figure 8). Anterior coverage can be assessed using the false profile view, on which an ACEA less than 20° is indicative of undercoverage (Figure 9). In some patients, including those with ligamentous hyperlaxity, more subtle signs of dysplasia (such as an LCEA less than 25°, uprising sourcil, ACEA less than 25°) may give rise to symptomatic instability.[30]

Magnetic Resonance Imaging

MRI can be helpful in assessing labral pathology. The sensitivity is significantly enhanced with intra-articular contrast dye, making magnetic resonance arthrography (MRA) with gadolinium the preferred imaging technique. If possible, all imaging should be performed using high-resolution 1.5 Tesla (or greater) MRI. True labral tears must be differentiated from naturally occurring clefts. Paralabral cysts and subchondral edema or cysts are indirect signs of labral and chondral injury, respectively. Labral hypertrophy can indicate underlying dysplasia. The addition of a long-acting anesthetic to the intra-articular gadolinium can provide additional diagnostic value. Temporary relief of symptoms verifies an intra-articular source of pain. The articular cartilage is poorly visualized with conventional MRI. Delayed gadolinium-enhanced

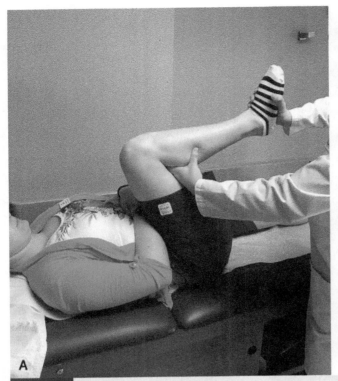
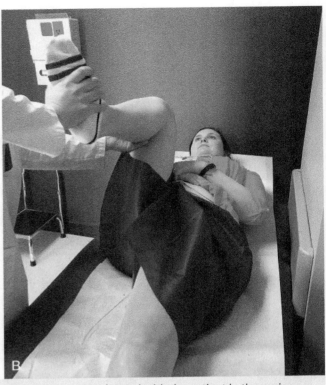

Figure 4   **A** and **B**, Photographs show the subspine impingement test, which is performed with the patient in the supine position. Maintaining neutral rotation and abduction, the hip is maximally flexed. In a patient with symptomatic subspine impingement, the anterior soft tissues become pinched between the inferior femoral neck and a prominent anterior inferior iliac spine (AIIS), causing pain.

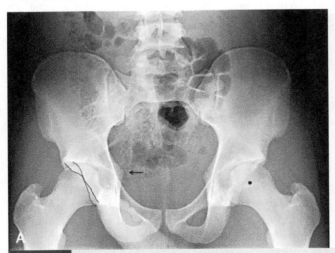
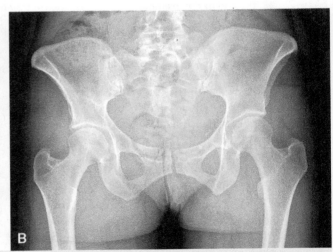

Figure 5   **A**, AP radiograph demonstrates true bilateral acetabular retroversion. Apparent are a crossover sign on the posterior wall (dashed line) and the anterior wall (solid line), a prominent ischial spine (black arrow), and a positive posterior wall sign where the posterior wall line lies medial to the midpoint of the femoral head (black dot). **B**, AP radiograph shows normal acetabulum.

MRI of cartilage (dGEMRIC) is a newer imaging technique that can detect early chondral degeneration by measuring the glycosaminoglycan content of the hyaline layer[32] (Figure 10). Patients receive intravenous contrast dye 30 minutes before imaging. This technique can be a useful adjunct when there is a concern for underlying osteoarthritis, because preexisting chondral degeneration is a known risk factor for poor outcomes following hip

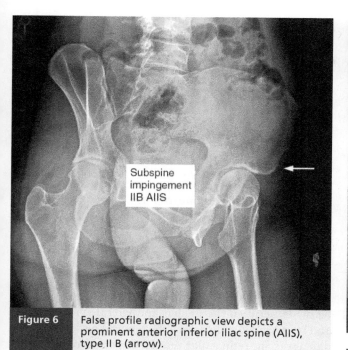

Figure 6   False profile radiographic view depicts a prominent anterior inferior iliac spine (AIIS), type II B (arrow).

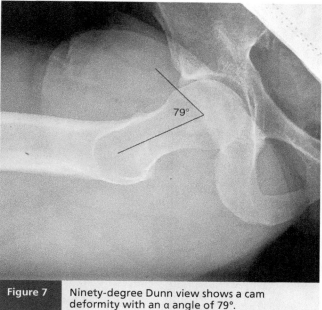

Figure 7   Ninety-degree Dunn view shows a cam deformity with an α angle of 79°.

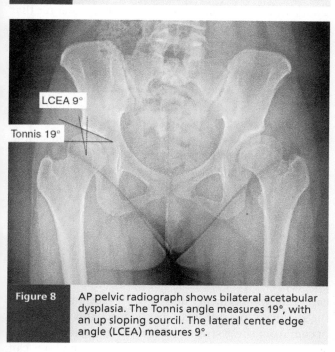

Figure 8   AP pelvic radiograph shows bilateral acetabular dysplasia. The Tonnis angle measures 19°, with an up sloping sourcil. The lateral center edge angle (LCEA) measures 9°.

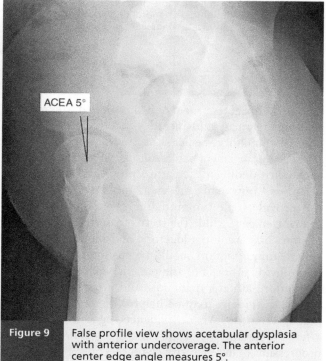

Figure 9   False profile view shows acetabular dysplasia with anterior undercoverage. The anterior center edge angle measures 5°.

arthroscopy and open hip preservation surgery.[33]

Three-Dimensional CT

Three-dimensional computed tomography (3D CT), which provides detailed information about the bony architecture, can be a helpful adjunct in planning bony resection. Although a crossover sign or ischial spine may alert the surgeon to pincer impingement, CT allows the direct assessment of acetabular version and depth. This can be especially helpful in identifying focal rim lesions, such as cephalad retroversion, and in differentiating them from true acetabular retroversion. CT is also invaluable to the assessment of AIIS morphology, which is poorly visualized on plain radiographs. Software programs can be applied to 3D CT images to model areas of impingement and plan sites of resection.

2: Hip and Pelvis

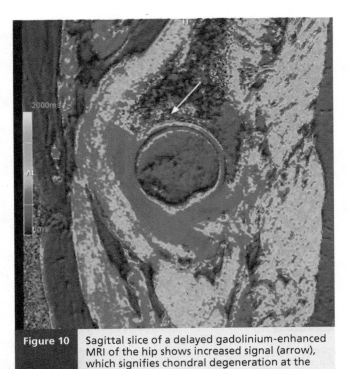

Figure 10 Sagittal slice of a delayed gadolinium-enhanced MRI of the hip shows increased signal (arrow), which signifies chondral degeneration at the superior acetabulum.

Nonsurgical Management

The nonsurgical treatment of FAI is limited to symptomatic management and includes activity modification, anti-inflammatory medications, and physical therapy.[34] Because impingement can result in compensatory injury to the surrounding musculature, physical therapy directed toward improving muscular mobility and strength can provide some symptomatic relief. Common areas of involvement include the rectus femoris, psoas muscle tendon complex, hip adductors, and hip abductors.[34,35] The therapy program should be customized to address the individual needs of the patient, including mobility restriction, athletic demands, and areas of weakness. Although therapy may be helpful in the symptomatic management of FAI, no evidence suggests that it will affect the natural history of the disease and/or alter the progression of degenerative changes.

Surgical Management

The decision to proceed to surgery is based on a combination of factors including the patient history, physical examination, imaging studies, failure of nonsurgical management, and temporary relief with injection. Although an open approach, such as the surgical hip dislocation described by Ganz, can be used, this chapter focuses on

the arthroscopic management of FAI. Successful treatment requires a comprehensive approach that addresses the osseous deformity and the resulting intra-articular damage. Incomplete decompression of the impinging lesion is the leading cause of recurrent pain in patients undergoing hip arthroscopy in the absence of substantial chondral injury.[33,36]

Hip arthroscopy proceeds via the standard technique, using a minimum of two arthroscopic portals. The procedure typically begins by addressing pathology in the central compartment, including the pincer and subspine deformity and the chondrolabral injury. Afterward, traction is released, and the arthroscope is advanced to the peripheral compartment for decompression of the cam deformity. An extensive capsulotomy (interportal, H-shaped, or T-shaped) has been described to improve access to pathology in the central and peripheral compartments. When performed, the capsulotomy should be made between the medial and lateral synovial folds and be extended in line with the femoral neck to prevent damage to the retinacular vessels. Capsular management remains an area of controversy. Some surgeons argue that anatomic closure is required to restore the stability and kinematics of the hip.

Central Compartment
Pincer Impingement
Acetabuloplasty or rim trimming involves removal of the pincer impingement. This can be performed with or without labral takedown. The extent of the resection should be determined preoperatively from the baseline imaging studies. Fluoroscopy can be used to assess progress intraoperatively. Care must be taken to prevent overresection and iatrogenic instability.

Labral Injuries
More than 90% of labral tears occur in conjunction with impingement deformity. The characteristics of labral injury depend on the type and duration of impingement. In early cam impingement, minimal intrasubstance injury to the labrum is present, because the mechanism of injury occurs from shear stress between the articular cartilage from the subchondral bone. Favorable healing rates can be achieved with labral refixation after rim trimming (Figure 11). In contrast, long-standing cam impingement and combined impingement typically lead to intrasubstance tearing and maceration of the labrum, which may present with an irreparable labrum. In the setting of an irreparable labrum, options include selective labral débridement and reconstruction.

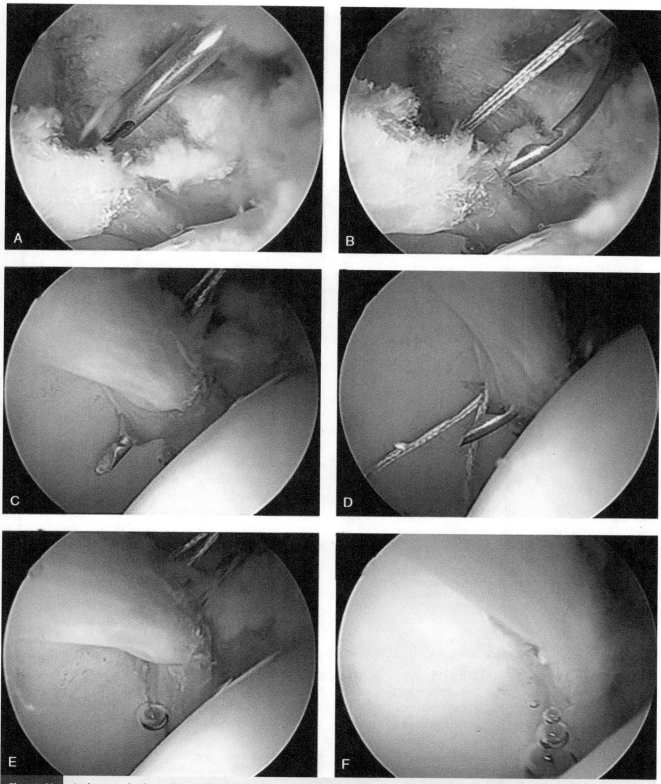

Figure 11 Arthroscopic views demonstrate labral repair using a suture passing device. **A,** A suture anchor is placed along the acetabular rim. **B,** A suture passing device is then introduced into the joint. A single limb of suture is grasped and passed through the labrum. **C,** An attempt is made to incorporate any chondral delamination into the repair. **D,** A second pass is made with the suture passer more peripheral to the first. **E,** The limbs are retrieved, and the repair is secured with an arthroscopic knot consisting of a series of alternating half-hitches. **F,** The repaired labrum and cartilage have been reapproximated to the subchondral bone.

2: Hip and Pelvis

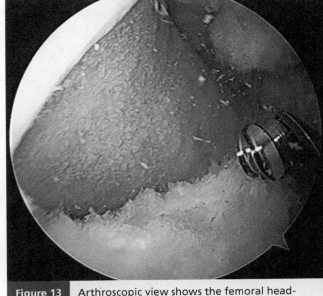

Figure 12 Arthroscopic view shows the peripheral compartment of the cam lesion following T-capsulotomy.

Figure 13 Arthroscopic view shows the femoral head-neck junction following completion of the osteochondroplasty.

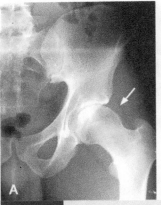 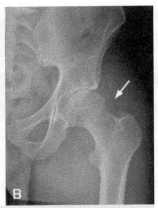

Figure 14 **A**, Preoperative AP radiograph depicts a typical cam deformity (arrow). **B**, Postoperative AP radiograph shows the restored femoral head-neck offset following decompression.

Chondral Injuries

The chondral injuries associated with FAI can range from delamination to full-thickness loss. In the setting of an intact chondrolabral junction, labral repair can serve to reapproximate the delaminated cartilage back to the subchondral bone. Detached and unstable flaps pose a clinical challenge. Débridement, refixation with fibrin glue, removal, and microfracture all have been described, but no gold standard treatment exists. In general, significant chondral injury is a poor prognostic factor for outcome and is one of the primary predictors of continued pain and reduced function postoperatively.

Peripheral Compartment

Failure to recognize and address osseous pathology is a prime factor contributing to treatment failure.[33] Comprehensive treatment of the cam deformity depends on the understanding of the deformity, adequate visualization, the ability to access the CAM deformity in its entirety, and capsular management. After the central compartment has been addressed, the hip traction is released, and the hip is placed in approximately 20° to 30° of flexion with neutral rotation. The author's preference is to use a T-capsulotomy perpendicular from the interportal capsulotomy and extended to the intertrochanteric line between the iliocapsularis and the gluteus minimus (Figure 12). The cam deformity is resected using a high-speed burr while using intraoperative fluoroscopy to confirm a comprehensive femoral osteochondroplasty (Figure 13). The hip must be positioned from complete hip extension and internal rotation to full flexion and external rotation to permit access to the entire cam deformity. After the dynamic examination and fluoroscopic evaluation confirm restoration of the head-neck offset, the capsule is completely closed by shuttling numerous high-strength sutures (Figure 14).

Outcomes

Proper patient selection is critical to the successful surgical treatment of FAI. Reduced pain and improved function are reported in 68% to 96% of patients.[37] Approximately 75% of athletes are able to return to competition at the same level or better.[38] The long-term effect of hip arthroscopy and its potential to alter the natural history of FAI and prevent early degenerative joint disease remain to be determined. The current literature does not support prophylactic cam or pincer decompression in asymptomatic patients.[39]

The presence of preoperative osteoarthritis (Tonnis grade greater than or equal to 2 or Outerbridge grade greater than or equal to 3) is the strongest predictor of poor outcome following hip arthroscopy. Other factors associated with a poorer outcome include older age, a longer duration of symptoms, more severe preoperative pain, and poorer functional scores.[37,40] In the absence of preexisting chondral disease, residual impingement is the leading cause of continued postoperative pain and revision surgery.[33,36]

Summary

Active adolescents and young adults who report hip and/or groin pain should be assessed for FAI. The presence of a cam and/or pincer deformity not only restricts motion, but also leads to joint degeneration over time. Patient history, physical examination, and radiographs are critical to the diagnosis of FAI and to the planning of surgical intervention. Hip arthroscopy is an effective treatment modality. Failure to address all the components of osseous impingement is a prime reason for continued pain and dysfunction following hip arthroscopy.

Key Study Points

- FAI results from a structural mismatch between the proximal femur (cam) and the acetabulum (pincer).
- Extra-articular impingement is a less common but increasingly recognized source of symptomatic impingement.
- Most patients with symptomatic impingement present with activity-related groin pain.
- Limited range of motion of the hip is one of the defining characteristics of FAI.
- FAI must be differentiated from dysplasia when evaluating a patient with hip pain. The two conditions may coexist.
- Both arthroscopic and open techniques are effective in the surgical management of FAI.
- Residual deformity is a leading cause of continued pain after the surgical management of FAI.
- Older age, preexisting osteoarthritis, and a longer duration of symptoms are risk factors for poor outcomes following surgical intervention.

Annotated References

1. Ganz R, Parvizi J, Beck M, Leunig M, Nötzli H, Siebenrock KA: Femoroacetabular impingement: A cause for osteoarthritis of the hip. *Clin Orthop Relat Res* 2003;417:112-120.

2. Beck M, Kalhor M, Leunig M, Ganz R: Hip morphology influences the pattern of damage to the acetabular cartilage: Femoroacetabular impingement as a cause of early osteoarthritis of the hip. *J Bone Joint Surg Br* 2005;87(7):1012-1018.

3. Tannast M, Goricki D, Beck M, Murphy SB, Siebenrock KA: Hip damage occurs at the zone of femoroacetabular impingement. *Clin Orthop Relat Res* 2008;466(2):273-280.

4. Hack K, Di Primio G, Rakhra K, Beaulé PE: Prevalence of cam-type femoroacetabular impingement morphology in asymptomatic volunteers. *J Bone Joint Surg Am* 2010;92(14):2436-2444.

   Two hundred asymptomatic volunteers underwent MRI of both hips. The images were examined for evidence of cam deformity (α angle greater than 50.5°). Cam deformity was found in 14% of asymptomatic volunteers (10.5% bilateral deformity and 3.5% unilateral deformity).

5. Kang AC, Gooding AJ, Coates MH, Goh TD, Armour P, Rietveld J: Computed tomography assessment of hip joints in asymptomatic individuals in relation to femoroacetabular impingement. *Am J Sports Med* 2010;38(6):1160-1165.

   One hundred hips in 50 patients with no history of hip dysfunction underwent CT for abdominal pain or trauma. The images were assessed for evidence of impingement pathology. At least one radiographic finding consistent with FAI was identified in 39% of hips.

6. Gosvig KK, Jacobsen S, Sonne-Holm S, Palm H, Troelsen A: Prevalence of malformations of the hip joint and their relationship to sex, groin pain, and risk of osteoarthritis: A population-based survey. *J Bone Joint Surg Am* 2010;92(5):1162-1169.

   This is a cross-sectional study of 4,151 individuals in the Copenhagen Osteoarthritis Study. Patient radiographs were assessed for evidence of osteoarthritis and hip deformity (impingement and dysplasia). The prevalence of osteoarthritis was 9.5% in men and 12.5% in women. Combined deformity and arthritis were found in 71% of men and 36% of women. A pistol-grip deformity was associated with an increased risk of osteoarthritis (risk ratio 2.2), as was a deep acetabular socket (risk ratio 2.4).

7. Laborie LB, Lehmann TG, Engesæter IØ, Eastwood DM, Engesæter LB, Rosendahl K: Prevalence of radiographic findings thought to be associated with femoroacetabular impingement in a population-based cohort of 2081 healthy young adults. *Radiology* 2011;260(2):494-502.

   This is a prospective study of 2,081 young adults (mean age, 18 years). Radiographs were reviewed for evidence of impingement pathology. A pistol-grip deformity was found in 21% of males and 3% of females. Pincer deformity was seen equally among the sexes (14% in men and 5% in women, $p < 0.001$).

8. Pollard TC, Villar RN, Norton MR, et al: Genetic influences in the aetiology of femoroacetabular impingement: A sibling study. *J Bone Joint Surg Br* 2010;92(2):209-216.

Ninety-six siblings of 64 patients treated for primary FAI were clinically and radiographically assessed for evidence of hip impingement. The siblings of patients with cam deformity had a 2.8 relative risk of having the same deformity. Compared with control patients, the siblings of affected individuals had a 2.5 relative risk of having impingement morphology.

9. Agricola R, Heijboer MP, Ginai AZ, et al: A cam deformity is gradually acquired during skeletal maturation in adolescent and young male soccer players: A prospective study with minimum 2-year follow-up. *Am J Sports Med* 2014;42(4):798-806.

This is a prospective cohort study of 63 preprofessional soccer players who were radiographically assessed before skeletal maturity and then reassessed over a 2.5-year period. The prevalence of a cam deformity increased from 2.1% to 17.7% during the time of physeal closure, with no additional increase in severity following physeal closure. The authors hypothesize that cam deformities develop slowly around the time of physeal closure and may be prevented by limiting athletic activity during this period of skeletal growth.

10. Carsen S, Moroz PJ, Rakhra K, et al: The Otto Aufranc Award. On the etiology of the cam deformity: A cross-sectional pediatric MRI study. *Clin Orthop Relat Res* 2014;472(2):430-436.

This is a cross-sectional cohort study of pediatric patients. MRI was used to evaluate 44 healthy volunteers (88 hips) before and after physeal closure. The images were assessed for evidence of a cam deformity (α angle greater than or equal to 50.5°), and volunteer activity level was collected. The mean α angles were 38° and 42° in the patients with open and closed physes, respectively. Although no patients with open physes had cam morphology, 3 of 21 (14%) of those with closed physes had at least one hip with cam morphology. These patients were all male and had a higher daily activity level.

11. Kapron AL, Anderson AE, Aoki SK, et al: Radiographic prevalence of femoroacetabular impingement in collegiate football players: AAOS Exhibit Selection. *J Bone Joint Surg Am* 2011;93(19):e111, 1-10.

This is a prospective study of 67 male collegiate football players (134 hips). Plain radiographs were obtained and assessed for evidence of FAI (cam α angle greater than or equal to 50° or head-neck offset less than 8 mm, pincer LCEA greater than 40°, Tonnis angle less than 0°, and/or positive crossover sign). At least one sign of cam or pincer impingement was present in 95% of hips. An abnormal α angle was found in 72% of hips, decreased femoral head-neck offset in 64%, a crossover sign in 61%, a reduced Tonnis angle in 16%, and an increased LCEA in 7%.

12. Siebenrock KA, Behning A, Mamisch TC, Schwab JM: Growth plate alteration precedes cam-type deformity in elite basketball players. *Clin Orthop Relat Res* 2013;471(4):1084-1091.

A case-control comparative analysis was performed on young (age 9 to 22 years) elite male basketball players. The proximal femoral physeal extension was measured using radial sequence MRI cuts and compared with an age-matched control group of nonathletes. In athletes with closed physes, epiphyseal extension occurred only at the 3 o'clock position and correlated with an α angle greater than 55°. The authors concluded that cam deformity develops in athletes as a consequence of alterations to the growth plate.

13. Siebenrock KA, Kaschka I, Frauchiger L, Werlen S, Schwab JM: Prevalence of cam-type deformity and hip pain in elite ice hockey players before and after the end of growth. *Am J Sports Med* 2013;41(10):2308-2313.

To assess for evidence of FAI, 77 elite male ice hockey players underwent physical examination and MRI. Of the athletes, 20% reported a history of hip pain and had a positive impingement test finding. Alpha angles were higher in athletes with closed physes than in those with open physes (58° versus 49°). The α angle was higher, and internal rotation was reduced in symptomatic patients versus asymptomatic patients.

14. Silvis ML, Mosher TJ, Smetana BS, et al: High prevalence of pelvic and hip magnetic resonance imaging findings in asymptomatic collegiate and professional hockey players. *Am J Sports Med* 2011;39(4):715-721.

This is a cross-sectional study of 21 professional and 18 collegiate asymptomatic ice hockey players. Athletes completed the modified Oswestry Disability Questionnaire and underwent MRI. Pathologic hip changes were seen in 64% of athletes, and MRI findings of common adductor-abdominal rectus dysfunction were seen in 36% of athletes.

15. Gerhardt MB, Romero AA, Silvers HJ, Harris DJ, Watanabe D, Mandelbaum BR: The prevalence of radiographic hip abnormalities in elite soccer players. *Am J Sports Med* 2012;40(3):584-588.

The authors retrospectively reviewed the pelvic radiographs of 95 elite male and female soccer players to assess for evidence of FAI. Symptomatic and asymptomatic athletes were included. Radiographic evidence of FAI was found in 72% of males and 50% of females. A cam lesion was found in 68% of males (77% bilateral) and 50% of females (90% bilateral). Pincer lesions were found in 27% of males and 10% of females.

16. Larson CM, Sikka RS, Sardelli MC, et al: Increasing alpha angle is predictive of athletic-related "hip" and "groin" pain in collegiate National Football League prospects. *Arthroscopy* 2013;29(3):405-410.

This is a cohort study involving 125 male collegiate football players (239 hips) undergoing physical and radiographic evaluation of the hip during the National Football League Scouting Combine. Symptomatic and asymptomatic athletes were included. Ninety percent of athletes had at least one radiographic finding consistent with FAI (pincer or cam deformity). An increased prevalence of cam deformity was found in the symptomatic group, and an increasing α angle was the only independent predictor of activity-related groin pain.

17. Clohisy JC, Baca G, Beaulé PE, et al; ANCHOR Study Group: Descriptive epidemiology of femoroacetabular impingement: A North American cohort of patients undergoing surgery. *Am J Sports Med* 2013;41(6):1348-1356.

    This a cross-sectional multicenter study assessing the epidemiology of FAI. A total of 1,076 consecutive patients (1,130 hips) undergoing surgical treatment of FAI were included. A primary cam deformity was the main pathology in 48% of hips; 45% had combined pincer/cam pathology; and 7.9% had isolated pincer pathology. Surgical intervention included a hip arthroscopy in 50% of patients, surgical dislocation in 34%, a reverse periacetabular osteotomy in 9.4%, a combined hip arthroscopy and limited open osteochondroplasty in 5.8%, and an isolated limited open osteochondroplasty in 1.5%. At the time of surgery, labral and chondral lesions were found in more than 90% of hips. A labral repair was performed in 48% of hips, a labral débridement in 16%, a rim trim in 37%, and a femoral osteochondroplasty in 92%.

18. Larson CM, Giveans MR: Arthroscopic management of femoroacetabular impingement: Early outcomes measures. *Arthroscopy* 2008;24(5):540-546.

19. Beck M, Leunig M, Parvizi J, Boutier V, Wyss D, Ganz R: Anterior femoroacetabular impingement: Part II. Midterm results of surgical treatment. *Clin Orthop Relat Res* 2004;418:67-73.

20. Johnston TL, Schenker ML, Briggs KK, Philippon MJ: Relationship between offset angle alpha and hip chondral injury in femoroacetabular impingement. *Arthroscopy* 2008;24(6):669-675.

21. Bedi A, Kelly BT, Khanduja V: Arthroscopic hip preservation surgery: Current concepts and perspective. *Bone Joint J* 2013;95-B(1):10-19.

    The study is a review of the epidemiology, etiology, diagnosis, and treatment of femoroacetabular impingement.

22. Larson CM, Kelly BT, Stone RM: Making a case for anterior inferior iliac spine/subspine hip impingement: Three representative case reports and proposed concept. *Arthroscopy* 2011;27(12):1732-1737.

    The study is a case report of three patients with symptomatic subspine impingement who were treated with arthroscopic decompression.

23. Hetsroni I, Larson CM, Dela Torre K, Zbeda RM, Magennis E, Kelly BT: Anterior inferior iliac spine deformity as an extra-articular source for hip impingement: A series of 10 patients treated with arthroscopic decompression. *Arthroscopy* 2012;28(11):1644-1653.

The study is a retrospective review of 10 patients with symptomatic subspine impingement. Of all patients, 90% had a coexisting cam lesion that also was addressed at the time of hip arthroscopy. The technique for arthroscopic subspine decompression is presented. Postoperatively, the mean patient hip range of motion improved from 99° ± 7° to 117° ± 8°. The modified Harris Hip Score improved from 64 to 98 at an average follow-up of 14.7 months.

24. Clohisy JC, Nunley RM, Curry MC, Schoenecker PL: Periacetabular osteotomy for the treatment of acetabular dysplasia associated with major aspherical femoral head deformities. *J Bone Joint Surg Am* 2007;89(7):1417-1423.

25. Siebenrock KA, Schöll E, Lottenbach M, Ganz R: Bernese periacetabular osteotomy. *Clin Orthop Relat Res* 1999;363:9-20.

26. Hammoud S, Bedi A, Voos JE, Mauro CS, Kelly BT: The recognition and evaluation of patterns of compensatory injury in patients with mechanical hip pain. *Sports Health* 2014;6(2):108-118.

    The study is a literature review of the compensatory injury patterns associated with intra-articular hip pathology, including osteitis pubis and dysfunction of the sacroiliac joint and/or lumbosacral spine.

27. Clohisy JC, Knaus ER, Hunt DM, Lesher JM, Harris-Hayes M, Prather H: Clinical presentation of patients with symptomatic anterior hip impingement. *Clin Orthop Relat Res* 2009;467(3):638-644.

    This is a prospective cohort study that evaluated the clinical presentation of patients with symptomatic FAI. Most patients reported an insidious onset of symptoms with a time of onset to definitive diagnosis beginning at 3.1 years. Eighty-eight patients reported pain in the anterior groin. Hip motion was limited to an average flexion of 97° and 9° of internal rotation at 90° of hip flexion.

28. Allen D, Beaulé PE, Ramadan O, Doucette S: Prevalence of associated deformities and hip pain in patients with cam-type femoroacetabular impingement. *J Bone Joint Surg Br* 2009;91(5):589-594.

    This is a cohort study of 113 patients with symptomatic FAI of at least one hip without evidence of concomitant dysplasia or osteoarthritis. Bilateral cam deformity was present in 78% of patients, but only 26% had bilateral hip pain. A higher α angle was found in symptomatic hips compared with asymptomatic hips (70° versus 63°, $p < 0.001$). The odds ratio of a painful hip was 2.59 in hips with an α angle greater than 60°.

29. Nepple JJ, Martel JM, Kim Y-J, Zaltz I, Clohisy JC; ANCHOR Study Group: Do plain radiographs correlate with CT for imaging of cam-type femoroacetabular impingement? *Clin Orthop Relat Res* 2012;470(12):3313-3320.

    This is a retrospective review of 41 surgical patients. Radial oblique reformats of preoperative CT scans were compared with plain radiographs. A standard radiographic hip series (AP pelvis, 45° Dunn, and frog-lateral views) has an 86% to 90% sensitivity in detecting an abnormal

2: Hip and Pelvis

α angle as seen on CT. The Dunn view was most sensitive in detecting a cam deformity (71% to 80%) but the frog-lateral view was the most specific (91% to 100%). The cross-table lateral view did not improve sensitivity.

30. Clohisy JC, Carlisle JC, Beaulé PE, et al: A systematic approach to the plain radiographic evaluation of the young adult hip. *J Bone Joint Surg Am* 2008;90(Suppl 4):47-66.

31. Meyer DC, Beck M, Ellis T, Ganz R, Leunig M: Comparison of six radiographic projections to assess femoral head/neck asphericity. *Clin Orthop Relat Res* 2006;445(445):181-185.

32. Zilkens C, Miese F, Kim Y-J, et al: Three-dimensional delayed gadolinium-enhanced magnetic resonance imaging of hip joint cartilage at 3T: A prospective controlled study. *Eur J Radiol* 2012;81(11):3420-3425.

    This is a case-control study of 40 patients with symptomatic FAI, dysplasia, or Legg-Calvé-Perthes disease who underwent high-resolution dGEMRIC MRI for evaluation of the hip articular cartilage. The patient imaging results were compared with those of a group of asymptomatic controls. The glycosaminoglycan content was significantly higher in the control group than in the patient group, corresponding to underlying chondral damage in the patients with FAI.

33. Bogunovic L, Gottlieb M, Pashos G, Baca G, Clohisy JC: Why do hip arthroscopy procedures fail? *Clin Orthop Relat Res* 2013;471(8):2523-2529.

    This is a prospective cohort study of 1,724 consecutive patients who underwent revision hip preservation surgery following prior hip arthroscopy. Residual FAI was the reason for failure in 68% of patients, and underlying acetabular dysplasia was the reason for failure in 24% of patients. Revision procedures included revision hip arthroscopy (42%), periacetabular osteotomy (24%), and surgical hip dislocation (32%).

34. Wall PD, Fernandez M, Griffin DR, Foster NE: Nonoperative treatment for femoroacetabular impingement: A systematic review of the literature. *PM R* 2013;5(5):418-426.

    This is a systematic review including five studies evaluating the nonsurgical treatment of FAI. Despite limited data in the included studies, the authors suggest that physical therapy and activity modification may confer some benefit to patients. Further research evaluating the outcome of nonsurgical management, especially physical therapy, is needed, however.

35. Yazbek PM, Ovanessian V, Martin RL, Fukuda TY: Nonsurgical treatment of acetabular labrum tears: A case series. *J Orthop Sports Phys Ther* 2011;41(5):346-353.

    This is a case series of four patients with a symptomatic labral tear treated with nonsurgical management. All patients underwent a three-phase physical therapy program progressing from pain control and trunk stabilization to muscular strengthening, sensory motor training, and sport specific progression. All patients reported reduced pain and improved function.

36. Ricciardi BF, Fields K, Kelly BT, Ranawat AS, Coleman SH, Sink EL: Causes and risk factors for revision hip preservation surgery. *Am J Sports Med* 2014;42(11):2627-2633.

    This is a cross-sectional study of 147 patients in whom prior hip arthroscopy had failed. Reasons for prior failure included residual femoroacetabular impingement (75%) and residual extra-articular impingement (9.5%). Approximately 80% of revision procedures were performed arthroscopically. Patients reported improved function following revision at an average of 15 months.

37. Clohisy JC, St John LC, Schutz AL: Surgical treatment of femoroacetabular impingement: A systematic review of the literature. *Clin Orthop Relat Res* 2010;468(2):555-564.

    This is a systematic review of 11 studies evaluating the surgical treatment of FAI. The mean follow-up was 3.2 years. All studies reported reduced pain and improved function in patients following surgery. Major complications occurred in zero to 18% of procedures.

38. Nho SJ, Magennis EM, Singh CK, Kelly BT: Outcomes after the arthroscopic treatment of femoroacetabular impingement in a mixed group of high-level athletes. *Am J Sports Med* 2011;39(Suppl):14S-19S.

    This is a case series of 47 high-level athletes who underwent arthroscopic treatment of symptomatic FAI. Follow-up was obtained in 70% of patients at 1 year. The average modified Harris Hip Score improved from 68 to 88, and the mean α angle improved from 76° to 51°. Of all patients, 79% were able to return to play at an average of 9 months postoperatively. At 2-year follow-up, 73% of patients continued to compete.

39. Collins JA, Ward JP, Youm T: Is prophylactic surgery for femoroacetabular impingement indicated? A systematic review. *Am J Sports Med* 2014;42(12):3009-3015.

    This is a systematic review performed to determine the efficacy of prophylactic surgery for FAI. No studies were identified to support treatment of an asymptomatic hip.

40. Saadat E, Martin SD, Thornhill TS, Brownlee SA, Losina E, Katz JN: Factors associated with the failure of surgical treatment for femoroacetabular impingement: Review of the literature. *Am J Sports Med* 2013;42(6):1487-1495.

    This is a systematic review of 13 studies evaluating the factors associated with failure of hip arthroscopy. Factors associated with poor postoperative outcome and conversion to hip arthroplasty included preoperative chondral damage, older age, a poor preoperative modified Harris Hip Score, and a longer duration of symptoms (more than 1.5 years). Preoperative osteoarthritis was the strongest predictor of postoperative conversion to hip arthroplasty.

2: Hip and Pelvis

Chapter 12

Extra-articular Hip Disorders

J.W. Thomas Byrd, MD   Guillaume D. Dumont, MD

Abstract

Extra-articular etiologies of pain represent an important subset of hip disorders. Physical examination and imaging modalities including radiographs, ultrasonography, and MRI are helpful in accurately identifying the pathology. Most hip pathologies can be treated initially with nonsurgical measures including rest, activity modification, NSAIDs, and physical therapy. Directed injections are helpful in the diagnosis and treatment of extra-articular pain. The surgical treatment of these disorders can be successful in cases that persist despite nonsurgical measures.

Keywords: greater trochanteric pain syndrome; trochanteric bursitis; hip abductor tears; piriformis syndrome; snapping hip

Introduction

Extra-articular hip disorders are common and can present a diagnostic and therapeutic dilemma. Treatment algorithms have evolved with the advent of modern arthroscopic and endoscopic techniques. Thorough directed history and physical examination techniques as well as patient selection for various nonsurgical and surgical treatment options remain paramount for the successful treatment of these disorders. This chapter discusses the scientific advances relating to greater trochanteric pain syndrome (GTPS), piriformis syndrome, external snapping hip, and internal snapping hip.

Greater Trochanteric Pain Syndrome

GTPS is a term that encompasses various possible etiologies of pain to the lateral hip, including trochanteric bursitis, tears or enthesopathy of the gluteus medius and minimus, and occasionally, friction of the iliotibial band over the greater trochanter. GTPS typically presents with pain or reproducible tenderness over the greater trochanter, buttock, or lateral thigh and is relatively common, affecting 10% to 25% of the general population.[1] The use of the term "trochanteric bursitis" has declined in recent years, after the realization that inflammation of the bursa typically is not identified in patients with lateral hip pain. More often, pathology involving the tendinous insertions to the greater trochanter appears to be culpable.

A retrospective study of the ultrasonograms of 877 patients with GTPS revealed that only 20.2% (177 patients) had sonographic evidence of bursitis. Of the remainder, 49.9% (438 patients) had gluteal tendinosis, 0.5% (4 patients) had gluteal tendon tears, and 28.5% (250 patients) had thickening of the iliotibial band.[2]

Although evidence is increasing for the importance of tendon injury versus bursal abnormality in patients with GTPS, the importance of the bursa in GTPS should not yet be discounted completely. A 2014 histologic study found that the presence of substance P was increased, or found more frequently, in the trochanteric bursa of patients with GTPS and control subjects, but no increase was noted within the gluteus medius tendon. The study group and control group showed little evidence of positive staining for inflammatory cells in the tendon or bursa, reinforcing the hypothesis that inflammation likely is not the main cause of GTPS. The increased presence of substance P also has been identified previously in the subacromial space of patients with rotator tendinopathy.[3]

Dr. Byrd or an immediate family member serves as an unpaid consultant to A3 Surgical; has stock or stock options held in A3 Surgical; serves as a paid consultant to or is an employee of Smith & Nephew; has received research or institutional support from Smith & Nephew; and serves as a board member, owner, officer, or committee member of the American Orthopaedic Society for Sports Medicine, the Arthroscopy Association of North America, and the International Society for Hip Arthroscopy. Neither Dr. Dumont nor any immediate family member has received anything of value from or has stock or stock options held in a commercial company or institution related directly or indirectly to the subject of this chapter.

2: Hip and Pelvis

Increasing evidence has shown an association between abnormal biomechanics and the development of GTPS. A 2015 study of 203 hip MRIs found a significant association between increased acetabular anteversion and the presence of gluteal tendinosis. The mean acetabular version in patients with gluteal tendinosis was 18.4° compared with 15.7° in those without gluteal pathology.[4]

Several muscles insert at or near the greater trochanter of the femur, including the gluteus medius and minimus, obturator internus, and obturator externus. The gluteus maximus has a broad origin from the ilium and sacrum and inserts on the iliotibial band and gluteal tuberosity of the lateral femur. The gluteus medius and minimus lie deep to the gluteus maximus, originating from the ilium and inserting at the greater trochanter. The tensor fascia latae originates from the iliac crest and inserts on the iliotibial tract. Figure 1 shows the close relationship of these structures. Several bursae surround the greater trochanter to protect it from the surrounding tendons. The subgluteus medius bursa lies superior to the greater trochanter, deep to the gluteus medius. The subgluteus maximus bursa lies between the gluteus maximus and the gluteus medius and lateral to the greater trochanter. A division of this bursa commonly is referred to as the trochanteric bursa.[5,6]

Patients typically present with hip pain. A careful history can help differentiate GTPS from pain originating from the lumbar spine or groin pain originating from intra-articular hip pathologies. Patients often report difficulty sleeping on the affected side and pain with increased periods of standing on the limb or with walking. Pain can radiate down the lateral thigh to the knee. A dermatomal distribution of pain or pain radiation distal to the knee should trigger the evaluation of lumbar spine radiculopathy.

The presence of GTPS was evaluated in members of the military, and its prevalence was found to be higher in individuals older than 40 years. Female sex had the largest association with the presence of GTPS, with a fivefold increase compared with males.[7] Another prospective cohort study of women treated for GTPS compared with an asymptomatic control group found that a lower femoral neck-shaft angle and adiposity were associated with GTPS.[8]

Pain from GTPS can cause substantial disability and, when chronic, can affect mental health, employment, and quality of life. One study found that patients with GTPS were the least likely to be working full time compared with patients with end-stage hip osteoarthritis and asymptomatic control patients. Otherwise, GTPS appeared to confer levels of disability and affect the quality of life similarly to end-stage hip osteoarthritis.[9]

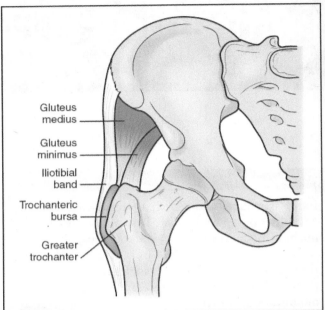

Figure 1 Drawing shows the anatomic insertion of the gluteus medius and the gluteus minimus on the greater trochanter in close proximity to the iliotibial band. The trochanteric bursa lies deep to the iliotibial band. All of these structures have been implicated in the development of symptoms of greater trochanteric pain syndrome.

Physical examination often shows tenderness with palpation of the greater trochanter. Patients may present with an antalgic gait or the classic Trendelenburg gait if weakness of the gluteus medius is pronounced. Manual muscle testing of the gluteus medius often demonstrates weakness and reproduces pain at the greater trochanter. A new physical examination finding, the hip lag sign, has been described, in which the examiner places the hip in 10° of extension, maximal abduction, and internal rotation. The patient's inability to actively maintain the position, with a noted drop of 10 cm at the foot, is considered a positive finding associated with hip abductor damage substantiated by MRI.[10]

Radiographs of the hip may show surface irregularities at the greater trochanter consistent with enthesopathy or calcific tendinosis. Radiographs are also useful in identifying possible coexisting disorders such as osteoarthritis of the hip and fractures. MRI has the ability to depict osseous and soft-tissue abnormalities, including peritrochanteric edema and tendinosis or tearing of the gluteus medius and gluteus minimus. The use of ultrasonography to aid in the diagnosis and management of gluteal tendon tears has evolved because of its low cost, availability, and ability to guide treatments such as anesthetic and corticosteroid injections.[11] A systematic review that compared the accuracy of ultrasonography and MRI in diagnosing gluteal tendon pathology with surgical findings of the same pathology found that MRI had a sensitivity of 33% to 100%, a specificity of 92% to 100%, and a positive predictive value of 71% to 100%, with a high rate of false-positive results. Ultrasonography had a sensitivity of 79% to 100% and a positive predictive value of 95% to 100%.[12] Although ultrasonography is dependent on technician proficiency, it may be a less costly and more effective imaging modality for gluteal tendon pathology.

Nonsurgical treatment is the mainstay of care and should begin with activity modification, NSAIDs, stretching, and physical therapy. Anesthetic and corticosteroid injections to the trochanteric bursa can be beneficial and can be performed with or without image guidance. Ultrasonographic guidance offers the advantage of providing visual evidence of damage to the gluteus medius tendon and can help accurately position the injectate adjacent to the damaged tissue to maximize efficacy.

Fluoroscopic guidance also has been used to direct injections in patients with GTPS. A multicenter double-blind, randomized controlled study showed no improvement in outcomes at 1-month or 3-month follow-up in patients who had received fluoroscopically guided injections compared with those who were administered injections without image guidance. The cost associated with fluoroscopically guided injections was significantly higher.[13] Given the lack of evidence supporting the use of fluoroscopically guided injections for the treatment of GTPS, ultrasonographic guidance can be considered instead, because it offers the ability to concomitantly assess the abductor tendons for structural damage.

A randomized controlled trial of patients with GTPS assigned to a group that received corticosteroid injections or a group that received nonsurgical care without injections showed clinically significant improvement at 3 months in the study group compared with the control group. The difference in outcomes was no longer present at 12 months, however.[14]

The authors of a 2014 study considered some pain relief from the first injection to be a positive indicator of complete remission, although pain reduction was maximal after the third injection to the region of the trochanteric bursa. The radiologic presence of isolated trochanteric bursitis, versus the presence of associated gluteus medius tendinopathy, was associated with greater pain reduction in the immediate postinjection phase and over the long term.[15]

A study comparing the efficacy of ultrasound-guided injections directed toward the trochanteric bursa with those administered in the subgluteus medius bursa found that those administered in the trochanteric bursa were most effective, eliciting a visual analog scale (VAS) score reduction of 3, compared with 0 in those given in the subgluteus medius bursa. No association was seen between demographic variables or ultrasound findings and pain relief.[16]

Extracorporeal shock wave therapy (ESWT) has been used to treat various tendinopathies, including GTPS. A systematic review examining the effectiveness of ESWT found moderate evidence that it was more effective than home physical therapy and corticosteroid injections at short-term (less than 12 months) and long-term (greater than 12 months) follow-up.[17] Its use in conjunction with other nonsurgical treatment methods is supported.

Surgical treatment typically is not required; however, in cases of recalcitrant pain with tearing of the abductor tendons, repair of the abductor tendons can be performed.[18] Various techniques can be used to repair the tendons to their insertion, including open transosseous or bone-anchored suture techniques, endoscopic techniques, and tendon augmentation for repair reinforcement.[19] Double-row fixation analogous to the repair of the rotator cuff has been described.[20] Other authors advocate the importance of iliotibial band release to reduce excessive tension between the iliotibial band and the greater trochanter and report a technique for endoscopic bursectomy and cruciate release of the iliotibial band.[21]

A study examining outcomes in 22 patients treated with open repair of the gluteus medius tendon through bone tunnels showed improvement in the mean Harris Hip Score from 53 preoperatively to 87 at 1-year follow-up and 88 at 5-year follow-up. No correlation was found between tear size or pattern and outcomes, but the three patients with poor results were in the group with larger tears. Most patients were satisfied and would undergo the procedure again if necessary.[22]

In a series of 23 patients with GTPS who underwent endoscopic cruciate release of the iliotibial band, substantial improvements were noted in the visual analog scale pain score, the modified Harris Hip Score, the Western Ontario and McMaster Universities Arthritis Index, and the Hip Outcome Score, at 3, 6, and 12 months, compared with preoperative scores. The mean VAS improved from 8.1 preoperatively to 0.48 at 12 months, whereas the modified Harris Hip score improved from 40.2 preoperatively to 86.29 at 12 months. No patients underwent additional surgical procedures to the hip within the follow-up period.[23]

A systematic review of treatment options for GTPS found that traditional nonsurgical methods, including physical therapy with stretching, low-energy shock wave therapy, and corticosteroid injections, help most patients. The efficacy of all surgical treatments studied, including bursectomy, longitudinal release of the iliotibial band, Z-plasty lengthening of the iliotibial band, osteotomy, and gluteal tendon repair, was superior to nonsurgical management; thus, these surgical treatments are worthy of consideration in refractory cases.[24]

Piriformis Syndrome

Piriformis syndrome is characterized by extrapelvic compression of the sciatic nerve by the piriformis muscle in the area of the greater sciatic notch. Symptoms include pain and dysthesthesias to the buttock, hip, or posterior thigh and pain distally as a result of radicular pain. Hypertrophy of the bands of the piriformis can compress the sciatic nerve or its branches. The sciatic nerve typically exits the greater sciatic foramen, passing deep to the belly of the piriformis and superficial to the superior and inferior gemelli and obturator internus (Figure 2). Several anatomic variants of this relationship have been noted and can contribute to undue compression of the sciatic nerve; however, the normal anatomic relationship is found in most cases. One cadaver study identified 275 of 294 specimens (93.6%) that had the typical anatomic pattern, with variations of the anatomy in the other 19 specimens (6.4%).[25] Other lesions such as soft-tissue masses, abscesses, aneurysms or aberrant veins, and myositis ossificans can contribute to compression of the sciatic nerve.

Diagnosis relies on a detailed history and clinical examination. Piriformis syndrome should be considered in cases of sciatica or posterior gluteal or thigh pain associated with nondiagnostic clinical evaluation and MRI of the spine. Palpation usually reveals tenderness of the piriformis muscle, where a sausage-shaped mass may be noted. Palpation may reproduce radicular pain. Passive straight leg raise (the Lasegue sign) and flexion, adduction, and internal rotation (FADIR) of the hip exacerbate the symptoms. Passive internal rotation of the hip in neutral extension and resisted flexion and external rotation place tension on the piriformis muscle and can reproduce symptoms. Neurologic examination findings such as abnormal reflexes, motor weakness, and sensory changes are possible but rare.

Diagnostic imaging is used to exclude other sources of symptoms, including the lumbar spine and hip joint. CT and MRI are useful for detecting space-occupying lesions that could produce symptoms of sciatic nerve compression. MRI also can identify the presence of a hypertrophied or damaged piriformis and can identify anomalous piriformis muscle anatomy or variations in the sciatic nerve.

Electrodiagnostic testing can be useful to localize an impingement of the sciatic nerve by the piriformis. The

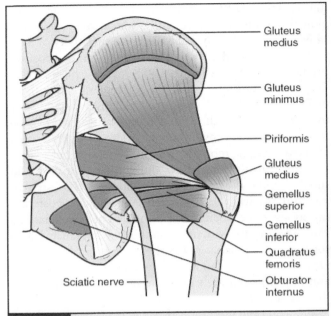

Figure 2   Drawing depicts the course of the sciatic nerve, which is typically deep to the piriformis muscle and superficial to the superior and inferior gemelli, the obturator internus, and the quadratus femoris. In patients with piriformis syndrome, the nerve is compressed by one or more of these structures.

H-reflex of the peroneal division of the sciatic nerve is substantially prolonged in affected patients when the limb is placed in the provocative FADIR position.[26] Injections of local anesthetic and steroid into the piriformis muscle can be useful to confirm the diagnosis.

One report suggested a diagnostic criteria for the diagnosis of piriformis syndrome that included (1) buttock or leg pain made worse by sitting, stair climbing, and/or leg crossing; (2) pain with palpation of the sciatic notch; (3) no evidence of axonal loss of the sciatic nerve on electrophysiologic testing; (4) no other imaging findings that could explain the presence of sciatica; and (5) reduction of symptoms by more than 60% with diagnostic injection under image guidance.[27]

The treatment algorithm of piriformis syndrome should begin with rest, anti-inflammatory medications, muscle relaxation, and physical therapy directed at stretching the piriformis muscle. Stretching positions should include the FADIR position. Therapeutic injections to the piriformis muscle using steroids, botulinum toxin, or pain-blocking agents have been used with success. Imaging guidance using CT or ultrasonography is acceptable. Several studies have verified the placement of ultrasound-guided injections using MRI or CT and found the technique reliable.[28,29] Caudal epidural steroid injections

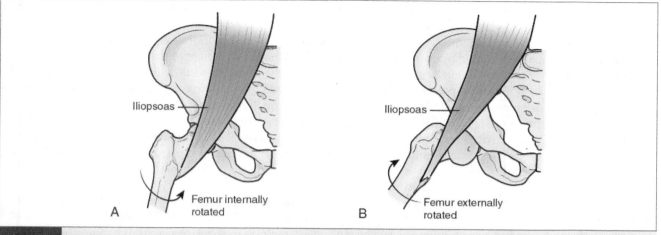

Figure 3 Drawings show the iliopsoas tendon, which produces a loud and sometimes painful snapping when it moves over the anterior hip capsule and femoral head as the hip is extended, internally rotated, and adducted (**A**) from an externally rotated, flexed, and abducted position (**B**).

also have been reported for the treatment of piriformis syndrome. Anesthetic and corticosteroid injections deposited into the caudal epidural space can be expected to course along the nerve root to the sciatic nerve and can provide substantial relief.

Surgical release of the piriformis tendon and neurolysis of the sciatic nerve can be performed using an open or endoscopic surgical approach. Only minimal functional loss occurs after release of the piriformis because of the contribution of the other external rotators of the hip. In properly selected patients in whom the piriformis is actually the impinging structure, immediate relief usually can be anticipated. In a series of patients treated with endoscopic decompression of the sciatic nerve, VAS scores for pain improved from a mean of 6.9 preoperatively to 2.4 at 12-month follow-up. Of all patients, 83% had no pain after sitting for more than 30 minutes at follow-up.[30]

In summary, emphasis should be placed on thorough evaluation of patients presenting with symptoms consistent with piriformis syndrome and on the importance of exhaustive nonsurgical management, including rest, activity modification, stretching, and physical therapy. Diagnostic and therapeutic injections can help confirm the diagnosis and provide substantial relief. Recalcitrant cases can be considered for surgical release of the piriformis and any other structures impinging on the sciatic nerve.

Coxa Saltans Interna

Coxa saltans interna, or internal snapping hip, is a syndrome caused by the snapping of the iliopsoas tendon over the structures lying deep to it. The iliacus and psoas combine to form one tendon as they pass between the anterior inferior iliac spine and the iliopectineal eminence. The tendon passes over the anterior hip capsule and courses posteriorly in its bursa to insert at the lesser trochanter. Patients typically report an audible, loud clunk, which they often can reproduce. With the hip in a flexed, abducted, and externally rotated position, the tendon assumes a lateral position on the iliopectineal eminence and moves from lateral to medial as the hip is moved to extension, adduction, and internal rotation. The snapping results from the movement of the tendon over the anterior hip capsule and femoral head (Figure 3). Bony variants or abnormalities of the anterior acetabulum, femoral head, or lesser trochanter also can contribute to the pathology. Inflammation of the large iliopsoas tendon bursa also has been implicated.[31]

Patients may present for evaluation of medial groin pain and with history of a hyperextension injury or groin strain. They may have noted clicking or popping of the hip that has worsened over time. The popping sound typically is audible to anyone near the patient, in contrast to the external snapping hip, which clearly is visible but not usually audible. Activities of daily living may not be painful; however, sports requiring hip flexion can aggravate the symptoms.

Physical examination of the hip must be thorough to rule outother pathologies than can present with medial groin pain, such as adductor strains, osteitis pubis, and intra-articular disorders such as femoroacetabular impingement. In the supine position, the patient often can reproduce the snapping by extending and adducting the flexed and abducted hip. The examiner can suppress the snapping by applying pressure over the anterior hip, thereby restricting the motion of the tendon.

Plain radiographs of the hip typically are normal but may show bony morphologic variants such as hip dysplasia or femoroacetabular impingement. MRI may show thickening of the tendon and fluid in its bursa.

A certain portion of the population has a painless snapping iliopsoas tendon. Without the presence of associated pain, the patient can be reassured, and no treatment is required. Initial treatment of the painful internal snapping hip should focus on rest, activity modification, stretching of the iliopsoas, and NSAIDs. Image-guided anesthetic injections can help to confirm the diagnosis but also can be therapeutic with the addition of a corticosteroid.

Surgical treatment involves the release or fractional lengthening of the tendon and can be performed through an open, endoscopic, or arthroscopic approach. The tendon can be released at its insertion at the lesser trochanter, from the peripheral compartment, or more proximally from an intra-articular approach.

Release both from the central compartment and at the lesser trochanter produced good results in a study comparing the two techniques in 20 patients with a minimum follow-up of 24 months.[32] A series of 55 patients undergoing fractional lengthening of the tendon from the central compartment reported 81.8% (45 patients) excellent or good outcomes and 81.8% resolution of the snapping. Resolution of the snapping was highly predictive of improved outcomes. The rate of persistent snapping at 2-year follow-up may be higher than previously thought.[33]

A 2014 case series described the release of the iliopsoas tendon from the central compartment for patients with symptomatic impingement of the anterior labrum by the iliopsoas tendon. Two of the patients underwent a second procedure to release the iliopsoas at the lesser trochanter for iliopsoas snapping. Of the remaining 28 patients, 23 had good or excellent results.[34]

A systematic review of reported outcomes for open versus arthroscopic techniques for the treatment of internal snapping hip reported a reduced failure rate, few complications, and reduced postoperative pain in patients undergoing arthroscopic treatment.[35]

A cadaver study found substantial variability in the number of distinct tendons of the iliopsoas at the level of the hip joint. The psoas major tendon consistently was found to be the most medial tendon, whereas the primary iliacus tendon was found immediately lateral to it. An accessory iliacus tendon sometimes was present adjacent and lateral to the primary iliacus. The presence of a single-banded, double-banded, and triple-banded iliopsoas tendon was found in 28.3%, 64.2%, and 7.5% of specimens, respectively. The study suggests that surgeons should be mindful of this anatomic variability when performing iliopsoas tendon releases.[36]

Patients with increased femoral anteversion may be at risk for poorer clinical outcomes after a release of the iliopsoas tendon. The iliopsoas may be an important passive and dynamic stabilizer of the anterior hip in this patient population, leading to alterations in kinematics, especially with the hip in terminal extension and external rotation, when the iliopsoas is most taut.[37] Serious complications, including anterior hip instability or dislocation, have been reported after iliopsoas release in the setting of increased femoral anteversion; therefore, caution is advised when considering the procedure in this patient population.

Coxa Saltans Externa

Coxa saltans externa, or external snapping hip, is a snapping of the iliotibial band over the greater trochanter of the femur. Most cases of external snapping hip are not associated with pain and can be treated with reassurance. Occasionally, when the snapping is painful, further investigation and treatment are warranted.

Proximally, the iliotibial band attaches to the gluteus maximus posteriorly, and the tensor fascia lata anteriorly. It courses down the lateral aspect of the thigh and has insertions on the linea aspera of the femur and on the Gerdy tubercle on the anterolateral tibia. The iliotibial band lies posterior to the greater trochanter when the hip is extended and translates anteriorly with flexion. In cases of external coxa saltans, snapping often is noted during internal or external rotation of the hip, with the hip in the extended position while standing.

Patients often report the ability to "dislocate" their hips with certain movements and have pain localized to the lateral hip at the greater trochanter. The pain is aggravated by the frequency of snapping episodes and may improve if activities are modified to avoid snapping. Repetitive snapping of the hip likely causes thickening and inflammation of the iliotibial band at the region of the greater trochanter.

The initial treatment should focus on physical therapy to stretch the iliotibial band and gluteus maximus, activity modification, and a course of NSAIDs. Pain refractory to these measures can be treated with selected anesthetic and corticosteroid injections to the trochanteric bursa. Nonsurgical treatment is the mainstay of care, and most patients will improve.

Surgical treatment occasionally is offered to patients who have exhausted nonsurgical options. An array of surgical procedures have been described to lengthen the iliotibial band or decompress it over the greater trochanter.

One retrospective study evaluated outcomes in 15 patients with external snapping hip at a mean of 33.8 months after endoscopic transverse iliotibial band release just distal to the greater trochanter. Of all patients, nine (60%) were pain free. Preoperative VAS pain scores improved from a mean of 5.5 to 0.53 postoperatively, and snapping symptoms were resolved in all patients postoperatively.[38] Another technique involving distal Z-plasty lengthening of the iliotibial band was presented in a series of five patients. Although the total number of patients was small, snapping resolved in all of them.[39] Techniques that involve release or Z-plasty lengthening of the gluteus maximus tendon also have been reported with good results.[40,41] Each of these techniques would benefit from longer term evaluation within a larger number of study patients.

Summary

Extra-articular hip disorders can present a diagnostic and therapeutic dilemma. Understanding of these disorders, including the anatomy involved, diagnostic algorithms, and treatment options, allows the physician to recommend effective treatment strategies. Directed anesthetic injections are useful in narrowing the differential diagnosis in many cases. Endoscopic surgical techniques continue to evolve in the treatment of extra-articular hip pathology.

Key Study Points

- Greater trochanteric pain syndrome encompasses various etiologies of pain at the greater trochanter of the femur, including trochanteric bursitis, gluteus medius or gluteus minimus tendon tears, and friction of the iliotibial band over the greater trochanter.
- Piriformis syndrome involves the extrapelvic compression of the sciatic nerve by the piriformis muscle or other adjacent structures.
- Internal snapping hip is the result of the iliopsoas tendon moving back and forth over the internally and externally rotated femoral head.
- External snapping hip is the result of the iliotibial band snapping over the greater trochanter of the femur.

Annotated References

1. Strauss EJ, Nho SJ, Kelly BT: Greater trochanteric pain syndrome. *Sports Med Arthrosc* 2010;18(2):113-119.

   This article reviews the concepts of GTPS, including its etiologies, diagnosis, and treatment.

2. Long SS, Surrey DE, Nazarian LN: Sonography of greater trochanteric pain syndrome and the rarity of primary bursitis. *AJR Am J Roentgenol* 2013;201(5):1083-1086.

   This article is a retrospective study examining the prevalence of gluteus tendon pathology, bursitis, and iliotibial band pathology on ultrasonography in patients with GTPS.

3. Fearon AM, Twin J, Dahlstrom JE, et al: Increased substance P expression in the trochanteric bursa of patients with greater trochanteric pain syndrome. *Rheumatol Int* 2014;34(10):1441-1448.

   This study examines the presence of substance P in the bursa and the abductor tendons in patients with GTPS.

4. Moulton KM, Aly AR, Rajasekaran S, Shepel M, Obaid H: Acetabular anteversion is associated with gluteal tendinopathy at MRI. *Skeletal Radiol* 2015;44(1):47-54.

   This MRI study evaluates the possible association between increased acetabular anteversion and gluteal tendinopathy, trochanteric bursitis, and subgluteal bursitis.

5. Mallow M, Nazarian LN: Greater trochanteric pain syndrome diagnosis and treatment. *Phys Med Rehabil Clin N Am* 2014;25(2):279-289.

   This review article describes the epidemiology, anatomy, diagnosis, and treatment of GTPS.

6. Flack NA, Nicholson HD, Woodley SJ: The anatomy of the hip abductor muscles. *Clin Anat* 2014;27(2):241-253.

   This cadaver study examines the anatomy of the hip abductors in 12 specimens.

7. Blank E, Owens BD, Burks R, Belmont PJ Jr: Incidence of greater trochanteric pain syndrome in active duty US military servicemembers. *Orthopedics* 2012;35(7):e1022-e1027.

   This study examines the epidemiology of GTPS in United States military service members.

8. Fearon A, Stephens S, Cook J, et al: The relationship of femoral neck shaft angle and adiposity to greater trochanteric pain syndrome in women. A case control morphology and anthropometric study. *Br J Sports Med* 2012;46(12):888-892.

   This case-controlled study found an association between increased femoral neck shaft angle and increased adiposity and the diagnosis of GTPS.

9. Fearon AM, Cook JL, Scarvell JM, Neeman T, Cormick W, Smith PN: Greater trochanteric pain syndrome negatively affects work, physical activity and quality of life: A case control study. *J Arthroplasty* 2014;29(2):383-386.

   This study found that GTPS affects quality of life scores and disability levels similarly to hip osteoarthritis.

10. Kaltenborn A, Bourg CM, Gutzeit A, Kalberer F: The Hip Lag Sign—prospective blinded trial of a new

clinical sign to predict hip abductor damage. *PLoS One* 2014;9(3):e91560.

This study introduces and validates a new physical examination finding, the Hip Lag Sign, which can be used to predict hip abductor damage.

11. Chowdhury R, Naaseri S, Lee J, Rajeswaran G: Imaging and management of greater trochanteric pain syndrome. *Postgrad Med J* 2014;90(1068):576-581.

This review article reviews the etiologies and diagnostic imaging options for GTPS.

12. Westacott DJ, Minns JI, Foguet P: The diagnostic accuracy of magnetic resonance imaging and ultrasonography in gluteal tendon tears—a systematic review. *Hip Int* 2011;21(6):637-645.

This systematic review compares MRI and ultrasonography as diagnostic imaging studies for GTPS, using surgical findings as the reference standard.

13. Cohen SP, Strassels SA, Foster L, et al: Comparison of fluoroscopically guided and blind corticosteroid injections for greater trochanteric pain syndrome: Multicentre randomised controlled trial. *BMJ* 2009;338:b1088.

This multicenter randomized controlled trial evaluates patient outcomes after injections for the treatment of GTPS with and without fluoroscopic guidance. It found no benefit to fluoroscopic guidance.

14. Brinks A, van Rijn RM, Willemsen SP, et al: Corticosteroid injections for greater trochanteric pain syndrome: A randomized controlled trial in primary care. *Ann Fam Med* 2011;9(3):226-234.

This randomized controlled trial compares outcomes in patients receiving injections for GTPS with those in patients not receiving injections. Patients receiving injections had improved outcomes at 3 months, but the improved outcomes were no longer present after 12 months.

15. Wilson SA, Shanahan EM, Smith MD: Greater trochanteric pain syndrome: Does imaging-identified pathology influence the outcome of interventions? *Int J Rheum Dis* 2014;17(6):621-627.

This retrospective study investigated the association between imaging-identified pathology (gluteal tendinopathy and/or trochanteric bursitis) and outcomes after anesthetic and corticosteroid injections to the area of the trochanteric bursa.

16. McEvoy JR, Lee KS, Blankenbaker DG, del Rio AM, Keene JS: Ultrasound-guided corticosteroid injections for treatment of greater trochanteric pain syndrome: Greater trochanter bursa versus subgluteus medius bursa. *AJR Am J Roentgenol* 2013;201(2):W313-7.

This study investigates the effectiveness of corticosteroid injections to the subgluteal bursa versus those administered to the trochanteric bursa. Injections to the trochanteric bursa resulted in greater pain relief.

17. Mani-Babu S, Morrissey D, Waugh C, Screen H, Barton C: The effectiveness of extracorporeal shock wave therapy in lower limb tendinopathy: A systematic review. *Am J Sports Med* 2015;43(3):752-761.

This article is a systematic review of the use and effectiveness of ESWT for lower-limb tendinopathies, including GTPS. The study found ESWT to be more effective than home training and corticosteroid injections in the treatment of GTPS.

18. Byrd JW: Peritrochanteric access and gluteus medius repair. *Arthrosc Tech* 2013;2(3):e243-e246.

This study describes a technique for gaining endoscopic access to the peritrochanteric space and gluteus medius tendon repair.

19. Ebert JR, Bucher TA, Ball SV, Janes GC: A review of surgical repair methods and patient outcomes for gluteal tendon tears. *Hip Int* 2015;25(1):15-23.

This article reviews various surgical repair techniques for gluteal tendon tears and their outcomes.

20. Domb BG, Carreira DS: Endoscopic repair of full-thickness gluteus medius tears. *Arthrosc Tech* 2013;2(2):e77-e81.

This article describes an endoscopic double-row technique for the repair of gluteus medius tendon tears.

21. Govaert LH, van Dijk CN, Zeegers AV, Albers GH: Endoscopic bursectomy and iliotibial tract release as a treatment for refractory greater trochanteric pain syndrome: A new endoscopic approach with early results. *Arthrosc Tech* 2012;1(2):e161-e164.

This article describes a surgical technique for endoscopic bursectomy and cross incision of the iliotibial band for the treatment of GTPS.

22. Davies JF, Stiehl JB, Davies JA, Geiger PB: Surgical treatment of hip abductor tendon tears. *J Bone Joint Surg Am* 2013;95(15):1420-1425.

This article reports the clinical outcomes of a series of patients with hip abductor tears who were treated with open surgical repair. The repair of higher-grade tears was augmented with acellular human dermal allograft.

23. Domínguez A, Seijas R, Ares O, Sallent A, Cuscó X, Cugat R: Clinical outcomes of trochanteric syndrome endoscopically treated. *Arch Orthop Trauma Surg* 2015;135(1):89-94.

This article presents the outcomes of a series of patients with GTPS treated with endoscopic iliotibial band release.

24. Lustenberger DP, Ng VY, Best TM, Ellis TJ: Efficacy of treatment of trochanteric bursitis: A systematic review. *Clin J Sport Med* 2011;21(5):447-453.

This article is a systematic review of treatment options for trochanteric bursitis. It found that nonsurgical modalities helped most patients and that surgery was effective in refractory cases. Surgical treatment resulted in greater improvements in VAS scores and Harris Hip Scores than did corticosteroid injections and physical therapy.

25. Natsis K, Totlis T, Konstantinidis GA, Paraskevas G, Piagkou M, Koebke J: Anatomical variations between the sciatic nerve and the piriformis muscle: A contribution to surgical anatomy in piriformis syndrome. *Surg Radiol Anat* 2014;36(3):273-280.

   In this cadaver study, 294 limbs were dissected to evaluate the relationship between the piriformis muscle and the sciatic nerve. Anatomic variations were present in 19 of the limbs examined (6.4%).

26. Jawish RM, Assoum HA, Khamis CF: Anatomical, clinical and electrical observations in piriformis syndrome. *J Orthop Surg Res* 2010;5:3.

   This article presents a series of patients treated for piriformis syndrome, including their outcomes from nonsurgical and surgical treatment. The authors identify new anatomic patterns of compression of the sciatic nerve and ascertain the diagnostic utility of the H-reflex of the peroneal nerve.

27. Miller TA, White KP, Ross DC: The diagnosis and management of Piriformis Syndrome: Myths and facts. *Can J Neurol Sci* 2012;39(5):577-583.

   This article discusses various diagnostic and treatment options for piriformis syndrome and proposes standardized criteria for its diagnosis, which include presenting signs and symptoms, imaging, and the response to injections.

28. Fabregat G, Roselló M, Asensio-Samper JM, et al: Computer-tomographic verification of ultrasound-guided piriformis muscle injection: A feasibility study. *Pain Physician* 2014;17(6):507-513.

   This study examines the accuracy of ultrasound-guided injections to the piriformis muscle by adding iodinated contrast to the botulinum toxin injection and then performing CT to assess intramuscular distribution.

29. Blunk JA, Nowotny M, Scharf J, Benrath J: MRI verification of ultrasound-guided infiltrations of local anesthetics into the piriformis muscle. *Pain Med* 2013;14(10):1593-1599.

   This study uses MRI to confirm the intramuscular injection of local anesthetic to the piriformis muscle using ultrasound guidance.

30. Martin HD, Shears SA, Johnson JC, Smathers AM, Palmer IJ: The endoscopic treatment of sciatic nerve entrapment/deep gluteal syndrome. *Arthroscopy* 2011;27(2):172-181.

   This article describes the presentation and evaluation of deep gluteal space syndrome and presents the surgical outcomes of endoscopic decompression of the sciatic nerve.

31. Ilizaliturri VM Jr, Camacho-Galindo J: Endoscopic treatment of snapping hips, iliotibial band, and iliopsoas tendon. *Sports Med Arthrosc* 2010;18(2):120-127.

   This review article discusses internal and external snapping hip syndromes and their surgical treatment options.

32. Ilizaliturri VM Jr, Buganza-Tepole M, Olivos-Meza A, Acuna M, Acosta-Rodriguez E: Central compartment release versus lesser trochanter release of the iliopsoas tendon for the treatment of internal snapping hip: A comparative study. *Arthroscopy* 2014;30(7):790-795.

   This retrospective study examines outcomes in a series of patients with snapping iliopsoas tendon treated with endoscopic release of the tendon at its insertion at the lesser trochanter or release through the central compartment of the hip. Patients in both groups had favorable outcomes.

33. El Bitar YF, Stake CE, Dunne KF, Botser IB, Domb BG: Arthroscopic Iliopsoas Fractional Lengthening for Internal Snapping of the Hip: Clinical Outcomes With a Minimum 2-Year Follow-up. *Am J Sports Med* 2014;42(7):1696-1703.

   This is a retrospective review of prospectively collected outcomes data in patients undergoing fractional lengthening of the iliopsoas tendon for painful internal snapping hip. Most patients experienced resolution of the painful snapping. Those with persistent snapping had poorer outcomes.

34. Nelson IR, Keene JS: Results of labral-level arthroscopic iliopsoas tenotomies for the treatment of labral impingement. *Arthroscopy* 2014;30(6):688-694.

   This case series reports the outcomes of patients treated with arthroscopic iliopsoas tendon release from the central compartment for the treatment of labral impingement from the iliopsoas.

35. Khan M, Adamich J, Simunovic N, Philippon MJ, Bhandari M, Ayeni OR: Surgical management of internal snapping hip syndrome: A systematic review evaluating open and arthroscopic approaches. *Arthroscopy* 2013;29(5):942-948.

   This systematic review compares the outcomes of open techniques and arthroscopic techniques in the management of internal snapping hips. A reduced failure rate, fewer complications, and less postoperative pain with arthroscopic management were noted.

36. Philippon MJ, Devitt BM, Campbell KJ, et al: Anatomic variance of the iliopsoas tendon. *Am J Sports Med* 2014;42(4):807-811.

   This cadaver study explores the anatomic variants of the iliopsoas tendon at the level of the hip joint. It was determined that presence of more than two distinct tendons is more common than previously thought.

37. Fabricant PD, Bedi A, De La Torre K, Kelly BT: Clinical outcomes after arthroscopic psoas lengthening: The effect of femoral version. *Arthroscopy* 2012;28(7):965-971.

   This study reports inferior outcomes in patients with increased femoral anteversion undergoing iliopsoas lengthening for internal snapping hip.

38. Zini R, Munegato D, De Benedetto M, Carraro A, Bigoni M: Endoscopic iliotibial band release in snapping hip. *Hip Int* 2013;23(2):225-232.

    This retrospective case series reports the outcomes after endoscopic transverse release of the iliotibial band for symptomatic external snapping hip.

39. Sayed-Noor AS, Pedersen E, Sjödèn GO: A new surgical method for treating patients with refractory external snapping hip: Pedersen-Noor operation. *J Surg Orthop Adv* 2012;21(3):132-135.

    This article presents a technique for lengthening of the iliotibial band by Z-plasty under local anesthesia on an outpatient basis. Snapping was resolved in the five patients in this series.

40. Polesello GC, Queiroz MC, Domb BG, Ono NK, Honda EK: Surgical technique: Endoscopic gluteus maximus tendon release for external snapping hip syndrome. *Clin Orthop Relat Res* 2013;471(8):2471-2476.

    This article describes a technique for the endoscopic release of the gluteus maximus tendon for external snapping hip and reports the results on a small series of patients.

41. Nam KW, Yoo JJ, Koo KH, Yoon KS, Kim HJ: A modified Z-plasty technique for severe tightness of the gluteus maximus. *Scand J Med Sci Sports* 2011;21(1):85-89.

    This article describes a technique for and presents the outcomes following lengthening of the iliotibial band by Z-plasty for treatment of external snapping hip caused by a tight gluteus maximus.

Chapter 13

Muscle Injuries of the Proximal Thigh

James T. Beckmann, MD, MS   Marc R. Safran, MD

Abstract

Muscle contusions, strains, and lacerations account for 10% to 55% of all sports-related injuries, with many occurring around the hip. Injuries to hip muscles often result in a substantial amount of time missed from competition. Muscle strains and contusions can usually be managed nonsurgically, but some tendon avulsions may require surgical reattachment. The hamstrings and quadriceps are susceptible to strain injury in sports requiring explosive movements and/or rapid changes in direction such as soccer, track, hockey, and football. Return-to-sport protocols are based on the range of motion of the joint spanned by the affected muscle, pain-free use of the injured muscle in basic movements, strength testing, and the willingness of the athlete to risk reinjury. Supervised rehabilitation comprising trunk stabilization, agility exercises, and eccentric strengthening is important in preventing reinjury.

Dr. Safran or an immediate family member has received royalties from DJ Orthopaedics and Stryker; is a member of a speakers' bureau or has made paid presentations on behalf of Smith & Nephew; serves as a paid consultant to ConMed Linvatec and Cool Systems; serves as an unpaid consultant to Cool Systems, Cradle Medical, Ferring Pharmaceuticals, Biomimedica, and Eleven Blade Solutions; has stock or stock options held in Cool Systems, Cradle Medical, Biomimedica, and Eleven Blade Solutions; has received research or institutional support from Ferring Pharmaceuticals and Smith & Nephew; and serves as a board member, owner, officer, or committee member of the American Orthopaedic Society for Sports Medicine, the International Society for Hip Arthroscopy, and the International Society of Arthroscopy, Knee Surgery, and Orthopaedic Sports Medicine. Neither Dr. Beckmann nor any immediate family member has received anything of value from or has stock or stock options held in a commercial company or institution related directly or indirectly to the subject of this chapter.

Keywords: hip; tendon; injury; hamstring; rectus; quadriceps; contusion; strain; avulsion; treatment

Introduction

Muscle injuries most often occur during athletic participation. Muscle contusions, strains, and lacerations account for 10% to 55% of all sports-related injuries, with many occurring around the hip.[1-3] Up to 35% of all collegiate football injuries[4] and 10% to 23% of all professional soccer injuries[5] involve hip muscle injuries, which can result in a substantial amount of time missed from competition.

Muscle strains and contusions are far more common than are lacerations. Contusions result from direct muscular trauma, which produces damage at the site of impact, and are frequently seen in contact sports. In contrast, muscle strains occur indirectly when tensile forces shear individual muscle fibers during eccentric loading. Strains around the hip most commonly affect the hamstrings and quadriceps in sports requiring explosive movements and/or rapid changes in direction such as soccer, track, hockey, and football. Muscle contusions and low-grade strains share similar treatment principles despite differing mechanistically. Most can be managed nonsurgically, but some tendon avulsions may require surgical reattachment.

Return-to-sport protocols are based on the range of motion of the joint spanned by the affected muscle, pain-free use of the injured muscle in basic movements, strength testing, and the willingness of the athlete to risk reinjury. In some situations, MRI can help to predict the degree of injury and the recovery time but has the same predictive value as clinical examination in terms of return to competitive sports.[6] Patients with a previous musculotendinous junction injury have a twofold increased risk (or greater) for recurrent strain.[7] Supervised rehabilitation that includes trunk stabilization, agility exercises, and eccentric strengthening has been shown to reduce the likelihood of

© 2016 American Academy of Orthopaedic Surgeons

2: Hip and Pelvis

subsequent events.[8,9] The focus of this chapter is on injuries to the quadriceps and hamstrings muscles.

Evaluation of Athletic Hip Injuries

Muscle injuries of the hip can occur in isolation but also may present with other sources of hip pathology. Up to 90% of patients with groin pain have been demonstrated to have more than one injury; therefore, consideration of less obvious sources of hip pain should not be overlooked simply because contusions and strains are common.[10] Considerable overlap exists among clinical signs and symptoms about the hip and pelvis region, necessitating a formulaic differential diagnosis addressing both intra-articular and extra-articular sources of hip pathology.

Common patterns of concomitant hip pathology include the "sports hip triad" of adductor, rectus abdominis, and labral tears; the "symphysis syndrome" of abdominal, groin, and adductor pain; and associations of muscle strains with labral tears and intra-articular hip pathology.[11-13] In addition, femoroacetabular impingement (FAI), hip dysplasia, and hip capsular microinstability increasingly have been recognized as sources of hip pain in athletes in whom only recurrent groin pulls and hip flexor strains have been diagnosed. The duration of symptomatic athletic participation with untreated FAI is associated with worsening, irreversible joint damage and should therefore be considered in the differential diagnosis of athletes in combination with muscular injuries.[14]

Treatment Principles of Muscle Strain Injuries

Strains are the most common injuries to the musculotendinous units of the proximal thigh. Muscles most at risk are fast-twitch muscles that span two or more joints,[15] including the quadriceps (particularly the rectus femoris) and hamstring muscles, which cross the hip and the knee. The most common mechanism of injury is eccentric contraction.[3,16] The location of injury tends to be at the musculotendinous junction. Clinically, the location of injury can range from mid-muscle belly to an eccentric position because some muscles have an elongated musculotendinous junction.

Muscle strains and contusions cause myofiber damage within the basal lamina, mysial sheaths, and associated blood vessels.[17] Avulsion injuries are associated with different outcomes, a different prognosis, and a different surgical recommendation and should be considered separately.[18] Symptoms and the clinical course following grade 1 or 2 muscle strains (Figure 1) or muscle contusion depend on the amount of muscle damage and the size of

| Figure 1 | Illustrations show the grading of musculotendinous strains. Grade 1, stretch, increased signal on MRI, less than 5% disrupted; grade 2, less than 50% disrupted; grade 3, completely disrupted macroscopically. |

the accumulated hematoma.

Initial treatment is aimed at reducing the size of the hematoma and producing a conductive environment for an optimal healing response. Hematoma formation is reduced through rest, ice, compression, and elevation (RICE). Compression and cryotherapy are associated with smaller hematoma formation. Elevation reduces hydrostatic pressure in the affected extremity and lessens the amount of interstitial fluid accumulation. Rest of the affected muscle is recommended to allow opposition of the muscle during early scar formation, which is allowed to mature until it can withstand the forces applied during rehabilitation without rerupture but should not exceed 1 week.[17] Prolonged immobilization has been associated with an increased risk of rerupture and large permanent scar formation.[19] After the acute phase, range of motion is initiated within the limits of pain. This phase is important to accelerate the regeneration process and properly orient the regenerating muscle tissue.[20,21]

The use of NSAIDs during the acute healing phase is controversial. NSAIDs can provide analgesia, reduce inflammation, and help prevent ectopic ossification, but concerns of delayed or weakened healing have been expressed.[22] Some studies have reported no adverse effects of short-term NSAID use on the healing process; evidence of later decreased growth and healing exists, however. Rarely is NSAID use needed for longer than 3 to 7 days following injury.

Muscle Contusions

Contusions causing significant muscle damage nearly always occur in one of four muscles: the quadriceps, hamstrings, adductors, or calf muscles. Contracted and stronger muscles will absorb force better and incur less severe injuries.[15] Quadriceps contusions should be braced in 120° of flexion for 24 hours to limit hematoma formation. Return to play from quadriceps contusions averaged 13 days for mild, 19 days for moderate, and 21 days for severe contusions in West Point cadets.[23] Myositis ossificans occurs in 9% to 17% of contusions.[1] Clinically, myositis ossificans should be considered if improvement is not seen in 1 week or if symptoms worsen in 2 to 3 weeks postinjury. Radiographic evidence can be present as early as 3 weeks post injury but may take as long as several months to become evident. NSAIDs can be used at the time of acute injury to reduce the possibility of myositis ossificans development. Rehabilitation for contusions should follow that of low-grade muscle strains, and should include trunk stabilization, agility exercises, and eccentric strengthening.

Hamstring Strains and Avulsions

Anatomy

The hamstrings are composed of three muscles: the semimembranosus, semitendinosus, and biceps femoris. The biceps is formed by a short head and a long head, which are innervated by the peroneal and tibial branches of the sciatic nerve, respectively. The long head of the biceps and semitendinosus join proximally to form a single conjoined tendon that inserts on the medial portion of the ischial tuberosity, but they separate into distinct tendons approximately 5 centimeters distally; the semimembranosus inserts on the lateral portion of the tuberosity. The hamstrings course medially to the sciatic nerve as they enter the thigh. This anatomic relationship is clinically significant, because it is common to have sciatic nerve irritation in chronic avulsions from traction injury or scarring.[24] Distally, the hamstring tendons cross the knee joint, where they serve as knee flexors. The hamstrings are maximally stretched with combined knee extension and hip flexion because they pass posteriorly to both the hip and the knee. Athletic maneuvers that require this simultaneous knee extension and hip flexion such as hurdling and water-skiing are common causes of hamstring strain.

History

In patients with hamstrings injuries, the history reveals posterior hip pain located deep in the buttocks. Patients will typically report that a pop, tearing, or pulling

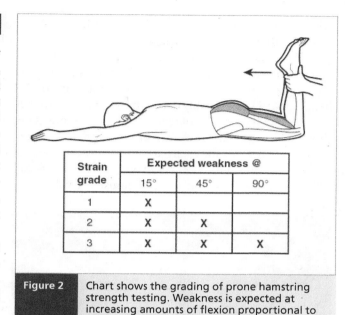

Strain grade	Expected weakness @		
	15°	45°	90°
1	X		
2	X	X	
3	X	X	X

Figure 2 Chart shows the grading of prone hamstring strength testing. Weakness is expected at increasing amounts of flexion proportional to the severity of the muscle strain.

occurred at the time of injury. With avulsion injuries, patients occasionally describe feeling a "gunshot" to the area of the ischial tuberosity. Sitting can be particularly painful.

Physical Examination

Inspection can show mild to severe ecchymosis over the posterior buttocks. An examination finding of ecchymosis is associated with a prolonged return to competition (more than 4 weeks). Palpation over the ischium or musculotendinous junction will reveal tenderness and a possible tendinous defect in avulsion injuries. Patients with hamstring strains will feel tenderness more in the mid-thigh, at the elongated musculotendinous junction of the biceps femoris. Patients with more severe injuries ambulate with a stiff-legged gait to avoid hip flexion. Range-of-motion and strength testing not only confirm the diagnosis, but also help determine when return to sporting activities is appropriate. Strength testing at 15°, 45°, and 90° can help determine the severity of the tear[25] (Figure 2). Knee extension is often limited compared with the opposite extremity. The sciatic nerve, particularly the peroneal division, should be examined by testing ankle dorsiflexion strength and performing a straight-leg raise for radicular pain.

Imaging

Plain radiography need not be routinely performed, but can be used to identify bony avulsion injuries. Bony hamstring avulsions from the ischial tuberosity (Figure 3) are common before the ischial apophysis closes during early adulthood (ages 20 to 25 years), but can occur as a bony avulsion after skeletal maturity.

MRI is useful in characterizing hamstring strains. Hamstring tears have intermediate signal intensity on T1-weighted imaging, and high signal intensity on T2 imaging. MRI can reliably determine the number of torn tendons and the amount of tendon retraction but was not shown in a systematic review of grade 1 and 2 injuries to predict reinjury[26] or the return to sport.[27] Chronic injuries can be delineated with MRI based on the presence of fatty infiltration, scarring, and reduced hamstring volume.

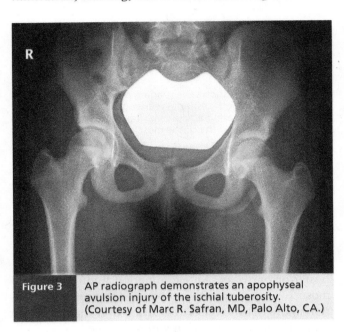

| Figure 3 | AP radiograph demonstrates an apophyseal avulsion injury of the ischial tuberosity. (Courtesy of Marc R. Safran, MD, Palo Alto, CA.) |

Classification

Proximal hamstring injuries can be divided broadly into musculotendinous junction (MTJ) or avulsion injuries. MTJ strains comprise most (up to 90%) of these injuries, and of the three hamstrings tendons, the long head of the biceps femoris is most commonly injured. Avulsion injuries from the ischial tuberosity comprise 12% of such injuries and are less common but are associated with a worse prognosis and different surgical recommendations than are MTJ injuries.[28] A treatment algorithm for hamstring injuries is shown in Figure 4.

Avulsion injuries can be strictly tendinous or contain an avulsed bony portion. Subclassification of proximal avulsions[18] is presented in Table 1. With single-tendon avulsions, retraction is unlikely because the torn tendon scars to the intact tendons, producing a functional musculotendinous unit; therefore, single-tendon avulsions rarely require surgery.[25] The potential for tendon retraction and impaired functional healing increases proportionally to the number of avulsed tendons. Retraction greater than 2 cm requires two or more completely torn tendons, and retraction greater than 5 cm is indicative of a three-tendon avulsion[25] (Figure 5). Strength deficits with nonsurgical treatment are clinically detectable when all three tendons are avulsed.

Treatment

MTJ injuries and single-tendon avulsions of the hamstrings can be treated successfully without surgical intervention. The initial 3 to 5 days following injury are devoted to rest, ice, relative immobilization, compression,

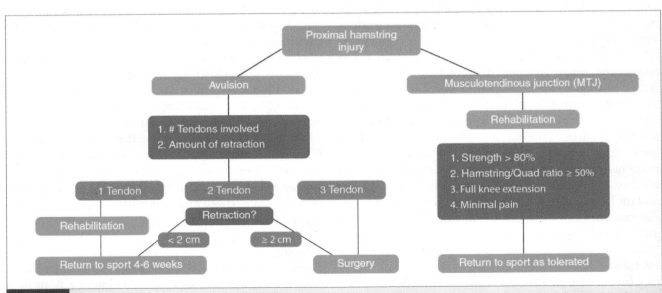

| Figure 4 | Algorithm shows the treatment protocol for a proximal hamstring injury. (Courtesy of Marc R. Safran, MD, Palo Alto, CA.) |

and analgesics. Weight bearing as tolerated with crutches is permitted until pain-free ambulation without a limp is achieved. The ability to ambulate unassisted without pain 1 day after injury is associated with a shorter recovery time than is an inability to do so. Clinical findings such as bruising/hematoma, tenderness to palpation, a lack of complete range of motion, and pain with isometric limb lengthening 3 to 5 days following injury are predictors of a prolonged recovery (more than 4 weeks).[29] Rehabilitation following the acute phase should focus on agility training and eccentric exercises, which have been shown in randomized trials to return athletes to competitive sport more quickly than traditional hamstring strengthening protocols.[9,30]

Table 1

Wood Classification of Hamstring Injuries

Type	Characteristic
1	Bone avulsion
2	Musculotendinous junction avulsion
3	Incomplete avulsion
4	Complete avulsion (no retraction)
5	Complete avulsion (retraction)

Corticosteroid and platelet-rich plasma (PRP) injections have been reported to expedite a return to play following hamstring injuries of the musculotendinous junction. Corticosteroid injections were reported to be safe in 58 National Football League (NFL) players with focal hamstring musculotendinous injuries. These players all had a significant hamstring injury evidenced by a palpable defect on physical examination, but over 80% were able to return to play within a week of injury.[31] Despite the beneficial effects found in this case series, concerns raised by experimental studies question the practice of corticosteroid injection for acute hamstring injuries. Delayed hematoma evacuation, skeletal muscle necrosis, and reduced biomechanical strength all have been found as a result of glucocorticoid injection. PRP injection for grade 2 MTJ injuries was compared with isolated rehabilitation in a recent nonblinded randomized trial. Patients receiving the PRP injection were able to return to sport an average of 6 days faster.[32] Additional studies have found better pain relief with PRP injection measured by visual analog scale. This contrasts with the findings of a 2014 study of 80 recreational athletes that showed no difference in return to play or reinjury in a double-blinded study comparing PRP with normal saline.[33]

Strength, range of motion, and pain are the typical criteria used to determine the timing of a return to sport.

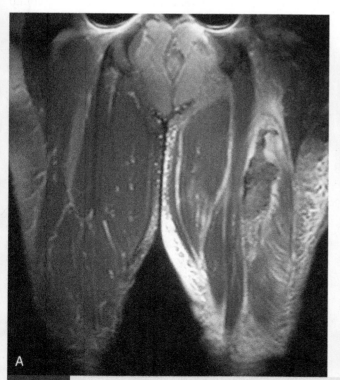
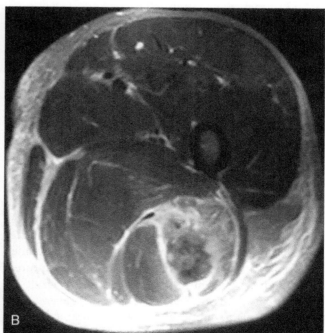

Figure 5 Coronal (**A**) and axial (**B**) MRI views depict the appearance of a hamstring avulsion injury with retraction. (Courtesy of Marc R. Safran, MD, Palo Alto, CA.)

Hamstring strength should be at least 80% of the contralateral side, and the hamstring/quadriceps ratio should exceed 50% but can vary significantly by sport and position played.[34] Clinical parameters including full knee extension, symmetric leg-extension strength at 15° of flexion, and minimal tenderness over the proximal hamstrings have been shown to be important predictors in preventing reinjury when returning to sport. The presence of pain at the time of the return to sport has been found to portend a fourfold increased risk of reinjury on return.[26]

Reinjury is common following proximal hamstring musculotendinous strains. Rates of reinjury have been reported in up to 48% of patients. Prior injury, reduced hamstring flexibility, strength asymmetry, and age have been reported as independent predictors of reinjury.[5,35] Reduced eccentric hamstring strength was found to increase the relative risk of hamstring injury 2.7-fold in a prospective study of Australian football players.[36] Athletes with prior hamstring injury have been shown to have smaller improvements with eccentric hamstring exercises in both the affected and unaffected limb[37] and may require more intense training to reduce the risk of reinjury. Inadequate warm-up or stretching also could predispose to re-strain. Previous studies have demonstrated that warmer muscles have muscle length to failure ratios.[15] Trunk stability and agility exercises have been shown to prevent reinjury compared with stretching and strengthening for grade 1 and 2 hamstring strains and should be included in rehabilitation protocols.[30]

Surgical Indications

Complete hamstring avulsions involving all three tendons or two tendons with significant retraction may benefit from early surgical repair.[25] Ischial apophyseal avulsions are treated with surgical repair only if they are displaced more than 1 to 2 centimeters. A systematic review of proximal hamstring avulsions found superior results in patients treated with acute repair compared with those treated with chronic repair or nonsurgical management. Acute surgical repair performed within 4 weeks of injury was found to have a higher return to preinjury levels of sport (96%) than chronic repair (75%) or nonsurgical management (14%). Acute surgery was associated with better patient satisfaction, subjective outcomes, pain relief, and strength and less chance of rerupture.[38] Selection bias inherent in the retrospective series design was present in all studies included in this review. Poor description of the number of avulsed tendons between groups also could bias these results and explain the differences found.

Postoperative Care

Preventing simultaneous hip flexion and knee extension protects the repair. Hip or knee braces can be used to prevent stress on the repair.[25] A knee brace locked in flexion may suffice to limit active knee flexion and is generally better tolerated. The brace is discontinued 6 weeks postoperatively. At 6 weeks, stretching and range-of-motion exercises are initiated. Strengthening is introduced 3 months postoperatively, with the goal of returning to sport at 6 to 9 months postoperatively.

Quadriceps Strains and Avulsions

Anatomy

The four quadriceps muscles are the rectus femoris, vastus medialis, vastus lateralis, and vastus intermedius. The bipennate rectus femoris is the most susceptible to strain or avulsion, because it is the only quadriceps muscle that crosses the hip joint and serves as a hip flexor, in addition to being a knee extensor.[16] As with the hamstrings, this anatomic relationship places the rectus femoris at increased risk for strain compared with the vastus muscles, which are purely knee extensors. In fact, only two cases of vastus lateralis avulsions have ever been reported. The direct head of the rectus femoris originates from the anterior inferior iliac spine (AIIS), whereas the indirect head originates more laterally from the supra-acetabular ridge adjacent to the acetabular labrum (**Figure 6**). The indirect head is more commonly injured. Distally, the indirect head extends nearly two-thirds the length of the entire muscle as a central intramuscular tendon, whereas fibers from the direct head blend anteriorly on the periphery of the muscle belly. This anatomy is important to appreciate because central tendon injuries of the indirect head are associated with a longer return to play than are peripheral injuries.[39]

Patient Evaluation

Quadriceps injuries occur during kicking or sudden deceleration from a sprint. Soccer players and football kickers typically are affected. Injury mechanisms include a sudden forcible block to a kicking motion, or kicking the air instead of the intended object. Risk factors include insufficient warm-up, poor muscle conditioning, and previous tears.

Physical examination demonstrates tenderness to palpation around the AIIS. Ecchymosis and palpable defects can be seen in more severe injuries. Rarely, in chronic cases, the avulsed proximal tendon can be palpated distally as a mass that can sometimes mimic a tumor, but a history of trauma helps to differentiate the two pathologies.[40]

Radiographs are not obtained routinely for isolated

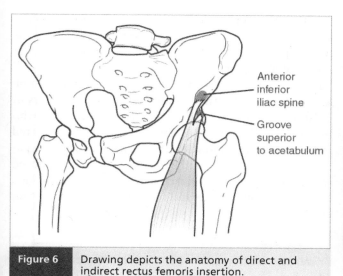

Figure 6 Drawing depicts the anatomy of direct and indirect rectus femoris insertion.

Anterior inferior iliac spine

Groove superior to acetabulum

injuries that follow the expected clinical course. A radiographic work-up should be considered for palpable defects near the AIIS, recurrent injuries, and young patients with risk for avulsions. MRI helps to characterize MTJ injuries and proximal avulsions. Increased signal on fluid-sensitive imaging within the indirect head is the most common MRI finding. Injuries of the indirect head can involve a long segment of the rectus muscle centrally that can result in a bulls-eye sign on axial imaging (Figure 7), longitudinal scarring, or pseudocyst/hematoma.

Classification

Proximal rectus femoris injuries are classified as either MTJ or avulsion injuries, similarly to proximal hamstring injuries. Musculotendinous injuries can involve the indirect head, the direct head, or the conjoined portion of the tendon. Avulsions occur with or without a bony portion of the AIIS. In skeletally immature patients, AIIS avulsions account for 20% to 25% of all avulsion injuries and nearly 50% of all pelvic apophyseal avulsions.[41] Proximal avulsion also can occur less commonly in skeletally mature individuals (Figure 8).

Treatment

Musculotendinous injuries are treated nonsurgically with a graduated rehabilitation program aimed at returning athletes to competition 6 to 10 weeks after injury (Table 2). Return to participation was shown to be proportional to the length of the central aponeurosis tear in Spanish soccer players. Every 1-cm increase in tear length greater than 4 cm resulted in an average 5-day increase in return to sport. Proximal injuries of the rectus femoris require a longer recovery period than do distal tears by an average of approximately 1 week.[42]

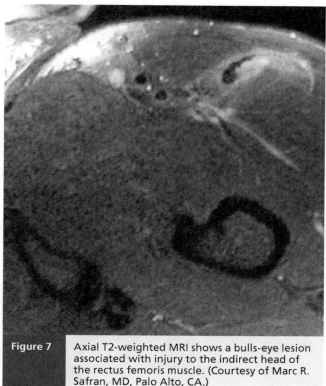

Figure 7 Axial T2-weighted MRI shows a bulls-eye lesion associated with injury to the indirect head of the rectus femoris muscle. (Courtesy of Marc R. Safran, MD, Palo Alto, CA.)

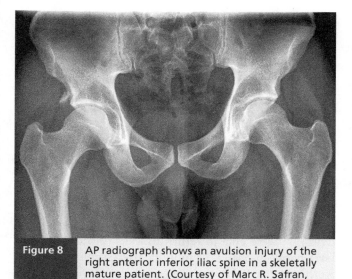

Figure 8 AP radiograph shows an avulsion injury of the right anterior inferior iliac spine in a skeletally mature patient. (Courtesy of Marc R. Safran, MD, Palo Alto, CA.)

AIIS avulsions with less than 2 centimeters of tendon retraction can be treated nonsurgically. Retractions of more than 2 centimeters are more likely to develop nonunions or cause subspinous impingement and should undergo internal fixation. Subspinous impingement can cause pain and reduced hip range of motion, because the femoral neck or greater trochanter impinges on a low-lying AIIS.[43] Subspinous impingement is most common

Table 2

Suggested Nonsurgical Rehabilitation for Rectus Femoris Injuries

Week 1:	Protected weight bearing with crutches
	Ice
	Anti-inflammatory medications
	Modalities
	Passive range of motion
Weeks 2-4:	Gait training
	Active range of motion
	Isometrics
Weeks 4-6:	Resisted strength training
	Running
	Functional drills
Weeks 6-10:	Return to play

when the AIIS extends to the level of the acetabular rim (type 2) or past the rim, which is seen most frequently as a sequelae of healed avulsion injuries (type 3). Surgical indications for chronic AIIS avulsions include reduction and internal fixation of symptomatic nonunited fragments, resection of exostoses that cause functional impairment, and painful subspinous impingement.[44]

Acute surgical reattachment of purely tendinous avulsions has been reported in several case series with good results; other studies have shown good results with nonsurgical management alone, however, even in high-level kicking athletes.[45] In a series of four soccer players and one hurdler treated with acute repair (at less than 102 days), all were able to return to their previous activity level between 5 and 10 months after surgical repair.[46] Authors of a 2012 study reported on 10 professional soccer players who underwent repair of an avulsed rectus injury with direct suture repair or bone anchors.[47] At a mean follow-up of 35 months, they found fewer reinjuries in the surgical repair group. In contrast, another study reported on 11 NFL players, including two punters who were treated nonsurgically.[45] The NFL players were able to return to professional football at a mean of 70 days. Studies between surgical repair and nonsurgical management are needed to compare the two treatment options.

Chronic injuries that fail to improve may require surgical management. A pain-free return to sport has been reported in a soccer player treated with surgical repair of a chronic musculotendinous junction injury.[48] Surgical débridement of the symptomatic tendon stump also can enable a return to high-level sport. Authors of a 2011 study reported on five collegiate athletes who underwent débridement of chronically painful retracted indirect heads.[49] Although all five improved, only one patient returned to sport without recurrent pain or reduced athletic ability. Symptomatic pseudocyst formation, which can occur around the central tendon of the indirect head, can be surgically excised with good results.[50]

Summary

Muscle injuries are common in sports and frequently involve areas around the hip. MTJ injuries can be treated nonsurgically, initially with RICE followed by rehabilitation focusing on agility training, trunk stabilization, and eccentric strengthening. The return to sport should be determined by physical examination criteria including minimal pain, full range of motion, and near-symmetric strength to prevent reinjury; full recovery may take several weeks in some cases. Avulsion injuries should be recognized and treated differently than low-grade strains or contusions according to specific guidelines for the affected muscle.

Key Study Points

- Hip muscle strains are commonly encountered in sports; treatment is largely nonsurgical with RICE acutely followed by rehabilitation focusing on agility training, trunk stabilization, and eccentric strengthening.
- Complete hamstring avulsions involving all three tendons or two tendons with significant retraction may benefit from early surgical repair.
- Rectus femoris strains and avulsions can both be managed successfully even in high-level kicking athletes with 6 to 10 weeks of rehabilitation. The length of the central aponeurosis tear in MTJ strains predicts return to play.

Annotated References

1. Beiner JM, Jokl P: Muscle contusion injuries: Current treatment options. *J Am Acad Orthop Surg* 2001;9(4):227-237.

2. Ekstrand J, Hägglund M, Waldén M: Epidemiology of muscle injuries in professional football (soccer). *Am J Sports Med* 2011;39(6):1226-1232.

Fifty-one soccer teams, comprising 2,299 players, were followed prospectively for 8 years, registering 2,908 muscle injuries. On average, a player sustained 0.6 muscle injuries per season. Of the injuries, 92% were sustained by the major muscles of the lower leg. Level of evidence: II.

3. Garrett WE Jr, Rich FR, Nikolaou PK, Vogler JB III: Computed tomography of hamstring muscle strains. *Med Sci Sports Exerc* 1989;21(5):506-514.

4. Woods C, Hawkins RD, Maltby S, Hulse M, Thomas A, Hodson A; Football Association Medical Research Programme: The Football Association Medical Research Programme: An audit of injuries in professional football—analysis of hamstring injuries. *Br J Sports Med* 2004;38(1):36-41.

5. Fousekis K, Tsepis E, Poulmedis P, Athanasopoulos S, Vagenas G: Intrinsic risk factors of non-contact quadriceps and hamstring strains in soccer: A prospective study of 100 professional players. *Br J Sports Med* 2011;45(9):709-714.

This cohort study of 100 professional soccer players found that players with eccentric hamstring-strength asymmetries and functional leg-length asymmetries were at greater risk for hamstring strain. Quadriceps strains were seen in players with eccentric strength and flexibility asymmetries.

6. Malliaropoulos N, Isinkaye T, Tsitas K, Maffulli N: Reinjury after acute posterior thigh muscle injuries in elite track and field athletes. *Am J Sports Med* 2011;39(2):304-310.

Return to sport in track and field athletes was lower for low-grade injuries: 7.4 days for grade 1, 12.9 days for grade 2, 29.5 days for grade 3, and 55.0 days for grade 4 injuries. Objective clinical findings accurately predicted the risk of reinjury.

7. Warren P, Gabbe BJ, Schneider-Kolsky M, Bennell KL: Clinical predictors of time to return to competition and of recurrence following hamstring strain in elite Australian footballers. *Br J Sports Med* 2010;44(6):415-419.

Australian footballers were 4 times more likely to have a prolonged recovery if they were unable to walk pain-free the day after injury. A 20-fold increased risk for recurrence was seen if the previous hamstring injury had occurred in the last 12 months.

8. Arnason A, Andersen TE, Holme I, Engebretsen L, Bahr R: Prevention of hamstring strains in elite soccer: An intervention study. *Scand J Med Sci Sports* 2008;18(1):40-48.

9. Askling CM, Tengvar M, Thorstensson A: Acute hamstring injuries in Swedish elite football: A prospective randomised controlled clinical trial comparing two rehabilitation protocols. *Br J Sports Med* 2013;47(15):953-959.

Professional soccer players were randomized to two rehabilitation protocols. Conventional rehabilitation was found to have a longer return to play (mean of 51 days) compared with a protocol emphasizing lengthening of the muscle group (mean of 28 days).

10. Morelli V, Weaver V: Groin injuries and groin pain in athletes: Part 1. *Prim Care* 2005;32(1):163-183.

11. Feeley BT, Powell JW, Muller MS, Barnes RP, Warren RF, Kelly BT: Hip injuries and labral tears in the national football league. *Am J Sports Med* 2008;36(11):2187-2195.

12. Gallo RA, Silvis ML, Smetana B, et al: Asymptomatic hip/groin pathology identified on magnetic resonance imaging of professional hockey players: Outcomes and playing status at 4 years' follow-up. *Arthroscopy* 2014;30(10):1222-1228.

Twenty-one asymptomatic hockey players underwent MRI and were followed for 4 years. Despite a high prevalence of muscle strains (10 of 21) and labral tears (15 of 21), only one player missed competition because of a hip/pelvis injury. Level of evidence: IV.

13. Foote CJ, Maizlin ZV, Shrouder J, Grant MM, Bedi A, Ayeni OR: The association between avulsions of the reflected head of the rectus femoris and labral tears: A retrospective study. *J Pediatr Orthop* 2013;33(3):227-231.

Seven of nine pediatric patients with sports-related rectus femoris avulsions also were found to have labral tears on magnetic resonance arthrography. The ages ranged from 8 to 17 years, with two patients requiring surgery. Level of evidence: IV.

14. Philippon MJ, Weiss DR, Kuppersmith DA, Briggs KK, Hay CJ: Arthroscopic labral repair and treatment of femoroacetabular impingement in professional hockey players. *Am J Sports Med* 2010;38(1):99-104.

Treatment of femoroacetabular impingement and labral lesions in professional hockey players resulted in successful outcomes, with high patient satisfaction and a prompt return to sport within a mean of 3.4 months. Level of evidence: IV.

15. Safran MR, Garrett WE Jr, Seaber AV, Glisson RR, Ribbeck BM: The role of warmup in muscular injury prevention. *Am J Sports Med* 1988;16(2):123-129.

16. Hughes C IV, Hasselman CT, Best TM, Martinez S, Garrett WE Jr: Incomplete, intrasubstance strain injuries of the rectus femoris muscle. *Am J Sports Med* 1995;23(4):500-506.

17. Järvinen TA, Järvinen M, Kalimo H: Regeneration of injured skeletal muscle after the injury. *Muscles Ligaments Tendons J* 2013;3(4):337-345.

This review focused on the basic biologic principles of skeletal muscle regeneration and healing processes. Clinical and animal studies were discussed, with recommendations provided to promote healing and return athletes safely to competition.

2: Hip and Pelvis

18. Wood DG, Packham I, Trikha SP, Linklater J: Avulsion of the proximal hamstring origin. *J Bone Joint Surg Am* 2008;90(11):2365-2374.

19. Järvinen M: Immobilization effect on the tensile properties of striated muscle: An experimental study in the rat. *Arch Phys Med Rehabil* 1977;58(3):123-127.

20. Aärimaa V, Rantanen J, Best T, Schultz E, Corr D, Kalimo H: Mild eccentric stretch injury in skeletal muscle causes transient effects on tensile load and cell proliferation. *Scand J Med Sci Sports* 2004;14(6):367-372.

21. Kannus P, Parkkari J, Järvinen TL, Järvinen TA, Järvinen M: Basic science and clinical studies coincide: Active treatment approach is needed after a sports injury. *Scand J Med Sci Sports* 2003;13(3):150-154.

22. Almekinders LC, Gilbert JA: Healing of experimental muscle strains and the effects of nonsteroidal antiinflammatory medication. *Am J Sports Med* 1986;14(4):303-308.

23. Ryan JB, Wheeler JH, Hopkinson WJ, Arciero RA, Kolakowski KR: Quadriceps contusions. West Point update. *Am J Sports Med* 1991;19(3):299-304.

24. Cross MJ, Vandersluis R, Wood D, Banff M: Surgical repair of chronic complete hamstring tendon rupture in the adult patient. *Am J Sports Med* 1998;26(6):785-788.

25. Cohen S, Bradley J: Acute proximal hamstring rupture. *J Am Acad Orthop Surg* 2007;15(6):350-355.

26. De Vos RJ, Reurink G, Goudswaard GJ, Moen MH, Weir A, Tol JL: Clinical findings just after return to play predict hamstring re-injury, but baseline MRI findings do not. *Br J Sports Med* 2014;48(18):1377-1384.

    This cohort study found no association between baseline MRI findings and hamstrings reinjury within 12 months; previous hamstring injuries and clinical signs (knee extension or isometric-force deficits and tenderness with palpation) were significant independent predictors of reinjury, however.

27. Moen MH, Reurink G, Weir A, Tol JL, Maas M, Goudswaard GJ: Predicting return to play after hamstring injuries. *Br J Sports Med* 2014;48(18):1358-1363.

    In 74 nonprofessional athletes, MRI findings were unable to predict return to play. Only a self-predicted time to return to play by the athlete and a passive straight leg raise deficit remained significantly associated with the time to return to sport.

28. Koulouris G, Connell D: Evaluation of the hamstring muscle complex following acute injury. *Skeletal Radiol* 2003;32(10):582-589.

29. Guillodo Y, Bouttier R, Saraux A: Value of sonography combined with clinical assessment to evaluate muscle injury severity in athletes. *J Athl Train* 2011;46(5):500-504.

    Ninety-three consecutive sports-related muscle injuries were analyzed. Physical examination findings (bruising, tenderness to palpation, limited range of motion, and pain with isometric contraction) and ultrasound findings including hematoma volume were found to predict the return to play following muscle strain.

30. Sherry MA, Best TM: A comparison of 2 rehabilitation programs in the treatment of acute hamstring strains. *J Orthop Sports Phys Ther* 2004;34(3):116-125.

31. Levine WN, Bergfeld JA, Tessendorf W, Moorman CT III: Intramuscular corticosteroid injection for hamstring injuries. A 13-year experience in the National Football League. *Am J Sports Med* 2000;28(3):297-300.

32. A Hamid MS, Mohamed Ali MR, Yusof A, George J, Lee LP: Platelet-rich plasma injections for the treatment of hamstring injuries: A randomized controlled trial. *Am J Sports Med* 2014;42(10):2410-2418.

    This randomized trial compared rehabilitation programs with and without a single platelet-rich plasma (PRP) injection on return to play following hamstring strain. Return to play was, on average, 15 days longer in the rehabilitation-only group. The study was not placebo controlled. Level of evidence: II.

33. Reurink G, Goudswaard GJ, Moen MH, et al; Dutch Hamstring Injection Therapy (HIT) Study Investigators: Platelet-rich plasma injections in acute muscle injury. *N Engl J Med* 2014;370(26):2546-2547.

    In a three-center randomized, placebo-controlled trial comparing PRP to isotonic saline, the investigators found an equal return-to-play time (mean of 42 days) for both groups. Two injections were given: one 5 days after injury, and the second at 10 to 12 days after injury.

34. Clanton TO, Coupe KJ: Hamstring strains in athletes: Diagnosis and treatment. *J Am Acad Orthop Surg* 1998;6(4):237-248.

35. Engebretsen AH, Myklebust G, Holme I, Engebretsen L, Bahr R: Intrinsic risk factors for hamstring injuries among male soccer players: A prospective cohort study. *Am J Sports Med* 2010;38(6):1147-1153.

    In a cohort of 508 professional soccer players, 76 hamstring injuries were identified. In multivariate analysis, previous hamstring injury was the most predictive factor for reinjury, more than doubling the risk of a new injury. Level of evidence: II.

36. Opar DA, Williams MD, Timmins RG, Hickey J, Duhig SJ, Shield AJ: Eccentric hamstring strength and hamstring injury risk in Australian footballers. *Med Sci Sports Exerc* 2015;47(4):857-865.

    Australian footballers with reduced preseason eccentric hamstring strength below a threshold value had a 2.7-fold increased risk of hamstring injury that season. Conversely, increased eccentric strength mitigated other risk factors, including increased age or previous injury.

37. Opar DA, Williams MD, Timmins RG, Hickey J, Duhig SJ, Shield AJ: The effect of previous hamstring strain injuries on the change in eccentric hamstring strength during preseason training in elite Australian footballers. *Am J Sports Med* 2015;43(2):377-384.

   Athletes with previous hamstring injuries showed a relatively reduced capacity for eccentric strengthening with exercise compared with those without previous injury. This finding was true for the affected and the nonaffected limb. Level of evidence: II.

38. Harris JD, Griesser MJ, Best TM, Ellis TJ: Treatment of proximal hamstring ruptures - A systematic review. *Int J Sports Med* 2011;32(7):490-495.

   This systematic review compared surgical treatment with nonsurgical treatment and acute repair timing of proximal hamstring avulsions with that of chronic repair. Nonsurgical and chronic repairs were found to have inferior outcomes in terms of patient satisfaction and return to the previous level of competition.

39. Cross TM, Gibbs N, Houang MT, Cameron M: Acute quadriceps muscle strains: Magnetic resonance imaging features and prognosis. *Am J Sports Med* 2004;32(3):710-719.

40. Hasselman CT, Best TM, Hughes C IV, Martinez S, Garrett WE Jr: An explanation for various rectus femoris strain injuries using previously undescribed muscle architecture. *Am J Sports Med* 1995;23(4):493-499.

41. Schuett DJ, Bomar JD, Pennock AT: Pelvic apophyseal avulsion fractures: A retrospective review of 228 cases. *J Pediatr Orthop* 2014.

   The authors identified 228 apophyseal avulsions. The mean age was 14, and 76% of injuries occurred in males. Most injuries occurred during sprinting or kicking. AIIS avulsions were most common (49%), followed by avulsions at the anterior superior iliac spine (30%), ischial tuberosity (11%), and iliac crest (10%). Level of evidence: IV.

42. Balius R, Maestro A, Pedret C, et al: Central aponeurosis tears of the rectus femoris: Practical sonographic prognosis. *Br J Sports Med* 2009;43(11):818-824.

43. Hetsroni I, Poultsides L, Bedi A, Larson CM, Kelly BT: Anterior inferior iliac spine morphology correlates with hip range of motion: A classification system and dynamic model. *Clin Orthop Relat Res* 2013;471(8):2497-2503.

   The authors reported a correlation between AIIS morphology and hip range of motion. A lower-hanging AIIS (at or below the level of the acetabular rim) correlated with decreased hip flexion and internal rotation on clinical examination. Level of evidence: III.

44. Hetsroni I, Larson CM, Dela Torre K, Zbeda RM, Magennis E, Kelly BT: Anterior inferior iliac spine deformity as an extra-articular source for hip impingement: A series of 10 patients treated with arthroscopic decompression. *Arthroscopy* 2012;28(11):1644-1653.

   The authors describe the arthroscopic technique and outcomes of AIIS decompression. At a mean of 14 months postoperatively, hip range of motion and modified Harris Hip scores improved significantly. Level of evidence: IV.

45. Gamradt SC, Brophy RH, Barnes R, Warren RF, Thomas Byrd JW, Kelly BT: Nonoperative treatment for proximal avulsion of the rectus femoris in professional American football. *Am J Sports Med* 2009;37(7):1370-1374.

46. Irmola T, Heikkilä JT, Orava S, Sarimo J: Total proximal tendon avulsion of the rectus femoris muscle. *Scand J Med Sci Sports* 2007;17(4):378-382.

47. García VV, Duhrkop DC, Seijas R, Ares O, Cugat R: Surgical treatment of proximal ruptures of the rectus femoris in professional soccer players. *Arch Orthop Trauma Surg* 2012;132(3):329-333.

   This study included ten proximal rectus avulsions in high-level athletes who underwent surgical repair. Six were repaired directly, whereas suture anchors were used in four cases. No recurrences occurred, and all athletes returned to the same level of competition.

48. Straw R, Colclough K, Geutjens G: Surgical repair of a chronic rupture of the rectus femoris muscle at the proximal musculotendinous junction in a soccer player. *Br J Sports Med* 2003;37(2):182-184.

49. Wittstein J, Klein S, Garrett WE: Chronic tears of the reflected head of the rectus femoris: Results of operative treatment. *Am J Sports Med* 2011;39(9):1942-1947.

   Five patients with chronic tears of the rectus femoris that failed nonsurgical therapy were treated with excision of the reflected head. All reported a reduction in pain severity, but four of five had mild residual symptoms with athletic participation. Level of evidence: IV.

50. Cicvarić T, Lucin K, Roth S, Ivancić A, Marinović M, Santić V: Giant pseudocyst of the rectus femoris muscle—repetitive strain injury in recreational soccer player. *Coll Antropol* 2010;34(Suppl 2):53-55.

Chapter 14

Athletic Pubalgia/Core Muscle Injury and Groin Pathology

Christopher M. Larson, MD   David M. Rowley, MD

Abstract

Hip and groin-related symptoms and disorders are increasingly recognized as a cause of significant disability in athletes. Hip and groin symptoms can be the result of extra-articular disorders (sports hernia/athletic pubalgia/core muscle injury, proximal adductor pathology, osteitis pubis) and or intra-articular disorders (labral tears, chondral pathology, femoroacetabular impingement). It is now recognized that there is a compensatory relationship between intra-articular and extra-articular hip and groin disorders, and a high index of suspicion is required to accurately diagnose these conditions. A thorough history and physical examination combined with appropriate imaging studies can lead to an accurate diagnosis and effective treatment recommendations. Ultimately, this can help to minimize disability duration and maximize return to athletic participation in this potentially challenging patient population.

Keywords: athletic pubalgia; groin injuries; hip injuries

Introduction

Hip and groin injuries are common problems that can lead to disability in athletes. The clinical and diagnostic presentations of the various potential entities can overlap, making diagnosis and treatment difficult. These challenges can lead to time lost from athletic participation and subsequent frustration for athletes with these conditions.[1] The differential diagnosis for activity-related groin pain has been described in broad categories as core muscle injury (athletic pubalgia or sports hernia), hip/joint pathology (intra-articular pathology), and other etiologies.[2] This chapter discusses extra-articular hip pathology with a focus on athletic pubalgia, proximal adductor injuries, and osteitis pubis.

The anatomic structures of the hip and pelvis have been described based on layers. Layer 1 consists of the osseous morphology, including the pelvic bones, acetabulum, and proximal femur. Layer 2 consists of soft tissue in and around the hip including the labrum, capsule, and ligaments, which add substantial stability to the hip. Layer 3 consists of the contractile layer around the hip including the adductors, abductors, flexors/extensors, and internal and external rotators of the hip. Layer 4 consists of the neurovascular structures that surround the hip. The main components of this layer are the lateral femoral cutaneous nerve, obturator nerve, inguinal nerve, sciatic nerve, and genitofemoral nerve.[3] It should be noted that all of these structures can be sources of pain when evaluating patients with lower abdominal/hip/groin pain. In addition, patients with extra-articular hip pathology can have concomitant femoroacetabular impingement (FAI) or intra-articular hip pathology.

Athletic Pubalgia

Pathoanatomy

The anterior bony pelvis, with its many muscle attachments and the pubic symphysis, forms the center of core injuries and sports hernia.[1] The abdominal wall musculature also has been described in layers. The layers, from superficial to deep, are the fascia, external oblique fascia and muscle, internal oblique fascia and muscle, transversus abdominis muscle, and transversalis fascia.[4] The rectus abdominis muscle, conjoint tendon (internal oblique and transversus abdominis fascia), and external

Dr. Larson or an immediate family member serves as a paid consultant to A3 Surgical and Smith & Nephew; has stock or stock options held in A3 Surgical; and has received research or institutional support from Smith & Nephew. Neither Dr. Rowley nor any immediate family member has received anything of value from or has stock or stock options held in a commercial company or institution related directly or indirectly to the subject of this chapter.

2: Hip and Pelvis

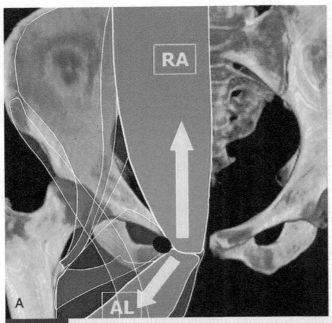
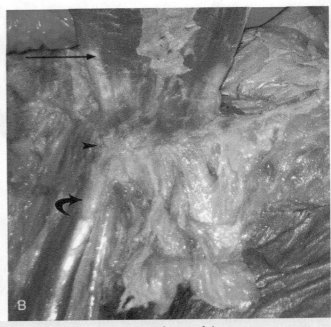

Figure 1 Images show the abdominal wall musculature. **A,** Illustration depicts the opposing forces of the rectus abdominis (RA) and the adductor longus muscles (AL) at the pubic tubercle. The rectus abdominis muscle creates superoposterior tension, whereas the adductor longus muscle creates inferoanterior tension. Disruption of either muscle leads to altered biomechanics. The black circle represents the superficial inguinal ring. **B,** Gross specimen demonstrates the rectus abdominis (straight arrow), the adductor longus (curved arrow), and the pubic tubercle attachment of the rectus abdominis/adductor aponeurosis (arrowhead). (Reproduced with permission from Palisch A, Zoga A, Meyers W: Imaging of athletic pubalgia and core muscle injuries: Clinical and therapeutic correlations. *Clin Sports Med* 2013;32[3]:427-447.)

oblique muscle merge to form the pubic aponeurosis, which inserts onto the pubic tubercle. The medial thigh compartment consists of the pectineus, the gracilis, and the adductor brevis, longus, and magnus muscles (Figure 1). The ligamentous complex at the pubic symphysis consists of the anterior, superior, posterior, and arcuate ligaments. The superior and arcuate ligaments are the main stabilizers of the pubic symphysis.[1]

The pubic symphysis is the center of the various forces generated at the anterior pelvis. Athletic pubalgia is defined as an injury to one of the previously described structures, as it inserts into the pubis, without the presence of a clinically recognizable hernia, so the term sports hernia is a misnomer.[5] Injury to or deconditioning of one of the anterior pelvic structures can result in increased stress and strain on the adjacent structures. This can lead to complete disruption of one of the musculotendinous origins/insertions or ligaments about the pelvis.

Clinical Presentation

Rapid lateral motion, acceleration, deceleration, hyperextension, or hyperabduction can lead to increased tension in the pubic region.[1] Athletic pubalgia is seen primarily in athletes who are involved in cutting and pivoting activities. In one study, 82% of patients who presented with

athletic pubalgia were athletes.[6] Patients typically present with exertional pain during activity without a specific injury or event causing the pain. They report anterior groin or lower abdominal pain that is brought on by physical activity and is usually relieved with rest.[7] The lower abdominal or groin pain often resumes with activity after a period of rest from vigorous activity. Coughing, sit-ups, and kicking can reproduce the symptoms. Occasionally, pain can radiate proximally into the abdominal musculature or distally into the thigh, groin region, or scrotum.[1]

Physical Examination

The physical examination should begin with palpation of the pubic symphysis, the rectus abdominis muscle, the internal/external oblique muscles, the origin of the adductor muscles, the pectineus and gracilis muscles, and the inguinal ring for areas of tenderness. Lower abdominal pain or groin pain, pain that is worse with sport-specific activities including kicking, cutting, sit-ups, and sprinting and that is relieved with rest, tenderness to palpation over the pubic ramus, pain with resisted hip adduction, and pain with resisted abdominal sit-ups are the five most common complaints or findings in patients with athletic pubalgia.[8] Evaluation of potential intra-articular hip pathology using the FADIR (flexion, adduction, internal rotation) test should be performed, because concomitant hip-joint pathology is not uncommon, and intra-articular and extra-articular hip and pelvis disorders often are related and compensatory in nature.

Imaging

Initial imaging begins with a well-centered AP pelvis and lateral hip radiograph.[9] These images are usually negative in patients with isolated athletic pubalgia but are used to rule out avulsion injuries about the pelvis, radiographic signs of bony impingement, stress fractures, osteitis pubis, sacralized lumbar vertebrae, and other potential sources of pain.

MRI is the current standard for evaluation of activity-related pelvic pain.[10] A dedicated athletic pubalgia MRI protocol, including large field-of-view and small field-of-view images focusing on the pubic symphysis, is useful for accurate diagnosis and location of the pathology.[1] MRI is 68% sensitive and 100% specific for rectus abdominis pathology compared with findings at surgery and is 86% sensitive and 89% specific for adductor pathology. It also is 100% sensitive for osteitis pubis.[11] MRI should be reviewed closely for osteitis pubis, rectus abdominis strain, adductor tendon injury, rectus abdominis or adductor aponeurotic injury or plate disruption, inguinal hernias, femoral stress fractures, and hip–joint-related pathology.[10] The most frequent finding on MRI is fluid signal extending from the anterior-inferior insertion of the rectus abdominis into the adductor origin, with corresponding fluid signal in the pubis[11,12] (Figure 2).

Diagnostic Injections

As described previously, several potential pain generators are present about the pelvis and groin. Diagnostic injections can help determine the etiology of pain when conflicting results appear on clinical examination. Administering an intra-articular injection of local anesthetic into the hip joint can be useful before having the athlete perform activities that typically provoke pain or re-examining the patient in the office. Persistent pain in the groin or lower abdominal regions after intra-articular injection can be consistent with concomitant or isolated athletic pubalgia. Anesthetic injection into the pubic symphysis, adductor cleft, or psoas bursa also can aid in diagnosis.

Treatment

Nonsurgical Treatment

Relative rest and avoidance of activities that provoke pain comprise the initial treatment. Physical therapy should focus on core strengthening as well as identifying areas of weakness or reduced range of motion. Therapy should

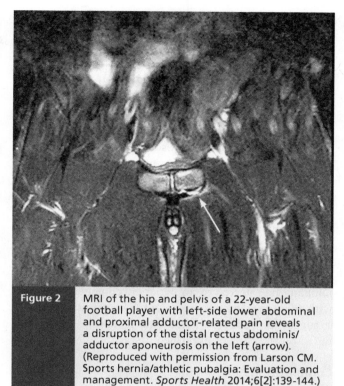

Figure 2 MRI of the hip and pelvis of a 22-year-old football player with left-side lower abdominal and proximal adductor-related pain reveals a disruption of the distal rectus abdominis/adductor aponeurosis on the left (arrow). (Reproduced with permission from Larson CM. Sports hernia/athletic pubalgia: Evaluation and management. *Sports Health* 2014;6[2]:139-144.)

focus on resolving imbalances between the pelvic and hip stabilizers.[7] NSAIDs and ice can be used to minimize swelling and pain during the rehabilitation period.

Patients generally are treated for at least 3 months with activity modification and physical therapy. If substantial improvement is achieved, nonsurgical treatment is continued with a gradual sport-specific activity progression. If no improvement is seen by 3 months, surgery might be considered.[7] Ultimately, the duration of nonsurgical treatment and the timing of potential surgery are variable, depending on the level of the athlete and the schedule of the sport season.

Surgical Treatment

Various surgical procedures have been described for the treatment of athletic pubalgia. Plication of the transversalis fascia, reapproximation of the conjoint tendon to the inguinal ligament, and approximation of the external oblique aponeurosis has been described.[13] Patients had a return-to-sport rate of 96% at 12 weeks. An open approach for the treatment of athletic pubalgia has been described, with reattachment of the anterior-inferior rectus abdominis with an adductor release;[7] 152 of 157 patients with athletic pubalgia who underwent primary pelvic floor repair were able to return to their preinjury level of competition. In a study examining results over

20 years, 95% of athletes were able to return to sports participation at 3 months postoperatively.[14] An open repair technique using mesh has been studied; all patients underwent bilateral mesh repairs with the mesh bridging from the pubis to the anterior superior iliac spine.[15] The peritoneum was closed over the mesh, and it was reported that all patients were able to return to full sports participation postoperatively. Multiple authors have published their experience with laparoscopic repair.[16,17] A recent randomized controlled trial compared patients with athletic pubalgia treated with a laparoscopic mesh technique with those who underwent nonsurgical treatment. At 3 months, 90% of the laparoscopic group returned to sport compared with 27% of the nonsurgical group. At 12 months, 97% of the surgical group had returned to sport compared with 50% of the nonsurgical group.[18]

It is recommended that patients with suspected athletic pubalgia be referred to an experienced general surgeon with an interest in groin pathology. There is little evidence to suggest that one repair technique is superior to another, based on the current published literature.

Complications

The most common postoperative complication is edema in the abdomen, thighs, genitals, and perineum. Wound infection is reported at 0.4%, and hematoma requiring reoperation has a rate of 0.3%. Nerve dysesthesia has a less than 1% occurrence rate and usually affects the anterior/lateral femoral cutaneous nerve distribution, the ilioinguinal nerve, or the genitofemoral nerve.[14] Penile vein thrombosis is reported in the literature but all cases resolved. The most common reason for reoperation is the development of athletic pubalgia on the contralateral side. The second most common reason for reoperation is inadequate adductor release or repair at the time of the athletic pubalgia repair.[14] Failure to address intra-articular pathology (FAI) is another reason for continued disability after repair.[19]

Rehabilitation

Most recent studies have reported a return to full activity 1 to 6 months after surgery, depending on the type of repair.[11,17] Patients may bear weight as tolerated postoperatively, with physical therapy starting at 1 to 14 days postoperatively. Physical therapy initially focuses on abdominal and adductor flexibility and targeted abdominal strengthening. A stepwise running program begins at 4 weeks after surgery, with sport-specific exercises starting at week 5.[8,11] Activity as tolerated is allowed around 6 weeks postoperatively.[8]

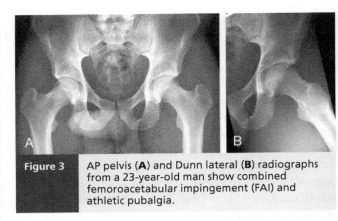

Figure 3 AP pelvis (**A**) and Dunn lateral (**B**) radiographs from a 23-year-old man show combined femoroacetabular impingement (FAI) and athletic pubalgia.

Combined Athletic Pubalgia and FAI

Overlap between intra-articular and extra-articular pathology often occurs in patients presenting with lower abdominal groin or hip pain. Recently, using a cadaver model, it has been shown that patients with FAI have increased stress placed on the pubic symphysis, which may predispose to combined FAI and athletic pubalgia.[20] It is imperative to determine the source of the pain so that proper expectations and treatment options can be presented. A subset of patients will present with combined FAI and athletic pubalgia. Clinical examination and detailed imaging can help to determine the combined diagnosis (Figure 3). Often, it is difficult to determine how much pain or disability results from each entity. In these cases, anesthetic intra-articular and extra-articular injections can aid in the diagnosis. When it is determined through a detailed examination, imaging, and possibly diagnostic injections that a combined process is occurring, treatment can be tailored for both entities. Treatment of only one of the pathologies can lead to a suboptimal result. In a study of patients with combined FAI and athletic pubalgia, patients who had athletic pubalgia surgery alone returned to their previous level of sport participation 25% of the time. Of patients who underwent arthroscopy for FAI only, 50% returned to their previous level. Of patients who had both athletic pubalgia surgery and hip arthroscopy, 85% to 91% returned to sport. No difference was seen, whether surgery was performed in a staged fashion or if both treatments were performed at the same time.[19]

Adductor Strain

Pathoanatomy

Myotendinous injuries and strains are more common when the muscle crosses two joints, and they usually result from eccentric contraction.[21] The injury usually occurs at the myotendinous junction. Adductor injures often occur at the origin onto the pelvis, however, and may be caused by a different mechanism than typical muscle strain[22] (Figure 4). Adductor strains are common in athletes who participate in pivoting and cutting activities and in kicking in soccer. The adductor group works in conjunction with the abdominal musculature to stabilize the pelvis during walking and running.[23] The adductor longus origin on the pelvis may be predisposed to injury because of its small cross-sectional area compared with the size of the muscle belly.[21] Another etiology for adductor strain is a muscle imbalance between the abductors and the adductors. It has been reported that professional hockey players are 17 times more likely to incur an adductor strain if their adductor strength was less than 80% of their abductor strength.[21] In a follow-up study, the authors showed a significant reduction in adductor strains in a similar population when a preventive adductor strengthening program was instituted.[24,25]

Clinical Presentation

Adductor strains are common in athletes participating in football, soccer, hockey, and dance.[21] These athletes often present with acute medial groin or proximal thigh pain. Adductor strains are usually self-limiting, requiring minimal treatment with very high rates of return to play. Chronic proximal adductor pain related to sports participation can be associated with athletic pubalgia or hip impingement, such as FAI. One study of athletes with proximal adductor pain reported underlying FAI in 94% of athletes, based on radiographs.[26] On examination, tenderness to palpation is present over the adductor longus tendon.[24] Patients experience pain with passive abduction, and a palpable defect sometimes will be present. Patients also have pain with resisted adduction. When evaluating patients with adductor injury, it is important to assess for athletic pubalgia and FAI.

Imaging

Imaging for adductor strains is usually not indicated, because many of these injuries are self-limiting. For patients experiencing chronic disability secondary to a groin injury or in patients with a palpable defect, imaging may be warranted. A well-centered AP pelvis radiograph should be obtained, with initial evaluation for apophyseal avulsions, osteitis pubis, pelvic stress fractures, or intra-articular findings that may explain continued disability. MRI is the next study for evaluation of musculotendinous injury, injury at the insertion site, and intra-articular hip pathology. MRI sequences that have been described for the evaluation of athletic pubalgia are indicated.[7] Muscle strains with a cross-sectional area involvement greater than 50% on MRI, fluid collections, and muscle tears are associated with longer recovery times. Adductor longus

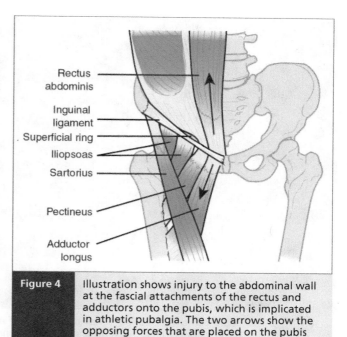

Labels: Rectus abdominis, Inguinal ligament, Superficial ring, Iliopsoas, Sartorius, Pectineus, Adductor longus

Figure 4 Illustration shows injury to the abdominal wall at the fascial attachments of the rectus and adductors onto the pubis, which is implicated in athletic pubalgia. The two arrows show the opposing forces that are placed on the pubis secondary to the rectus and adductors.

tears with a palpable defect usually show a 3-cm or greater retraction of the tendon on MRI[1,27] (Figure 5).

Treatment

Activity modification, ice, compression, NSAIDs, and gentle range-of-motion exercises are the mainstay of initial treatment after adductor injury. When pain decreases, formal physical therapy can begin using a variety of modalities, including static stretching, massage, tissue mobilizations, and proprioceptive neuromuscular facilitation. Cryotherapy may be helpful for the reduction of swelling and pain relief.[25] Electrical stimulation may be used to prevent muscle atrophy. External wraps can limit the amount of active and passive hip abduction and can provide comfort in the acute setting.

When pain is manageable, gentle range-of-motion exercises can begin, including exercise-bike riding and pool exercises. After full range of motion is achieved, a strengthening program is instituted focusing on core strengthening, plyometrics, and gentle running straight ahead.[21] The patients' activities are gradually advanced with sport-specific drills. Patients are able to return to play after full strength and pain-free motion are achieved, with a mean return to play of 6 weeks.[21]

For patients in whom nonsurgical treatment has failed, injections may be warranted. Platelet-rich plasma (PRP), corticosteroid, and simple anesthetic injections have been described for adductor strains. Injections into the adductor enthesis have shown some success in competitive and recreational athletes.[8]

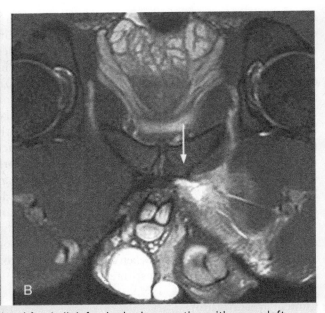

Figure 5 MRI depicts an anterior adductor avulsion in a professional football defensive back presenting with severe left-side groin pain. Right-side defensive backs often injure their left rectus abdominis/adductor aponeurosis when transitioning during pass coverage. **A,** Large field-of-view coronal short tau inversion-recovery (STIR) image of the bony pelvis shows detachment of the left adductor origin from the aponeurosis (arrow) with the retracted tendon fibers (arrowhead). The distance of retraction often is measured best on the coronal STIR images. **B,** Small field-of-view coronal oblique T2-weighted fat-saturated fast spin-echo image using a pubalgia protocol demonstrates the detachment of the left anterior adductor origin from the aponeurotic plate (arrow). Often, the pectineus and adductor longus muscles detach together. This condition is referred to as an anterior adductor avulsion because these muscles are the two most anterior muscles at the pubic attachment. (Reproduced with permission from Palisch A, Zoga A, Meyers W: Imaging of athletic pubalgia and core muscle injuries: Clinical and therapeutic correlations. *Clin Sports Med* 2013;32[3]:427-447.)

If nonsurgical treatment of 3 to 6 months has failed, surgical treatment may be considered. In a case series of 16 competitive athletes with chronic isolated adductor pathology, nonsurgical measures including rest, physical therapy, NSAIDs, and corticosteroid injections failed in all patients.[28] Surgical treatment consisted of open tenotomy 1 cm from the adductor longus origin. All patients improved and were able to return to sports activities. At final follow-up, 10 of 16 patients were pain free. Adduction strength was weaker after full recovery. One of the authors of this chapter (CML) prefers a fractional lengthening 3 cm distal to the origin to minimize postoperative weakness. Caution should be exercised when considering a release in soccer strikers, because this procedure might lead to detrimental adductor weakness.[27] In a 2009 study of 19 National Football League (NFL) players who sustained a rupture of the adductor longus, 14 were treated nonsurgically, and 9 underwent surgical repair.[27] The nonsurgical group returned to play at 6 weeks, compared with 12 weeks in the surgical group. No strength deficits were present in either group. Of the surgical group, 20% experienced wound complications, a fact that favors nonsurgical treatment in these instances.

Complications

Injury to the spermatic cord can occur during surgical lengthening of the adductor longus if dissection is carried medial to the gracilis origin on the pubis.[29,30]

Rehabilitation

Postoperatively, patients can bear weight as tolerated with crutches until a nonantalgic gait is achieved. Gentle range-of-motion exercises may begin as tolerated. Strengthening exercises may begin at 6 to 8 weeks, with a mean return to play of 12 weeks.

Osteitis Pubis

Pathoanatomy

Osteitis pubis is thought to be a stress injury of the parasymphyseal pubic bones secondary to increased strain on the anterior pelvis.[31] It is described secondary to chronic overuse, resulting in a stress reaction adjacent to the pubic symphysis and later leads to symphyseal pathology.[32] This was demonstrated in a study of pubic rami bone biopsies of athletes in whom osteitis pubis had been diagnosed.[33] The specimens showed formation of new woven bone,

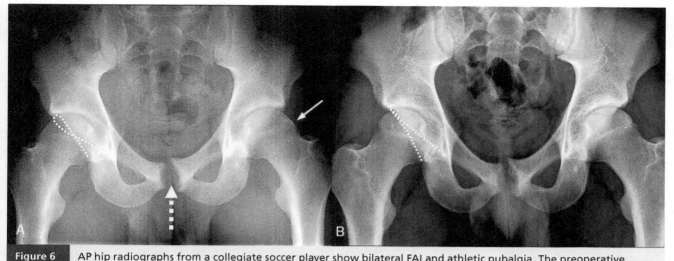

Figure 6 AP hip radiographs from a collegiate soccer player show bilateral FAI and athletic pubalgia. The preoperative radiograph (**A**) shows a crossover sign (dotted line) indicative of pincer-type impingement, cam impingement (solid arrow), and lytic changes at the pubic symphysis (dashed arrow) consistent with osteitis pubis. After rim resection and femoral resection osteoplasty (**B**), an improved relation can be seen between the anterior and posterior acetabular walls, and removal of the crossover sign (dotted lines) is seen. (Reproduced with permission from Larson CM, Pierce BR, Giveans M: Treatment of athletes with symptomatic intra-articular hip pathology and athletic pubalgia/sports hernia: A case series. *Arthroscopy* 2011; 27[6]:768-775.)

osteoblasts, and neovascularization, with an absence of inflammatory cells and no signs of osteonecrosis. Osteitis pubis is seen most commonly in athletes participating in soccer, Australian-rules football, rugby, ice hockey, American football, and distance running.[34]

Clinical Presentation

Patients often present with lower abdominal pain, bilateral or unilateral groin pain, and/or pain over the anterior pelvis. Initial symptoms are similar to those in patients who present with athletic pubalgia or adductor strains. Patients also have tenderness to palpation over the pubic symphysis and adjacent rami.[34] Pain also can be experienced in the perineal, inguinal, and scrotal regions.[33] Patients may report a clicking sensation over the anterior pelvis with activity. Pain is usually aggravated by running or cutting activities, loading of the rectus abdominis, and resisted hip flexion and adduction. Osteitis pubis is often a chronic condition that can result in an inability to compete in athletics secondary to pain and discomfort.[33] This presentation is distinctly different from the osteitis pubis presenting with disability during daily activities and a waddling gait, which is seen more typically in females.

Physical Examination

Examination findings commonly overlap with athletic pubalgia and adductor strains and include tenderness to palpation over the pubic symphysis and pubic tubercle, adductor origin tenderness, and pain during resisted adduction.[33] Patients may have apprehension during hip range of motion. Patients with reduced hip range of motion are also more likely to have osteitis pubis, because it is thought to cause compensatory stress at the pubic symphysis.[20]

Imaging

The initial imaging study for the evaluation of osteitis pubis is plain radiography. A well-centered AP pelvis radiograph will be normal in acute cases. Chronic cases (those lasting more than 6 months) of osteitis pubis can present with cystic changes, sclerosis, or widening of the symphysis. A single-leg stance AP flamingo view of the pelvis can be used to evaluate for pubic instability. Widening greater than 7 mm or vertical shift greater than 2 mm indicates instability at the pubic symphysis.[35] Radiographs also should be evaluated for the presence of FAI, stress fractures, and avulsion injuries[19] (**Figure 6**).

MRI will show subchondral bone marrow edema similar to that seen in osteoarthritis of other joints. The edema is usually bilateral but often will be asymmetric, with increased signal intensity on the more symptomatic side (**Figure 7**). The bone marrow edema will encompass the entire subchondral region of the symphysis from anterior to posterior, thus differentiating it from isolated edema related to an avulsion injury. Subchondral cysts and resorption of the subchondral bone also can be present on MRI.[10] A severe episode of osteitis pubis can show articular erosion in addition to subchondral edema similar to that seen in patients with osteolysis at the acromioclavicular joint. Healing can be protracted in these more advanced cases.[36]

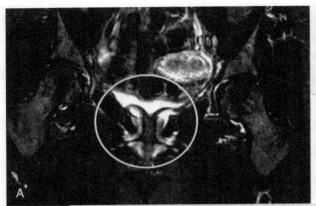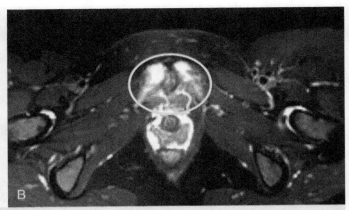

Figure 7 Coronal (**A**) and axial (**B**) MRI scans show chronic osteitis pubis (circled areas). (Courtesy of Dr. Ira Zaltz, Royal Oak, MI.)

Treatment

Nonsurgical Treatment

Nonsurgical management consists of rest, ice, NSAIDs, activity modification, corticosteroid or PRP injections, and physical therapy focusing on core strengthening. Currently, the evidence for nonsurgical treatment of osteitis pubis is level IV. In a prospective cohort study, osteitits pubis was diagnosed by physical examination and MRI in 27 professional Australian-rules football players. Treatment consisted of swimming and upper-body activities as tolerated. Core strengthening and cycling were started at 3 weeks in patients who were relatively pain free. Stair stepping was started at 6 weeks, with a graduated running program instituted at 12 weeks. Using this protocol, 89% of the athletes returned to their sport at 1 year, and 100% returned at 2 years.[34] It is not uncommon in the chapter authors' practice for osteitis symptoms subside after 1 to 2 years regardless of treatment.

Surgical Treatment

The surgical treatment of osteitis pubis is indicated primarily for demonstrable instability on radiographs or failure of prolonged nonsurgical management. Techniques that are described in the literature for the treatment of osteitis pubis include curettage of the symphysis, wedge resection, mesh reinforcement of the symphysis, arthrodesis of the symphysis using compression plating, and broad pelvic-floor core-muscle procedures.[34,35,37]

Complications

Complications after surgical treatment of osteitis pubis include hemospermia, scrotal swelling, continued symphyseal instability, and chronic anterior groin pain.[31]

Rehabilitation

Postoperatively, patients are initially kept nonweight bearing. Gentle range-of-motion exercises and stretching are instituted once pain allows. Patients progress through a graduated strengthening program with return to activity as tolerated at 6 weeks.

Summary

The understanding of athletic pubalgia and groin pathology is constantly expanding. Previously, they were seen as several isolated pathologies, but substantial evidence now supports the overlap of intra-articular and extra-articular hip and pelvis disorders as well as other compensatory disorders up and down the kinetic chain in patients presenting with groin pain. As the ability to diagnose specific groin-related pathology improves, precise treatment of these disorders will help to optimize results and minimize disability times in this challenging and demanding patient population. Based on the evidence supporting an overlap between athletic pubalgia and FAI, athletes presenting with groin or pelvic pain should be evaluated for both entities. A critical aspect of treating patients with combined intra-articular hip pathology and athletic pubalgia, adductor strain, or osteitis pubis is deciding whether patients require treatment for both entities. This is a challenging scenario, because a point likely exists at which treating FAI alone is inadequate secondary to advanced injury to the anterior pelvic musculature and/or structures.

Key Study Points

- The key anatomic structures involved in extra-articular hip pain should be identified.
- An understanding of the diagnosis and treatment of the various causes of extra-articular hip pain is imperative.
- Key physical examination findings differentiate intra-articular and extra-articular hip pain.

Annotated References

1. Palisch A, Zoga AC, Meyers WC: Imaging of athletic pubalgia and core muscle injuries: Clinical and therapeutic correlations. *Clin Sports Med* 2013;32(3):427-447.

This article highlights several common causes of groin pain in the athlete. The article describes the clinical presentation and MRI findings of these common causes of groin pain. It also highlights the overlap of symptoms and presentations that these conditions share.

2. Meyers W, Zoga A, Joseph T, et al: Current understanding of core muscle injuries (athletic pubalgia, "sports hernia"), in Thomas Byrd JW, ed: *Operative Hip Arthroscopy*. New York, Springer, 2013, pp 67-77.

This chapter aims to clarify soft-tissue injuries in the pelvis. It explains why sports hernia is a misnomer and describes the complex anatomy of the pelvis. The chapter also stresses the importance of correctly identifying the injured area as intra-articular or extra-articular.

3. Draovitch P, Edelstein J, Kelly BT: The layer concept: Utilization in determining the pain generators, pathology and how structure determines treatment. *Curr Rev Musculoskelet Med* 2012;5(1):1-8.

This article discusses the complex anatomy of the pelvis in layers. Layer 1 is the osseous layer, layer 2 is the tissue layer, layer 3 is the contractile layer, and layer 4 is the neuromechanical layer. Level of evidence: V.

4. Birmingham PM, Larson CM: Medial soft tissue injuries of the hip: Adductor strains and athletic pubalgia, in Kelly BT, Larson CM, Bedi A, eds: *Sports Hip Injuries: Diagnosis and Management*. New Jersey. SLACK Inc. 2013.

This review highlights common extra-articular causes of groin pain, focusing on athletic pubalgia and adductor injuries.

5. Farber AJ, Wilckens JH: Sports hernia: Diagnosis and therapeutic approach. *J Am Acad Orthop Surg* 2007;15(8):507-514.

6. Taylor DC, Meyers WC, Moylan JA, Lohnes J, Bassett FH, Garrett WE Jr: Abdominal musculature abnormalities as a cause of groin pain in athletes. Inguinal hernias and pubalgia. *Am J Sports Med* 1991;19(3):239-242.

7. Meyers WC, Foley DP, Garrett WE, Lohnes JH, Mandlebaum BR; PAIN (Performing Athletes with Abdominal or Inguinal Neuromuscular Pain Study Group): Management of severe lower abdominal or inguinal pain in high-performance athletes. *Am J Sports Med* 2000;28(1):2-8.

8. Litwin DE, Sneider EB, McEnaney PM, Busconi BD: Athletic pubalgia (sports hernia). *Clin Sports Med* 2011;30(2):417-434.

This article provides an approach for the diagnosis and treatment of athletic pubalgia. It also instructs clinicians how to use the current information and understanding of groin pathology to accurately diagnose the cause of lower abdominal pain syndrome in the athlete. Level of evidence: V.

9. Nofsinger C, Kelly BT: Methodical approach to the history and physical exam of athletic groin pain. *Oper Tech Sports Med* 2007;15(4):152-156.

10. Mullens FE, Zoga AC, Morrison WB, Meyers WC: Review of MRI technique and imaging findings in athletic pubalgia and the "sports hernia". *Eur J Radiol* 2012;81(12):3780-3792.

This article presents a comprehensive, current review of common and uncommon MRI findings in patients with athletic pubalgia. It also explains an MRI protocol specifically devised for the diagnosis of athletic pubalgia. Level of evidence: V.

11. Zoga AC, Kavanagh EC, Omar IM, et al: Athletic pubalgia and the "sports hernia": MR imaging findings. *Radiology* 2008;247(3):797-807.

12. Larson CM: Sports hernia/athletic pubalgia: Evaluation and management. *Sports Health* 2014;6(2):139-144.

This article provides up-to-date information on the overlap of athletic pubalgia and FAI. It highlights that patients with combined intra-articular and extra-articular pathology have improved outcomes when both are addressed. Level of evidence: V.

13. Gilmore OJA: Gilmore's groin: Ten years experience of groin disruption–a previously unsolved problem in sportsmen. *Sports Med Soft Tissue Trauma* 1991;1(3):12-14.

14. Meyers WC, McKechnie A, Philippon MJ, Horner MA, Zoga AC, Devon ON: Experience with "sports hernia" spanning two decades. *Ann Surg* 2008;248(4):656-665.

15. Genitsaris M, Goulimaris I, Sikas N: Laparoscopic repair of groin pain in athletes. *Am J Sports Med* 2004;32(5):1238-1242.

16. Kluin J, den Hoed PT, van Linschoten R, IJzerman JC, van Steensel CJ: Endoscopic evaluation and treatment of groin pain in the athlete. *Am J Sports Med* 2004;32(4):944-949.

17. Ingoldby CJ: Laparoscopic and conventional repair of groin disruption in sportsmen. *Br J Surg* 1997;84(2):213-215.

18. Paajanen H, Brinck T, Hermunen H, Airo I: Laparoscopic surgery for chronic groin pain in athletes is more effective than nonoperative treatment: A randomized clinical trial with magnetic resonance imaging of 60 patients with sportsman's hernia (athletic pubalgia). *Surgery* 2011;150(1):99-107.

This prospective randomized trial compared nonsurgical treatment with surgical treatment of athletic pubalgia. Thirty patients were randomized into each group after nonsurgical treatment of at least 3 months duration failed. Of surgical patients, 90% returned to sports at 3 months, compared with 27% of the nonsurgical patients at 3 months. Level of evidence: II.

19. Larson CM, Pierce BR, Giveans MR: Treatment of athletes with symptomatic intra-articular hip pathology and athletic pubalgia/sports hernia: A case series. *Arthroscopy* 2011;27(6):768-775.

This case series presents 37 patients who had combined femoroacetabular impingement (FAI) and athletic pubalgia. Of patients who underwent hip arthroscopy for FAI and athletic pubalgia surgery, 89% were able to return to sport, compared with 25% who had isolated athletic pubalgia surgery and 50% who had isolated hip arthroscopy. Level of evidence: IV.

20. Birmingham PM, Kelly BT, Jacobs R, McGrady L, Wang M: The effect of dynamic femoroacetabular impingement on pubic symphysis motion: A cadaveric study. *Am J Sports Med* 2012;40(5):1113-1118.

This cadaveric study looked at pubic symphysis motion in specimens with FAI. Cam lesions led to increased motion at the pubic symphysis and were proposed to contribute to athletic pubalgia in patients with FAI. Controlled laboratory study.

21. Anderson K, Strickland SM, Warren R: Hip and groin injuries in athletes. *Am J Sports Med* 2001;29(4):521-533.

22. Larson CM, Birmingham PM, Oliver SM: Athletic pubalgia, in *Delee & Drez's Orthopaedic Sports Medicine: Principles and Practice, 4th Edition.* Philadelphia, PA, Elsevier, 2015, pp 966-974.

This book chapter is dedicated to the anatomy, diagnosis and treatment of athletic pubalgia. It discusses key imaging findings of athletic pubalgia. It also discusses nonsurgical and surgical treatment of athletic pubalgia.

23. Mann RA, Moran GT, Dougherty SE: Comparative electromyography of the lower extremity in jogging, running, and sprinting. *Am J Sports Med* 1986;14(6):501-510.

24. Tyler TF, Nicholas SJ, Campbell RJ, McHugh MP: The association of hip strength and flexibility with the incidence of adductor muscle strains in professional ice hockey players. *Am J Sports Med* 2001;29(2):124-128.

25. Strauss EJ, Campbell K, Bosco JA: Analysis of the cross-sectional area of the adductor longus tendon: A descriptive anatomic study. *Am J Sports Med* 2007;35(6):996-999.

26. Weir A, de Vos RJ, Moen M, Hölmich P, Tol JL: Prevalence of radiological signs of femoroacetabular impingement in patients presenting with long-standing adductor-related groin pain. *Br J Sports Med* 2011;45(1):6-9.

This case series looked at 34 patients with long-standing adductor-related groin pain. Pelvis/hip radiographs were taken of each patient. Of all patients, 94% had radiographic signs of FAI. Level of evidence: IV.

27. Schlegel TF, Bushnell BD, Godfrey J, Boublik M: Success of nonoperative management of adductor longus tendon ruptures in National Football League athletes. *Am J Sports Med* 2009;37(7):1394-1399.

This case series presents 19 National Football League (NFL) players with documented proximal adductor longus tendon ruptures. Nonsurgical treatment led to a faster return to play with fewer complications than did surgical repair. All players were able to return to play in the NFL. Level of evidence: IV.

28. Akermark C, Johansson C: Tenotomy of the adductor longus tendon in the treatment of chronic groin pain in athletes. *Am J Sports Med* 1992;20(6):640-643.

29. Rizio L III, Salvo JP, Schürhoff MR, Uribe JW: Adductor longus rupture in professional football players: Acute repair with suture anchors: A report of two cases. *Am J Sports Med* 2004;32(1):243-245.

30. Robertson IJ, Curran C, McCaffrey N, Shields CJ, McEntee GP: Adductor tenotomy in the management of groin pain in athletes. *Int J Sports Med* 2011;32(1):45-48.

In this case series, 109 male athletes underwent unilateral tenotomy for the treatment of chronic adductor pain. Of all patients, 91% reported improvement after tenotomy. The procedure was most successful for patients who presented with severe preoperative pain and disability. Level of evidence: IV.

31. Hiti CJ, Stevens KJ, Jamati MK, Garza D, Matheson GO: Athletic osteitis pubis. *Sports Med* 2011;41(5):361-376.

This article presents the current understanding of and various treatment options for osteitis pubis. The authors emphasize the need for future research to determine the optimal treatment of this pathology. Level of evidence: IV.

32. Gamble JG, Simmons SC, Freedman M: The symphysis pubis. Anatomic and pathologic considerations. *Clin Orthop Relat Res* 1986;203:261-272.

33. Verrall GM, Henry L, Fazzalari NL, Slavotinek JP, Oakeshott RD: Bone biopsy of the parasymphyseal pubic bone region in athletes with chronic groin injury demonstrates new woven bone formation consistent with a diagnosis of pubic bone stress injury. *Am J Sports Med* 2008;36(12):2425-2431.

34. Radic R, Annear P: Use of pubic symphysis curettage for treatment-resistant osteitis pubis in athletes. *Am J Sports Med* 2008;36(1):122-128.

35. Williams PR, Thomas DP, Downes EM: Osteitis pubis and instability of the pubic symphysis. When nonoperative measures fail. *Am J Sports Med* 2000;28(3):350-355.

36. Cunningham PM, Brennan D, O'Connell M, MacMahon P, O'Neill P, Eustace S: Patterns of bone and soft-tissue injury at the symphysis pubis in soccer players: Observations at MRI. *AJR Am J Roentgenol* 2007;188(3):W291-296.

37. Grace JN, Sim FH, Shives TC, Coventry MB: Wedge resection of the symphysis pubis for the treatment of osteitis pubis. *J Bone Joint Surg Am* 1989;71(3):358-364.

Section 3

Knee and Leg

SECTION EDITOR

David R. McAllister, MD

Chapter 15

Cruciate Ligament Injuries

Lucas S. McDonald, MD, MPH&TM   Nathan Coleman, MD   Andrew D. Pearle, MD

Abstract

Anterior cruciate ligament (ACL) injuries and their treatment continue to be intensively studied. Isolated injury to the posterior cruciate liagement (PCL) is rare. A low-grade injury can be successfully managed nonsurgically. The discussion includes the anatomy and function of the ACL and PCL, the evaluation of injuries, surgical techniques for ACL reconstruction and revision including tunnel placement and graft choice, surgical management of the PCL including surgical techniques, and the association of the PCL with multiligamentous knee injury.

Keywords: anterior cruciate ligament reconstruction; posterior cruciate ligament reconstruction; revision anterior cruciate ligament reconstruction

Introduction

Cruciate ligament injuries of the knee are common, and their incidence continues to increase. Current research focuses on anatomic evaluation, the biomechanics of injury, and reconstruction techniques. Outcome studies can guide treatment, but ideal graft locations and surgical techniques have not yet been identified.

Dr. Pearle or an immediate family member has received royalties from Biomet; serves as a paid consultant to Biomet and MakoSurgical; has stock or stock options held in Bluebelt Technologies; and serves as a board member, owner, officer, or committee member of Bluebelt Technologies. Neither of the following authors nor any immediate family member has received anything of value from or has stock or stock options held in a commercial company or institution related directly or indirectly to the subject of this chapter: Dr. McDonald and Dr. Coleman.

Anterior Cruciate Ligament Injury

The rate of anterior cruciate ligament (ACL) reconstructions in the United States increased from 32.9 to 43.5 per 100,000 person-years from 1994 to 2006 because of an increased number of reconstructions in patients who were women, were younger than 20 years, or were older than 40 years.[1] High rates of radiographic osteoarthritis have been reported after ACL reconstruction, with recent long-term outcomes data demonstrating a threefold increase in prevalence.[2] Predictors for the development of radiographic knee osteoarthritis after ACL reconstruction include a prior medial or lateral meniscectomy, medial meniscectomy at the time of reconstruction, elevated body mass index, and a relatively long time from injury to surgery.[2,3] Nonsurgical management of ACL-deficient knees in active patients does not lead to a satisfactory result, and a delay of more than 12 months before reconstruction is associated with meniscal and chondral injuries.[4] The cost-effectiveness of early ACL reconstruction is an additional argument for surgical treatment. The cost to society is $1,500 lower, and there is an increase in the patient's quality-adjusted life-years when surgical stabilization was performed within 1 year rather than 2 years after injury.[5]

Anatomy and Biomechanics

The anatomy of the ACL footprint and the ideal surgical graft position remain areas of active research. Macroscopically, the ACL consists of anteromedial and posterolateral functional bundles (Figure 1). The anteromedial bundle is tighter in knee flexion, but the posterolateral bundle is tighter in extension. Both bundles are under tension during loading with anterior translation or combined anterior translation and internal rotation, with the anteromedial bundle maintaining tension throughout knee flexion.

The native ACL inserts on the tibia just anterior to the posterior part of the anterior horn of the lateral meniscus. Tibial tunnel placement should include a portion of the anteromedial bundle footprint to provide optimal graft obliquity. Graft placement anterior to the footprint notch can cause impingement in extension or posteriorly can cause impingement on the posterior cruciate ligament (PCL).

3: Knee and Leg

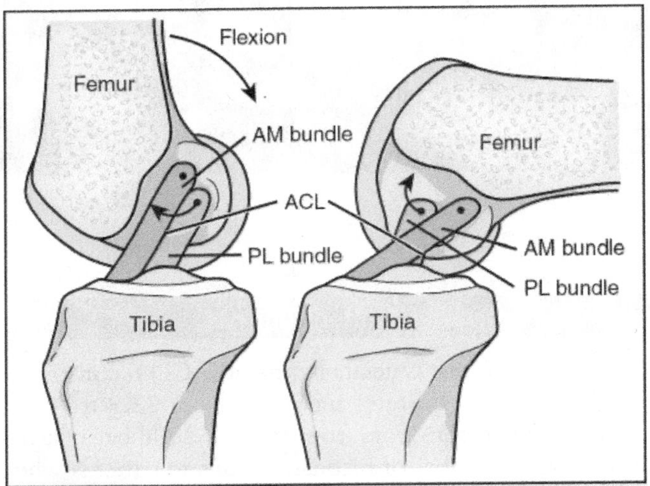

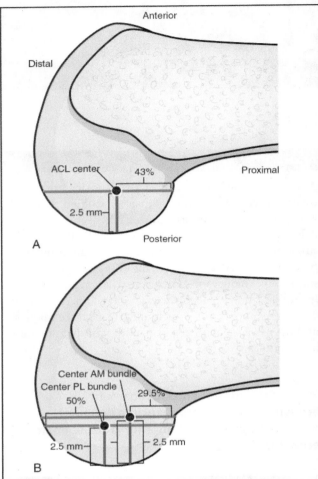

Figure 1 Schematic drawings showing the anteromedial (AM) and posterolateral (PL) macroscopic bundles of the anterior cruciate ligament (ACL). **A,** The posterolateral bundle (in blue) is tighter than the anteromedial bundle in extension, although it is less isometric than in flexion. **B,** The anteromedial bundle (in red) is tighter than the posterolateral bundle in flexion.

A systematic review based on all studies published since 2000 reported radiographic findings and arthroscopic landmarks related to ACL femoral anatomy.[6] The center of the ACL femoral footprint is 43% of the distance from the proximal to distal articular cartilage margin. The center of the anteromedial bundle is 29.5% of the proximal to distal distance of the lateral femoral intercondylar notch, and the center of the posterolateral bundle is 50% of the same distance. The posterior edge of the ACL is 2.5 mm from the posterior articular cartilage border[6] (Figure 2).

Histologic evaluation of ACL femoral footprint anatomy is defined by direct and indirect insertion fibers. Direct insertion fibers are more critical than indirect insertion fibers in the process of linking ligaments to bone, and the placement of reconstruction tunnels may produce a more anatomic ACL reconstruction. A correlation of histologic and macroscopic findings of ACL femoral insertion anatomy found that the ACL inserts more anteriorly on a macroscopic than on a histologic level.[7] The direct insertion is in a narrow area extending from the intercondylar ridge to a second osseous ridge 4 mm posterior. The direct fibers do not continue to the posterior articular cartilage. Posterior fibers that extend to the articular cartilage are indirect fibers with a fanlike attachment[7] (Figure 3). Further research is necessary to determine the best location for graft placement based on macroscopically visible bundles or histologic principles.

Figure 2 Schematic drawings representing the anterior cruciate ligament (ACL) femoral footprint. The posterior edge of the ACL is 2.5 mm from the posterior articular cartilage (purple lines). **A,** The center of the ACL femoral footprint (black dot along the red line), is 43% of the distance from the proximal to the distal articular cartilage margin. **B,** The center of the anteromedial (AM) bundle (black dot along the blue line) is 29.5% of the distance from the proximal to the distal articular margin. The center of the posterolateral (PL) bundle (black dot along the red line) is 50% of the distance from the proximal to the distal articular margin.

Diagnosis

The diagnosis of an ACL rupture is made from patient history, physical examination findings, and imaging studies. The Lachman test remains the most clinically sensitive in-office examination for diagnosing an acute, complete ACL rupture. The sensitivity of the in-office pivot shift test is not as high. During an examination under anesthesia, the Lachman test remains more sensitive but the sensitivity of the pivot shift test improves, and it is the most specific physical examination finding for ACL tears.[8]

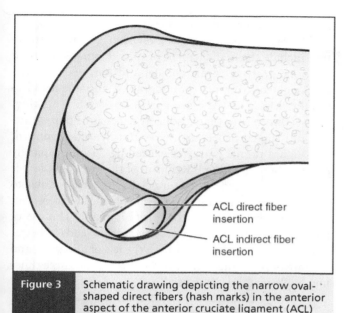

Figure 3 Schematic drawing depicting the narrow oval-shaped direct fibers (hash marks) in the anterior aspect of the anterior cruciate ligament (ACL) insertion and the fan-shaped indirect fibers (dots) in the posterior aspect.

MRI can be useful for the diagnosis of ACL disruption or associated meniscal, osteochondral, or collateral ligament injury.

A delay in ACL reconstruction is correlated with an increased likelihood of meniscal injury or chondral damage.[9] Medial collateral ligament (MCL) injuries are commonly associated with ACL disruptions. Grade I and II (MCL) injuries are treated nonsurgically, but distal grade III injuries may be best treated with surgical repair or reconstruction. Missed or untreated fibular collateral ligament or posterolateral corner knee injuries, which increase the stress on the ACL graft, are common reasons ACL reconstruction is unsuccessful.[10]

Surgical Treatment

Outcomes

Only 65% of patients return to their preinjury level of sports after ACL reconstruction, and only 55% return to a competitive level.[11] Factors having a positive association with return to a preinjury level of participation include relatively young age, symmetric hopping ability, male sex, and sports participation at an elite level.[11] The desire to return to sports soon after ACL reconstruction is not always realistic. A 33% rate of successful return to competitive sports was reported 12 months after ACL reconstruction with hamstring autograft.[12]

Although women are at a greater risk than men for primary ACL disruption, a recent systematic review found no greater risk among women than men for graft failure, contralateral ACL rupture, or postoperative knee laxity

as determined on physical examination or by patient-reported outcomes.[13]

Cigarette smoking negatively affects the outcome of ACL reconstruction. Patients who smoked had an increased risk of postoperative anterior translation and knee instability after ACL reconstruction with bone–patellar tendon–bone (BPTB) autograft.[14] Patients who stopped smoking at least 1 month before ACL reconstruction had no difference in outcome from patients who had never smoked. Surgeons should consider delaying reconstruction until patients have stopped smoking tobacco.

Tunnel Placement

Multiple techniques exist for drilling ACL tunnels. With the traditional transtibial endoscopic single-bundle technique from the early 1990s, in some knees the tibial bone tunnel was placed in the posterior portion of the native ACL footprint at the posterolateral bundle insertion. This placement can result in a malpositioned femoral tunnel, with vertical graft placement and femoral insertion superior to and outside of the native footprint. A cadaver comparison of transtibial and independent femoral drilling techniques found that a smaller portion of the tunnel aperture was contained within the anatomic tibial footprint during transtibial drilling.[15]

Evaluations of femoral tunnel placement with transtibial and anteromedial drilling techniques found that anteromedial techniques created a more anatomic femoral tunnel position and improved postreconstruction stability on the anterior drawer, Lachman, and pivot shift tests.[16,17] A systematic review found mixed results; in some cadaver and clinical studies rotational stability was superior when the anteromedial technique was used, but in other studies there was no difference based on the use of a transtibial or anteromedial technique.[18] One registry-based study demonstrated slightly higher failure rates 4 years following ACL reconstruction with transtibial techniques than with anteromedial techniques, hypothesizing a greater force placed on this anatomically placed graft.[19] Although debate exists as to the ideal method for creation of the femoral tunnel, the goal is to be in the correct position.

The use of flexible guide pins and reamers can be advantageous because they permit transtibial drilling of femoral tunnels to the anatomic ACL femoral footprint.[20] Although anatomic tunnel placement is possible using anteromedial techniques with rigid instruments, the use of flexible instruments results in longer femoral tunnels that exit further from the posterior femoral cortex.[20]

Biomechanical evidence supports the importance of an anatomic ACL reconstruction. ACL reconstruction in the center-center position (anatomic) was compared with reconstruction in the posterolateral-to-anteromedial

3: Knee and Leg

(nonanatomic) position.[21] With an instrumented Lachman examination, the use of the center-center position reduced anterior tibial translation from 4.7 mm to 2.0 mm following ACL reconstruction.

Video 15.1: Arthroscopic Double-Bundle ACL Reconstruction Using Quadriceps Tendon Autograft. Sung-Jae Kim, MD; Sul-Gee Kim, MD; Sung-Hwan Kim, MD; Dae-Young Lee, MD; In-Kee Jo, MD; and Yong-Min Chun, MD (10 min)

Double-Bundle Reconstruction

A meta-analysis of randomized controlled studies comparing clinical outcomes of ACL reconstruction using single-bundle or double-bundle techniques found that double-bundle techniques may improve rotational stability without adding a substantial clinical benefit.[22] Any benefit of an anatomic double-bundle ACL reconstruction is limited to biomechanical findings rather than clinical outcomes, and it is not known which patients will benefit from this reconstruction technique.

Video 15.2: Revision Single Bundle ACL Reconstruction Using BPTB Autograft part 1. Bernard R. Bach, Jr, MD (21 minutes)

Video 15.3: Revision Single Bundle ACL Reconstruction Using BPTB Autograft part 2. Bernard R. Bach, Jr, MD (18 min)

Revision Surgery

Causes of failure following ACL reconstruction include recurrent instability, postoperative complications including infection, or loss of motion and comorbidity from concomitant pathology such as a meniscus deficiency. A graft rupture rate of 4.5% and a contralateral ACL injury rate of 7.5% were reported at 3-year follow-up.[23] There was an increased risk for injury to either knee in patients who were younger than 20 years or who had returned to sports requiring cutting and pivoting. A longer term study reported a 23% rate of graft rupture or contralateral ACL rupture at a minimum 15-year follow-up.[24] The 93% rate of expected graft survival at 5 years decreased to 89% at 15 years.

The reasons an ACL reconstruction was unsuccessful must be determined before a revision reconstruction is attempted. Early recurrent instability results from poor surgical technique, failure of graft incorporation, or premature return to high-demand activities. Late recurrent instability usually is the result of trauma, poor graft

placement, or failure to treat concomitant pathology.[10]

Technical challenges during revision ACL reconstruction include the management of tunnel expansion, need for bone grafting, graft choice, and hardware removal. Weight-bearing plain radiographs, alignment radiographs, MRI, and CT are useful in decision making. Tunnel dimensions that absolutely necessitate bone grafting and staged procedures have not been determined, although a tunnel diameter exceeding 16 mm typically requires bone grafting.[10] Removal of the initial implant is not always required during tunnel drilling; it is possible to avoid a metallic implant located outside the new footprint or to drill through a biocomposite implant. The use of autograft for revision ACL reconstruction leads to better outcome and activity scores than the use of allograft, and the rate of subsequent graft rupture is almost three times lower when autograft is used.[25]

Video 15.4: Pitfalls in ACL Reconstruction. Darren L. Johnson, MD (12 minutes)

Video 15.5: Anatomic ACL Reconstruction--All Comers. Mark D. Miller, MD; Joseph Hart, PhD, ATC; and Gregory Kurkis, Medical Student (20 min)

Video 15.6: Anatomical Rectangular Tunnel ACL Reconstruction Using BTB Graft. Konsei Shino, MD, PhD (17 min)

Video 15.7: ACL Reconstruction Using a Free-Tendon Quadriceps Autograft. John P. Fulkerson, MD (21 min)

Video 15.8: Technique for Harvesting Hamstring Tendons for ACL Reconstruction. Stephen M. Howell, MD (8 min)

Video 15.9: Tips for Harvesting BTB Autograft. K. Donald Shelbourne, MD (13 min)

Graft Selection

Several studies have compared hamstring to BPTB autografts and compared the use of autografts or allografts. The graft choice should be individual to the patient, with consideration of the research literature. At 15-year follow-up of ACL reconstruction, hamstring autografts had an overall survival rate of 83%, and BPTB autografts

© 2016 American Academy of Orthopaedic Surgeons

had a similar survival rate.[24,26] The size of the hamstring graft may play a role in the outcome; grafts smaller than 8 mm in diameter have a relatively high risk of failure.[27] Large Scandinavian and Danish studies found that the overall risk of revision after ACL surgery was less than 5% but was significantly higher after hamstring autograft reconstruction than after BPTB autograft reconstruction.[28,29] A comparison of outcomes after BPTB or hamstring autograft reconstruction in young athletes found no difference in return to preinjury activity levels at 2- to 10-year follow-up, although hamstring autografts were associated with more complete restoration of knee extension, less radiographic osteoarthritis, and better patient outcomes scores.[30] Hamstring autograft reconstruction is more likely to lead to deep surgical site infection than BPTB autograft or allograft reconstruction.[31]

Video 15.10: ACL Reconstruction Using Achilles Allograft and Interference Screws. Colin G. Looney, MD, and William I. Sterett, MD (7 min)

Video 15.11: Anatomic Single Bundle ACL Reconstruction without Roof and PCL Impingement - Tibialis Allograft. Stephen M. Howell, MD, and Oscar Andres, MD (20 min)

Randomized controlled studies comparing hamstring autograft and soft-tissue allograft reported no differences for any outcome measures, although one study found increased laxity with irradiated allograft than with autograft.[32] These results were in patients with an average age older than 30 years and may not be applicable in younger patients. In skeletally mature patients younger than 18 years, BPTB allografts failed 15 times more often than BPTB autografts; all failures occurred within the first year after ACL reconstruction.[33] BPTB autograft reconstruction led to less anterior knee pain and better overall International Knee Documentation Committee scores, pivot shift test results, and return to preinjury activity levels than BPTB allograft.[34] The rates of graft rupture and knee laxity were higher and overall patient satisfaction was lower with BPTB allograft, however. Systematic reviews comparing the outcomes of ACL reconstruction with autograft, nonirradiated allograft tissue, and nonirradiated, nonchemically treated allograft tissue found no difference on any outcome measure.[35,36] Finally, a comparison of Achilles tendon with anterior tibial tendon allograft found no differences in clinical or laxity testing after ACL reconstruction.[37]

Rehabilitation and Return to Sport

A wide variety of criteria are used to determine readiness for return to unrestricted sports activities after ACL reconstruction, and no consensus criteria exist. However, many surgeons require full motion and normal Lachman, pivot shift, anterior drawer, and proprioception tests without using specific clinical scores as return-to-play criteria.[38] Objective data on testing and return-to-play criteria are not yet available, although most researchers recommend at least 6 months of rehabilitation, an absence of knee effusion, full knee motion, symmetry greater than 90% with single-leg hop, and quadriceps strength of 85% compared with the contralateral side.[39]

Posterior Cruciate Ligament Injury

No recent studies have defined the incidence of isolated PCL injury, but it is less common than ACL injury. Emergency department studies report PCL injury in 37% to 44% of knees affected by trauma and in 1% to 3% of all injured knees.[40,41] PCL injury is often associated with other pathology, with concomitant ligament injury in up to 95% of high-energy PCL injuries. The most common causes of PCL injury are motor vehicle crashes involving a motorcycle or dashboard impact, followed by sports-related injuries such as falls onto a flexed knee with a plantar flexed foot.[42] Prospective data collected an average 8 years after injury indicated that 40% of patients had an excellent result with nonsurgical management of an isolated PCL-deficient knee.[43,44] Functional knee scores had not deteriorated at an average 14-year follow-up, but 11% of patients had moderate to severe radiographic osteoarthritis.

Anatomy and Biomechanics

The PCL is stronger than the ACL, has a broader femoral attachment, and because of its extrasynovial location, it has better healing potential. The primary function of the PCL is to resist posterior displacement of the tibia in all knee flexion angles. The PCL is also a secondary varus, valgus, and rotational stabilizer, and it facilitates internal rotation of the tibia at higher flexion angles.[45,46] The PCL has two functional components, the anterolateral and posteromedial bundles (Figure 4). The anterolateral bundle carries more load in flexion, and the posteromedial bundle carries more load in extension (Figure 5). The PCL is associated with the meniscofemoral ligaments of Humphrey (anterior) and Wrisberg (posterior).

The femoral insertion of the PCL extends more than 20 mm from anterior to posterior. The anterolateral bundle is more vertical than the posteromedial bundle and inserts on the anterior roof of the intercondylar notch. The

3. Knee and Leg

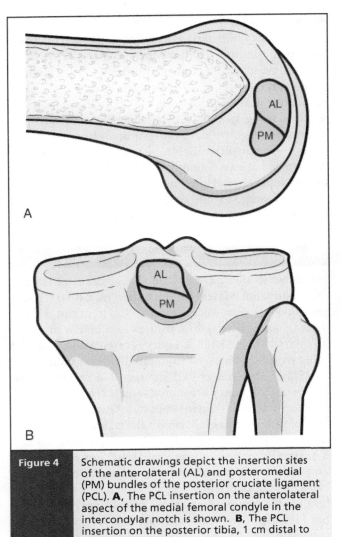

Figure 4 Schematic drawings depict the insertion sites of the anterolateral (AL) and posteromedial (PM) bundles of the posterior cruciate ligament (PCL). **A,** The PCL insertion on the anterolateral aspect of the medial femoral condyle in the intercondylar notch is shown. **B,** The PCL insertion on the posterior tibia, 1 cm distal to the joint line, is shown.

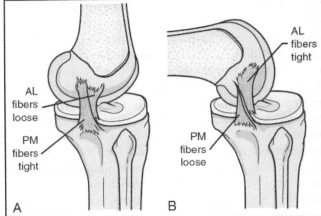

Figure 5 Schematic drawings depicting tensioning patterns of the anterolateral (AL) and posteromedial (PM) bundles of the posterior cruciate ligament through a range of motion. **A,** The PM bundle with a greater load than the AL bundle with knee extension is shown. **B,** The AL bundle with a greater load than the PM bundle with knee flexion is shown.

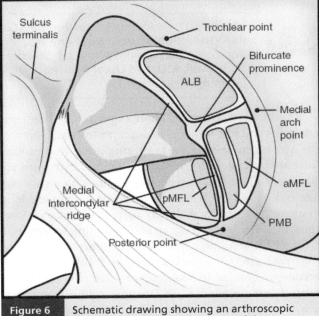

Figure 6 Schematic drawing showing an arthroscopic view of the femoral attachment of the posterior cruciate ligament (PCL) in a right knee. ALB = the anterolateral bundle, aMFL = the anterior meniscofemoral ligament, PMB = the posteromedial bundle, pMFL = the posterior meniscofemoral ligament. The PCL and meniscofemoral ligaments cover most of the intercondylar notch anterior to the medial intercondylar ridge.

posteromedial bundle is more oblique, inserting posteriorly on the lateral wall of the medial femoral condyle. The PCL and meniscofemoral ligaments cover almost all of the medial aspect of the intercondylar notch anterior to the medial intercondylar ridge. The anterior margin of the PCL is 2 mm from the articular cartilage, and the bundle centers are an average of 12 mm apart[47,48] (Figure 6).

The tibial insertion of the PCL is narrower than the femoral insertion and is in the posterior intercondylar fossa of the proximal tibia. The PCL footprint extends anteriorly and proximally from the medial meniscus root and the edge of the lateral plateau articular cartilage to a point 1 to 1.5 cm below the joint line and distal to the posterior osseous ridge of the tibial plateau.[47-49] The most posterior distal fibers consist of the thicker posteromedial bundle, and they blend with the periosteum and posterior

capsule to insert distal to the osseous ridge cradling the anterior proximal fibers of the anterolateral bundle. The centers of these bundles on average are 9 mm apart.[48]

Diagnosis

A PCL injury can be diagnosed from the patient history and physical examination. Examination maneuvers specific to the PCL include the posterior drawer and quadriceps active tests. The posterior sag sign indicates a PCL injury. The accuracy, sensitivity, and specificity of the clinical examination findings for PCL injury are greater than 90%.[50] Assessment of tibial station is useful for determining the severity of a PCL injury. In the intact state, the medial tibial plateau is approximately 1 cm anterior to the medial femoral condyle. In a grade I injury there is 0.5 cm of posterior tibial translation, a grade II injury is flush with the femoral condyles, and a grade III injury causes tibial translation posterior to the femoral condyles. Determining the amount of posterior translation is challenging, however, and a simplified grading system has been developed for PCL injuries.[51] With the knee in 90° of flexion, a posterior force is applied to the tibia. The result is no tibial offset in a normal knee, a slight loss of anterior tibial offset in a grade A injury, a tibia flush with the femoral condyles in a grade B injury, and tibial displacement posterior to the femoral condyles in a grade C injury. Grades A, B, and C injuries correlate with grades I, II and III injuries when considering treatment options and outcomes.

A complete series of plain radiographs should be obtained if knee ligament injury is suspected. Radiographs can reveal PCL tibial avulsion injury, capsular avulsion, or associated fracture as well as resting position and any posterior subluxation of the tibia. Stress radiographs also can be used to assess PCL disruption.[52,53] MRI is used to determine the location and severity of PCL disruption and shows concomitant meniscal, osteochondral, chondral, and ligament injuries. If grade III posterior tibial laxity is present and radiographs show more than 10 mm of posterior subluxation, a combined PCL and posterolateral corner injury should be suspected.[54,55]

Treatment and Outcomes

Nonsurgical treatment is recommended for a patient with an isolated grade I or II injury. The program includes extension bracing, protected weight bearing, and quadriceps strengthening rehabilitation. Return to sport can be considered as early as 2 to 4 weeks after injury. Two natural history studies of nonsurgically treated isolated grade I or II PCL injuries found good subjective and objective outcomes with no functional deterioration and 97% quadriceps and 93% hamstring strength.[43,44] A 7-year follow-up study reported that based on Tegner Activity Level Scale and Lysholm-II Knee Questionnaire scores, 92% of patients with grade I or II injuries had a good to excellent result after nonsurgical management.[56]

The treatment of isolated grade III PCL injuries is controversial. Some experts recommend acute reconstruction of grade III injuries in young athletes or if normal tibial station cannot be maintained in the presence of a so-called peel-off lesion. Surgical treatment is recommended for a chronic grade III lesion if the patient is symptomatic.[49,51,54] There is no consensus on graft choice or technique for repair or reconstruction of the PCL.[57]

Avulsion of the PCL usually occurs at the femoral attachment and can be repaired using suture anchors or femoral bone tunnels. Large osseous avulsion fragments from the tibial attachment can be repaired with open reduction and screw-and-washer fixation.

Various surgical techniques permit reconstruction of the PCL. The tibial inlay technique is usually performed through an open posterior approach. The bone block is recessed and fixed with an interference screw at the posterior tibia, ensuring to avoid graft protrusion. The advantages of the tibial inlay technique include osseous graft healing, avoidance of so-called killer turn stresses, decreased graft wear, and improved graft biomechanics. An arthroscopic inlay technique using suture button fixation over the tibial-side bone block has been described as combining the advantages of arthroscopic and inlay techniques.[58,59] In the transtibial technique, the tibial tunnel is reamed from anterior to posterior through the tibia under direct arthroscopic and fluoroscopic visualization. The tibial footprint is approximately 7 mm anterior to the posterior tibial cortex as seen on a perfect lateral image.[55] Cadaver biomechanical data revealed no difference between transtibial and tibial inlay techniques when grafts were appropriately pretensioned before insertion.[60] Multiple studies report no difference in functional, radiographic, or clinical outcomes between transtibial and tibial inlay techniques or between arthroscopic and open techniques.[49,59,61-64]

Biomechanical comparison studies of double-bundle and single-bundle PCL reconstruction techniques concluded that double-bundle reconstruction is preferable for decreasing posterior tibial translation and improving rotational restraint.[65-67] Biomechanical advantages were not correlated with superior clinical outcomes, however, and isolated single-bundle reconstruction yields good long-term results without functional differences in comparison with double-bundle reconstruction.[68,69]

Summary

Although ACL injury is among the most commonly studied orthopaedic injuries, many questions remain unanswered. Irrespective of technique, the goals of ACL reconstruction include an anatomic tunnel position for

3: Knee and Leg

optimal biomechanical and clinical outcomes. Return-to-play profiles are similar after ACL reconstruction with hamstring or BPTB autograft, although lower rates of revision surgery and lower infection rates were observed with the use of BPTB autograft. Allograft use is an option but requires caution in young athletes. Further study of long-term outcomes is needed to determine the optimal patient age ranges and activity levels for each graft choice. Most PCL injuries can be managed nonsurgically, although surgical reconstruction is preferable for some higher grade injuries. Differences exist between the biomechanical advantages and patient outcomes of specific surgical techniques.

Key Study Points

- ACL anatomy has both macroscopic and microscopic definitions, and the choice of the best location for reconstruction after injury should consider the native anatomy.

- The specifics of ACL reconstruction, including the method of tunnel drilling and the graft choice, remain debatable. It is important that the tunnels be placed correctly. The use of autograft may be preferable to allograft in young athletes.

- Most isolated PCL injuries can be nonsurgically managed, though some higher grade injuries benefit from surgical reconstruction. Optimal graft choice and methods of tibial graft attachment remain debatable.

Annotated References

1. Mall NA, Chalmers PN, Moric M, et al: Incidence and trends of anterior cruciate ligament reconstruction in the United States. *Am J Sports Med* 2014;42(10):2363-2370.

   An epidemiologic study described an increase in the number of ACL reconstructions in the United States between 1994 and 2006, particularly in women and in patients younger than 20 years or older than 40 years.

2. Barenius B, Ponzer S, Shalabi A, Bujak R, Norlén L, Eriksson K: Increased risk of osteoarthritis after anterior cruciate ligament reconstruction: A 14-year follow-up study of a randomized controlled trial. *Am J Sports Med* 2014;42(5):1049-1057.

   A threefold increased incidence of osteoarthritis was found after ACL reconstruction compared with the contralateral knee. Level of evidence: I.

3. Li RT, Lorenz S, Xu Y, Harner CD, Fu FH, Irrgang JJ: Predictors of radiographic knee osteoarthritis after anterior cruciate ligament reconstruction. *Am J Sports Med* 2011;39(12):2595-2603.

   Despite decreased instability and improved activity levels, patients undergoing ACL reconstruction were at increased risk for knee osteoarthritis. Level of evidence: III.

4. Fok AW, Yau WP: Delay in ACL reconstruction is associated with more severe and painful meniscal and chondral injuries. *Knee Surg Sports Traumatol Arthrosc* 2013;21(4):928-933.

   Delay before ACL reconstruction was associated with an increased incidence of articular cartilage and meniscus pathology. Level of evidence: III.

5. Mather RC III, Hettrich CM, Dunn WR, et al: Cost-effectiveness analysis of early reconstruction versus rehabilitation and delayed reconstruction for anterior cruciate ligament tears. *Am J Sports Med* 2014;42(7):1583-1591.

   An economic and decision analysis study found that early ACL reconstruction improved quality-adjusted life-years at a lower cost than delayed ACL reconstruction after rehabilitation and from a health system perspective was the preferred treatment. Level of evidence: II.

6. Piefer JW, Pflugner TR, Hwang MD, Lubowitz JH: Anterior cruciate ligament femoral footprint anatomy: Systematic review of the 21st century literature. *Arthroscopy* 2012;28(6):872-881.

   A systematic review of basic science studies concluded that the center of the ACL footprint is 43% of the proximal-to-distal length of the femoral intercondylar notch wall and the radius of the femoral socket is 2.5 mm anterior to the posterior articular margin.

7. Sasaki N, Ishibashi Y, Tsuda E, et al: The femoral insertion of the anterior cruciate ligament: Discrepancy between macroscopic and histological observations. *Arthroscopy* 2012;28(8):1135-1146.

   A basic science study defined the direct and indirect femoral insertions of the ACL as they correspond to macroscopic appearance.

8. van Eck CF, van den Bekerom MP, Fu FH, Poolman RW, Kerkhoffs GM: Methods to diagnose acute anterior cruciate ligament rupture: A meta-analysis of physical examinations with and without anaesthesia. *Knee Surg Sports Traumatol Arthrosc* 2013;21(8):1895-1903.

   A meta-analysis of diagnostic test accuracy concluded that the Lachman test is most sensitive for diagnosing acute ACL disruption in an office setting. With the patient under anesthesia, the Lachman test remained the most sensitive, but the pivot-shift test was most specific. Level of evidence: II.

9. Sri-Ram K, Salmon LJ, Pinczewski LA, Roe JP: The incidence of secondary pathology after anterior cruciate ligament rupture in 5086 patients requiring ligament reconstruction. *Bone Joint J* 2013;95-B(1):59-64.

A retrospective review to determine the incidence of secondary pathology with respect to time between injury and reconstruction found an increased incidence of medial meniscal tears and chondral damage. Level of evidence: III.

10. Kamath GV, Redfern JC, Greis PE, Burks RT: Revision anterior cruciate ligament reconstruction. *Am J Sports Med* 2011;39(1):199-217.

A clinical update on revision ACL reconstruction reviewed diagnostic and surgical challenges as well as causes of failure to provide decision-making guidance.

11. Ardern CL, Taylor NF, Feller JA, Webster KE: Fifty-five per cent return to competitive sport following anterior cruciate ligament reconstruction surgery: An updated systematic review and meta-analysis including aspects of physical functioning and contextual factors. *Br J Sports Med* 2014;48(21):1543-1552.

A systematic review reported varied return-to-sports rates after ACL reconstruction; 81% of patients returned to some sport, but only 55% returned to a competitive-level sport.

12. Ardern CL, Webster KE, Taylor NF, Feller JA: Return to the preinjury level of competitive sport after anterior cruciate ligament reconstruction surgery: Two-thirds of patients have not returned by 12 months after surgery. *Am J Sports Med* 2011;39(3):538-543.

A case study found that patients may require longer than the typically reported 12-month return to sports after ACL reconstruction. Level of evidence: IV.

13. Ryan J, Magnussen RA, Cox CL, Hurbanek JG, Flanigan DC, Kaeding CC: ACL reconstruction: Do outcomes differ by sex? A systematic review. *J Bone Joint Surg Am* 2014;96(6):507-512.

A systematic review and meta-analysis found no difference in graft failure risk, contralateral ACL rupture risk, or postoperative knee laxity based on the sex of the patient. Level of evidence: II.

14. Kim S-J, Lee S-K, Kim S-H, Kim S-H, Ryu S-W, Jung M: Effect of cigarette smoking on the clinical outcomes of ACL reconstruction. *J Bone Joint Surg Am* 2014;96(12):1007-1013.

A prognostic study found that cigarette smoking had a negative effect on the outcome of ACL reconstruction. Level of evidence: III.

15. Keller TC, Tompkins M, Economopoulos K, et al: Tibial tunnel placement accuracy during anterior cruciate ligament reconstruction: Independent femoral versus transtibial femoral tunnel drilling techniques. *Arthroscopy* 2014;30(9):1116-1123.

A cadaver study suggested that transtibial drilling had deleterious effects on tibial tunnel position and aperture. Independent femoral drilling was associated with a higher percentage of placements of the tibial tunnel in an anatomic position.

16. Bedi A, Musahl V, Steuber V, et al: Transtibial versus anteromedial portal reaming in anterior cruciate ligament reconstruction: An anatomic and biomechanical evaluation of surgical technique. *Arthroscopy* 2011;27(3):380-390.

A cadaver study found that, compared with transtibial techniques, anteromedial portal drilling allowed placement of the femoral socket central in the native footprint, thus improving time-zero tibial translation and pivot shift testing.

17. Tompkins M, Milewski MD, Brockmeier SF, Gaskin CM, Hart JM, Miller MD: Anatomic femoral tunnel drilling in anterior cruciate ligament reconstruction: Use of an accessory medial portal versus traditional transtibial drilling. *Am J Sports Med* 2012;40(6):1313-1321.

A cadaver study found that anteromedial drilling placed the femoral tunnel in the native femoral footprint more often than transtibial drilling.

18. Chalmers PN, Mall NA, Cole BJ, Verma NN, Bush-Joseph CA, Bach BR Jr: Anteromedial versus transtibial tunnel drilling in anterior cruciate ligament reconstructions: A systematic review. *Arthroscopy* 2013;29(7):1235-1242.

A systematic review with a review of cadaver studies compared anteromedial and transtibial drilling techniques for ACL reconstruction. Some studies found superiority of anteromedial techniques, and others found no differences. Level of evidence: III.

19. Rahr-Wagner L, Thillemann TM, Pedersen AB, Lind MC: Increased risk of revision after anteromedial compared with transtibial drilling of the femoral tunnel during primary anterior cruciate ligament reconstruction: Results from the Danish Knee Ligament Reconstruction Register. *Arthroscopy* 2013;29(1):98-105.

A registry-based study comparing revision rates following ACL reconstruction with femoral tunnels drilled through transtibial and anteromedial approaches that demonstrated higher revision rates with the anteromedial approach.

20. Steiner ME, Smart LR: Flexible instruments outperform rigid instruments to place anatomic anterior cruciate ligament femoral tunnels without hyperflexion. *Arthroscopy* 2012;28(6):835-843.

A cadaver study found that the ability to obtain an anatomic femoral tunnel with transtibial drilling was improved by the use of flexible instruments and longer tunnel length when compared with use of the same instruments in an anteromedial drilling technique.

21. Bedi A, Maak T, Musahl V, et al: Effect of tunnel position and graft size in single-bundle anterior cruciate ligament reconstruction: An evaluation of time-zero knee stability. *Arthroscopy* 2011;27(11):1543-1551.

A cadaver study found that increased graft size does not compensate for nonanatomic tunnel position or improve time-zero stability of the knee after ACL reconstruction.

3: Knee and Leg

22. Li Y-L, Ning G-Z, Wu Q, et al: Single-bundle or double-bundle for anterior cruciate ligament reconstruction: A meta-analysis. *Knee* 2014;21(1):28-37.

A meta-analysis comparing single- and double-bundle ACL reconstruction techniques found better outcomes for rotational laxity with double-bundle techniques, but there were no functional between-group differences. Level of evidence: II.

23. Webster KE, Feller JA, Leigh WB, Richmond AK: Younger patients are at increased risk for graft rupture and contralateral injury after anterior cruciate ligament reconstruction. *Am J Sports Med* 2014;42(3):641-647.

A case-control study determined that patients younger than 20 years are at higher risk for graft rupture and contralateral ACL injury than older patients after ACL reconstruction. Level of evidence: III.

24. Bourke HE, Salmon LJ, Waller A, Patterson V, Pinczewski LA: Survival of the anterior cruciate ligament graft and the contralateral ACL at a minimum of 15 years. *Am J Sports Med* 2012;40(9):1985-1992.

A case study reported an 89% survival rate of ACL grafts 15 years after surgery. The expected survival rate for the contralateral ACL was 87%. Level of evidence: IV.

25. MARS Group: Effect of graft choice on the outcome of revision anterior cruciate ligament reconstruction in the Multicenter ACL Revision Study (MARS) Cohort. *Am J Sports Med* 2014;42(10):2301-2310.

A cohort study reported improved sports function and patient-reported outcomes with decreased graft rerupture rates when autograft rather than allograft was used for revision ACL reconstruction. Level of evidence: II.

26. Bourke HE, Gordon DJ, Salmon LJ, Waller A, Linklater J, Pinczewski LA: The outcome at 15 years of endoscopic anterior cruciate ligament reconstruction using hamstring tendon autograft for 'isolated' anterior cruciate ligament rupture. *J Bone Joint Surg Br* 2012;94(5):630-637.

At 15-year follow-up after ACL reconstruction using hamstring tendon autograft, graft survival was 83%, and 7% of patients had osteoarthritic changes. Level of evidence: IV.

27. Conte EJ, Hyatt AE, Gatt CJ Jr, Dhawan A: Hamstring autograft size can be predicted and is a potential risk factor for anterior cruciate ligament reconstruction failure. *Arthroscopy* 2014;30(7):882-890.

A systematic review found decreased failure rates in quadrupled hamstring autograft with a diameter of more than 8 mm. Level of evidence: IV.

28. Gifstad T, Foss OA, Engebretsen L, et al: Lower risk of revision with patellar tendon autografts compared with hamstring autografts: A registry study based on 45,998 primary ACL reconstructions in Scandinavia. *Am J Sports Med* 2014;42(10):2319-2328.

In a cohort study of Scandinavian patients, ACL reconstruction with patellar tendon autograft led to a lower rate of revision than ACL reconstruction with hamstring autograft. Level of evidence: II.

29. Rahr-Wagner L, Thillemann TM, Pedersen AB, Lind M: Comparison of hamstring tendon and patellar tendon grafts in anterior cruciate ligament reconstruction in a nationwide population-based cohort study: Results from the Danish registry of knee ligament reconstruction. *Am J Sports Med* 2014;42(2):278-284.

A population-based cohort study reported an increased percentage of ACL reconstruction using hamstring autograft and overall good outcomes with both patellar tendon and hamstring autograft. There was an increased relative risk of revision ACL reconstruction surgery with hamstring autograft. Level of evidence: II.

30. Mascarenhas R, Tranovich MJ, Kropf EJ, Fu FH, Harner CD: Bone-patellar tendon-bone autograft versus hamstring autograft anterior cruciate ligament reconstruction in the young athlete: A retrospective matched analysis with 2-10 year follow-up. *Knee Surg Sports Traumatol Arthrosc* 2012;20(8):1520-1527.

A case-controlled therapeutic study comparing hamstring and BPTB autograft ACL reconstruction techniques found that 70% of patients returned to sports. Only 50% returned to their preinjury activity level. Hamstring graft reconstruction yielded better motion and outcomes scores, and it led to less radiographic osteoarthritis than BPTB graft reconstruction. Level of evidence: III.

31. Maletis GB, Inacio MC, Reynolds S, Desmond JL, Maletis MM, Funahashi TT: Incidence of postoperative anterior cruciate ligament reconstruction infections: Graft choice makes a difference. *Am J Sports Med* 2013;41(8):1780-1785.

A cohort study reported a 0.48% rate of surgical site infection after ACL reconstruction. The risk was 8.2 times higher after hamstring tendon autograft than after BPTB autograft reconstruction. Level of evidence: II.

32. Cvetanovich GL, Mascarenhas R, Saccomanno MF, et al: Hamstring autograft versus soft-tissue allograft in anterior cruciate ligament reconstruction: A systematic review and meta-analysis of randomized controlled trials. *Arthroscopy* 2014;30(12):1616-1624.

A systematic review and meta-analysis reported no significant difference between ACL reconstruction with hamstring autograft or soft-tissue allograft in patients with an average age older than 30 years. Level of evidence: II.

33. Ellis HB, Matheny LM, Briggs KK, Pennock AT, Steadman JR: Outcomes and revision rate after bone-patellar tendon-bone allograft versus autograft anterior cruciate ligament reconstruction in patients aged 18 years or younger with closed physes. *Arthroscopy* 2012;28(12):1819-1825.

A retrospective comparative study found no differences in function, activity, or satisfaction between BPTB allograft and autograft for ACL reconstruction in young patients, although allograft reconstruction had a 15 times higher failure rate than autograft reconstruction. Level of evidence: III.

34. Kraeutler MJ, Bravman JT, McCarty EC: Bone-patellar tendon-bone autograft versus allograft in outcomes of anterior cruciate ligament reconstruction: A meta-analysis of 5182 patients. *Am J Sports Med* 2013;41(10):2439-2448.

   A meta-analysis concluded that patients who underwent ACL reconstruction with BPTB autografts had lower rates of graft rupture or knee laxity and better satisfaction than those who underwent ACL reconstruction with BPTB allograft.

35. Mariscalco MW, Magnussen RA, Mehta D, Hewett TE, Flanigan DC, Kaeding CC: Autograft versus non-irradiated allograft tissue for anterior cruciate ligament reconstruction: A systematic review. *Am J Sports Med* 2014;42(2):492-499.

   A systematic review compared autografts with nonirradiated allografts for ACL reconstruction in patients in their late 20s to early 30s. No differences were reported in graft failure rate, postoperative knee laxity, or outcome scores. Level of evidence: III.

36. Lamblin CJ, Waterman BR, Lubowitz JH: Anterior cruciate ligament reconstruction with autografts compared with non-irradiated, non-chemically treated allografts. *Arthroscopy* 2013;29(6):1113-1122.

   A systematic review compared outcomes after autograft or non–chemically treated, nonirradiated allograft tissue was used for ACL reconstruction. No statistically significant differences were found. Level of evidence: III.

37. Kim S-J, Bae J-H, Lim H-C: Comparison of Achilles and tibialis anterior tendon allografts after anterior cruciate ligament reconstruction. *Knee Surg Sports Traumatol Arthrosc* 2014;22(1):135-141.

   An outcome study found no significant differences between outcomes of ACL reconstruction using Achilles tendon or anterior tibial allograft. Level of evidence: III.

38. Petersen W, Zantop T: Return to play following ACL reconstruction: Survey among experienced arthroscopic surgeons (AGA instructors). *Arch Orthop Trauma Surg* 2013;133(7):969-977.

   Surgeons were surveyed on the outcome measures they used to determine readiness for return to play after ACL reconstruction. Most surgeons relied primarily on physical examination and motion while considering other factors to a lesser degree.

39. Mueller LM, Bloomer BA, Durall CJ: Which outcome measures should be utilized to determine readiness to play after ACL reconstruction? *J Sport Rehabil* 2014;23(2):158-164.

   Outcome measures to determine readiness for return to play after ACL reconstruction were discussed.

40. Fanelli GC: Posterior cruciate ligament injuries in trauma patients. *Arthroscopy* 1993;9(3):291-294.

41. Fanelli GC, Edson CJ: Posterior cruciate ligament injuries in trauma patients: Part II. *Arthroscopy* 1995;11(5):526-529.

42. Schulz MS, Russe K, Weiler A, Eichhorn HJ, Strobel MJ: Epidemiology of posterior cruciate ligament injuries. *Arch Orthop Trauma Surg* 2003;123(4):186-191.

43. Shelbourne KD, Muthukaruppan Y: Subjective results of nonoperatively treated, acute, isolated posterior cruciate ligament injuries. *Arthroscopy* 2005;21(4):457-461.

44. Shelbourne KD, Clark M, Gray T: Minimum 10-year follow-up of patients after an acute, isolated posterior cruciate ligament injury treated nonoperatively. *Am J Sports Med* 2013;41(7):1526-1533.

   Sixty-eight patients treated nonsurgically for isolated PCL injury were followed prospectively with subjective and objective outcome measures. At an average 14-year follow-up, 44 patients had good strength, remained active, and had full knee motion. The rate of osteoarthritis was 11%. Level of evidence: IV.

45. Li G, Papannagari R, Li M, et al: Effect of posterior cruciate ligament deficiency on in vivo translation and rotation of the knee during weightbearing flexion. *Am J Sports Med* 2008;36(3):474-479.

46. Kennedy NI, Wijdicks CA, Goldsmith MT, et al: Kinematic analysis of the posterior cruciate ligament: Part 1. The individual and collective function of the anterolateral and posteromedial bundles. *Am J Sports Med* 2013;41(12):2828-2838.

   A controlled cadaver biomechanics laboratory study evaluated knees at different flexion angles in the intact, PCL-deficient, and PCL-reconstructed state after a single-bundle graft fixed in the anterolateral position. A single-bundle graft was found to reduce knee laxity at all angles but not to the intact state.

47. Amis AA, Gupte CM, Bull AM, Edwards A: Anatomy of the posterior cruciate ligament and the meniscofemoral ligaments. *Knee Surg Sports Traumatol Arthrosc* 2006;14(3):257-263.

48. Anderson CJ, Ziegler CG, Wijdicks CA, Engebretsen L, LaPrade RF: Arthroscopically pertinent anatomy of the anterolateral and posteromedial bundles of the posterior cruciate ligament. *J Bone Joint Surg Am* 2012;94(21):1936-1945.

   A cadaver dissection study described the anatomy of the PCL in relation to relevant anatomic landmarks.

49. MacGillivray JD, Stein BE, Park M, Allen AA, Wickiewicz TL, Warren RF: Comparison of tibial inlay versus transtibial techniques for isolated posterior cruciate ligament reconstruction: Minimum 2-year follow-up. *Arthroscopy* 2006;22(3):320-328.

50. Rubinstein RA Jr, Shelbourne KD, McCarroll JR, VanMeter CD, Rettig AC: The accuracy of the clinical

J: Knee and Leg

examination in the setting of posterior cruciate ligament injuries. *Am J Sports Med* 1994;22(4):550-557.

51. Marx RG, Shindle MK, Warren RF: Management of posterior cruciate ligament injuries. *Oper Tech Sports Med* 2009;17:162-166.

    Institutional preferences for treatment of PCL injury to include patient selection, surgical timing, preferred surgical technique, graft selection, rehabilitation and return to sport were reviewed. Additionally, previously published literature on outcomes was reviewed.

52. Jackman T, LaPrade RF, Pontinen T, Lender PA: Intraobserver and interobserver reliability of the kneeling technique of stress radiography for the evaluation of posterior knee laxity. *Am J Sports Med* 2008;36(8):1571-1576.

53. Schulz MS, Steenlage ES, Russe K, Strobel MJ: Distribution of posterior tibial displacement in knees with posterior cruciate ligament tears. *J Bone Joint Surg Am* 2007;89(2):332-338.

54. Harner CD, Höher J: Evaluation and treatment of posterior cruciate ligament injuries. *Am J Sports Med* 1998;26(3):471-482.

55. Voos JE, Mauro CS, Wente T, Warren RF, Wickiewicz TL: Posterior cruciate ligament: Anatomy, biomechanics, and outcomes. *Am J Sports Med* 2012;40(1):222-231.

    The literature on the anatomy and biomechanics of the PCL as well as its diagnosis and treatment was reviewed.

56. Patel DV, Allen AA, Warren RF, Wickiewicz TL, Simonian PT: The nonoperative treatment of acute, isolated (partial or complete) posterior cruciate ligament-deficient knees: An intermediate-term follow-up study. *HSS J* 2007;3(2):137-146.

57. Hammoud S, Reinhardt KR, Marx RG: Outcomes of posterior cruciate ligament treatment: A review of the evidence. *Sports Med Arthrosc* 2010;18(4):280-291.

    A systematic review of databases evaluating treatment outcomes of isolated PCL injury and multiligament injury knee injury found no consensus on treatment of isolated PCL injury or reconstruction technique. The results of nonsurgical and surgical treatment generally are good.

58. Jordan SS, Campbell RB, Sekiya JK: Posterior cruciate ligament reconstruction using a new arthroscopic tibial inlay double-bundle technique. *Sports Med Arthrosc* 2007;15(4):176-183.

59. Campbell RB, Jordan SS, Sekiya JK: Arthroscopic tibial inlay for posterior cruciate ligament reconstruction. *Arthroscopy* 2007;23(12):1356.e1-1356.e4.

60. McAllister DR, Markolf KL, Oakes DA, Young CR, McWilliams J: A biomechanical comparison of tibial inlay and tibial tunnel posterior cruciate ligament reconstruction techniques: Graft pretension and knee laxity. *Am J Sports Med* 2002;30(3):312-317.

61. Zehms CT, Whiddon DR, Miller MD, et al: Comparison of a double bundle arthroscopic inlay and open inlay posterior cruciate ligament reconstruction using clinically relevant tools: A cadaveric study. *Arthroscopy* 2008;24(4):472-480.

62. Song E-K, Park H-W, Ahn Y-S, Seon J-K: Transtibial versus tibial inlay techniques for posterior cruciate ligament reconstruction: Long-term follow-up study. *Am J Sports Med* 2014;42(12):2964-2971.

    A cohort study found that the outcomes of the transtibial and tibial inlay techniques for PCL reconstruction were comparable. Level of evidence: III.

63. May JH, Gillette BP, Morgan JA, Krych AJ, Stuart MJ, Levy BA: Transtibial versus inlay posterior cruciate ligament reconstruction: An evidence-based systematic review. *J Knee Surg* 2010;23(2):73-79.

    Studies comparing tibial inlay to transtibial PCL reconstruction were reviewed. No differences were found in clinical results.

64. Panchal HB, Sekiya JK: Open tibial inlay versus arthroscopic transtibial posterior cruciate ligament reconstructions. *Arthroscopy* 2011;27(9):1289-1295.

    A systematic review of biomechanical and clinical studies compared open tibial inlay and arthroscopic transtibial techniques for PCL reconstruction. Level of evidence: IV.

65. Markolf KL, Feeley BT, Jackson SR, McAllister DR: Biomechanical studies of double-bundle posterior cruciate ligament reconstructions. *J Bone Joint Surg Am* 2006;88(8):1788-1794.

66. Markolf KL, Jackson SR, McAllister DR: Single- versus double-bundle posterior cruciate ligament reconstruction: Effects of femoral tunnel separation. *Am J Sports Med* 2010;38(6):1141-1146.

    A controlled laboratory cadaver study evaluated the biomechanics of double-bundle femoral reconstruction of the PCL. The posteromedial bundle carries a high load in full extension.

67. Markolf KL, Feeley BT, Jackson SR, McAllister DR: Where should the femoral tunnel of a posterior cruciate ligament reconstruction be placed to best restore anteroposterior laxity and ligament forces? *Am J Sports Med* 2006;34(4):604-611.

68. Hermans S, Corten K, Bellemans J: Long-term results of isolated anterolateral bundle reconstructions of the posterior cruciate ligament: A 6- to 12-year follow-up study. *Am J Sports Med* 2009;37(8):1499-1507.

    The medium- to long-term outcomes of 25 patients with isolated single-bundle PCL reconstruction were evaluated. Level of evidence: IV.

69. Kohen RB, Sekiya JK: Single-bundle versus double-bundle posterior cruciate ligament reconstruction. *Arthroscopy* 2009;25(12):1470-1477.

3: Knee and Leg

A systematic review of studies comparing single- and double-bundle PCL reconstruction did not find either to be superior. Level of evidence: IV.

Video References

15.1: Kim SJ, Kim SG, Kim SH, Lee DY, Jo IK: *Arthroscopic Double-Bundle ACL Reconstruction Using Quadriceps Tendon Autograft* [video excerpt]. Rosemont, IL, American Academy of Orthopaedic Surgeons, 2010.

15.2: Bach Jr BR: *Revision Single Bundle ACL Reconstruction Using BPTB Autograft, part 1* [video excerpt]. River Forest, IL, 2010.

15.3: Bach Jr BR: *Revision Single Bundle ACL Reconstruction Using BPTB Autograft, part 2* [video excerpt]. River Forest, IL, 2010.

15.4: Johnson DH: *Pitfalls in ACL Reconstruction* [video excerpt]. Rosemont, IL, American Academy of Orthopaedic Surgeons, 2010.

15.5: Miller MD, Hart J, Kurkis G: *Anatomic ACL Reconstruction--All Comers* [video excerpt]. Charlottesville, VA, 2013.

15.6: Shino K: *Anatomical Rectangular Tunnel ACL Reconstruction Using BTB Graft* [video excerpt]. Osaka, Japan, 2010.

15.7: Fulkerson JP: *ACL Reconstruction Using a Free-Tendon Quadriceps Autograft* [video excerpt]. Farmington, CT, 2010.

15.8: Howell SM: *Technique for Harvesting Hamstring Tendons for ACL Reconstruction* [video excerpt]. Sacramento, CA, 2010.

15.9: Shelbourne KD: *Tips for Harvesting BTB Autograft* [video excerpt]. Indianapolis, IN, 2010.

15.10: Looney CG, Sterett WI: *ACL Reconstruction Using Achilles Allograft and Interference Screws* [video excerpt]. Franklin, TN, 2010.

15.11: Howell SM, Andres O: *Anatomic Single Bundle ACL Reconstruction without Roof and PCL Impingement - Tibialis Allograft* [video excerpt]. Sacramento, CA, 2010.

Chapter 16

Collateral Ligament Injuries

Eduard Alentorn-Geli, MD, MSc, PhD, FEBOT   Joseph J. Stuart, MD   J.H. James Choi, MD   Claude T. Moorman III, MD

Abstract

The most important research related to the medial collateral ligament, posteromedial corner, lateral collateral ligament, and posterolateral corner during the past 5 years includes more than 50 studies related to the basic science, anatomy, biomechanics, diagnosis, and treatment of these structures. Most of the studies involved anatomy or biomechanics (25 studies) or injury treatment (19 studies). The most important advances in research into collateral ligament injuries of the knee have involved anatomic identification, biomechanical testing, and clinical outcomes of anatomic reconstruction of ligament injuries.

Keywords: lateral collateral ligament; medial collateral ligament; posterolateral corner; posteromedial corner

Introduction

Collateral ligament injuries of the knee are common and challenging to treat. Medial collateral ligament (MCL) and lateral collateral ligament (LCL) injuries often occur with cruciate ligament injury, and the combined injury is even more complex to treat. The number of original investigations related to collateral ligament injuries has increased in recent years. This chapter reviews the most important recent research related to the MCL, posteromedial corner (PMC), LCL, and posterolateral corner (PLC) and provides clinical recommendations for treatment of these injuries.

The Medial Collateral Ligament

Basic Science

The healing potential of the MCL is greater than that of the anterior cruciate ligament (ACL). An in vitro investigation found differences in the stem cell characteristics of the MCL and ACL.[1] Specifically, the size and number of ACL-derived stem cell colonies were smaller, and they grew at a slower rate than MCL-derived stem cell colonies. The ACL-derived stem cells expressed lower levels of stem cell marker genes than the MCL-derived stem cells. ACL-derived cells had less potential for adipogenesis, chondrogenesis, and osteogenesis. Another recent investigation found that gene expression of lysyl oxidases was higher in MCL fibroblasts than in ACL fibroblasts.[2] These enzymes are important for cross-linking between collagen and elastin during injury healing. In response to transforming growth factor–β1, which is an important mediator of ligament healing, MCL fibroblasts had a higher expression of lysyl oxidases; ACL fibroblasts had a higher expression of matrix metalloproteinases, which increase the degradation of extracellular matrix.[3] The same results were observed when the expression of lysyl oxidases and matrix metalloproteinases was compared in response to interleukin-1β, which is an important chemical mediator of acute inflammatory response in injured ligaments.[4] Together, these results show that the MCL has good healing potential because of the growth rate and functioning of its stem cells and the expression of important enzymes for ligament healing. These results may explain why isolated MCL injuries have a better response to nonsurgical treatment than isolated ACL injuries.

Dr. Moorman serves as a paid consultant to or is an employee of HeadTrainer; has stock or stock options held in HeadTrainer, PrivIT, and Regado; has received research or institutional support from Tornier, Moximed, Zetroz, HeadTrainer, and Histogenics; and serves as a board member, owner, officer, or committee member of the Atlantic Coast Conference Team Physicians Society and the American Orthopaedic Society for Sports Medicine. None of the following authors or any immediate family member has received anything of value from or has stock or stock options held in a commercial company or institution related directly or indirectly to the subject of this article: Dr. Alentorn-Geli, Dr. Stuart, and Dr. Choi.

3: Knee and Leg

Anatomy and Biomechanics

Three studies recently were published on MCL anatomy.[5-7] The perpendicular mean distance from the saphenous nerve to the adductor tubercle or the medial epicondyle was found to be 5 cm or 6.1 cm, respectively.[5] The perpendicular mean distance of the sartorial branch of the saphenous nerve to the anterior aspect of the superficial MCL was 4.8 cm at a point 2 cm distal to the joint line, 4.1 cm at 4 cm distal to the joint line, and 3.8 cm at 6 cm distal to the joint line. A comparison of displacement of the meniscus in a healthy MCL and an MCL detached from the femoral insertion found that only a few fibers of the ligament radiated to the medial meniscus and that the displacement did not significantly differ between the healthy and the detached MCL.[6] The femoral insertion site of the superficial MCL was found to be a mean 1.6 mm posterior and 4.9 mm proximal to the intersection between a line paralleling the posterior femoral cortex and a line drawn perpendicular to the posterior femoral cortex, where it intersects the Blumensaat line.[7] Thus, intraoperative fluoroscopy can be valuable in treating a chronic tear with an absence of ligament footprint or bony attrition.

Several MCL biomechanical studies have investigated aspects of MCL injury diagnosis, tensile properties, length patterns during gait, structural properties of the individual components of the medial complex, and biomechanical characteristics of several surgical procedures in cadavers.[8-15] Isolated grade III superficial MCL injury in a cadaver model resulted in a mean increase of 3.2 mm in medial joint line opening; in the intact state, the opening increased to 8.8 mm when the deep MCL and posterior oblique ligament (POL) were injured and to 13.8 mm when ACL injury was added.[8] A cutoff distance of 3.2 mm of medial joint line opening was established as the basis for suspecting an isolated grade III superficial MCL injury. In another biomechanical study, the MCL and LCL showed no significant difference in stiffness, but the ultimate tensile strength of the MCL was twice that of the LCL.[9] The MCL was most commonly torn at the femoral insertion site, and the LCL failed at the fibular attachment (60%) or midsubstance (40%). In a healthy knee the anterior bundles of both the superficial and deep MCL were elongated in flexion during gait, and the posterior bundles were distended with knee flexion angles.[10] The elongation of the posterior bundles peaked at midstance and the terminal extension–preswing stance phase.

The structural properties of the individual components of the medial knee ligaments (superficial MCL, deep MCL, and POL) were investigated in a controlled laboratory study.[11] The superficial MCL with intact femoral and distal tibial attachments had the highest load to failure and stiffness, followed by the POL and the deep MCL. A significant increase in displacement was observed after all medial knee structures were sectioned for valgus angulation, external rotation, internal rotation (from 0° to 60° only), anterior tibial translation (from 20° to 90° only), and posterior tibial translation (from 0° to 30° only).[12] The optimal position for MCL reconstruction to reproduce native knee kinematics was found at the center of the femoral attachment and the center of the superficial MCL attachment (the most isometric point).[13] Minor variations of the insertion sites were found to significantly modify the graft excursion. The anatomic MCL reconstruction (superficial MCL and POL; Figure 1) completely restored stability for valgus angulation as well as external and internal rotation but did not restore anterior and posterior tibial translation[13] (Figure 1). A subsequent cadaver study compared superficial MCL anatomic repair augmented using ipsilateral semitendinosus graft with anatomic reconstruction using bovine digital extensor tendon graft.[14] Both techniques significantly reduced medial joint space gapping and valgus rotation compared with the sectioned state of the MCL, with no significant differences based on surgical technique. Neither technique was able to reproduce the behavior of the native intact MCL. Nonanatomic MCL reconstruction using a shorter graft technique produced greater tibial external rotation during active knee extension and passive stability testing conditions, in comparison with anatomic superficial MCL reconstruction, which restored normal knee kinematics and stability.[15]

Treatment of Injuries

A recent large epidemiologic study of 346 MCL injuries in soccer players found that the mean return-to-play time was 23 days.[16] This time did not significantly differ between players with an index injury (18 days) or a reinjury (13 days). Whether patients underwent nonsurgical or surgical treatment was not specified, but it can be assumed that almost all patients received nonsurgical treatment. The outcomes of nonsurgical treatment of recalcitrant MCL injuries recently were published.[17] The therapy consisted of an image-guided injection of anesthetic and hydrocortisone beneath the periosteal attachment of the MCL. A significant improvement in pain and function was observed at a mean 9-month follow-up, and 66% of athletes returned to the previous level of sports competition, including professional sports.

Recent studies related to the surgical treatment of isolated MCL injuries were based on modifications of the surgical technique[18-21] (Table 1). In the MCL recession technique for treating symptomatic chronic MCL laxity, a bone block of the medial epicondyle containing

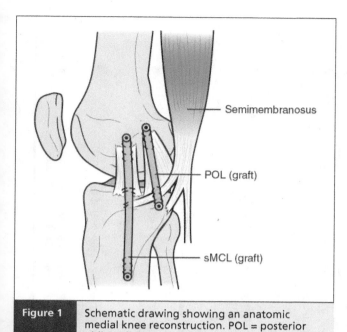

Figure 1 Schematic drawing showing an anatomic medial knee reconstruction. POL = posterior oblique ligament, sMCL = superficial medial collateral ligament.

Labels in figure: Semimembranosus, POL (graft), sMCL (graft)

the ligament insertion was obtained.[18] The bone was removed from the bone window to a depth that would create sufficient tension on the MCL. The bone block was fixed with a cancellous screw and spiked washer.[18] The results of using this technique were not reported. Another nonanatomic MCL reconstruction procedure used a triangular double-bundle allograft. The anterior bundle was placed 4.5 cm distal to the joint line, and the posterior bundle was placed 2 cm below the joint line with the same femoral fixation site in anatomic position[21] (Figure 2). The medial joint line opening and anteromedial rotatory stability improved after the reconstruction. The International Knee Documentation Committee (IKDC) Subjective Knee Evaluation Form scores (grade A in 59% and grade B in 36%) represented a significant improvement over scores from the preoperative period. These parameters did not significantly differ between patients who underwent isolated MCL reconstruction and those who underwent MCL plus ACL reconstruction.[21] Another study reported the outcomes of the surgical treatment of MCL injuries.[20] Anatomic medial knee reconstruction led to a significant increase in subjective IKDC scores and a significant decrease in medial compartment gapping on valgus stress radiographs.[12,20] The natural history and outcomes of surgical repair of proximal deep MCL injuries have been described.[19] This subgroup of injuries did not respond well to nonsurgical treatment. Most injuries were caused by a combined valgus stress and external tibial rotation during sports participation. MRI revealed edema

in the proximal insertion of the deep MCL. None of the patients had improvement with nonsurgical treatment. Surgery revealed lack of healing as well as retraction. The surgical repair elicited good results; all patients returned to sports and remained asymptomatic at a mean 48-week follow-up.[19]

Posteromedial Corner and Other Combined Injuries
Anatomic and Biomechanical Studies
An MRI-based retrospective study found that 81% of patients with a confirmed knee dislocation or a knee dislocatable under anesthesia had an injury to the PMC, and 63% had a superficial MCL tear alone.[22] All patients with injury to the posterior horn of the medial meniscus had concomitant meniscotibial ligament injury, and 67% had a tear of the POL. All patients with grade III laxity of the MCL had a complete tear of the POL and meniscotibial ligament. The researchers concluded that high-grade medial instability or an MCL tear with an associated tear of the posterior horn of the medial meniscus should raise suspicion for PMC instability.[22] A biomechanical study compared injured and intact knees for PCL or POL injury alone or in combination, before and after reconstruction.[23] Reconstruction of the POL was found to significantly contribute to a decrease in the posterior tibial translation of knees with associated PCL injury and applied valgus and internal rotation moments. The addition of MCL reconstruction did not improve knee kinematics. A nonanatomic reconstruction of the PMC was done using a double-strand semitendinosus graft.[23]

Surgical Treatment
Although most MCL injuries do not require surgical treatment because of the great healing potential of the MCL, some injuries need to be surgically fixed, particularly if other ligaments also are injured. The outcomes of surgical treatment of the PMC, with or without injury to the MCL and cruciate ligaments, generally are good (Table 1). In a study of a minimally invasive reconstruction of medial structures with ACL reconstruction, MCL and POL repair was done through advancement and retensioning of both ligaments proximal to the medial epicondyle.[24] Improvement in subjective and functional outcomes as well as stability in valgus stress and external rotation was reported in the postoperative period compared with the preoperative period. A similar surgical technique was used in patients with acute or chronic grade III ACL or medial knee injury.[25] Medial knee injuries were treated with proximal advancement of the superficial and deep MCL, POL, and joint capsule (Figure 3). Of the 18 patients, 7 needed double semitendinosus tendon augmentation to achieve adequate medial-side knee stability.[25] The researchers

Table 1

Outcomes of the Surgical Treatment of Isolated and Combined Medial Collateral Ligament Injuries

Study	Number of Patients With Injury Characteristics Mean Age (Range), in Months	Treatment	Mean Follow-up, in Months	Outcomes	Complications
Narvani et al[19] (2010)	17 men with proximal deep MCL injury 29 (18 to 44)	Deep MCL repair	12	100% returned to preinjury sport 100% were asymptomatic	Sensory deficit (infrapatellar branch of saphenous nerve) in 11.7%
LaPrade and Wijdicks[20] (2012)	28 patients (19 men, 9 women); 8 with acute, 20 with chronic MCL injury 32 (16 to 56)	Anatomic medial knee reconstruction (superficial MCL with both proximal and distal tibial attachments plus POL reconstruction using two separate grafts)	18	IKDC subjective score: 43.5 before, 76.2 after surgery Valgus stress on radiographs: 6.2 mm opening before, 1.3 mm opening after surgery	Wound infection in 3.5%
Dong et al[21] (2012)	56 patients; 27 with isolated MCL, 29 with MCL-ACL injury 36 (18 to 60)	Isolated MCL reconstruction (nonanatomic triangular double-bundle allograft) Combined injury reconstruction (nonanatomic triangular double-bundle allograft for MCL and double-bundle allograft for ACL)	33	Medial opening: 10.1 mm before, 2.9 mm after surgery Anteromedial instability: 67.9% incidence before, 9.4% incidence after surgery IKDC subjective score: grade A 59% before, grade B 36% after surgery IKDC symptom score: 84% normal or almost normal No difference after MCL or MCL-ACL treatment	ROM: >6° loss of extension in 7%, >25° loss of flexion in 3.6% Knee stiffness in 1.7% Medial meniscus tear in 7% MCL graft failure in 1.7%
Canata et al[24] (2012)	36 patients with ACL or MCL-POL tear 37 (15 to 70)	ACL reconstruction and mini-invasive MCL-POL repair with retensioning sutures	24	IKDC subjective score: 36 before, 94 after surgery (significant) KOOS score: 45 before, 93 after surgery (significant) Lysholm score: 40 before, 93 after surgery (significant) 100% had negative valgus and external rotatory tests	NR

ACL = anterior cruciate ligament, IKDC = International Knee Documentation Committee, KOOS = Knee Injury and Osteoarthritis Outcome Score, MCL = medial collateral ligament, NR = not reported, PCL = posterior cruciate ligament, PLC = posterolateral corner, PMC = posteromedial corner, POL = posterior oblique ligament, ROM = range of motion.

Table 1 (continued)

Outcomes of the Surgical Treatment of Isolated and Combined Medial Collateral Ligament Injuries

Study	Number of Patients With Injury Characteristics Mean Age (Range), in Months	Treatment	Mean Follow-up, in Months	Outcomes	Complications
Koga et al[25] (2012)	18 patients (9 women, 9 men) with ACL and medial knee injury 24 (17 to 44)	ACL reconstruction plus proximal advancement of superficial and deep MCL, POL, and capsule	26	Valgus stress on radiographs: 6 mm before, 1 mm after surgery (significant) Lysholm score: 81 before, 91 after surgery (significant)	Loss of 15° of flexion in 11%
Marx and Hetsroni[26] (2012)	14 patients with MCL and ACL and/or PCL injury 34 (19 to 60)	MCL reconstruction with Achilles tendon allograft plus ACL or/or PCL reconstruction	36	Symmetric valgus stability in 78% IKDC subjective score after surgery: mean, 91 Lysholm score after surgery: mean, 92 KOOS score after surgery: mean, 93.	ROM: 15° loss in 14% Valgus instability: grade 1 asymmetry in 22% Pivot instability in 14%
Liu et al[27] (2013)	16 patients (12 men, 4 women) with MCL and ACL, PCL and/or PLC injury 37 (19 to 53)	Superficial MCL reconstruction with Achilles tendon allograft plus other ligament reconstruction	34 (median)	Valgus stability (side-to-side): 8.9 mm before, 1.1 mm after surgery (significant) IKDC subjective score: 50 before, 84 after surgery (significant) Lysholm score: 69 before, 88 after surgery (significant)	ROM: ≥10° loss of flexion in 25%
Stannard et al[29] (2012)	73 patients (45 men, 26 women) with PMC and other ligament injury 36 (17 to 63)	PMC repair or reconstruction (MCL and POL with autograft or allograft) plus other ligament reconstruction	43	Failure rate 20% after repair, 4% after reconstruction IKDC subjective scores: repair, 57; autograft reconstruction, 42; allograft reconstruction, 37 (significance NR)	Arthrofibrosis in 17% Infection in 4% Hematoma in 5% No between-group differences
Kitamura et al[28] (2013)	30 patients (24 men, 6 women) with multiligament injury 28 (16 to 60)	Superficial MCL reconstruction with hybrid technique plus ACL and/or PCL reconstruction	NR (range, 2 to 12 years)	Lysholm score after surgery: 94 IKDC score: grade A, 9; grade B, 17; grade C, 3; grade D, 1 Mean medial joint opening: 8.5 mm in surgically treated, 8 mm in healthy knees (nonsignificant)	ROM: >3° loss of knee extension in 1; 6° to 15° loss of knee flexion in 5; 16° to 25° loss of knee flexion in 2

ACL = anterior cruciate ligament, IKDC = International Knee Documentation Committee, KOOS = Knee Injury and Osteoarthritis Outcome Score, MCL = medial collateral ligament, NR = not reported, PCL = posterior cruciate ligament, PLC = posterolateral corner, PMC = posteromedial corner, POL = posterior oblique ligament, ROM = range of motion.

3: Knee and Leg

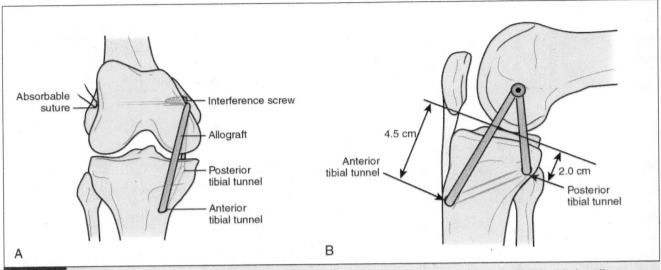

Figure 2 Schematic drawings showing frontal (**A**) and lateral (**B**) views of the knee after a triangular, double-bundle reconstruction of the medial collateral ligament.

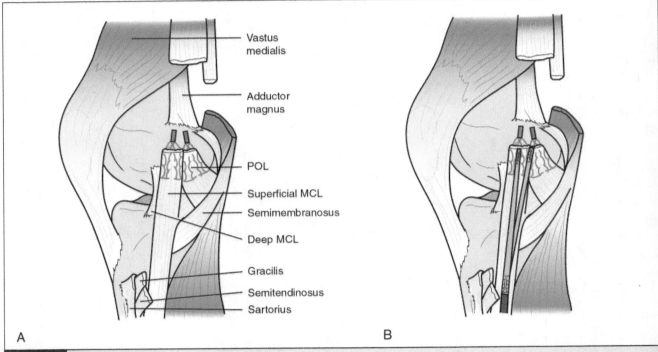

Figure 3 Schematic medial-view drawings showing the proximal advancement procedure for posteromedial corner repair alone (**A**) and with double semitendinosus tendon augmentation (**B**). MCL = medial collateral ligament, POL = posterior oblique ligament.

reported significant improvement in radiographically assessed valgus laxity as well as adequate function, sports performance, and satisfaction with surgery. Both studies found good results after surgical treatment of medial knee injury in patients with a concomitant ACL tear.

Two studies reported the outcomes of surgical treatment of MCL injury using Achilles tendon allograft in the context of combined ligament injury[26,27] (Table 1). The MCL was reconstructed by fixing the bone block of the Achilles tendon allograft into anatomic position in the femur and fixing the tendon part into the tibia with a cortical screw and spiked washer.[26] The MCL was fixed at 20° of flexion and slight varus after reconstruction of the ACL. The 14 patients had good functionality, stability, and return to preinjury activity level. A similar technique was used to correct subacute and chronic valgus instability in multiligament-injured knees through superficial MCL reconstruction.[27] Valgus laxity and functional outcomes significantly improved after surgery on the superficial MCL with the other injured ligaments. Because of concerns related to the difficulty of the surgical technique, the risk of infection, and the loss of motion, some surgeons prefer to use Achilles tendon allograft only if multiple ligaments are involved and not for isolated MCL injury. The surgical outcomes of MCL reconstruction were reported when a novel hybrid technique was used in multiligament-injured knees.[28] The MCL was reconstructed using both semitendinosus tendon autograft and a polyester tape (Neoligaments). The tibial tape portion of the graft was reflected to the anteromedial tibia under the subcutaneous tissue after being passed though the tibial tunnel (Figure 4). This reconstruction has biomechanical properties comparable to those of a bone–patellar tendon–bone graft fixed with an interference screw, allows anatomic tunnel placement, and has good length and thickness adaptability. Function and stability were satisfactory at an average 2-year follow-up.

A study of the surgical treatment of PMC injuries included a comparison of repair and reconstruction of both the MCL and POL.[29] The repair was done with suture

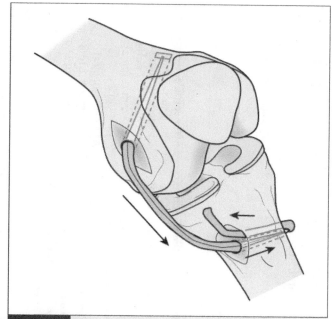

Figure 4 Schematic drawing showing an anatomic medial collateral ligament reconstruction using a hybrid technique with semitendinosus tendon autograft and a polyester tape. The arrows demonstrate the direction of the construct, which is anchored in the lateral aspect of the distal humerus (dashed lines).

Video 16.1: Medial Collateral Ligament (MCL) Acute Meniscotibial Repair. David Gordon, MB, ChB, MD; Leo Pinczewski, FRACS (9.04 min)

anchors in injuries less than 4 weeks old. Repairs of PMC injury had a higher failure rate than reconstruction with autograft or allograft. Therefore, reconstruction may be preferable to repair of PMC injury.

The recommended surgical technique for PMC injuries is the modified Bosworth technique, with plicature of the posterior capsule to treat injury to the POL.

The Lateral Collateral Ligament

Anatomy and Biomechanics
In an anatomic study, the LCL femoral insertion site was identified after anatomic dissection and correlated with the radiographic location.[30] The LCL was found to be located at 58% of the width of the condyle from the anterior aspect and at 2.3 mm distal to the Blumensaat line, and there was less than 5 mm variance from mean values. Another study determined the relationship between the

LCL femoral insertion site and the physis of skeletally immature cadaver knees.[31] The midpoint of the femoral origin of the LCL in infants and children was 6.3 mm or 5.9 mm distal to the physis, respectively. LCL reconstruction is uncommon in patients with open physes, but this study allows prevention of iatrogenic injury by improving the understanding of the spatial relationship between the LCL femoral origin and the distal femoral physis.

A biomechanical study using a finite element analysis determined the stress changes of the LCL at several knee flexion angles (0°, 30°, 60°, 90°, and 120°) and translation forces (anterior-posterior, varus rotation, and internal-external rotation).[32] The LCL was found to shorten with increasing knee flexion and to be most vulnerable with varus motion in almost all evaluated knee flexion angles. The stress on the LCL increased with anterior-posterior translation and internal-external rotation at 30° of knee flexion. A biomechanical cadaver study compared the varus stability of isolated LCL tears after figure-of-8 reconstruction or biceps femoris tenodesis.[33] Nine knees were loaded at 10 N·m (0° and 30° of knee flexion) in three states: with an intact LCL, with a sectioned LCL, and after reconstruction. Both techniques restored varus stability at least to baseline values. The normalized varus displacement was significantly lower after tenodesis than after figure-of-8 reconstruction. The advantage of this

Table 2

Outcomes of Surgical Treatment of Isolated and Combined Lateral Collateral Ligament Injuries

Study	Number of Patients With Injury Characteristics Mean Age (Range), in Months	Treatment	Mean Follow-up, in Months	Outcomes	Complications
LCL Injuries					
Bushnell et al[34] (2010)	9 men with isolated grade III LCL tear NR	Surgical repair, 4 Nonsurgical treatment, 5	NR (minimum, 1 year)	Missed weeks of play: 14.5 after surgical treatment, 2 after nonsurgical treatment (significant) Return to play during same season: 0 patients after surgery, 4 after nonsurgical treatment Mean additional seasons played: 2.8 after surgical treatment, 4.4 after nonsurgical treatment	After surgical treatment: mild subjective instability (but returned to play) in 1 patient; 1 to 3 mm residual varus laxity in 2 After nonsurgical treatment: 1 to 3 mm residual varus laxity in 5
PLC and Combined Injuries					
Jakobsen et al[47] (2010)	27 patients (16 men, 11 women) with PLC injury 29 (13 to 57)	Anatomic PLC reconstruction (LCL, PT, PFL) with hamstring autograft (semitendinosus tendon for LCL injury, gracilis tendon for PT and PFL)	46 (median)	Positive dial test: 60% before, 5% after surgery (significant) IKDC subjective score of grade C or D: 60% before, 28% after surgery (significant) KOOS subscores after surgery: pain, 75; symptoms, 77; ADL, 83; sports, 55; QoL, 59 Tegner score after surgery (mean): 4.6	10° loss of flexion in 7% 5° loss of flexion in 7% Deep infection in 3.7% Persistent pain in 11%
von Heideken et al[48] (2011)	6 pediatric patients (5 boys, 1 girl) with acute avulsion fracture of LCL–PT femoral attachment 13.3 (12.6 to 13.7)	Open reduction and internal fixation of bony fragment, 5 Nonsurgical treatment, 1	60	Lysholm score (mean) after surgery, 98; KOOS QoL score (mean) after surgery, 80 Lysholm score (mean) after nonsurgical treatment, 80; KOOS QoL score (mean) after nonsurgical treatment, 25 Normal stability and ROM	Growth arrest, 5° extension deficit, 10° flexion deficit in 1 nonsurgically treated patient

ACL = anterior cruciate ligament, ADL = activities of daily living, IKDC = International Knee Documentation Committee, KOOS = Knee Injury and Osteoarthritis Outcome Score, LCL = lateral collateral ligament, NR = not reported, PCL = posterior cruciate ligament, PFL = popliteofibular ligament, PLC = posterolateral corner, PT = popliteus tendon, QoL = quality of life, ROM = range of motion.

Table 2 (continued)

Outcomes of Surgical Treatment of Isolated and Combined Lateral Collateral Ligament Injuries

Study	Number of Patients With Injury Characteristics Mean Age (Range), in Months	Treatment	Mean Follow-up, in Months	Outcomes	Complications
Cartwright-Terry et al[49] (2014)	125 patients: 25 (22 men, 3 women) with PLC injury, 100 with isolated ACL injury 34 (23 to 50)	PLC injury treated with split biceps tenodesis technique	85	ACL-PLC injury: IKDC score (mean) after surgery, 90; overall KOOS score (mean), 40 before, 82 after surgery; Lysholm score, 35 before, 77 after surgery Return to sports: 92%	PLC injury: hardware intolerance in 4%, reconstruction failure in 4%, superficial infection in 8%
Zorzi et al[50] (2013)	19 patients (13 men, 6 women) with PLC and PCL injury 29 (17 to 41)	PLC injury treated with modified Larsson technique (LCL and PFL)	38	Stability: 100% had <5 mm posterior drawer step-off, negative dial test, 89% varus stress ROM: mean 10° less than contralateral side Mean Tegner score: 2 before, 6 after surgery	NR
Kim et al[51] (2011)	46 patients (36 men, 10 women) with PCL and PLC injury 35 (19 to 60)	PLC reconstructed with anatomic (LCL and PT) technique with posterior tibial tendon allograft (A) or with split biceps tenodesis technique (B)	24	Pre-postop differences (all significant): Dial test: A 16°, B 13°; Varus stress A 3.6mm, B 2.5mm; Lysholm A 29, B 22; Flexion loss A 4°, B 8.8°	Anatomic technique: fibular tunnel break in 5% Split biceps tenodesis technique: transient peroneal nerve injury in 4%, biceps tendon pressure necrosis in 8%
Zhang et al[52] (2010)	18 patients (13 men, 5 women) with PCL and PLC injury 33 (15 to 47)	PLC reconstruction Miniopen PFL reconstruction with anterior tibial tendon allograft (PCL with Achilles tendon allograft)	42	Stability: posterior tibial translation 17 mm before, 4.6 mm after surgery (significant); tibial external rotation 14° before, -3° after surgery (significant) IKDC score: 100% grade D before surgery; 28% grade A, 44% grade B, 28% grade C after surgery	>10° limitation of tibial external rotation in 16%

ACL = anterior cruciate ligament, ADL = activities of daily living, IKDC = International Knee Documentation Committee, KOOS = Knee Injury and Osteoarthritis Outcome Score, LCL = lateral collateral ligament, NR = not reported, PCL = posterior cruciate ligament, PFL = popliteofibular ligament, PLC = posterolateral corner, PT = popliteus tendon, QoL = quality of life, ROM = range of motion.

3: Knee and Leg

nonanatomic reconstruction technique is that it is simple and does not require allograft or autograft.

Treatment of Injuries

The only recent study of the treatment of isolated LCL injuries evaluated return to play in professional American football players after nonsurgical or surgical treatment of an isolated grade III LCL injury[34] (Table 2). The four surgically treated patients missed an average 14.5 weeks of play and did not return to play until the next season. In contrast, the five nonsurgically treated patients missed only an average 2 weeks of play. Four patients returned to play at an average of 10 days, and the remaining patient returned to play the next season. Although the study's sample size was limited, the data warrant further research.

Posterolateral Corner and Other Combined Injuries
Anatomic and Biomechanical Studies

Anatomic studies have been based on identification of ligaments involved in the PLC and the intertunnel relationships in multiligament-injured knees.[35-38] A recent study detailed the anatomy of all structures of the PLC.[35] The LCL was found to be more proximal to the lateral femoral epicondyle (mean, 3.6 mm) than the popliteus tendon (PT) insertion, which was more anterior to the LCL footprint (mean, 5.7 mm) than previously reported. The study also specified the length and diameter of the fabellofibular, arcuate, oblique popliteal, posterior meniscofemoral, and popliteomeniscal ligaments. The intertunnel relationship in multiligament knee surgery was investigated in three studies. The most adequate tunnel angles for anatomic PLC reconstruction were determined in CT-assessed, multiligament-injured cadaver knees.[36] To avoid collision with ACL and PCL tunnels, the safest femoral tunnel drilling angles for anatomic PLC reconstruction were found to be PT drilling at 30° of angulation in both axial and coronal planes and LCL drilling at 30° angulation in the axial plane and 0° angulation in the coronal plane. A study of the violation of the intercondylar notch and potential tunnel collision in single-bundle or double-bundle ACL reconstruction found that the safest angles for the LCL and PT tunnels were 20° anterior and 10° proximal to the transepicondylar axis.[37] Detailed data were provided on distances and angulations in ACL reconstruction based on single-bundle or double-bundle reconstruction and anteromedial or transtibial femoral tunnel drilling. In a similar study, the safest angulations to prevent intersection of LCL and ACL tunnels were 40° anterior angulation in the axial plane and 0° proximal angulation in the coronal plane.[38] However, at these angles two of six specimens for the axial plane and two of five specimens for the coronal plane had a trochlea violation without a tunnel collision. It is likely that small variations in the LCL femoral origin may explain differences in angles related to tunnel collision. This study determined that the LCL femoral insertion site was 1.4 mm proximal and 3.1 mm posterior to the lateral epicondyle.[38]

Several recent biomechanical studies were related to PLC reconstruction.[39-43] The LCL and popliteofibular ligament (PFL) were found to equally limit tibial external rotation at low flexion angles (0° and 30°), and the PFL was more important than the LCL for limiting external rotation at 60° and 90° of knee flexion.[42] These results suggest that PLC knee injuries occurring at a high knee flexion angle may have more involvement of the PFL (and probably the PT) than the LCL. Four biomechanical studies compared reconstruction techniques. Varus and external rotatory laxity were compared in PT and LCL reconstruction using the posterior tibial tendon, PT and PFL reconstruction using patellar tendon and bone, and PFL and LCL reconstruction using the semitendinosus tendon.[40] No significant differences were found in varus and tibial external rotation at 0°, 30°, 60°, and 90° of knee flexion. None of the three techniques could achieve the strength of the native knee. Tibial external rotation depended on whether the PT, PFL, or both were reconstructed (in an intact LCL model).[43] Sectioning both structures significantly increased external rotation. The PFL reconstruction restored external rotation to that of the intact knee at 30° and 90° of knee flexion. However, the PT and PT plus PFL reconstruction techniques overconstrained external rotation at 0°, 30°, 45°, 60°, 90°, and 120° of knee flexion. Varus and tibial external rotation at 0°, 30°, and 60° of knee flexion were compared in several fibula-based reconstruction techniques: femoral attachment with a single-tunnel or double-tunnel technique and fibular attachment with an anterior-posterior or oblique tunnel technique.[39] All reconstruction techniques restored varus and external rotation compared with the ligament-deficient state, but the double femoral tunnel (one tunnel for the PT and another for the LCL) with an oblique fibular tunnel was the best technique for restoring native knee kinematics. None of the reconstruction techniques overconstrained the knee at the evaluated knee flexion angles. However, drilling more than one tunnel in the femur may increase the complexity of a revision surgery, especially if tunnel communication develops, and can increase the risk of tunnel collision if there is associated ACL injury.[44] Varus and tibial external rotation were compared in a fibula-based figure-of-8 technique alone and a combined PT and fibula-based figure-of-8 technique.[41] These techniques similarly restored varus and tibial external rotation stability at 30° and 90° compared with the intact state. Varus stability at 30° in the fibula-based reconstruction technique was significantly lower than in the combined procedure, although it was not significantly different from that of the intact knee.

Diagnostic Studies

An MRI-based study determined the location of bone bruises in PLC injuries.[45] In 28 patients with an isolated grade III PLC injury and 74 with a combined ligament injury, the most common bone bruise location was in the medial compartment. Specifically, bone bruises were located in the anteromedial femoral condyle in 60% of patients with an isolated injury and 52% of patients with a combined injury. Bone bruise of the posteromedial tibial plateau also was found in 29% of patients with PLC and ACL injury. Another diagnostic study classified the peel-off type of acute grade III PLC injury using both MRI and intraoperative arthroscopy in 48 patients.[46] A peel-off injury was found in 19 patients (40%), of whom 4 (21%) had a type I isolated PT injury, 8 (42%) had a type II combined PT and LCL tear, and 7 (37%) had a type III complex tear involving intrasubstance-based and/or fibula-based injury. Peel-off injury led to tibial external rotation of more than 10° in 84% of patients and to positive varus instability in 73% of patients. These injuries could be diagnosed with visualization of the lateral gutter during arthroscopy in 94% of patients.[46]

Surgical Treatment

Two recent studies evaluated the results of surgical treatment of isolated PLC injuries[47,48] (Table 2). In a study of 27 patients with this injury who were treated with anatomic reconstruction of the PLC (LCL, PT, and PFL) with hamstring autograft, 26 (95%) achieved adequate rotatory stability, and 19 (71%) had a normal or near-normal IKDC score.[47] Five of six pediatric patients (mean age, 13.3 years) were surgically treated with fragment fixation after an acute avulsion fracture of the femoral attachment of the LCL and PT.[48] At a mean 5-year follow-up, the patients had a mean Lysholm Knee Questionnaire score of 98, a mean Knee Injury and Osteoarthritis Outcome Score (KOOS) quality of life score of 80, and normal knee stability and range of motion.

A study of PLC injuries associated with other ligament injuries compared the surgical outcomes of ACL and PLC reconstruction with those of ACL reconstruction alone[49] (Table 2). All PLC injuries were treated with the split biceps tenodesis technique. At a mean 85-month follow-up, all patients had a negative dial test, and the Lysholm, IKDC, and KOOS scores had significantly improved compared with preoperative values. Several parameters were lower after a combination of procedures than after ACL reconstruction alone, but the patients who underwent a combined procedure had excellent return to work and sporting activity outcomes. Three studies reported the outcomes of surgical treatment of PLC injuries associated with PCL.[50-52] The outcomes of patients who underwent PCL reconstruction in combination with anatomic PLC reconstruction (LCL and PT) were compared with those of patients who underwent posterior tibial tendon allograft or the split biceps tenodesis technique[51] (Figure 5). The anatomic PLC reconstruction technique led to significantly better results in terms of rotatory stability, varus stability, Lysholm score, IKDC score, and range of motion than the biceps tenodesis technique. A study of 19 patients with PLC and PCL injuries surgically treated with a single-bundle reconstruction of the PCL and a modified Larsson technique for LCL and PFL reconstruction found excellent results in terms of absence of complications, dial test and varus stress stability, range of motion, and function.[50] A comparison of the results of single-bundle PCL reconstruction with Achilles tendon allograft combined with a miniopen PFL reconstruction using anterior tibial tendon allograft found significant improvement in posterior tibial translation, tibial external rotation, and function (as measured using IKDC scores) at a minimum 2-year follow-up.[52]

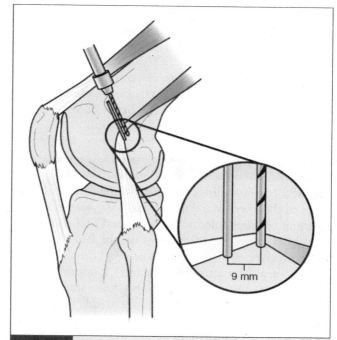

Figure 5 Schematic lateral-view drawing showing the modified biceps femoris rerouting technique for posterolateral corner insufficiency. After confirming the isometric point, a 3.2-mm hole was created proximally from the isometric point as long as the radius of a screw and washer (9 mm) used for fixation.

The recommended surgical technique for treating PLC injuries is the fibula-based, single-bundle, figure-of-8 semitendinosus autograft reconstruction.

Video 16.2: Posterolateral Corner Primary Repair and Reconstruction. Case Based. Mark D. Miller, MD; Brian C. Werner, MD; Sean Higgins (17:45 min)

Summary

The most recent findings on injury to the collateral ligaments of the knee are related to the basic science, anatomy, and biomechanics of the MCL and LCL. Many of the studies correspond to studies on the PMC or PLC. These injuries clearly impair knee stability and may warrant surgical treatment. In general, anatomic reconstruction is recommended to achieve knee stability and function. However, clinical studies are needed to compare anatomic and nonanatomic PMC or PLC reconstruction before definitive conclusions can be drawn.

Key Study Points

- The MCL has good healing potential thanks to greater growth and function of stem cells and expression of important enzymes for ligament healing, as compared with the ACL.
- Most MCL injuries can be treated nonsurgically, especially if they are incomplete or isolated (not associated with PMC or multiligament knee injury).
- More than 3.2 mm of medial joint line opening should raise suspicion for a grade III complete tear in a superficial MCL injury.
- The MCL and LCL have similar stiffness, but the ultimate tensile strength of the MCL is twice that of the LCL.
- Isolated anatomic MCL reconstruction, PMC reconstruction, and MCL reconstruction associated with cruciate ligament reconstruction have good results in terms of knee stability (valgus angulation and external and internal rotation) and function.
- The drilling angles in an anatomic PLC reconstruction to avoid tunnel collision with cruciate ligament reconstruction are the PT drilled at 30° of angulation in both axial and coronal planes and the LCL drilled at 30° angulation in the axial plane and 0° angulation in the coronal plane.
- The fibula-based and combined fibular and tibial PLC reconstruction techniques allow adequate restoration of knee varus and tibial external rotation.

Key Study Points (continued)

- Isolated PLC reconstruction and PLC reconstruction associated with cruciate ligament reconstruction lead to good outcomes in terms of stability and function at short-term and midterm follow-up.

Annotated References

1. Zhang J, Pan T, Im HJ, Fu FH, Wang JH: Differential properties of human ACL and MCL stem cells may be responsible for their differential healing capacity. *BMC Med* 2011;9:68.

   An in vitro study found differences in the stem cell characteristics of the human ACL and MCL, which are related to differences in healing potential.

2. Xie J, Huang W, Jiang J, et al: Differential expressions of lysyl oxidase family in ACL and MCL fibroblasts after mechanical injury. *Injury* 2013;44(7):893-900.

   An in vitro study found higher expression of lysyl oxidase in the human MCL than in the ACL, which is related to greater healing potential in the MCL.

3. Xie J, Wang C, Huang DY, et al: TGF-beta1 induces the different expressions of lysyl oxidases and matrix metalloproteinases in anterior cruciate ligament and medial collateral ligament fibroblasts after mechanical injury. *J Biomech* 2013;46(5):890-898.

   An in vitro study found that transforming growth factor–β1 induces higher expression of lysyl oxidase in the human MCL than in the ACL. There is higher expression of matrix metalloproteinases in the human ACL than in the MCL. These findings are related to a lower healing potential in the ACL than in the MCL.

4. Xie J, Wang C, Yin L, Xu C, Zhang Y, Sung KL: Interleukin-1 beta influences on lysyl oxidases and matrix metalloproteinases profile of injured anterior cruciate ligament and medial collateral ligament fibroblasts. *Int Orthop* 2013;37(3):495-505.

   An in vitro study found that interleukin-1 induces higher expression of lysyl oxidase in the human MCL and higher expression of matrix metalloproteinases in the human ACL, which are related to a lower healing potential in the ACL than in the MCL.

5. Wijdicks CA, Westerhaus BD, Brand EJ, Johansen S, Engebretsen L, LaPrade RF: Sartorial branch of the saphenous nerve in relation to a medial knee ligament repair or reconstruction. *Knee Surg Sports Traumatol Arthrosc* 2010;18(8):1105-1109.

   A human cadaver study reported the anatomic relationships between the surgical approach for MCL injuries and the saphenous nerve with its sartorial branch.

6. Stein G, Koebke J, Faymonville C, Dargel J, Müller LP, Schiffer G: The relationship between the medial collateral ligament and the medial meniscus: A topographical and biomechanical study. *Surg Radiol Anat* 2011;33(9):763-766.

   A human cadaver study found that the deep MCL had no relevant influence on the stability of the medial meniscus.

7. Hartshorn T, Otarodifard K, White EA, Hatch GF III: Radiographic landmarks for locating the femoral origin of the superficial medial collateral ligament. *Am J Sports Med* 2013;41(11):2527-2532.

   A human cadaver anatomic and radiographic study reported the exact location of the femoral attachment of the superficial MCL using true lateral radiographs.

8. LaPrade RF, Bernhardson AS, Griffith CJ, Macalena JA, Wijdicks CA: Correlation of valgus stress radiographs with medial knee ligament injuries: An in vitro biomechanical study. *Am J Sports Med* 2010;38(2):330-338.

   A human cadaver anatomic and radiographic study quantified medial compartment gapping with valgus stress tests based on types of medial knee injuries.

9. Wilson WT, Deakin AH, Payne AP, Picard F, Wearing SC: Comparative analysis of the structural properties of the collateral ligaments of the human knee. *J Orthop Sports Phys Ther* 2012;42(4):345-351.

   A human cadaver study compared the structural properties of the LCL and MCL. Differences were found in geometry and strength but not stiffness.

10. Liu F, Gadikota HR, Kozánek M, et al: In vivo length patterns of the medial collateral ligament during the stance phase of gait. *Knee Surg Sports Traumatol Arthrosc* 2011;19(5):719-727.

    A human biomechanical study found differences in the elongation of anterior and posterior bundles of the superficial and deep MCL during gait.

11. Wijdicks CA, Ewart DT, Nuckley DJ, Johansen S, Engebretsen L, LaPrade RF: Structural properties of the primary medial knee ligaments. *Am J Sports Med* 2010;38(8):1638-1646.

    A human biomechanical cadaver study investigated load to failure and stiffness of the superficial and deep MCL and the POL.

12. Coobs BR, Wijdicks CA, Armitage BM, et al: An in vitro analysis of an anatomical medial knee reconstruction. *Am J Sports Med* 2010;38(2):339-347.

    A human biomechanical cadaver study found that anatomic medial knee reconstruction completely restored valgus and internal-external rotation instability.

13. Feeley BT, Muller MS, Allen AA, Granchi CC, Pearle AD: Isometry of medial collateral ligament reconstruction. *Knee Surg Sports Traumatol Arthrosc* 2009;17(9):1078-1082.

    A human cadaver biomechanical study investigated the isometry of anatomic MCL reconstruction. The lowest graft excursion was found when the graft was fixed in the center of the MCL femoral attachment and the center of the superficial MCL attachment.

14. Wijdicks CA, Michalski MP, Rasmussen MT, et al: Superficial medial collateral ligament anatomic augmented repair versus anatomic reconstruction: An in vitro biomechanical analysis. *Am J Sports Med* 2013;41(12):2858-2866.

    A human cadaver study compared superficial MCL anatomic repair and anatomic reconstruction. Both techniques significantly reduced medial joint space gapping and valgus rotation compared with intact knees.

15. Van den Bogaerde JM, Shin E, Neu CP, Marder RA: The superficial medial collateral ligament reconstruction of the knee: Effect of altering graft length on knee kinematics and stability. *Knee Surg Sports Traumatol Arthrosc* 2011;19(Suppl 1):S60-S68.

    A human biomechanical cadaver study found that nonanatomic superficial MCL reconstruction led to higher values of tibial external rotation than anatomic reconstruction.

16. Lundblad M, Waldén M, Magnusson H, Karlsson J, Ekstrand J: The UEFA injury study: 11-year data concerning 346 MCL injuries and time to return to play. *Br J Sports Med* 2013;47(12):759-762.

    A prospective cohort study of 346 MCL injuries in European soccer players found that the mean time to return to play was 23 days. Level of evidence: II.

17. Drumm O, Chan O, Malliaras P, Morrissey D, Maffulli N: High-volume image-guided injection for recalcitrant medial collateral ligament injuries of the knee. *Clin Radiol* 2014;69(5):e211-e215.

    A retrospective case study reported good results after image-guided anesthetic and hydrocortisone injection for recalcitrant MCL injuries. Level of evidence: IV.

18. Backes JR, Wiltfong RE, Steensen RN: Medial collateral ligament recession for chronic medial knee laxity. *J Knee Surg* 2013;26(3):179-183.

    A surgical technique for chronic isolated MCL laxity consisted of MCL recession. Bone block was obtained from the femoral origin of the superficial MCL, bone was removed from the depth of the window, and bone block fixation was done in a more lateral position to increase tension.

19. Narvani A, Mahmud T, Lavelle J, Williams A: Injury to the proximal deep medial collateral ligament: A problematical subgroup of injuries. *J Bone Joint Surg Br* 2010;92(7):949-953.

    In a retrospective case study, injury to the proximal deep MCL was identified as having a poor prognosis. This injury may not heal easily and may be best treated surgically. Level of evidence: IV.

3: Knee and Leg

20. LaPrade RF, Wijdicks CA: Surgical technique: Development of an anatomic medial knee reconstruction. *Clin Orthop Relat Res* 2012;470(3):806-814.

A prospective case study of patients with anatomic MCL reconstruction (superficial MCL and POL) found good outcomes related to stability and function. Level of evidence: IV.

21. Dong JT, Chen BC, Men XQ, et al: Application of triangular vector to functionally reconstruct the medial collateral ligament with double-bundle allograft technique. *Arthroscopy* 2012;28(10):1445-1453.

A retrospective case study compared patients with isolated MCL injury to those with MCL and ACL injury. Triangular vector reconstruction of the MCL led to good stability and function. Level of evidence: IV.

22. Chahal J, Al-Taki M, Pearce D, Leibenberg A, Whelan DB: Injury patterns to the posteromedial corner of the knee in high-grade multiligament knee injuries: A MRI study. *Knee Surg Sports Traumatol Arthrosc* 2010;18(8):1098-1104.

A retrospective diagnostic study correlated MRI-assessed injury patterns in the PMC in multiligament knee injuries with examination under anesthesia. Level of evidence: IV.

23. Weimann A, Schatka I, Herbort M, et al: Reconstruction of the posterior oblique ligament and the posterior cruciate ligament in knees with posteromedial instability. *Arthroscopy* 2012;28(9):1283-1289.

A human biomechanical cadaver study reported good stability after reconstruction of the POL in knees with injury to the PMC and PCL.

24. Canata GL, Chiey A, Leoni T: Surgical technique: Does mini-invasive medial collateral ligament and posterior oblique ligament repair restore knee stability in combined chronic medial and ACL injuries? *Clin Orthop Relat Res* 2012;470(3):791-797.

A prospective case study found that a novel technique consisting of minimally invasive MCL and POL repair in patients with chronic medial laxity led to good stability and function. Level of evidence: IV.

25. Koga H, Muneta T, Yagishita K, Ju YJ, Sekiya I: Surgical management of grade 3 medial knee injuries combined with cruciate ligament injuries. *Knee Surg Sports Traumatol Arthrosc* 2012;20(1):88-94.

A retrospective case study of proximal advancement of both the superficial MCL and the POL with the underlying deep MCL and joint capsule in patients with combined cruciate ligament injuries reported reasonable restoration of medial knee stability. Level of evidence: IV.

26. Marx RG, Hetsroni I: Surgical technique: Medial collateral ligament reconstruction using Achilles allograft for combined knee ligament injury. *Clin Orthop Relat Res* 2012;470(3):798-805.

A retrospective case study in which patients with MCL and combined knee ligament injuries were treated with Achilles tendon allograft reported good medial stability at 2- to 5-year follow-up. Level of evidence: IV.

27. Liu X, Feng H, Zhang H, et al: Surgical treatment of subacute and chronic valgus instability in multiligament-injured knees with superficial medial collateral ligament reconstruction using Achilles allografts: A quantitative analysis with a minimum 2-year follow-up. *Am J Sports Med* 2013;41(5):1044-1050.

A retrospective case study of patients with a multiligament knee injury treated with Achilles tendon allograft reconstruction of the superficial MCL reported good functional and valgus stability. Level of evidence: IV.

28. Kitamura N, Ogawa M, Kondo E, Kitayama S, Tohyama H, Yasuda K: A novel medial collateral ligament reconstruction procedure using semitendinosus tendon autograft in patients with multiligamentous knee injuries: Clinical outcomes. *Am J Sports Med* 2013;41(6):1274-1281.

A retrospective case study of patients with a multiligament knee injury treated with a novel superficial MCL reconstruction technique combining semitendinosus tendon autograft and synthetic tape reported good functional and stability outcomes. Level of evidence: IV.

29. Stannard JP, Black BS, Azbell C, Volgas DA: Posteromedial corner injury in knee dislocations. *J Knee Surg* 2012;25(5):429-434.

A retrospective case study of patients with a knee dislocation compared repair and reconstruction of the PMC. Reconstruction led to better stability than repair. Level of evidence: IV.

30. Kamath GV, Redfern JC, Burks RT: Femoral radiographic landmarks for lateral collateral ligament reconstruction and repair: A new method of reference. *Am J Sports Med* 2010;38(3):570-574.

A human anatomic and radiographic cadaver study identified the femoral origin of the LCL. Intraoperative fluoroscopy can be used to determine femoral tunnel placement during posterolateral or LCL reconstruction.

31. Shea KG, Polousky JD, Jacobs JC Jr, Ganley TJ: Anatomical dissection and CT imaging of the posterior cruciate and lateral collateral ligaments in skeletally immature cadaver knees. *J Bone Joint Surg Am* 2014;96(9):753-759.

A human anatomic and radiographic cadaver study in skeletally immature knees described the relationship of the PCL and LCL to the physeal structures.

32. Zhong YL, Wang Y, Wang HP, Rong K, Xie L: Stress changes of lateral collateral ligament at different knee flexion with or without displaced movements: A 3-dimensional finite element analysis. *Chin J Traumatol* 2011;14(2):79-83.

A biomechanical study investigated stress changes of the LCL at different knee flexion angles, with or without displacement movements. The LCL was vulnerable to varus force and susceptible to anterior-posterior translation and internal-external rotation at 30° of knee flexion.

© 2016 American Academy of Orthopaedic Surgeons

33. Beiro C, Parks BG, Tsai M, Hinton RY: Biceps tenodesis versus allograft reconstruction for varus instability. *J Knee Surg* 2014;27(2):133-137.

A human biomechanical cadaver study found that both biceps tenodesis and allograft reconstruction restored varus stability to baseline values.

34. Bushnell BD, Bitting SS, Crain JM, Boublik M, Schlegel TF: Treatment of magnetic resonance imaging-documented isolated grade III lateral collateral ligament injuries in National Football League athletes. *Am J Sports Med* 2010;38(1):86-91.

A cross-sectional study of grade III LCL injuries found that nonsurgical treatment led to more rapid return to play than surgical treatment, with an equal likelihood of returning to professional-level play. Level of evidence: III.

35. Osti M, Tschann P, Künzel KH, Benedetto KP: Posterolateral corner of the knee: Microsurgical analysis of anatomy and morphometry. *Orthopedics* 2013;36(9):e1114-e1120.

A human cadaver study detailed the anatomy of structures of the PMC, with emphasis on the LCL.

36. Gelber PE, Erquicia JI, Sosa G, et al: Femoral tunnel drilling angles for the posterolateral corner in multiligamentary knee reconstructions: Computed tomography evaluation in a cadaveric model. *Arthroscopy* 2013;29(2):257-265.

A human anatomic cadaver study of intertunnel relationships in PLC and cruciate ligament reconstruction found that the safest angulation for avoiding tunnel collision was 30° axial and 0° coronal angulation for the LCL and 30° angulation for both axial and coronal planes for the PT.

37. Kim SJ, Chang CB, Choi CH, et al: Intertunnel relationships in combined anterior cruciate ligament and posterolateral corner reconstruction: An in vivo 3-dimensional anatomic study. *Am J Sports Med* 2013;41(4):849-857.

A human anatomic cadaver study reported intertunnel relationships in combined PLC and cruciate ligament reconstruction. The safest angulations to avoid tunnel collision of the LCL and PT tunnels were 20° anterior and 10° proximal to the transepicondylar axis.

38. Narvy SJ, Hall MP, Kvitne RS, Tibone JE: Tunnel intersection in combined anatomic reconstruction of the ACL and posterolateral corner. *Orthopedics* 2013;36(7):529-532.

A human anatomic cadaver study of intertunnel relationships in LCL and ACL reconstruction found that the safest angulation to avoid tunnel collision for the LCL was 40° anterior angulation in the axial plane and 0° proximal angulation in the coronal plane.

39. Feeley BT, Muller MS, Sherman S, Allen AA, Pearle AD: Comparison of posterolateral corner reconstructions using computer-assisted navigation. *Arthroscopy* 2010;26(8):1088-1095.

A human biomechanical cadaver study compared several fibula-based techniques for PLC injuries. The double femoral tunnel with an oblique fibular tunnel was the best technique for restoring native knee kinematics.

40. Kim SJ, Kim HS, Moon HK, Chang WH, Kim SG, Chun YM: A biomechanical comparison of 3 reconstruction techniques for posterolateral instability of the knee in a cadaveric model. *Arthroscopy* 2010;26(3):335-341.

A human biomechanical cadaver study compared varus and external rotation laxity in PT-LCL, PT-PFL, and PFL-LCL reconstruction techniques. There were no differences in varus and external rotation laxity.

41. Rauh PB, Clancy WG Jr, Jasper LE, Curl LA, Belkoff S, Moorman CT III: Biomechanical evaluation of two reconstruction techniques for posterolateral instability of the knee. *J Bone Joint Surg Br* 2010;92(10):1460-1465.

A human biomechanical cadaver study compared fibula-based and combined tibial and fibular tunnel reconstruction techniques. Both techniques restored varus and tibial external rotation stability at 30° and 90° of knee flexion.

42. Lim HC, Bae JH, Bae TS, Moon BC, Shyam AK, Wang JH: Relative role changing of lateral collateral ligament on the posterolateral rotatory instability according to the knee flexion angles: A biomechanical comparative study of role of lateral collateral ligament and popliteofibular ligament. *Arch Orthop Trauma Surg* 2012;132(11):1631-1636.

A human biomechanical cadaver study found that the PFL and LCL equally restored tibial external rotation at low knee flexion angles but that the PFL was more important than the LCL at limiting this movement at 60° and 90°.

43. Zhang H, Zhang J, Liu X, et al: In vitro comparison of popliteus tendon and popliteofibular ligament reconstruction in an external rotation injury model of the knee: A cadaveric study evaluated by a navigation system. *Am J Sports Med* 2013;41(9):2136-2142.

A human biomechanical cadaver study compared PT, PFL, and PT-PFL surgical reconstruction techniques for PLC injuries. All techniques restored external rotation, but PT and PT-PFL techniques overconstrained the external rotation.

44. Shuler MS, Jasper LE, Rauh PB, Mulligan ME, Moorman CT III: Tunnel convergence in combined anterior cruciate ligament and posterolateral corner reconstruction. *Arthroscopy* 2006;22(2):193-198.

A human cadaver anatomic study of tunnel collision in combined PLC and ACL reconstruction found that tunnel collision is common and that the surgeon should keep a neutral alignment in the coronal plane, avoid long tunnels, and direct the lateral tunnel anteriorly in the axial plane no more than 40°.

45. Geeslin AG, LaPrade RF: Location of bone bruises and other osseous injuries associated with acute grade III isolated and combined posterolateral knee injuries. *Am J Sports Med* 2010;38(12):2502-2508.

A retrospective case study described the location of bone bruises in PLC injuries. Most bone bruises were located in the medial compartment in both isolated and combined PLC corner injuries. Level of evidence: IV.

46. Feng H, Zhang H, Hong L, Wang XS, Cheng KB, Zhang J: Femoral peel-off lesions in acute posterolateral corner injuries: Incidence, classification, and clinical characteristics. *Arthroscopy* 2011;27(7):951-958.

A retrospective diagnostic study described the peel-off type of injury, which represents 40% of PLC injuries. Level of evidence: IV.

47. Jakobsen BW, Lund B, Christiansen SE, Lind MC: Anatomic reconstruction of the posterolateral corner of the knee: A case series with isolated reconstructions in 27 patients. *Arthroscopy* 2010;26(7):918-925.

A retrospective case study of patients with an isolated PLC injury treated with anatomic reconstruction with hamstring autograft found good function and stability outcomes. Level of evidence: IV.

48. von Heideken J, Mikkelsson C, Boström Windhamre H, Janarv PM: Acute injuries to the posterolateral corner of the knee in children: A case series of 6 patients. *Am J Sports Med* 2011;39(10):2199-2205.

A retrospective case study of acute PLC injuries (acute femoral avulsions) in children found good functional and stability outcomes after fragment reattachment. Level of evidence: IV.

49. Cartwright-Terry M, Yates J, Tan CK, Pengas IP, Banks JV, McNicholas MJ: Medium-term (5-year) comparison of the functional outcomes of combined anterior cruciate ligament and posterolateral corner reconstruction compared with isolated anterior cruciate ligament reconstruction. *Arthroscopy* 2014;30(7):811-817.

A cross-sectional study of surgical treatment of PLC injuries found that the split biceps tenodesis technique plus ACL reconstruction improved functional and stability outcomes. Level of evidence: III.

50. Zorzi C, Alam M, Iacono V, Madonna V, Rosa D, Maffulli N: Combined PCL and PLC reconstruction in chronic posterolateral instability. *Knee Surg Sports Traumatol Arthrosc* 2013;21(5):1036-1042.

A retrospective case study of patients treated using the modified Larsson technique for PLC reconstruction and PCL reconstruction reported good results in terms of stability and range of motion. Level of evidence: IV.

51. Kim SJ, Kim TW, Kim SG, Kim HP, Chun YM: Clinical comparisons of the anatomical reconstruction and modified biceps rerouting technique for chronic posterolateral instability combined with posterior cruciate ligament reconstruction. *J Bone Joint Surg Am* 2011;93(9):809-818.

A cross-sectional study compared the results of anatomic and biceps tenodesis techniques for PLC injuries associated with PCL reconstruction. Anatomic reconstruction had better functional and stability outcomes than the biceps tenodesis technique. Level of evidence: III.

52. Zhang H, Hong L, Wang XS, et al: Single-bundle posterior cruciate ligament reconstruction and mini-open popliteofibular ligament reconstruction in knees with severe posterior and posterolateral rotation instability: Clinical results of minimum 2-year follow-up. *Arthroscopy* 2010;26(4):508-514.

A cross-sectional study reported the results of PCL and miniopen PFL reconstruction. This technique provided good posterior and posterolateral rotatory stability. Level of evidence: III.

Video References

16.1: Gordon D, Pinczewski L: Video. *Medial Collateral Ligament (MCL) Acute Meniscotibial Repair.* Sydney, Austalia, 2012.

16.2: Miller MD, Werner BD, Higgins S: Video. *Posterolateral Corner Primary Repair and Reconstruction. Case Based.* Charlottesville, VA, 2014.

Chapter 17

Patellofemoral Joint Disorders

Miho J. Tanaka, MD   John J. Elias, PhD   Andrew J. Cosgarea, MD

Abstract

The evaluation and treatment of patellofemoral disorders requires a thorough understanding of the multiple factors that can contribute to these conditions. Treatments should be individualized to address the specific anatomic or functional deficits of a patient, while taking care to avoid the commonly reported complications that can occur with these procedures.

Keywords: patellofemoral instability; medial patellofemoral ligament; tibial tuberosity osteotomy

Introduction

The patellofemoral joint is a complex structure in which the patella articulates with the femoral trochlea. The patella serves as a fulcrum for the extensor mechanism, and as a result, high loads are transmitted across the patellofemoral joint. Disorders of the patellofemoral joint typically arise from joint overload or instability. Joint overload can be caused by overuse or excessive force and

Dr. Elias or an immediate family member has received research or institutional support from MedShape and has received nonincome support (such as equipment or services), commercially derived honoraria, or other non–research-related funding (such as paid travel) from Mitek and Synthes. Dr. Cosgarea or an immediate family member has received research support from Toshiba and serves as a board member, owner, officer, or committee member of the American Academy of Orthopaedic Surgeons, the American Orthopaedic Society for Sports Medicine, and the Patellofemoral Foundation. Neither Dr. Tanaka nor any immediate family member has received anything of value from or has stock or stock options held in a commercial company or institution related directly or indirectly to the subject of this chapter.

often is exacerbated by mechanical or structural variations that contribute to kinematic alterations within the joint. In contrast, patellar instability is a partial or complete displacement of the patella from the trochlear groove. The stability of the patellofemoral joint is influenced by the interaction of multiple anatomic factors that generally are categorized as static soft-tissue restraints, osteochondral constraints, dynamic restraints, and lower extremity alignment.

Anatomy and Biomechanics

The medial patellofemoral ligament (MPFL) is the primary static restraint to lateral patellar translation within the first 30° of knee flexion. A cadaver dissection study described the femoral origin of the MPFL as 9.5 mm distal and 9.5 mm anterior to the adductor tubercle.[1] The femoral origin was radiographically described as a point 1 mm anterior to a line that extends along the posterior cortex, 2.5 mm distal to the posterior origin of the medial femoral condyle, and proximal to the posterior aspect of the Blumensaat line.[2] On its patellar insertion, the MPFL typically merges with the attachment of the vastus medialis obliquus (VMO) and vastus intermedius tendons and extends to the medial border of the patella.[1,3] The average width of the MPFL is 17 mm at its insertion on the proximal two-thirds of the medial border of the patella. The MPFL remains relatively isometric between 0° and 70° of knee flexion and tension decreases with greater knee flexion.[4]

At a flexion angle greater than 30°, the osteochondral constraint of the trochlea provides primary stability to the patellofemoral joint (Figure 1). An MRI study of patients with normal anatomy found that the mean depth of the trochlea was 4.0 mm. This value differed significantly by sex (3.4 mm in women and 4.2 mm in men).[5] The medial facet contributed to 37.4% of the width of the cartilage covering the trochlea, and the lateral facet contributed to 62.6%. Decreased trochlear depth can reduce the effectiveness of the osteochondral restraint of the patella and contribute to patellar instability. A recent study using a created cadaver model found that elevating

3: Knee and Leg

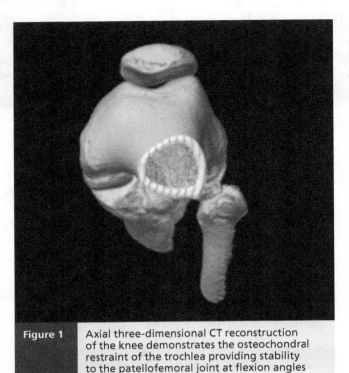

Figure 1 Axial three-dimensional CT reconstruction of the knee demonstrates the osteochondral restraint of the trochlea providing stability to the patellofemoral joint at flexion angles greater than 30°.

the floor of the trochlea simulated trochlear dysplasia.[6] Biomechanical studies found that measurements of trochlear dysplasia are significantly correlated with increased lateral patellar displacement and tilt across a range of knee flexion angles.[7,8]

The VMO provides a dynamic restraint to lateral translation. In vitro studies found that increasing the force applied by the VMO decreases the maximum lateral patellofemoral contact pressure and lateral patellar shift at multiple flexion angles.[9,10] Conversely, a study using dynamic cine phase-contrast MRI found that administering a motor branch block to the VMO increased lateral patellar shift during knee extension.[11] The morphology of the VMO was found to be correlated with its function. A sonography-based study found a significant difference in the characteristics of the VMO based on whether a patient had patellofemoral pain.[12] The insertion level of the VMO (measured as distance to the proximal pole of the patella), the medial orientation of the VMO muscle fibers, and VMO muscle volume were lower in those with patellofemoral pain. The role of the VMO in patellar stability can be assessed in terms of its relationship to the vastus lateralis. A prospective study of men undergoing military training found a significant delay in activation of the VMO with respect to the vastus lateralis in those who later experienced patellofemoral pain.[13] A biomechanical study using weight-bearing MRI found

that measurements of lateral patellar translation and tilt were correlated with a delay in the activation of the VMO in patients with pain and that an increase in the activation ratio of the vastus lateralis to the vastus medialis was associated with increased lateral patellar tilt.[14]

Abnormalities in lower extremity alignment can influence the kinematics of the patellofemoral joint. An MRI-based study found that measurements of femoral anteversion and genu valgum were greater in knees with patellar instability than in healthy control knees.[15] Increased lateralization of the tibial tuberosity relative to the trochlear groove is a common type of lower extremity malalignment. Recent studies have documented the relationship of radiographic measurements of malalignment with patellar position. A study of patellar kinematics based on MRI at multiple knee flexion angles found that a radiographic measurement of malalignment was significantly correlated with increased lateral shift and tilt of the patella in patients with patellar instability.[6] An in vitro study found that reducing tuberosity lateralization with a tibial tuberosity osteotomy (TTO) decreased the lateral shift and tilt of the patella.[16]

The patellar height type of malalignment influences patellofemoral kinematics by increasing the extent of knee flexion before the patella can engage within the trochlear groove. A study evaluating topographic differences on MRI between patients with or without patellar instability found that radiographic measurements of patellar height were significantly greater in those with patellar instability.[17] An earlier biomechanical study also found a relationship between patellar height and abnormal patellar tracking, with greater lateral shift and tilt of the patella in subjects with an increased patellar height index (patella alta).[18]

Clinical Evaluation

History and Physical Examination
The primary objective in evaluating patellofemoral dysfunction is to differentiate between pain and instability. A clear description of the patient's symptoms can be helpful when distinguishing patellar subluxation from symptoms such as giving way of the knee because of pain or weakness. The mechanism of injury and the chronicity, number, and type of episodes (dislocation versus subluxation) are important elements of the patient's history. Knowledge of earlier treatments and surgical procedures can aid in determining treatment options.

A systematic examination that extends beyond the patellofemoral joint can identify multiple factors contributing to a patient's symptoms. General ligamentous laxity has been associated with an increased risk of patellar instability[19] and can be identified using criteria such as the Beighton hypermobility score. The assessment of alignment begins with the patient in a standing position. Alignment of the lower extremity traditionally has been quantified with the Q angle, but this measurement should be used with caution because its reliability and validity have not been established. The lateralization of the tibial tuberosity is assessed relative to the axis of the femur. Abnormalities in alignment such as external tibial torsion and a greater than normal valgus angle at the knee, as well as the presence of increased femoral anteversion, can effectively increase lateralizing forces on the extensor mechanism. Rotational malalignment in particular was found to be a risk factor in patellar instability.[15] Excessive femoral anteversion often can be detected in hip range of motion, and often so-called squinting patellae are present when the patient stands in neutral position (Figure 2).

Dynamic assessment of the lower extremity includes quadriceps strength. Quadriceps weakness is associated with the presence of patellofemoral pain. In unilateral limb-loading tests such as single-leg squatting and landing from a single-leg hop, greater dynamic knee valgus was found to be present in patients with patellofemoral pain than in control subjects.[20] Patients with unilateral symptoms had increased dynamic knee valgus angles in the symptomatic knee compared with the normal contralateral knee. Deficits in hip strength, particularly in hip abduction and external rotation, also were associated with the presence of symptoms.[21] Women with patellofemoral pain had less activation of the gluteus medius than control subjects during single-leg squat testing. Lack of flexibility of the hamstring musculature and tightness of the iliotibial band (detected using the Ober test) also are associated with the presence of symptoms. Iliotibial band tightness can lead to excessive lateral retinacular tightness and decreased medial patellar mobility.

Patellar mobility is assessed using the glide test. A force is applied in both medial and lateral directions, and the translation is quantified based on patellar quadrants (25% of the width of the patella) (Figure 3). The presence of two quadrants of patellar motion is normal, with variation in some individuals. Comparison to the contralateral side is useful for gauging normal patellar motion in patients with unilateral symptoms. The patellar tilt test is used to assess lateral retinacular tightness. A recent study found that patients with unilateral patellar instability had increased lateral patellar translation and tilt in both knees, and they had greater lateral patellar translation and tilt than patients with normal knees.[22] In patients with patellar instability, the apprehension sign can be elicited using a manually directed lateral force on the patella. Patellar tracking is observed as the patient

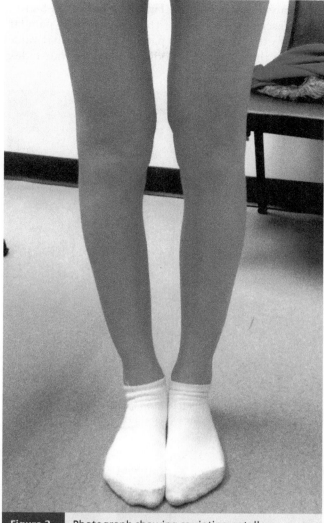

Figure 2   Photograph showing squinting patellae, which are associated with excessive femoral anteversion and tibial torsion.

actively extends the knee from a flexed position. Increased lateralization during terminal extension, called the J sign, may indicate loss of the medial soft-tissue checkreins. A positive apprehension test and J sign in the setting of increased lateral glide can represent a loss of patellar stability. Not all patients with these clinical signs have instability episodes, however. Findings should be correlated with the patient's description of symptoms to determine whether the patellofemoral joint is functionally unstable.

Imaging

Radiography
The radiographic assessment of the patellofemoral joint includes AP, lateral, and axial views. Patellar height is assessed on lateral radiographs using several different

radiographic measurements (**Figure 4**). The Insall-Salvati index describes the ratio of the length of the patellar tendon to the length of the patella; an abnormal value is greater than 1.2. The modified Insall-Salvati index adjusts for differences in patellar morphology by measuring the length of the articular surface of the patella relative to the length of the patellar tendon (from the inferior articular surface to the tuberosity); an abnormal value is greater than 2. The Caton-Deschamps index allows assessment of patellar height regardless of patellar tendon length and can be helpful if the patient has had a TTO. The Caton-Deschamps index is calculated by dividing the distance from the inferior articular surface of the patella to the anterosuperior margin of the tibial plateau by the length of the patellar articular surface. Normal values are less than 1.3. In a lateral radiograph used for determining patellar height, the knee should be positioned in 30° of flexion to allow appropriate tension on the patellar tendon.

Trochlear dysplasia is assessed on lateral radiographs using the Dejour classification (**Figure 5**). The severity of trochlear dysplasia is classified as mild (type A) to severe (type D), based on the appearance of the anterior femoral condyles. Type A dysplasia is described as a crossing sign at the superior margin of the trochlea, which corresponds to the presence of a shallow trochlea. Type B is described as a crossing sign with a supratrochlear spur, indicating a flat trochlea. Type C is characterized by the presence of a double-contour sign in addition to the crossing sign; the double contour indicates medial condylar hypoplasia. Type D dysplasia has all three components (the crossing

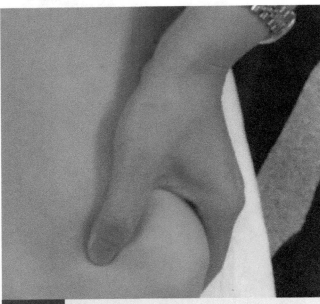

Figure 3 Photograph showing the glide test, in which force is applied in both medial and lateral directions to assess patellar mobility.

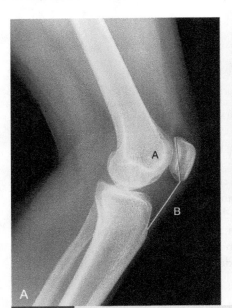
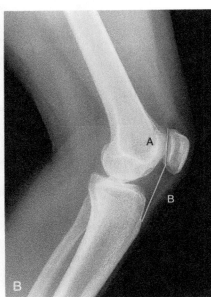
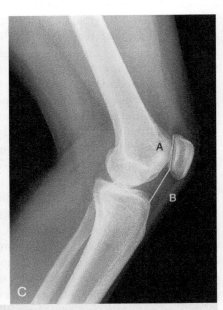

Figure 4 Lateral radiographs showing measurements of patellar height with the knee in 30° of flexion. **A,** The Insall-Salvati index describes the ratio of the length of the patellar tendon to the length of the patella (B/A). A value greater than 1.2 is abnormal. **B,** The modified Insall-Salvati index adjusts for differences in patellar morphology by measuring the length of articular surface of the patella relative to the length of the patellar tendon (B/A). A value greater than 2 is abnormal. **C,** The Caton-Deschamps index divides the distance from the inferior articular surface of the patella to the anterosuperior margin of the tibial plateau by the length of the patellar articular surface (B/A). A value greater than 1.3 is pathologic.

© 2016 American Academy of Orthopaedic Surgeons

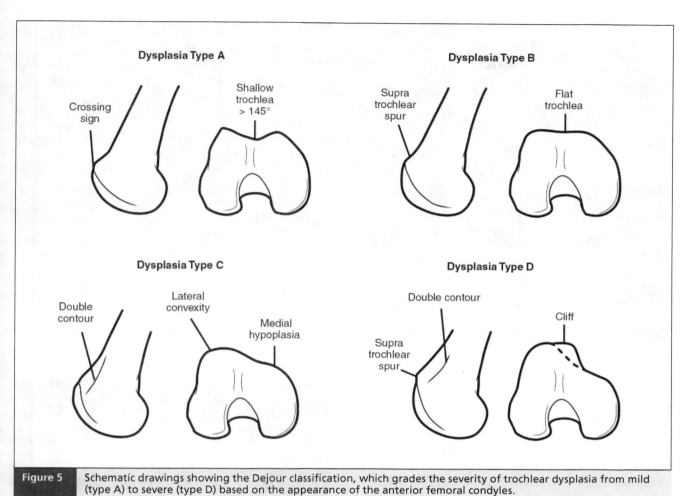

Dysplasia Type A

Crossing sign

Shallow trochlea > 145°

Dysplasia Type B

Supra trochlear spur

Flat trochlea

Dysplasia Type C

Double contour

Lateral convexity

Medial hypoplasia

Dysplasia Type D

Double contour

Supra trochlear spur

Cliff

Figure 5   Schematic drawings showing the Dejour classification, which grades the severity of trochlear dysplasia from mild (type A) to severe (type D) based on the appearance of the anterior femoral condyles.

sign, supratrochlear spur, and double-contour sign) and is correlated with a so-called cliff pattern, which is a prominence at the junction of the medial and lateral margins of the trochlea.

CT and MRI

MRI is comparable to CT in its ability to show patellofemoral morphology and in particular allows measurement of patellar tilt and the patellar height index.[17] MRI has two advantages over CT: it allows chondral lesions and the location of MPFL injury to be identified, and it carries no radiation risk. After an acute patellar dislocation episode, bony edema on the lateral femoral condyle and medial patella may be seen on MRI, as is typical with a relocation event. The presence of a large chondral fragment may suggest the necessity of an early surgical repair. MPFL injury is identified in most patients who have had a patellar dislocation event. Skeletally immature patients are most likely to sustain a patellar-side injury. Those with femoral-based ruptures of the MPFL have been found to be older (25.7 +/- 9.2 versus 19.7 +/- 6.1

years) than those with patellar-based ruptures after a patellar dislocation event.[23,24]

Axial CT or MRI studies are used to measure the sulcus angle and trochlear inclination in trochlear dysplasia (Figure 6). The sulcus angle is measured by determining the angle formed by the two lines that connect the anteriormost points of the medial and lateral femoral condyles to the deepest point of the trochlear groove. An angle greater than 144° is considered pathologic. Trochlear inclination is determined by measuring the angle between the line through the posterior condylar axis and a second line along the lateral trochlear wall. An angle of less than 11° indicates trochlear dysplasia. Lateral patellar tilt is determined by measuring the angle between the posterior condylar axis and the midpatellar line. An angle greater than 20° is pathologic and may indicate lateral retinacular tightness.

The distance between the tibial tuberosity and trochlear groove (the TTTG distance) is measured as the lateral distance between the deepest portion of the trochlear groove and the apex of the tibial tuberosity, on a line

3: Knee and Leg

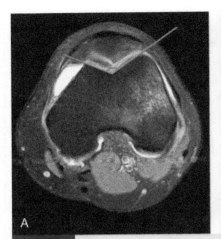
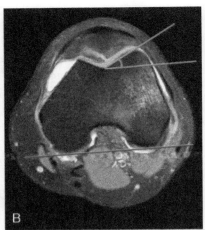
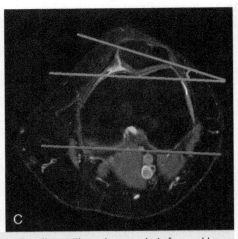

Figure 6 Axial view on MRI showing measurements of trochlear dysplasia and patellar tilt. **A,** The sulcus angle is formed by two lines that connect the anteriormost points of the medial and lateral femoral condyles to the deepest portion of the trochlear groove. An angle greater than 144° is considered pathologic. **B,** Lateral trochlear inclination is determined by the angle between two red lines, one parallel to the line through the posterior condylar axis (blue line), and a second line along the lateral trochlear wall. An angle of less than 11° is indicative of trochlear dysplasia. **C,** Lateral patellar tilt is a measurement of patellar position that is determined by the angle (in red) between the line parallel to the posterior condylar axis (blue line) and the midpatellar line. An angle greater than 20° is considered abnormal.

parallel to the posterior condylar axis (**Figure 7**). CT traditionally is used for this measurement, but MRI also has been used. However, MRI may underestimate the TTTG distance by 2.3 mm, and this possibility should be considered when determining surgical treatment.[25] Variability in the TTTG distance has been identified based on differences in measurement techniques. An MRI study of patients without patellar instability found that the TTTG distance decreased as patients flexed the knee.[26] Patient-specific factors also have an influence. A correlation was reported between TTTG distance and the age and height of the patient.[27] TTTG distance increased as a function of height regardless of whether the patient had patellar instability. The TTTG distance was found to decrease with increasing age in patients with instability. Because of the variability in TTTG distances, the distance from the tibial tuberosity to the medial border of the posterior cruciate ligament has been proposed as an alternative measurement for determining malalignment.[28] This technique uses two landmarks on the tibia and thereby eliminates the influence of the knee flexion angle as well as the difficulty of measuring TTTG distance in patients with severe trochlear dysplasia. Further study is needed to validate the applicability of the tibial tuberosity–posterior cruciate ligament distance in determining indications for tuberosity osteotomy (TTO).

Dynamic CT and MRI recently have been used to allow objective evaluation of patellofemoral motion and tracking. Dynamic kinematic MRI was used in a study of patients with or without patellar instability, in which

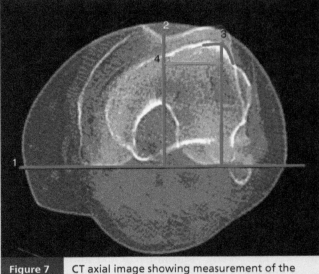

Figure 7 CT axial image showing measurement of the tibial tuberosity and trochlear groove distance (in mm, denoted in red (4) between the deepest portion of the trochlear groove (2) to the apex of the tibial tuberosity (3), on a line parallel to the posterior condylar axis (1).

those with unilateral patellar instability were found to have abnormal patellar subluxation and tilt in both the affected and the asymptomatic knee.[22] Another study used preoperative and postoperative dynamic CT to create a computational reconstruction of in vivo knee function and applied this technique to the assessment of patellar kinematics.[16] Surgical patellar stabilization with tuberosity medialization was found to decrease lateral patellar shift and tilt, particularly at low knee flexion angles.

Patellofemoral Pain Syndrome

Patellofemoral pain syndrome is a nonspecific diagnosis traditionally used to describe anterior knee pain without overt instability. Patients often describe pain with running, jumping, climbing stairs, or prolonged sitting with the knee in a flexed position. Although many theories have been proposed, the cause of patellofemoral pain most often is multifactorial.

An association between joint overload and pain in the patellofemoral joint has been supported by finite element analysis studies that used computational modeling to predict stress distributions within the joint. One study reported greater peak and average strain levels within the joint during squatting maneuvers in women with patellofemoral pain, compared with control subjects.[29] Increased joint stresses and altered contact forces within the patellofemoral joint also may be the result of patellar maltracking. A kinematic study using a three-dimensional optical motion capture system compared patellofemoral kinematics during squatting maneuvers in patients with or without patellofemoral pain.[30] The patients with symptoms had more lateral rotation and lateral translation of the patella at 90° of knee flexion.

Chondral damage in the patellofemoral joint has been implicated in the development of anterior knee pain, although this finding often is nonspecific. A comparison of women with patellofemoral pain and control subjects identified a negative relationship between cartilage thickness and computationally determined strain magnitude within the patellofemoral joint. This relationship was constant in both groups. Those in the group with symptoms had significant reduction in patellar cartilage thickness in comparison with those in the control group.[29]

The mainstay treatment of patellofemoral pain is an exercise program emphasizing strengthening of the quadriceps, core, and hip muscles. A multicenter randomized study found that adding hip- and core-strengthening exercises to an exercise program focused on the knee led to an earlier resolution of pain and increased gains in strength.[31] A systematic review found several factors that significantly predicted successful management of patellar pain with exercise treatment, including negative patellar apprehension, lack of patellar chondral defects, and tibial tuberosity deviation of less than 14.6 mm; in comparison with other patients, these patients also had symptoms less often and of shorter duration, were younger, had a faster VMO response time, and had a larger quadriceps cross-sectional area on MRI.[32]

Patellar taping was found to alter patellofemoral biomechanics, specifically by correcting lateralization and increasing the posterodistal position of the patella.[33] Earlier and increased muscle activity in the vastus medialis was reported when McConnell taping was used during squatting activities.[34] Foot orthoses are used as an adjunct treatment because altered mechanics in the foot affect tibial rotation; orthoses can be used to correct forefoot valgus, rearfoot eversion, and pronation.[32] In a study of foot orthosis use in patients with patellofemoral pain, only 25% reported a marked improvement in pain after 12 weeks of use. In comparison with all patients in the study, those who had a favorable response wore relatively unsupportive footwear, reported a low initial level of pain, had decreased ankle dorsiflexion, and reported an immediate reduction in pain during single-leg squatting while wearing foot orthoses.[35]

Surgical treatment rarely is indicated for patellofemoral pain syndrome. Although lateral retinacular release or lengthening can be used to treat isolated lateral patellofemoral compression syndrome, the indications are limited, and it is critical that patellar instability be ruled out before the procedure is considered. Lateral retinacular release should not be used as an isolated treatment of instability because it can lead to disastrous medial and lateral patellar instability.

Patellofemoral Instability

Most patients who have had a first patellar instability episode can be successfully treated without surgery. Recurrent episodes of instability occur in fewer than half of these patients.[36] Small loose bodies are commonly found but often are asymptomatic.

First Dislocation

The initial goals after an acute patellar dislocation are to control pain, manage swelling, and protect the knee while the symptoms and function gradually improve. Pain and swelling can be treated using a combination of cryotherapy, over-the-counter analgesic medications, and compression. Most patients benefit from using crutches to limit weight bearing. Those whose knee is unstable or uncomfortable should use a knee immobilizer, followed by a functional hinged brace as they gradually return to recreational and occupational activities. Knee aspiration helps to relieve pain in patients with a tense hemarthrosis. Heel slide and quadriceps activation exercises are initiated within a few days of the injury and are followed by a supervised rehabilitation program. Physical therapy allows the patient to progress to light activities within days to weeks and to athletic activities within weeks to a few months.

3: Knee and Leg

Radiographs should be obtained to assess for the presence of a fracture or large osteochondral loose bodies. MRI can be selectively used to assess the status of the extensor mechanism and rule out concomitant intra-articular pathology. Loose bodies are commonly found after dislocation but usually are small, asymptomatic, and not amenable to fixation. The primary indications for surgery after a first-time dislocation are the presence of repairable osteochondral loose bodies or large chondral loose bodies that are or are likely to become symptomatic. Other indications include a concomitant injury such as a meniscal tear, anterior cruciate ligament tear, or persistent subluxation. Many clinicians consider primary repair of the torn MPFL after a first-time dislocation if surgery is necessary for another reason. In the absence of another indication, MPFL repair has not been shown to be beneficial for restoring function or avoiding recurrence. Isolated lateral retinacular release is not effective in treating patellar instability.

Recurrent Instability

The reported incidence of recurrent instability after a first dislocation is 15% to 44%.[36,37] Surgical stabilization is indicated if the patient has recurrent instability and nonsurgical treatment has not been successful. A rehabilitation program often can be considered successful if the patient is willing to modify athletic activities. A patient with substantial malalignment is relatively likely to have ongoing instability episodes, however. Physical examination and imaging studies are used to identify the anatomic and biomechanical factors that created a predisposition to instability and to develop a patient-specific surgical treatment plan. The three main stabilizers of the patellofemoral joint are the muscles that provide dynamic stability (the VMO, hip external rotators, and core), the medial soft-tissue restraints (MPFL and medial retinaculum) and the osteochondral constraints. Weakness of the dynamic stabilizers is treated through rehabilitation. If medial soft-tissue insufficiency is identified, a procedure such as MPFL reconstruction can stabilize the patella by reestablishing the deficient medial soft-tissue checkrein. If the primary deficiency involves the osteochondral restraints, a soft-tissue procedure alone often is insufficient to correct the underlying pathoanatomy, and a TTO may be necessary.

Medial Patellofemoral Ligament Reconstruction

The MPFL provides the primary restraint to pathologic lateral translation. Repair of the MPFL is a good option after an acute first-time dislocation if the location of the tear can be identified. The results are inferior to those of MPFL reconstruction in a patient with recurrent instability. A case study of isolated MPFL repair for recurrent instability found that 8 of 29 knees (28%) had a later recurrence.[38] Numerous techniques for MPFL reconstruction have been described, using a variety of different graft sources and fixation methods, but no one technique is clearly superior. Although the graft tissue is much stronger than the native tissue, MPFL reconstruction alone may not be enough to stabilize the patellofemoral joint in a patient with substantial malalignment. The initial enthusiasm for MPFL reconstruction has been moderated by recognition of the difficulty of the surgical technique and the frequency of complications.[39,40]

Studies of MPFL reconstruction reported success rates of 80% to 96%, with few occurrences of recurrent instability.[41] In general, excellent outcomes were reported, with a high likelihood of resumption of activities of daily living. MPFL reconstruction had a good outcome in 31 knees with recurrent patellar instability.[42] Range of motion, Kujala Anterior Knee Pain Scale scores, and radiographic indexes improved after surgery, and only one patient showed signs of apprehension at follow-up. Studies reporting the results of MPFL reconstruction generally are limited by small sample sizes, short-term follow-up, and the use of concomitant procedures as well as limited information on rehabilitation and return to sports. The largest study to date included 240 consecutive MPFL reconstructions at a single clinic. The mean Kujala score improved from 62.5 to 80.4 at a minimum 1-year follow-up. A concomitant TTO was done in 23% of patients.[43]

The most common complications of MPFL reconstruction are recurrent instability, loss of motion, painful hardware, and patellar fracture. The largest study to date reported a 4.6% rate of recurrent dislocation.[43] In addition, 14% of patients had a positive apprehension sign, and 12% had a flexion deficit of 10° or more. A meta-analysis of 25 studies reporting on a total of 629 knees found that a complication occurred in 164 knees (26.1%).[44] The most common of these complications were recurrent apprehension (52/164 knees), loss of knee flexion (22), painful hardware (19) and patellar fracture (4) (Figure 8). The risk of patellar fracture from violation of the anterior patellar cortex or large-diameter transverse patellar tunnels has led to the development of numerous alternative graft fixation techniques. Appropriate positioning of the bony tunnels and tensioning of the graft are thought to be crucial to the success of MPFL reconstruction. Malpositioning of the femoral tunnel and securing of the graft with excessive tension are associated with medial patellofemoral articular overload, iatrogenic medial subluxation, and recurrent lateral instability.[39,45] Proper positioning of the femoral tunnel

© 2016 American Academy of Orthopaedic Surgeons

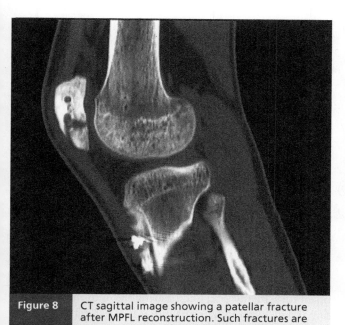

Figure 8 CT sagittal image showing a patellar fracture after MPFL reconstruction. Such fractures are most common with surgical violation of the anterior cortex or creation of large patellar tunnels.

can be difficult, even for experienced surgeons. In a study of MPFL reconstructions, 10 of the 29 femoral tunnels were malpositioned.[40] Intraoperative fluoroscopy is useful for achieving optimal tunnel positioning. Confirmation of normal patellar translation and full knee range of motion is recommended before final graft fixation to prevent overtensioning of the graft.

Tibial Tuberosity Osteotomy

TTO procedures correct malalignment by permanently realigning the abnormal bony anatomy. Modification of the position of the patellar tendon attachment on the tibia changes the forces applied to the patellofemoral joint. A variety of TTO procedures have been described for use with different types of malalignment. A medializing osteotomy such as the Elmslie-Trillat osteotomy is used to correct maltracking caused by a lateralized tuberosity (an increased TTTG distance). A distalizing osteotomy is used to treat patella alta. An anteriorizing (Maquet) or anteromedializing (Fulkerson) osteotomy is used to unload specific areas of articular cartilage wear. Complex distalizing osteotomies incorporate medial or anteromedial displacement of the tuberosity shingle. Medializing osteotomy is indicated if the TTTG distance is greater than 15 to 20 mm. The TTO is modified to the patient's needs by adjusting the amount of medialization, the amount of distalization, and the slope of the osteotomy to achieve the desired degree of correction. Surgeons often combine a TTO with soft-tissue release, repair, or reconstruction.

A study of 34 athletes found that excellent overall results were achieved by anteromedialization combined with lateral retinacular release. Distalization also was used in the patients with patella alta.[46] There is no consensus as to when distalizing osteotomies should be included.

Good to excellent outcomes were reported in 63% to 95% of patients, with modest deterioration of results caused by patellofemoral pain and arthritis.[47] The overall rate of recurrent patellar instability after TTO ranged from 0% to 15%. Male sex, predominant instability symptoms, and low-grade cartilage lesions were generally positive prognostic factors.[47] The location of chondral lesions was found to be correlated with clinical results after anteromedialization.[48] Patients with distal or lateral lesions had improvement after surgery, but patients with medial, proximal, or diffuse lesions had little to no improvement. Postoperative decrease in lateral patellar shift and tilt was reported in a small group of patients who underwent successful TTO.[16]

The most common complications of TTO include painful screws, loss of motion, proximal tibial fracture, shingle fracture, delayed union, nonunion, neurovascular injury, thromboembolic events, and overcorrection. In one study, 49% of patients required screw removal.[46] Painful hardware after TTO is more common with the use of 6.5- or 4.5-mm screws than with 3.5-mm screws. Postoperative fracture of the proximal tibia and tibial tuberosity shingle can be prevented by optimal screw fixation and 6 weeks of postoperative protected weight bearing (**Figure 9**). Patients with proximal patellar lesions may be adversely affected by anteriorization. Overmedialization of the tuberosity increases patellofemoral contact pressures in the medial patellofemoral compartment and may lead to patellofemoral osteoarthritis.[49] Anteromedialization also can cause postoperative changes in the tibiofemoral compartment loading, with unknown long-term consequences.[9]

Trochleoplasty

Trochlear dysplasia is found in 85% of patients with recurrent patellar instability.[50] The goal of a trochleoplasty procedure is to correct the shape of the deficient distal femoral articular constraint. A sulcus-deepening trochleoplasty is preferable to elevation of the lateral condyle to avoid the risk of increasing the lateral patellofemoral joint forces. Trochleoplasty is contraindicated in patients with patellofemoral arthritis, open physes, or isolated anterior knee pain without instability. The procedure generally is performed through an arthrotomy, is technically challenging, and carries a significant risk of cartilage damage, osteoarthritis, and arthrofibrosis. Trochleoplasty almost always is done with a concomitant soft-tissue procedure

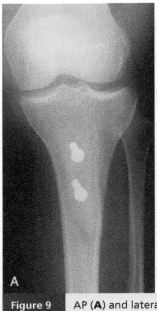
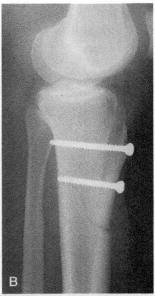

Figure 9 AP (**A**) and lateral (**B**) radiographs showing a tibial fracture that occurred as a complication of tibial tuberosity osteotomy. (Reproduced with permission from Luhmann SJ, Fuhrhop S, O'Donnell JC, Gordon JE: Tibial fractures after tibial tubercle osteotomies for patellar instability: A comparison of three osteotomy configurations. *J Child Orthop* 2011;5[1]:19-26.)

(especially lateral release and MPFL reconstruction) and often with TTO with anteromedialization or distalization. As a result, it is difficult to determine the efficacy of trochleoplasty as an isolated procedure. Recommendations for optimal surgical treatment are elusive because of the variable pathology as well as the variety of procedures described in the literature. Trochleoplasty usually is not necessary to achieve patellar stability, even in the presence of a dysplastic trochlea.[51] Because of the relatively rare indications and the technical difficulty of trochleoplasty, it should be routinely performed only by surgeons with extensive experience in the procedure.

Studies of trochleoplasty combined with MPFL reconstruction found excellent results at a minimum 2-year follow-up.[52,53] The incidence of postoperative pain and radiographic arthrosis was low, especially in those with minimal degenerative changes at the time of the index surgery. Patients with substantial preoperative pain, unsuccessful earlier patellar stabilization, and chondral degenerative changes had the poorest results. Very good results can be obtained even in patients who had undergone unsuccessful patellar stabilization surgery.[54]

A systematic review of studies of patients with severe trochlear dysplasia found a complication rate of 13.4% in those who underwent trochleoplasty compared with 19.2% of those who underwent a nontrocheoplasty procedure.[55]

None of the analyzed studies directly compared the two procedures, and there was no strong evidence of superior clinical outcomes after a trochleoplasty procedure. The patients treated with trochleoplasty had a lower redislocation rate (0.9% vs 16.2%) but a higher rate of deficits in range of motion than those treated with a nontrochleoplasty procedure. The most common complications of trochleoplasty were arthrofibrosis, persistent pain, and osteoarthritis. Postoperative continuous passive motion often is recommended to reduce the risk of stiffness.

Summary

Multiple factors contribute to the stability of the patellofemoral joint, including static restraints, dynamic restraints, osteochondral constraints, and lower extremity alignment. Patellofemoral disorders appear as pain or instability. Identifying and treating the anatomic or functional deficits specific to the individual patient are crucial for directing nonsurgical and surgical treatments. Surgery may be indicated in patients with recurrent instability after unsuccessful nonsurgical treatment. The surgical procedure should be tailored to the specific dynamic and anatomic variations contributing to the patient's instability. Future directions in patellofemoral research include quantification and standardization of the measurements of contributing factors to determine the appropriate indications for surgical correction.

Key Study Points

- The clinician should differentiate between patellofemoral pain and instability based on the patient's history and physical examination.
- The etiology of patellar instability is multifactorial, and successful surgical management requires identifying and considering the contributing factors.
- The complications of patellofemoral instability surgery often can be avoided by using appropriate surgical techniques.

Annotated References

1. Placella G, Tei MM, Sebastiani E, et al: Shape and size of the medial patellofemoral ligament for the best surgical reconstruction: A human cadaveric study. *Knee Surg Sports Traumatol Arthrosc* 2014;22(10):2327-2333.

Analysis of 20 cadaver knees revealed that the MPFL attaches on the proximal third of the patella. On the femur, the attachment was on average 9.5 mm distal and anterior to the adducter tubercle.

2. Schöttle PB, Schmeling A, Rosenstiel N, Weiler A: Radiographic landmarks for femoral tunnel placement in medial patellofemoral ligament reconstruction. *Am J Sports Med* 2007;35(5):801-804.

3. Mochizuki T, Nimura A, Tateishi T, Yamaguchi K, Muneta T, Akita K: Anatomic study of the attachment of the medial patellofemoral ligament and its characteristic relationships to the vastus intermedius. *Knee Surg Sports Traumatol Arthrosc* 2013;21(2):305-310.

Analysis of 16 cadaver knees revealed that the proximal fibers of the MPFL are attached to the vastus intermedius tendon and that the distal fibers are interdigitated with the medial retinaculum attached to the medial margin of the patellar tendon.

4. Smirk C, Morris H: The anatomy and reconstruction of the medial patellofemoral ligament. *Knee* 2003;10(3):221-227.

5. Hasler RM, Gal I, Biedert RM: Landmarks of the normal adult human trochlea based on axial MRI measurements: A cross-sectional study. *Knee Surg Sports Traumatol Arthrosc* 2014;22(10):2372-2376.

In an MRI study of 53 patients without trochlear dysplasia, the mean trochlear depth was 4.0 mm (3.4 mm in women, 4.2 mm in men). The lateral facet contributed 62.6% of the width of the cartilage, and the medial facet contributed 37.4%. Level of evidence: II.

6. Latt LD, Christopher M, Nicolini A, et al: A validated cadaveric model of trochlear dysplasia. *Knee Surg Sports Traumatol Arthrosc* 2014;22(10):2357-2363.

A model of trochlear dysplasia was created in a cadaver study by elevating the floor of the trochlear groove and comparing radiographic markers of dysplasia before and after modification. Decreased trochlear depth, increased sulcus angle, and positive crossing signs were noted.

7. Biyani R, Elias JJ, Saranathan A, et al: Anatomical factors influencing patellar tracking in the unstable patellofemoral joint. *Knee Surg Sports Traumatol Arthrosc* 2014;22(10):2334-2341.

Computational models were created using MRI to represent knees with patellar instability when flexed and loaded to multiple flexion angles. The patellar bisect offset index and lateral tilt were significantly correlated with the lateral trochlear inclination and the distance between the tibial tuberosity and trochlear groove. Level of evidence: II.

8. Teng HL, Chen YJ, Powers CM: Predictors of patellar alignment during weight bearing: An examination of patellar height and trochlear geometry. *Knee* 2014;21(1):142-146.

MRI of the patellofemoral joint at multiple flexion angles in 36 participants indicated that lateral trochlear inclination was the best predictor of lateral patellar displacement and that patellar height was the best predictor of patellar tilt at 0°. Level of evidence: III.

9. Elias JJ, Kilambi S, Goerke DR, Cosgarea AJ: Improving vastus medialis obliquus function reduces pressure applied to lateral patellofemoral cartilage. *J Orthop Res* 2009;27(5):578-583.

A biomechanical study assessed changes in patellofemoral cartilage pressures with VMO loading. Increasing the VMO force significantly decreased the maximum lateral pressure and increased the maximum medial pressure at different knee flexion angles.

10. Shalhoub S, Maletsky LP: Variation in patellofemoral kinematics due to changes in quadriceps loading configuration during in vitro testing. *J Biomech* 2014;47(1):130-136.

In vitro kinematic simulation of 14 knees indicated that a weak vastus medialis increased patellar lateral shift and abduction rotation and that a weak vastus lateralis increased patellar medial shift and adduction rotation.

11. Sheehan FT, Borotikar BS, Behnam AJ, Alter KE: Alterations in in vivo knee joint kinematics following a femoral nerve branch block of the vastus medialis: Implications for patellofemoral pain syndrome. *Clin Biomech (Bristol, Avon)* 2012;27(6):525-531.

In kinematic analysis of asymptomatic knees of women using dynamic cine phase-contrast MRI, administering a motor branch block to the VMO increased patellar lateral shift, tibiofemoral lateral shift, and tibiofemoral external rotation.

12. Jan MH, Lin DH, Lin JJ, Lin CH, Cheng CK, Lin YF: Differences in sonographic characteristics of the vastus medialis obliquus between patients with patellofemoral pain syndrome and healthy adults. *Am J Sports Med* 2009;37(9):1743-1749.

Sonographic analysis of the VMO in 54 patients revealed that insertion level, fiber angle, and muscle volume were significantly smaller in those with patellofemoral pain than in control subjects. Level of evidence: III.

13. Van Tiggelen D, Cowan S, Coorevits P, Duvigneaud N, Witvrouw E: Delayed vastus medialis obliquus to vastus lateralis onset timing contributes to the development of patellofemoral pain in previously healthy men: A prospective study. *Am J Sports Med* 2009;37(6):1099-1105.

Surface electromyographic analysis of the VMO and vastus lateralis in 79 healthy men before 6 weeks of military basic training found a significant delay in VMO activity in those who later had patellofemoral pain. Level of evidence: II.

14. Pal S, Draper CE, Fredericson M, et al: Patellar maltracking correlates with vastus medialis activation delay in patellofemoral pain patients. *Am J Sports Med* 2011;39(3):590-598.

Based on weight-bearing MRI, patellar lateral tilt was correlated with an increase in the ratio of vastus lateralis to vastus medialis activation. Lateral translation and tilt were correlated with vastus medialis delay in patients with pain arising from maltracking. Level of evidence: III.

15. Diederichs G, Köhlitz T, Kornaropoulos E, Heller MO, Vollnberg B, Scheffler S: Magnetic resonance imaging analysis of rotational alignment in patients with patellar dislocations. *Am J Sports Med* 2013;41(1):51-57.

MRI of 30 patients with patellar instability and 30 control subjects revealed that symptomatic knees had approximately 1.6 times more femoral antetorsion and knee rotation than knees of control subjects and almost three times more mechanical axis deviation. Level of evidence: III.

16. Elias JJ, Carrino JA, Saranathan A, Guseila LM, Tanaka MJ, Cosgarea AJ: Variations in kinematics and function following patellar stabilization including tibial tuberosity realignment. *Knee Surg Sports Traumatol Arthrosc* 2014;22(10):2350-2356.

Computational models of six knees based on dynamic CT were used to quantify lateral shift and tilt of the patella at varying flexion angles. Comparison of CT before and after stabilization surgery showed decreased shift and tilt at low flexion angles. Level of evidence: II.

17. Charles MD, Haloman S, Chen L, Ward SR, Fithian D, Afra R: Magnetic resonance imaging-based topographical differences between control and recurrent patellofemoral instability patients. *Am J Sports Med* 2013;41(2):374-384.

A retrospective review of MRI of 40 patients with recurrent patellar instability and 81 control subjects showed that the symptomatic knees had more patellar tilt, patellar height, and trochlear dysplasia. Level of evidence: III.

18. Ward SR, Terk MR, Powers CM: Patella alta: Association with patellofemoral alignment and changes in contact area during weight-bearing. *J Bone Joint Surg Am* 2007;89(8):1749-1755.

19. Arnbjörnsson A, Egund N, Rydling O, Stockerup R, Ryd L: The natural history of recurrent dislocation of the patella. Long-term results of conservative and operative treatment. *J Bone Joint Surg Br* 1992;74(1):140-142.

20. Herrington L: Knee valgus angle during single leg squat and landing in patellofemoral pain patients and controls. *Knee* 2014;21(2):514-517.

Twelve women with unilateral patellofemoral pain and 30 asymptomatic control subjects were assessed for frontal plane projection angle during single-leg squatting and single-leg hopping. Patients in the symptomatic group had significantly greater frontal plane angles in both tests.

21. Nakagawa TH, Moriya ET, Maciel CD, Serrão FV: Trunk, pelvis, hip, and knee kinematics, hip strength, and gluteal muscle activation during a single-leg squat in males and females with and without patellofemoral pain syndrome. *J Orthop Sports Phys Ther* 2012;42(6):491-501.

A study of 80 patients found that patients with patellar pain had greater trunk lean and contralateral pelvic drop and knee abduction as well as 17% less hip adduction and 17% less hip external rotation strength on single-leg squat testing than those without pain.

22. Regalado G, Lintula H, Eskelinen M, et al: Dynamic KINE-MRI in patellofemoral instability in adolescents. *Knee Surg Sports Traumatol Arthrosc* 2014;22(11):2795-2802.

Kinematic MRI was used to compare patients with patellar instability and control subjects. A significant difference was noted in bisect offset, lateral patellar displacement and patellar tilt angles between the affected knees, unaffected knees in patients, and healthy knees in control subjects. Level of evidence: II.

23. Felus J, Kowalczyk B: Age-related differences in medial patellofemoral ligament injury patterns in traumatic patellar dislocation: Case series of 50 surgically treated children and adolescents. *Am J Sports Med* 2012;40(10):2357-2364.

The locations of MPFL injuries in first-time traumatic patellar dislocations were compared using sonography. Forty-six percent of patients had injury in more than one location. Skeletally immature patients had a greater incidence of patellar-side injury than skeletally mature patients (79% versus 54%). Level of evidence: IV.

24. Petri M, von Falck C, Broese M, et al: Influence of rupture patterns of the medial patellofemoral ligament (MPFL) on the outcome after operative treatment of traumatic patellar dislocation. *Knee Surg Sports Traumatol Arthrosc* 2013;21(3):683-689.

A retrospective study of 40 patients who underwent MRI after first-time traumatic patellar dislocation found that patients with patellar-based MPFL rupture were comparatively young (mean age, 19.5 years) and that older patients were more likely to sustain femoral-side ruptures (mean age, 25.4 years). Level of evidence: IV.

25. Camp CL, Stuart MJ, Krych AJ, et al: CT and MRI measurements of tibial tubercle-trochlear groove distances are not equivalent in patients with patellar instability. *Am J Sports Med* 2013;41(8):1835-1840.

A randomized, blinded study used CT and MRI of patients with patellar instability to determine TTTG distances. The mean TTTG distance was 16.9 mm on CT and 14.7 mm on MRI. Interrater reliability was excellent for each modality but only fair when the two modalities were compared. Level of evidence: II.

26. Dietrich TJ, Betz M, Pfirrmann CW, Koch PP, Fucentese SF: End-stage extension of the knee and its influence on tibial tuberosity-trochlear groove distance (TTTG) in asymptomatic volunteers. *Knee Surg Sports Traumatol Arthrosc* 2014;22(1):214-218.

Thirty asymptomatic individuals underwent MRI at 0°, 15°, and 30° of knee flexion. Mean TTTG distances were found to significantly decrease with increasing knee flexion.

27. Pennock AT, Alam M, Bastrom T: Variation in tibial tubercle-trochlear groove measurement as a function of age, sex, size, and patellar instability. *Am J Sports Med* 2014;42(2):389-393.

TTTG distance was measured on MRI, and normal values were reported. TTTG distance increased with overall height in patients with patellar instability and control subjects, and it decreased with age in those with instability. Level of evidence: III.

28. Seitlinger G, Scheurecker G, Högler R, Labey L, Innocenti B, Hofmann S: Tibial tubercle-posterior cruciate ligament distance: A new measurement to define the position of the tibial tubercle in patients with patellar dislocation. *Am J Sports Med* 2012;40(5):1119-1125.

A new tibial tubercle–posterior cruciate ligament distance measurement was described as an alternative to TTTG distance. Mean values were 18.4 mm in control subjects and 21.9 mm in patients with patellar dislocation. A value greater than 24 mm was considered abnormal. Level of evidence: II.

29. Ho KY, Keyak JH, Powers CM: Comparison of patella bone strain between females with and without patellofemoral pain: A finite element analysis study. *J Biomech* 2014;47(1):230-236.

Finite element analysis of 10 patients with symptoms and 10 control subjects showed that the patients had greater peak and average principal strain in the patella. Patellar cartilage thickness was negatively associated with peak minimum and maximum principal patellar strain.

30. Wilson NA, Press JM, Koh JL, Hendrix RW, Zhang LQ: In vivo noninvasive evaluation of abnormal patellar tracking during squatting in patients with patellofemoral pain. *J Bone Joint Surg Am* 2009;91(3):558-566.

An optoelectronic motion capture system was used to record three-dimensional patellar kinematics in 9 patients with patellofemoral pain syndrome and 10 control subjects. At 90° of knee flexion, the patients had increased lateral spin and lateral translation.

31. Ferber R, Bolgla L, Earl-Boehm JE, Emery C, Hamstra-Wright K: Strengthening of the hip and core versus knee muscles for the treatment of patellofemoral pain: A multicenter, randomized controlled trial. *J Athl Train* [Published online ahead of print November 3, 2014].

Patients with patellofemoral pain were assigned to a 6-week knee- or hip-exercise protocol. Visual analog scale scores improved in patients in both groups but improved 1 week earlier in those in the hip protocol, who also had greater overall gains in strength.

32. Lack S, Barton C, Vicenzino B, Morrissey D: Outcome predictors for conservative patellofemoral pain management: A systematic review and meta-analysis. *Sports Med* 2014;44(12):1703-1716.

A systematic review of outcome predictors in nonsurgical management of patellofemoral pain found that several factors were associated with successful exercise intervention: absence of chondromalacia patella and TTTG distance of less than 14.6 mm, as well as a relatively short symptom duration, low frequency of pain, young age, fast VMO reflex response time, and large cross-sectional area of the quadriceps on MRI.

33. Song CY, Huang HY, Chen SC, Lin JJ, Chang AH: Effects of femoral rotational taping on pain, lower extremity kinematics, and muscle activation in female patients with patellofemoral pain. *J Sci Med Sport* 2014.

Electromyelography was performed in 16 patients with patellofemoral pain and 8 control subjects during single-leg squatting after random assignment to kinesiotaping, sham taping, or no taping. In the patients with symptoms, kinesiotaping shifted the patella posteriorly and distally.

34. Lee SE, Cho SH: The effect of McConnell taping on vastus medialis and lateralis activity during squatting in adults with patellofemoral pain syndrome. *J Exerc Rehabil* 2013;9(2):326-330.

Sixteen patients with patellofemoral pain received no taping, placebo taping, or McConnell taping. Vastus medialis activity and its ratio to vastus lateralis activity were greater after McConnell taping than no taping.

35. Barton CJ, Menz HB, Crossley KM: Clinical predictors of foot orthoses efficacy in individuals with patellofemoral pain. *Med Sci Sports Exerc* 2011;43(9):1603-1610.

Twenty-five percent of patients reported improvement in patellofemoral pain after 12 weeks of wearing foot orthoses. The percentage increased to 78% if three of these criteria were met: use of relatively unsupportive footwear, visual analog pain scale score lower than 22, weight-bearing ankle dorsiflexion of less than 41°, and reduced pain during single-leg squatting while wearing the orthoses.

36. Cofield RH, Bryan RS: Acute dislocation of the patella: Results of conservative treatment. *J Trauma* 1977;17(7):526-531.

37. Fithian DC, Paxton EW, Stone ML, et al: Epidemiology and natural history of acute patellar dislocation. *Am J Sports Med* 2004;32(5):1114-1121.

38. Camp CL, Krych AJ, Dahm DL, Levy BA, Stuart MJ: Medial patellofemoral ligament repair for recurrent patellar dislocation. *Am J Sports Med* 2010;38(11):2248-2254.

Retrospective review a minimum of 2 years after 27 patients (29 knees) underwent MPFL repair for recurrent dislocation found that 28% of patients had a recurrent dislocation. The only significant risk factor was nonanatomic MPFL repair at the medial femoral condyle. Level of evidence: IV.

39. Bollier M, Fulkerson J, Cosgarea A, Tanaka M: Technical failure of medial patellofemoral ligament reconstruction. *Arthroscopy* 2011;27(8):1153-1159.

Five patients with malpositioned femoral tunnels and disabling symptoms required revision MPFL reconstruction. The effects of a malpositioned femoral graft were described, with strategies to identify the femoral insertion during surgery. Level of evidence: IV.

40. Servien E, Fritsch B, Lustig S, et al: In vivo positioning analysis of medial patellofemoral ligament reconstruction. *Am J Sports Med* 2011;39(1):134-139.

5: Knee and Leg

A prospective study of 29 patients undergoing MPFL reconstruction found that that 19 femoral tunnels were in the proper location and 10 were in an anterior and/or high position. This study highlighted the difficulty of reproducible anatomic femoral tunnel positioning. Level of evidence: IV.

41. Buckens CF, Saris DB: Reconstruction of the medial patellofemoral ligament for treatment of patellofemoral instability: A systematic review. *Am J Sports Med* 2010;38(1):181-188.

    A systematic review of 14 studies found generally excellent functional outcomes after MPFL reconstruction. Most studies were small, had limited follow-up, and encompassed additional procedures. As a result, it was difficult to distinguish the determining factors in the outcomes. Level of evidence: IV.

42. Deie M, Ochi M, Adachi N, Shibuya H, Nakamae A: Medial patellofemoral ligament reconstruction fixed with a cylindrical bone plug and a grafted semitendinosus tendon at the original femoral site for recurrent patellar dislocation. *Am J Sports Med* 2011;39(1):140-145.

    Thirty-one knees in 29 patients with recurrent patellar dislocation were treated with MPFL reconstruction. At a minimum 2-year follow-up, the mean Kujala Anterior Knee Pain Scale score had improved from 64 to 94.5 points. One patient had residual apprehension, but there were no redislocations. Level of evidence: IV.

43. Enderlein D, Nielsen T, Christiansen SE, Faunø P, Lind M: Clinical outcome after reconstruction of the medial patellofemoral ligament in patients with recurrent patella instability. *Knee Surg Sports Traumatol Arthrosc* 2014;22(10):2458-2464.

    A prospective study of 224 patients undergoing MPFL reconstruction with a gracilis tendon autograft found improvement in mean Kujala score from 62.5 to 80.4 at 1-year follow-up. The revision rate was 2.8%. MPFL reconstruction consistently normalized patella stability and improved knee function. Age greater than 30 years, obesity, cartilage injury, and female sex were predictors of a poor subjective outcome. Level of evidence: IV.

44. Shah JN, Howard JS, Flanigan DC, Brophy RH, Carey JL, Lattermann C: A systematic review of complications and failures associated with medial patellofemoral ligament reconstruction for recurrent patellar dislocation. *Am J Sports Med* 2012;40(8):1916-1923.

    A systematic review of 25 articles on MPFL reconstruction found a total of 164 complications in 629 knees (26.1%). The rate of recurrent subluxation was 4.3%, and 7.7% of patients had continued apprehension without subluxation.

45. Elias JJ, Cosgarea AJ: Technical errors during medial patellofemoral ligament reconstruction could overload medial patellofemoral cartilage: A computational analysis. *Am J Sports Med* 2006;34(9):1478-1485.

46. Tjoumakaris FP, Forsythe B, Bradley JP: Patellofemoral instability in athletes: Treatment via modified Fulkerson osteotomy and lateral release. *Am J Sports Med* 2010;38(5):992-999.

    Forty-one knees in 34 athletes underwent Fulkerson osteotomy and lateral retinacular release for patellofemoral instability. One patient had recurrent instability at a minimum 22-month follow-up. Seventeen patients had symptomatic hardware removed. Level of evidence: IV.

47. Naveed MA, Ackroyd CE, Porteous AJ: Long-term (ten- to 15-year) outcome of arthroscopically assisted Elmslie-Trillat tibial tubercle osteotomy. *Bone Joint J* 2013;95-B(4):478-485.

    In a study of patients who underwent an Elmslie-Trillat TTO, 19 knees (79.2%) had a good or excellent outcome at 4-year follow-up, and 15 knees (62.5%) had a good or excellent outcome at a minimum 10-year follow-up. Intraoperative chondral damage created a predisposition to the development of patellofemoral osteoarthritis. Level of evidence: IV.

48. Pidoriano AJ, Weinstein RN, Buuck DA, Fulkerson JP: Correlation of patellar articular lesions with results from anteromedial tibial tubercle transfer. *Am J Sports Med* 1997;25(4):533-537.

49. Kuroda R, Kambic H, Valdevit A, Andrish JT: Articular cartilage contact pressure after tibial tuberosity transfer: A cadaveric study. *Am J Sports Med* 2001;29(4):403-409.

50. Dejour H, Walch G, Nove-Josserand L, Guier C: Factors of patellar instability: An anatomic radiographic study. *Knee Surg Sports Traumatol Arthrosc* 1994;2(1):19-26.

51. Thaunat M, Bessiere C, Pujol N, Boisrenoult P, Beaufils P: Recession wedge trochleoplasty as an additional procedure in the surgical treatment of patellar instability with major trochlear dysplasia: Early results. *Orthop Traumatol Surg Res* 2011;97(8):833-845.

    Seventeen patients (19 knees) with severe trochlear dysplasia and patellofemoral instability underwent recession wedge trochleoplasty. At a minimum 1-year follow-up, the trochlear prominence was reduced from a mean 4.8 mm to –0.8 mm. Two patients had instability, and three required further surgery. Level of evidence: IV.

52. Nelitz M, Dreyhaupt J, Lippacher S: Combined trochleoplasty and medial patellofemoral ligament reconstruction for recurrent patellar dislocations in severe trochlear dysplasia: A minimum 2-year follow-up study. *Am J Sports Med* 2013;41(5):1005-1012.

    Twenty-three consecutive patients (26 knees) with patellofemoral instability and severe trochlear dysplasia underwent combined trochleoplasty and MPFL reconstruction. At a minimum 2-year follow-up, there was significant improvement in Kujala, International Knee Documentation Committee Subjective Knee Evaluation Form, and visual analog scale scores. No dislocations occurred, and 22 patients (95.7%) were satisfied or very satisfied. Level of evidence: III.

53. Ntagiopoulos PG, Byn P, Dejour D: Midterm results of comprehensive surgical reconstruction including sulcus-deepening trochleoplasty in recurrent patellar dislocations with high-grade trochlear dysplasia. *Am J Sports Med* 2013;41(5):998-1004.

Twenty-seven patients (31 knees) with recurrent patellar dislocation and high-grade trochlear dysplasia without previous surgery underwent sulcus-deepening trochleoplasty combined with additional bone or soft-tissue surgery. There were no postoperative dislocations or radiographic evidence of patellofemoral osteoarthritis at a minimum 2-year follow-up. The mean Kujala score improved from 59 to 87. The apprehension sign remained positive in 19.3% of patients. Level of evidence: IV.

54. Dejour D, Byn P, Ntagiopoulos PG: The Lyon's sulcus-deepening trochleoplasty in previous unsuccessful patellofemoral surgery. *Int Orthop* 2013;37(3):433-439.

Twenty-two patients (24 knees) who had undergone unsuccessful patellofemoral surgery underwent sulcus-deepening trochleoplasty combined with additional soft-tissue and bony surgery. At a minimum 2-year follow-up, Kujala scores had improved, and no patient had postoperative instability or patellofemoral arthritis. Level of evidence: IV.

55. Song GY, Hong L, Zhang H, et al: Trochleoplasty versus nontrochleoplasty procedures in treating patellar instability caused by severe trochlear dysplasia. *Arthroscopy* 2014;30(4):523-532.

A systematic review of 17 studies of patients with patellar instability and severe trochlear dysplasia treated with trochleoplasty (329 patients) or a nontrochleoplasty procedure (130 patients) found lower redislocation and osteoarthritis rates but poorer range of motion after trochleoplasty. Level of evidence: IV.

Chapter 18

Articular Cartilage of the Knee

Andreas H. Gomoll, MD   Brian J. Chilelli, MD

Abstract

Injuries to articular cartilage of the knee are increasingly common. Chondral lesions may involve only the superficial layer of articular cartilage or may extend more deeply to affect the underlying subchondral bone, leading to an injury to the entire osteochondral unit. Symptomatic defects are often associated with injury to other structures of the knee and can lead to significant pain and dysfunction. Management of these conditions continues to be challenging despite recent advances in surgical technique and cartilage repair technology. It is crucial for the surgeon to evaluate the articular cartilage and subchondral bone as an intimately related unit. Several procedures are available to treat both the chondral and subchondral components of the osteochondral unit.

Keywords: articular cartilage; cartilage repair; cartilage restoration; chondral defect; osteochondral defect

Introduction

Articular cartilage injuries are common and may be idiopathic, associated with repetitive microtrauma, or traumatic in etiology. Defects that extend beyond the superficial chondral surface have the potential to affect the underlying subchondral bone. Careful attention to articular cartilage and subchondral bone pathology should

Dr. Gomoll or an immediate family member serves as a paid consultant to Aesculap/B. Braun, Cartiheal, Geistlich, Genzyme, Novartis, and Science for BioMaterials and serves as a board member, owner, officer, or committee member of the American Orthopaedic Society for Sports Medicine and the International Cartilage Repair Society. Neither Dr. Chilelli nor any immediate family member has received anything of value from or has stock or stock options held in a commercial company or institution related directly or indirectly to the subject of this chapter.

be given and articular cartilage and subchondral bone should be viewed as a closely related osteochondral unit. Any disturbance of this osteochondral unit can lead to altered biomechanics and abnormal joint contact pressures, leading to an inflammatory response. This response may result in pain and dysfunction with the theoretical risk of widespread joint degeneration. An initial trial of nonsurgical management is usually warranted in the form of rest, activity modification, anti-inflammmatory medications, physical therapy, bracing, or injections. Patients who do not respond to conservative measures may benefit from surgical intervention. Surgical management should focus on removing inflammatory mediators and restoring the osteochondral unit. Surgical options include arthroscopic débridement, bone marrow stimulation, osteochondral autograft transfer, osteochondral allograft transplantation, autologous chondrocyte implantation, as well as various newer, emerging techniques. This chapter will concentrate on the evaluation, diagnosis, and management of injuries to the interrelated osteochondral unit of articular cartilage and subchondral bone in the knee.

Basic Science

Articular cartilage is a complex and highly organized structure. The primary component of articular cartilage is type II hyaline cartilage, which decreases force through the joint by dissipating stress to the subchondral bone and facilitating low-friction motion. Articular cartilage is aneural, alymphatic, and lacks a blood supply. These characteristics contribute to the poor healing potential of articular cartilage and its inability to restore its structure after injury. Chondral defects have little potential for self-repair or spontaneous healing.[1-3] A full-thickness defect that penetrates the subchondral bone may release bone marrow content, mesenchymal cells, and growth factors. An intralesional clot may then form, followed by a fibrocartilaginous scar primarily composed of type I collagen.[4] The biomechanical properties and wear characteristics of this fibrocartilage were found to be inferior to those of hyaline cartilage, which is primarily composed of type II collagen.[5,6]

3: Knee and Leg

Epidemiology and Natural History

Chondral or osteochondral lesions were found in 61% to 66% of patients undergoing knee arthroscopy.[7-9] A recent systematic review estimated a 36% prevalence of focal chondral defects of the knee in athletes.[10] The true incidence and prevalence are difficult to determine because many defects are asymptomatic. A cartilage defect can be idiopathic, traumatic, and/or associated with repetitive microtrauma. Cartilage damage is often associated with injury to another anatomic structure of the knee and sometimes occurs in conjunction with malalignment. Acute anterior cruciate ligament tears and meniscal derangement are highly correlated with chondral defects.[11,12] A chondral or osteochondral lesion was found in more than 90% of patients with a patellar dislocation.[13] The natural history of articular cartilage defects is not completely understood, but any disruption of the osteochondral unit can alter its biomechanics and increase the joint contact forces to the surrounding chondral surfaces and subchondral bone. The resulting mechanical wear and loose body formation can lead to an inflammatory response, and subsequent release of cartilage-degrading enzymes potentially causing joint degeneration. If left untreated, chondral defects can lead to osteoarthritis.[14,15]

Clinical Evaluation

Patients with a symptomatic chondral defect typically have knee pain and swelling. Instability and mechanical symptoms such as catching and locking may be present. A traumatic etiology is often associated with a specific event such as a fall or a twisting injury while playing sports. The patient may not recall a specific event preceding the insidious onset of an idiopathic lesion or a lesion associated with repetitive microtrauma. A detailed history as to the onset of symptoms should be followed by a comprehensive physical examination, although neither the history nor examination is sensitive or specific for a cartilage defect compared with another type of intra-articular derangement. The physical examination begins with a gait analysis and continues with an assessment for effusion, deformity, contracture, malalignment, range of motion, ligament stability, and patellar maltracking, with close attention to the possible presence of a mechanical blockage or crepitus.

The routine radiographic studies include the standing AP, lateral, Merchant, and 45° flexion PA views. The radiographs are scrutinized for fractures, loose bodies, osteophytes, and joint space narrowing. Full–limb length radiographs may be helpful to determine mechanical alignment in a patient with a known chondral defect. MRI is effective for evaluating the articular cartilage and detecting subchondral edema. Determining the size of the lesion on imaging is helpful for prognostic purposes and can help guide surgical decision making. The size of a lesion is often underestimated by more than 60% on MRI, however.[16] Ligamentous and meniscal structures should be assessed for any evidence of injury. CT can provide fine anatomic detail of subchondral bone if a bone injury is suspected, as after subchondral drilling, bone grafting, or osteochondral allograft transplantation, for example. The addition of intra-articular gadolinium to CT allows excellent visualization of the articular cartilage. The distance from the tibial tubercle to the trochlear groove or from the tibial tubercle to the posterior cruciate ligament can be determined from axial MRI or CT in patients with patellofemoral instability or a patellofemoral chondral defect.

Nonsurgical Treatment

Most articular cartilage lesions are initially managed with rest, activity modification, anti-inflammatory medications, and physical therapy. Steroid or viscosupplementation (hyaluronic acid) injection may decrease inflammation and improve symptoms, especially in a patient who is sedentary or older than 55 years. However, physiologic age is often more important than chronologic age when determining treatment options. The use of an unloader brace can be effective in a patient with unilateral compartment overload, in which a chondral defect is exposed to excessive forces as a result of malalignment or meniscal deficiency.

 Video 18.1: Combined Cartilage Restoration and Distal Realignment for Patellar and Trochlear Chondral Lesions. Peter Chalmers, MD; Adam Yanke, MD; Seth Sherman, MD; Vasili Karas, BS; Brian J. Cole, MD, MBA (24 min)

Surgical Treatment

Patients whose symptoms are not relieved by nonsurgical measures should be considered for surgical intervention. The patient's age, activity level, expectations, defect size, and associated injuries are important factors in determining whether surgery is appropriate. A patient who is considered to be a candidate for surgery must understand that many cartilage-restoring procedures require extensive rehabilitation, a return to activity will not be possible for an extended period, and high-impact activity such as running or basketball is discouraged.

© 2016 American Academy of Orthopaedic Surgeons

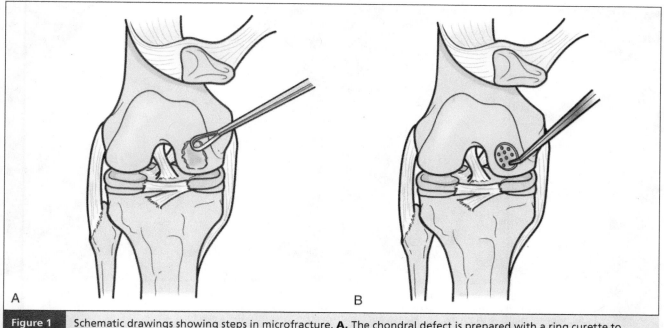

Figure 1 Schematic drawings showing steps in microfracture. **A,** The chondral defect is prepared with a ring curette to create stable borders. **B,** The subchondral plate is penetrated multiple times 2 to 3 mm apart to a depth of 2 to 4 mm.

Arthroscopic Débridement

Arthroscopic débridement is commonly done as a first-line procedure. The goal of the surgery is to remove inflammatory mediators, loose bodies, and unstable chondral or meniscal flaps. Arthroscopic débridement can be useful for a patient who is not a good candidate for cartilage restoration (older than 55 years, advanced degenerative changes, high BMI), or a patient who is unwilling to adhere to a strict postoperative rehabilitation protocol. Data are lacking to support the long-term efficacy of arthroscopic débridement, however.

Bone Marrow Stimulation

Bone marrow stimulation using microfracture, intralesional drilling, or abrasion arthroplasty is commonly done to treat a full-thickness chondral defect. A review of more than 163,000 cartilage procedures in the knee over a 6-year period found that 98% consisted of microfracture or chondroplasty.[17] Bone marrow stimulation can be done arthroscopically, through a miniopen approach, or through an open medial or lateral parapatellar approach. The arthroscopic and miniopen methods most frequently are used.

The microfracture technique involves preparing the lesion with an arthroscopic shaver or curette to remove loose chondral flaps and create a contained lesion with stable borders of healthy cartilage (**Figures 1** and **2**). The subchondral plate is penetrated multiple times to recruit mesenchymal stem cells from the bone marrow into the defect; penetration is done 2 to 3 mm apart and 2 to 4 mm deep perpendicular to the surface.[18] A microfracture awl is traditionally used to penetrate the subchondral plate, but recent investigations found that drilling provides a superior result.[19-22] Bone marrow stimulation causes formation of an intralesional clot with the potential to form fibrocartilage repair tissue (type I cartilage). Focal lesions smaller than 4 cm^2 in patients younger than 30 years were found to be most amenable to this technique.[23] Microfracture should be avoided if subchondral bone deficiency is present.

Postoperative rehabilitation generally involves a prolonged period of non–weight bearing or partial weight bearing. The use of passive motion is recommended beginning immediately after surgery, generally by using a continuous passive motion (CPM) machine for a period of 6 weeks. The goal is to return the patient to sports activity 6 to 9 months after surgery.

Osteochondral Autograft Transfer

Osteochondral autograft transfer (OAT), also called mosaicplasty, involves harvesting one or more osteochondral cylinders from a minimally weight-bearing area of the femur for transfer to a defect in a more heavily weight-bearing area (**Figures 3** and **4**). OAT can be done as an arthroscopic, open, or miniopen procedure. The miniopen procedure is increasingly recognized as a useful compromise offering minimal morbidity and maximal precision.

3: Knee and Leg

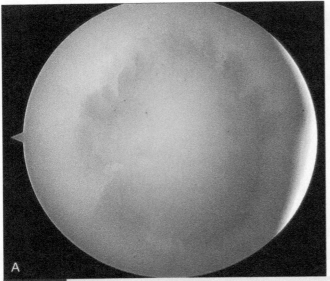
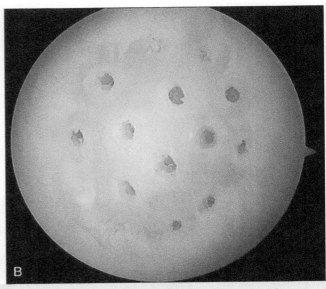

Figure 2 Arthroscopic views shows steps in microfracture. **A,** The chondral defect as prepared for microfracture, with loose chondral flaps removed to create a healthy, stable rim of articular cartilage. **B,** Multiple penetration of the subchondral plate with an awl to release bone marrow contents into the defect is shown.

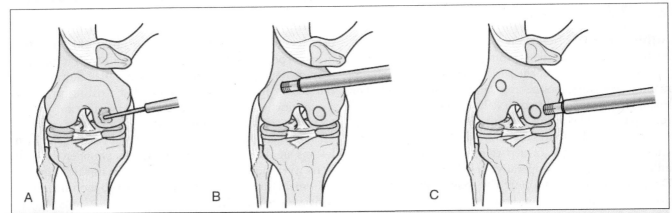

Figure 3 Schematic drawings showing steps in osteochondral autograft transfer. **A,** The size and shape of the chondral defect are determined, and the defect is prepared using proprietary equipment. **B,** The donor osteochondral cylinder is obtained from the intercondylar region of the peripheral trochlea. **C,** The osteochondral cylinder is inserted into the prepared recipient tunnel using a press fit.

Most commonly, diagnostic arthroscopy is followed by OAT through a miniopen approach. The size and shape of the defect are determined, and the defect is prepared with the use of proprietary equipment. The femoral donor site is selected based on the size and contour of the recipient defect. The recommended donor sites include the intercondylar notch region or the peripheral trochlea (medial or lateral) above the level of the sulcus terminalis. The lateral trochlea is larger than the medial trochlea, but the medial trochlea has lower contact pressures.[24] The osteochondral cylinder is obtained using a harvesting chisel. To obtain an even chondral surface, it is important to ensure that the harvesting chisel remains perpendicular to the articular cartilage.[25] The graft is inserted into the prepared recipient tunnel using a press-fit technique. Aggressive impaction of the chondral surface of the graft should be avoided to minimize chondrocyte death.[26-28] Contact pressures and forces are normal when grafts are placed flush with the surrounding articular cartilage. Small incongruities, especially if the graft is proud, can increase contact pressures.[29]

One of the main advantages of this procedure is that it provides hyaline cartilage at the defect site.[25,30] In addition, OAT can be successfully used in the setting of subchondral bone loss or abnormality. The drawbacks of OAT include possible donor site morbidity and the

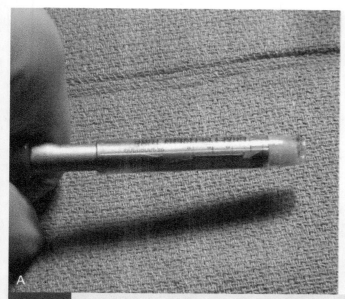
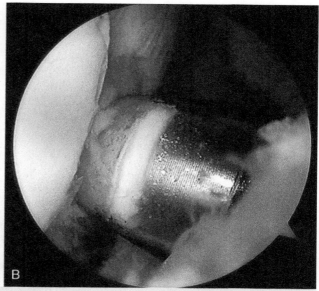

Figure 4 Photographs showing steps in osteochondral autograft transfer. **A,** An osteochondral cylinder has been harvested and is ready to be inserted into the prepared recipient site. **B,** The osteochondral cylinder is inserted into the recipient site using a press fit.

limited amount of graft material that can be harvested. As a result, OAT is ideal for chondral or osteochondral defects smaller than 2 cm².

Postoperative rehabilitation includes toe-touch weight bearing for 4 to 8 weeks, depending on the size of the lesion and the number of osteochondral cylinders used. Early progressive motion is encouraged with use of a CPM machine. A return to athletic activity is delayed for 4 to 6 months.

Osteochondral Allograft Transplantation

Osteochondral allograft transplantation is an excellent option for chondral or osteochondral defects larger than 2 to 4 cm². This procedure also can be used as a salvage option after an unsuccessful cartilage repair surgery. The defects most commonly treated are in the weight-bearing medial or lateral femoral condyle. Tibial and patellofemoral defects can be treated with this procedure, but tibial access requires extensive surgical dissection. The complex patellar and trochlear surface geometry presents challenges for graft matching and preparation. Fresh refrigerated allografts are used rather than frozen or freeze-dried specimens to ensure the highest level of chondrocyte viability.[31] The recommended time from graft harvest to transplantation is no more than 28 days because at that time at least 70% of chondrocytes are viable.[32] Ideally the graft is from the same side and compartment as the recipient defect and is size matched.

The technique is similar to that for OAT except that the cylinder obtained from the donor cadaver hemicondyle is larger than can be obtained in an autograft (Figures 5 and 6). A medial or lateral parapatellar arthrotomy is performed, and the lesion is identified. A guidewire is placed in the center of the defect for sizing. When the size has been determined, the defect is prepared using proprietary equipment. The defect is reamed to remove the abnormal cartilage and approximately 8 to 10 mm of subchondral bone. The recipient tunnel is created, and the donor osteochondral cylinder is taken from the fresh allograft specimen. An attempt is made to harvest from a matching area of the allograft specimen so that the contour will match the recipient area. The donor cylindrical plug is inserted into the recipient tunnel with a press fit. As in OAT, the use of a mallet should be avoided during insertion to minimize chondrocyte death.

Postoperative rehabilitation includes toe-touch weight bearing for 6 to 12 weeks. Early progressive motion is encouraged with use of a CPM machine. Some surgeons recommend limiting flexion to 45° during the first 4 to 6 weeks in patients treated for a patellofemoral lesion. High-loading activities such as running and jumping should be avoided for 6 to 12 months after surgery.

Autologous Chondrocyte Implantation

Autologous chondrocyte implantation (ACI) is an articular cartilage–restoring procedure used to treat 2 to 4 cm² or larger full-thickness chondral defects of the knee (**Figures 7** and **8**). ACI is a two-stage procedure in which an initial arthroscopic cartilage biopsy is followed by 4 to 6 weeks of in vitro chondrocyte expansion and

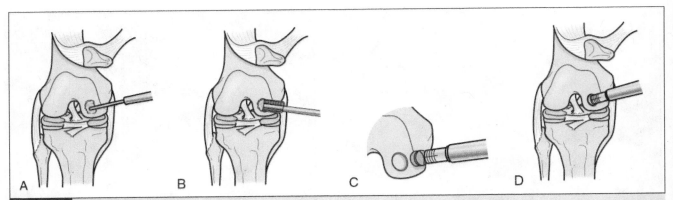

Figure 5 Schematic drawings show steps in osteochondral allograft transplantation. **A,** The size and shape of the chondral defect are determined. **B,** The defect is reamed to remove abnormal cartilage and 8 to 10 mm of subchondral bone. **C,** The donor osteochondral cylinder is obtained from the fresh allograft specimen. **D,** The donor cylindrical plug is inserted into the recipient tunnel using a press fit.

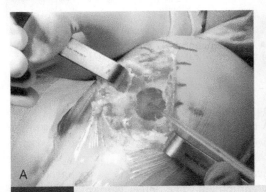
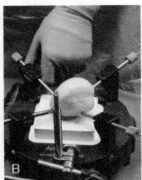
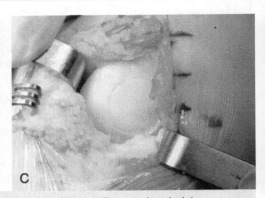

Figure 6 Photographs show steps in osteochondral allograft transplantation. **A,** Unhealthy cartilage and underlying subchondral bone have been removed in preparation for insertion of the osteochondral allograft cylinder. **B,** The fresh femoral hemicondyle is prepared for obtaining the donor osteochondral cylinder. **C,** The osteochondral allograft cylinder has been placed into the recipient tunnel using a press fit.

reimplantation. The first-generation technique required harvesting of proximal tibia periosteum for use as a patch to contain the chondrocyte suspension within the defect. Second-generation techniques use a synthetic type I/III collagen membrane. The advantages of using the type I/III collagen membrane include shorter surgical time, less morbidity, and fewer postsurgical complications such as graft patch hypertrophy.[33] A third-generation technique is being used in Europe but has not yet been approved for use in the United States.

The purposes of the initial arthroscopy are to evaluate the size and location of the defect and determine whether the lesion has a stable rim of surrounding healthy cartilage. If the defect is determined to be amenable to ACI, a full-thickness 200- to 300-mg cartilage biopsy is taken from the superolateral intercondylar notch or the periphery of the trochlea. The biopsy material is transported in special medium for expansion in the laboratory. After 4 to 6 weeks, the cells usually are ready to be reimplanted. For most patients, however, a cryopreservation stage is added that allows implantation to be delayed as much as 2 years. The reimplantation procedure requires a medial or lateral parapatellar arthrotomy. The defect is identified and outlined using a scalpel to contain the defect by establishing a stable rim of surrounding cartilage. Ring curettes are used to remove all remaining unhealthy cartilage in the contained defect while avoiding penetration of the subchondral plate. The defect is traced onto sterile glove paper or foil to create a template for the type I/III collagen membrane. The membrane is trimmed to the desired size and shape and sutured to the stable rim of cartilage using a 6-0 polyglycolic acid suture in a simple interrupted fashion. A small opening is left so that an 18-gauge plastic angiocatheter can be inserted beneath the membrane. Before inserting the cells, fibrin glue is applied to the perimeter of the membrane except for the area to be used for cell insertion. After cell injection, this small opening is closed using an additional suture and fibrin glue to create a watertight seal. One of the advantages of this technique is that there is no limit to the size or shape

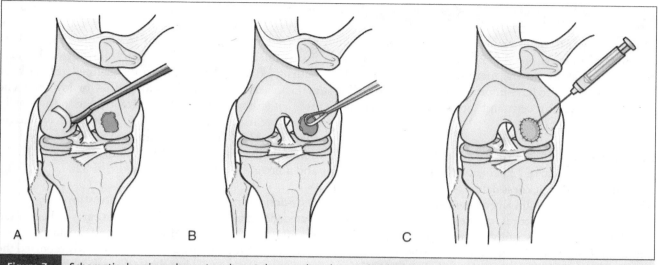

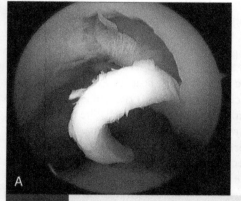
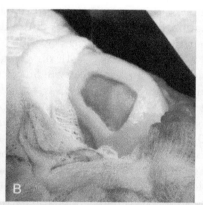
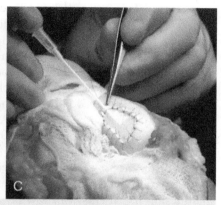

Figure 7 Schematic drawings show steps in autologous chondrocyte implantation. **A,** Cartilage biopsy tissue is obtained from the intercondylar region of the lateral trochlea. **B,** The chondral defect is prepared with a ring curette to create stable borders. **C,** Type I/III collagen membrane has been secured in place, and chondrocytes are injected beneath the membrane.

Figure 8 Steps in autologous chondrocyte implantation. **A,** Arthroscopic view shows cartilage biopsy tissue taken from the intercondylar region of the femur. **B,** Photograph shows the defect prepared by removing unhealthy cartilage and creating a contained lesion with stable borders of healthy cartilage. **C,** Photograph shows injection of chondrocytes beneath the membrane that has been sutured into place using multiple interrupted sutures. (Panel **A** reproduced from Gomoll AH: Autologous chondrocyte implantation, in Amendola A, Gomoll AH, eds: *Let's Discuss: Joint Preservation of the Knee*. Rosemont, IL, American Academy of Orthopaedic Surgeons, 2015, in press.)

of the lesion treated as long as the defect is contained. Any location in the knee can be treated, although the US FDA does not consider patellar or tibial lesions to be approved indications.

The most current technique is cell-seeded ACI, in which the collagen patch is sized and cut to shape while dry and subsequently seeded with the chondrocyte suspension in the operating room. Within 5 to 10 minutes, the cells attach themselves to the membrane, which is placed into the defect and secured circumferentially with a running 6-0 resorbable suture. The suture line is waterproofed with fibrin glue, but no additional injection of cells is required. This technique is less invasive than standard ACI and decreases the surgical time, but it has not been approved for use in the United States. The results appear to be comparable to those of standard ACI.[34]

Rehabilitation after ACI begins with immediate motion. A CPM machine is used 6 to 8 hours a day for the first 6 weeks with progression toward 90° of knee flexion. After treatment of a defect in the femoral condyle, toe-touch weight bearing is used for 6 weeks, after which the patient progresses toward weight bearing as tolerated. After treatment of a patellofemoral defect, the patient can bear weight from the beginning as tolerated in full extension. Running is not allowed for 12 months, and other strenuous sports activity is restricted for 18 months.

Outcomes

Until recently, little high-quality evidence was available on articular cartilage surgery. In 2013, a review of cartilage surgery studies found the methodologic quality to be generally poor but to have improved within the preceding 10 years.[35] Several recent high-quality studies were not included in the review.[36,37]

Microfracture

At 11-year follow-up of 72 patients who underwent microfracture for a full-thickness defect of the knee, substantial improvement in Lysholm Knee Questionnaire and Tegner Activity Level Scale scores was reported, and scores on the Medical Outcomes Study 36-Item Short Form Health Survey and Western Ontario and McMaster Universities Osteoarthritis Index were good to excellent.[38] At 7-year follow-up, 80% of patients reported improvement. A review of the results after treatment of 53 athletes with a mean 4-cm² defect found that 70% had a normal or near-normal International Knee Documentation Committee (IKDC) Subjective Knee Evaluation Form score at 6-year follow-up.[23] Patients younger than 40 years and with a lesion smaller than 2 cm² were most likely to return to high-impact sports. Another study also reported that patients had improved clinical scores after microfracture surgery.[39] However, the results of microfracture may deteriorate with time. A systematic review of 28 studies involving more than 3,000 patients reported improved knee function at 24-month follow-up, but data were insufficient for evaluating longer term outcomes.[40] A systematic review reported that microfracture for a small lesion in patients with low physical demands had good outcomes at short-term follow-up but that treatment failure could be expected after 5 years, regardless of lesion size.[41] Similarly, microfracture for small lesions improved symptoms, but deterioration of clinical outcomes was found to be expected 2 to 5 years after surgery.[42] Even with proper surgical technique and appropriate patient selection, the results of microfracture were found to deteriorate over time.[43]

Osteochondral Autograft Transfer

At an average 9.6-year follow-up of patients treated with OAT (mosaicplasty), good to excellent outcomes were found in 91% of those with a femoral condyle lesion, 86% of those with a tibial lesion, and 74% of those with a patellofemoral lesion.[44] Patellofemoral pain related to graft harvest was found in 5% of patients. These data suggest that OAT should be considered for competitive athletes with a 1- to 4-cm² lesion. Another study reported that at an average 7-year follow-up, 61 of 69 patients who

underwent OAT (88%) said that they would choose to undergo the surgery again.[45] However, a deterioration of results was observed from the 12-month to the 5- to 9-year follow-up. At 10- to 14-year follow-up of the same patients, 40% had a poor outcome (defined as later knee arthroplasty or a Lysholm score of 64 or lower).[46] The poor outcomes were associated with patient age older than 40 years (59%), female sex (61%), and a defect larger than 3 cm² (57%). Patients younger than 40 years with a defect smaller than 3 cm² had a failure rate of only 12.5% and a favorable mean Lysholm score of 82.

Osteochondral Allograft Transplantation

Osteochondral allograft transplantation has been used for 40 to 50 years. Several studies found satisfactory outcomes.[47-49] A recent long-term outcome study reported the results of fresh osteochondral allograft transplantation in 58 patients at a mean 22-year follow-up.[50] At the time of surgery, the patients were younger than 50 years and had a unipolar osteochondral or osteochondritis dissecans defect of the distal femur larger than 3 cm in diameter and 1 cm in depth. Graft survival at 10, 15, 20, or 25 years was 91%, 84%, 69%, or 59% respectively. Patients with surviving grafts had a mean modified Hospital for Special Surgery score of 86.

A systematic review of 19 studies evaluated the outcomes of osteochondral allograft transplantation in 644 knees at a mean 58-month follow-up.[51] The mean patient age was 37 years, and the mean defect size was 6.3 cm². The defects were idiopathic or related to trauma, osteochondritis dissecans, or osteonecrosis. The overall patient satisfaction rate was 86%, and 65% of patients had little or no osteoarthritis. The short-term complication rate was 2.4%, and the overall failure rate was 18%.

Despite the complexity of osteochondral allograft transplantation in the patellofemoral joint, encouraging outcomes have been documented. A retrospective review of 14 fresh patellofemoral allograft transplantations in 11 patients found that at an average 10-year follow-up (range, 2.5 to 17.5 years), 8 grafts were in place.[52] Four grafts survived longer than 10 years, and 2 survived longer than 5 years. Three allografts survived more than 10 years but did not survive until final follow-up. Ten of the 11 patients stated that they would undergo the procedure again. Another study found that 5 of 20 fresh osteochondral allografts used to treat patellofemoral lesions in 18 patients did not survive at an average follow-up of 94 months.[26]

Autologous Chondrocyte Implantation

Since the first description of ACI in 1994, short- to immediate-term studies have found favorable outcomes.[53-56] Several long-term studies have recently become available. At a mean 12.8-year follow-up, 74% of patients reported their status as better than or unchanged from that of preceding years.[57] Ninety-two percent were satisfied and would have the procedure again. In a 12-year study of 210 patients, the average defect size was 8.4 cm^2.[58] At 10-year follow-up, graft survivorship was 71%, and 75% of patients reported improved function. At least one graft had failed in 53 of the patients (25%). A subgroup analysis revealed that concurrent osteotomy significantly increased graft survivorship (88% with osteotomy, 66% without osteotomy). A study of the results of ACI for chronic chondral and osteochondral defects followed 104 patients (mean age, 30.2 years) for an average 10.4 years.[59] The patients were considered difficult to treat; their mean duration of symptoms was 7.8 years, and they had undergone an average 1.3 cartilage procedures before ACI. Twenty-seven patients (26%) had graft failure at a mean 5.7 years. Of the 73 patients with surviving grafts, 64 (88%) reported a good to excellent result.

Until recently, no outcome data have been available to support the use of ACI in the patella. In a large multicenter study, 110 patients were treated with ACI for a cartilage defect of the patella and were followed for at least 4 years.[60] There were statistically significant and clinically important improvements in all physical outcome scales; IKDC scores improved from 40 to 69, modified Cincinnati Knee Rating System scores improved from 3.2 to 6.2, and Western Ontario and McMaster Universities Osteoarthritis Index scores improved from 50.4 to 28.6. One hundred one patients (92%) stated they would undergo the procedure again, and 95 (86%) rated their knees as good or excellent at final follow-up.

Newer data suggested that earlier bone marrow stimulation procedures such as microfracture may have a detrimental effect on outcomes after ACI. A review of more than 300 consecutive patients compared outcomes based on whether the patient had undergone a bone marrow stimulation procedure before ACI.[36] Graft failure occurred in 26% of patients who had undergone earlier bone marrow stimulation compared with 8% of patients who had not had a bone marrow stimulation procedure.

Similar results were found in a comparison study of ACI after unsuccessful microfracture or as a first-line procedure.[61] Significantly more graft failures were associated with ACI after microfracture (7 of 28) than with ACI as a first-line treatment (1 of 28). Inferior clinical outcome also was associated with ACI after microfracture.

Comparative Outcome Studies

Microfracture Versus OAT

A level I randomized controlled study of 60 patients compared microfracture to OAT in athletes (mean age, 24.3 years).[62] After 37.1 months, patients in both groups had significant clinical improvement. However, at 12, 24, and 36 months, those treated with OAT had statistically significantly better Hospital for Special Surgery and International Cartilage Repair Society scores than those treated with microfracture. In addition, 93% of patients treated with OAT were able to return to sports activity at the preinjury level at an average 6.5-month follow-up, compared with 52% of patients who underwent microfracture. In 10-year follow-up data, the same patients had significant clinical improvement in follow-up International Cartilage Repair Society scores compared with scores before surgery.[63] However, patients in the OAT group had significantly better scores compared with patients in the microfracture group. Similar trends were found in patient activity levels. Fifteen of 20 patients in the OAT group (75%) were able to maintain the same preinjury activity level compared with 8 of 22 patients in the microfracture group (37%). In patients who underwent OAT, lesions smaller than 2 cm^2 were associated with a significantly higher rate of return to sports compared with larger lesions. No difference was found between OAT and microfracture in muscle strength, patient-reported outcomes, and radiographic outcomes at a mean 9.8-year follow-up.[64] This study involved only 25 patients, and therefore it is difficult to draw firm conclusions from the data.

Microfracture Versus ACI

Because few high-powered studies have compared ACI and microfracture, outcome data conflict. A randomized study of 80 patients found no difference in clinical outcomes at 2- and 5-year follow-up.[65,66] However, defects larger than 4 cm^2 were associated with a worse outcome after microfracture than smaller lesions. A similar trend was not observed after ACI, and ACI was recommended for treatment of large lesions. This study was criticized because most of the involved surgeons had little or no prestudy experience with ACI. A randomized controlled study with 2-year follow-up compared matrix-applied ACI with microfracture in 144 patients with a mean lesion size of 4.8 cm^2.[67] The important exclusion criteria included malalignment requiring osteotomy. The assessed outcomes included the Knee Injury and Osteoarthritis Outcome Score, knee-related quality of life, and repair tissue quality as based on histologic and MRI findings. For cartilage defects larger than 3 cm^2, treatment with

3: Knee and Leg

matrix-applied ACI was statistically and clinically better than microfracture, with similar structural repair tissue and safety outcomes.

ACI Versus OAT

A prospective study of 40 patients compared ACI to OAT.[37] Meyers, Lysholm, and Tegner activity scores were obtained at 3, 6, 12, and 24 months, and biopsy specimens were obtained for histomorphologic evaluation. Both surgical procedures led to improvement in symptoms, but recovery after ACI was slower than after OAT, as indicated by Lysholm scores. After ACI, biopsied tissue primarily was filled with fibrocartilage, but after OAT, hyalinelike tissue with an interface between the transplanted and original cartilage was maintained. This study lacked a preoperative radiographic evaluation of mechanical alignment. Seven of the 20 patients who underwent ACI had undergone earlier abrasion arthroplasty, compared with 4 of the 20 patients who underwent OAT. Cell culturing was done by the investigators rather than a commercial entity with experience in chondrocyte culture processes.

At a mean 1.7-year follow-up, a prospective randomized study of 100 patients with an osteochondral defect found that 88% of those treated with ACI had good to excellent modified Cincinnati and Stanmore Functional Rating scores compared with 69% of those treated with mosaicplasty.[68] In addition, arthroscopy at 1 year found that 82% of the patients treated with ACI had a good or excellent repair compared with 34% of those treated with mosaicplasty. The long-term outcomes of the same patients were reported at a minimum 10-year follow-up.[69] Graft failure had occurred in 10 of the 58 patients treated with ACI (17%) and 23 of the 42 patients treated with mosaicplasty (55%). None of the five patellar mosaicplasty procedures were successful.

Biologic Techniques

Each of the available articular cartilage–restoring procedures is hampered by specific limitations, and this factor has led to increased interest in new biologic techniques using allografts, stem cells, and scaffolds.

Particulated Juvenile Cartilage

It has been proved in animal and human models that juvenile cartilage is superior to adult cartilage in chondrocytic activity, cell density, and healing potential.[70,71] DeNovo NT Natural Tissue Graft (Zimmer) was commercially introduced recently as a particulated juvenile allograft cartilage from donors age 13 years or younger. The surgical technique requires a medial or lateral parapatellar arthrotomy, identification of the defect, and initial preparation similar to the ACI technique. In a multicenter prospective study, 25 patients treated with juvenile particulated cartilage had statistically significant improvements in IKDC and Knee Injury and Osteoarthritis Outcome Score at 2-year follow-up.[72] Histologic analysis of biopsied material from eight patients revealed a mixture of hyaline cartilage and fibrocartilage with more type II than type I collagen.

Platelet-Rich Plasma

Autologous platelet-rich plasma (PRP) has been used to treat musculoskeletal conditions such as lateral epicondylitis and rotator cuff tears. Animal studies have identified potential uses for PRP alone or as an augmentation of other biologic treatments for repairing hyaline cartilage.[73,74] However, uncertainty remains as to the in vivo efficacy of PRP. A systematic review of 10 studies of PRP used in degenerative knee and hip disease did not find evidence of a short-term clinical benefit.[75] High-quality comparative studies with longer term follow-up are needed to determine whether PRP could be efficacious for treatment of articular cartilage conditions.

Cord Blood Stem Cell Transplants

Cartistem (Medipost) is a stem cell drug used to treat articular cartilage defects and osteoarthritis. This drug contains mesenchymal stem cells derived from umbilical cord blood. In 2012, Cartistem was approved for clinical use by the Food and Drug Administration of Korea, and it has been approved for clinical study at certain US institutions.

Amniotic Stem Cell Transplants

The use of amniotic tissues has attracted considerable attention. Amnionic stem cell transplants are routinely used in the treatment of eye and diabetic foot disease and are being investigated for use in cartilage repair and osteoarthritis applications.

Next-Generation Chondrocyte Implantation

The currently used chondrocyte implants consist of autologous cells, but concern as to cell quality variability among donors has led to investigation of allogeneic chondrocyte products. Allogeneic implants could be derived from donor chondrocytes that express high levels of chondrogenic potential.

Summary

Articular cartilage repair is a rapidly developing orthopaedic subspecialty. The rate of positive outcomes generally exceeds 80% if the technique is carefully matched to specific patient and defect characteristics. Débridement is useful for temporary pain relief and reduction of mechanical symptoms. Microfracture is indicated for treating a small acute femoral condyle defect in a young patient. OAT has better outcomes than microfracture but is limited by donor site morbidity. Osteochondral allograft transplantation can be used to treat large osteochondral defects and revise an unsuccessful earlier cartilage repair procedure, but its use in the patellofemoral compartment is complicated by the difficulty of matching the varied anatomy. ACI can more easily be used to treat multiple patellofemoral defects, but it requires intact subchondral bone. Numerous techniques and products are under development and are expected to be ready for clinical use within 5 to 10 years.

Key Study Points

- Initial evaluation of chondral defects requires a thorough history, physical examination, and radiographic assessment.
- Associated injuries, malalignment, age, activity level, and expectations should all be considered when formulating a definitive treatment plan.
- For patients on whom nonsurgical treatment fails and who are candidates for cartilage repair and/or restoration surgery, OAT or microfracture should be considered for smaller lesions (< 2-4 cm^2) and ACI or osteochondral allograft transplantation for larger lesions (> 2-4 cm^2).
- Lesions resulting in abnormal or deficient subchondral bone may be best treated with procedures that address the entire osteochondral unit, such as OAT or osteochondral allograft transplantation.

Annotated References

1. Newman AP: Articular cartilage repair. *Am J Sports Med* 1998;26(2):309-324.

2. O'Driscoll SW: The healing and regeneration of articular cartilage. *J Bone Joint Surg Am* 1998;80(12):1795-1812.

3. Shapiro F, Koide S, Glimcher MJ: Cell origin and differentiation in the repair of full-thickness defects of articular cartilage. *J Bone Joint Surg Am* 1993;75(4):532-553.

4. Furukawa T, Eyre DR, Koide S, Glimcher MJ: Biochemical studies on repair cartilage resurfacing experimental defects in the rabbit knee. *J Bone Joint Surg Am* 1980;62(1):79-89.

5. Heath CA, Magari SR: Mini-review: Mechanical factors affecting cartilage regeneration in vitro. *Biotechnol Bioeng* 1996;50(4):430-437.

6. Ahsan T, Lottman LM, Harwood F, Amiel D, Sah RL: Integrative cartilage repair: Inhibition by beta-aminopropionitrile. *J Orthop Res* 1999;17(6):850-857.

7. Curl WW, Krome J, Gordon ES, Rushing J, Smith BP, Poehling GG: Cartilage injuries: A review of 31,516 knee arthroscopies. *Arthroscopy* 1997;13(4):456-460.

8. Arøen A, Løken S, Heir S, et al: Articular cartilage lesions in 993 consecutive knee arthroscopies. *Am J Sports Med* 2004;32(1):211-215.

9. Hjelle K, Solheim E, Strand T, Muri R, Brittberg M: Articular cartilage defects in 1,000 knee arthroscopies. *Arthroscopy* 2002;18(7):730-734.

10. Flanigan DC, Harris JD, Trinh TQ, Siston RA, Brophy RH: Prevalence of chondral defects in athletes' knees: A systematic review. *Med Sci Sports Exerc* 2010;42(10):1795-1801.

    A systematic review of 11 level IV studies determined the prevalence of full-thickness chondral defects in athletes' knees to be 36%. Patellofemoral defects accounted for 37%, femoral condyle defects for 35%, and tibial plateau defects for 25%.

11. Brophy RH, Zeltser D, Wright RW, Flanigan D: Anterior cruciate ligament reconstruction and concomitant articular cartilage injury: Incidence and treatment. *Arthroscopy* 2010;26(1):112-120.

    A systematic review of five studies revealed a 16% to 46% incidence of severe articular cartilage injury in acute anterior cruciate ligament tears.

12. Lewandrowski KU, Müller J, Schollmeier G: Concomitant meniscal and articular cartilage lesions in the femorotibial joint. *Am J Sports Med* 1997;25(4):486-494.

13. Nomura E, Inoue M, Kurimura M: Chondral and osteochondral injuries associated with acute patellar dislocation. *Arthroscopy* 2003;19(7):717-721.

14. Lefkoe TP, Trafton PG, Ehrlich MG, et al: An experimental model of femoral condylar defect leading to osteoarthrosis. *J Orthop Trauma* 1993;7(5):458-467.

15. Messner K, Maletius W: The long-term prognosis for severe damage to weight-bearing cartilage in the knee: A 14-year clinical and radiographic follow-up in 28 young athletes. *Acta Orthop Scand* 1996;67(2):165-168.

16. Gomoll AH, Yoshioka H, Watanabe A, Dunn JC, Minas T: Preoperative measurement of cartilage defects by MRI underestimates lesion size. *Cartilage* 2011;2(4):389-393.

    Seventy-seven patients had knee MRI before arthroscopic surgery for a cartilage defect. Defect size was determined on MRI and at time of arthroscopy. MRI underestimated the defect area an average 65% of the time compared with arthroscopic visualization. Level of evidence: II.

17. Montgomery SR, Foster BD, Ngo SS, et al: Trends in the surgical treatment of articular cartilage defects of the knee in the United States. *Knee Surg Sports Traumatol Arthrosc* 2014;22(9):2070-2075.

    Microfracture and chondroplasty accounted for more than 98% of 163,448 knee articular cartilage procedures over a 6-year period, usually in patients age 40 to 59 years. Other procedures were more often done in patients younger than 40 years. Level of evidence: IV.

18. Williams RJ III, Harnly HW: Microfracture: Indications, technique, and results. *Instr Course Lect* 2007;56:419-428.

19. Chen H, Chevrier A, Hoemann CD, Sun J, Ouyang W, Buschmann MD: Characterization of subchondral bone repair for marrow-stimulated chondral defects and its relationship to articular cartilage resurfacing. *Am J Sports Med* 2011;39(8):1731-1740.

    Bone marrow stimulation procedures were done on 16 skeletally mature rabbits. Repair led to an average bone volume density similar to that of control subjects but the repaired bone was more porous and branched. Relatively deep drilling induced a larger region of repairing and remodeling of subchondral bone that was positively correlated with cartilage repair.

20. Chen H, Hoemann CD, Sun J, et al: Depth of subchondral perforation influences the outcome of bone marrow stimulation cartilage repair. *J Orthop Res* 2011;29(8):1178-1184.

    This study used a rabbit model to compare depth (6 mm versus 2 mm) and type of marrow stimulation (drilling versus microfracture) on cartilage defects. Outcomes included quantitative histomorphometry and histologic scoring. Results demonstrated that deeper versus shallow drilling produced a greater fill of the cartilage defect with a more hyaline-like repair tissue. Microfracture and drilling to 2 mm resulted in similar quantity and quality of cartilage repair.

21. Chen H, Sun J, Hoemann CD, et al: Drilling and microfracture lead to different bone structure and necrosis during bone-marrow stimulation for cartilage repair. *J Orthop Res* 2009;27(11):1432-1438.

    Chondral defects were treated with bone marrow stimulation in a mature rabbit model. Microfracture was found to produce fractured and compacted bone around holes, sealing them off from bone marrow content. Drilling cleanly removed bone from the holes and provided access channels to marrow content. Microfracture was associated with more osteocyte death than drilling.

22. Eldracher M, Orth P, Cucchiarini M, Pape D, Madry H: Small subchondral drill holes improve marrow stimulation of articular cartilage defects. *Am J Sports Med* 2014;42(11):2741-2750.

    Subchondral drilling was done in 13 adult sheep. Osteochondral repair was assessed at 6 months. Compared with 1.8-mm drill holes, the application of 1.0-mm subchondral drill holes led to significantly better histologic matrix staining, cellular morphologic characteristics, subchondral bone reconstitution, average total histologic score, immunoreactivity to type II collagen, and immunoreactivity to type I collagen in the repair tissue.

23. Gobbi A, Nunag P, Malinowski K: Treatment of full thickness chondral lesions of the knee with microfracture in a group of athletes. *Knee Surg Sports Traumatol Arthrosc* 2005;13(3):213-221.

24. Garretson RB III, Katolik LI, Verma N, Beck PR, Bach BR, Cole BJ: Contact pressure at osteochondral donor sites in the patellofemoral joint. *Am J Sports Med* 2004;32(4):967-974.

25. Hangody L, Ráthonyi GK, Duska Z, Vásárhelyi G, Füles P, Módis L: Autologous osteochondral mosaicplasty: Surgical technique. *J Bone Joint Surg Am* 2004;86(Suppl 1):65-72.

26. Jamali AA, Emmerson BC, Chung C, Convery FR, Bugbee WD: Fresh osteochondral allografts: Results in the patellofemoral joint. *Clin Orthop Relat Res* 2005;437:176-185.

27. Pylawka TK, Wimmer M, Cole BJ, Virdi AS, Williams JM: Impaction affects cell viability in osteochondral tissues during transplantation. *J Knee Surg* 2007;20(2):105-110.

28. Görtz S, Bugbee WD: Allografts in articular cartilage repair. *Instr Course Lect* 2007;56:469-480.

29. Koh JL, Wirsing K, Lautenschlager E, Zhang LO: The effect of graft height mismatch on contact pressure following osteochondral grafting: A biomechanical study. *Am J Sports Med* 2004;32(2):317-320.

30. Hangody L, Kish G, Kárpáti Z, Udvarhelyi I, Szigeti I, Bély M: Mosaicplasty for the treatment of articular cartilage defects: Application in clinical practice. *Orthopedics* 1998;21(7):751-756.

31. Bugbee WD, Convery FR: Osteochondral allograft transplantation. *Clin Sports Med* 1999;18(1):67-75.

32. LaPrade RF, Botker J, Herzog M, Agel J: Refrigerated osteoarticular allografts to treat articular cartilage defects of the femoral condyles: A prospective outcomes study. *J Bone Joint Surg Am* 2009;91(4):805-811.

    Twenty-three consecutive patients were treated with refrigerated osteochondral allografts for chondral defects. The average age of implanted graft was 20.3 days. At 3-year follow-up, modified Cincinnati and IKDC scores revealed a statistically significant improvement. There were no graft failures. Level of evidence: IV.

33. Gomoll AH, Probst C, Farr J, Cole BJ, Minas T: Use of a type I/III bilayer collagen membrane decreases reoperation rates for symptomatic hypertrophy after autologous chondrocyte implantation. *Am J Sports Med* 2009;37(Suppl 1):20S-23S.

In a multicenter comparison study of 300 patients treated with periosteum-covered ACI and 101 patients treated with collagen membrane–covered ACI, the 1-year failure rates were similar but there was a significantly higher reoperation rate for graft hypertrophy after periosteum-covered ACI (25.7%) than after collagen membrane–covered ACI (5%).

34. Niemeyer P, Lenz P, Kreuz PC, et al: Chondrocyte-seeded type I/III collagen membrane for autologous chondrocyte transplantation: Prospective 2-year results in patients with cartilage defects of the knee joint. *Arthroscopy* 2010;26(8):1074-1082.

   A prospective study of 59 patients treated with ACI using a collagen membrane to seed the chondrocytes found that the percentage of patients with knees rated normal or near normal increased from 33.9% before surgery to 92.5% at 24-month follow-up on the objective International Cartilage Repair Society rating. IKDC and Lysholm scores increased from 50.1 points and 60.5 points, respectively, to 76.1 points (*P* < 0.001) and 82.5 points (*P* < 0.001). Level of evidence: IV.

35. Harris JD, Erickson BJ, Abrams GD, et al: Methodologic quality of knee articular cartilage studies. *Arthroscopy* 2013;29(7):1243-1252.e5.

   A review of 194 level I to IV studies found that ACI was the most commonly reported technique (62% of studies). The most common study weaknesses were related to blinding, subject selection process, study type, sample size calculation, and outcome measures and assessment. There was improvement in study quality after 2004.

36. Minas T, Gomoll AH, Rosenberger R, Royce RO, Bryant T: Increased failure rate of autologous chondrocyte implantation after previous treatment with marrow stimulation techniques. *Am J Sports Med* 2009;37(5):902-908.

   In a study of 321 consecutive patients treated with ACI, 26% of grafts were unsuccessful among those who had undergone an earlier bone marrow stimulation procedure compared with 8% among those who had not had a bone marrow stimulation procedure.

37. Horas U, Pelinkovic D, Herr G, Aigner T, Schnettler R: Autologous chondrocyte implantation and osteochondral cylinder transplantation in cartilage repair of the knee joint: A prospective, comparative trial. *J Bone Joint Surg Am* 2003;85(2):185-192.

38. Steadman JR, Briggs KK, Rodrigo JJ, Kocher MS, Gill TJ, Rodkey WG: Outcomes of microfracture for traumatic chondral defects of the knee: Average 11-year follow-up. *Arthroscopy* 2003;19(5):477-484.

39. Mithoefer K, Williams RJ III, Warren RF, et al: The microfracture technique for the treatment of articular cartilage lesions in the knee: A prospective cohort study. *J Bone Joint Surg Am* 2005;87(9):1911-1920.

40. Mithoefer K, McAdams T, Williams RJ, Kreuz PC, Mandelbaum BR: Clinical efficacy of the microfracture technique for articular cartilage repair in the knee: An evidence-based systematic analysis. *Am J Sports Med* 2009;37(10):2053-2063.

   A systematic review of 28 studies including 3,122 patients who underwent microfracture for cartilage injury (average follow-up, 41 months) found that microfracture provides effective short-term improvement of knee function but that insufficient data were available on long-term results.

41. Goyal D, Keyhani S, Lee EH, Hui JH: Evidence-based status of microfracture technique: A systematic review of level I and II studies. *Arthroscopy* 2013;29(9):1579-1588.

   A systematic review of 15 level I or II studies compared the clinical outcomes of microfracture with those of ACI and osteochondral cylinder transfers. Most studies reported poor clinical outcomes. Two studies reported the absence of any significant difference in the results. Small lesions and relatively young patients had good short-term results, but at 5- to 10-year follow-up there was a high rate of osteoarthritis.

42. Gobbi A, Karnatzikos G, Kumar A: Long-term results after microfracture treatment for full-thickness knee chondral lesions in athletes. *Knee Surg Sports Traumatol Arthrosc* 2014;22(9):1986-1996.

   Sixty-one of 67 patients (91%) were available at an average final 15.1-year follow-up after microfracture. Pain and swelling during strenuous activity was reported by 9 patients at 2-year follow-up and 35 patients at final follow-up. Outcome scores deteriorated over time. The conclusion was that deterioration of the clinical outcome should be expected after 2 to 5 years. Level of evidence: IV.

43. Bedi A, Feeley BT, Williams RJ III: Management of articular cartilage defects of the knee. *J Bone Joint Surg Am* 2010;92(4):994-1009.

   This review article focused on management and outcomes related to articular cartilage defects of the knee.

44. Hangody L, Dobos J, Baló E, Pánics G, Hangody LR, Berkes I: Clinical experiences with autologous osteochondral mosaicplasty in an athletic population: A 17-year prospective multicenter study. *Am J Sports Med* 2010;38(6):1125-1133.

   In a multicenter study, 354 of 383 patients who underwent mosaicplasty were followed for an average of 9.6 years. Good to excellent results were found after 91% of femoral, 86% of tibial, and 74% of patellofemoral mosaicplasties. Patellofemoral pain related to graft harvest was observed in 5% of patients. Level of evidence: IV.

45. Solheim E, Hegna J, Øyen J, Austgulen OK, Harlem T, Strand T: Osteochondral autografting (mosaicplasty) in articular cartilage defects in the knee: Results at 5 to 9 years. *Knee* 2010;17(1):84-87.

   Sixty-nine patients (median age, 33 years) were available after mosaicplasty for a full-thickness chondral defect. Mean Lysholm and visual analog scale pain scores improved from 48 and 62, respectively, at the time of surgery to 81 and 24 at 12-month follow-up (*P* < 0.001).

3: Knee and Leg

Scores deteriorated to 68 and 32 at 5- to 9-year follow-up ($P < 0.001$).

46. Solheim E, Hegna J, Øyen J, Harlem T, Strand T: Results at 10 to 14 years after osteochondral autografting (mosaicplasty) in articular cartilage defects in the knee. *Knee* 2013;20(4):287-290.

Seventy-three patients (median age, 34 years) were available after mosaicplasty for a full-thickness chondral defect. Baseline mean Lysholm and visual analog scale pain scores improved significantly at mid- and long-term follow-up. Forty percent of patients had a poor outcome at long-term follow-up; most of these patients were age 40 years or older (59%), were women (61%), or had a defect of 3 cm² or larger (57%). In men younger than 40 years with a defect smaller than 3 cm², the failure rate was 12.5% and the mean Lysholm score was 82.

47. Gross AE, Shasha N, Aubin P: Long-term followup of the use of fresh osteochondral allografts for posttraumatic knee defects. *Clin Orthop Relat Res* 2005;435:79-87.

48. Gross AE, Kim W, Las Heras F, Backstein D, Safir O, Pritzker KP: Fresh osteochondral allografts for posttraumatic knee defects: Long-term followup. *Clin Orthop Relat Res* 2008;466(8):1863-1870.

49. Bakay A, Csönge L, Papp G, Fekete L: Osteochondral resurfacing of the knee joint with allograft: Clinical analysis of 33 cases. *Int Orthop* 1998;22(5):277-281.

50. Raz G, Safir OA, Backstein DJ, Lee PT, Gross AE: Distal femoral fresh osteochondral allografts: Follow-up at a mean of twenty-two years. *J Bone Joint Surg Am* 2014;96(13):1101-1107.

In a study of long-term outcomes after fresh allograft transplantation for posttraumatic osteochondral and osteochondritis dissecans defects of the distal aspect of the femur, 58 patients were followed for a mean 21.8 years. Thirteen patients required further surgery, three underwent graft removal, nine underwent conversion to total knee arthroplasty, and one underwent multiple débridements followed by amputation above the knee.

51. Chahal J, Gross AE, Gross C, et al: Outcomes of osteochondral allograft transplantation in the knee. *Arthroscopy* 2013;29(3):575-588.

Nineteen studies of a total of 644 knees (mean follow-up, 58 months) were included in a systematic review. All patients underwent osteochondral allograft transplantation. Forty-six percent of patients had concomitant procedures, and the mean defect size was 6.3 cm². The overall satisfaction rate was 86%.

52. Torga Spak R, Teitge RA: Fresh osteochondral allografts for patellofemoral arthritis: Long-term followup. *Clin Orthop Relat Res* 2006;444:193-200.

53. Peterson L, Minas T, Brittberg M, Nilsson A, Sjögren-Jansson E, Lindahl A: Two- to 9-year outcome after autologous chondrocyte transplantation of the knee. *Clin Orthop Relat Res* 2000;374:212-234.

54. Peterson L, Brittberg M, Kiviranta I, Akerlund EL, Lindahl A: Autologous chondrocyte transplantation: Biomechanics and long-term durability. *Am J Sports Med* 2002;30(1):2-12.

55. Minas T: Autologous chondrocyte implantation for focal chondral defects of the knee. *Clin Orthop Relat Res* 2001;391(Suppl):S349-S361.

56. McNickle AG, L'Heureux DR, Yanke AB, Cole BJ: Outcomes of autologous chondrocyte implantation in a diverse patient population. *Am J Sports Med* 2009;37(7):1344-1350.

After 137 patients (140 knees) underwent ACI for a knee defect (mean size, 5.2 cm²), outcomes were assessed at 4.3-year follow-up. A significant improvement after surgery was observed on all outcome measures. Level of evidence: IV.

57. Peterson L, Vasiliadis HS, Brittberg M, Lindahl A: Autologous chondrocyte implantation: A long-term follow-up. *Am J Sports Med* 2010;38(6):1117-1124.

Questionnaires with outcome measures were sent to 341 patients who also were asked to grade their status during the past 10 years as better, worse, or unchanged; 224 patients replied. At an average of 12.8 years after surgery 74% of the patients reported their status as better or the same as in previous years, and 92% were satisfied and would have the ACI again.

58. Minas T, Von Keudell A, Bryant T, Gomoll AH: A minimum 10-year outcome study of autologous chondrocyte implantation. *Clin Orthop Relat Res* 2014;472(1):41-51.

At final 12-year follow-up after ACI for a symptomatic cartilage defects, 53 of 210 patients (25%) had at least one failed ACI graft. Nineteen patients went on to arthroplasty, 27 patients had revision cartilage repair, 7 patients declined further treatment, and 3 patients were lost to follow-up. ACI provided durable outcomes with a survivorship of 71% at 10 years and improved function in 75% of patients. A history of bone marrow stimulation or treatment of a very large defect was associated with an increased risk of failure.

59. Biant LC, Bentley G, Vijayan S, Skinner JA, Carrington RW: Long-term results of autologous chondrocyte implantation in the knee for chronic chondral and osteochondral defects. *Am J Sports Med* 2014;42(9):2178-2183.

In 104 patients who underwent ACI for a symptomatic cartilage lesion, the mean duration of symptoms before surgery was 7.8 years. The mean number of previous surgical procedures on the cartilage defect was 1.3, and the mean defect size was 477.1 mm². Twenty-seven patients (26%) had graft failure at a mean 5.7 years after ACI. Of the remaining 73 patients, 46 (63% of patients with a surviving graft) had an excellent result, 18 (25%) had a good result, 6 (8%) had a fair result, and 3 (4%) had a poor result; 98 of the 100 were satisfied and would undergo the procedure again.

60. Gomoll AH, Gillogly SD, Cole BJ, et al: Autologous chondrocyte implantation in the patella: A multicenter experience. *Am J Sports Med* 2014;42(5):1074-1081.

In a multicenter study of 110 patients treated for a cartilage defect of the patella and followed at least 4 years, outcome scores improved, 92% of patients would choose to undergo ACI again, and 86% of patients rated the knee as good or excellent.

61. Pestka JM, Bode G, Salzmann G, Südkamp NP, Niemeyer P: Clinical outcome of autologous chondrocyte implantation for failed microfracture treatment of full-thickness cartilage defects of the knee joint. *Am J Sports Med* 2012;40(2):325-331.

Patients treated with ACI after unsuccessful microfracture had significantly more failures (7 of 28 patients) than those who received ACI as a first-line treatment (1 of 28 patients).

62. Gudas R, Kalesinskas RJ, Kimtys V, et al: A prospective randomized clinical study of mosaic osteochondral autologous transplantation versus microfracture for the treatment of osteochondral defects in the knee joint in young athletes. *Arthroscopy* 2005;21(9):1066-1075.

63. Gudas R, Gudaite A, Pocius A, et al: Ten-year follow-up of a prospective, randomized clinical study of mosaic osteochondral autologous transplantation versus microfracture for the treatment of osteochondral defects in the knee joint of athletes. *Am J Sports Med* 2012;40(11):2499-2508.

In a randomized controlled study, 60 athletes (mean age, 24.3 years) underwent OAT or microfracture. Statistically significantly better results were detected in patients in the OAT group at 10-year follow-up (*P* < 0.005). OAT failed in 4 patients (14%), and microfracture failed in 11 (38%) (*P* < 0.05). Level of evidence: I.

64. Ulstein S, Årøen A, Røtterud JH, Løken S, Engebretsen L, Heir S: Microfracture technique versus osteochondral autologous transplantation mosaicplasty in patients with articular chondral lesions of the knee: A prospective randomized trial with long-term follow-up. *Knee Surg Sports Traumatol Arthrosc* 2014;22(6):1207-1215.

Eleven of 25 patients with a full-thickness chondral lesion of the femur were randomly assigned to microfracture, and 14 were assigned to mosaicplasty. At a median 9.8-year follow-up, there were no significant between-group differences in outcome measures, isokinetic muscle strength, or radiographic osteoarthritis. Level of evidence: II.

65. Knutsen G, Engebretsen L, Ludvigsen TC, et al: Autologous chondrocyte implantation compared with microfracture in the knee: A randomized trial. *J Bone Joint Surg Am* 2004;86(3):455-464.

66. Knutsen G, Drogset JO, Engebretsen L, et al: A randomized trial comparing autologous chondrocyte implantation with microfracture: Findings at five years. *J Bone Joint Surg Am* 2007;89(10):2105-2112.

67. Saris D, Price A, Widuchowski W, et al: Matrix-applied characterized autologous cultured chondrocytes versus microfracture: Two-year follow-up of a prospective randomized trial. *Am J Sports Med* 2014;42(6):1384-1394.

In a randomized controlled study comparing the use of microfracture and matrix-applied ACI for symptomatic cartilage defects, the 2-year assessment was completed by 137 of the 144 patients (mean age, 33.8 years; mean lesion size, 4.8 cm²). Outcomes scores favored matrix-applied ACI. Repair tissue quality was good but did not vary by treatment. The rates of treatment failure were 12.5% after matrix-applied ACI and 31.9% after microfracture. Level of evidence: I.

68. Bentley G, Biant LC, Carrington RW, et al: A prospective, randomised comparison of autologous chondrocyte implantation versus mosaicplasty for osteochondral defects in the knee. *J Bone Joint Surg Br* 2003;85(2):223-230.

69. Bentley G, Biant LC, Vijayan S, Macmull S, Skinner JA, Carrington RW: Minimum ten-year results of a prospective randomised study of autologous chondrocyte implantation versus mosaicplasty for symptomatic articular cartilage lesions of the knee. *J Bone Joint Surg Br* 2012;94(4):504-509.

A randomized study followed 100 patients (mean age, 31.3 years) for at least 10 years after ACI or mosaicplasty. Ten of 58 patients (17%) had failure of ACI, and 23 of 42 (55%) had failure of mosaicplasty (*P* < 0.001). Patients with a surviving graft had significantly better function after ACI than mosaicplasty (*P* = 0.02). Level of evidence: I.

70. Liu H, Zhao Z, Clarke RB, Gao J, Garrett IR, Margerrison EE: Enhanced tissue regeneration potential of juvenile articular cartilage. *Am J Sports Med* 2013;41(11):2658-2667.

In a laboratory study, articular cartilage was harvested from juvenile and adult bovine femoral condyles and cultured for 4 weeks to monitor chondrocyte migration, glycosaminoglycan content conservation, new tissue formation, cartilage cell density, and proliferative activity. Compared with adult cartilage, juvenile bovine cartilage had significantly greater cell density, cell proliferation rate, cell outgrowth, glycosaminoglycan content, and matrix metallopeptidase-2 activity. Only juvenile cartilage was able to generate new cartilaginous tissues in culture.

71. Adkisson HD IV, Martin JA, Amendola RL, et al: The potential of human allogeneic juvenile chondrocytes for restoration of articular cartilage. *Am J Sports Med* 2010;38(7):1324-1333.

In a laboratory study, cartilage samples were obtained from juvenile and adult human donors. The chondrogenic activity of chondrocytes and expanded cells after monolayer culture was measured by proteoglycan assay, gene expression analysis, and histology. Juvenile human chondrocytes were found to have greater potential to restore articular cartilage than adult cells and can be transplanted without fear of rejection.

3: Knee and Leg

72. Farr J, Tabet SK, Margerrison E, Cole BJ: Clinical, radiographic, and histological outcomes after cartilage repair with particulated juvenile articular cartilage: A 2-year prospective study. *Am J Sports Med* 2014;42(6):1417-1425.

Twenty-five patients (mean age, 37.0 years; mean lesion size, 2.7cm^2) were treated with particulated juvenile articular cartilage for a symptomatic chondral defect. Clinical outcomes were significantly improved 2 years after surgery compared with baseline. T2-weighted MRI suggested that cartilage was approaching a normal level. The repair tissue in biopsy samples from 8 patients was composed of a mixture of hyaline and fibrocartilage. Staining revealed a higher content of type II than type I cartilage. Level of evidence: IV.

73. Milano G, Deriu L, Sanna Passino E, et al: Repeated platelet concentrate injections enhance reparative response of microfractures in the treatment of chondral defects of the knee: An experimental study in an animal model. *Arthroscopy* 2012;28(5):688-701.

A full-thickness chondral lesion on the medial femoral condyle was created in 30 sheep and treated with microfracture. One group of animals received five postoperative weekly injections of autologous conditioned plasma. The postoperatively treated animals had significantly better macroscopic, histologic, and biomechanical results than the nontreated animals at 3, 6, and 12 months.

74. Milano G, Deriu L, Sanna Passino E, et al: The effect of autologous conditioned plasma on the treatment of focal chondral defects of the knee: An experimental study. *Int J Immunopathol Pharmacol* 2011;24(1, Suppl 2)117-124.

The effect of local application of autologous conditioned plasma on full-thickness knee cartilage was investigated in 30 sheep. One group of animals received five postoperative weekly injections of autologous conditioned plasma. Histologic evaluation at 3 and 6 months showed that these animals had significantly better total scores than the untreated animals. At 12 months, there was no significant between-group difference. The local injections did not produce hyaline cartilage but did promote a reparative response of the cartilage defect until 6 months after treatment.

75. Dold AP, Zywiel MG, Taylor DW, Dwyer T, Theodoropoulos J: Platelet-rich plasma in the management of articular cartilage pathology: A systematic review. *Clin J Sport Med* 2014;24(1):31-43.

Analysis of 10 studies found that most assessed the use of PRP in the treatment of degenerative osteoarthritis of the knee or hip. Most patients were treated with intra-articular injections, but two studies used PRP as an adjunct to surgical treatment. Significant improvements in joint-specific clinical scores, general health scores, and pain scores were reported at 6-month follow-up, but few studies provided longer term data. No studies reported worse scores compared with baseline at final follow-up.

Video Reference

18.1: Chalmers P, Yanke A, Sherman S, Karas V, Cole BJ: Video. *Combined Cartilage Restoration and Distal Realignment for Patellar and Trochlear Chondral Lesions.* Chicago, IL, 2012.

Chapter 19

Nonarthroplasty Management of Osteoarthritis of the Knee

Ljiljana Bogunovic, MD   Charles A. Bush-Joseph, MD

Abstract

The knee is the most common site of osteoarthritis. With an aging population, the prevalence of this progressive disease is increasing. The management of symptomatic osteoarthritis of the knee can be challenging. Although joint arthroplasty generally is effective after unsuccessful nonsurgical management, several other treatment modalities can be successfully implemented before joint arthroplasty is considered.

Keywords: osteoarthritis of the knee; nonarthroplasty management of osteoarthritis

Introduction

Osteoarthritis of the knee is a common source of pain and disability in adults who are middle aged or older. According to 2008 estimates, knee osteoarthritis affected 33% of people older than 65 years in the United States.[1] Lifestyle changes such as weight loss and exercise as well as medications, injections, and, in some patients, joint-preserving surgery can help minimize the progress of knee osteoarthritis, manage pain, and delay the need for joint arthroplasty.

Patient Evaluation

History and Physical Examination

The evaluation of symptomatic osteoarthritis of the knee begins with a detailed patient history and physical examination. The patient's symptoms and response to

Neither of the following authors nor any immediate family member has received anything of value from or has stock or stock options held in a commercial company or institution related directly or indirectly to the subject of this chapter: Dr. Bogunovic and Dr. Bush-Joseph.

Table 1
Key Information From the Patient History
Current medications
History of injury or prior surgery
Instability
Mechanical symptoms
Medical comorbidities
Location of pain (unicompartmental or global)
Response to previous treatments
Swelling
Symptom duration

previous therapy will help guide future treatment and allow an accurate prognosis to be determined (Table 1). A patient who is overweight should be asked about any recent weight gain or loss and current weight-maintenance strategy. A comorbidity such as renal or peptic ulcer disease and social factors that could affect the treatment strategy, such as residence in a nursing home, also should be determined.

The patient's gait as well as lower body alignment, range of motion, and ligamentous stability should be assessed and documented (Table 2). Catching or locking, instability, or an effusion can signal the presence of a mechanical pathology warranting surgical treatment. The lumbar spine and hips should be examined because pathology in one of these locations often appears as pain referred to the knee. The lower extremities should be examined for evidence of muscular atrophy or weakness, with particular attention to hip abductor and quadriceps strength. Distal sensation and vascular perfusion (peripheral pulses) should be assessed in all patients, and any abnormalities should be documented.

Imaging

Baseline weight-bearing radiographs should be obtained in all patients with symptomatic osteoarthritis of the

3: Knee and Leg

knee. A standing PA view obtained with the patient's knee in 45° of flexion often is preferred over the standard standing AP view.[2] The flexion view allows better evaluation of the posterior femoral condyles and earlier detection of subtle joint-space loss than the AP view[2] (Figure 1). Additional radiographs should include a lateral view of the affected side and a Merchant or sunrise view of the patellofemoral joint.

Nonsurgical Management

Weight Loss
Maintenance of a healthy body weight is effective for decreasing the severity of symptoms and slowing the

Table 2

Key Information From the Physical Examination

Alignment (varus or valgus, rigid or flexible)

Effusion
Instability
Ipsilateral hip comparison
Joint line tenderness
Lower extremity strength (quadriceps, gluteus)

Peripheral pulses and sensation
Previous incision(s)
Range of motion

progression of osteoarthritis of the knee.[3-7] Obesity has been identified as an independent risk factor for osteoarthritis of the knee; it increases the likelihood of symptomatic disease as much as threefold.[5,8] Patients with coexisting knee malalignment, particularly genu varum, have an even greater susceptibility to the negative effect of excessive body weight.[3] A clinical practice guideline of the American Academy of Orthopaedic Surgeons (AAOS) recommends weight loss for patients who have symptomatic osteoarthritis of the knee and are overweight (defined as a body mass index above 25 kg/m[2])[9] (Table 3). Forces at the knee are magnified to three to seven times the actual body weight, and therefore even a small change in body weight can have a significant effect on joint loading at the knee.[3] At a minimum, the patient who is overweight should strive to lose 5% of his or her current body weight and to maintain the decreased weight with a combination of diet and exercise.[10-12]

Exercise and Activity
Regular physical activity was found to improve physical function and quality of life in patients with symptomatic osteoarthritis of the knee.[1,13,14] AAOS strongly recommends patient participation in a self-management program such as the Arthritis Foundation exercise program.[9,15] Such programs typically extend over 6 to 8 weeks, are offered at a local hospital or community center, and focus on lower extremity and core musculature strengthening, low-impact aerobic activity, and

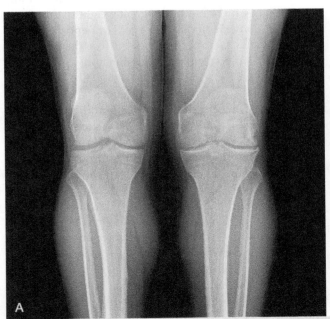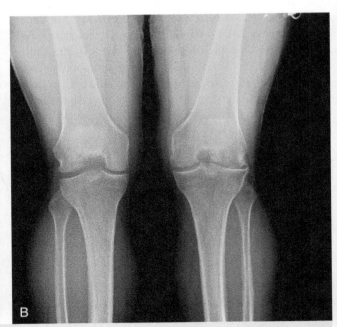

Figure 1 Standing AP (**A**) and 45° flexion PA weight-bearing (Rosenberg) (**B**) radiographs of a patient with osteoarthritis. Wear on the left posterior lateral condyle can be seen in **B**.

Table 3

Summary of AAOS Clinical Practice Guideline Recommendations

Modality	Recommendation	Strength[a]
Activity and lifestyle		
Lateral wedge insole for medial osteoarthritis	Cannot suggest	Moderate
Physical activity	Recommend	Strong
Unloader bracing for medial osteoarthritis	Unable to recommend	Inconclusive
Weight loss (patient with body mass index of 25 kg/m² or higher)	Suggest	Moderate
Medications and supplements		
Acetaminophen	Unable to recommend	Inconclusive
Glucosamine and/or chondroitin	Cannot recommend	Strong
NSAIDs (oral and topical)	Recommend	Strong
Opioids or pain patches	Unable to recommend	Inconclusive
Tramadol	Recommend	Strong
Alternative treatments		
Acupuncture	Cannot recommend	Strong
Electrotherapeutic and manual therapy	Unable to recommend	Inconclusive
Intra-articular injections		
Corticosteroids	Unable to recommend	Inconclusive
Growth factors, platelet-rich plasma	Unable to recommend	Inconclusive
Hyaluronic acid	Cannot recommend	Strong
Needle lavage	Cannot suggest	Moderate
Surgical treatments		
Arthroscopic lavage and/or débridement	Cannot recommend	Strong
Arthroscopic partial meniscectomy	Unable to recommend	Inconclusive
Valgus proximal tibial osteotomy for medial compartment osteoarthritis	Might recommend	Limited

[a] Inconclusive = A lack of compelling evidence has resulted in an unclear balance between the benefits and potential harm; practitioners should not be constrained from following the recommendation. Limited = The quality of the supporting evidence is unconvincing, or well-conducted studies show little clear advantage to one approach over another; practitioners should exercise clinical judgment when following the recommendation. Moderate = The benefits exceed the potential harm (or the potential harm clearly exceeds the benefit in a negative recommendation), but the quality or applicability of the supporting evidence is not strong; practitioners generally should follow the recommendation but remain alert to new information and be sensitive to patient preferences. Strong = The quality of the supporting evidence is high; practitioners should follow this recommendation unless there is a clear and compelling rationale for an alternative approach.

Data from American Academy of Orthopaedic Surgeons: *Treatment of Osteoarthritis of the Knee: Evidence-based Guidelines,* ed 2. Rosemont, IL, American Academy of Orthopaedic Surgeons, 2013. http://www.aaos.org/Research/guidelines/TreatmentofOsteoarthritisoftheKneeGuideline.pdf. Accessed October 31, 2014.

neuromuscular training. Patients receive information on activity modification, healthy eating, stress management, and disease progression.[9,16,17]

General activity recommendations for patients with osteoarthritis of the knee include avoidance of high-impact activities and repetitive heavy lifting, squatting, crouching, or climbing.[18] Patients can safely undertake at least 150 minutes of moderate activity each week with no risk of worsening the disease progression.[18,19] Activities such as water aerobics, walking, swimming, cycling, and tai chi can increase cardiovascular endurance, lower extremity strength, mobility, and balance, with minimal impact on the knees.[20-22]

Physical Therapy

A patient who is sedentary or has a persistent deficit in strength or mobility after completion of a self-management program can benefit from a course of prescribed

3: Knee and Leg

Table 4

Summary of AAOS Appropriate Use Criteria Recommendations

Modality	Recommendation[a]
Activity and lifestyle	
Hinged knee brace and/or unloading brace	May be appropriate
Prescribed physical therapy	Appropriate
Self-management program	Appropriate
Medications	
Acetaminophen	Appropriate
Intra-articular corticosteroid	Appropriate
Narcotic for refractory pain	Rarely appropriate
NSAIDs (topical or oral)	Appropriate
Tramadol	May be appropriate
Surgical treatments	
Meniscectomy or loose body removal	Rarely appropriate[b]
Realignment osteotomy	Rarely appropriate

[a] Appropriate = The treatment is generally acceptable, reasonable for the indications, and likely to improve the patient's health outcome or survival. May be appropriate = The treatment may be acceptable and reasonable for the indication, but uncertainty implies that more research and/or patient information is needed to further classify the indication. Rarely appropriate = The treatment rarely is appropriate for patients with symptomatic osteoarthritis of the knee because of the lack of a clear benefit-risk advantage; the clinical reasons for proceeding with the treatment should be documented in case of an exception.

[b] May be appropriate for patients with mechanical symptoms.

Data from American Academy of Orthopaedic Surgeons: *Appropriate Use Criteria for Non-arthroplasty Treatment of Osteoarthritis of the Knee.* Rosemont, IL, American Academy of Orthopaedic Surgeons, 2013. http://www.aaos.org/Research/Appropriate_Use/oakaucfull.pdf. Accessed October 31, 2014.

---

physical therapy.[7,15] Extensor mechanism weakness is common in patients with symptomatic osteoarthritis of the knee and has been associated with exacerbation of symptoms and disease progression.[23-25] Therapist-supervised exercises directed at quadriceps strengthening can be helpful in alleviating pain, decreasing subjective instability, and improving overall function.[26] Physical therapy also can be helpful in improving proprioception and neuromuscular control. Only limited data support the use of physical therapy to improve range of motion and flexibility in patients with osteoarthritis of the knee.[10] If possible, a prescribed physical therapy program should include a transition to a patient-directed home program at the completion of formal therapy.

Bracing

The routine use of a brace is not recommended for managing the symptoms of osteoarthritis of the knee, but in some patients the use of an unloader brace was found to decrease pain and improve function.[9,15,27-29] According to the 2013 AAOS Appropriate Use Criteria (Table 4), treatment with a valgus- or varus-producing unloader brace may be appropriate for a patient with symptomatic unicompartmental medial or lateral osteoarthritis, respectively.[3,15] Unloader braces exert an external moment at the joint during gait and thereby shift axial joint forces preferentially toward the normal compartment[28] (Figure 2). A biomechanical study found that the greatest load reduction occurred during stair ascending and descending.[28] An unloader brace can be helpful for an active patient who wants to delay surgical treatment (osteotomy or arthroplasty).

Pain relief during a trial of brace wearing was found to predict a favorable outcome of realignment osteotomy.[30] Medial-side disease was found to be more responsive to bracing than lateral-side disease.[27] Bracing can be effective in the setting of fixed deformity, but most brace manufacturers recommend bracing only for patients with no more than 10° of varus or valgus deformity.[31] Instability, especially excessive medial or lateral collateral laxity in the affected compartment, is a contraindication to unloader bracing. Concomitant arthritis of the patellofemoral joint is not considered a contraindication.[31] Custom braces were found to be slightly more effective than off-the-shelf braces, and a custom brace may be required to achieve the desired fit and force generation

© 2016 American Academy of Orthopaedic Surgeons

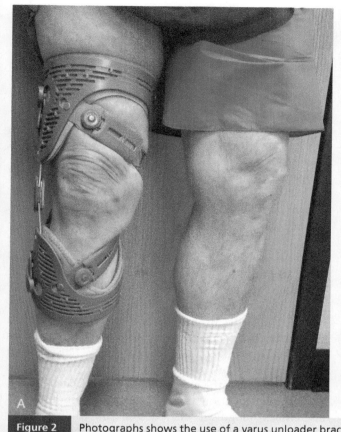 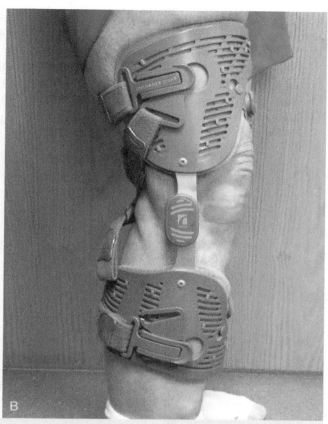

Figure 2 Photographs shows the use of a varus unloader brace to treat valgus malalignment (**A**) and lateral compartment osteoarthritis (**B**).

for a patient who is obese.[29] Patient tolerance is one of the main limitations of unloader bracing. The load distribution depends on the stiffness and angulation of the brace, and the brace specifications required to achieve a load reduction of more than 25% are not well tolerated by most patients.[28]

Taping and Insoles

Therapeutic taping can be helpful in managing the symptoms of patellofemoral osteoarthritis.[32,33] The use of a taping technique such as McConnell taping generates a medially directed force across the patella, provides short-term pain relief, and improves function.[32,33] The use of a lateral heel-wedge insole for symptomatic medial compartment osteoarthritis was not found to be effective and is not recommended.[9,34]

Alternative Therapy

High-quality studies did not find acupuncture to be beneficial in the treatment of symptomatic osteoarthritis of the knee, and it should not be recommended.[9] Little or no benefit was documented when an electrotherapeutic modality such as electrical stimulation was used.[35,36] The

risks and benefits of manual therapy and ultrasonography have not been established.[9,35,37]

Medications

Nonsteroidal Anti-inflammatory Drugs

NSAIDs are recommended as a first-line treatment for patients with osteoarthritis of the knee. Both oral and topical NSAID preparations are effective in alleviating pain and swelling.[7] Because of their possible renal, cardiovascular, and gastrointestinal adverse effects, NSAIDs should be used with caution in patients older than 60 years and those with a medical comorbidity. The gastrointestinal effects of a nonselective oral NSAID can be minimized in patients with moderate risk factors by coprescribing a proton-pump inhibitor or substituting a selective cyclo-oxygenase-2 inhibitor.[35] Complete avoidance of all oral NSAIDs is recommended for patients at significant risk for an adverse effect.[35]

Acetaminophen

The 2013 AAOS clinical practice guideline on managing osteoarthritis of the knee reported a lack of compelling available evidence to support acetaminophen use.[9]

Nonetheless, AAOS still considered treatment with acetaminophen to be appropriate for patients with osteoarthritis of the knee because of its favorable safety profile and potential analgesic effects.[7,15] Acetaminophen can be particularly helpful in patients who are older than 60 years or have a comorbidity that precludes long-term NSAID use. Treatment and dosage should be maintained within the prescribed limits to prevent hepatotoxicity.[38]

Tramadol

Tramadol was found to be as effective as NSAIDs for alleviating the pain associated with osteoarthritis of the knee.[7,15,39] This atypical opioid analgesic medication can be particularly useful in patients who are older than 60 years or have a medical comorbidity because it has no cardiovascular, renal, or gastrointestinal adverse effects. Unlike NSAIDs, tramadol has no effect on the inflammation associated with osteoarthritis.[39]

Opioids

The routine use of oral or transdermal narcotic medications is not recommended for patients with osteoarthritis of the knee.[9,35] A recent systematic review found a significant risk of adverse events that far outweighed the relatively insignificant pain control benefit.[40]

Nutritional Supplements

Data from several high-quality studies showed no benefit from the use of a daily glucosamine and/or chondroitin sulfate supplement.[9,15,35,41] Ginger was found to be moderately effective in alleviating arthritis pain.[42] Avocado soybean unsaponifiables also had moderate to high efficacy for short-term pain relief in osteoarthritis of the knee, but a long-term effect has not been established.[35,43]

Injections

Corticosteroids

Intra-articular corticosteroid injection is effective for managing the symptoms of osteoarthritis of the knee, and the AAOS considers it to be an appropriate treatment option.[15] Corticosteroid injection can be a helpful treatment adjunct after unsuccessful nonpharmacologic or oral NSAID or analgesic therapy. Reliable pain relief lasting approximately 4 weeks can be expected after injection.[44,45] Treatment with corticosteroid injection can reduce symptoms sufficiently to allow initiation of lifestyle changes such as increased activity. The minimal interval between injections is 3 months; if more frequent pain relief is needed, other treatments should be considered.[45] Comparisons of intra-articular hyaluronic acid and corticosteroid injections found that corticosteroid was more effective in alleviating pain.[44,46]

Hyaluronic Acid

The benefit of intra-articular hyaluronic acid remains debatable. Several studies found that viscosupplementation led to a statistically significant improvement in pain, but recent analysis, including an evidence-based review by AAOS, suggested that treatment with hyaluronic acid did not meet the threshold for a minimum clinically important difference.[9,35,46] Reliance on this criterion as a primary metric for treatment efficacy is controversial, however, and the AAOS guideline was criticized for relying on it.[47] The effect of intra-articular hyaluronic acid probably depends on several factors including the severity of osteoarthritis, the patient's age, and limb alignment. In a comparison of intra-articular corticosteroid and hyaluronic acid injections, corticosteroid appeared to be more effective in alleviating pain during the first 4 weeks after injection, but hyaluronic acid was more effective beyond 8 weeks after injection.[46] A recent systematic review reported a small and clinically irrelevant improvement in pain after hyaluronic acid injection as well as a significant increase in the risk of serious adverse events including a postinjection flare reaction.[37] The addition of corticosteroid to a viscosupplementation injection was found to decrease the postinjection pain associated with viscosupplementation alone.[48] Practitioners should exercise clinical judgment when considering this treatment modality by weighing the potential for improving the patient's pain against the risk of adverse events.

Growth Factors and Platelet-Rich Plasma

The benefits of using growth factors or a biologic agent such as platelet-rich plasma (PRP) or mesenchymal stem cells in treating osteoarthritis has not been established. In theory, these agents provide biologic stimulation for articular cartilage maintenance and possibly repair. A systematic review of level I and II studies found a short-term (6-month) beneficial effect of PRP treatment on subjective outcomes in patients with mild to moderate osteoarthritis, but the risk of nonspecific adverse events was increased.[49] A randomized controlled study comparing treatment with PRP and treatment with hyaluronic acid found no significant between-group difference in patient-rated outcomes at 12-month follow-up.[50] Subgroup analysis revealed a trend toward better patient function after PRP treatment in patients with mild osteoarthritis (defined as Kellgren-Lawrence grade 1 or 2). The rate of adverse reactions, particularly postinjection pain, was higher in patients who received PRP than in those who received hyaluronic acid.[50] The use of PRP for the treatment of osteoarthritis of the knee is not currently approved by the US FDA, and its off-label use typically is not covered by insurance plans. More investigation into the efficacy, safety, and optimal preparation of PRP is needed before it can be routinely used for the treatment of osteoarthritis of the knee.

Surgical Treatment

Arthroscopic Débridement and Lavage

Arthroscopic débridement and lavage of the knee is not recommended for a patient with a primary diagnosis of osteoarthritis.[9,15] One high-level study found no benefit to using this treatment modality.[51] In patients with mechanical symptoms secondary to the presence of a loose body, knee arthroscopy with loose body removal may be beneficial, especially if the patient has mild to moderate osteoarthritis.

Arthroscopic Meniscectomy

The effectiveness of arthroscopic partial meniscectomy for patients with osteoarthritis of the knee and a concomitant meniscal tear remains an area of debate. In a randomized controlled study comparing partial arthroscopic meniscectomy with physical therapy, an intention-to-treat analysis found no between-group differences in patient-rated outcomes at 12-month follow-up.[52] There was a 35% crossover from the physical therapy group to the surgery group, however. A second randomized controlled study compared arthroscopic partial meniscectomy with diagnostic arthroscopy and found no difference in patient-rated outcomes at 12-month follow-up.[53] Exclusion of patients with a traumatic meniscal tear, lateral tear, acute tear, acute-on-chronic tear, or radiographic evidence of osteoarthritis limited the relevance of the study results for the general population of patients with osteoarthritis of the knee.[53] Additional data suggested that the benefits of partial meniscectomy may be limited to patients with mild to moderate osteoarthritis who have a large, unstable meniscal tear and mechanical symptoms.[51,54] These patients may experience symptomatic improvement after partial meniscectomy. Given the limited indications, nonsurgical treatment including physical therapy, NSAIDs, and injection should be tried before surgical intervention is considered for patients with osteoarthritis and meniscal pathology.[55]

Realignment Osteotomy

Knee malalignment is a known risk factor for the development and progression of osteoarthritis.[56,57] Realignment osteotomy rarely is indicated but can be considered for a patient who is active, younger than 55 years, and not obese and who has moderate varus or valgus deformity, mild to moderate unicompartmental disease, stable collateral ligaments, and a near-normal range of motion[9,58-61] (Table 5). A trial of unloader bracing can be helpful in

Table 5	
Contraindications to Realignment Osteotomy for Symptomatic Osteoarthritis of the Knee	
Relative Contraindications	**Absolute Contraindications**
Obesity	Contralateral compartment osteoarthritis
Moderate to severe osteoarthritis of the knee	
Age older than 50 years	Flexion of less than 100°
Patellofemoral arthritis	
Collateral laxity	Flexion contracture of more than 10°

predicting response to surgical realignment.[30] Arthroscopy before osteotomy often is recommended to confirm the absence of osteoarthritis in the remaining compartments and to allow any concomitant meniscal or chondral pathology to be treated.

A medial opening wedge high-tibial osteotomy is becoming the preferred realignment technique for isolated medial compartment disease[61-63] (Figure 3). A randomized controlled study comparing medial opening wedge and lateral closing wedge high-tibial osteotomies found no differences in patient-rated outcomes or maintenance of alignment at 6-year follow-up.[62] At 6-year follow-up, the medial opening wedge technique was associated with more postoperative complications but 14% fewer conversions to total knee arthroplasty than the lateral closing wedge technique (8% versus 22%). The medial opening wedge technique is more sensitive to sagittal plane alterations of the tibial slope than closing wedge techniques (Figure 4). Overall survivorship of a high-tibial osteotomy for medial compartment disease was found to range from 88% to 96% at 5-year follow-up, from 63% to 97% at 10-year follow-up, and from 57% to 90% at 15-year follow-up.[60,64] Neither medial nor lateral high-tibial osteotomy affected the functional outcomes or survivorship of a subsequent total knee arthroplasty.[65]

In patients with lateral compartment disease and valgus deformity, a lateral opening wedge distal femoral osteotomy can be used.[66] The outcome of the varus-producing osteotomy appears to be less affected by concomitant patellofemoral arthritis than patients with medial compartment arthritis undergoing a valgus producing osteotomy.[67] A 50% conversion rate to total knee arthroplasty was reported within 15 years.[67,68]

Summary

The nonarthroplasty treatment of symptomatic osteoarthritis of the knee is a common clinical challenge.

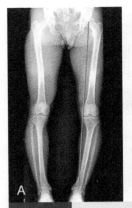
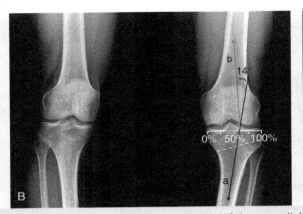
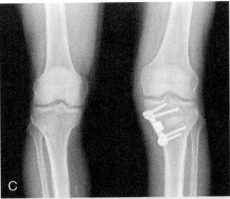

Figure 3 Full-length standing AP radiographs of a patient with left knee medial compartment osteoarthritis and varus alignment. **A,** The mechanical axis is drawn from the center of the femoral head to the center of the ankle. The line passes through the medial compartment, indicating varus alignment. **B,** Preoperative templating for a high-tibial osteotomy of the left leg. The goal is to shift the mechanical axis to a point at 62.5% of the width of the tibial plateau, as measured from the medial edge. A line is drawn from the center of the ankle (a) to this point and from the center of the femoral head (b) to this point. The angle formed by the intersection of these two lines represents the angle of correction (14°). The osteotomy cut (dashed line) starts on the medial cortex at a point approximately 4 mm from the joint line and continues laterally to the level of the fibular head. The lateral cortex is left intact. One millimeter of opening corresponds to one degree of correction. **C,** The left knee after a medial opening wedge high-tibial osteotomy.

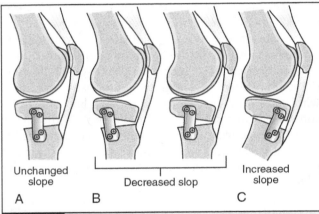

Figure 4 Schematic drawings show alteration of the tibial slope with plate positioning in a medial opening wedge osteotomy. **A,** Direct medial placement of a rectangular wedge plate does not change the slope. **B,** In a knee with a deficiency in the anterior cruciate ligament, anterior translation of the tibia can be reduced by decreasing the tibial slope with posteromedial placement of a rectangular wedge plate (left) or with a taper wedge plate (right). **C,** Increasing the tibial slope with anteromedial placement of a rectangular wedge plate can decrease posterior tibial translation in a knee with a deficiency in the posterior cruciate ligament.

of biologic therapies such as PRP is under investigation. In selected patients, nonarthroplasty surgical procedures such as realignment osteotomy can help to alleviate symptoms. In the absence of mechanical symptoms, arthroscopic débridement has not been shown to be an effective treatment strategy.

Key Study Points

- A variety of nonsurgical treatment modalities can be used to treat the symptoms and decrease the progression of symptomatic osteoarthritis of the knee.
- Weight loss for patients with a body mass index above 25 kg/m² is effective in decreasing pain and minimizing the progression of symptomatic osteoarthritis of the knee.
- Intra-articular corticosteroid injections are effective for symptomatic management of osteoarthritis of the knee.
- Oral supplementation with glucosamine and/or chondroitin sulfate has no benefit for management of symptomatic osteoarthritis of the knee.
- Continued study is needed to identify the benefits of PRP and stem cell therapy in the treatment of osteoarthritis of the knee.
- In the absence of mechanical symptoms, knee arthroscopy with débridement is not effective in treating osteoarthritis of the knee.

Patients may experience substantial pain and disability. Lifestyle modifications including weight loss and exercise as well as the use of NSAIDs or intra-articular injections can reliably decrease pain and improve function. The role

Annotated References

1. Helmick CG, Felson DT, Lawrence RC, et al; National Arthritis Data Workgroup: Estimates of the prevalence of arthritis and other rheumatic conditions in the United States: Part I. *Arthritis Rheum* 2008;58(1):15-25.

2. Rosenberg TD, Paulos LE, Parker RD, Coward DB, Scott SM: The forty-five-degree posteroanterior flexion weight-bearing radiograph of the knee. *J Bone Joint Surg Am* 1988;70(10):1479-1483.

3. Yates AJ Jr, McGrory BJ, Starz TW, Vincent KR, McCardel B, Golightly YM: AAOS appropriate use criteria: Optimizing the non-arthroplasty management of osteoarthritis of the knee. *J Am Acad Orthop Surg* 2014;22(4):261-267.

   The 2013 AAOS appropriate use criteria for the nonarthroplasty management of osteoarthritis of the knee were reviewed and applied to examples.

4. Changulani M, Kalairajah Y, Peel T, Field RE: The relationship between obesity and the age at which hip and knee replacement is undertaken. *J Bone Joint Surg Br* 2008;90(3):360-363.

5. Blagojevic M, Jinks C, Jeffery A, Jordan KP: Risk factors for onset of osteoarthritis of the knee in older adults: A systematic review and meta-analysis. *Osteoarthritis Cartilage* 2010;18(1):24-33.

   A systematic review found an increased risk of osteoarthritis of the knee with obesity (odds ratio, 2.63) and previous trauma (odds ratio, 3.86). Level of evidence: V.

6. Gandhi R, Wasserstein D, Razak F, Davey JR, Mahomed NN: BMI independently predicts younger age at hip and knee replacement. *Obesity (Silver Spring)* 2010;18(12):2362-2366.

   A retrospective review of patients undergoing hip and knee replacement found that obesity (body mass index greater than 25) was associated with significantly decreased age at the time of hip or knee arthroplasty. Level of evidence: IV.

7. Bruyère O, Cooper C, Pelletier J-P, et al: An algorithm recommendation for the management of knee osteoarthritis in Europe and internationally: A report from a task force of the European Society for Clinical and Economic Aspects of Osteoporosis and Osteoarthritis (ESCEO). *Semin Arthritis Rheum* 2014;44(3):253-263.

   Guidelines for the nonarthroplasty management of osteoarthritis of the knee were established by the European Society for Clinical and Economic Aspects of Osteoporosis and Osteoarthritis, which is composed of rheumatologists, clinical epidemiologists, and clinical scientists.

8. Sowers M: Epidemiology of risk factors for osteoarthritis: Systemic factors. *Curr Opin Rheumatol* 2001;13(5):447-451.

9. American Academy of Orthopaedic Surgeons: *Treatment of Osteoarthritis of the Knee: Evidence-based Guidelines*, ed 2. Rosemont, IL, American Academy of Orthopaedic Surgeons, 2013. http://www.aaos.org/Research/guidelines/TreatmentofOsteoarthritisoftheKneeGuideline.pdf. Accessed October 31, 2014.

   The AAOS evidence-based guidelines included methodology and guidance for the nonarthroplasty management of osteoarthritis of the knee.

10. Richmond J, Hunter D, Irrgang J, et al; American Academy of Orthopaedic Surgeons: American Academy of Orthopaedic Surgeons clinical practice guideline on the treatment of osteoarthritis (OA) of the knee. *J Bone Joint Surg Am* 2010;92(4):990-993.

    The first edition of the American Academy of Orthopaedic Surgeons evidence-based guidelines for the nonarthroplasty management of osteoarthritis of the knee was reviewed.

11. Christensen R, Bartels EM, Astrup A, Bliddal H: Effect of weight reduction in obese patients diagnosed with knee osteoarthritis: A systematic review and meta-analysis. *Ann Rheum Dis* 2007;66(4):433-439.

12. Felson DT, Zhang Y, Anthony JM, Naimark A, Anderson JJ: Weight loss reduces the risk for symptomatic knee osteoarthritis in women: The Framingham Study. *Ann Intern Med* 1992;116(7):535-539.

13. Messier SP, Mihalko SL, Legault C, et al: Effects of intensive diet and exercise on knee joint loads, inflammation, and clinical outcomes among overweight and obese adults with knee osteoarthritis: The IDEA randomized clinical trial. *JAMA* 2013;310(12):1263-1273.

    A randomized controlled study of adults who were overweight and had osteoarthritis of the knee found that combined diet and exercise led to improved weight loss, reduction of interleukin-6 levels, and improved quality-of-life scores compared with diet or exercise alone. Level of evidence: I.

14. Messier SP, Loeser RF, Miller GD, et al: Exercise and dietary weight loss in overweight and obese older adults with knee osteoarthritis: The Arthritis, Diet, and Activity Promotion Trial. *Arthritis Rheum* 2004;50(5):1501-1510.

15. American Academy of Orthopaedic Surgeons: *Appropriate use criteria for non-arthroplasty treatment of osteoarthritis of the knee*. Rosemont, IL, American Academy of Orthopaedic Surgeons, 2013. http://www.aaos.org/Research/Appropriate_Use/oakaucfull.pdf. Accessed October 31, 2014.

    The AAOS appropriate use criteria included methodology and guidance for the nonarthroplasty management of osteoarthritis of the knee.

16. Coleman S, Briffa NK, Carroll G, Inderjeeth C, Cook N, McQuade J: A randomised controlled trial of a self-management education program for osteoarthritis of the knee delivered by health care professionals. *Arthritis Res Ther* 2012;14(1):R21.

3: Knee and Leg

A randomized controlled study found better patient-reported outcomes in patients with osteoarthritis who underwent a self-management program, in comparison with control subjects. Level of evidence: II.

17. Jevsevar DS: Treatment of osteoarthritis of the knee: Evidence-based guideline, 2nd edition. *J Am Acad Orthop Surg* 2013;21(9):571-576.

The second edition of the AAOS evidence-based clinical practice guideline on the nonarthroplasty treatment of osteoarthritis of the knee was reviewed.

18. Buckwalter JA, Lane NE: Athletics and osteoarthritis. *Am J Sports Med* 1997;25(6):873-881.

19. Barbour KE, Hootman JM, Helmick CG, et al: Meeting physical activity guidelines and the risk of incident knee osteoarthritis: A population-based prospective cohort study. *Arthritis Care Res (Hoboken)* 2014;66(1):139-146.

A retrospective review of 1,522 adults found no association between high levels of physical activity and the development of symptomatic osteoarthritis of the knee. Level of evidence: IV.

20. Fransen M, McConnell S: Exercise for osteoarthritis of the knee. *Cochrane Database Syst Rev* 2008;8(4):CD004376.

21. Bartels EM, Lund H, Hagen KB, Dagfinrud H, Christensen R, Danneskiold-Samsøe B: Aquatic exercise for the treatment of knee and hip osteoarthritis. *Cochrane Database Syst Rev* 2007;4:CD005523.

22. Kang JW, Lee MS, Posadzki P, Ernst E: T'ai chi for the treatment of osteoarthritis: A systematic review and meta-analysis. *BMJ Open* 2011;1(1):e000035.

A systematic review of randomized clinical studies investigated the use of tai chi as a treatment of osteoarthritis and identified evidence of effectiveness in controlling pain and improving physical function. Level of evidence: III.

23. Hortobágyi T, Garry J, Holbert D, Devita P: Aberrations in the control of quadriceps muscle force in patients with knee osteoarthritis. *Arthritis Rheum* 2004;51(4):562-569.

24. Segal NA, Glass NA, Torner J, et al: Quadriceps weakness predicts risk for knee joint space narrowing in women in the MOST cohort. *Osteoarthritis Cartilage* 2010;18(6):769-775.

A prospective longitudinal study found an association between quadriceps weakness and tibiofemoral joint space narrowing in women over time. Level of evidence: III.

25. Segal NA, Glass NA, Felson DT, et al: Effect of quadriceps strength and proprioception on risk for knee osteoarthritis. *Med Sci Sports Exerc* 2010;42(11):2081-2088.

A prospective study of 1,829 patients found that quadriceps muscle strength had a protective effect against the development of symptomatic osteoarthritis of the knee. Level of evidence: II.

26. Deyle GD, Henderson NE, Matekel RL, Ryder MG, Garber MB, Allison SC: Effectiveness of manual physical therapy and exercise in osteoarthritis of the knee: A randomized, controlled trial. *Ann Intern Med* 2000;132(3):173-181.

27. Huleatt JB, Campbell KJ, Laprade RF: Nonoperative treatment approach to knee osteoarthritis in the master athlete. *Sports Health* 2014;6(1):56-62.

The management of active patients with symptomatic osteoarthritis of the knee was reviewed.

28. Kutzner I, Küther S, Heinlein B, et al: The effect of valgus braces on medial compartment load of the knee joint: In vivo load measurements in three subjects. *J Biomech* 2011;44(7):1354-1360.

An in vivo biomechanical study found significant reductions in joint loading in stair ascending (26%) and stair descending (24%) with the use of a valgus unloader brace.

29. Draganich L, Reider B, Rimington T, Piotrowski G, Mallik K, Nasson S: The effectiveness of self-adjustable custom and off-the-shelf bracing in the treatment of varus gonarthrosis. *J Bone Joint Surg Am* 2006;88(12):2645-2652.

30. Minzlaff P, Saier T, Brucker PU, Haller B, Imhoff AB, Hinterwimmer S: Valgus bracing in symptomatic varus malalignment for testing the expectable "unloading effect" following valgus high tibial osteotomy. *Knee Surg Sports Traumatol Arthrosc* 2015;23(7):1964-1970.

A prospective study of 48 patients with medial compartment osteoarthritis found that temporary relief with unloader bracing could predict pain relief after valgus-producing high-tibial osteotomy. Level of evidence: III.

31. Pollo FE, Jackson RW: Knee bracing for unicompartmental osteoarthritis. *J Am Acad Orthop Surg* 2006;14(1):5-11.

32. Hinman RS, Crossley KM, McConnell J, Bennell KL: Efficacy of knee tape in the management of osteoarthritis of the knee: Blinded randomised controlled trial. *BMJ* 2003;327(7407):135.

33. Warden SJ, Hinman RS, Watson MA Jr, Avin KG, Bialocerkowski AE, Crossley KM: Patellar taping and bracing for the treatment of chronic knee pain: A systematic review and meta-analysis. *Arthritis Rheum* 2008;59(1):73-83.

34. Malvankar S, Khan WS, Mahapatra A, Dowd GS: How effective are lateral wedge orthotics in treating medial compartment osteoarthritis of the knee? A systematic review of the recent literature. *Open Orthop J* 2012;6:544-547.

A systematic review found no long-term benefit of using lateral shoe wedge orthoses for the symptomatic treatment of medial compartment osteoarthritis. Level of evidence: IV.

35. McAlindon TE, Bannuru RR, Sullivan MC, et al: OARSI guidelines for the non-surgical management of knee osteoarthritis. *Osteoarthritis Cartilage* 2014;22(3):363-388.

The Osteoarthritis Research Society International established guidelines for the nonsurgical treatment of symptomatic osteoarthritis of the knee.

36. Yilmaz OO, Senocak O, Sahin E, et al: Efficacy of EMG-biofeedback in knee osteoarthritis. *Rheumatol Int* 2010;30(7):887-892.

A randomized clinical study of patients with osteoarthritis found improvement in functional outcomes and reported pain with regular lower extremity strengthening exercise but no additional benefit of electromyographic biofeedback therapy. Level of evidence: II.

37. Rutjes AW, Jüni P, da Costa BR, Trelle S, Nüesch E, Reichenbach S: Viscosupplementation for osteoarthritis of the knee: A systematic review and meta-analysis. *Ann Intern Med* 2012;157(3):180-191.

A systematic review of randomized clinical studies found a small, clinically irrelevant benefit of intra-articular viscosupplementation for the symptomatic treatment of osteoarthritis of the knee.

38. Craig DG, Bates CM, Davidson JS, Martin KG, Hayes PC, Simpson KJ: Staggered overdose pattern and delay to hospital presentation are associated with adverse outcomes following paracetamol-induced hepatotoxicity. *Br J Clin Pharmacol* 2012;73(2):285-294.

A retrospective review of 663 patients with paracetamol-induced liver injury emphasized the danger of staggered dosing in older patients.

39. Cepeda MS, Camargo F, Zea C, Valencia L: Tramadol for osteoarthritis: A systematic review and metaanalysis. *J Rheumatol* 2007;34(3):543-555.

40. da Costa BR, Nüesch E, Kasteler R, et al: Oral or transdermal opioids for osteoarthritis of the knee or hip. *Cochrane Database Syst Rev* 2014;9:CD003115.

A systematic review found a significantly increased risk of adverse events with the use of nontramadol opioids for the treatment of osteoarthritis of the knee compared with a small, possibly clinically irrelevant reduction in patient-reported pain. Level of evidence: II.

41. Yang S, Eaton CB, McAlindon TE, Lapane KL: Effects of glucosamine and chondroitin supplementation on knee osteoarthritis: An analysis with marginal structural models. *Arthritis Rheumatol* 2015;67(3):714-723.

A systematic review found no benefit to glucosamine-chondroitin supplementation for relieving patient symptoms or modifying disease progression. Level of evidence: I.

42. Bartels EM, Folmer VN, Bliddal H, et al: Efficacy and safety of ginger in osteoarthritis patients: A meta-analysis of randomized placebo-controlled trials. *Osteoarthritis Cartilage* 2015;23(1):13-21.

A systematic review found modest pain reduction in patients with osteoarthritis who were treated with supplemental ginger. Level of evidence: II.

43. Cameron M, Chrubasik S: Oral herbal therapies for treating osteoarthritis. *Cochrane Database Syst Rev* 2014;5:CD002947.

A systematic review found a pain-relieving benefit from supplementation with avocado-soybean unsaponifiables for symptomatic treatment of osteoarthritis of the knee compared with placebo. Level of evidence: I.

44. Cheng OT, Souzdalnitski D, Vrooman B, Cheng J: Evidence-based knee injections for the management of arthritis. *Pain Med* 2012;13(6):740-753.

A systematic review found benefit in intra-articular steroid injections for relief of symptoms in osteoarthritis of the knee. Level of evidence: II.

45. Bellamy N, Campbell J, Robinson V, Gee T, Bourne R, Wells G: Intraarticular corticosteroid for treatment of osteoarthritis of the knee. *Cochrane Database Syst Rev* 2006;2(2):CD005328.

46. Bannuru RR, Natov NS, Obadan IE, Price LL, Schmid CH, McAlindon TE: Therapeutic trajectory of hyaluronic acid versus corticosteroids in the treatment of knee osteoarthritis: A systematic review and meta-analysis. *Arthritis Rheum* 2009;61(12):1704-1711.

A systematic review compared hyaluronic acid to corticosteroids for the treatment of osteoarthritis of the knee. Pain relief was better at 4 weeks after steroid treatment but better beyond 8 weeks after hyaluronic acid treatment. Level of evidence: I.

47. Bannuru RR, Vaysbrot EE, McIntyre LF: Did the American Academy of Orthopaedic Surgeons osteoarthritis guidelines miss the mark? *Arthroscopy* 2014;30(1):86-89.

Commentary on the 2013 AAOS clinical practice guideline argued against the use of the minimum clinically important improvement criterion in assessing the efficacy of viscosupplementation for the treatment of osteoarthritis of the knee.

48. de Campos GC, Rezende MU, Pailo AF, Frucchi R, Camargo OP: Adding triamcinolone improves viscosupplementation: A randomized clinical trial. *Clin Orthop Relat Res* 2013;471(2):613-620.

A prospective cohort study of 104 patients found improvement in patient-rated outcomes during the first week after corticosteroid injection combined with viscosupplementation compared with viscosupplementation alone. Level of evidence: II.

49. Khoshbin A, Leroux T, Wasserstein D, et al: The efficacy of platelet-rich plasma in the treatment of symptomatic knee osteoarthritis: A systematic review with quantitative synthesis. *Arthroscopy* 2013;29(12):2037-2048.

A systematic review found improved patient-rated function with intra-articular PRP injection compared with normal saline or hyaluronic acid injection in patients with osteoarthritis of the knee. Level of evidence: II.

3: Knee and Leg

50. Filardo G, Kon E, Di Martino A, et al: Platelet-rich plasma vs hyaluronic acid to treat knee degenerative pathology: Study design and preliminary results of a randomized controlled trial. *BMC Musculoskelet Disord* 2012;13:229.

A prospective study of 109 patients found a trend toward clinical improvement 1 year after PRP injection compared with hyaluronic acid injection in patients with mild osteoarthritis of the knee, but there was no difference in outcomes in patients with moderate disease. Level of evidence: III.

51. Siparsky P, Ryzewicz M, Peterson B, Bartz R: Arthroscopic treatment of osteoarthritis of the knee: Are there any evidence-based indications? *Clin Orthop Relat Res* 2007;455(455):107-112.

52. Katz JN, Brophy RH, Chaisson CE, et al: Surgery versus physical therapy for a meniscal tear and osteoarthritis. *N Engl J Med* 2013;368(18):1675-1684.

A multicenter prospective study found no difference in outcomes in patients with osteoarthritis and a degenerative meniscal tear based on treatment with physical therapy or arthroscopic meniscectomy. Level of evidence: I.

53. Sihvonen R, Paavola M, Malmivaara A, et al; Finnish Degenerative Meniscal Lesion Study (FIDELITY) Group: Arthroscopic partial meniscectomy versus sham surgery for a degenerative meniscal tear. *N Engl J Med* 2013;369(26):2515-2524.

A multicenter prospective study found no difference in patient-rated outcomes at 1-year follow-up in patients with osteoarthritis and a degenerative medial meniscal tear based on treatment with sham surgery or arthroscopic medial meniscectomy. Level of evidence: I.

54. Dervin GF, Stiell IG, Rody K, Grabowski J: Effect of arthroscopic débridement for osteoarthritis of the knee on health-related quality of life. *J Bone Joint Surg Am* 2003;85-A(1):10-19.

55. Khan M, Evaniew N, Bedi A, Ayeni OR, Bhandari M: Arthroscopic surgery for degenerative tears of the meniscus: A systematic review and meta-analysis. *CMAJ* 2014;186(14):1057-1064.

A systematic review found no benefit to arthroscopic meniscal débridement for degenerative meniscal tears compared with nonsurgical treatment or sham surgery. Level of evidence: I.

56. Brouwer GM, van Tol AW, Bergink AP, et al: Association between valgus and varus alignment and the development and progression of radiographic osteoarthritis of the knee. *Arthritis Rheum* 2007;56(4):1204-1211.

57. Sharma L, Song J, Felson DT, Cahue S, Shamiyeh E, Dunlop DD: The role of knee alignment in disease progression and functional decline in knee osteoarthritis. *JAMA* 2001;286(2):188-195.

58. Bonasia DE, Dettoni F, Sito G, et al: Medial opening wedge high tibial osteotomy for medial compartment overload/arthritis in the varus knee: Prognostic factors. *Am J Sports Med* 2014;42(3):690-698.

A study of 123 patients found that patient age older than 56 years and postoperative flexion of less than 120° were risk factors for a poor outcome after high-tibial osteotomy for medial compartment arthritis. Level of evidence: V.

59. Flecher X, Parratte S, Aubaniac JM, Argenson JN: A 12-28-year followup study of closing wedge high tibial osteotomy. *Clin Orthop Relat Res* 2006;452:91-96.

60. Akizuki S, Shibakawa A, Takizawa T, Yamazaki I, Horiuchi H: The long-term outcome of high tibial osteotomy: A ten- to 20-year follow-up. *J Bone Joint Surg Br* 2008;90(5):592-596.

61. Amendola A, Bonasia DE: Results of high tibial osteotomy: Review of the literature. *Int Orthop* 2010;34(2):155-160.

A review of the long-term survival of high-tibial osteotomy found that the factors associated with a successful outcome in patients younger than 60 years were isolated medial compartment osteoarthritis, good range of motion, and ligamentous stability.

62. Duivenvoorden T, Brouwer RW, Baan A, et al: Comparison of closing-wedge and opening-wedge high tibial osteotomy for medial compartment osteoarthritis of the knee: A randomized controlled trial with a six-year follow-up. *J Bone Joint Surg Am* 2014;96(17):1425-1432.

A randomized study compared medial opening wedge high-tibial osteotomy with lateral closing wedge osteotomy and found no difference in clinical outcome or radiographic alignment at 6-year follow-up. Medial opening wedge osteotomy was associated with a lower rate of conversion to total knee arthroplasty but a higher rate of early complications. Level of evidence: II.

63. Rossi R, Bonasia DE, Amendola A: The role of high tibial osteotomy in the varus knee. *J Am Acad Orthop Surg* 2011;19(10):590-599.

The indications, surgical technique, and complications of high-tibial osteotomy in the varus knee were reviewed.

64. Yasuda K, Majima T, Tsuchida T, Kaneda K: A ten- to 15-year follow-up observation of high tibial osteotomy in medial compartment osteoarthrosis. *Clin Orthop Relat Res* 1992;282:186-195.

65. Preston S, Howard J, Naudie D, Somerville L, McAuley J: Total knee arthroplasty after high tibial osteotomy: No differences between medial and lateral osteotomy approaches. *Clin Orthop Relat Res* 2014;472(1):105-110.

A retrospective review of 265 patients found no difference in functional outcome or survivorship in patients who had undergone a medial opening wedge or lateral closing wedge high-tibial osteotomy before total knee arthroplasty. Level of evidence: IV.

© 2016 American Academy of Orthopaedic Surgeons

66. Backstein D, Morag G, Hanna S, Safir O, Gross A: Long-term follow-up of distal femoral varus osteotomy of the knee. *J Arthroplasty* 2007;22(4, Suppl 1):2-6.

67. Wang JW, Hsu CC: Distal femoral varus osteotomy for osteoarthritis of the knee. *J Bone Joint Surg Am* 2005;87(1):127-133.

68. Kosashvili Y, Safir O, Gross A, Morag G, Lakstein D, Backstein D: Distal femoral varus osteotomy for lateral osteoarthritis of the knee: A minimum ten-year follow-up. *Int Orthop* 2010;34(2):249-254.

A retrospective review of survivorship and outcome after distal femoral varus osteotomy for lateral compartment osteoarthritis and valgus alignment found that at 15-year follow-up approximately half of patients had undergone conversion to total joint arthroplasty. Level of evidence: IV.

3: Knee and Leg

Chapter 20

Meniscal Injuries

Stephanie W. Mayer, MD   Johnathan A. Bernard, MD, MPH   Scott A. Rodeo, MD

Abstract

The menisci are fibrocartilaginous structures with gross and microscopic structural properties that provide load distribution, lubrication, and stability to the knee joint. Diagnosis of a symptomatic meniscal tear requires a thorough patient history, a physical examination with meniscus-specific tests, and often, imaging studies. The anatomy, function, and vascular supply of the menisci have implications for the treatment of a meniscal tear. The long-term outcome after a total or subtotal meniscectomy is likely to include osteoarthritis. Biomechanical studies found an increase in contact pressure after subtotal meniscectomy or a high-grade radial tear causing loss of the ability to absorb hoop stresses. Strain on the anterior cruciate ligament (ACL) in medial meniscus–deficient knees and strain on the medial meniscus in ACL-deficient knees proves the important stabilizing function of the meniscus. These results have led to an increase in the number of meniscal repairs performed to preserve load absorption and stabilization. Clinical and radiographic healing rates of 60% to 85% have been reported after repair. Meniscal repair with concomitant ACL surgery leads to a higher rate of healing than isolated meniscal repair, probably because of the release of bone marrow–derived stem cells during tunnel reaming. Irreparable tears and post-meniscectomy pain syndrome are common in young patients and are difficult to treat. Collagen scaffold implants and synthetic polyurethane scaffolds have had promising results in animal and human studies for filling large defects after partial meniscectomy. Relatively young patients who need to undergo total or subtotal meniscectomy as a primary procedure may be candidates for meniscal allograft transplantation. Biomechanical studies found that strain on the ACL is reduced and knee kinematics and contact pressures are improved to near-baseline levels after transplantation.

Keywords: meniscus; meniscal transplant

Introduction

The medial and lateral menisci have important roles in the knee joint. Their unique anatomic structure provides both static and dynamic stability to the knee. The histologic and biologic composition of the menisci allows load distribution, proprioception, and lubrication, and biomechanical and clinical results have confirmed the

Dr. Rodeo or an immediate family member serves as a paid consultant to Rotation Medical and has stock or stock options held in Cayenne Medical. Neither of the following authors nor any immediate family member has received anything of value from or has stock or stock options held in a commercial company or institution related directly or indirectly to the subject of this chapter: Dr. Mayer and Dr. Bernard.

importance of radial, horizontal, and root tears of the meniscus. Advances in imaging have improved the characterization of normal and pathologic menisci. Research into biologic and meniscal collagen implants is expanding the treatment options for patients with meniscal pathology. Short-term and long-term studies of meniscal allograft transplantation have led to improvements in this technique for carefully selected patients.

Anatomy

The menisci are wedge-shaped fibrocartilaginous structures situated between the femoral condyles and the tibial plateau. These structures have many functions in the knee including proprioceptive feedback, load distribution during physiologic loading, joint lubrication during motion, and maintenance of tibiofemoral joint stability and congruity.[1,2] The substance of the menisci is a solid extracellular matrix and water. Fibrochondrocytes are the predominant meniscal cell type, and they produce the

3: Knee and Leg

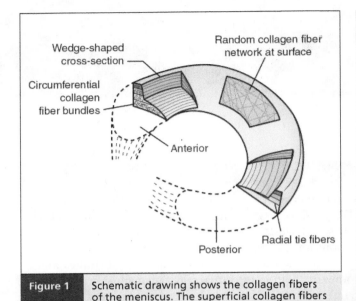

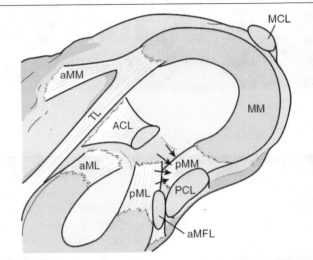

Figure 1	Schematic drawing shows the collagen fibers of the meniscus. The superficial collagen fibers are randomly oriented to resist sheer stress. The deeper fibers are oriented circumferentially to dissipate loads as hoop stresses. The circumferential fibers are secured by radially oriented tie fibers.

Figure 2	Illustration shows the menisci and the proximal tibial plateau. The medial meniscus (MM) is C shaped. The insertion of the posteromedial meniscal root (pMM) (arrows) is shown just anterior to the posterior cruciate ligament (PCL). The insertion of the anteromedial meniscal root (aMM) is shown on the anterior tibial plateau extending down the anterior proximal tibia. The lateral meniscus is more circular in shape than the medial meniscus, and the anterolateral meniscal root (aML) inserts just lateral to the anterior cruciate ligament (ACL) on the tibial plateau. The posterior lateral meniscal root (pML) is shown with its anterior meniscofemoral ligament (ligament of Humphrey) (aMFL). The most common intermeniscal ligament, the transverse ligament (TL), is shown connecting the anterior horns of the medial and lateral menisci. MCL = medial collateral ligament.

extracellular matrix. Type I collagen comprises most of the extracellular matrix; smaller amounts of types II, III, V, and VI collagen also are present. Other components are proteoglycans such as aggrecan. Proteoglycans consist of a protein core covalently bound to negatively charged glycosaminoglycan polysaccharides. Proteoglycans attract and bond to water, which comprises 65% to 75% of the meniscal volume. Type I collagen is most abundant in the superficial zones of the menisci to provide tensile strength. Proteoglycans and water are found in the deeper zones and provide compressive strength.

The collagen fibers are randomly oriented on the superficial aspects of the menisci. In the deeper zones the collagen fibers are oriented in a circumferential pattern and stabilized by intermittent radially oriented tie fibers that anchor the circumferential fibers (**Figure 1**). This orientation provides tensile strength superficially as well as absorption and dissipation of the hoop stresses from axial loading during weight bearing by 50% in knee extension and as much as 85% in flexion. In these ways the menisci protect the articular cartilage from excessive loads and contribute to joint congruity during weight bearing.

The medial and lateral menisci have different gross anatomic features (**Figure 2**). Each has an anterior horn, a body, and a posterior horn. The medial meniscus is semicircular or C shaped, and it covers 50% to 60% of the medial tibial plateau. The posterior horn is approximately 11 mm wide, and the anterior horn is slightly smaller. The

medial meniscus is attached to the deep medial collateral ligament fibers and the joint capsule, and its mobility therefore is limited. The inferior aspect of the posterior horn also is attached to the tibia by the meniscotibial ligament or coronary ligament.[3] The lateral meniscus is more circular in shape than the medial meniscus, and it has equal-size anterior and posterior horns. At the posterior lateral meniscal attachment the popliteomeniscal fascicles extend from the meniscus to the posterior capsule and create the popliteal hiatus as the popliteus tendon becomes intra-articular. The meniscofemoral ligaments connect the posterior horn of the lateral meniscus and the medial femoral condyle. The anterior meniscofemoral ligament of Humphrey courses anterior to the posterior cruciate ligament, and the posterior meniscofemoral ligament of Wrisberg courses posterior to the posterior cruciate ligament. Because the lateral meniscus has less continuous attachment to the capsule than the medial meniscus it has more mobility, which may confer a protective effect. The most common connection between the medial and lateral menisci is the transverse intermeniscal ligament, which is present in 60% to 94% of knees. A posterior and medial or lateral oblique intermeniscal ligament also can be present.[3]

The vascular supply of the menisci comes from the superior, middle, and inferior geniculate arteries. The peripheral 10% to 30% of the meniscus is well vascularized by synovial and capsular branches (Figure 3). The anterior and posterior root attachments are well vascularized by synovial branches.[4] Zones of the menisci are described based on this vascular anatomy. The outer third, the well-vascularized region, is called the red-red zone. The middle third is the border between the vascularized and avascular zones and is called the red-white zone. The inner third is devoid of a vascular supply and is called the white-white zone. The location of a meniscal tear through the zones partly determines the treatment because the potential for healing increases with vascularity. The portion of the menisci that is not well vascularized receives nutrition through diffusion during loading. Neural elements are found mostly in the periphery of the anterior and posterior horns. The menisci are believed to have a role in proprioception because of this configuration.

The Role of the Menisci in Load Sharing

During weight bearing, the menisci offset and diffuse the load between the femur and tibia through development of hoop stresses that rely on intact circumferential collagen fibers. Biomechanical studies found that a partial meniscectomy necessitated by the presence of a bucket-handle or peripheral longitudinal tear increases peak tibiofemoral contact pressure by 65% to 110% and that a total meniscectomy increases the pressure by as much as 235%.[5] In a cadaver study, an incremental increase in peak contact stress and a decrease in contact area were found as the size of radial tears increased and as a larger amount of meniscal tissue was removed.[6] A radial tear 50% or 75% of the width of the medial meniscus and a partial or total meniscectomy caused a substantial change from the intact state. Only a radial tear more than 90% of the width of the medial meniscus or a partial meniscectomy of such a radial tear substantially increased peak contact pressure and caused the peak contact to shift to a more posterior location.[7] A lateral radial meniscal tear 90% of the width of the lateral meniscus and a partial meniscectomy were found to significantly increase contact pressures.[8] These biomechanical data explain the clinical observation of meniscal extrusion and progressive degenerative osteoarthritis in knees with a radial or

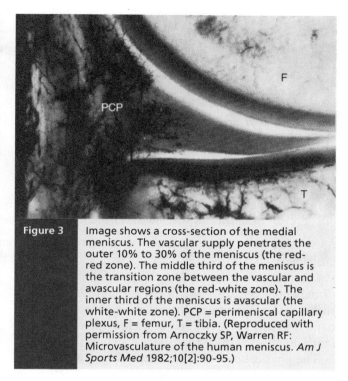

Figure 3 Image shows a cross-section of the medial meniscus. The vascular supply penetrates the outer 10% to 30% of the meniscus (the red-red zone). The middle third of the meniscus is the transition zone between the vascular and avascular regions (the red-white zone). The inner third of the meniscus is avascular (the white-white zone). PCP = perimeniscal capillary plexus, F = femur, T = tibia. (Reproduced with permission from Arnoczky SP, Warren RF: Microvasculature of the human meniscus. *Am J Sports Med* 1982;10[2]:90-95.)

complex meniscus tear.[9]

The Medial and Lateral Menisci as Stabilizers

Biomechanical studies have contributed to insight into the function of the menisci as dynamic stabilizers under specific conditions.[1,2] Sectioning of the medial meniscus led to increased tibial translation and strain on the ACL during anterior tibial translation that occurs with Lachman testing.[2] Another sectioning study found that in the absence of an intact ACL, the medial meniscus acts as a secondary stabilizer during anterior tibial translation.[1] The lateral meniscus was found to be an important stabilizer for rotatory and valgus loads during the pivot shift maneuver in ACL-deficient knees.[1] The anterior translational stability conferred by the ACL protects the posterior horn of the medial meniscus. These results emphasize the important static and dynamic role of the menisci in knee kinematics.

Diagnosis

A thorough patient history is important for both the diagnosis of a meniscal tear and treatment decision making. The patient's demographic profile, preinjury level of activity, earlier symptoms or injuries, and mechanism of injury can guide the examiner toward an accurate diagnosis and an appropriate treatment plan. Patients with a traumatic tear may have pain onset during a twisting mechanism or deep flexion. Occasionally a popping sensation is reported. Approximately one-half to two-thirds

3. Knee and Leg

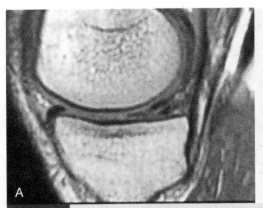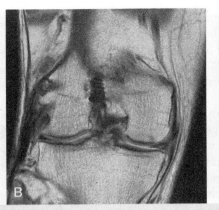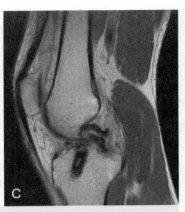

Figure 4 Proton density–weighted magnetic resonance images show meniscal tears. **A,** Sagittal view shows a complex medial meniscal tear; the signal extends to the articular surface. **B,** Coronal view shows a horizontal cleavage tear of the medial meniscus at the junction of the body and posterior horn. **C,** Sagittal view shows the double–posterior cruciate ligament sign, which is consistent with a bucket-handle tear with the fragment displaced into the notch.

of patients have knee swelling. Mechanical symptoms such as catching or frank locking were observed in 12% to 69% of patients in two recent studies; these are important symptoms because they suggest an unstable tear.[10,11]

The physical examination should begin with assessment of overall lower limb alignment and inspection for external signs of trauma or the presence of an effusion. Active and passive range of motion is recorded with a notation of any mechanical block to motion. The status of the collateral and cruciate ligaments is important to test because the presence of an injury affects treatment decision making. Palpation of the joint line may elicit tenderness in the region of a tear. Posterior horn tears are most prevalent, and therefore the posterior joint line is a common location for tenderness. The meniscus-specific McMurray, Apley, and Thessaly tests should be interpreted for pain as well as mechanical signs. The McMurray test involves taking the knee through a range of motion while internally and externally rotating the tibia relative to the femur and applying an axial load. For the Apley test, the patient is prone with the knee flexed to 90°; the examiner applies an axial load while the tibia is rotated internally and externally. For the Thessaly test, the patient stands on the affected leg and performs a one-legged squat of approximately 20°. During flexion and extension the patient also rotates the torso to create internal and external rotation of the tibiofemoral joint. Each of these functional tests is designed to trap the pathologic meniscus under axial load and rotation, and pain and/or mechanical symptoms should be re-created. In a patient with an isolated meniscal tear, joint line tenderness was found to be an accurate test in 81% to 90% of patients compared with 57% to 77% for the McMurray test and 61% to 80% for the Thessaly test.[10,11] With associated ligamentous or chondral injury, the physical examination can be particularly challenging because the tests lose their accuracy for meniscal pathology.[10,12] However, the combination of joint line tenderness and a positive McMurray or Thessaly test has sensitivity and specificity approaching those of an isolated meniscal tear.[10]

Radiographic evaluation of a patient with knee pain should begin with weight-bearing radiographs including AP in extension, lateral, and PA 45° flexion views in addition to a Merchant view of the patellofemoral joint. Signs of osteoarthritis or trauma can provide clues to the internal environment of the knee and the status of the meniscus before the onset of acute pain. Osteoarthritis can signify a degenerative meniscal tear, and trauma can be associated with an acute tear. MRI is useful for confirming a clinical suspicion of a meniscal tear. Meniscal tears can be well evaluated with proton density–weighted MRI. A tear can be described as longitudinal (vertical), horizontal, radial, flap, parrot beak, bucket-handle, degenerative, or complex. The criteria for MRI diagnosis of a meniscal tear include increased signal intensity extending to the articular surface from within the normally low-signal meniscal substance; distortion of the shape or size of the meniscus, which signifies missing meniscal tissue; or a displaced meniscal fragment[13] (Figure 4). The sensitivity and specificity of 1.5-Tesla (T) and 3.0-T MRI diagnosis of medial meniscal tears, as confirmed with arthroscopy, were found to be 93% to 96% and 88% to 90%, respectively.[13] MRI was less sensitive (77% to 82%) but more specific (98% to 99%) for lateral meniscal tears. In general, 1.5-T MRI was slightly less sensitive and specific than 3.0-T MRI, but the difference did not reach significance. A report of 3.0-T MRI for detecting posterior meniscal root tears found sensitivity of 77% and specificity of 73%.[14] These findings may be attributable to the radial orientation of many posterior root tears, which makes them more difficult to see on MRI. The patient history and physical examination remain the most important diagnostic tools. To be considered a pertinent finding, a meniscal tear seen on MRI should correspond to the patient's history and positive clinical examination findings.

Treatment

The treatment options following diagnosis of a symptomatic meniscal tear include observation, excision (a partial meniscectomy), repair, and replacement. The treatment should be tailored to the patient and the type of tear. Observation can be chosen for stable peripheral tears smaller than 5 to 10 mm, some degenerative tears that do not cause mechanical symptoms, and tears in the setting of substantial osteoarthritis. Unstable tears causing mechanical symptoms; tears in the avascular zone, such as radial or flap tears; and degenerative tears without substantial osteoarthritis can be treated with partial meniscectomy. During partial meniscectomy, the unstable portion of the meniscus is identified and excised, and the adjacent tissue is shaped into a smooth and stable contour leading into the excised segment. The surgeon should preserve as much meniscal tissue as possible and avoid creating a defect traversing the entire width of the meniscus. Clinical studies with long-term follow-up of partial meniscectomy for the treatment of meniscal tears found an increase in osteoarthritic changes within the affected compartment. Partial meniscectomy for the treatment of radial tears that were within 1 cm of the posterior horn insertion led to progression of osteoarthritis in 35% of patients at a mean 77-month follow-up.[15] At 5- to 7-year follow-up of 46 patients, one-third had progression of Kellgren-Lawrence grade 0 to 2 osteoarthritis to grade 3 or 4 osteoarthritis. Although the modified Lysholm Knee Questionnaire score often significantly improved after partial meniscectomy, only 56% of patients reported pain improvement.

In a systematic review of treatment for traumatic meniscal tears, both the short- and long-term reoperation rates were higher after meniscal repair than after meniscectomy (16.5% versus 1.4% and 20.7% versus 3.9%, respectively).[16] However, there were no plain radiographic degenerative changes in 78% of knees after meniscal repair, compared with 64% of knees after meniscectomy. These results were corroborated by another study that compared partial meniscectomy and inside-out repair of longitudinal tears.[17] Almost 80% of patients with arthroscopic meniscal repair had no osteoarthritis progression compared with only 40% of patients with meniscectomy at 8- to 10-year follow-up. More than 96% of the patients who underwent arthroscopic meniscal repair returned to

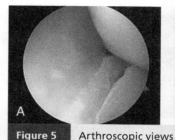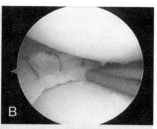

Figure 5 Arthroscopic views showing a longitudinal tear in the vascular red-red zone of the medial meniscus (**A**) and repair of the tear with vertical mattress sutures (**B**).

their preinjury level of sports activity compared with only half of those who underwent a partial meniscectomy.[17] Similarly, at 4-year follow-up, patients who underwent repair of a medial meniscal root tear had less progression of osteoarthritis and better clinical scores than those who underwent partial medial meniscectomy.[18] Preservation of the integrity of the articular cartilage on quantitative MRI has been associated with healed meniscal repairs.[19] This finding supports the reported clinical results.

With increasing evidence that both meniscal injury and partial meniscectomy are linked to the development of osteoarthritis, there has been a shift toward meniscal repair as the treatment of choice for meniscal tears. The goal of meniscal repair is to provide the meniscus with structural support and the ability to heal and therefore to preserve its integrity and function. In general, traumatic longitudinal tears occurring in the red-red (vascular) zone in patients younger than 30 years age are believed to be most amenable to a successful repair, although good results also were found in red-white zone repairs in young patients[19] (Figure 5). Because of their blood supply, tears in the red-red zone are most likely to heal, followed by tears in the red-white zone.[4] White-white zone tears are avascular and thus have limited potential for healing. The failure and reoperation rate was found to be higher for medial than lateral meniscal repairs at short- and medium-term follow-up.[16,20-22] Concomitant ACL reconstruction positively correlated with healing,[21,23] and age younger than 30 years trended toward a positive correlation with healing.[23] Tears longer than 2 cm and tobacco smoking negatively affect healing rates.[23]

 Video 20.1: All-Inside Meniscus Repair - FAST-FIX. Walter R. Shelton, MD (12 min)

 Video 20.2: All-Inside Meniscus Repair - MaxFire MarXmen. Keith W. Lawhorn, MD (8 min)

Open repair has largely been replaced by arthroscopic repair unless an arthrotomy is needed for another injury, such as a tibial plateau fracture. Arthroscopic repair can be done using an outside-in, inside-out, or all-inside technique. Outside-in repair often is chosen for an anterior horn or meniscal body tear, which is difficult to reach using an inside-out or all-inside technique. Spinal needles are placed from outside the joint through the meniscal tear, and suture is shuttled through the needles under arthroscopic observation. A small skin incision is made, and a knot is tied directly on the outside of the capsule with care to avoid entrapping any superficial soft tissue. An inside-out repair commonly is used for a posterior horn or posterior meniscal body tear. Long, flexible needles are placed with the use of specialized guides through the meniscal tear and are retrieved outside the joint. Suture is shuttled through the tear and tied over the capsule through the open posterior incision. Accessory incisions are necessary for needle retrieval and knot tying. Retractors are used in the accessory incisions to protect the popliteal neurovascular structures as well as the saphenous nerve and vein medially or the peroneal nerve laterally. MRI at an average 48-month follow-up after inside-out meniscal repair with vertical mattress suturing showed a 100% healing rate for partial tears and a 80.3% rate for full-thickness tears.[23] All-inside meniscal repair has the advantage of being less invasive than inside-out or outside-in techniques, with no required accessory portal and therefore less risk of superficial vessel or nerve injury. Multiple devices are on the market, each of which is inserted through a standard anterior portal using a guide. The trajectories possible through an anterior portal make the all-inside devices most suitable for tears in the posterior horn or midbody of the meniscus. Despite the small risk of injury to popliteal fossa structures if the device penetrates the posterior capsule too deeply, a recent review of patients treated with second-generation all-inside devices reported no neurovascular complications.[24] The second-generation insertion devices currently on the market mimic inside-out suture configurations to make the device more user-friendly and safe for the articular cartilage. The improved suture fixation mechanism reduces the risk of device migration or loosening. Midterm outcomes are promising; at an average 7-year follow-up of 83 all-inside meniscal repairs, 84% were healed according to clinical criteria.[24]

Biomechanical studies comparing the strength of inside-out and outside-in all-suture repairs had conflicting findings. A systematic review of 41 studies on the load to failure of suture repairs compared with repairs using all-inside devices found a higher load to failure with suture repairs.[25] A vertical mattress suture configuration was found to have a greater load to failure than

a horizontal mattress configuration. Another study simulated inside-out vertical mattress suture fixation and compared it with fixation using several available all-inside devices; inside-out repair had a failure load of 73 to 88 N and a mean displacement of 2.58 to 2.75 mm after 100 cycles, and all except one all-inside device had comparable performance.[26] The clinical results of all-suture and all-inside techniques were generally equivalent in several recent systematic reviews and meta-analyses. A systematic review of heterogeneous meniscal repairs with or without concomitant ACL reconstruction found that 61.7% of repairs completely healed.[16] The complete healing rate was 62% for inside-out repairs, 56% for outside-in repairs, and 83% for all-inside repairs. A meta-analysis of studies with more than 5 years of outcome data reported a success rate of 76.1% when the outside-in technique was used for isolated meniscal repairs.[22] Inside-out repairs of ACL-intact and ACL-reconstructed knees had a 77.7% success rate, and all-inside repairs had a 75.7% success rate. A systematic review of inside-out and all-inside repairs of isolated bucket-handle meniscal tears without concomitant ACL reconstruction found clinical healing rates of 83% and 81% for inside-out and all-inside repairs, respectively.[27] All-inside repairs led to more local soft-tissue irritation and implant migration, and inside-out repairs had a higher rate of nerve injury.

The ability to return to sports after meniscal repair has been investigated. A study of elite athletes found that 81% were able to return to sports an average of 5.6 months after surgery.[20] In this active population, the failure rate was 26.7% at an average of 41.7 months. A study of high-level soccer players found that 89.6% were able to return to the same activity level an average of 4.3 months after surgery. At 5-year follow-up, 45% were still participating in soccer.[28]

It can be difficult to interpret imaging after meniscectomy or meniscal repair. The diagnostic criteria for a retear after a meniscectomy in which less than 25% of the native meniscus was removed are the same as for a primary tear, and the diagnostic accuracy is similar. Tears requiring a more extensive meniscectomy or a meniscal repair may reach the vascular zone of the meniscus, and these tears heal with fibrovascular tissue that can mimic the hyperintense signal of a retear. Based on MRI appearance, tears are classified as fully healed if there is no fluid signal in the repair site, partially healed if fluid extends into less than 50% of the width of the repair site, and not healed if fluid extends into more than 50% of the repair site width.

Failure of meniscal repair can be attributed to inadequate meniscus fixation strength, poor vascular supply at the repair site, or concomitant knee instability caused by ligamentous laxity. The medial and lateral menisci have a secondary role in stabilizing the knee, and repairing a posterior horn meniscal tear in an ACL-deficient knee without correcting anterior laxity can lead to a retear or compromised healing.[1] The reason for the failure should be considered in deciding whether a revision meniscal repair or a partial meniscectomy is preferable. Revision meniscal repair was evaluated in 15 patients who had undergone primary repair using different techniques.[29] The revision repair failed in five patients at an average of 25 months after surgery. The presence of degenerative changes at all five revision repair sites suggested that avascularity or instability played a role in the degeneration of the meniscal tissue. In the patients who did not have a retear after the revision repair, the average Lysholm score improved to 97.4 of 100.

 Video 20.3: Posterior Horn Medial Meniscus Root Repair. Dharmesh Vyas, MD, and Christopher D. Harner, MD (14 min)

Root Tears

The role of the posterior meniscal root attachment and the underestimated prevalence of this injury have received attention recently. Both degenerative and traumatic tears can occur. A traumatic tear often is associated with multiligamentous knee injury or injury occurring during deep knee flexion. The medial posterior root is less mobile than the lateral root and therefore is more susceptible to isolated injury; in contrast, a lateral root tear is most common in association with ligamentous injury. Tears of the posterior medial meniscal root can increase contact pressure, external rotation, and lateral tibial translation, which are corrected with repair of the posterior medial meniscal root.[30,31] Similarly, a lateral root avulsion or a radial tear within 9 mm of the root substantially decreases the contact area and increases contact pressure in the lateral compartment.[32,33] Repair of medial and lateral root tears substantially decreases the contact pressures within the medial and lateral compartments.

Biologic Treatments

The mechanism of healing in the vascular portion of the meniscus involves an initial inflammatory response and fibrin clot formation followed by migration of undifferentiated mesenchymal cells from the vasculature, which leads to new matrix formation and healing through fibrous scar tissue. Synovial cells also can participate in the repair response. This process has led to a recommendation that trephination of the peripheral meniscus and capsule and synovial abrasion should be done during meniscal repair to increase vascularity and resulting migration of vascular-derived undifferentiated cells to the repair site. There also is interest in the direct application of pluripotent stem cells into the joint for augmentation of healing in meniscal repair.[34] In animal models, synovial mesenchymal stem cells injected intra-articularly during meniscal repair adhered well to sites of meniscal injury and differentiated into meniscal fibrochondrocytes, thus improving the amount of meniscal tissue formation 1 to 4 months later.[34] A human study of intra-articular injection of bone marrow–derived mesenchymal stem cells found that the meniscal volume substantially increased in 24% of patients within 1 week of meniscectomy.[35] Patients who also had osteoarthritis had substantial improvement in pain. In a rabbit model, adipose-derived stem cells delivered to the site of a longitudinal meniscal tear were found to improve the healing rate and amount of regenerated meniscus in both the vascular and avascular zones.[36] The effect of adipose-derived stem cells was most apparent after acute repairs.

Concomitant ACL reconstruction was found to be positively correlated with meniscal healing rates, probably because bone marrow–derived mesenchymal cells were released during tunnel reaming.[21,23] Bone marrow stimulation achieved by drilling a 5-mm hole into the intercondylar notch recently was reported for augmentation of healing of avascular horizontal cleavage tears.[37] The clinical healing rate was 91%, and 73% of patients had complete healing at second-look arthroscopy. A relatively short duration of meniscal symptoms was associated with a superior clinical outcome score.

 Video 20.4: All-Arthroscopic Meniscus Repair with Biological Augmentation. Nicholas A. Sgaglione, MD, and Eric Chen, MD (28 min)

Platelet-rich plasma (PRP) is a source of anabolic growth factors such as insulin-like growth factor–1, vascular endothelial growth factor, fibroblast growth factor–2, transforming growth factor–β, and platelet-derived growth factor–AB, all of which have been isolated from meniscal repair tissue.[38] There is evidence that PRP application at the site of meniscal repair increases the adherence and content of fibroblasts and chondrocytes and improves the histologic appearance of the healing meniscus both in vitro and in vivo.[39] Only small retrospective studies have compared meniscal repair with and without the application of PRP.[40,41] One study found no between-group difference in clinical outcomes scores, reoperation rate, or the proportion of patients who returned to work or sports.[40] Another study reported no difference in reoperation rate or overall clinical outcome scores but did find improvement in pain and sports parameters in patients who received PRP. Improvement in the MRI appearance of PRP-treated repairs also was reported; 0 of 17 control patients and 5 of 17 repairs supplemented with PRP had a normal meniscus signal intensity.[41]

Collagen Implants

For patients with irreparable meniscal injury and substantial meniscal loss, synthetic scaffolds may provide a new treatment option. A composite type I bovine collagen–glycosaminoglycan scaffold was found to support the formation of meniscus-like tissue when attached to a meniscal rim.[42] The scaffold was infiltrated by synovial and/or vascular-derived cells and replaced by host meniscuslike tissue. Long-term clinical data are promising. A retrospective review found that patients treated with collagen meniscal implants for an irreparable medial meniscal tear had better clinical, radiologic, and functional outcomes at 10-year follow-up than patients treated with partial medial meniscectomy alone.[42] A prospective cohort study of 33 patients compared a medial collagen meniscal implant with a partial meniscectomy. At an average 133-month follow-up, patients who received the medial meniscal implant had substantially better visual analog scale pain scores as well as significantly higher functional outcomes as measured using the Tegner Activity Level Scale, International Knee Documentation Committee Subjective Knee Evaluation Form, and Medical Outcomes Study 36-Item Short Form Health Survey scores.[42] Patients with an irreparable lateral meniscus tear or a history of partial lateral meniscectomy also had substantial improvement in clinical outcome scores at 2-year follow-up, with no progressive cartilage degeneration.[43] In a prospective randomized study of the use of collagen implants, patients with no history of surgery and patients who had undergone previous meniscal surgery received a collagen scaffold implant or a partial meniscectomy.[44] Patients who received the collagen implant had significantly increased meniscal volume at second-look arthroscopy, compared with baseline. Patients with a history of meniscal surgery gained 42% of lost activity 5 years after collagen scaffold implantation, which was substantially more than those who received meniscectomy alone.[44]

An acellular, biodegradable, synthetic polyurethane scaffold has been developed for medial and lateral meniscal defects. This scaffold is highly porous and allows vascular and fibrochondrocyte ingrowth. In animal models there was vascular ingrowth and matrix deposition onto the scaffold at 2 weeks, and by 3 months the pores were filled with fibrovascular tissue.[45] At 2-year follow-up patients who were treated with the polyurethane scaffold

for postmeniscectomy syndrome after medial or lateral partial meniscectomy had significant improvement in all clinical outcome scores, and 92.5% had stable or improved International Cartilage Repair Society cartilage status.[46] In 9 of 52 patients (17.3%) treatment failed, but 2 of these patients were asymptomatic and the failure was discovered during protocol-stipulated second-look arthroscopy. Six of the nine treatment failures were a lateral tear, where mobility and the complex anatomy of the meniscal attachments create a biomechanically challenging procedure. Another recent study on the use of a polyurethane scaffold for lateral meniscal defects and postmeniscectomy pain found substantial improvement in pain and clinical outcome scores at 24-month follow-up.[47] Three of the 54 patients (5.5%) required reoperation because of persistent pain, and 2 of these patients were found to have a small tear at the edge of the scaffold.

Meniscal Allograft Transplantation

Meniscus replacement with allograft tissue appears to be a viable treatment for patients younger than 50 years with pain and dysfunction from meniscal pathology warranting subtotal or total meniscectomy. A biomechanical study found that meniscal allograft transplantation restores normal knee contact mechanics and restores strain on the ACL with anterior translation to baseline.[2,48] The described techniques include arthroscopically assisted and open procedures as well as methods of fixation such as transplantation with bone plugs attached to the anterior and posterior horns, a common bone bridge attached to both horns, and suture fixation only (Figure 6).

Video 20.5: Lateral Meniscus Transplantation. Benjamin S. Shaffer, MD (6 min)

Video 20.6: Lateral Meniscus Transplantation - Bridge-in-Slot. Brian J. Cole, MD, MBA (15 min)

Video 20.7: Medial Meniscus Transplantation - Double Bone Plug. Thomas R. Carter, MD (11 min)

Video 20.8: Medial Meniscus Transplantation During ACL Repair. John C. Richmond, MD (7 min)

Three- to 4-year outcomes were reported for medial and lateral meniscal allograft transplantation in patients with or without a history of meniscal surgery.[49,50] After

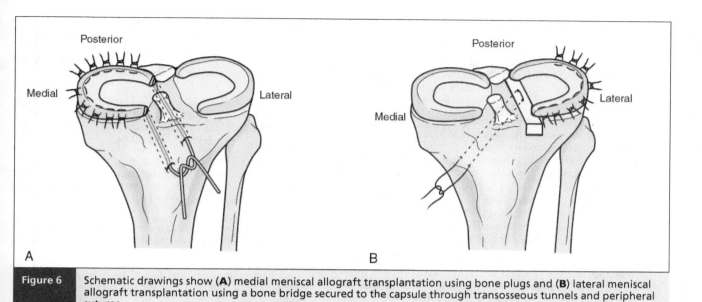

Figure 6 Schematic drawings show (**A**) medial meniscal allograft transplantation using bone plugs and (**B**) lateral meniscal allograft transplantation using a bone bridge secured to the capsule through transosseous tunnels and peripheral sutures.

meniscal allograft transplantation, patients had substantial improvement in clinical outcome scores on the mean Lysholm, Knee Injury and Osteoarthritis Outcome Score, International Knee Documentation Committee, Tegner, and Knee Society Score measures as well as radiographic measures of osteoarthritis.[49,50] Seventy-seven percent of high school and higher level athletes were able to return to sports activity.[49] Based on second-look arthroscopy and MRI, 81.8% of patients had a satisfactory outcome. Midterm follow-up of arthroscopically assisted meniscal allograft transplantation also found promising results.[51] Patients had improvement over baseline scores on the Knee Injury and Osteoarthritis Outcome Score subscores for pain, other symptoms, activities of daily living, sports activity, and quality of life as well as the visual analog pain scale, Medical Outcomes Study Short Form-36, and Lysholm scores. Long-term follow-up on open meniscal allograft transplantation using cryopreserved allograft found a 29% failure rate.[52] Short-term outcome scores were better than baseline scores but deteriorated at long-term follow-up. The most important factor determining outcome was the extent of concomitant articular cartilage degeneration; better results were reported in patients with minimal degenerative changes.

Summary

The menisci have been shown to provide load distribution, lubrication, and both translational and rotatory stability to the knee joint. Studies showing an increase in contact pressure on the articular cartilage and increased strain on

the ACL following subtotal meniscectomy or high-grade radial tear have led to an increase in the number of meniscal repairs performed to preserve the load absorption and stabilization properties of the menisci. Clinical and radiographic healing rates of 60% to 85% are reported after repair. Meniscal repair with concomitant ACL surgery leads to a higher rate of healing than isolated meniscal repair, and tears repaired in smokers and tears larger than 20 mm have a lower rate of healing. Irreparable tears and postmeniscectomy pain syndrome are common in young patients and are difficult to treat. Collagen scaffold implants and synthetic polyurethane scaffolds have had promising results in animal and human studies for filling large defects after partial meniscectomy. Relatively young patients who undergo total or subtotal meniscectomy as a primary procedure may be candidates for meniscal allograft transplantation. Biomechanical studies found that strain on the ACL is reduced and knee kinematics and contact pressures are improved to near-baseline levels after transplantation.

Key Study Points

- The menisci are important load-distributing and stabilizing structures in the knee.
- Repairs of tears in the red-red zone and repairs with concomitant ACL reconstruction are the most likely to completely heal.
- Results of meniscal scaffold implantation and allograft transplantation have shown promising results.

Annotated References

1. Musahl V, Citak M, O'Loughlin PF, Choi D, Bedi A, Pearle AD: The effect of medial versus lateral meniscectomy on the stability of the anterior cruciate ligament-deficient knee. *Am J Sports Med* 2010;38(8):1591-1597.

   A biomechanical study evaluated the effect of the medial and lateral menisci on ACL-deficient knees. The medial meniscus was found to be a secondary stabilizer to anterior translation, but the lateral meniscus was a more important stabilizer during the pivot shift test.

2. Spang JT, Dang AB, Mazzocca A, et al: The effect of medial meniscectomy and meniscal allograft transplantation on knee and anterior cruciate ligament biomechanics. *Arthroscopy* 2010;26(2):192-201.

   A biomechanical study evaluated strain at the ACL with tibial displacement in intact, total meniscectomy, and medial allograft transplantation conditions. Medial meniscectomy produced the greatest tibial displacement and strain on the ACL. Medial meniscal allograft transplantation restored normal conditions.

3. Śmigielski R, Becker R, Zdanowicz U, Ciszek B: Medial meniscus anatomy: From basic science to treatment. *Knee Surg Sports Traumatol Arthrosc* 2015;23(1):8-14.

   This anatomic study of the medial meniscus focuses on the peripheral attachments of the medial meniscus to divide it into five distinct zones. An understanding of the peripheral anatomy of the meniscus is important during meniscal repair.

4. Arnoczky SP, Warren RF: Microvasculature of the human meniscus. *Am J Sports Med* 1982;10(2):90-95.

5. Baratz ME, Fu FH, Mengato R: Meniscal tears: The effect of meniscectomy and of repair on intraarticular contact areas and stress in the human knee. A preliminary report. *Am J Sports Med* 1986;14(4):270-275.

6. Lee SJ, Aadalen KJ, Malaviya P, et al: Tibiofemoral contact mechanics after serial medial meniscectomies in the human cadaveric knee. *Am J Sports Med* 2006;34(8):1334-1344.

7. Bedi A, Kelly NH, Baad M, et al: Dynamic contact mechanics of the medial meniscus as a function of radial tear, repair, and partial meniscectomy. *J Bone Joint Surg Am* 2010;92(6):1398-1408.

   A biomechanical study found that radial tears involving 90% of the width of the meniscus caused an increase in peak contact pressure and alteration of its location. Partial meniscectomy further increased pressures. Inside-out repair reduced pressures to a level similar to that of the intact state.

8. Bedi A, Kelly N, Baad M, et al: Dynamic contact mechanics of radial tears of the lateral meniscus: Implications for treatment. *Arthroscopy* 2012;28(3):372-381.

   A biomechanical study found that a radial tear of the posterior root 90% of the width of the meniscus or a partial meniscectomy of such a tear significantly increased contact pressures and decreased contact area. Repair significantly decreased peak contact pressure.

9. Badlani JT, Borrero C, Golla S, Harner CD, Irrgang JJ: The effects of meniscus injury on the development of knee osteoarthritis: Data from the osteoarthritis initiative. *Am J Sports Med* 2013;41(6):1238-1244.

   A case control study found that medial meniscus extrusion, complex tears, and large radial tears were more common in patients with osteoarthritis than in control subjects. Level of evidence: III.

10. Konan S, Rayan F, Haddad FS: Do physical diagnostic tests accurately detect meniscal tears? *Knee Surg Sports Traumatol Arthrosc* 2009;17(7):806-811.

    Joint line tenderness was found to be superior to the McMurray or Thessaly test for the diagnosis of isolated meniscal tears confirmed at arthroscopy. The combination of joint line tenderness and one other test improved diagnostic accuracy.

11. Goossens P, Keijsers E, van Geenen RJ, et al: Validity of the Thessaly test in evaluating meniscal tears compared with arthroscopy: A diagnostic accuracy study. *J Orthop Sports Phys Ther* 2015;45(1):18-24, B1.

    For the evaluation of possible meniscal tears the Thessaly test had sensitivity of 64% and specificity of 53%, the McMurray test had sensitivity of 70% and specificity of 45%, and combined testing had sensitivity of 53% and specificity of 62%. These values were lower than reported in the original description.

12. Mirzatolooei F, Yekta Z, Bayazidchi M, Ershadi S, Afshar A: Validation of the Thessaly test for detecting meniscal tears in anterior cruciate deficient knees. *Knee* 2010;17(3):221-223.

    In patients with combined ACL and meniscal injury, joint line tenderness was most sensitive and the McMurray test was most specific for diagnosis of the meniscal tear.

13. Van Dyck P, Vanhoenacker FM, Lambrecht V, et al: Prospective comparison of 1.5 and 3.0-T MRI for evaluating the knee menisci and ACL. *J Bone Joint Surg Am* 2013;95(10):916-924.

    Sensitivity and specificity for diagnosis of medial and lateral meniscal tears was higher when 3.0-T MRI was used rather than 1.5-T MRI, but the difference was not significant. Sensitivity was higher for medial tears, and specificity was higher for lateral tears. Level of evidence: I.

14. LaPrade RF, Ho CP, James E, Crespo B, LaPrade CM, Matheny LM: Diagnostic accuracy of 3.0 T magnetic resonance imaging for the detection of meniscus posterior root pathology. *Knee Surg Sports Traumatol Arthrosc* 2015;23(1):152-157.

Moderate sensitivity and specificity was found for MRI diagnosis of meniscal root tears confirmed at arthroscopy. Level of evidence: II.

15. Han SB, Shetty GM, Lee DH, et al: Unfavorable results of partial meniscectomy for complete posterior medial meniscus root tear with early osteoarthritis: A 5- to 8-year follow-up study. *Arthroscopy* 2010;26(10):1326-1332.

At a mean 5-year follow-up, a retrospective study of 46 patients who underwent arthroscopic partial menis-cectomy of a posterior medial meniscal root tear found improvement in clinical parameters after arthroscopic meniscectomy but a 35% radiographic progression of osteoarthritis. Level of evidence: IV.

16. Paxton ES, Stock MV, Brophy RH: Meniscal repair versus partial meniscectomy: A systematic review comparing reoperation rates and clinical outcomes. *Arthroscopy* 2011;27(9):1275-1288.

A systematic review of partial meniscectomy and menis-cal repair found that partial meniscectomy resulted in a lower reoperation rate but a higher rate of progression of radiographic degeneration. Meniscal repairs concomitant with ACL reconstruction had a lower failure rate. Level of evidence: IV.

17. Stein T, Mehling AP, Welsch F, von Eisenhart-Rothe R, Jäger A: Long-term outcome after arthroscopic meniscal repair versus arthroscopic partial meniscec-tomy for traumatic meniscal tears. *Am J Sports Med* 2010;38(8):1542-1548.

A cohort study compared the outcomes of arthroscopic meniscal repair and arthroscopic partial meniscectomy in 81 patients. At mid- and long-term follow up, patients who underwent repair had better sports activity and no osteo-arthritic progression compared with those who underwent partial meniscectomy. Level of evidence: III.

18. Kim SB, Ha JK, Lee SW, et al: Medial meniscus root tear refixation: Comparison of clinical, radiologic, and arthroscopic findings with medial meniscectomy. *Arthros-copy* 2011;27(3):346-354.

A retrospective study compared medial meniscus re-pair and partial meniscectomy in 58 consecutive patients. At a mean 48.5-month follow-up, arthroscopic repair yielded better clinical and radiographic results than partial meniscectomy. Level of evidence: III.

19. Noyes FR, Chen RC, Barber-Westin SD, Potter HG: Great-er than 10-year results of red-white longitudinal meniscal repairs in patients 20 years of age or younger. *Am J Sports Med* 2011;39(5):1008-1017.

The success rate was 62% after repair of longitudinal tears extending into the red-white zone in patients age 20 years or younger. In healed repairs, quantitative cartilage scores on MRI were not significantly different from those of the uninjured knee. Level of evidence: IV.

20. Logan M, Watts M, Owen J, Myers P: Meniscal repair in the elite athlete: Results of 45 repairs with a minimum 5-year follow-up. *Am J Sports Med* 2009;37(6):1131-1134.

After meniscal repair 81% of elite athletes were able to return to sports at a preinjury level, despite a 24% retear rate. Medial repairs had the highest failure rate. Level of evidence: IV.

21. Lyman S, Hidaka C, Valdez AS, et al: Risk factors for meniscectomy after meniscal repair. *Am J Sports Med* 2013;41(12):2772-2778.

The overall rate of meniscectomy after meniscal repair was 8.9%. A regression analysis found that concomitant ACL reconstruction was a risk factor for meniscectomy after repair. Patients who underwent isolated meniscal repair were at lower risk if they were older than 40 years or had undergone lateral repair or if the surgeon had performed a large number of meniscal repairs. Level of evidence: III.

22. Nepple JJ, Dunn WR, Wright RW: Meniscal repair outcomes at greater than five years: A systematic liter-ature review and meta-analysis. *J Bone Joint Surg Am* 2012;94(24):2222-2227.

A systematic review of studies reporting outcomes of me-niscal repair with a minimum 5-year follow-up found that the overall rate of failure was 23.1% There was no statistical difference in outcomes among patients who underwent medial or lateral repair, and simultaneous ACL reconstruction did not affect results. Level of evidence: IV.

23. Haklar U, Donmez F, Basaran SH, Canbora MK: Results of arthroscopic repair of partial- or full-thickness longi-tudinal medial meniscal tears by single or double vertical sutures using the inside-out technique. *Am J Sports Med* 2013;41(3):596-602.

A retrospective review of inside-out repair of longitudinal medial meniscal tears with or without ACL reconstruction found that at an average 49.3-month follow-up, 88.4% were healed by clinical and radiographic analysis. Patients who had undergone ACL reconstruction or had a tear smaller than 2 cm or who did not smoke tobacco had a higher rate of healing. Level of evidence: IV.

24. Bogunovic L, Kruse LM, Haas AK, Huston LJ, Wright RW: Outcome of all-inside second-generation meniscal repair: Minimum five-year follow-up. *J Bone Joint Surg Am* 2014;96(15):1303-1307.

A retrospective review of the 5-year outcomes of 75 pa-tients treated with the all-inside FAST-FIX meniscal repair system (Smith & Nephew) found a 16% failure rate. There was no difference between isolated meniscal repairs and repairs with concomitant ACL reconstruction. Level of evidence: IV.

25. M Buckland D, Sadoghi P, Wimmer MD, et al: Meta-anal-ysis on biomechanical properties of meniscus repairs: Are devices better than sutures? *Knee Surg Sports Traumatol Arthrosc* 2015;23(1):83-89.

Meta-analysis of biomechanical studies comparing all-su-ture meniscal repairs and all-inside devices found that all-suture devices had a higher load to failure and stiff-ness than all-inside devices. Vertical mattress suture con-figuration was stronger than horizontal mattress suture configuration.

3: Knee and Leg

26. Barber FA, Herbert MA, Bava ED, Drew OR: Biomechanical testing of suture-based meniscal repair devices containing ultrahigh-molecular-weight polyethylene suture: Update 2011. *Arthroscopy* 2012;28(6):827-834.

A biomechanical study of the load to failure of all-suture constructs and all-inside devices found that vertical mattress sutures were stronger than all-inside devices, but there was no significant difference between all-suture devices and all except one all-inside device.

27. Grant JA, Wilde J, Miller BS, Bedi A: Comparison of inside-out and all-inside techniques for the repair of isolated meniscal tears: A systematic review. *Am J Sports Med* 2012;40(2):459-468.

A systematic review of 19 studies comparing inside-out and all-inside repairs found a 17% rate of clinical failure for inside-out repairs and a 19% rate for all-inside repairs. Patient-reported outcomes were similar. Nerve irritation was more prevalent with inside-out repairs, and implant-related complications were more prevalent with all-inside repairs. Level of evidence: IV.

28. Alvarez-Diaz P, Alentorn-Geli E, Llobet F, Granados N, Steinbacher G, Cugat R: Return to play after all-inside meniscal repair in competitive football players: A minimum 5-year follow-up. *Knee Surg Sports Traumatol Arthrosc* 2014.

A retrospective review of the rate of return to sport of 29 male soccer players who underwent all-inside repair of a complete longitudinal tear found that 89.6% returned to the same level after initial recovery and 6.7% required meniscectomy before return to sport. At 5-year follow-up, 45% continued to play soccer, of whom 28% were playing at the same level. Level of evidence: IV.

29. Imade S, Kumahashi N, Kuwata S, Kadowaki M, Ito S, Uchio Y: Clinical outcomes of revision meniscal repair: A case series. *Am J Sports Med* 2014;42(2):350-357.

A retrospective study compared 15 revision meniscal repairs and 96 primary repairs. Five revision repairs were unsuccessful, but patients with a successful revision had significant improvement in their clinical outcome scores. Degenerative meniscal tissue was found at the repair site in all unsuccessful revision repairs. Level of evidence: IV.

30. Allaire R, Muriuki M, Gilbertson L, Harner CD: Biomechanical consequences of a tear of the posterior root of the medial meniscus: Similar to total meniscectomy. *J Bone Joint Surg Am* 2008;90(9):1922-1931.

31. Muriuki MG, Tuason DA, Tucker BG, Harner CD: Changes in tibiofemoral contact mechanics following radial split and vertical tears of the medial meniscus an in vitro investigation of the efficacy of arthroscopic repair. *J Bone Joint Surg Am* 2011;93(12):1089-1095.

A controlled laboratory study compared knee contact pressures in intact medial menisci and medial menisci with a radial split tear, vertical tear, or repaired tear. Repair of a meniscal tear created contact pressure and area similar to that of the intact meniscus.

32. LaPrade CM, Jansson KS, Dornan G, Smith SD, Wijdicks CA, LaPrade RF: Altered tibiofemoral contact mechanics due to lateral meniscus posterior horn root avulsions and radial tears can be restored with in situ pull-out suture repairs. *J Bone Joint Surg Am* 2014;96(6):471-479.

A cadaver biomechanical study compared contact area and pressures in intact lateral menisci, lateral menisci with a footprint tear, root avulsion, or radial tear 3 mm or 6 mm from the posterior root, with repair of each of the injured states. Avulsion of the root and the radial tears significantly decreased the contact area and increased the peak pressure. In situ pullout suture repair decreased peak pressures.

33. Padalecki JR, Jansson KS, Smith SD, et al: Biomechanical consequences of a complete radial tear adjacent to the medial meniscus posterior root attachment site: In situ pull-out repair restores derangement of joint mechanics. *Am J Sports Med* 2014;42(3):699-707.

A cadaver biomechanical study compared contact area and pressures in intact lateral menisci, lateral menisci with a footprint tear, root avulsion, or radial tear 3 mm, 6 mm, or 9 mm from the posterior root, with repair of each of the injured states. Avulsion of the root and the radial tears significantly decreased the contact area and increased the peak pressure. In situ pullout suture repair decreased peak pressures and increased contact area to a level similar to that of the intact meniscus.

34. Horie M, Driscoll MD, Sampson HW, et al: Implantation of allogenic synovial stem cells promotes meniscal regeneration in a rabbit meniscal defect model. *J Bone Joint Surg Am* 2012;94(8):701-712.

Injection of synovial stem cells into meniscal defects in rabbits increased the quantity of regenerated meniscal tissue 4 and 12 weeks after implantation. Tissue quality scores were improved 12 and 24 weeks after implantation. Implanted cells adhered to the defects and became differentiated into type I and II collagen–expressing cells.

35. Vangsness CT Jr, Farr J II, Boyd J, Dellaero DT, Mills CR, LeRoux-Williams M: Adult human mesenchymal stem cells delivered via intra-articular injection to the knee following partial medial meniscectomy: A randomized, double-blind, controlled study. *J Bone Joint Surg Am* 2014;96(2):90-98.

A randomized, controlled study found that 6% to 24% of patients who received one of two different concentrations of allogeneic stem cells had a 15% or greater increase in meniscal volume after partial medial meniscectomy. None of the control subjects reached this level. Patients with osteoarthritis had a significant reduction in pain. Level of evidence: I.

36. Ruiz-Ibán MA, Díaz-Heredia J, García-Gómez I, Gonzalez-Lizán F, Elías-Martín E, Abraira V: The effect of the addition of adipose-derived mesenchymal stem cells to a meniscal repair in the avascular zone: An experimental study in rabbits. *Arthroscopy* 2011;27(12):1688-1696.

An animal study found that the addition of adipose-derived allogeneic stem cells to acutely repaired longitudinal

3: Knee and Leg

tears in the avascular zone of the medial meniscus significantly improved histologic properties at 12 weeks compared with those of control animals. The difference was less robust after delayed repair.

37. Ahn JH, Kwon OJ, Nam TS: Arthroscopic repair of horizontal meniscal cleavage tears with marrow-stimulating technique. *Arthroscopy* 2015;31(1):92-98.

In a retrospective review, 32 horizontal cleavage tears extending into the avascular zone were treated with repair and augmentation with bone marrow stimulation through drill holes in the intercondylar notch. Clinical outcomes scores improved, and 91% of patients were clinically healed. At second-look arthroscopy 73% were healed and 18% were partially healed. Level of evidence: IV.

38. Braun HJ, Kim HJ, Chu CR, Dragoo JL: The effect of platelet-rich plasma formulations and blood products on human synoviocytes: Implications for intra-articular injury and therapy. *Am J Sports Med* 2014;42(5):1204-1210.

This review article on the current use of PRP discusses its use in tendinopathy as well as the early results of use in meniscal and ligament healing. Although there are promising results in preliminary studies, no conclusive evidence on the use of PRP for meniscal or ligament healing has been proven.

39. Kwak HS, Nam J, Lee JH, Kim HJ, Yoo JJ: Meniscal repair in vivo using human chondrocyte-seeded PLGA mesh scaffold pretreated with platelet-rich plasma. *J Tissue Eng Regen Med* [Published online ahead of print June 19, 2014]. http://dx.doi.org/10.1002/term.1938

PRP pretreatment on a poly(lactic-*co*-glycolic acid) mesh scaffold enhanced the healing capacity of the meniscus with human chondrocyte–seeded scaffolds in an animal model. Six of 16 menisci healed and 9 partially healed when implanted with the PRP-treated scaffold.

40. Griffin JW, Hadeed MM, Werner BC, Diduch DR, Carson EW, Miller MD: Platelet-rich plasma in meniscal repair: Does augmentation improve surgical outcomes? *Clin Orthop Relat Res* 2015;473(5):1665-1672.

A retrospective comparative study found no between-group differences in reoperation rate, functional outcomes scores, return to work, or return to sports in patients treated with or without PRP during meniscal repair. Level of evidence: III.

41. Pujol N, Salle De Chou E, Boisrenoult P, Beaufils P: Platelet-rich plasma for open meniscal repair in young patients: Any benefit? *Knee Surg Sports Traumatol Arthrosc* 2015;23(1):51-58.

A case-control study found that patients treated with repair of a horizontal cleavage tear augmented with PRP injection had higher Knee Injury and Osteoarthritis Outcome Score (KOOS), and KOOS pain and sports subscores were significantly higher. Five patients treated with PRP had complete resolution of MRI findings of meniscal injury. Level of evidence: III.

42. Zaffagnini S, Marcheggiani Muccioli GM, Lopomo N, et al: Prospective long-term outcomes of the medial collagen meniscus implant versus partial medial meniscectomy: A minimum 10-year follow-up study. *Am J Sports Med* 2011;39(5):977-985.

A prospective cohort study compared the results of medial meniscal collagen implantation and partial meniscectomy. Clinical outcome scores and MRI findings were better after medial meniscal collagen implantation at 10-year follow-up.

43. Zaffagnini S, Marcheggiani Muccioli GM, Bulgheroni P, et al: Arthroscopic collagen meniscus implantation for partial lateral meniscal defects: A 2-year minimum follow-up study. *Am J Sports Med* 2012;40(10):2281-2288.

A case study evaluated 2-year outcomes of lateral meniscal collagen implantation. Pain was decreased pain and function was improved compared with preoperative levels without significant change to cartilage in the lateral compartment. Level of evidence: IV.

44. Rodkey WG, DeHaven KE, Montgomery WH III, et al: Comparison of the collagen meniscus implant with partial meniscectomy: A prospective randomized trial. *J Bone Joint Surg Am* 2008;90(7):1413-1426.

45. Maher SA, Rodeo SA, Doty SB, et al: Evaluation of a porous polyurethane scaffold in a partial meniscal defect ovine model. *Arthroscopy* 2010;26(11):1510-1519.

Lateral meniscal defects were created in sheep, and a polyurethane scaffold was implanted into half of the animals. There was no significant chondral damage beneath the scaffold. Fibrochondrocytes were well integrated into the scaffold within 3 months.

46. Verdonk P, Beaufils P, Bellemans J, et al; Actifit Study Group: Successful treatment of painful irreparable partial meniscal defects with a polyurethane scaffold: Two-year safety and clinical outcomes. *Am J Sports Med* 2012;40(4):844-853.

A retrospective review of patients with postmeniscectomy syndrome who were treated with polyurethane scaffold implantation found clinically and significant improvement in clinical outcomes. Implantation failure occurred in 17.3%, and stable or improved cartilage grading was noted in 92.5% of patients. Level of evidence: IV.

47. Bouyarmane H, Beaufils P, Pujol N, et al: Polyurethane scaffold in lateral meniscus segmental defects: Clinical outcomes at 24 months follow-up. *Orthop Traumatol Surg Res* 2014;100(1):153-157.

A prospective multicenter study of 54 patients with lateral postmeniscectomy syndrome who were treated with polyurethane scaffold implantation found significant improvements in clinical outcome scores. Level of evidence: IV.

48. Paletta GA Jr, Manning T, Snell E, Parker R, Bergfeld J: The effect of allograft meniscal replacement on intraarticular contact area and pressures in the human knee: A biomechanical study. *Am J Sports Med* 1997;25(5):692-698.

3: Knee and Leg

49. Chalmers PN, Karas V, Sherman SL, Cole BJ: Return to high-level sport after meniscal allograft transplantation. *Arthroscopy* 2013;29(3):539-544.

A retrospective case study evaluated return to sports of 13 patients after meniscal allograft transplantation. At a mean 3.3-year follow-up, 77% had returned to their approved level of return to play and had concomitant improvement in clinical outcome scores. Level of evidence: IV.

50. Kim JM, Lee BS, Kim KH, Kim KA, Bin SI: Results of meniscus allograft transplantation using bone fixation: 110 cases with objective evaluation. *Am J Sports Med* 2012;40(5):1027-1034.

A retrospective case study of 115 knees after meniscal allograft transplantation found significant clinical and functional outcome improvements at 49.4-month follow-up. Level of evidence: IV.

51. Vundelinckx B, Bellemans J, Vanlauwe J: Arthroscopically assisted meniscal allograft transplantation in the knee: A medium-term subjective, clinical, and radiographical outcome evaluation. *Am J Sports Med* 2010;38(11):2240-2247.

A case study of 50 meniscal allograft transplantations found improvement in measured clinical outcome scores and function. There was no increase in osteoarthritis in 58% of patients. Level of evidence: IV.

52. van der Wal RJ, Thomassen BJ, van Arkel ER: Long-term clinical outcome of open meniscal allograft transplantation. *Am J Sports Med* 2009;37(11):2134-2139.

A case study of 63 open meniscal allograft transplantations evaluated the clinical outcomes and failure rate at 13.8-year follow-up. The poorest results were observed after medial allograft transplantation and in women. Level of evidence: IV.

Video References

20.1: Shelton WR: *All-Inside Meniscus Repair - FAST-FIX* [video excerpt]. Jackson, MS, 2011.

20.2: Lawhorn KW: *All-Inside Meniscus Repair - MaxFire MarXmen* [video excerpt]. Fairfax, VA, 2011.

20.3: Vyas D, Harner CD: *Posterior Horn Medial Meniscus Root Repair* [video excerpt]. Blawnox, PA, 2011.

20.4: Sgaglione NA, Chen E: *All-Arthroscopic Meniscus Repair with Biological Augmentation* [video excerpt]. Rosemont, IL, American Academy of Orthopaedic Surgeons, 2011.

20.5: Shaffer BS: *Lateral Meniscus Transplantation* [video excerpt]. Rosemont, IL, American Academy of Orthopaedic Surgeons, 2011.

20.6: Cole BJ: *Lateral Meniscus Transplantation - Bridge-in-Slot* [video excerpt]. Rosemont, IL, American Academy of Orthopaedic Surgeons, 2011.

20.7: Carter TR: *Medial Meniscus Transplantation - Double Bone Plug* [video excerpt]. Pheonix, AZ, 2011.

20.8: Richmond JC: *Medial Meniscus Transplantation During ACL Repair* [video excerpt]. Boston, MA, 2011.

© 2016 American Academy of Orthopaedic Surgeons

Chapter 21

Leg Pain Disorders

Justin Shu Yang, MD   Thomas M. DeBerardino, MD

Abstract

Exertional leg pain can be a difficult spectrum of disorders to diagnose and treat. Medial tibial stress syndrome, tibial stress reaction, and tibial stress fractures are overuse disorders that can cause substantial time away from competition. The keys to preventing stress fracture include adequate dietary consumption of calcium and vitamin D, and other targeted interventions in at-risk populations. Nonsurgical management usually allows patients to return to their earlier activity level, although prolonged rest often is needed. Surgical intervention can be considered for a patient with a recalcitrant stress fracture or a high-risk fracture of the anterior tibia or an athlete who needs to return to sports quickly. Current diagnostic criteria for chronic exertional compartment syndrome can lead to high rates of false-positive results. Criteria using improved standardized exercise testing may have greater sensitivity and specificity. Surgical release is successful for pain relief in chronic exertional compartment syndrome but may not lead to a return to full sports activity or active military duty. Early recognition and treatment of popliteal artery syndrome is critical to a good outcome.

Keywords: chronic exertional compartment syndrome; leg pain; medial tibial stress syndrome; popliteal artery entrapment syndrome; tibial stress fracture; tibial stress reaction

Dr. DeBerardino or an immediate family member has received royalties from Arthrex; serves as a paid consultant to Arthrex; has received research or institutional support from Arthrex, Histogenics, and the Musculoskeletal Transplant Foundation; and serves as a board member, owner, officer, or committee member of the American Orthopaedic Society for Sports Medicine. Neither Dr. Yang nor any immediate family member has received anything of value from or has stock or stock options held in a commercial company or institution related directly or indirectly to the subject of this chapter.

Introduction

Exertion-related leg pain is common among people who are physically active. As many as 80% of collegiate athletes seek health care for leg pain.[1] Leg pain can present a clinical conundrum because the symptoms of several disorders are similar, and a meticulous workup is required to reach the correct diagnosis. Medial tibial stress syndrome (MTSS), stress reaction and fracture, chronic exertional compartment syndrome (CECS), and popliteal artery entrapment syndrome (PAES) should be considered in the differential diagnosis. Recent research has examined the clinical characteristics, risk factors, diagnostic modalities, treatment options, and outcomes of conditions causing leg pain.

Medial Tibial Stress Syndrome

MTSS, often called shin splints, is a common cause of leg pain. The incidence in athletic and military populations is 20% to 44%.[2-4] MTSS is characterized by pain on the medial border of the tibia, typically near the origin of the soleus, posterior tibial tendon, and flexor digitorum longus.[4,5] This posterior medial pain has led some authors to conclude that traction of these muscles leads to an enthesopathy, periostitis, and pain.[6,7] However, in some patients dual-energy x-ray absorptiometry and CT reveal relative osteopenia of the anterior tibia.[8,9] This finding suggests that MTSS is on a spectrum of tibial stress injuries that includes tendinopathy, periostitis, periosteal remodeling, and tibial stress reaction.[5] Pain with palpation and the presence of edema are highly sensitive for this spectrum of disorders.[10]

Although MTSS is common in running and jumping athletes, the pool of at-risk individuals has been expanded. A prospective study of naval recruits found that MTSS was twice as likely to develop in women as in men.[4] Excessive pronation of the foot was found to be a key risk factor in two biomechanical studies of foot posture during walking and running.[11,12] Patients with MTSS had greater medial longitudinal arch deformation while walking or standing than healthy control subjects. Early heel rise, forefoot abduction, and apropulsive gait were significantly different in patients with MTSS. Relatively small internal and external hip range of motion, high body mass index, and lean calf girth as well as a history of MTSS also have been identified as risk factors.[4,13] Anthropometric parameters including thigh length, leg length, foot length, and leg circumference as well as limb length alignment had no association with MTSS.[14,15] Individuals who had participated in an athletic activity for fewer than 5 years were found to be substantially more likely to have MTSS than those who had participated for a longer period of time.[2] Individuals who used a foot orthosis were found to be at increased risk for MTSS.[2] Multivariate analysis found that tobacco smoking conferred a ninefold increased risk of MTSS.[16]

MTSS is self-limiting with proper treatment. In a prospective cohort study, 37 of 38 runners with MTSS had complete recovery at an average of 72 days (range, 16 to 582 days).[17] Recovery from injury was defined as absence of pain in the affected anatomic location after two consecutive sessions of running at least 500 m. In a study of Dutch military recruits, the average time to recovery was 58 days.[13] Most treatment regimens consist of active rest followed by a gradual return to running, which begins only when low-impact activity such as walking or cycling produces no pain.[18] Return-to-running programs vary, but implementation should be gradual. Running distance should increase no more than 10% per week and should be immediately decreased if symptoms return. In a randomized controlled study, no benefit was found to adding calf strengthening and stretching or the use of compression stockings to a return-to-running program.[19] Rehabilitation taping was found to decrease loading of the foot in patients with MTSS, although it did not relieve the symptoms.[20] Using a foot orthosis was found to be helpful during a 3-week study period.[21] Pain was reduced by 50% in 15 of 20 runners with MTSS, but this effect might have been produced by rest alone. Low-energy extracorporeal shock wave therapy (ESWT) was found to be a treatment option for patients with MTSS of more than 6 months' duration.[22] ESWT is believed to induce periosteal detachment and microfractures of the trabeculae, which can stimulate healing. At 15-month follow-up of 47 patients with chronic MTSS who underwent ESWT in addition to a home therapy program, 40 had returned to sports at the preinjury level. In comparison, only 22 of 47 patients who underwent home therapy alone had returned to the preinjury sport level.

Tibial Stress Reaction

On the spectrum of tibial stress disorders, the severity of tibial stress reaction is between that of MTSS and

Table 1

The Fredericson MRI Grading System for Bone Stress Reaction and Fracture

MRI Grade	Description
0	Normal MRI findings
1	Mild to moderate periosteal edema on T2-weighted images only
	No focal bone marrow abnormality
2	Severe periosteal edema and bone marrow edema on T2-weighted images only
3	Moderate to severe edema of both the periosteum and bone marrow on T1- and T2-weighted images
4	Low-signal fracture line on all sequences
	Severe bone marrow edema on both T1- and T2-weighted images

Adapted with permission from Fredericson M, Bergman AG, Hoffman KL, Dillingham MS: Tibial stress reaction in runners: Correlation of clinical symptoms and scintigraphy with a new magnetic resonance imaging grading system. *Am J Sports Med* 1995;23(4):472-481.

tibial stress fracture. Radiographs may show a periosteal reaction and cortical thickening.[23] An MRI study identified a progression of injury from periosteal edema to progressive bone marrow involvement and ultimately to cortical stress fracture[24] (Table 1). Osteopenia in the anterior cortex of patients with MTSS also may be part of the progression.[8,9] The etiology is believed to be inadequate bone remodeling after damage. Figure 1 shows a theoretic cascade of events.[23]

Tibial stress reactions often are asymptomatic. A study of 21 collegiate long-distance runners who were asymptomatic found that 9 (43%) had grade 1, 2, or 3 MRI changes indicative of a tibial stress injury.[25] None had grade 4 changes. Five patients had bilateral involvement. The most common finding was severe periosteal edema and bone marrow edema with T2 weighting, as is consistent with a grade 2 injury. None of the patients became symptomatic during the subsequent year. This study highlights the value of the clinical history and physical examination in treating tibial stress reaction (Figure 2).

Tibial Stress Fracture

Stress fractures are the most severe bone stress injuries. The history and physical examination are characteristic,

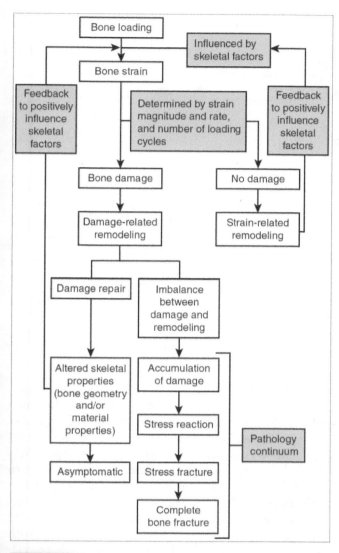

Figure 1   Proposed pathophysiology of tibial stress injury.

and the diagnosis is made with radiographs, CT, bone scan, and MRI. Approximately half of all stress fractures occur in the tibia.[23] The reported incidence of tibial stress fractures was found to range from 4% to 20% based on the population; those at risk typically include long-distance runners, track and field athletes, jumping athletes, and military recruits.[26-28] A year-long prospective study of elite Israeli military recruits found that almost all tibial stress fractures occurred during the first 6 months of training.[28] In contrast, stress fractures of the metatarsal were most likely to occur during the second 6 months of training.

Low bone mineral density, low body mass in the lower extremities, menstrual imbalance, and a low-fat diet are associated with stress fractures as well as MTSS in women.[18,23,26,29] The Female Athlete Triad Coalition and the International Olympic Committee recently proposed guidelines for the evaluation of risk factors, treatment, and return to play for at-risk female athletes.[30,31] The Female Athlete Triad Coalition Consensus Statement includes a scoring system for an athlete's diet, body mass index, age of first menarche, menses regularity, bone mineral density, and previous stress fractures.[30] The resulting score can guide the physician in deciding whether the athlete should be returned to play. The International Olympic Committee guideline is similar in that it includes many aspects of the athlete's health by calculating the so-called relative energy deficiency (which emphasizes maintaining energy availability by the following formula: energy availability = energy intake − exercise energy expenditure), but it is related to both male and female athletes.[31] A similar model has been created for predicting the risk of stress fracture in military recruits.[32]

A study of 891 recruits at the United States Military Academy found that the incidence of stress fracture was almost four times higher in women than in men.[29] Having a relatively small tibia and femur increased the risk of stress fracture. A history of physical training lowered the risk, particularly in men. Women with a relatively short time since menarche had an increased risk of stress fracture. In a biomechanical study, runners who had an earlier tibial stress fracture had greater peak hip adduction and rearfoot eversion angles during the stance phase of running than healthy control subjects. These factors may lead to altered loading within the lower extremity and thus predispose the person to stress fracture.[33] Similar biomechanical studies found that varying fatigue patterns in long-distance runners contribute to a reduced tolerance for impact.[34] Psychological stressors also were found to increase the risk of tibial stress fracture.[35]

The shock-absorbing effect of the foot may have a role in tibial stress fracture. Runners who had an earlier stress fracture were found to have greater plantar flexor musculotendinous stiffness, greater Achilles tendon stiffness, and less Achilles tendon elongation during maximal isometric contraction in comparison with healthy runners.[36] The use of a treadmill for running and increased foot pronation may reduce the risk of tibial stress fracture.[37,38] However, a systematic review found that the use of foot insoles were of no benefit in preventing tibial stress fracture.[39]

Recent research has emphasized the importance of calcium and vitamin D homeostasis in preventing and treating stress fractures. High levels of circulating parathyroid hormone with subsequent bone turnover is an established risk factor for osteoporotic fracture, and a high parathyroid level may be an independent risk factor for stress fracture.[40] Several randomized placebo-controlled

3: Knee and Leg

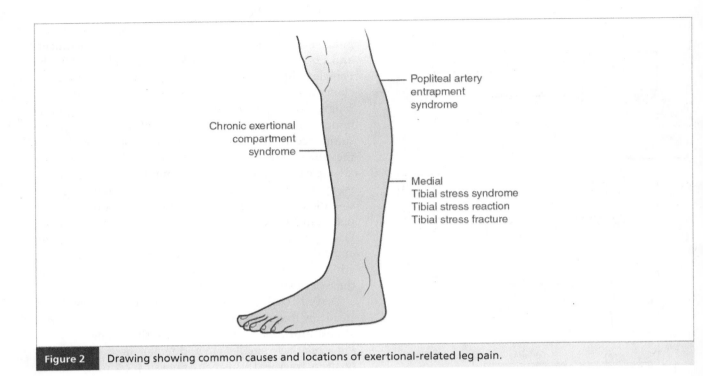

Chronic exertional
compartment
syndrome

Popliteal artery
entrapment
syndrome

Medial
Tibial stress syndrome
Tibial stress reaction
Tibial stress fracture

Figure 2 Drawing showing common causes and locations of exertional-related leg pain.

studies suggested that daily consumption of 2,000 mg of supplemental calcium and 1,000 IU of vitamin D reduces the risk of stress fracture by 20% and improves bone mineral density.[41,42] Some bone remodeling was found to be critical to repairing accumulated microdamage; pharmacologic inhibition of bone turnover did not reduce the incidence of stress fractures.[43] These studies suggest that military recruits and running athletes age 14 to 50 years should ensure sufficient calcium and vitamin D intake to meet or exceed the currently recommended dietary allowances (1,000 to 1,300 mg and 600 IU, respectively).[44]

The use of rest, restricted weight bearing, and immobilization has led to good long-term results. Of 26 military recruits with a tibial stress fracture who were treated with rest and immobilization, 13 were available 10 years after initial injury to answer questions on the long-term consequences of the fracture. None reported any limitation of active military duty or separation from the military as a result of the stress fracture.[45] Modalities such as pulsed ultrasound have been proposed for managing stress fractures. Although the exact mechanism of pulsed ultrasound is unknown, it is believed to induce aggrecan and proteoglycan synthesis in chondrocytes, leading to increased endochondral ossification. However, in a randomized double-blind study, 43 patients with tibial stress fracture were assigned to pulsed ultrasound or placebo treatment. There was no significant between-group difference in healing time.[46] Further study of this modality may be needed.

ESWT has been effective in treating athletes with a recalcitrant stress fracture. A study of five athletes treated with ESWT for a stress fracture of more than 6 months' duration reported that ESWT was effective.[47] A randomized placebo-controlled comparison study of capacitively coupled electric field stimulation used 15 hours a day to stimulate bone growth after acute stress fracture found no between-group difference in time to healing.[48] However, compliance with rest was associated with reduced time to healing, and noncompliance with rest was associated with increased time to healing. The study suggested that capacitively coupled electric field stimulation can be indicated for a severely injured or elite athlete or military recruit who is motivated to rest by a desire to return to activity.

Surgical intervention has been suggested to treat a high-risk stress fracture in athletes who must return to sport quickly. An anterior tibial stress fracture is less common but carries greater risk than a posteromedial tibial stress fracture. Nonunion rates higher than 60% and healing delayed as much as 12 months have been reported.[49,50] Such a difficult or long recovery can be career ending for a professional athlete. Intramedullary nailing of chronic anterior tibial stress fractures often is effective for relieving pain and increasing healing, but the associated complications include infection and insertion site pain.[51]

Recent studies focused on anterior tension-band plating with a compression plate at the anterolateral tibial surface. The theoretic advantage of this technique over the use of an intramedullary device is that the plate placed anterior to the central axis of the bone has a mechanical advantage in neutralizing tensile forces and fracture micromotion. Full healing and return to activities was reported at an average of 10 weeks to 3 months after surgery.[52,53] Drilling and anterior laminofixation also were reported, with healing rates of 50% and 93%, respectively.[54]

Chronic Exertional Compartment Syndrome

CECS is a relatively common cause of leg pain. The annual incidence of CECS ranges from 27% to 33% and is second only to that of MTSS (13% to 42%).[1] A patient with CECS usually reports pain during exercise that is relieved by rest, and subsequent examination of the patient typically is normal. The symptoms commonly are bilateral. CECS has been defined as a painful condition in which exercise induces high pressure within a closed myofascial space, with a resulting decrease in tissue perfusion and ischemia. CECS sometimes is accompanied by temporary neurologic impairments. A biopsy examination of the stiffness and thickness of leg fascia in patients with CECS and normal control subjects detected no between-group differences.[55] This finding suggests that CECS is not determined by structural and mechanical properties of the leg. In the military population, an elevated risk of CECS was correlated with increasing age, female sex, white race, junior enlisted rank, and Army service.[56] Women and running athletes are at particular risk in the civilian population.[57] CECS in the anterior or lateral compartment is most common and has the best treatment and recovery prognosis. The deep posterior compartment can be involved, but the results of surgery are likely to be inferior compared with those of CECS in other compartments.[58]

The most common diagnostic tool for CECS is measurement of intramuscular compartment pressure (IMCP). Invasively measured IMCP rose with a typical clinical picture of CECS in 45 of 131 patients (34%) with exercise-induced leg pain. The widely used Pedowitz criteria for the diagnosis of CECS are based on IMCP measured with the patient supine at discrete time points before and after an exercise challenge. A positive test is defined as a pressure measurement above 15 mm Hg before exercise, above 30 mm Hg 1 minute after exercise, and above 20 mm Hg 5 minutes after exercise.[59] Recent systematic reviews questioned the validity of these criteria for confirming a diagnosis of CECS because of a lack of control and normative IMCP data.[60-62] In a recent comparison of patients with CECS and normal control subjects, the diagnostic usefulness of IMCP was improved when it was measured continuously during exercise. The greatest between-group difference occurred while patients and control patients carried a 15-kg backpack, the treadmill incline was increased to 5%, and the treadmill walking pace was set at 6.5 km/h for 5 minutes.[63] A cutoff of 105 mm Hg during this specific treadmill exercise had better diagnostic accuracy than the Pedowitz criteria.

The use of MRI and ultrasound has been suggested for supporting a CECS diagnosis. In a study of 79 consecutive patients, abnormal signal on postexercise T2-weighted MRI was well correlated with increased intracompartmental pressures, with 96% sensitivity and 87% specificity.[64] An ultrasound study found an increase in anterior compartment fascial thickness during exercise in patients with CECS compared with normal control patients.[65] Ultrasound does not appear to be necessary for guiding routine deep or superficial posterior leg compartment pressure testing because direct palpation is similarly accurate for needle tip placement.[66]

The symptoms of CECS appear to be persistent. At an average 4-year follow-up of 12 military recruits in whom CECS was diagnosed and managed nonsurgically, the initial ICMP measurements (taken immediately after exercise) remained elevated in 16 of the 21 affected legs, and all 12 patients still had typical symptoms.[67] Nonsurgical treatment with botulinum toxin A injection recently had good short-term results in 16 patients with CECS.[68] Injection into the anterior and lateral compartments led to an IMCP reduction of approximately 60% at an average 4-month follow-up. Exertional pain was completely eliminated in 15 of 16 patients (94%), but there was a statistically significant decrease in muscle strength. It is unknown whether the strength reduction was clinically significant.

Surgical release of the compartment affected by CECS has been the treatment of choice, although its effectiveness has been questioned. In a retrospective study of 611 patients with CECS in a military population, 44.7% reported symptom recurrence and 27.7% were unable to return to full activity.[69] Documented surgical complications occurred in 15.7%, 17.3% were referred for medical discharge because of CECS, and 5.9% required surgical revision or repeat release.[69] These data were consistent with earlier studies that found a 20% to 30% rate of inability to return to active duty among military recruits.[70-72] In a study of 13 elite athletes, 11 (84%) were able to return to their sport at the same level at a mean of 10.6 weeks after surgical fasciotomy. Patients who had a four-compartment release required more than 3.5 weeks longer to return to full sports activity. Surgical technique may play a role. A recent study in a swine model found a strong correlation between fasciotomy length and reduction in intracompartmental pressure. The

3: Knee and Leg

researchers suggested that a 90% or greater fascial release is necessary to return the intracompartmental pressure to a value at or near its baseline.[73] However, other experts have recommended a limited release in some patients.[74] In a retrospective study of 73 patients with CECS, those younger than 23 years (high school or college athletes) had a better surgical result than older patients. In addition, an isolated anterior compartment release led to greater patient satisfaction and a better functional outcome than a combined anterior and lateral release.[75]

Popliteal Artery Entrapment Syndrome

PAES is a rare but painful and potentially limb-threatening disorder that predominantly occurs in athletes younger than 30 years. The popliteal artery becomes compressed by the various soft tissue against the medial femoral condyle during ankle plantar flexion. Over time, the intimal wall of the popliteal artery can be damaged, leading to aneurysms or stenotic lesions. Several anatomical variations can cause PAES, the most common being an abnormal attachment of the medial head of the gastrocnemius muscle; other variations include a medial course of the popliteal artery, medial gastrocnemius hypertrophy, and aberrant fibrous bands.[76,77] PAES and CECS occur in the same patient populations, and they must be differentiated with compartment pressure testing.[78,79] The diagnosis most often is based on provocative testing.[80-82] Forced ankle plantar flexion and a single-leg hop can reproduce the symptoms. These tests also can reveal a decrease in arterial blood flow with direct palpation, duplex ultrasound, angiography, or the ankle-brachial index.[82]

Early detection and intervention can limit the progress of PAES and lead to a more favorable outcome by minimizing arterial damage.[83] At 2-year follow-up, botulinum toxin A injection into the medial head of the gastrocnemius was found to lead to complete resolution of symptoms in a patient with an earlier bilateral popliteal arteriolysis without resection of the medial gastrocnemius head.[84] Surgical intervention is the standard treatment of patients with ischemic symptoms, although the rarity of the condition means that no high-level outcome studies exist. Decompression of the lesion by releasing the medial head of the gastrocnemius often is necessary to prevent recurrence.[82] In patients with long-standing entrapment, the popliteal artery may have irreversible damage and atherosclerosis, aneurysm, and thrombosis can develop. In these patients, bypass grafting is the treatment of choice among vascular surgeons. With bypass grafting, long-term arterial patency from 75% to 100% has been reported, and results are best after isolated popliteal artery occlusion.[85,86] Many patients return to their previous activities after surgical intervention; those who undergo decompression alone tend to have better outcomes than those who undergo decompression plus bypass.[82,85,86]

Summary

The spectrum of tibial stress disorders can be distinguished by history, examination, and imaging. Nonsurgical management usually allows patients to return to their earlier activity level, although prolonged rest often is needed. The widely used Pedowitz criteria for the diagnosis of CECS may have a high false-positive rate; a walking treadmill test on an inclined surface while carrying a 15-kg weight may have better diagnostic accuracy. Surgical release of the compartment affected by CECS has been the treatment of choice, although its effectiveness has been questioned in the military population. Early detection and intervention can limit the progress of PAES and lead to a more favorable outcome by minimizing arterial damage. Decompression alone is often enough if diagnosed early; and bypass grafting is often needed in the chronic setting.

Key Study Points

- MTSS, tibial stress reaction, and tibial stress fractures are overuse disorders that particularly affect women, endurance athletes, and military recruits. The keys to preventing stress fracture include adequate dietary consumption of calcium and vitamin D. Nonsurgical management usually allows patients to return to their earlier activity level, although prolonged rest often is needed. Surgical intervention can be considered for a patient with a recalcitrant stress fracture or a high-risk fracture of the anterior tibia or an athlete who needs to return to sports quickly.

- Current diagnostic criteria for CECS use IMCP and can lead to high rates of false-positive results. Criteria using improved standardized exercise testing may have greater sensitivity and specificity. Surgical release is successful for pain relief in CECS but may not lead to a return to full sports activity or active military duty.

- Early detection and treatment of PAES are critical for preventing chronic vascular disease and relieving symptoms.

Annotated References

1. George CA, Hutchinson MR: Chronic exertional compartment syndrome. *Clin Sports Med* 2012;31(2):307-319.

   The literature on the epidemiology, diagnosis, and treatment of CECS was reviewed.

2. Hubbard TJ, Carpenter EM, Cordova ML: Contributing factors to medial tibial stress syndrome: A prospective investigation. *Med Sci Sports Exerc* 2009;41(3):490-496.

   The factors most influencing the development of MTSS were found to be a history of MTSS and stress fracture, years of running experience, and use of orthoses. Level of evidence: III.

3. Yagi S, Muneta T, Sekiya I: Incidence and risk factors for medial tibial stress syndrome and tibial stress fracture in high school runners. *Knee Surg Sports Traumatol Arthrosc* 2013;21(3):556-563.

   A significant relationship was found between body mass index, internal hip rotation angle, and MTSS in female athletes. Level of evidence: II.

4. Yates B, White S: The incidence and risk factors in the development of medial tibial stress syndrome among naval recruits. *Am J Sports Med* 2004;32(3):772-780.

5. Galbraith RM, Lavallee ME: Medial tibial stress syndrome: Conservative treatment options. *Curr Rev Musculoskelet Med* 2009;2(3):127-133.

   The literature on nonsurgical treatment options for MTSS was reviewed.

6. Moen MH, Tol JL, Weir A, Steunebrink M, De Winter TC: Medial tibial stress syndrome: A critical review. *Sports Med* 2009;39(7):523-546.

   The literature on MTSS was reviewed.

7. Bouché RT, Johnson CH: Medial tibial stress syndrome (tibial fasciitis): A proposed pathomechanical model involving fascial traction. *J Am Podiatr Med Assoc* 2007;97(1):31-36.

8. Gaeta M, Minutoli F, Scribano E, et al: CT and MR imaging findings in athletes with early tibial stress injuries: Comparison with bone scintigraphy findings and emphasis on cortical abnormalities. *Radiology* 2005;235(2):553-561.

9. Magnusson HI, Westlin NE, Nyqvist F, Gärdsell P, Seeman E, Karlsson MK: Abnormally decreased regional bone density in athletes with medial tibial stress syndrome. *Am J Sports Med* 2001;29(6):712-715.

10. Newman P, Adams R, Waddington G: Two simple clinical tests for predicting onset of medial tibial stress syndrome: Shin palpation test and shin oedema test. *Br J Sports Med* 2012;46(12):861-864.

    The relationship between two clinical test results and a future diagnosis of MTSS in military recruits was examined. Level of evidence: II.

11. Tweed JL, Campbell JA, Avil SJ: Biomechanical risk factors in the development of medial tibial stress syndrome in distance runners. *J Am Podiatr Med Assoc* 2008;98(6):436-444.

12. Bandholm T, Boysen L, Haugaard S, Zebis MK, Bencke J: Foot medial longitudinal-arch deformation during quiet standing and gait in subjects with medial tibial stress syndrome. *J Foot Ankle Surg* 2008;47(2):89-95.

13. Moen MH, Bongers T, Bakker EW, et al: Risk factors and prognostic indicators for medial tibial stress syndrome. *Scand J Med Sci Sports* 2012;22(1):34-39.

    Risk factors and prognostic indicators for MTSS were examined. Decreased hip internal range of motion, increased ankle plantar flexion, and positive navicular drop were associated with MTSS. A higher body mass index was associated with an increased time to full recovery. Level of evidence: II.

14. Sabeti V, Khoshraftar Yazdi N, Bizheh N: The relationship between shin splints with anthropometric characteristics and some indicators of body composition. *J Sports Med Phys Fitness* [published online ahead of print October 6, 2014].

    Anthropometric characteristics and body composition indicators may not be risk factors for shin splints. Level of evidence: III.

15. Raissi GR, Cherati AD, Mansoori KD, Razi MD: The relationship between lower extremity alignment and medial tibial stress syndrome among non-professional athletes. *Sports Med Arthrosc Rehabil Ther Technol* 2009;1(1):11.

    A significant relationship was found between navicular drop and MTSS. There was no significant relationship between lower extremity alignment and MTSS. Level of evidence: II.

16. Sharma J, Golby J, Greeves J, Spears IR: Biomechanical and lifestyle risk factors for medial tibia stress syndrome in army recruits: A prospective study. *Gait Posture* 2011;33(3):361-365.

    An imbalance in foot pressure with greater pressure on the medial side than on the lateral side was the primary risk factor for MTSS. Level of evidence: II.

17. Nielsen RO, Rønnow L, Rasmussen S, Lind M: A prospective study on time to recovery in 254 injured novice runners. *PLoS One* 2014;9(6):e99877.

    MTSS was the most common injury among runners, followed by patellofemoral pain, medial meniscal injury, and Achilles tendinopathy. Half of the patients were unable to run 500 m twice without pain 10 weeks after injury. Almost 5% of patients received surgical treatment.

18. Gallo RA, Plakke M, Silvis ML: Common leg injuries of long-distance runners: Anatomical and biomechanical approach. *Sports Health* 2012;4(6):485-495.

19. Moen MH, Holtslag L, Bakker E, et al: The treatment of medial tibial stress syndrome in athletes: A randomized clinical trial. *Sports Med Arthrosc Rehabil Ther Technol* 2012;4:12.

    A comparison of three functional rehabilitation programs for MTSS (a graded running program alone, with stretching and strengthening exercises for the calves, or with a sports compression stocking) found no outcome differences. Level of evidence: I.

20. Griebert MC, Needle AR, McConnell J, Kaminski TW: Lower-leg Kinesio tape reduces rate of loading in participants with medial tibial stress syndrome. *Phys Ther Sport* 2014 Jan 29. Epub ahead of print. pii: S1466-853X(14)00002-9.

    Rehabilitation taping decreases the rate of medial loading in patients with MTSS and may be a useful adjunctive treatment. Level of evidence: III.

21. Loudon JK, Dolphino MR: Use of foot orthoses and calf stretching for individuals with medial tibial stress syndrome. *Foot Ankle Spec* 2010;3(1):15-20.

    Off-the-shelf orthoses and calf stretching may be effective in the initial treatment of runners with MTSS.

22. Rompe JD, Cacchio A, Furia JP, Maffulli N: Low-energy extracorporeal shock wave therapy as a treatment for medial tibial stress syndrome. *Am J Sports Med* 2010;38(1):125-132.

    Forty of 47 patients who received ESWT for MTSS were able to return to their sport at the preinjury level 15 months after injury, compared with 22 of 47 control subjects. Level of evidence: III.

23. Warden SJ, Davis IS, Fredericson M: Management and prevention of bone stress injuries in long-distance runners. *J Orthop Sports Phys Ther* 2014;44(10):749-765.

    The literature on management and prevention of bone stress injuries in long-distance runners was reviewed.

24. Fredericson M, Bergman AG, Hoffman KL, Dillingham MS: Tibial stress reaction in runners: Correlation of clinical symptoms and scintigraphy with a new magnetic resonance imaging grading system. *Am J Sports Med* 1995;23(4):472-481.

25. Bergman AG, Fredericson M, Ho C, Matheson GO: Asymptomatic tibial stress reactions: MRI detection and clinical follow-up in distance runners. *AJR Am J Roentgenol* 2004;183(3):635-638.

26. Tenforde AS, Sayres LC, McCurdy ML, Sainani KL, Fredericson M: Identifying sex-specific risk factors for stress fractures in adolescent runners. *Med Sci Sports Exerc* 2013;45(10):1843-1851.

    Earlier fracture is the most robust predictor of stress fractures in both women and men. Low body mass index, late menarche, and earlier participation in gymnastics or dance were identifiable risk factors for stress fractures in girls. Participation in basketball appeared to be protective in boys and may represent a modifiable risk factor for stress fracture. Level of evidence: III.

27. McCarthy MM, Voos JE, Nguyen JT, Callahan L, Hannafin JA: Injury profile in elite female basketball athletes at the Women's National Basketball Association Combine. *Am J Sports Med* 2013;41(3):645-651.

    The percentage of players at the Women's National Basketball Association Combine who reported a history of stress fracture was 7.3%. Level of evidence: III.

28. Finestone A, Milgrom C, Wolf O, Petrov K, Evans R, Moran D: Epidemiology of metatarsal stress fractures versus tibial and femoral stress fractures during elite training. *Foot Ankle Int* 2011;32(1):16-20.

    The incidence of stress fracture among military recruits was highest during the first 6 months of training but decreases after 6 months, possibly because of individual adaptations. Level of evidence: III.

29. Cosman F, Ruffing J, Zion M, et al: Determinants of stress fracture risk in United States Military Academy cadets. *Bone* 2013;55(2):359-366.

    Earlier physical training in men, length of estrogen exposure in women, and leg bone dimensions in both sexes were found to have only a minor role in the development of stress fractures in physically fit military cadets. Level of evidence: III.

30. De Souza MJ, Nattiv A, Joy E, et al; Female Athlete Triad Coalition; American College of Sports Medicine; American Medical Society for Sports Medicine; American Bone Health Alliance: 2014 Female Athlete Triad Coalition consensus statement on treatment and return to play of the female athlete triad: 1st International Conference held in San Francisco, CA, May 2012, and 2nd International Conference held in Indianapolis, IN, May 2013. *Clin J Sport Med* 2014;24(2):96-119.

    A scoring system was presented in which a female athlete's diet, body mass index, age of first menarche, menses regularity, bone mineral density, and history of stress fracture were tabulated. Level of evidence: II.

31. Mountjoy M, Sundgot-Borgen J, Burke L, et al: The IOC consensus statement: Beyond the female athlete triad. Relative energy deficiency in sport (RED-S). *Br J Sports Med* 2014;48(7):491-497.

    The International Olympic Committee guideline calculated the so-called relative energy deficiency to assess risk factors in female athletes. Level of evidence: II.

32. Moran DS, Finestone AS, Arbel Y, Shabshin N, Laor A: A simplified model to predict stress fracture in young elite combat recruits. *J Strength Cond Res* 2012;26(9):2585-2592.

A young male recruit for an elite combat unit was at a greater risk of developing stress fracture if he had a history of aerobic training less than 2 times per week for more than 40 minutes per session and had a waist circumference smaller than 75 cm. Level of evidence: III.

33. Milner CE, Hamill J, Davis IS: Distinct hip and rearfoot kinematics in female runners with a history of tibial stress fracture. *J Orthop Sports Phys Ther* 2010;40(2):59-66.

Runners with a history of tibial stress fracture had greater peak hip adduction and rearfoot eversion angles during the stance phase of running than healthy control subjects. A consequence may be altered load distribution within the lower extremity, creating a predisposition to stress fracture. Level of evidence: III.

34. Clansey AC, Hanlon M, Wallace ES, Lake MJ: Effects of fatigue on running mechanics associated with tibial stress fracture risk. *Med Sci Sports Exerc* 2012;44(10):1917-1923.

The identified risk factors for impact-related injuries such as tibial stress fracture are modified by fatigue, which is associated with a reduced tolerance for impact. These findings are important for identifying individuals at risk for injury from lower limb impact loading during running. Level of evidence: III.

35. Moran DS, Evans R, Arbel Y, et al: Physical and psychological stressors linked with stress fractures in recruit training. *Scand J Med Sci Sports* 2013;23(4):443-450.

Psychological factors may have a role in predicting stress fracture development. Level of evidence: IV.

36. Pamukoff DN, Blackburn JT: Comparison of plantarflexor musculotendinous stiffness, geometry, and architecture in male runners with and without a history of tibial stress fracture. *J Appl Biomech* 2015;31(1):41-47.

Runners with a history of stress fracture had greater plantar flexor musculotendinous stiffness, greater Achilles tendon stiffness, and less Achilles tendon elongation during maximal isometric contraction than healthy runners. Level of evidence: IV.

37. Hetsroni I, Finestone A, Milgrom C, et al: The role of foot pronation in the development of femoral and tibial stress fractures: A prospective biomechanical study. *Clin J Sport Med* 2008;18(1):18-23.

38. Milgrom C, Finestone A, Segev S, Olin C, Arndt T, Ekenman I: Are overground or treadmill runners more likely to sustain tibial stress fracture? *Br J Sports Med* 2003;37(2):160-163.

39. Snyder RA, DeAngelis JP, Koester MC, Spindler KP, Dunn WR: Does shoe insole modification prevent stress fractures? A systematic review. *HSS J* 2009;5(2):92-98.

The use of shoe insoles for prevention of stress fracture was systematically reviewed.

40. Välimäki VV, Alfthan H, Lehmuskallio E, et al: Risk factors for clinical stress fractures in male military recruits: A prospective cohort study. *Bone* 2005;37(2):267-273.

41. Lappe J, Cullen D, Haynatzki G, Recker R, Ahlf R, Thompson K: Calcium and vitamin D supplementation decreases incidence of stress fractures in female Navy recruits. *J Bone Miner Res* 2008;23(5):741-749.

42. Gaffney-Stomberg E, Lutz LJ, Rood JC, et al: Calcium and vitamin D supplementation maintains parathyroid hormone and improves bone density during initial military training: A randomized, double-blind, placebo controlled trial. *Bone* 2014;68:46-56.

Calcium and vitamin D supplementation can maintain and improve bone health during periods of elevated bone turnover such as initial military training. Level of evidence: I.

43. Milgrom C, Finestone A, Novack V, et al: The effect of prophylactic treatment with risedronate on stress fracture incidence among infantry recruits. *Bone* 2004;35(2):418-424.

44. Institute of Medicine: *Dietary Reference Intakes for Calcium and Vitamin D*. Washington, DC, National Academy of Sciences, 2010.

Dietary intake of calcium should be 1,000 to 1,300 mg and dietary intake of vitamin D should be 600 IU according to current guidelines.

45. Kilcoyne KG, Dickens JF, Rue JP: Tibial stress fractures in an active duty population: Long-term outcomes. *J Surg Orthop Adv* 2013;22(1):50-53.

Tibial stress fractures in military recruits most often were isolated, and they did not affect the ability to complete military training or lead to decreased physical activity at 10-year follow-up. Level of evidence: IV.

46. Rue JP, Armstrong DW III, Frassica FJ, Deafenbaugh M, Wilckens JH: The effect of pulsed ultrasound in the treatment of tibial stress fractures. *Orthopedics* 2004;27(11):1192-1195.

47. Taki M, Iwata O, Shiono M, Kimura M, Takagishi K: Extracorporeal shock wave therapy for resistant stress fracture in athletes: A report of 5 cases. *Am J Sports Med* 2007;35(7):1188-1192.

48. Beck BR, Matheson GO, Bergman G, et al: Do capacitively coupled electric fields accelerate tibial stress fracture healing? A randomized controlled trial. *Am J Sports Med* 2008;36(3):545-553.

49. Beals RK, Cook RD: Stress fractures of the anterior tibial diaphysis. *Orthopedics* 1991;14(8):869-875.

50. Batt ME, Kemp S, Kerslake R: Delayed union stress fractures of the anterior tibia: Conservative management. *Br J Sports Med* 2001;35(1):74-77.

51. Young AJ, McAllister DR: Evaluation and treatment of tibial stress fractures. *Clin Sports Med* 2006;25(1):117-128, x.

52. Borens O, Sen MK, Huang RC, et al: Anterior tension band plating for anterior tibial stress fractures in high-performance female athletes: A report of 4 cases. *J Orthop Trauma* 2006;20(6):425-430.

53. Cruz AS, de Hollanda JP, Duarte A Jr, Hungria Neto JS: Anterior tibial stress fractures treated with anterior tension band plating in high-performance athletes. *Knee Surg Sports Traumatol Arthrosc* 2013;21(6):1447-1450.

    Anterior tibial tension-band plating was found to lead to prompt fracture consolidation and was a good alternative treatment of anterior tibial cortex stress fractures. Bone grafting was found to be unnecessary. Level of evidence: IV.

54. Liimatainen E, Sarimo J, Hulkko A, Ranne J, Heikkilä J, Orava S: Anterior mid-tibial stress fractures: Results of surgical treatment. *Scand J Surg* 2009;98(4):244-249.

    Surgical treatment of nonunited tibial stress fractures with laminofixation may be superior to tibial fracture site drilling. Level of evidence: IV.

55. Dahl M, Hansen P, Stål P, Edmundsson D, Magnusson SP: Stiffness and thickness of fascia do not explain chronic exertional compartment syndrome. *Clin Orthop Relat Res* 2011;469(12):3495-3500.

    No difference was found in fascial thickness and stiffness between patients with CECS, with or without diabetes, compared with healthy individuals. This finding suggests that structural and mechanical properties are unlikely to explain CECS. Level of evidence: II.

56. Waterman BR, Liu J, Newcomb R, Schoenfeld AJ, Orr JD, Belmont PJ Jr: Risk factors for chronic exertional compartment syndrome in a physically active military population. *Am J Sports Med* 2013;41(11):2545-2549.

    The epidemiology of CECS was examined in a physically active military population. Sex, age, race, military rank, and branch of service were important factors associated with the incidence of CECS in this at-risk population. Level of evidence: II.

57. Davis DE, Raikin S, Garras DN, Vitanzo P, Labrador H, Espandar R: Characteristics of patients with chronic exertional compartment syndrome. *Foot Ankle Int* 2013;34(10):1349-1354.

    The average age of patients with CECS was 24 years. Women accounted for 60.1% of those with elevated pressures. Anterior and lateral compartment pressures were elevated in 42.5% and 35.5% of patients, respectively. Level of evidence: III.

58. Winkes MB, Hoogeveen AR, Houterman S, Giesberts A, Wijn PF, Scheltinga MR: Compartment pressure curves predict surgical outcome in chronic deep posterior compartment syndrome. *Am J Sports Med* 2012;40(8):1899-1905.

    Preoperative intracompartmental pressures measured at rest and after a standard exercise test may predict the success of surgery for deep posterior compartment CECS of the lower limb. Level of evidence: IV.

59. Pedowitz RA, Hargens AR, Mubarak SJ, Gershuni DH: Modified criteria for the objective diagnosis of chronic compartment syndrome of the leg. *Am J Sports Med* 1990;18(1):35-40.

60. Tiidus PM: Is intramuscular pressure a valid diagnostic criterion for chronic exertional compartment syndrome? *Clin J Sport Med* 2014;24(1):87-88.

    A systematic review concluded that use of the currently accepted diagnostic criteria for anterior tibial intramuscular pressure before, during, and after exercise would include many individuals without symptoms of CECS.

61. Roberts A, Franklyn-Miller A: The validity of the diagnostic criteria used in chronic exertional compartment syndrome: A systematic review. *Scand J Med Sci Sports* 2012;22(5):585-595.

    In a systematic review of the validity of diagnostic criteria for CECS, the use of protocol-specific upper confidence limits was recommended to guide the diagnosis after unsuccessful nonsurgical management.

62. Aweid O, Del Buono A, Malliaras P, et al: Systematic review and recommendations for intracompartmental pressure monitoring in diagnosing chronic exertional compartment syndrome of the leg. *Clin J Sport Med* 2012;22(4):356-370.

    A systematic review concluded that new diagnostic criteria should be established for CECS.

63. Roscoe D, Roberts AJ, Hulse D: Intramuscular compartment pressure measurement in chronic exertional compartment syndrome: New and improved diagnostic criteria. *Am J Sports Med* 2015;43(2):392-398.

    In patients with symptoms consistent with CECS, the diagnostic utility of IMCP was improved with continuous measurement during exercise. Level of evidence: II.

64. Ringler MD, Litwiller DV, Felmlee JP, et al: MRI accurately detects chronic exertional compartment syndrome: A validation study. *Skeletal Radiol* 2013;42(3):385-392.

    Exercise-based MRI was moderately reliable and reproducible as a noninvasive screening test for CECS. Level of evidence: III.

65. Rajasekaran S, Beavis C, Aly AR, Leswick D: The utility of ultrasound in detecting anterior compartment thickness changes in chronic exertional compartment syndrome: A pilot study. *Clin J Sport Med* 2013;23(4):305-311.

    Patients with CECS had an increase in anterior compartment fascial thickness on ultrasound compared with control subjects. It is unclear whether this finding can be used for reliable noninvasive screening. Level of evidence: III.

66. Peck E, Finnoff JT, Smith J, Curtiss H, Muir J, Hollman JH: Accuracy of palpation-guided and ultrasound-guided needle tip placement into the deep and superficial posterior leg compartments. *Am J Sports Med* 2011;39(9):1968-1974.

Needle tip placement into the deep and superficial posterior leg compartments was relatively accurate with palpation guidance, regardless of the practitioner's level of experience, and accuracy did not improve with the use of ultrasound guidance. Level of evidence: II.

67. Van der Wal WA, Heesterbeek PJ, Van den Brand JG, Verleisdonk EJ: The natural course of chronic exertional compartment syndrome of the lower leg. *Knee Surg Sports Traumatol Arthrosc* 2015;23(7):2136-2141.

The natural course of CECS appears to include persistent symptoms. Level of evidence: IV.

68. Isner-Horobeti ME, Dufour SP, Blaes C, Lecocq J: Intramuscular pressure before and after botulinum toxin in chronic exertional compartment syndrome of the leg: A preliminary study. *Am J Sports Med* 2013;41(11):2558-2566.

Injection with botulinum toxin A reduced intramuscular pressure and eliminated exertional pain in patients with anterior or anterolateral CECS as long as 9 months later. The mode of action of botulinum toxin A is unclear. Level of evidence: IV.

69. Waterman BR, Laughlin M, Kilcoyne K, Cameron KL, Owens BD: Surgical treatment of chronic exertional compartment syndrome of the leg: Failure rates and postoperative disability in an active patient population. *J Bone Joint Surg Am* 2013;95(7):592-596.

CECS is a substantial contributor to the rate of lower extremity disability in the military population. Almost half of all service members undergoing fasciotomy reported persistent symptoms, and one in five had unsuccessful surgical treatment. Level of evidence: IV.

70. Dunn JC, Waterman BR: Chronic exertional compartment syndrome of the leg in the military. *Clin Sports Med* 2014;33(4):693-705.

Clinical success has been documented in civilian patients treated for CECS, but surgical treatment in military service members has not been reliably successful. Only half of military service members had complete resolution of symptoms, and at least 25% were unable to return to full active duty. Level of evidence: IV.

71. McCallum JR, Cook JB, Hines AC, Shaha JS, Jex JW, Orchowski JR: Return to duty after elective fasciotomy for chronic exertional compartment syndrome. *Foot Ankle Int* 2014;35(9):871-875.

A return to full military duty was reported for 41% of patients who underwent elective fasciotomy for CECS. Overall, 78% of patients remained in the military, and the subjective satisfaction rate was 71%. Level of evidence: IV.

72. Roberts AJ, Krishnasamy P, Quayle JM, Houghton JM: Outcomes of surgery for chronic exertional compartment syndrome in a military population. *J R Army Med Corps* 2015;161(1):42-45.

Many miliary patients with CECS do not return to full fitness after fasciectomy. The lack of a relationship between intramuscular pressure and outcome calls into question the role of pressure in CECS. Level of evidence: IV.

73. Mathis JE, Schwartz BE, Lester JD, Kim WJ, Watson JN, Hutchinson MR: Effect of lower extremity fasciotomy length on intracompartmental pressure in an animal model of compartment syndrome: The importance of achieving a minimum of 90% fascial release. *Am J Sports Med* 2015;43(1):75-78.

This study found a strong correlation between fasciotomy length and a reduction in intracompartmental pressures in a swine model. A 90% fascial release may represent a possible watershed zone for returning intracompartmental pressure to its baseline. Level of evidence: II.

74. Finestone AS, Noff M, Nassar Y, Moshe S, Agar G, Tamir E: Management of chronic exertional compartment syndrome and fascial hernias in the anterior lower leg with the forefoot rise test and limited fasciotomy. *Foot Ankle Int* 2014;35(3):285-292.

Selected patients with CECS were found to benefit from a limited fasciotomy. Level of evidence: IV.

75. Packer JD, Day MS, Nguyen JT, Hobart SJ, Hannafin JA, Metzl JD: Functional outcomes and patient satisfaction after fasciotomy for chronic exertional compartment syndrome. *Am J Sports Med* 2013;41(2):430-436.

Age younger than 23 years and isolated anterior compartment release were factors associated with improved subjective function and satisfaction after fasciotomy. Lateral release should be avoided unless symptoms or postexertion compartment pressures clearly indicate lateral compartment involvement. Level of evidence: III.

76. Pillai J, Levien LJ, Haagensen M, Candy G, Cluver MD, Veller MG: Assessment of the medial head of the gastrocnemius muscle in functional compression of the popliteal artery. *J Vasc Surg* 2008;48(5):1189-1196.

77. Aktan Ikiz ZA, Ucerler H, Ozgur Z: Anatomic variations of popliteal artery that may be a reason for entrapment. *Surg Radiol Anat* 2009;31(9):695-700.

Anomalous anatomic relationships between muscle and arteries in the popliteal fossa were found to lead to arterial compression.

78. Politano AD, Bhamidipati CM, Tracci MC, Upchurch GR Jr, Cherry KJ: Anatomic popliteal entrapment syndrome is often a difficult diagnosis. *Vasc Endovascular Surg* 2012;46(7):542-545.

In the diagnostic algorithm for four patients with PAES, angiography with forced plantar flexion against resistance was useful for eliciting pathognomonic images of arterial occlusion. Level of evidence: IV.

© 2016 American Academy of Orthopaedic Surgeons

3: Knee and Leg

79. Turnipseed WD: Functional popliteal artery entrapment syndrome: A poorly understood and often missed diagnosis that is frequently mistreated. *J Vasc Surg* 2009;49(5):1189-1195.

    PAES and CECS occur in the same populations and have similar symptoms, but they require different treatments.

80. Anil G, Tay KH, Howe TC, Tan BS: Dynamic computed tomography angiography: Role in the evaluation of popliteal artery entrapment syndrome. *Cardiovasc Intervent Radiol* 2011;34(2):259-270.

    Dynamic CT angiography is a useful tool for diagnosing PAES.

81. Zhong H, Gan J, Zhao Y, et al: Role of CT angiography in the diagnosis and treatment of popliteal vascular entrapment syndrome. *AJR Am J Roentgenol* 2011;197(6):W1147-W1154.

    Digital subtraction angiography was found to have limited value in the evaluation of PAES and has been replaced by noninvasive imaging techniques such as Doppler sonography, CT angiography, MRI, and magnetic resonance angiography.

82. Lane R, Nguyen T, Cuzzilla M, Oomens D, Mohabbat W, Hazelton S: Functional popliteal entrapment syndrome in the sportsperson. *Eur J Vasc Endovasc Surg* 2012;43(1):81-87.

    PAES can be characterized by provocative noninvasive clinical tests, particularly hopping. A positive clinical outcome of surgery can be predicted by abnormal presurgical ultrasonic findings and confirmed by a similar normal postsurgical study. While standing, patients may have concomitant venous compression related to muscle hypertrophy. Level of evidence: IV.

83. Zünd G, Brunner U: Surgical aspects of popliteal artery entrapment syndrome: 26 years of experience with 26 legs. *Vasa* 1995;24(1):29-33.

84. Isner-Horobeti ME, Muff G, Masat J, Daussin JL, Dufour SP, Lecocq J: Botulinum toxin as a treatment for functional popliteal artery entrapment syndrome. *Med Sci Sports Exerc* 2015;47(6):1124-1127.

    Botulinum toxin treatment could be an alternative to surgery for patients with functional PAES. Botulinum toxin could reduce functional compression and consequently reduce exercise-induced pain by decreasing gastrocnemius muscle volume. Level of evidence: IV.

85. Kim SY, Min SK, Ahn S, Min SI, Ha J, Kim SJ: Long-term outcomes after revascularization for advanced popliteal artery entrapment syndrome with segmental arterial occlusion. *J Vasc Surg* 2012;55(1):90-97.

    After surgery for advanced PAES, a relatively long arterial bypass with superficial femoral artery inflow had poor long-term graft patency. Graft patency was excellent in patients with popliteal artery occlusion only after popliteal interposition graft with a reversed saphenous vein. A longer bypass extending beyond the popliteal artery may be indicated in patients with critical limb ischemia only if the extent of disease does not allow a short interposition graft. Level of evidence: IV.

86. Yamamoto S, Hoshina K, Hosaka A, Shigematsu K, Watanabe T: Long-term outcomes of surgical treatment in patients with popliteal artery entrapment syndrome. *Vascular* 2014 Nov 17 [Epub ahead of print].

    The 10-year cumulative patency of 13 limbs treated with bypass for PAES was 100%, although 2 of these limbs had an occlusion that occurred 12 or 23 years after surgery. Level of evidence: IV.

© 2016 American Academy of Orthopaedic Surgeons

Chapter 22

Ankle and Foot Injuries and Other Disorders

Thomas O. Clanton, MD   Norman E. Waldrop III, MD   Nicholas S. Johnson, MD   Scott R. Whitlow, MD

Abstract

The most common foot and ankle injuries and other conditions in athletes are ankle sprains, syndesmosis injuries, osteochondral injuries, ankle impingement, heel pain, Lisfranc injuries, turf toe, stress fractures, and Achilles tendon disorders. The diagnostic and treatment recommendations are based on a review of the current research.

Keywords: Achilles tendon; ankle; ankle sprain; ankle impingement; foot; heel pain; Lisfranc injury; osteochondral lesion; sesamoid; stress fracture; syndesmosis; turf toe

Introduction

The foot and ankle are the most commonly injured body parts in athletics, and these injuries often result in loss of playing time.[1,2] A study of intercollegiate football

Dr. Clanton or an immediate family member is a member of a speakers' bureau or has made paid presentations on behalf of Arthrex, Small Bone Innovations, Stryker, and Wright Medical Technology; serves as a paid consultant to Arthrex, Small Bone Innovations, Stryker, and Wright Medical Technology; has received research or institutional support from Arthrex; and serves as a board member, owner, officer, or committee member of the American Orthopaedic Foot and Ankle Society. Dr. Waldrop or an immediate family member is a member of a speakers' bureau or has made paid presentations on behalf of Arthrex and Wright Medical Technology and serves as a paid consultant to Arthrex. Neither of the following authors nor any immediate family member has received anything of value from or has stock or stock options held in a commercial company or institution related directly or indirectly to the subject of this chapter: Dr. Johnson and Dr. Whitlow.

players in the National Football League Scouting Combine found that 72% had a history of foot or ankle injury, the most common of which were lateral ankle sprain (40%), syndesmosis sprain (17%), metatarsophalangeal (MTP) joint injury (13%), and fibula fracture (9%).[3] Such findings have led to increased interest in the diagnosis, treatment, and rehabilitation of these injuries. Acute traumatic and chronic overuse athletic injuries can often be treated nonsurgically, though many of these disorders are often challenging for both the athlete and physician. Nevertheless, it is imperative for the physician to quickly recognize a pathology or circumstance that requires surgical intervention.

Ankle Injuries

The incidence of ankle sprains in the United States was reported as 2.15 per 1,000 person-years.[4] Almost half of all sprains occurred during athletic activity; basketball (41.1%), football (9.3%), and soccer (7.9%) were responsible for the most ankle sprains. In contrast, a similar study found an ankle sprain rate of 58.4 per 1,000 person-years; 64.1% of the sprains occurred during an athletic activity, most commonly men's rugby, women's cheerleading, men's and/or women's basketball, soccer, and lacrosse.[2] Lateral ankle sprains account for 85% of ankle sprains, syndesmosis sprains account for 10%, and medial sprains account for 5%.[5]

Ankle stability is a function of extrinsic elements such as ligaments and tendons and intrinsic elements such as the geometry of the articular surface. The contribution of each element varies with the load level, the direction in which force is applied, and the integrity of the ligaments. In general, the ankle is most stable in dorsiflexion and when loaded and is least stable in plantar flexion and when unloaded. When the ankle is loaded, articular geometry provides 100% of translational stability and 60% of rotational stability. The unloaded ankle, however, relies on the ligaments. Between 70% and 80% of anterior stability is provided by the lateral ligaments, 50% to 80%

3: Knee and Leg

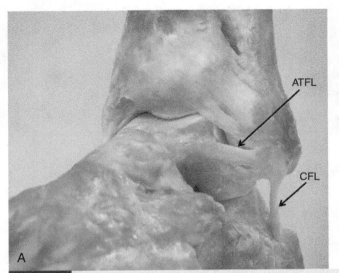
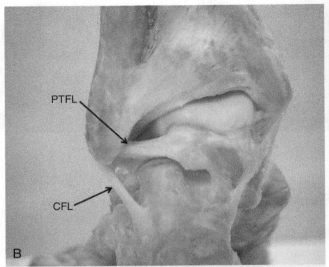

Figure 1   Photographs show the primary lateral ankle ligaments in anterolateral **(A)** and posterolateral **(B)** views of a left ankle. ATFL = anterior talofibular ligament, CFL = calcaneofibular ligament, PTFL = posterior talofibular ligament.

of posterior stability is provided by the deltoid ligaments, and 50% to 80% of rotational stability is provided by the lateral and deltoid ligaments.[6]

Lateral Ankle Injury

The lateral ligamentous complex of the ankle joint includes the anterior talofibular ligament (ATFL), the calcaneofibular ligament (CFL), and the posterior talofibular ligament (PTFL) (Figure 1). Relatively recent anatomic research provided important information on the qualitative and quantitative characteristics of these ligaments.[7] The ATFL, which is the primary restraint to inversion in plantar flexion and has the least strength of the lateral ligaments (138.9 N), resists anterior translation and internal rotation of the talus in the mortise[8] (Figure 2). When the ankle is in neutral position or dorsiflexion, the CFL is the primary restraint to inversion; its average strength is 345.7 N[8] (Figure 3). The CFL spans the tibiotalar and subtalar joints, thereby restraining subtalar inversion. The PTFL, which is the largest of the lateral ligaments, rarely is injured.[7, 9] Radiographic parameters have been defined to quantitatively describe these anatomic origins and insertions of the lateral ankle ligaments.[10]

Injury to the lateral ankle ligaments typically occurs during plantar flexion and supination, which combine inversion and adduction. In this type of injury, the anterolateral joint capsule tears first, followed by rupture of the ATFL and CFL as the force of injury progresses laterally. The ATFL is injured in 85% of lateral ankle sprains, and the CFL is injured in 20% to 40%. A grade I lateral ankle injury involves stretching of the ATFL with mild tenderness, no evidence of mechanical instability, and

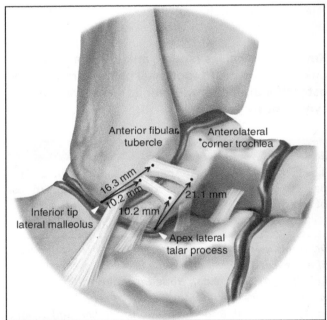

Figure 2   Schematic drawing shows the origin and insertion sites of a two-band anterior talofibular ligament in a right ankle, with the distances from landmarks. (Reproduced with permission from Clanton TO, Campbell KJ, Wilson KJ, et al: Qualitative and quantitative anatomic investigation of the lateral ankle ligaments for surgical reconstruction procedures. *J Bone Joint Surg Am* 2014;96[12]:e98.)

ability to bear weight with minimal discomfort. A grade II injury is a complete tear of the ATFL, usually accompanied by a partial injury of the CFL. A grade III injury is complete rupture of the ATFL and CFL. Symptoms of severe tenderness and pain are common, and weight bearing is difficult.[9]

In an effort to reduce the incidence and severity of lateral ankle sprains, numerous studies of varying quality have focused on identifying the risk factors. A level II study identified age, sex, race, and athletic involvement as risk factors.[4] The highest risk of ankle sprains was 10 to 14 years old in females and 15 to 19 years old in males. Boys and men age 15 to 24 years had a higher incidence of lateral ankle injury than their female counterparts. Women age 30 to 99 years had a higher incidence than men in that age range. Athletic involvement was responsible for 45% to 50% of ankle sprains. The same database showed a race-based disparity; the incidence was substantially higher among those identified as black or white than among those identified as Hispanic. Several factors may be related to the race-based differences in injury rate, including obesity, exposure to high-risk athletic activity, connective tissue properties, and skeletal foot morphology (specifically as related to the cavovarus foot). Additional risk factors assumed to be important include strength, proprioception, range of motion, and balance, but there is no high-quality evidence to support these assumptions.[11] The best evidence supports the belief that an earlier ankle injury is a significant risk factor for a second ankle sprain in the same or the contralateral ankle.[12]

Extrinsic risk factors are related to specific sport participation, level of competitiveness, playing surface, and shoe wear. According to level II evidence, sports injury to the lateral ankle is most common during wall climbing, rock climbing, indoor volleyball, basketball, women's cheerleading, and field sports such as rugby, soccer, lacrosse, and American football. Game competition places an athlete at greater risk for an ankle sprain than practice participation.[2,11]

Meta-analyses have evaluated the optimal treatment of acute lateral ankle sprains.[11,13] Current opinion, practice patterns, and research studies support functional nonsurgical management as the preferred method of treating all lateral ankle sprains. This conclusion is well supported for grade I and II sprains, but many variables can affect the outcome and cost-benefit ratio for a severe grade III sprain. Surgery for a severe sprain leads to a slightly better functional outcome than nonsurgical treatment. However, surgery is more costly and has a higher complication rate than nonsurgical treatment, with a slightly higher risk of osteoarthritic change on MRI. Functional nonsurgical treatment leads to a higher incidence of reinjury; however, rates of return to preinjury status are similar after surgical or nonsurgical treatment.[14] Nonsurgical treatment was unsuccessful in 10% of Japanese athletes, and athletes

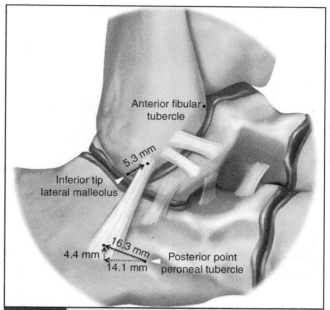

Figure 3 Schematic drawing shows the calcaneofibular ligament origin and insertion sites in a right ankle, with the distances from landmarks. (Reproduced with permission from Clanton TO, Campbell KJ, Wilson KJ, et al: Qualitative and quantitative anatomic investigation of the lateral ankle ligaments for surgical reconstruction procedures. *J Bone Joint Surg Am* 2014;96[12]:e98.)

who underwent surgery had a more rapid return to athletic activity.[15] Only level V evidence suggests that surgical treatment is preferable for professional or elite athletes.[16]

In patients who received nonsurgical treatment for a severe sprain, the outcome was better after cast immobilization for 10 days than after use of a rigid stirrup brace or walking boot.[17] Other evidence-based treatments of ankle sprains include supervised early exercise, unsupervised balance-board training, NSAIDs, and the traditional rest-ice-compression-elevation program.[11] No scientific evidence supports the use of ultrasound, laser therapy, electrotherapy, manual mobilization, extracorporeal shock wave therapy (ESWT), hyperbaric oxygenation, or platelet-rich plasma (PRP).[11] Evidence exists to support bracing or taping during the postinjury period until rehabilitation is complete.[13]

Acute surgical repair of a lateral ligament rupture of the ankle is not always controversial. The indications include an open injury, a large avulsion, or another associated pathology such as dislocated peroneal tendon, osteochondral fracture, or bimalleolar fracture variant with a complete tear of the medial and lateral ligaments. Even an avulsion fracture of the distal fibula heals readily without late instability compared with a purely ligamentous injury.[18] Some evidence supports surgical treatment of a

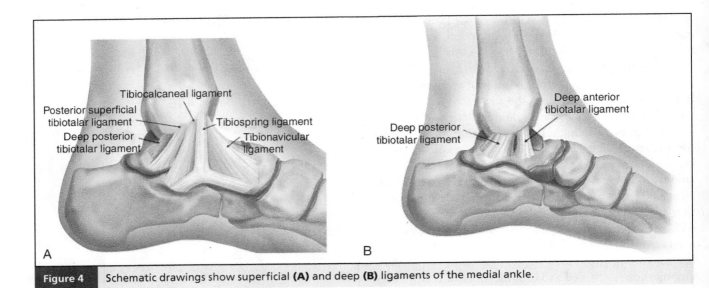

Figure 4 Schematic drawings show superficial (A) and deep (B) ligaments of the medial ankle.

severe lateral ankle sprain, particularly in an elite athlete or a patient who does hazardous work and cannot risk persistent instability or reinjury.[14,15]

Evidence from high-level randomized studies confirms that the use of lace-up ankle braces reduces the incidence but not the severity of acute ankle sprains in basketball and football players.[19,20] Evidence also supports the value of neuromuscular education and balance training in reducing the incidence of recurrent ankle sprains.[11,13] Residual disability after ankle sprain is reported to be present in 32% to 76% of patients.[5,21-23] The disability usually is in the form of residual swelling, pain, and/or instability. Elucidating the cause of disability can be a complex and challenging process requiring a history and physical examination as well as stress radiography, CT, MRI, or ankle arthroscopy.

A disability resulting from instability must be identified as functional or mechanical. Functional instability has been defined as "the occurrence of recurrent joint instability and the sensation of joint instability due to the contributions of any neuromuscular deficits."[24] The primary cause is injury to the joint mechanoreceptors and afferent nerves resulting in impaired balance, reduced joint position sense, slowed firing of the peroneal muscles in response to inversion stress, slowed nerve conduction velocity, impaired cutaneous sensation, strength deficits, and decreased ankle dorsiflexion. Functional instability typically improves in response to a well-designed rehabilitation program. Mechanical instability, however, is "laxity of a joint due to structural damage to ligamentous tissues which support the joint."[24] Mechanical instability can lead to altered joint kinematics and arthritic changes, which often require surgical correction.[25, 26]

Both anatomic and nonanatomic surgical techniques are used for treating recurrent instability. The standard treatment of chronic lateral ankle instability has been the Gould modification of the Broström procedure, which is an anatomic reconstruction of the ATFL and CFL that has had good long-term results.[9] This procedure has limitations related to poor tissue quality, hyperflexibility, the stresses imposed by large or elite athletes, and aggressive early rehabilitation.[27] Several modifications or recommendations should be considered when the Broström-Gould procedure is used, such as the use of an augmentation method for reinforcement and protection, anatomic allograft reconstruction if local tissue is inadequate, and immobilization for an adequate period of time before aggressive rehabilitation.[28-30]

Medial Ankle Injury

The deltoid ligament on the medial side of the ankle is composed of distinct superficial and deep layers. The ligament consists of a maximum of six bands, of which only the tibionavicular ligament, tibiospring ligament, and deep posterior tibiotalar ligament are constant. The superficial layer is a broad, band-like structure that originates from the anterior colliculus and fans out to insert into the navicular, neck of the talus, sustentaculum tali, and posteromedial talar tubercle (Figure 4). The deep portion of the deltoid is the primary medial stabilizer of the ankle joint. Unlike the superficial portion, the deep portion is organized into two short, thick, discrete bands: the deep anterior tibiotalar ligament and deep posterior tibiotalar ligament, which are intra-articular but extrasynovial. The deep posterior tibiotalar ligament is the largest band of the deltoid complex.[31]

The primary function of the deltoid ligament as a whole, and specifically the tibiospring and tibiocalcaneal ligaments, is to prohibit eversion and abduction. The deep deltoid, primarily the deep posterior tibiotalar ligament, also resists external rotation when the foot is dorsiflexed, and it is responsible for the greatest restraint against lateral translation. Valgus tilting of the talus within the mortise requires complete rupture of both the superficial and deep deltoid. As a multicomponent ligament, the deltoid requires considerable force for disruption. The deep deltoid ligament was found to have a greater load to failure (713.8 N [± 69.3 N]) than the lateral collateral ligaments.[32] The dominant mode of failure of the deep deltoid ligament is an intrasubstance rupture near the talar insertion; the superficial deltoid ligament most commonly fails at its insertion into the anterior colliculus.[33]

Rupture of the deltoid ligament is rare in the absence of lateral ligamentous or fibula injury. In all patients, the physical examination must exclude associated syndesmosis injury, lateral ligamentous injury, or fibula fracture (including high fibula fracture or proximal tibiofibular joint injury). The posterior tibial, flexor digitorum longus, and flexor hallucis longus tendons also must be evaluated. Any associated neurologic pathology such as tibial or saphenous nerve injury should be noted.

Anterior and posterior translation, medial and lateral translation, internal and external rotational instability, and varus-valgus instability should be carefully evaluated. The patient can be seated, supine, or prone, but it is beneficial to test in more than one position and to be certain the patient is fully relaxed. Comparison with the normal contralateral extremity is key to appreciating subtle differences. The criteria for the diagnosis of medial instability are medial ankle joint pain, a subjective feeling of giving way, and a valgus or pronation deformity that is correctable with posterior tibial muscle activation.[34] The diagnosis is reinforced by an examination indicating excess motion in external rotation, eversion, valgus, or posterior translation.

Radiographs may suggest deltoid ligament injury, especially if there is an associated syndesmosis injury or fibula fracture. The presence of small avulsion fragments at the tip of the medial malleolus may indicate an acute injury in association with the history and physical examination findings. In a complete deltoid ligament injury, a valgus AP stress radiograph shows a talar tilt. Most such injuries are incomplete, and standard radiographs appear normal. As a result, the traditional gold standard for evaluating medial ankle instability is stress radiography.[35] A gravity stress radiograph may be useful in the office setting for detecting an acute injury. MRI increasingly is the imaging modality of choice for defining injury to the deltoid ligaments and associated structures.[36]

Most deltoid ligament injuries can be treated nonsurgically. Treatment is dictated by the associated injuries. Usually there is no need to repair the injured deltoid ligament because stabilization of the concomitant injuries stabilizes the ankle and allows the deltoid ligament to heal. Functional management of grade I and most grade II isolated deltoid sprains with a pneumatic brace, a walking boot, or rarely, a walking cast is sufficient for adequate healing, although the delay before return to sports usually is greater than after a lateral ankle sprain. A grade II or III medial sprain does not require surgery if an anatomic reduction can be maintained by immobilization in a cast or walking boot.[37]

After the repair of an associated injury, such as fibula fracture or syndesmosis rupture, stress fluoroscopy occasionally reveals persistent medial instability. Primary repair of the deltoid ligament is warranted in this circumstance. The use of suture anchors or a suture-only construct often is sufficient to stabilize the medial side of the ankle.

Syndesmosis Injury

The ankle syndesmosis is continuous with the interosseous membrane proximally and is located at the level of the tibial plafond. In most patients, the ankle syndesmosis forms a synovium-lined joint space. Several recent studies clarified the important anatomic features of this region of the ankle and provided valuable information related to injury interpretation, method of treatment, and anatomic reconstruction.[38-41] Although the distal fibula and tibia are congruent, most of the stability in the syndesmosis comes from its ligamentous support, which includes three well-defined ligaments: the anteroinferior tibiofibular ligament (AITFL), the posteroinferior tibiofibular ligament, and the interosseous tibiofibular ligament (Figure 5).

The motion that occurs between the distal tibia and distal fibula is limited but includes an increase in the intermalleolar distance of approximately 1.5 mm as the ankle moves from plantar flexion to dorsiflexion, rotational movement in the horizontal plane of approximately 12° to 17°, and an average 2.4 mm of distal migration of the fibula. When a force overstresses these limits of motion, ligaments tear and/or the bone fractures. Several mechanisms can produce such an injury, the most common of which is internal rotation of the leg and body on a foot that is firmly planted, causing an external rotatory force on the fibula.

The wide spectrum of injuries to the syndesmosis complex ranges from subtle sprain to complete diastasis and instability (Figure 6). Local swelling and tenderness

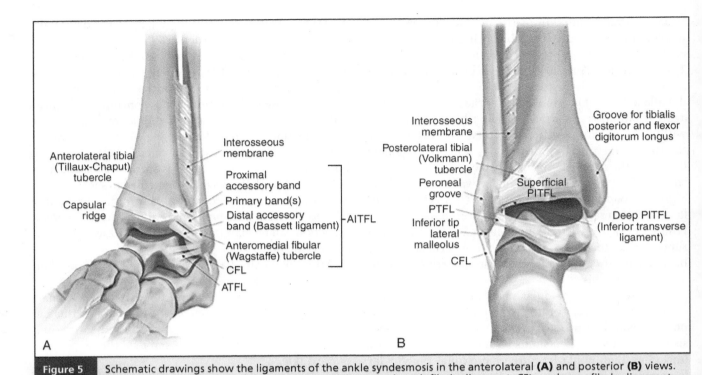

Figure 5 Schematic drawings show the ligaments of the ankle syndesmosis in the anterolateral (A) and posterior (B) views. AITFL = anteroinferior tibiofibular ligament, ATFL = anterior talofibular ligament, CFL = calcaneofibular ligament, PITFL = posteroinferior tibiofibular ligament, PTFL = posterior talofibular ligament. (Reproduced with permission from Williams BT, Ahrberg AB, Goldsmith MT, et al: Ankle syndesmosis: A qualitative and quantitative anatomic analysis. *Am J Sports Med* 2015;43[1]:88-97.)

after the acute injury quickly give way to diffuse signs and symptoms that make the diagnosis less obvious. The Cotton, proximal fibular squeeze, external rotation stress, hop, weighted rotation, and crossed-leg gravity stress tests specifically are designed to detect syndesmosis injury and instability, but neither these tests nor the standard imaging methodologies (plain and stress radiographs, CT, ultrasound, and MRI) are completely reliable. More than 6 mm of widening of the tibiofibular clear space on the AP radiograph indicates a syndesmosis injury, but significant injury can be present in the absence of this finding. MRI has become the preferred diagnostic study for a suspected syndesmosis injury in a professional or collegiate athlete in the United States.[41] MRI is useful for correlating physical examination findings with syndesmosis injury and predicting time missed from sports based on the severity of findings.[42]

Nonsurgical treatment is preferred for a stable syndesmosis injury. Rest, immobilization, NSAIDs, and ice are used. PRP was found to be a useful additional treatment for stable injuries.[43] A syndesmosis injury requires almost twice as much time before return to play as a severe lateral ankle sprain. A systematic review of the literature found that time lost from sports after a syndesmosis sprain ranged from 0 to 137 days and that the average

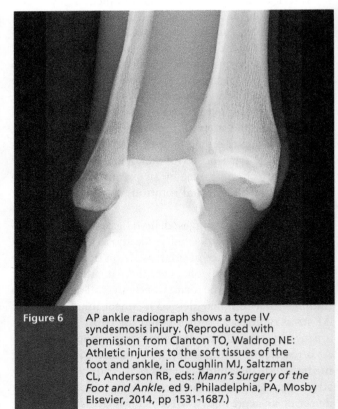

Figure 6 AP ankle radiograph shows a type IV syndesmosis injury. (Reproduced with permission from Clanton TO, Waldrop NE: Athletic injuries to the soft tissues of the foot and ankle, in Coughlin MJ, Saltzman CL, Anderson RB, eds: *Mann's Surgery of the Foot and Ankle,* ed 9. Philadelphia, PA, Mosby Elsevier, 2014, pp 1531-1687.)

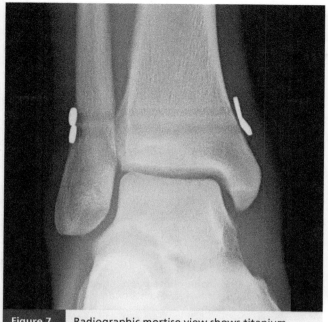

Figure 7 Radiographic mortise view shows titanium button stabilization of a type IV syndesmosis injury. (Reproduced with permission from Clanton TO, Waldrop NE: Athletic injuries to the soft tissues of the foot and ankle, in Coughlin MJ, Saltzman CL, Anderson RB, eds: *Mann's Surgery of the Foot and Ankle,* ed 9. Philadelphia, PA, Mosby Elsevier, 2014, pp 1531-1687.)

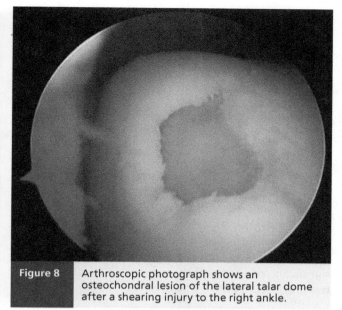

Figure 8 Arthroscopic photograph shows an osteochondral lesion of the lateral talar dome after a shearing injury to the right ankle.

loss ranged from 10 to 52 days.[44] Residual symptoms are not uncommon. One study found good to excellent ankle function in 86% of patients at an average 47-month follow-up, although one-third of patients had mild stiffness and one-fourth had mild activity-related pain.[45]

Surgical treatment is indicated for patients who have obvious diastasis on plain or stress radiographs or who have undergone unsuccessful rehabilitation. High-level athletes with subtle diastasis and/or an MRI-confirmed tear of syndesmotic ligaments may benefit from surgical stabilization, although this treatment is controversial. Ankle arthroscopy usually is warranted to inspect the joint and evaluate it for cartilage lesions. After the joint is débrided, it is stabilized with a screw or a suture-button construct. There is mounting evidence that suture-button stabilization is more beneficial than screw fixation[46,47] (Figure 7). A screw typically is removed 3 to 4 months after implantation, although the need for screw removal has been questioned by recent studies.[48,49] Nevertheless, screw removal has been shown to improve a malreduced syndesmosis and improve pain and function.[50,51] Despite considerable research related to syndesmosis injury and treatment, significant controversy remains, and there is a lack of high-level evidence on optimal methods for

diagnosis and treatment.

Osteochondral Lesions of the Talus and Distal Tibia

An osteochondral lesion of the talus (OLT) is a common injury that is challenging to treat because of the poor healing capability of articular cartilage and the difficulty of access to all areas of the ankle joint (Figure 8). Talar cartilage is thinner than articular cartilage in the hip and knee ("0.89 mm thick, compared with 2.0, 3.33, or 2.92 mm thick for the femur, patella, or tibial plateau, respectively").[48] The mechanical properties of talar articular cartilage make it more resistant to the effects of aging, including development of stiffness and osteoarthritis, in comparison with hip or knee cartilage.[52]

The characteristic finding in an OLT is pain aggravated by weight-bearing exertion. A history of prior injury is common in the diagnosis of OLT. It is important to define the OLT as the source of the pain through a thorough history and physical examination, diagnostic imaging, and occasionally an anesthetic injection to the ankle joint.[53]

Staging of the lesion is helpful in determining the treatment. The Berndt-Hardy-Loomer radiographic system is commonly used.[54,55] Type I is subchondral compression, type II is a partially detached osteochondral fragment, type III is completely detached, type IV is a completely detached and displaced osteochondral fragment, and type V is a cystic lesion.[54,55] CT- and MRI-based classification systems also have been described. MRI is helpful in identifying additional pathology, but it tends to exaggerate the extent of the OLT. CT does not define soft-tissue pathology but provides an accurate picture of the structural character of the OLT and any cystic dimensions.[53]

The arthroscopic classification of OLTs follows the system established by the International Cartilage Research Society.[56] The combined use of radiographs, CT and/or MRI, and arthroscopy is essential for optimal treatment of these lesions.

Articular cartilage injuries are common in both severe sprains (acute or chronic) and fractures of the ankle. The incidence of articular cartilage injuries ranged from 63% to 95% in studies of both acute and chronic lateral ankle sprains and was as high as 80% in unstable ankle fractures.[57,58] If an OLT is left untreated, the risk of posttraumatic ankle osteoarthritis increases significantly; approximately 50% of untreated OLTs were found to have later degenerative changes within the ankle joint.[59,60] Nonsurgical treatment of OLTs is successful in fewer than 50% of patients, and this factor as well as the risk of significant long-term effects requires an effective surgical treatment strategy.[61]

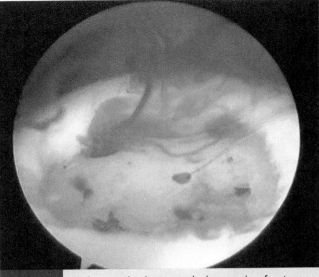

Figure 9 Arthroscopic photograph shows microfracture treatment of an osteochondral lesion of the talar dome.

Video 22.1: Autologous Chrondrocyte Implantation. Richard D. Ferkel, MD, and Kyle David Stuart, MD (13 min)

Video 22.2: Conventional Treatment - Débridement Abrasion Microfracture Drilling. Mark Glazebrook, MD (4 min)

Video 22.3: OATS Procedure. Laszlo Hangody, MD, PhD, DSc (10 min)

Arthroscopic drilling or curettage, bone marrow stimulation using microfracture, mosaicplasty, osteochondral autograft or allograft transplantation, and autologous chondrocyte implantation have been used to treat OLTs[62,63] (**Figure 9**). A systematic review of 52 studies compared the outcomes of treatments of articular cartilage lesions of the talus including nonsurgical treatment, excision, curettage, bone marrow stimulation (microfracture), autogenous bone graft, transmalleolar drilling, osteochondral autologous transplantation, autologous chondrocyte implantation, retrograde drilling, and fixation. The primary outcome measure was the American Orthopaedic Foot and Ankle Society hindfoot score.[64] Curettage had a 77% success rate, and drilling had an approximately 66% success rate for the treatment of OLTs. In addition, 18 studies reported that 85% of patients had an excellent outcome after bone marrow stimulation. Osteochondral autologous transplantation had a good to excellent outcome in approximately 87% of patients, and autologous chondrocyte implantation had a 76% success rate. Bone marrow stimulation was recommended as the first-line treatment because of its high success rate, low morbidity rate, and relatively low cost. Supplementation of bone marrow stimulation with viscosupplementation, PRP, micronized cartilage allograft, or mesenchymal stem cells had better results than bone marrow stimulation alone.[65-68]

Several factors may have a role in the success of treatment for OLT. Talar defects larger than 150 mm^2 were found to be relatively unlikely to have a satisfactory outcome, as indicated by an American Orthopaedic Foot and Ankle Society score lower than 80.[69] The location of the lesion as well as the patient's age, sex, body mass index, history of trauma, and duration of symptoms also can affect the clinical outcome, but discrepancies in results have made it difficult to confirm other predictors of the success or failure of OLT treatment.[63]

A large lesion, including a lesion with a large cystic area, typically requires complex treatment such as autologous chondrocyte implantation with or without simultaneous bone graft, autologous osteochondral transplantation with single or multiple plugs, or fresh talar osteochondral allograft[53] (**Figure 10**). Treating an OLT after unsuccessful bone marrow stimulation can be challenging, but autologous chondrocyte implantation was reported to be successful in 23 of 29 patients at a mean 8.3-year follow-up, and osteochondral autologous transplantation was effective in 18 of 22 patients who had undergone earlier treatment of an OLT.[70, 71] Double-plug osteochondral autologous transplantation and mosaicplasty were found to be effective for large lesions,

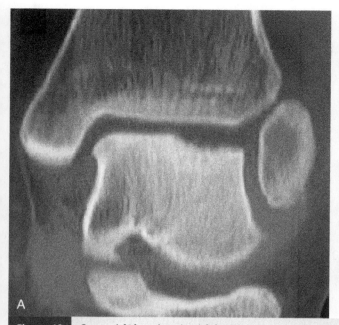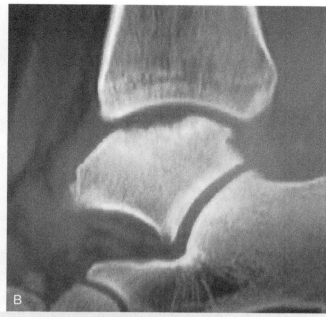

Figure 10 Coronal **(A)** and sagittal **(B)** CT images of a large osteochondral lesion of the talar dome.

in comparison with fresh talar osteochondral allograft, which often leads to osteolysis, subchondral cysts, and degenerative changes.[72]

Tibial osteochondral lesions are much less common than talar lesions; only one tibial lesion occurs for every 14 to 20 talar lesions.[73] No single area of the plafond is a particularly common site for these lesions.[74] The limited available reports suggest that techniques similar to those used for the talus are effective.[73] Many patients in the study had a concomitant procedure such as removal of soft tissue or osseous anterior impingement without a substantial reported change in outcome.

Ankle Impingement Syndromes

Anterior Bony Impingement

Anterior ankle impingement is a common source of pain in athletes and is related to osteophytes on the dorsomedial aspect of the talar neck and the anterolateral aspect of the distal tibia. Athletes often have a palpable spur of bone that is painful to palpation and interferes with performance, particularly during cutting, push-off, and maximum dorsiflexion, which can be critical in sports such as alpine skiing. It is believed that bony impingement in the anterior ankle is a consequence of athletic activity that consistently places the ankle in extreme positions over a long period of time. A laboratory study of 150 kicking actions by 15 elite football players found that maximal plantar flexion and stretching of the capsule occurred in only 39% of the kicks but that direct trauma

to the anteromedial tibia occurred in 76%.[75] A cadaver study found that the anterior capsule attaches to the distal tibia on average 6 mm proximal to the anterior cartilage rim rather than near the spurring at the distalmost tibia.[76]

Lateral radiographs of the ankle reveal osteophytes on the anterior tibia and talar neck, often described as kissing lesions, although CT studies found that these osteophytes usually do not contact one another during dorsiflexion.[77] Chronic changes in the talar surface can be caused by osteophytes. A divot sign of the talar neck and a tram track fissure of the talar dome articular cartilage surface were found to correspond to the offending spurs.[78] The Scranton-McDermott classification of ankle bony impingement is based on the radiographic size and location of the spurs, and the van Dijk classification is based on the extent of osteoarthritis.[79] MRI can be used to define additional pathology, articular cartilage injury, intra-articular effusion, and bone contusions.

 Video 22.4: Anterior Ankle Impingement. J. Chris Coetzee, MD (7 min)

The treatment includes rest, ice, range-of-motion exercises, and corticosteroid injections for van Dijk grade I impingement (osteophytes without joint space narrowing). If nonsurgical measures are unsuccessful, arthroscopic débridement of the ankle is recommended. According to one study, 90% of patients without joint space narrowing (van Dijk grade I, II, or III) and 73% of patients with pain

3: Knee and Leg

of less than 2 years' duration improved significantly.[80] These patients typically do not have osteoarthritic ankles and therefore have a good response to arthroscopic treatment with spur excision. However, the presence of other symptoms, such as those from an OLT, can affect long-term outcome. The outcome most commonly is related to the age of the patient, size of the osteophyte, ankle morphology, or an associated condition such as a chondral lesion.[81] Although osteophyte lesions commonly recur, the improvement in function remains.[82]

Posterior Bony Ankle Impingement

Posterior ankle impingement is caused by irritation of the posterior structures of the ankle, usually as a result of compression in maximum plantar flexion. The bony impingement may involve the posterior malleolus, the posterolateral talar process (trigonal or Stieda process), an os trigonum, the posterior subtalar joint, or the posterior calcaneal tuberosity. The os trigonum, which is an ununited lateral tubercle of the posterior process of the talus, and the posterolateral tubercle are most commonly involved in the impingement syndrome.[83]

Posterior impingement is seen in athletes who extensively use the extreme plantarflexed position, as is common in dance as well as kicking and jumping sports. The athlete reports a deep pain anterior to the Achilles tendon during specific activities such as jumping, kicking, or a push-off maneuver. A traumatic incident can be an inciting event, as in fracture of the os trigonum or posterior talar process, but usually the symptoms are caused by overuse. The initial diagnosis is based on the patient history and physical examination. The standard workup includes radiographs, which may reveal the presence of an os trigonum or posterior talar process. MRI can detect the soft-tissue and bony edema that commonly occurs with posterior ankle impingement.

Video 22.5: Posterior Ankle Arthroscopy - Impingement Os Trigonum FHL Tenosynovitis. Johannes J. Wiegerinck, MSc, PhD; Peter de Leeuw, MD; and C. Niek van Dijk, MD (8 min)

The treatment of posterior ankle impingement begins with rest, ice, NSAIDs, and avoidance of extreme plantar flexion. Physical therapy can be useful, as can selective posterior injections to calm the local inflammation. Nonsurgical treatment was successful in 60% of patients with posterior impingement symptoms, and 85% of patients who received an injection reported pain relief.[84,] [85] Surgical treatment is indicated after 3 to 6 months of unsuccessful nonsurgical treatment. The traditional procedure involves open excision of the trigonal process or os trigonum through a posteromedial or posterolateral approach. Although open surgery has been successful, arthroscopic excision and decompression of the posterior ankle has become popular during the past decade and is as successful as open surgery. All 16 patients who underwent posterior ankle arthroscopy had good to excellent health-related quality of life and functional outcome scores at a mean 32-month follow-up, and 93% had returned to their preinjury athletic level.[86] High-level athletes had a significant decrease in visual analog pain scale scores, with an average return to the preinjury level 46.9 days after arthroscopic decompression surgery.[87]

Soft-Tissue Impingement of the Ankle

Inflammation within the ankle joint is common after injury and often becomes chronic as a result of repeated injury. Recurrent ankle sprains can cause repeated hemorrhage into the joint, leading to synovitis and subsequent scarring of the ligaments. This often leads to soft-tissue impingement in the ankle. Although impingement lesions most commonly are found in the anterior ankle, they can occur in almost any part of the ankle.

Ankle impingement most commonly is anterolateral. Thickening of the ATFL or the inferiormost portion of the AITFL and the surrounding soft tissues is the most common cause. The Bassett ligament, a well-described accessory band of the AITFL, and the extensor tendons can be the source of soft-tissue impingement in the anterior ankle. Posterior soft-tissue impingement results from repeated plantar flexion that traps the tissue between the calcaneus and the tibia. Stenosing tenosynovitis of the flexor hallucis longus, hypertrophy of the posterior capsule, and enlargement of the posterior intermalleolar ligament also are common causes of soft-tissue impingement in the posterior ankle. Medial impingement is less common but was found to affect athletes.[88] The patient history and physical examination play an important role in the diagnosis of soft-tissue impingement. Patients report a history of chronic injury to the ankle or participation in a sport that predisposes them to impingement, such as basketball, volleyball, or gymnastics. Typically, there is tenderness to palpation along the anterolateral gutter or the inferior aspect of the AITFL. In posterior impingement, maximum plantar flexion reproduces the symptoms. Radiographs are necessary to rule out bony pathology but rarely reveal positive findings. MRI is more useful than radiographs for detecting soft-tissue impingement.

Nonsurgical treatment is unlikely to be successful in athletes. A regimen of rest, ice, and NSAIDs is the starting point, but immobilization with a controlled ankle movement walking boot can be used to prevent the extremes of motion that elicit symptoms. Intra-articular steroid injections also can provide relief. After unsuccessful nonsurgical treatment, arthroscopy is the surgical treatment of choice.

Foot Disorders

Heel Pain and Plantar Fasciitis

The plantar fascia is dense connective tissue that supports the arch of the foot. The medial and lateral bands, the two main bands of the plantar fascia, run from the calcaneal tuberosity and insert on the plantar plates of the MTP joints and the base of the proximal phalanges. This strong band of tissue provides stabilization for the plantar arch of the foot as well as the first MTP joint through the windlass mechanism. The aponeurosis functions from heel strike to toe-off in the normal gait cycle to achieve hindfoot inversion, tibial external rotation, and transverse tarsal joint stabilization.

In athletes, the plantar fascia is susceptible to injury primarily through overuse. Long-distance running and prolonged training regimens can lead to repetitive, chronic trauma that can damage the plantar fascia. Acute injury also is possible and results in a partial or complete tear of the plantar fascia that can lead to chronic injury. Patients typically report morning or activity-related pain specific to the plantarmedial aspect of the heel at the origin of the medial band of the plantar fascia. Pain is aggravated by direct palpation or by initial weight bearing and stretching of the plantar arch.

Cavovarus foot deformity and Achilles tendon contracture are believed to have a role in the pathology of plantar fasciitis. Obesity and work-related weight bearing were found to be independent variables contributing to plantar fasciitis.[89] In evaluating a patient with heel pain, it is important to keep in mind the numerous conditions that must be considered in the differential diagnosis (Table 1). Calcaneal stress fracture and tarsal tunnel syndrome are the conditions most likely to mimic plantar fasciitis. A calcaneal stress fracture should be suspected with an acute exacerbation of heel pain or pain elicited by compression of the heel. The diagnosis is confirmed by heel radiographs on which the classic findings of a stress fracture can be seen after several weeks. A bone scan or MRI often is indicated to rule out stress fracture and help in determining the severity of plantar fasciitis.

Tarsal tunnel syndrome or nerve entrapment of the first branch of the lateral plantar nerve also should be ruled out. Patients with tarsal tunnel syndrome report radiating pain and paresthesia, and they often have a positive Tinel sign. The most commonly involved nerve

Table 1
Differential Diagnosis for Plantar Fasciitis

Skeletal Disorders
Calcaneal cyst
Calcaneal epiphysitis
Calcaneal stress fracture
Infection
Subtalar osteoarthritis
Systemic arthritis (lupus, psoriatic, rheumatoid)

Neurologic Disorders
Abductor digiti quinti nerve entrapment
Lumbar spine pathology
Neuropathy
Tarsal tunnel syndrome

Soft-Tissue Disorders
Fat pad atrophy
Flexor hallucis brevis tear
Heel pad atrophy
Plantar fascia rupture
Retrocalcaneal bursitis

Other Disorders
Gout
Osteomalacia
Paget disease
Tumor
Vascular disorder

is the Baxter nerve (the first branch of the lateral plantar nerve), which is a mixed motor and sensory nerve to the abductor digiti quinti and the lateral border of the plantar surface of the foot. Most commonly, the nerve becomes entrapped between the deep fascia of the abductor hallucis and the quadratus plantae. The workup typically involves electromyographic or nerve conduction velocity studies to confirm the diagnosis.

Nonsurgical treatment is the mainstay for almost all forms of heel pain. The treatment of plantar fasciitis focuses on NSAIDs, activity modification, and a dedicated stretching program of the plantar fascia and Achilles tendon complex. A custom-made or off-the-shelf cushioned in-shoe orthosis is used to control heel motion and prevent splaying of the heel pad, along with a dorsiflexion night

3: Knee and Leg

splint. More invasive treatments include iontophoresis, corticosteroid or PRP injections, and ESWT. High-quality studies have supported use of NSAIDs, plantar fascia stretching without weight bearing, calcaneal taping, and a night splint.[90-95] ESWT, corticosteroid injection, and PRP injection also were supported by research evidence, but little support was found for the long-term use of an orthosis in treating plantar fasciitis.[96-99]

Medial plantar fasciotomy typically is recommended after unsuccessful nonsurgical treatment. The medial third of the plantar fascia is excised, with maintenance of the lateral band to prevent collapse of the arch. The benefits of open and endoscopic release have been debated, but some surgeons prefer endoscopic surgery to decrease recovery time and lower associated morbidity.[100] Recently, other surgeons have become proponents of gastrocnemius recession alone as a treatment of chronic plantar fasciitis because it has better outcomes than traditional fasciotomy.[101] Most evidence supporting the efficacy of surgical treatment of plantar fasciitis is of only fair quality, and no randomized controlled study results are available.

Rupture of the plantar fascia reportedly occurs after sudden acceleration during an athletic activity. This injury typically is painful. Patients report a loud, painful popping sensation in the arch of the foot. Little evidence is available to guide treatment, although the injury usually is managed nonsurgically. Two to 3 weeks of immobilization with a non–weight-bearing cast or boot with arch support allows the inflammation and pain to subside. Gradual weight bearing is initiated with a return to activity as pain and swelling allow. One study found that none of the 18 patients with a plantar fascia rupture who were treated with this regimen sustained reinjury, had postinjury sequelae, or needed surgery.[102]

Lisfranc Fracture-Dislocation

The Lisfranc or tarsometatarsal (TMT) joint is the articulation between the base of the five metatarsals and the three cuneiforms and cuboid. Stability primarily is provided by the bone and ligament anatomy. There is no ligament between the bases of the first and second metatarsals, and stability in this area mostly depends on the recessed base of the second metatarsal, the Roman arch wedged shape of the midfoot arch, and the strong Lisfranc ligament, which connects the medial cuneiform to the base of the second metatarsal.

Injuries to the TMT joint are caused by indirect or direct forces. The indirect forces involve axial loading or twisting on a plantarflexed foot, and direct injury occurs when a load is applied to the midfoot. Ligamentous Lisfranc injury commonly occurs in athletes as an injury to the ligaments of the TMT joints that may extend to the intertarsal joints. These injuries range from a sprain to an avulsion fracture but usually are not the types of fractures or dislocations that occur in high-energy injury from a motor vehicle crash or a fall from a height. The spectrum of sprains in athletes ranges from a stable sprain without radiographic displacement to a severe sprain with obvious widening between the base of the first and second metatarsals or further into the midfoot. A classification system described in a 2002 study has been found to be useful in treating athletes with a relatively mild injury.[103] In a stage I injury, the patient is unable to participate in sports because of pain in the Lisfranc joint; weight-bearing radiographs show no displacement, and bone scan or MRI findings may be negative. A stage II injury has first to second metatarsal diastases of 1 to 5 mm but no evidence of loss of arch on weight-bearing radiographs. Stage III injury has first to second metatarsal diastases of more than 5 mm and evidence of loss of arch on weight-bearing radiographs. The common radiographic appearance of the misalignment can be classified as transverse or longitudinal, depending on whether the Lisfranc ligament is torn and whether the pathology extends horizontally across the MTP joints or vertically into the intercuneiform space and perhaps through the naviculocuneiform joint.[104]

Injuries to the TMT joint often are misdiagnosed, and therefore a high index of suspicion is required. The diagnosis of a severe injury with displacement usually is obvious, but a ligamentous injury with minimal displacement is likely to be missed. Pain with weight bearing should be the first sign if it is accompanied by local swelling and tenderness at the midfoot. Even with a mild injury, the athlete has difficulty pushing off. Pronation-abduction or supination-adduction stress usually is painful. The physical examination should include evaluation of the dorsalis pedis pulse and deep peroneal nerve function as well as assessment for a foot compartment syndrome in severe Lisfranc fracture-dislocation. Predisposing factors for Lisfranc injury include a ratio of second metatarsal length to foot length of less than 29% and a greater second metatarsal length relative to the depth of the mortise formed by the cuneiforms.[105]

Diagnostic imaging of a foot with a suspected Lisfranc fracture-dislocation begins with AP weight-bearing radiographs as well as oblique and lateral views (Figure 11). Comparison with a weight-bearing AP radiograph of the uninjured foot often is helpful. Ten common radiographic findings are indicative of midfoot injury[106] (Table 2).

If a Lisfranc injury is suspected and plain radiographs are not diagnostic, CT or MRI is useful. If routine radiographs are not diagnostic in a mild injury, stress radiographs taken with the patient under anesthesia may be helpful.

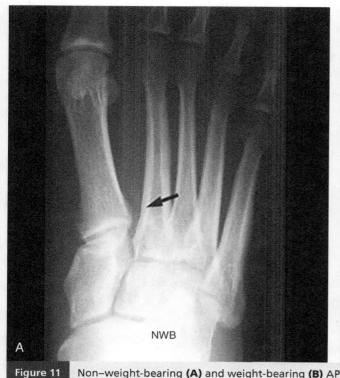
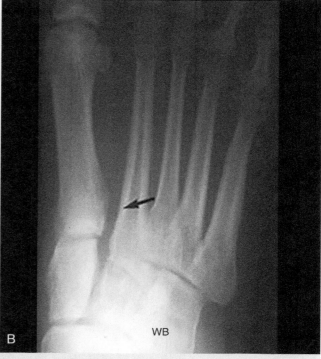

| Figure 11 | Non–weight-bearing (A) and weight-bearing (B) AP radiographs show a subtle Lisfranc injury (arrow). (Reproduced with permission from Haytmanek CT, Clanton TO: Ligamentous Lisfanc injuries in the athlete. *Oper Tech Sports Med* 2014;22[4]:313-320.) |

Table 2

Radiographic Findings Indicative of Midfoot Injury

Diastasis of first and second metatarsal bones

First and second cuneiform diastasis

Widening between second and third metatarsals

Widening between middle and lateral cuneiforms

Avulsion fracture at the base of the second metatarsal on CT or other advanced imaging (Fleck sign), representing Lisfranc ligament avulsion

Misalignment of tarsometatarsal joints on lateral images

Misalignment of second metatarsal medial border to align with medial border of middle cuneiform

Misalignment of fourth metatarsal medial border to align with medial edge of cuboid

Loss of congruity of metatarsal bases

Compression fracture of the lateral edge of the cuboid

Anatomic reduction is the key to a good outcome in a Lisfranc injury. A short leg non–weight-bearing cast is effective in patients with a truly nondisplaced, stable Lisfranc sprain until tenderness resolves at approximately 6 weeks, with subsequent functional rehabilitation. If displacement is present, rigid internal fixation is recommended for the first through third TMT joints as necessary for stability. Temporary stabilization in an anatomic alignment is preferable for the fourth and fifth TMT joints to preserve their mobility. There is little debate about the need to perform an arthrodesis in TMT joints with significant articular damage or preexisting arthritis, but controversy remains as to the treatment of young athletes with purely ligamentous injury to the Lisfranc joint (Figure 12). At least two high-quality studies suggested that arthrodesis is preferable for purely ligamentous Lisfranc injuries, but a systematic review of studies including 193 patients found no statistical difference in outcomes after open reduction and internal fixation or arthrodesis.[107-109]

Other points of discussion in the treatment of Lisfranc fracture-dislocations relate to methods of fixation and the timing or necessity of hardware removal. Lisfranc fracture-dislocations traditionally have been rigidly fixed with transarticular screws, but bridge plating to immobilize the TMT joints is gaining favor because the articular cartilage is preserved. The standard method for restabilizing the first and second TMT joints is the placement of a so-called Lisfranc screw between the medial cuneiform and the base of the second MT. The newer use of a suture button device has had good results, may provide a more

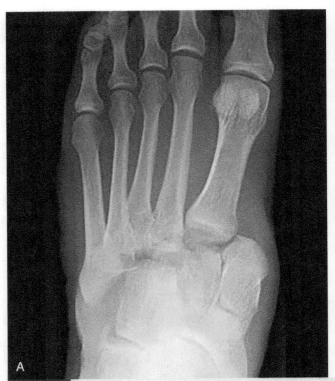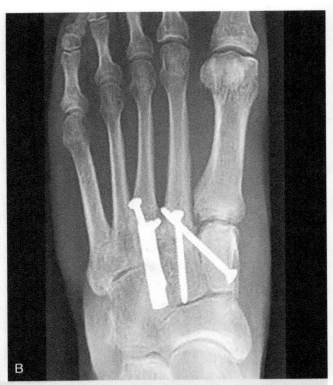

Figure 12   Radiographs show a severe Lisfranc injury with articular damage before **(A)** and after **(B)** arthrodesis. (Reproduced with permission from Haytmanek CT, Clanton TO: Ligamentous Lisfanc injuries in the athlete. *Oper Tech Sports Med* 2014;22[4]:313-320.)

physiologic fixation than screw fixation, and does not necessitate removal.[110] Regardless of other factors, however, it appears that the most important negative prognostic factors in these injuries are severe soft-tissue injury and nonanatomic reduction.

Turf Toe

Turf toe originally was described as a hyperextension injury to the first MTP joint caused by wearing flexible shoes on hard artificial surfaces, but the definition has evolved to encompass almost any injury to the first MTP joint caused by sports participation. The primary injury involves the plantar plate, or capsuloligamentous complex of the first MTP joint, which typically is injured in skill-position football players who axially load their heels when the forefoot is fixed on the turf.[111] Varus and valgus forces also can contribute to a turf toe injury, further destabilizing the joint with loss of integrity of the collateral ligaments.

After an acute injury, the athlete has pain, swelling, ecchymosis, and stiffness at the first MTP joint, which are classified by their severity[112] (Table 3). The initial radiographs are standing weight-bearing AP and lateral views of the foot, which often appear normal. The radiographic position of the sesamoids should be compared

with the contralateral normal side to detect any retraction. An avulsion fracture, sesamoid fracture, or diastasis of bipartite sesamoids also may be found. MRI is reliable for assessing the extent of soft-tissue injury[113] (Figure 13). Biomechanical studies found that stress fluoroscopy is reliable for diagnosing an unstable injury. Injury to at least three of the four ligaments is indicated by a 3-mm difference in sesamoid excursion compared with the uninjured side on stress dorsiflexion fluoroscopy.[114]

Nonsurgical treatment of a turf toe injury begins with the rest-ice-compression-elevation protocol. Immobilization is used to control acute swelling and rest the toe. However, early joint mobilization is essential because stiffness is a common sequela of this injury. Further treatment includes restricting dorsiflexion of the first MTP joint by stiffening the shoe or using carbon fiber or graphite inserts to reduce the amount of energy transfer from the foot during push-off. Taping of the hallux also is useful.

As soon as symptoms allow, the rehabilitation program begins with active and passive non–weight-bearing and weight-bearing range-of-motion exercises for the foot and ankle. The ability to return to play is dictated by symptoms and function. The use of anesthetics or steroid injections to allow the athlete to return to play is not

Table 3

Classification of Turf Toe Injury

Grade	Objective Findings	Activity Level	Pathology	Treatment
I	Local plantar or medial tenderness Minimal swelling No ecchymosis	Continued athletic participation	Stretching of capsuloligamentous complex	Symptomatic
II	More diffuse, intense tenderness Mild to moderate swelling Mild to moderate ecchymosis Painful, restricted range of motion	Loss of 3 to 14 days of playing time	Partial tear of capsuloligamentous complex No articular injury	Walking boot and crutches as needed
III	Severe, diffuse tenderness Marked swelling Moderate to severe ecchymosis Extremely painful, limited range of motion	Loss of 2 to 6 weeks of playing time	Complete tear of capsuloligamentous complex	Long-term boot or cast immobilization or surgical repair

Adapted from Clanton TO, Butler JE, Eggert A: Injuries to the metatarsophalangeal joints in athletes. *Foot Ankle* 1986;7(3):162-176; Coughlin ME: Biomechanics of the foot and ankle linkage in DeLee JC, Drez D Jr, eds: *Orthopaedic Sports Medicine*. Philadelphia, PA, WB Saunders, 1994, p 1862; Rodeo SA, Warren RF, O'Brien SJ, et al: Diastasis of bipartite sesamoids of the first metatarsophalangeal joint. *Foot Ankle* 1993;14:425-434.

recommended because of the potential for further joint deterioration or injury.

If the injury is severe, first MTP joint stability is compromised. A complete plantar plate tear, sesamoid retraction, sesamoid fracture or diastasis, traumatic bunion, progressive hallux valgus or varus, or dislocation of the MTP joint can indicate instability that requires surgical intervention. The joint is stabilized by repairing the pathology, including associated chondral lesions, fractures, and torn ligaments as well as removal of loose bodies. Only limited evidence is available on the outcomes of surgical treatment of these injuries.

Sesamoid Disorders

The sesamoids of the great toe, which are part of the plantar plate complex, often are involved in acute traumatic and overuse injuries. These two small bones undergo considerable force with weight bearing and can be a source of pain from traumatic fracture with displacement, stress reaction or fracture, sesamoiditis, osteonecrosis, or osteoarthritis. Radiographs, including weight-bearing AP comparison views, should be obtained and can be useful in acute injury. A dedicated bone scan and MRI can confirm the diagnosis and determine the site and extent of the injury.

Treatment of a sesamoid disorder can be difficult. Activity and shoe wear modifications are used, with an orthosis if necessary. Shock-absorbing shoes with dancer pads can be used to offload the stresses on the sesamoids

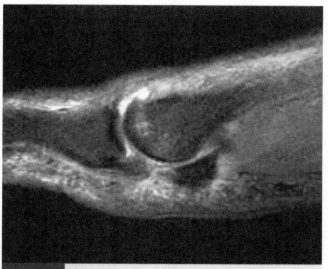

Figure 13 Sagittal MRI shows a plantar plate tear. (Courtesy of Jana Crain, MD, Atherton, CA.)

and can provide the patient with significant relief. These modifications are used with NSAIDs, physical therapy, and perhaps anesthetic and steroid injections to provide significant pain relief. If necessary, immobilization with a controlled ankle movement walking boot or toe spica cast can be used.[115] Surgery is the last resort, although satisfactory outcomes have been reported, especially among athletes.[116]

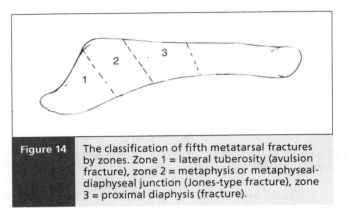

Figure 14 The classification of fifth metatarsal fractures by zones. Zone 1 = lateral tuberosity (avulsion fracture), zone 2 = metaphysis or metaphyseal-diaphyseal junction (Jones-type fracture), zone 3 = proximal diaphysis (fracture).

Stress Fractures

Stress fractures are considered to be the result of "excessive, repetitive, submaximal loads on bones that cause an imbalance between bone resorption and formation" and are a common overuse foot and ankle injury in athletes.[117] These injuries typically occur after a change in footwear or training (such as an increase in intensity) or use of a hard playing or running surface. Pain is generally insidious at onset and can be vague or point specific in the location of the stress fracture. Initial radiographs often are negative, and a high index of suspicion should be maintained so the injury can be diagnosed and treated in a timely fashion.

Stress fractures have been described in most bones of the foot and ankle, and most heal with rest and weight-bearing limitations. Three specific stress fractures are particularly problematic: stress fracture of the proximal fifth metatarsal (a Jones fracture), the tarsal navicular, and the medial malleolus. These areas are considered to be high-risk stress fractures that often progress to complete fracture, leading to delayed union or nonunion, and occurring along the tension side of the bone. These injuries necessitate aggressive treatment in the form of surgery or strict non–weight bearing.[118] A delay in diagnosis can exacerbate the risks associated with these fractures.

Fifth Metatarsal Fracture

Fractures of the base of the fifth metatarsal are classified by zone[119] (Figure 14). Zone 1 represents an avulsion fracture of the lateral tuberosity, zone 2 is a Jones-type fracture of the metaphysis or the metaphyseal-diaphyseal junction, and zone 3 is a proximal diaphyseal fracture. A stress fracture can occur in zone 2 or 3, and some experts recommend combining these two zones because they carry a similar risk of delayed union or nonunion and refracture, and the surgical treatment and outcomes

are similar.[120, 121] Proximal fifth metatarsal stress fractures are most common in athletes who participate in a sport such as basketball, football, or soccer. The patient has worsening activity-related pain along the lateral aspect of the midfoot over a period of several weeks. Physical examination may reveal point tenderness over the base of the fifth metatarsal as well as pain with passive inversion of the foot. The fracture often is apparent on radiographs and can be classified based on appearance as an acute traumatic fracture, stress-related fracture, delayed union, or nonunion.[122]

Treatment selection often is guided by the Torg classification of fractures in zones 2 and 3 as well as by the patient's goals and athletic participation.[122] Although nonsurgical management with strict non–weight bearing in a short leg cast for 6 to 8 weeks is an option for a Torg type I fracture (an acute fracture with sharp fracture line margins and no sclerosis), many active individuals and elite athletes opt for surgical fixation. The goals of early surgical fixation include minimizing the risk of nonunion and refracture as well as allowing a more rapid return to sport. If there is evidence of delayed union or nonunion (Torg type II or III), surgical fixation generally is recognized as the standard of care with selective open débridement and bone grafting. Fixation usually is done with an intramedullary screw and has a good to excellent result (Figure 15).

The challenges of intramedullary screw fixation primarily are related to the shape and contour of the bone itself. A recent radiographic study examined the fifth metatarsal in great detail using three-dimensional CT of 119 patients.[123] The average straight-segment length was found to be 52 mm, which was 68% of the overall length of the metatarsal from the proximal end; the medullary canal was found to be elliptical; the average coronal canal diameter at the isthmus was 5 mm; and in 81% of men the diameter was greater than 4.5 mm. The use of a solid, partially threaded screw with a 4.5-, 5.5-, or 6.5-mm diameter was recommended. The partially threaded configuration was found to provide compression across the fracture site. Headed screws were recommended over headless screws because of their superior pullout strength and easier removal.

The so-called plantar gap is a possible prognostic indicator, according to a study that found a significantly increased time to bony union in fractures with at least 1 mm of fracture margin separation, regardless of Torg classification.[124] A recent systematic review of surgical and nonsurgical treatment of high-risk stress fractures of the lower leg concluded that additional prospective research on fifth-metatarsal base fractures would be of great use in treatment decision making.[125] In addition,

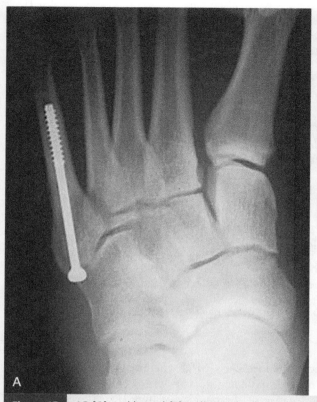
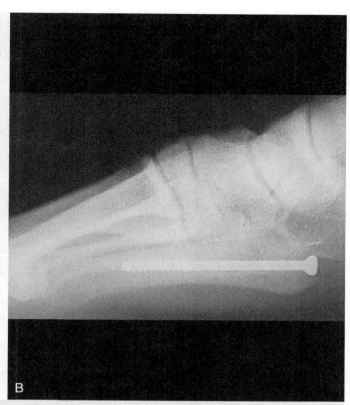

Figure 15 AP **(A)** and lateral **(B)** radiographs show intramedullary screw fixation of a fifth metatarsal fracture.

the review found a weighted mean return to sport of 14 weeks after surgical treatment and 19 weeks after non-surgical treatment.

Tarsal Navicular Fracture

Stress fractures of the navicular are most common in patients who participate in explosive running and jumping activities, as in basketball or track and field. Non-sports related factors that may play a role in the development of navicular stress fracture include the presence of a long second metatarsal or a short first metatarsal, anterior ankle impingement, or decreased ankle motion. The symptoms are similar to those of other stress fractures; the pain often is vague, insidious in onset, exacerbated by activity, and relieved with rest. Although the usual location of the pain is at the dorsal aspect of the midfoot, the patient may describe ankle pain and this may be tender to palpation during physical examination. The relatively avascular central third of the navicular bone predisposes it to stress fracture and subsequent nonunion or osteonecrosis. The use of a local vascularized pedicle bone graft for fractures with evidence of delayed union, nonunion, or osteonecrosis has had encouraging results.[126] Negative initial radiographs and vague initial symptoms were reported to lead to a 1- to 7-month delay in diagnosis.[127] A high

index of suspicion as well as MRI, CT, or bone scanning is useful in the diagnosis (**Figure 16**).

The traditional treatment of a stress fracture of the navicular is non–weight-bearing cast immobilization for 6 to 8 weeks. Attempts at limited weight bearing and shorter periods of immobilization have led to persistent pain and inability to return to activity.[128] The threshold for surgical treatment has decreased in the hope of allowing a more rapid return to play, especially in high-level athletes. Unfortunately, no high-quality studies have investigated the treatment of navicular stress fractures. A CT-based study reported that 8 of 10 surgically treated fractures went on to bony union and that complete, displaced fractures had an increased risk of nonunion.[127] A meta-analysis of surgical and nonsurgical treatment of complete, nondisplaced navicular stress fractures found no statistically significant differences related to time to return to activity or successful outcome rates, but the likelihood of a successful result was decreased after early weight bearing.[129] The methodologic flaws of this analysis were pointed out in a more recent systematic review of navicular stress fractures that used the 27-item Preferred Reporting Items for Systematic Reviews checklist for the content of a systematic review or meta-analysis.[130] A systematic review of surgical and nonsurgical treatment

© 2016 American Academy of Orthopaedic Surgeons

3: Knee and Leg

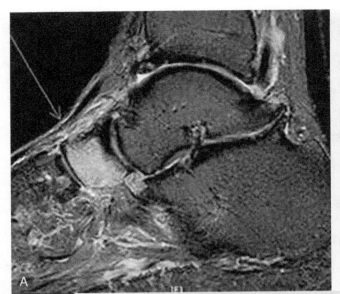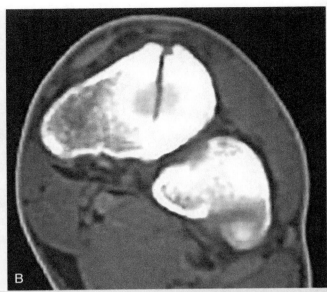

Figure 16 Advanced imaging for navicular fracture. **A,** MRI short tau inversion recovery sequence shows increased signal in the navicular. **B,** Coronal CT image shows fracture nonunion of the dorsal navicular extending into the body.

of high-risk stress fractures of the lower leg concluded that no strong recommendations could be made for the treatment of navicular stress fractures based on the literature.[125] The weighted mean return to sport was 16 weeks after surgical treatment and 22 weeks after nonsurgical management.[125]

Medial Malleolus Fracture

Stress fractures of the medial malleolus represent only 0.6% to 4.0% of all lower extremity stress fractures.[131] These injuries most often occur in athletes who participate in a running, jumping, or high-impact sport such as track and field or gymnastics. Several intrinsic factors are believed to predispose individuals to medial malleolar stress fracture (although none have been proved) including the presence of a narrow tibia, increased external hip rotation, forefoot varus, subtalar varus, limb-length discrepancy, tibial varus, pes cavus, and anteromedial osteophytes.[132] Patients often report medial ankle pain during activity. The onset of pain is gradual, but the pain may acutely worsen after a period of chronic medial ankle pain. Physical examination may reveal an effusion as well as pain on palpation along the anteromedial tibial plafond. Diagnosis can be challenging; only 30% of stress fractures of the medial malleolus are identified on initial radiographs, and CT, MRI, or a bone scan may be helpful.[133] A study of medial malleolar stress fracture diagnosis and surgical treatment found that initial radiographs were negative in all 10 patients.[134] MRI did reveal the fracture line in all patients, however, and the study

recommended early MRI whenever there is suspicion of a medial malleolar stress fracture.

Because of the paucity of high-quality research and the relative rarity of medial malleolar stress fracture, no treatment method is clearly preferred. Several factors should be considered in deciding whether nonsurgical or surgical treatment is preferable: the presence of a fracture line, cyst, or local osteopenia on radiographs; fracture displacement; level of athletic participation; and the timing of injury (in season or off season).[132] Nonsurgical management often consists of 6 weeks of non–weight-bearing cast immobilization followed by progressive weight bearing and a gradual return to activity. Surgical treatment consists of compression screw fixation perpendicular across the fracture as well as removal of any anteromedial osteophytes. A recent literature review included studies that recommended both nonsurgical and surgical management. A study that compared nonstandardized groups of patients suggested that those who were surgically treated had an earlier return to sport (4.5 weeks versus 7 weeks) and more rapid union (4.2 months versus 6.7 months) than those who were nonsurgically treated.[132]

Achilles Tendon Disorders

As the largest tendon arising from both the soleus and gastrocnemius muscles, the Achilles tendon can be affected by pathology ranging from acute or chronic rupture to overuse injury or insertional tendinopathy. Any of these conditions can result in create serious athletic limitation and loss of playing time.

Acute Rupture

Despite considerable published research, there is little consensus on the optimal treatment of Achilles tendon ruptures. The injury is most common in men who are so-called weekend warrior athletes in their third through fifth decades of life, but it can affect individuals regardless of age, sex, or level of athletic participation (including nonparticipation).

The mechanism of injury most commonly involves a sharp dorsiflexion force onto a tensioned tendon, which typically creates a rupture through an area of preexisting degenerative change in the watershed area between 2 cm and 6 cm from its insertion.[135] The diagnosis of acute rupture was missed in 24% of patients, many of whom were elderly or had a high body mass index.[136] With a careful history and physical examination findings including an abnormal Thompson test, decreased resting tension, and a palpable gap within the tendon, the diagnosis can reliably be made without the need for more sophisticated studies[137] (**Figure 17**). Ultrasound and MRI can be useful in patients who have ambiguous examination findings, a chronic rupture, or a need for objective confirmation of the injury.

The treatment of acute rupture of the Achilles tendon is controversial. A meta-analysis found a significant decrease in the rerupture rate after surgical repair of the Achilles tendon, whether open or percutaneous (4.4% compared with 10.6% after nonsurgical treatment).[138] The rate of complications was higher after open surgery than after nonsurgical treatment (27% versus 6%). Percutaneous fixation had a lower risk of infection than open repair (relative risk = 9.32) but carried a 1.1% risk of sural nerve injury. No solid conclusions about functional outcomes could be reached because of the studies' varied scoring tools, inconsistent definitions, and incomplete data acquisition, all of which highlighted the need for greater standardization in future studies.[138] A second meta-analysis found similar rerupture rates among patients treated nonsurgically using functional bracing and early range-of-motion exercises and patients treated surgically.[139] A Swedish study that compared surgical treatment with nonsurgical treatment using functional bracing also reported similar rerupture rates but found a significant improvement in single heel rise test and calf circumference in surgically treated patients.[140] Nonsurgical treatment with immediate weight bearing, which improves the patient's quality of life during the healing process, and dynamic rehabilitation can be recommended without concern for increasing the risk of rerupture or functional outcome deficits.[141]

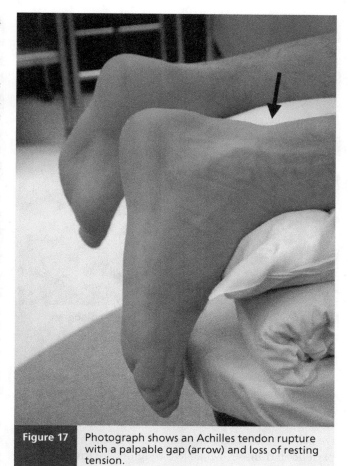

| Figure 17 | Photograph shows an Achilles tendon rupture with a palpable gap (arrow) and loss of resting tension. |

Video 22.6: Haglund Deformity, Achilles Problems. Johannes J. Wiegerinck, MSc, PhD; Peter de Leeuw, MD; and C. Niek van Dijk, MD (3 min)

Overuse Injuries

Overuse injuries related to the Achilles tendon are common and include tendinosis, paratenonitis, superficial and retrocalcaneal bursitis, and insertional Achilles tendinopathy. Achilles tendinosis is a noninflammatory condition that involves intratendinous degeneration and atrophy, initially is asymptomatic, and results from repetitive microtrauma or aging. Pain may represent partial tearing in an area of degenerative tendon and warrants evaluation and initiation of nonsurgical management consisting of rest, the use of a small heel lift or Achilles tendon heel pad, correction of hindfoot misalignment, physical therapy, and correction of training errors. Ultrasound and MRI can be used to evaluate the extent of tendon involvement. Eccentric training was found to be effective in reducing pain in male patients but may be significantly less effective

3: Knee and Leg

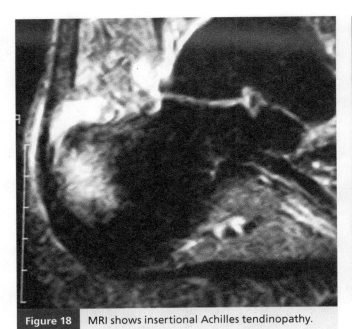

Figure 18   MRI shows insertional Achilles tendinopathy.

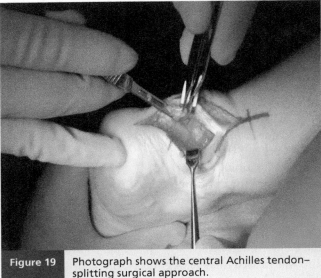

Figure 19   Photograph shows the central Achilles tendon–splitting surgical approach.

in women.[142] Surgical management involves débridement of diseased tissue through a medial or lateral approach, although the central tendon-splitting approach has gained favor as a more direct access to the pathology. Involvement of more than 50% of the tendon or advanced patient age necessitated augmentation with a flexor hallucis longus tendon transfer, which led to significant improvement in Achilles tendon function, physical function, and pain in patients who were older than 44 years and relatively inactive.[143]

Paratenonitis is an inflammation of the paratenon that in most patients can be successfully treated with the measures used for tendinosis. Surgery is considered after 3 to 6 months of unsuccessful nonsurgical treatment. Open or endoscopic débridement and lysis of adhesions are the procedures of choice.

Superficial bursitis often is associated with a posterolateral bony prominence at the lateral calcaneal ridge, which often is called Haglund deformity and may be mistaken for insertional Achilles tendinopathy.[144] Retrocalcaneal bursitis is characterized by tenderness both medially and laterally anterior to the Achilles insertion but not directly at the bone-tendon interface. Both forms of bursitis can occur in association with insertional Achilles tendinopathy but are separate entities that can be treated nonsurgically with rest, shoe wear modification, NSAIDs, physical therapy, and activity modification. In some patients, immobilization in a short leg cast or endoscopic surgical excision may be necessary. A systematic review found that patients were more satisfied after endoscopic excision of the retrocalcaneal bursa than after an open procedure.[145]

Insertional Achilles Tendinopathy

Insertional Achilles tendinopathy appears as pain at the bone-tendon junction and is common in men age 35 to 45 years who are recreational runners as well as elderly women, those who are overweight, sedentary or have multiple medical comorbidities. Nonsurgical management should be attempted but often is unsuccessful. Radiographs may show calcification at the Achilles tendon insertion or a posterosuperior calcaneal prominence. MRI is valuable for evaluating the extent of diseased tendon and allows the success of nonsurgical treatment to be predicted (Figure 18).[146] ESWT is more beneficial than other nonsurgical treatments and should be used before surgical treatment is considered.[147,148] Surgical treatment usually is successful, although no single method or approach appears to be more beneficial than others.[148] However, the central tendon-splitting approach has gained popularity because of its direct approach to the area of pathology (Figure 19).

Summary

Injuries and disorders of the foot and ankle are common among athletes and active individuals. Although both lateral and medial ankle sprains are most common, other subtle injuries will often occur. These can often be challenging to diagnose and treat. Clinicians must be vigilant and perform a thorough history and physical examination. The use of advanced imaging is often helpful in diagnosis when combined with a thorough clinical examination. Many of these conditions can be treated nonoperatively, though surgical management is sometimes indicated. With the appropriate treatments outlined in this chapter, good outcomes can be achieved.

Key Study Points

- Ankle sprains represent one of the most common athletic injuries. Good evidence from high-level studies is available to guide management and treatment decision making.

- Osteochondral lesions of the ankle respond poorly to nonsurgical management, and surgical treatment continues to evolve. The surgical options have different indications.

- The causes and locations of ankle impingement are numerous, and both open and arthroscopic procedures are used.

- Plantar fasciitis can be mimicked by calcaneal stress fracture or tarsal tunnel syndrome.

- Anatomic reduction is the most important factor in achieving a good outcome after a Lisfranc injury.

- A high index of suspicion should be maintained to diagnose a high-risk stress fracture of the foot or ankle. A prolonged recovery and delayed union or nonunion are common after these injuries.

Annotated References

1. Fernandez WG, Yard EE, Comstock RD: Epidemiology of lower extremity injuries among U.S. high school athletes. *Acad Emerg Med* 2007;14(7):641-645.

2. Waterman BR, Belmont PJ Jr, Cameron KL, Deberardino TM, Owens BD: Epidemiology of ankle sprain at the United States Military Academy. *Am J Sports Med* 2010;38(4):797-803.

   Among military cadets, 614 new ankle sprains were reported during 10,511 person-years (58.4 per 1,000 person-years). Level of evidence: II.

3. Kaplan LD, Jost PW, Honkamp N, Norwig J, West R, Bradley JP: Incidence and variance of foot and ankle injuries in elite college football players. *Am J Orthop (Belle Mead NJ)* 2011;40(1):40-44.

   A study of 320 intercollegiate football players found that 231 (72%) had a history of foot or ankle injury (1.24 injuries per injured player). Lateral ankle sprains were most common, followed by syndesmosis sprain, MTP dislocation, and fibula fracture.

4. Waterman BR, Owens BD, Davey S, Zacchilli MA, Belmont PJ Jr: The epidemiology of ankle sprains in the United States. *J Bone Joint Surg Am* 2010;92(13):2279-2284.

   The estimated incidence of ankle sprains was 2.15 per 1,000 person-years in the United States, and the peak incidence was at age 15 to 19 years. Most ankle sprains were in basketball, football, and soccer players. Level of evidence: II.

5. Gerber JP, Williams GN, Scoville CR, Arciero RA, Taylor DC: Persistent disability associated with ankle sprains: A prospective examination of an athletic population. *Foot Ankle Int* 1998;19(10):653-660.

6. Watanabe K, Kitaoka HB, Berglund LJ, Zhao KD, Kaufman KR, An KN: The role of ankle ligaments and articular geometry in stabilizing the ankle. *Clin Biomech (Bristol, Avon)* 2012;27(2):189-195.

   The contributions of the lateral ligaments, the deltoid ligament, and articular geometry in ankle stabilization were investigated. In the unloaded state, the lateral ligaments accounted for 70% to 80% of anterior stability and the deltoid ligament accounted for 50% to 80% of posterior stability. Both ligaments contributed 50% to 80% of rotational stability. In the loaded state, articular geometry accounted for 100% of translation and 60% of rotational stability.

7. Clanton TO, Campbell KJ, Wilson KJ, et al: Qualitative and quantitative anatomic investigation of the lateral ankle ligaments for surgical reconstruction procedures. *J Bone Joint Surg Am* 2014;96(12):e98.

   Anatomic study of the lateral ligaments of the ankle and subtalar joint found that the ATFL can be found as one to three bands, with the single band originating an average 13.8 mm above the inferior tip of the lateral malleolus on the anterior fibular border and attaching along the anterior border of the talar lateral articular facet an average 17.8 mm superior to the apex of the lateral talar process. The CFL originates from the fibula an average 5.3 mm anterior to the inferior tip of the lateral malleolus and courses posteroinferior to insert on the calcaneus an average 16.3 mm from the posterior point of the peroneal tubercle.

8. Attarian DE, McCrackin HJ, Devito DP, McElhaney JH, Garrett WE Jr: A biomechanical study of human lateral ankle ligaments and autogenous reconstructive grafts. *Am J Sports Med* 1985;13(6):377-381.

9. Reed ME, Feibel JB, Donley BG, Giza E: Athletic ankle injuries, in Kibler WB, ed: *Orthopaedic Knowledge Update: Sports Medicine, ed 4.* Rosemont, IL, American Academy of Orthopaedic Surgeons, 2010, pp 199-214.

   This chapter discusses various topics related to athletic ankle injuries and provides further insight into management of these conditions.

10. Haytmanek CT, Williams BT, James EW, et al: Radiographic identification of the primary lateral ankle structures. *Am J Sports Med* 2015;43(1):79-87.

    An anatomic study quantitatively described the anatomic attachments sites of the ATFL, CFL, and PTFL in relation to reproducible osseous landmarks.

11. Kerkhoffs GM, van den Bekerom M, Elders LA, et al: Diagnosis, treatment and prevention of ankle sprains:

An evidence-based clinical guideline. *Br J Sports Med* 2012;46(12):854-860.

A literature review provided an evidence-based guideline for the prevention, prediction, diagnosis, surgical treatment, and prognosis of lateral ankle injury.

12. Kofotolis ND, Kellis E, Viachopoulos SP: Ankle sprain injuries and risk factors in amateur soccer players during a 2-year period. *Am J Sports Med* 2007;35(3):458-466.

13. Petersen W, Rembitzki IV, Koppenburg AG, et al: Treatment of acute ankle ligament injuries: A systematic review. *Arch Orthop Trauma Surg* 2013;133(8):1129-1141.

    Analysis of 17 randomized controlled studies and three meta-analyses found that most grade I, II, and III lateral ankle ligament ruptures can be managed without surgery. A semirigid brace should be used, although grade III injuries may benefit from short-term immobilization before brace use. Level of evidence: I.

14. Pihlajamäki H, Hietaniemi K, Paavola M, Visuri T, Mattila VM: Surgical versus functional treatment for acute ruptures of the lateral ligament complex of the ankle in young men: A randomized controlled trial. *J Bone Joint Surg Am* 2010;92(14):2367-2374.

    All 51 active Finnish men with an acute grade III lateral ligament rupture reportedly returned to previous activity level after surgical or functional nonsurgical treatment. There was no significant difference in ankle scores, though the prevalence of reinjury was higher after functional treatment. Level of evidence: I.

15. Takao M, Miyamoto W, Matsui K, Sasahara J, Matsushita T: Functional treatment after surgical repair for acute lateral ligament disruption of the ankle in athletes. *Am J Sports Med* 2012;40(2):447-451.

    After 78 feet were treated nonsurgically and 54 were treated with primary surgical repair followed by nonsurgical treatment, 8 nonsurgically treated feet (10.3%) had a fair to poor result, and all surgically treated feet had a good to excellent result. Level of evidence: III.

16. van den Bekerom MP, Kerkhoffs GM, McCollum GA, Calder JD, van Dijk CN: Management of acute lateral ankle ligament injury in the athlete. *Knee Surg Sports Traumatol Arthrosc* 2013;21(6):1390-1395.

17. Lamb SE, Marsh JL, Hutton JL, Nakash R, Cooke MW; Collaborative Ankle Support Trial (CAST Group): Mechanical supports for acute, severe ankle sprain: A pragmatic, multicentre, randomised controlled trial. *Lancet* 2009;373(9663):575-581.

    A randomized trial of 584 subjects with severe ankle sprain showed that primary outcome was function at 3 months with Foot and Ankle Score (FAS). Patients who received the below-knee cast had a more rapid recovery than those treated with the tubular compression bandage.

18. Haraguchi N, Toga H, Shiba N, Kato F: Avulsion fracture of the lateral ankle ligament complex in severe inversion injury: Incidence and clinical outcome. *Am J Sports Med* 2007;35(7):1144-1152.

19. McGuine TA, Brooks A, Hetzel S: The effect of lace-up ankle braces on injury rates in high school basketball players. *Am J Sports Med* 2011;39(9):1840-1848.

    After 1,460 high school basketball players with ankle injury were randomly assigned to a lace-up ankle brace or a control group, lace-up ankle braces were found to reduce the incidence but not the severity of acute ankle injuries. Level of evidence: I.

20. McGuine TA, Hetzel S, Wilson J, Brooks A: The effect of lace-up ankle braces on injury rates in high school football players. *Am J Sports Med* 2012;40(1):49-57.

    After 2,081 high school football players with ankle injury were randomly assigned to a lace-up ankle brace or a control group, lace-up ankle braces were found to reduce the incidence but not the severity of acute ankle injuries. Level of evidence: I.

21. Bosien WR, Staple OS, Russell SW: Residual disability following acute ankle sprains. *J Bone Joint Surg Am* 1955;37:1237-1243.

22. Jackson DW, Ashley RL, Powell JW: Ankle sprains in young athletes: Relation of severity and disability. *Clin Orthop Relat Res* 1974;101:201-215.

23. Lentell G, Baas B, Lopez D, McGuire L, Sarrels M, Snyder P: The contributions of proprioceptive deficits, muscle function, and anatomic laxity to functional instability of the ankle. *J Orthop Sports Phys Ther* 1995;21:206-215.

24. Hertel J: Functional instability following lateral ankle sprain. *Sports Med* 2000;29(5):361-371.

25. Clanton TO, Waldrop NE: Athletic injuries to the soft tissues of the foot and ankle, in Coughlin MJ, Saltzman CL, Anderson RB, eds: *Mann's Surgery of the Foot and Ankle*, ed 9. Philadelphia, PA, Mosby Elsevier, 2014, pp 1531-1687.

26. Caputo AM, Lee JY, Spritzer CE, et al: In vivo kinematics of the tibiotalar joint after lateral ankle instability. *Am J Sports Med* 2009;37(11):2241-2248.

    Nine ankles with unilateral ATFL injuries were biomechanically studied and compared as they stepped on a level surface. A statistically significant increase in internal rotation, anterior translation, and superior translation of the talus was measured in ATFL-deficient ankles compared with the intact contralateral controls.

27. Maffulli N, Del Buono A, Maffulli GD, et al: Isolated anterior talofibular ligament Broström repair for chronic lateral ankle instability: 9-year follow-up. *Am J Sports Med* 2013;41(4):858-864.

    Long-term outcomes were reported for 38 of 42 patients who underwent Broström ATFL repair. Twenty-two patients (58%) returned to their preinjury activity level, 6

(16%) were at a lower activity level but still active, and 10 (26%) abandoned active sports but were still physically active. Level of evidence: IV.

28. Waldrop NE III, Wijdicks CA, Jansson KS, LaPrade RF, Clanton TO: Anatomic suture anchor versus the Broström technique for anterior talofibular ligament repair: A biomechanical comparison. *Am J Sports Med* 2012;40(11):2590-2596.

A cadaver study of 24 fresh-frozen ankles revealed significantly lower strength and stiffness in all three repair groups compared with the native, intact ATFL. It was determined that repairs must be sufficiently protected to avoid premature failure.

29. Viens NA, Wijdicks CA, Campbell KJ, Laprade RF, Clanton TO: Anterior talofibular ligament ruptures: Part 1. Biomechanical comparison of augmented Broström repair techniques with the intact anterior talofibular ligament. *Am J Sports Med* 2014;42(2):405-411.

A cadaver study of 18 fresh-frozen ankles compared ankles with an intact ATFL to those with suture tape augmentation or Broström repair with suture tape augmentation. Strength and stiffness were greater after Broström repair with suture tape augmentation in comparison to the intact ATFL or the Broström alone.

30. Clanton TO, Viens NA, Campbell KJ, Laprade RF, Wijdicks CA: Anterior talofibular ligament ruptures. Part 2. Biomechanical comparison of anterior talofibular ligament reconstruction using semitendinosus allografts with the intact ligament. *Am J Sports Med* 2014;42(2):412-416.

Allograft reconstruction of the ATFL led to no significant difference in strength or stiffness compared with the intact ATFL.

31. Campbell KJ, Michalski MP, Wilson KJ, et al: The ligament anatomy of the deltoid complex of the ankle: A qualitative and quantitative anatomical study. *J Bone Joint Surg Am* 2014;96(8):e62.

A cadaver anatomic study detailed the specific components of the deltoid ligament complex, their prevalence, and their relationships to nearby anatomic structures.

32. Attarian DE, McCrackin HJ, DeVito DP, McElhaney JH, Garrett WE Jr: Biomechanical characteristics of human ankle ligaments. *Foot Ankle* 1985;6(2):54-58.

33. Jeong MS, Choi YS, Kim YJ, Kim JS, Young KW, Jung YY: Deltoid ligament in acute ankle injury: MR imaging analysis. *Skeletal Radiol* 2014;43(5):655-663.

An MRI study of 36 patients with acute deltoid injury detailed patterns of deltoid injury for the superficial and deep deltoid and how they related to concomitant associated ankle pathologies.

34. Femino JE, Vaseenon T, Phisitkul P, Tochigi Y, Anderson DD, Amendola A: Varus external rotation stress test for radiographic detection of deep deltoid ligament disruption with and without syndesmotic disruption: A cadaveric study. *Foot Ankle Int* 2013;34(2):251-260.

Varus external rotation stress was more effective than valgus external rotation stress displacement of markers at the medial gutter and on AP and mortise radiographs of the deep deltoid ligament. This finding may improve detection of associated pathology and instability.

35. Beals TC, Crim J, Nickisch F: Deltoid ligament injuries in athletes: Techniques of repair and reconstruction. *Oper Tech Sports Med* 2010;18(1):11-17.

Deltoid ligament injuries are a source of valgus and rotational ankle instability and often occur as a result of athletic injury. The anatomy of the medial ankle ligament complex was reviewed, with emphasis on pertinent radiologic findings.

36. Chhabra A, Subhawong TK, Carrino JA: MR imaging of deltoid ligament pathologic findings and associated impingement syndromes. *Radiographics* 2010;30(3):751-761.

MRI technique for the deltoid ligament was reviewed, with the normal and abnormal appearances of its components.

37. Savage-Elliott I, Murawski CD, Smyth NA, Golanó P, Kennedy JG: The deltoid ligament: An in-depth review of anatomy, function, and treatment strategies. *Knee Surg Sports Traumatol Arthrosc* 2013;21(6):1316-1327.

The anatomy and biology of the medial ankle ligament complex and treatment strategies were reviewed.

38. Golanó P, Vega J, de Leeuw PA, et al: Anatomy of the ankle ligaments: A pictorial essay. *Knee Surg Sports Traumatol Arthrosc* 2010;18(5):557-569.

This article is an illustrative review of ankle ligament anatomy. Several annotated photographs and diagrams of ankle ligaments in various views are presented.

39. Williams BT, Ahrberg AB, Goldsmith MT, et al: Ankle syndesmosis: A qualitative and quantitative anatomic analysis. *Am J Sports Med* 2015;43(1):88-97.

The anteroinferior, posteroinferior, and interosseous tibiofibular ligaments were described in relation to osseous landmarks.

40. Williams GN, Jones MH, Amendola A: Syndesmotic ankle sprains in athletes. *Am J Sports Med* 2007;35(7):1197-1207.

41. Clanton TO, Ho CP, Williams BT, et al: Magnetic resonance imaging characterization of individual ankle syndesmosis structures in asymptomatic and surgically treated cohorts. *Knee Surg Sports Traumatol Arthrosc* 2014; Nov 15. [Published online ahead of print]

Preoperative 3-Tesla MRI had excellent accuracy in the diagnosis of syndesmotic ligament tears and allowed visualization of relevant individual syndesmosis structures. Associated ligament injuries could be readily identified.

42. Sikka RS, Fetzer GB, Sugarman E, et al: Correlating MRI findings with disability in syndesmotic sprains of NFL players. *Foot Ankle Int* 2012;33(5):371-378.

3: Knee and Leg

MRI findings consistent with increasing grade of injury can helped predict number of games missed in National Football League players. Level of evidence: IV.

43. Laver L, Carmont MR, McConkey MO, et al: Plasma rich in growth factors (PRGF) as a treatment for high ankle sprain in elite athletes: A randomized control trial. *Knee Surg Sports Traumatol Arthrosc* [published online ahead of print June 18, 2014].

Sixteen elite athletes with an AITFL tear and dynamic syndesmosis instability were randomly assigned to a PRP treatment or a control group. The treated patients returned to play at 40.8 days compared with 59.6 days for those in the control group, and they had significantly less residual pain upon return to activity. Level of evidence: II.

44. Jones MH, Amendola A: Syndesmosis sprains of the ankle: A systematic review. *Clin Orthop Relat Res* 2007;455(455):173-175.

45. Taylor DC, Englehardt DL, Bassett FH III: Syndesmosis sprains of the ankle: The influence of heterotopic ossification. *Am J Sports Med* 1992;20(2):146-150.

46. Degroot H, Al-Omari AA, El Ghazaly SA: Outcomes of suture button repair of the distal tibiofibular syndesmosis. *Foot Ankle Int* 2011;32(3):250-256.

Titanium button fixation of the syndesmosis was effective in maintaining reduction in 20 patients throughout an almost 2-year follow-up period. Device removal was more common than anticipated. Level of evidence: IV.

47. Naqvi GA, Cunningham P, Lynch B, Galvin R, Awan N: Fixation of ankle syndesmotic injuries: Comparison of tightrope fixation and syndesmotic screw fixation for accuracy of syndesmotic reduction. *Am J Sports Med* 2012;40(12):2828-2835.

A study of 46 patients included 23 who received tightrope fixation and 23 who received syndesmosis screw fixation. Level of evidence: II.

48. Hamid N, Loeffler BJ, Braddy W, Kellam JF, Cohen BE, Bosse MJ: Outcome after fixation of ankle fractures with an injury to the syndesmosis: The effect of the syndesmosis screw. *J Bone Joint Surg Br* 2009;91(8):1069-1073.

The authors present a comparative study of syndesmosis screws after ankle fracture with associated syndesmotic injury. American Orthopaedic Foot and Ankle Society score was 83.07 in the intact screw group, 92.40 in the broken screw group, and 85.80 in the removed screw group (*P* = 0.0466). No difference in clinical outcome of patients with intact or removed syndesmotic screws was found.

49. Manjoo A, Sanders DW, Tieszer C, MacLeod MD: Functional and radiographic results of patients with syndesmotic screw fixation: Implications for screw removal. *J Orthop Trauma* 2010;24(1):2-6.

A total of 76 patients underwent functional testing and radiographic review after syndesmosis screw fixation. Patients with a fractured, loosened, or removed screw had a better functional outcome than those with an intact screw. Level of evidence: III.

50. Song DJ, Lanzi JT, Groth AT, et al: The effect of syndesmosis screw removal on the reduction of the distal tibiofibular joint: A prospective radiographic study. *Foot Ankle Int* 2014;35(6):543-548.

Syndesmosis screw removal can lead to the spontaneous reduction of a malreduced syndesmosis. Almost 90% of the malreduced ankles were spontaneously reduced with screw removal. Level of evidence: IV.

51. Miller AN, Barei DP, Iaquinto JM, Ledoux WR, Beingessner DM: Iatrogenic syndesmosis malreduction via clamp and screw placement. *J Orthop Trauma* 2013;27(2):100-106.

A cadaver study of 14 dissected legs with complete syndesmosis disruption concluded intraoperative clamping and fixation could cause statistically significant syndesmosis malreduction.

52. Mitchell ME, Giza E, Sullivan MR: Cartilage transplantation techniques for talar cartilage lesions. *J Am Acad Orthop Surg* 2009;17(7):407-414.

This review article discusses the anatomy of talar cartilage and surgical treatment options. The article focuses especially on autologous chondrocyte implantation and matrix-induced autologous chondrocyte implantation.

53. Easley ME, Latt LD, Santangelo JR, Merian-Genast M, Nunley JA II: Osteochondral lesions of the talus. *J Am Acad Orthop Surg* 2010;18(10):616-630.

A review of management of OLTs included indications and contraindications, preoperative evaluation, arthroscopic procedures (débridement, drilling, microfracture, and bone grafting), medial and lateral open approaches, open procedures (osteochondral autograft transfer, autologous chondrocyte implantation, structural allograft transplantation), and complications and results.

54. Berndt AL, Harty M: Transchondral fractures (osteochondritis dissecans) of the talus. *J Bone Joint Surg Am* 1959;40:115-120.

55. Loomer R, Fisher C, Lloyd-Smith R, Sisler J, Cooney J: Osteochondral lesions of the talus. *Am J Sports Med* 1993;21(1):13-19.

56. Brittberg M, Aglietti P, Gambardella R, et al: ICRS Cartilage Injury Evaluation Package. Third ICRS Symposium, Göteborg, Sweden, April 28, 2000. Available at http://www.cartilage.org.

57. Hintermann B, Regazzoni P, Lampert C, Stutz G, Gächter A: Arthroscopic findings in acute fractures of the ankle. *J Bone Joint Surg Br* 2000;82(3):345-351.

58. Sugimoto K, Takakura Y, Okahashi K, Samoto N, Kawate K, Iwai M: Chondral injuries of the ankle with recurrent

3: Knee and Leg

lateral instability: An arthroscopic study. *J Bone Joint Surg Am* 2009;91(1):99-106.

The authors presented a cross-sectional study of 93 patients undergoing ankle arthroscopy for recurrent instability. The relationship between chondral damage, patient factors, injury patterns, alignment, and other variables was studied.

59. McGahan PJ, Pinney SJ: Current concept review: Osteochondral lesions of the talus. *Foot Ankle Int* 2010;31(1):90-101.

The etiology, clinical presentation, imaging, and classification of OLTs as well as treatment with bone marrow stimulation, osteochondral autografts, osteochondral allografts, autologous chondrocyte implantation, and autogenous bone grafting were reviewed.

60. Stufkens SA, Knupp M, Horisberger M, Lampert C, Hintermann B: Cartilage lesions and the development of osteoarthritis after internal fixation of ankle fractures: A prospective study. *J Bone Joint Surg Am* 2010;92(2):279-286.

At long-term follow-up of 109 patients who underwent surgical treatment of an ankle fracture, initial cartilage damage seen during arthroscopy was an independent predictor of posttraumatic osteoarthritis. Level of evidence: II.

61. Tol JL, Struijs PA, Bossuyt PM, Verhagen RA, van Dijk CN: Treatment strategies in osteochondral defects of the talar dome: A systematic review. *Foot Ankle Int* 2000;21(2):119-126.

62. Deol PP, Cuttica DJ, Smith WB, Berlet GC: Osteochondral lesions of the talus: Size, age, and predictors of outcomes. *Foot Ankle Clin* 2013;18(1):13-34.

The historical perspective, predictors of outcomes, and nonsurgical and surgical treatment options were presented for osteochondral lesions of the talus. Lesion size, presence of edema on MRI, and patient age were discussed as factors in patient care and outcomes.

63. Yoshimura I, Kanazawa K, Takeyama A, et al: Arthroscopic bone marrow stimulation techniques for osteochondral lesions of the talus: Prognostic factors for small lesions. *Am J Sports Med* 2013;41(3):528-534.

Fifty patients with OLTs smaller than 150 mm² underwent arthroscopic bone marrow stimulation. Deep lesions and lesions in patients older than 40 years had inferior clinical outcomes. Level of evidence: IV.

64. Zengerink M, Struijs PA, Tol JL, van Dijk CN: Treatment of osteochondral lesions of the talus: A systematic review. *Knee Surg Sports Traumatol Arthrosc* 2010;18(2):238-246.

A systematic review of treatment strategies for OLTs found success rates of 87% for osteochondral autologous transplantation, 85% for bone marrow stimulation, 76% for autologous chondrocyte implantation, 88% for retrograde drilling, and 89% for fixation. Because of its relatively low cost and morbidity, bone marrow stimulation was identified as the treatment of choice for primary OLTs.

65. Clanton TO, Johnson NS, Matheny LM: Use of cartilage extracellular matrix and bone marrow aspirate concentrate in treatment of osteochondral lesions of the talus. *Tech Foot Ankle Surg* 2014;13(4):212-220.

Surgical technique and preliminary results were presented for the use of micronized cartilage allograft extracellular matrix and bone marrow aspirate concentrate as a source of mesenchymal stem cells to augment standard microfracture technique.

66. Doral MN, Bilge O, Batmaz G, et al: Treatment of osteochondral lesions of the talus with microfracture technique and postoperative Hyaluronan injection. *Knee Surg Sports Traumatol Arthrosc* 2012;20(7):1398-1403.

A prospective randomized study of 16 patients who received débridement and microfracture alone and 41 patients who received débridement and microfracture as well as a postoperative intra-articular hyaluronan injection found a significant increase from preoperative to postoperative scores among those who received injection. Level of evidence: I.

67. Guney A, Akar M, Karaman I, Oner M, Guney B: Clinical outcomes of platelet rich plasma (PRP) as an adjunct to microfracture surgery in osteochondral lesions of the talus. *Knee Surg Sports Traumatol Arthrosc* 2014; Nov 30 [published online ahead of print].

In a study of 16 patients who underwent microfracture alone and 19 who underwent microfracture plus PRP, those who received PRP had significantly better functional scores. Level of evidence: II.

68. Kim YS, Lee HJ, Choi YJ, Kim YI, Koh YG: Does an injection of a stromal vascular fraction containing adipose-derived mesenchymal stem cells influence the outcomes of marrow stimulation in osteochondral lesions of the talus? A clinical and magnetic resonance imaging study. *Am J Sports Med* 2014;42(10):2424-2434.

MRI of 26 ankles after bone marrow stimulation alone and 24 after bone marrow stimulation plus stromal vascular fraction injection containing mesenchymal stem cells revealed significantly better clinical outcomes in the latter group of ankles. Level of evidence: III.

69. Choi WJ, Park KK, Kim BS, Lee JW: Osteochondral lesion of the talus: Is there a critical defect size for poor outcome? *Am J Sports Med* 2009;37(10):1974-1980.

This cohort study of 120 ankles examined osteochondral lesion size on the talus and clinical outcome following arthroscopic marrow stimulation. Initial defect size was found to be an important prognostic factor.

70. Kwak SK, Kern BS, Ferkel RD, Chan KW, Kasraeian S, Applegate GR: Autologous chondrocyte implantation of the ankle: 2- to 10-year results. *Am J Sports Med* 2014;42(9):2156-2164.

3: Knee and Leg

At long-term follow-up, 29 of 32 patients who underwent autologous chondrocyte implantation of the talus had significant improvement in outcomes scores. Level of evidence: IV.

71. Yoon HS, Park YJ, Lee M, Choi WJ, Lee JW: Osteochondral autologous transplantation is superior to repeat arthroscopy for the treatment of osteochondral lesions of the talus after failed primary arthroscopic treatment. *Am J Sports Med* 2014;42(8):1896-1903.

 After unsuccessful bone marrow stimulation, 22 patients underwent osteochondral autologous transplantation and 22 underwent repeat arthroscopy. At a mean 50-month follow-up, results were better in the patients who underwent osteochondral autologous transplantation. Level of evidence: III.

72. Haleem AM, Ross KA, Smyth NA, et al: Double-plug autologous osteochondral transplantation shows equal functional outcomes compared with single-plug procedures in lesions of the talar dome: A minimum 5-year clinical follow-up. *Am J Sports Med* 2014;42(8):1888-1895.

 Fourteen patients with a large OLT treated with double-plug autologous osteochondral transplantation were compared with 28 patients treated with single-plug autologous osteochondral transplantation. No statistically significant differences were noted in outcomes scores at a mean 85-month follow-up. Level of evidence: III.

73. Ross KA, Hannon CP, Deyer TW, et al: Functional and MRI outcomes after arthroscopic microfracture for treatment of osteochondral lesions of the distal tibial plafond. *J Bone Joint Surg Am* 2014;96(20):1708-1715.

 After 31 osteochondral lesions of the distal tibia were treated with microfracture, patient outcomes were improved but MRI revealed increased lesion size. Level of evidence: IV.

74. Elias I, Raikin SM, Schweitzer ME, Besser MP, Morrison WB, Zoga AC: Osteochondral lesions of the distal tibial plafond: Localization and morphologic characteristics with an anatomical grid. *Foot Ankle Int* 2009;30(6):524-529.

 Using a nine-zone grid system for the articular surface of the distal tibia, MRI scans from 38 patients were reviewed and locations were assigned for osteochondral lesions of the distal tibial plafond. No location had a predominant incidence, and so-called kissing lesions were rare. Level of evidence: II.

75. Tol JL, Slim E, van Soest AJ, van Dijk CN: The relationship of the kicking action in soccer and anterior ankle impingement syndrome: A biomechanical analysis. *Am J Sports Med* 2002;30(1):45-50.

76. Tol JL, van Dijk CN: Etiology of the anterior ankle impingement syndrome: A descriptive anatomical study. *Foot Ankle Int* 2004;25(6):382-386.

77. Elias I, Zoga AC, Morrison WB, Besser MP, Schweitzer ME, Raikin SM: Osteochondral lesions of the talus: Localization and morphologic data from 424 patients using a novel anatomical grid scheme. *Foot Ankle Int* 2007;28(2):154-161.

78. Kim SH, Ha KI, Ahn JH: Tram track lesion of the talar dome. *Arthroscopy* 1999;15(2):203-206.

79. van Dijk CN, Verhagen RA, Tol JL: Arthroscopy for problems after ankle fracture. *J Bone Joint Surg Br* 1997;79(2):280-284.

80. van Dijk CN, Tol JL, Verheyen CC: A prospective study of prognostic factors concerning the outcome of arthroscopic surgery for anterior ankle impingement. *Am J Sports Med* 1997;25(6):737-745.

81. Parma A, Buda R, Vannini F, et al: Arthroscopic treatment of ankle anterior bony impingement: The long-term clinical outcome. *Foot Ankle Int* 2014;35(2):148-155.

 A new classification of ankle impingement has long-term predictive value for the success of arthroscopic débridement. Associated pathology (including chondral lesions), advanced age, ankle morphology, and previous trauma were relevant prognostic factors. Level of evidence: IV.

82. Walsh SJ, Twaddle BC, Rosenfeldt MP, Boyle MJ: Arthroscopic treatment of anterior ankle impingement: A prospective study of 46 patients with 5-year follow-up. *Am J Sports Med* 2014;42(11):2722-2726.

 Functional outcomes of 46 patients with arthroscopic anterior ankle decompression remained high at 5-year follow-up despite radiographic recurrence of the lesions. Level of evidence: IV.

83. Giannini S, Buda R, Mosca M, Parma A, Di Caprio F: Posterior ankle impingement. *Foot Ankle Int* 2013;34(3):459-465.

 Treatment algorithms for posterior soft-tissue and bony impingement were presented, including workup and treatment options.

84. Hedrick MR, McBryde AM: Posterior ankle impingement. *Foot Ankle Int* 1994;15(1):2-8.

85. Mouhsine E, Crevoisier X, Leyvraz PF, Akiki A, Dutoit M, Garofalo R: Post-traumatic overload or acute syndrome of the os trigonum: A possible cause of posterior ankle impingement. *Knee Surg Sports Traumatol Arthrosc* 2004;12(3):250-253.

86. Willits K, Sonneveld H, Amendola A, Giffin JR, Griffin S, Fowler PJ: Outcome of posterior ankle arthroscopy for hindfoot impingement. *Arthroscopy* 2008;24(2):196-202.

87. López Valerio V, Seijas R, Alvarez P, et al: Endoscopic repair of posterior ankle impingement syndrome due to os trigonum in soccer players. *Foot Ankle Int* 2015;36(1):70-74.

 The posterior impingement syndrome associated with an os trigonum was described. Twenty soccer players underwent posterior ankle arthroscopy with excision of the os trigonum. Pain scores significantly decreased 1 month after surgery, and patients returned to preinjury levels 46.9 days after surgery. Level of evidence: IV.

88. Murawski CD, Kennedy JG: Anteromedial impingement in the ankle joint: Outcomes following arthroscopy. *Am J Sports Med* 2010;38(10):2017-2024.

89. Lareau CR, Sawyer GA, Wang JH, DiGiovanni CW: Plantar and medial heel pain: Diagnosis and management. *J Am Acad Orthop Surg* 2014;22(6):372-380.

   Anatomy, etiology, treatment options, and outcomes of plantar fasciitis were reviewed.

90. Donley BG, Moore T, Sferra J, Gozdanovic J, Smith R: The efficacy of oral nonsteroidal anti-inflammatory medication (NSAID) in the treatment of plantar fasciitis: A randomized, prospective, placebo-controlled study. *Foot Ankle Int* 2007;28(1):20-23.

91. Digiovanni BF, Nawoczenski DA, Malay DP, et al: Plantar fascia-specific stretching exercise improves outcomes in patients with chronic plantar fasciitis: A prospective clinical trial with two-year follow-up. *J Bone Joint Surg Am* 2006;88(8):1775-1781.

92. Radford JA, Landorf KB, Buchbinder R, Cook C: Effectiveness of calf muscle stretching for the short-term treatment of plantar heel pain: A randomised trial. *BMC Musculoskelet Disord* 2007;8:36.

93. Hyland MR, Webber-Gaffney A, Cohen L, Lichtman PT: Randomized controlled trial of calcaneal taping, sham taping, and plantar fascia stretching for the short-term management of plantar heel pain. *J Orthop Sports Phys Ther* 2006;36(6):364-371.

94. Crawford F, Thomson C: Interventions for treating plantar heel pain. *Cochrane Database Syst Rev* 2003;3:CD000416.

95. Lee WC, Wong WY, Kung E, Leung AK: Effectiveness of adjustable dorsiflexion night splint in combination with accommodative foot orthosis on plantar fasciitis. *J Rehabil Res Dev* 2012;49(10):1557-1564.

   The use of dorsiflexion night splints in conjunction with foot orthoses for the treatment of chronic plantar fasciitis is more effective in relieving heel pain than the use of foot orthoses alone.

96. Wang CJ, Wang FS, Yang KD, Weng LH, Ko JY: Long-term results of extracorporeal shockwave treatment for plantar fasciitis. *Am J Sports Med* 2006;34(4):592-596.

97. Porter MD, Shadbolt B: Intralesional corticosteroid injection versus extracorporeal shock wave therapy for plantar fasciopathy. *Clin J Sport Med* 2005;15(3):119-124.

98. Monto RR: Platelet-rich plasma efficacy versus corticosteroid injection treatment for chronic severe plantar fasciitis. *Foot Ankle Int* 2014;35(4):313-318.

   Forty patients with plantar fasciitis were randomly assigned to corticosteroid injection or PRP injection. Those who received the PRP injection had a more durable and effective response than those who received the steroid injection. Level of evidence: I.

99. Landorf KB, Keenan AM, Herbert RD: Effectiveness of foot orthoses to treat plantar fasciitis: A randomized trial. *Arch Intern Med* 2006;166(12):1305-1310.

100. Bader L, Park K, Gu Y, O'Malley MJ: Functional outcome of endoscopic plantar fasciotomy. *Foot Ankle Int* 2012;33(1):37-43.

   Patients had rapid improvement in chronic symptoms with low morbidity after undergoing endoscopic plantar fasciotomy. Level of evidence: IV.

101. Monteagudo M, Maceira E, Garcia-Virto V, Canosa R: Chronic plantar fasciitis: Plantar fasciotomy versus gastrocnemius recession. *Int Orthop* 2013;37(9):1845-1850.

   Thirty patients underwent partial plantar fasciotomy, and 30 underwent proximal medial gastrocnemius release. The result was satisfactory in 60% after partial plantar fasciotomy compared with 95% after proximal medial gastrocnemius release. Patients in the gastrocnemius release group had much-improved functional and pain outcome scores and fewer complications. Level of evidence: IV.

102. Saxena A, Fullem B: Plantar fascia ruptures in athletes. *Am J Sports Med* 2004;32(3):662-665.

103. Nunley JA, Vertullo CJ: Classification, investigation, and management of midfoot sprains: Lisfranc injuries in the athlete. *Am J Sports Med* 2002;30(6):871-878.

104. Kaar S, Femino J, Morag Y: Lisfranc joint displacement following sequential ligament sectioning. *J Bone Joint Surg Am* 2007;89(10):2225-2232.

105. Gallagher SM, Rodriguez NA, Andersen CR, Granberry WM, Panchbhavi VK: Anatomic predisposition to ligamentous Lisfranc injury: A matched case-control study. *J Bone Joint Surg Am* 2013;95(22):2043-2047.

   A retrospective case-control study of 26 patients with ligamentous Lisfranc injury and 52 control subjects found that the patients with Lisfranc injury had a significantly smaller ratio of second metatarsal length to foot length. Level of evidence: III.

106. Haytmanek CT, Clanton TO: Ligamentous Lisfranc injuries in the athlete. *Oper Tech Sports Med* 2014;22(4):313-320.

   Mechanism of injury, clinical decision making, radiographic evaluation, treatment options, and surgical approach were reviewed for ligamentous Lisfranc injuries.

107. Henning JA, Jones CB, Sietsema DL, Bohay DR, Anderson JG: Open reduction internal fixation versus primary arthrodesis for Lisfranc injuries: A prospective randomized study. *Foot Ankle Int* 2009;30(10):913-922.

5: Knee and Leg

A prospective randomized trial of surgical treatment options for Lisfranc injuries is presented. Forty patients underwent open reduction and internal fixation or primary arthrodesis. Arthrodesis was associated with significantly fewer secondary surgeries. There was no difference in 36-Item Short Form or Short Form Musculoskeletal Functional Assessment scores between cohorts.

108. Ly TV, Coetzee JC: Treatment of primarily ligamentous Lisfranc joint injuries: Primary arthrodesis compared with open reduction and internal fixation. A prospective, randomized study. *J Bone Joint Surg Am* 2006;88(3):514-520.

109. Sheibani-Rad S, Coetzee JC, Giveans MR, DiGiovanni C: Arthrodesis versus ORIF for Lisfranc fractures. *Orthopedics* 2012;35(6):e868-e873.

    A systematic review pertaining to primary arthrodesis and open reduction and internal fixation of Lisfranc fractures found that both procedures provided equivalent satisfactory results, although clinical outcomes may be slightly better after primary arthrodesis.

110. Marsland D, Belkoff SM, Solan MC: Biomechanical analysis of endobutton versus screw fixation after Lisfranc ligament complex sectioning. *Foot Ankle Surg* 2013;19(4):267-272.

    In a cadaver study, 24 fresh-frozen feet were assigned to titanium button or screw fixation and subsequently were loaded to 343 N and subjected to 10,000 cycles. After initial loading, 1.0 mm of diastasis was observed in the button group compared with no diastasis in the screw group. After cyclic loading, diastasis in the button group decreased to 0.7 mm, and the screw group was unchanged.

111. George E, Harris AH, Dragoo JL, Hunt KJ: Incidence and risk factors for turf toe injuries in intercollegiate football: Data from the National Collegiate Athletic Association injury surveillance system. *Foot Ankle Int* 2014;35(2):108-115.

    Turf toe is a common football injury that usually affects skill-position players. Appropriate acute and long-term management is required. Level of evidence: IV.

112. Clanton TO, Butler JE, Eggert A: Injuries to the metatarsophalangeal joints in athletes. *Foot Ankle* 1986;7(3):162-176.

113. Crain JM, Phancao JP, Stidham K: MR imaging of turf toe. *Magn Reson Imaging Clin N Am* 2008;16(1):93-103, vi.

114. Waldrop NE III, Zirker CA, Wijdicks CA, Laprade RF, Clanton TO: Radiographic evaluation of plantar plate injury: An in vitro biomechanical study. *Foot Ankle Int* 2013;34(3):403-408.

    Historical evaluation of turf toe injury has been qualitative. This study provided quantifiable data on the severity of plantar plate injuries, which may provide guidance to physicians. Three millimeters of difference in excursion from the intact state indicated a three-ligament injury.

115. Cohen BE: Hallux sesamoid disorders. *Foot Ankle Clin* 2009;14(1):91-104.

    This review article of hallux sesamoid disorders outlined treatment of several sesamoid pathologies, including acute fractures, stress fractures, nonunions, osteonecrosis, and chondromalacia.

116. Bichara DA, Henn RF III, Theodore GH: Sesamoidectomy for hallux sesamoid fractures. *Foot Ankle Int* 2012;33(9):704-706.

    Sesamoid resection is a good option after unsuccessful nonsurgical treatment. Twenty-two of 24 patients returned to full activity at a mean 11.6 weeks after surgery. Hallux valgus occurred in one patient. Pain levels significantly improved as patients returned to full activity. Level of evidence: IV.

117. Maquirriain J, Ghisi JP: The incidence and distribution of stress fractures in elite tennis players. *Br J Sports Med* 2006;40(5):454-459, discussion 459.

118. Kaeding CC, Spindler KP, Amendola A: Management of troublesome stress fractures. *Instr Course Lect* 2004;53:455-469.

119. Lawrence SJ, Botte MJ: Jones' fractures and related fractures of the proximal fifth metatarsal. *Foot Ankle* 1993;14(6):358-365.

120. Carreira DS, Sandilands SM: Radiographic factors and effect of fifth metatarsal Jones and diaphyseal stress fractures on participation in the NFL. *Foot Ankle Int* 2013;34(4):518-522.

    A study of the effect of proximal fifth metatarsal fractures on the number of games played, number of games started, and number of years played in the National Football League found no statistically significant differences between players with a fracture and those in the control group. Level of evidence: III.

121. Chuckpaiwong B, Queen RM, Easley ME, Nunley JA: Distinguishing Jones and proximal diaphyseal fractures of the fifth metatarsal. *Clin Orthop Relat Res* 2008;466(8):1966-1970.

122. Torg JS, Balduini FC, Zelko RR, Pavlov H, Peff TC, Das M: Fractures of the base of the fifth metatarsal distal to the tuberosity: Classification and guidelines for non-surgical and surgical management. *J Bone Joint Surg Am* 1984;66(2):209-214.

123. Ochenjele G, Ho B, Switaj PJ, Fuchs D, Goyal N, Kadakia AR: Radiographic study of the fifth metatarsal for optimal intramedullary screw fixation of Jones fracture. *Foot Ankle Int* 2015;36(3):293-301.

    In a retrospective review, 119 patients underwent three-dimensional CT of the foot to determine measurements of the fifth metatarsal.

© 2016 American Academy of Orthopaedic Surgeons

124. Lee KT, Park YU, Young KW, Kim JS, Kim JB: The plantar gap: Another prognostic factor for fifth metatarsal stress fracture. *Am J Sports Med* 2011;39(10):2206-2211.

In 75 patients with fifth metatarsal stress fracture treated with tension-band wiring, factors such as the plantar gap may help guide treatment, especially in patients at high risk for nonunion. Level of evidence: III.

125. Mallee WH, Weel H, van Dijk CN, van Tulder MW, Kerkhoffs GM, Lin CW: Surgical versus conservative treatment for high-risk stress fractures of the lower leg (anterior tibial cortex, navicular and fifth metatarsal base): A systematic review. *Br J Sports Med* 2015;49(6):370-376.

A systematic review of the literature pertaining to three stress fractures of the lower extremity included eight studies (246 fractures) on proximal fifth metatarsal stress fracture. Pooled results produced a weighted mean time to return to sport of 13.8 weeks after surgical treatment and 19.2 weeks after nonsurgical treatment. For navicular stress fracture, eight studies (200 fractures) had a weighted mean time to return to sport of 16.4 weeks after surgical treatment and 21.7 weeks after nonsurgical treatment. Because of the low-quality evidence and high risk of bias, recommendations for standard of care could not be made. Level of evidence: IV.

126. Fishman FG, Adams SB, Easley ME, Nunley JA II: Vascularized pedicle bone grafting for nonunions of the tarsal navicular. *Foot Ankle Int* 2012;33(9):734-739.

The limited blood supply of the navicular and difficulty in treating nonunion or osteonecrosis led to a technique using vascularized bone graft from the cuboid, second cuneiform, or third cuneiform to aid navicular healing. In seven patients with a mean 40-month radiographic follow-up, no cystic change or collapse was noted, although dorsal fragmentation or exostosis at the graft site occurred in four patients. Level of evidence: IV.

127. McCormick JJ, Bray CC, Davis WH, Cohen BE, Jones CP III, Anderson RB: Clinical and computed tomography evaluation of surgical outcomes in tarsal navicular stress fractures. *Am J Sports Med* 2011;39(8):1741-1748.

Healing and bony union of navicular stress fractures were evaluated with CT in 10 patients an average 42.4 months after surgery. Eight had bony union, of whom 6 had residual lucency of 1 to 2 mm, although it proved clinically insignificant. Both patients with nonunion had a complete, displaced fracture on preoperative imaging. Level of evidence: IV.

128. Khan KM, Fuller PJ, Brukner PD, Kearney C, Burry HC: Outcome of conservative and surgical management of navicular stress fracture in athletes: Eighty-six cases proven with computerized tomography. *Am J Sports Med* 1992;20(6):657-666.

129. Torg JS, Moyer J, Gaughan JP, Boden BP: Management of tarsal navicular stress fractures: conservative versus surgical treatment: A meta-analysis. *Am J Sports Med* 2010;38(5):1048-1053.

A meta-analysis included 313 tarsal navicular stress fractures from 23 different reports. No statistically significant difference was noted in terms of successful outcome and time to return to sport between non–weight-bearing nonsurgical management and surgical fixation. Nonsurgical management with weight bearing was statistically inferior to non–weight-bearing management.

130. Moher D, Liberati A, Tetzlaff J, Altman DG; PRISMA Group: Preferred reporting items for systematic reviews and meta-analyses: The PRISMA statement. *Int J Surg* 2010;8(5):336-341.

A review and guidelines statement for conducting ethical and high-quality systematic reviews is presented. The article specifically reviews the history of QUOROM and its subsequent evolution to PRISMA.

131. Gross CE, Nunley JA: Medial-sided stress fractures: Medial malleolus and navicular stress fractures. *Oper Tech Sports Med* 2014;22(4):296-304.

This article reviews the diagnosis and treatment of medial-sided stress fractures of the foot and ankle, as well as specific surgical techniques.

132. Caesar BC, McCollum GA, Elliot R, Williams A, Calder JD: Stress fractures of the tibia and medial malleolus. *Foot Ankle Clin* 2013;18(2):339-355.

The incidence, pathophysiology, clinical presentation, diagnosis, and treatment options for stress fractures of the medial malleolus and tibia were reviewed.

133. Steinbronn DJ, Bennett GL, Kay DB: The use of magnetic resonance imaging in the diagnosis of stress fractures of the foot and ankle: Four case reports. *Foot Ankle Int* 1994;15(2):80-83.

134. Lempainen L, Liimatainen E, Heikkilä J, et al: Medial malleolar stress fracture in athletes: Diagnosis and operative treatment. *Scand J Surg* 2012;101(4):261-264.

In a retrospective review of medial malleolar stress fracture in 10 patients, 5 patients initially were managed with pain-free limited weight bearing, though all 5 proceeded to surgical fixation after no radiographic signs of healing 4 to 6 months after diagnosis. Five patients underwent surgical fixation because of small diastasis on MRI or long-standing symptoms. In all 10 patients, no fracture was visible on initial plain radiographs although subsequent MRI revealed the fracture and discontinuity of the cortex. All 10 fractures were clinically healed 3 to 4 months after surgery. Level of evidence: IV.

135. Maffulli N, Longo UG, Maffulli GD, Rabitti C, Khanna A, Denaro V: Marked pathological changes proximal and distal to the site of rupture in acute Achilles tendon ruptures. *Knee Surg Sports Traumatol Arthrosc* 2011;19(4):680-687.

Microscopic analysis of the histopathologic features of tendon tissue samples from 29 patients with an Achilles tendon rupture and 11 control subjects who had died of cardiovascular causes found that patients with a rupture had profound histopathologic changes throughout the tendon and the control subjects had little pathologic change.

136. Raikin SM, Garras DN, Krapchev PV: Achilles tendon injuries in a United States population. *Foot Ankle Int* 2013;34(4):475-480.

A retrospective review of 406 patients with Achilles tendon rupture found that 275 ruptures (68%) were the result of sports activity. The most commonly involved sport was basketball. Injuries in patients older than 55 years and patients with a high body mass index were more likely to occur in nonsports activities, and the diagnosis was more likely to be initially unrecognized. Level of evidence: II.

137. Garras DN, Raikin SM, Bhat SB, Taweel N, Karanjia H: MRI is unnecessary for diagnosing acute Achilles tendon ruptures: Clinical diagnostic criteria. *Clin Orthop Relat Res* 2012;470(8):2268-2273.

A retrospective comparison of 66 patients with a surgically confirmed acute Achilles tendon rupture on MRI and 66 patients without a preoperative MRI found that three clinical findings (an abnormal Thompson test, decreased resting tension, and palpable defect) were present in all patients and were 100% sensitive. MRI was less sensitive and was read as inconclusive in two patients. Level of evidence: II.

138. Jones MP, Khan RJ, Carey Smith RL: Surgical interventions for treating acute achilles tendon rupture: Key findings from a recent Cochrane review. *J Bone Joint Surg Am* 2012;94(12):e88.

A Cochrane review of 14 studies compared surgical and nonsurgical treatment of acute Achilles tendon rupture. The results supported surgical treatment, although it was associated with more infections than nonsurgical treatment. The risk was reduced with percutaneous techniques.

139. Soroceanu A, Sidhwa F, Aarabi S, Kaufman A, Glazebrook M: Surgical versus nonsurgical treatment of acute Achilles tendon rupture: A meta-analysis of randomized trials. *J Bone Joint Surg Am* 2012;94(23):2136-2143.

A meta-analysis of 10 studies comparing surgical and nonsurgical treatment of acute Achilles tendon rupture found that functional rehabilitation with early range-of-motion exercises decreased the risk of rerupture to close to that of surgery, with fewer complications. Level of evidence: I.

140. Bergkvist D, Åström I, Josefsson PO, Dahlberg LE: Acute Achilles tendon rupture: A questionnaire follow-up of 487 patients. *J Bone Joint Surg Am* 2012;94(13):1229-1233.

A records review of 487 patients with an acute Achilles tendon rupture found that the rerupture rate was 3% after surgical treatment compared with 6.6% after functional nonsurgical treatment. Level of evidence: III.

141. Barfod KW, Bencke J, Lauridsen HB, Ban I, Ebskov L, Troelsen A: Nonoperative dynamic treatment of acute Achilles tendon rupture: The influence of early weight-bearing on clinical outcome. A blinded, randomized controlled trial. *J Bone Joint Surg Am* 2014;96(18):1497-1503.

Patients received nonsurgical functional treatment for acute Achilles tendon rupture based on full weight bearing (29 patients) or non–weight bearing (27 patients). There were no between-group heel-rise test or mean score differences. The patients who were weight bearing had a better health-related quality of life. Level of evidence: I.

142. Knobloch K, Schreibmueller L, Kraemer R, Jagodzinski M, Vogt PM, Redeker J: Gender and eccentric training in Achilles mid-portion tendinopathy. *Knee Surg Sports Traumatol Arthrosc* 2010;18(5):648-655.

In 63 patients who underwent eccentric training for treatment of midportion Achilles tendinopathy, men with symptoms had significantly better reduction in pain and improvement in scores than women with symptoms at 12-week follow-up. Level of evidence: III.

143. Schon LC, Shores JL, Faro FD, Vora AM, Camire LM, Guyton GP: Flexor hallucis longus tendon transfer in treatment of Achilles tendinosis. *J Bone Joint Surg Am* 2013;95(1):54-60.

A study of 46 sedentary patients (average age, 54 years) who underwent flexor hallucis longus tendon transfer for treatment of insertional or midsubstance Achilles tendinosis found significant improvement in Achilles tendon function, physical function, and pain intensity at 24-month follow-up. Level of evidence: IV.

144. van Dijk CN, van Sterkenburg MN, Wiegerinck JI, Karlsson J, Maffulli N: Terminology for Achilles tendon related disorders. *Knee Surg Sports Traumatol Arthrosc* 2011;19(5):835-841.

Inconsistencies in terminology used for Achilles tendon pathology were outlined. The preferred terminology and classifications of Achilles tendon and related disorders were presented.

145. Wiegerinck JI, Kok AC, van Dijk CN: Surgical treatment of chronic retrocalcaneal bursitis. *Arthroscopy* 2012;28(2):283-293.

A systematic review of surgical treatment of chronic retrocalcaneal bursitis reported on 547 procedures in 461 patients. Patient satisfaction and complication rates favored endoscopic surgery over open surgery. Level of evidence: IV.

146. Nicholson CW, Berlet GC, Lee TH: Prediction of the success of nonoperative treatment of insertional Achilles tendinosis based on MRI. *Foot Ankle Int* 2007;28(4):472-477.

147. Al-Abbad H, Simon JV: The effectiveness of extracorporeal shock wave therapy on chronic Achilles tendinopathy: A systematic review. *Foot Ankle Int* 2013;34(1):33-41.

A report of four randomized controlled studies concluded there was satisfactory evidence for the effectiveness of low-energy ESWT at a minimum 3-month follow-up. A combination of ESWT and eccentric loading had superior results. Level of evidence: I.

148. Wiegerinck JI, Kerkhoffs GM, van Sterkenburg MN, Sierevelt IN, van Dijk CN: Treatment for insertional Achilles tendinopathy: A systematic review. *Knee Surg Sports Traumatol Arthrosc* 2013;21(6):1345-1355.

A systematic review of surgical and nonsurgical treatment of insertional Achilles tendinopathy reported on 452 procedures in 433 patients. Patient satisfaction was high in all surgical studies, ESWT appeared effective in noncalcific insertional tendinopathy, and floor-level eccentric exercises had higher patient satisfaction than full range-of-motion eccentric exercises. Level of evidence: III.

Video References

22.1: Ferkel RD, Stuart KD: *Autologous Chrondrocyte Implantation* [video excerpt]. Van Nuys, CA, 2011.

22.2: Glazebrook M: Conventional Treatment - Debridement Abrasion Microfracture Drilling [video excerpt]. Halifax, Nova Scotia, 2011.

22.3: Hangody L: *OATS Procedure* [video excerpt]. Budapest, Hungary, 2011.

22.4: Coetzee JC: *Anterior Ankle Impingement* [video excerpt]. Edina, MN, 2011.

22.5: Wiegerinck JI, de Leeuw PA, van Dijk CN: *Posterior Ankle Arthroscopy - Impingement Os Trigonum FHL Tenosynovitis* [video excerpt]. Amsterdam, Netherlands, 2011.

22.6: Wiegerinck JI, de Leeuw PA, van Dijk CN: *Haglund Deformity, Achilles Problems*. [video excerpt]. Amsterdam, Netherlands, 2011.

3: Knee and Leg

Rehabilitation

SECTION EDITORS

James J. Irrgang, PhD, PT, ATC, FAPTA

Kevin Wilk, PT, DPT, FAPTA

Chapter 23

Current Concepts in Rehabilitation of Rotator Cuff Pathology: Nonsurgical and Postoperative Considerations

Todd S. Ellenbecker, DPT, MS, SCS, OCS, CSCS   George J. Davies, MD, DPT, MEd, PT, SCS, ATC, LAT, CSCS, PES, FAPTA

Abstract

Rehabilitation of the patient with rotator cuff pathology requires a comprehensive physical examination and evidence-based rehabilitation focusing on restoring normal joint motion, scapular stabilization, and rotator cuff strength. Many patients with rotator cuff tendinitis, impingement, and partial- and full-thickness tears can return to full activity by means of a complete rehabilitation program. Patients who ultimately undergo rotator cuff repair benefit from early range of motion and progression of rehabilitation exercises to treat both range of motion and strength deficiencies.

Keywords: shoulder; rotator cuff; rehabilitation

Introduction

Shoulder pain and conditions comprise one of the more common musculoskeletal problems that occur and can affect 16% to 21% of the population.[1] Rotator cuff pathology can comprise up to 60% of all shoulder conditions. Although several mechanisms have been reported to produce rotator cuff injury, one of the more commonly described mechanisms is shoulder impingement, or compression.

Dr. Ellenbecker or an immediate family member serves as an unpaid consultant to Thera-Band Hygenic. Neither Dr. Davies nor any immediate family member has received anything of value from or has stock or stock options held in a commercial company or institution related directly or indirectly to the subject of this chapter.

Several types of shoulder impingement have been defined in the literature, including primary, secondary, and internal impingement syndromes. The history, mechanism of injury, subjective comments by the patient, examination, and imaging studies all are used to identify the specific condition, and most important, the causative factors of the impingement.[2] Primary impingement usually results from three major causes: encroachment of the rotator cuff in the subacromial space because of swelling or scarring of the pain-generating structures, acromial morphologies (type II or type III acromion), or a selective hypomobility of noncontractile tissues such as the capsule, capsular ligaments, and fascial tissue. Secondary impingement usually results from microinstability of the glenohumeral joint, often because of acquired ligamentous laxity, inadequate dynamic muscular stabilization, and scapular dysfunction.[3] Internal impingement is commonly involved in overhead athletes or when the arm is used in an abducted, externally rotated, and horizontally extended position.[4] In addition to the listed conditions that can cause impingement, most patients will also have neuromuscular dynamic stability deficits of the scapulothoracic and glenohumeral musculature.

Nonsurgical Treatment

When treating patients with subacromial impingement syndrome, a multimodal approach is usually performed that includes, but is not limited to, physical therapy modalities, postural exercises, stretching for tight contractile musculotendinous units, mobilization for tight noncontractile tissue, taping techniques, movement reeducation of the entire kinematic chain, and strengthening of the entire kinematic chain including legs, core, scapulothoracic, and glenohumeral links. This includes rotator cuff,

© 2016 American Academy of Orthopaedic Surgeons

scapular, and total arm strengthening, neuromuscular dynamic stabilization exercises, and advanced functional specificity exercises.[5] Clinicians have an ethical obligation to do everything appropriate to help the patient recover and return to activity. However, because of this multimodal approach and the potential interaction of various interventions, it is not clear which are most effective and which may be unnecessary. Because no high-level evidence indicates the best practice pattern during the early phases of rehabilitation, many of the aforementioned treatment interventions that customize specific interventions to the patient and the cause of the problem can be applied.

The section of this chapter discussing nonsurgical treatment primarily focuses on the application of therapeutic exercises including neuromuscular dynamic stability and outcomes related to treating patients with neuromuscular dynamic stability deficits of the scapulothoracic and/or rotator cuff muscles. These also have exceptional application for postoperative rotator cuff rehabilitation. Numerous studies,[6-11] systematic reviews,[12-16] and meta-analyses[17,18] demonstrate the effectiveness of exercise for patients with subacromial impingement syndrome. Most of these studies demonstrated decreased pain, increased strength, improved movement patterns, and improved functional outcomes in patients following therapeutic exercise for shoulder impingement. Authors of a 2009 study performed a systematic review of 12,428 articles and identified only 11 that had good methodology.[13] Exercise strongly decreased the patients' symptoms and led to significant improvements in functional measures. However, one conclusion of the analysis was the lack of consensus on an ideal treatment program for patients with rotator cuff disease. A 2011 meta-analysis demonstrated the effectiveness of therapeutic exercises on patients with shoulder dysfunction.[17] Another meta-analysis of the effectiveness of therapeutic exercises for treatment of painful shoulder conditions evaluated 19 articles, 17 of which had a rating of 6 or better on the PEDro scale.[18] Therapeutic exercise had a greater positive effect on pain and function than all other interventions; however, subsequent research is necessary for translation to clinical practice.

Therapeutic exercises are usually performed as a combination of isolated and multiple-joint exercises. Most clinicians think that multiple-joint exercises must be performed because they are functional to improve performance. However, other studies have demonstrated that isolated rotator cuff exercises carry over to improving functional movements such as throwing and serving.[19-21]

A group of healthy, uninjured subjects in a training study performed isolated shoulder rehabilitation exercises for each muscle group in the shoulder complex.[22]

After training, functional test outcomes increased during both a closed kinetic chain (weight bearing) test and an open kinetic chain (throwing) test. This study found that subjects who never performed functional multiple-joint movement activity during training demonstrated improvements in these functional outcome measurements. One conclusion from these studies is that performing isolated shoulder exercises without multiple-joint exercises can still improve multiple-joint functional movement activities.

Exercise to Treat Rotator Cuff Pathology

The current review of literature supports the use of exercise to treat rotator cuff pathology. A therapeutic exercise program usually progresses through four stages: (1) muscle activation/motor learning/motor control, (2) muscle strengthening/power/endurance, (3) neuromuscular dynamic stability exercises, and (4) functional specificity exercises. Despite the forthcoming focus on rotator cuff and scapular exercise training, total-body training, including the legs and core muscles, should be performed and is recommended during a comprehensive rehabilitation program. Many training techniques can be used for these areas, but these are beyond the scope of this chapter. The authors of this chapter recommend working each link in the kinematic chain first to establish a good foundation with each muscle group and add the advanced neuromuscular dynamic stability and functional exercises after establishing the "basics."

Scapulothoracic Exercises

The following scapulothoracic exercises are supported by electromyographic (EMG) research and involve movement patterns appropriate for patients with rotator cuff pathology.[23-25]

Scapular Plane Elevation

Scapular plane elevation (scaption with the thumb pointing up) creates a functional strengthening of the force couple with the upper trapezius, lower trapezius, and serratus anterior. In most patients with shoulder dysfunction, the upper trapezius is hypertonic and does not need isolated strengthening. Consequently, this exercise activates both the upper trapezius in the scapula and the glenohumeral muscles. The patient moves through the range of motion (ROM) appropriate to his or her particular shoulder condition (typically limited to less than 90° of elevation to minimize the effects of subacromial contact). Alternating arm motions to prevent compensation and recruit core stabilization are also recommended[26] (Figure 1).

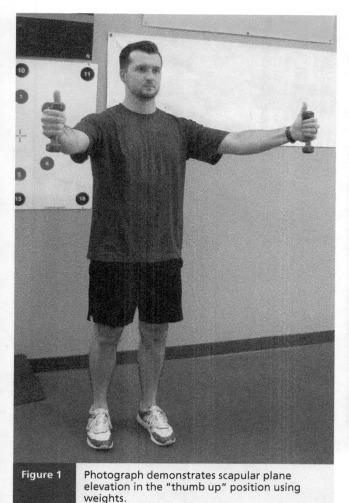

Figure 1 Photograph demonstrates scapular plane elevation in the "thumb up" position using weights.

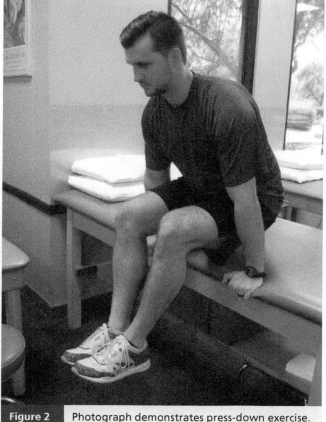

Figure 2 Photograph demonstrates press-down exercise.

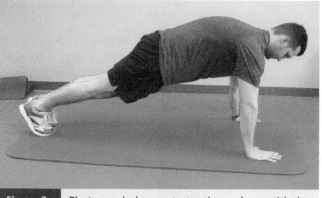

Figure 3 Photograph demonstrates the push-up with the plus position exercise.

Press Down/Up

Many muscle groups are recruited, but the lower trapezius muscles and scapular depressors are substantially activated (Figure 2).

Push-Up With Plus Position and Protraction

The push-up with the plus position is designed to recruit the serratus anterior muscle using the "plus" position, which encourages maximal scapular protraction. If a "hug motion" is used, such as in the dynamic hug exercise,[27] patients are recommended to have their palms face each other (thumbs pointed to the ceiling) to prevent internal rotation at the end of the plus maneuver. If the hands internally rotate, it causes the greater tuberosity to compress the pain generators in the subacromial space and can iatrogenically result in problems or continue aggravating the condition (Figures 3 and 4).

Rowing Motions and Scapular Retraction

The rowing motions activate the middle and lower trapezius muscles as well as the rhomboids. Scapular retraction exercises such as the robbery (Figure 5) and lawnmower exercises (Figure 6) use retraction to activate the muscles.[25,28] Additionally, exercises with elastic resistance such as external rotation with retraction[29] (Figure 7) combine the movements of external rotation with scapular retraction, and EMG research has shown the lower

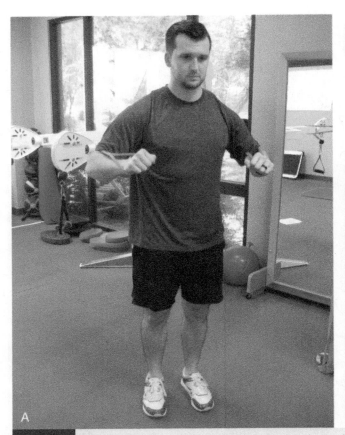 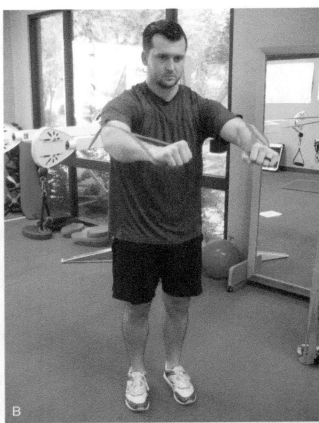

Figure 4 **A** and **B**, Photographs demonstrate dynamic hug using an elastic band.

trapezius is recruited at a 3.3-fold greater rate than the upper trapezius, forming a favorable lower trapezius–to–upper trapezius ratio. This ratio is important when reviewing EMG research of scapular stabilization exercises because many exercise movement patterns produce abnormally high upper trapezius muscle activity, which is unwanted and can result in abnormal motor patterns and recruitment strategies.[30] A 2012 study demonstrated that scapular exercises using a lower resistance level (Borg scale 3 versus Borg scale 8) produce higher lower trapezius–to–upper trapezius ratios, which are beneficial for the rehabilitation of shoulder pathology.[31]

Glenohumeral Exercises for the Rotator Cuff
Internal and External Rotation
Glenohumeral exercises include internal and external rotation exercises starting at 30° abduction/30° forward flexion into scaption/30° diagonal movement, also called the 30/30/30 position (Figures 8 and 9), and progressing the patient to the 90/90 position in the scapular plane (Figure 10), if appropriate.[32,33] The 30/30/30 position is the initial starting position for the rotator cuff strengthening exercises for several reasons. Using 30° of abduction prevents the wringing-out effect on the rotator cuff, speeds the healing process by means of increased blood flow to increase the oxygen and nutrients to the tendon, and decreases the strain on the rotator cuff tendon.[34,35] Using 30° of scapular plane elevation stress shields the antero-inferior capsule and prestretches the posterior shoulder muscles, which increases their length-tension ratio to improve power.[36] In the 30/30/30 position, a bolster is placed under the arm for the aforementioned reasons, but also for research-based reasons. Placing a bolster under the arm and adducting the muscles to hold the bolster in place creates a synergistic overflow (cocontraction/irradiation) to the posterior muscle groups.[32,37] These are the weakest muscles in the shoulder complex, and using the bolster enhances the muscles' ability to generate more power. Moreover, using the bolster and adducting the arm with 15 N of force increased the subacromial space in all arm positions: 30°, 60°, 90°, 120°, and 150° of abduction.[38,39] Because this area of the shoulder is the most vulnerable to impingement, this technique can help minimize subacromial contact stress in this area.

© 2016 American Academy of Orthopaedic Surgeons

Jobe Exercises

Prone horizontal abduction (Figure 11), prone extension (Figure 12), and prone external rotation with 90° of abduction (Figure 13), commonly referred to as Jobe exercises, have been studied extensively since their introduction in 1982.[40] Extensive EMG and research analysis have been performed on these movement patterns (exercises), the exact position of the extremity (thumb pointed out/in and so forth), and their inherent activation levels of the rotator cuff and surrounding musculature.[32,41-45] These exercises collectively report high levels of EMG activation in the rotator cuff including the supraspinatus while decreasing the level of activation of the surrounding deltoid and upper trapezius to minimize or quiet compensation. Additionally, a low-load, high-repetition format is used and recommended to decrease large muscle recruitment during humeral rotation and/or rotator cuff exercises.[46]

Additional Concepts of Exercise for Rotator Cuff Pathology

The 10 upper extremity exercises described for rehabilitation exercises of the shoulder complex should be performed using the following guidelines to establish the foundation by working each link in the kinematic chain. The American College of Sports Medicine and others[47] provide guidelines for designing exercise programs based on more than 700 references. The American College of

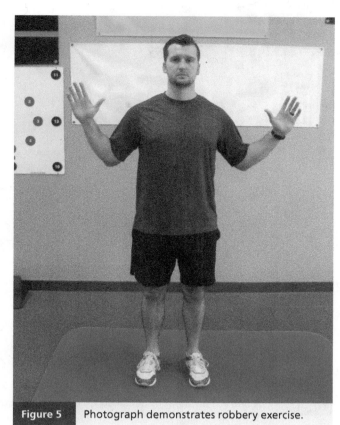

Figure 5 Photograph demonstrates robbery exercise.

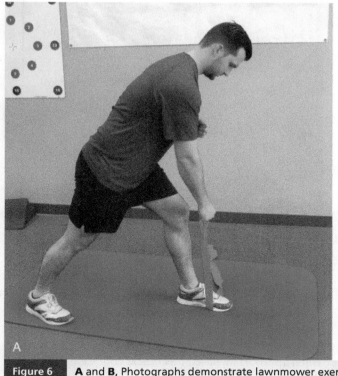

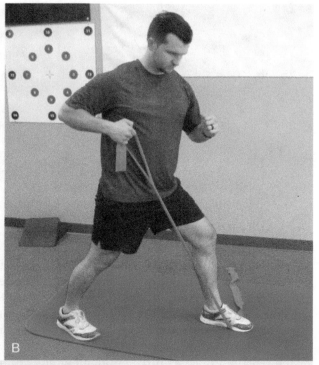

Figure 6 **A** and **B**, Photographs demonstrate lawnmower exercise using an elastic band.

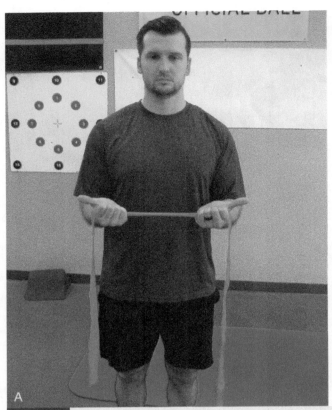
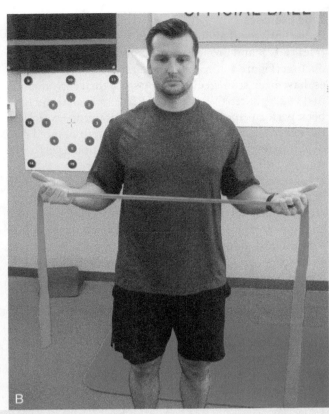

Figure 7　**A** and **B**, Photographs demonstrate external rotation with retraction using an elastic band.

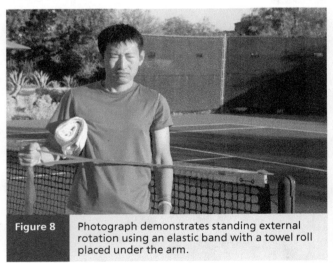

Figure 8　Photograph demonstrates standing external rotation using an elastic band with a towel roll placed under the arm.

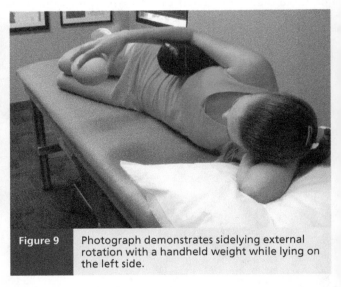

Figure 9　Photograph demonstrates sidelying external rotation with a handheld weight while lying on the left side.

Sports Medicine and others[47] recommend training 3 to 4 days per week with a day of rest and recovery between resistance training workouts. Patients who are untrained should perform one set of exercises; patients who are trained should perform three sets to optimize gains in total work, peak torque, and average power.[48]

Ten repetitions per set is the optimum number to increase strength in the beginning of an exercise program. As the exercise program progresses, the specificity of volume of training (the specific needs and functional demands of the patient) determines the number of repetitions. The rotator cuff muscles are predominantly fast-twitch muscle fibers; therefore, it is important to exercise the muscles when appropriate based on clinical conditions. To recruit the fast-twitch fibers, one must exercise at least 60% of

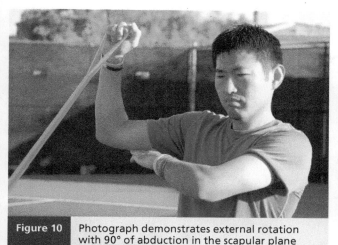

Figure 10 Photograph demonstrates external rotation with 90° of abduction in the scapular plane using an elastic band.

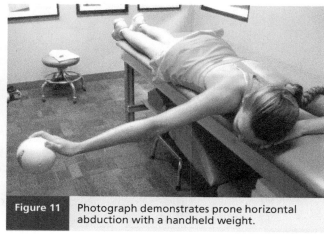

Figure 11 Photograph demonstrates prone horizontal abduction with a handheld weight.

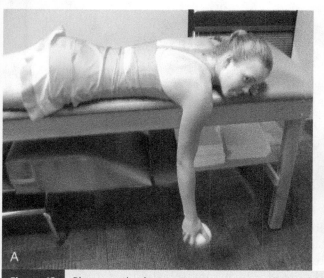

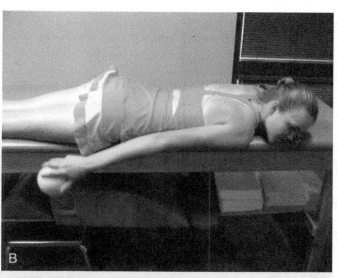

A

B

Figure 12 Photographs demonstrate prone extension with a handheld weight.

the maximal volitional contraction or repetition maximum.[49] The resistance should be established at 60% to 80% of the subject's one-repetition maximal contraction, allowing the subject to complete the exercises through full range of motion (ROM) without deviating from correct technique. The OMNI-Resistance Exercise Scale can be used as a guideline for the patients[50,51] (Figure 14). The patients should use a superset format in which the agonist muscle is trained followed immediately by the antagonist muscle. Supersets were used to improve muscle balance, save time in the clinic, and provide the muscle with recovery time to achieve efficiency of workouts.

After the basic exercises are performed to establish a solid foundation, the advanced neuromuscular dynamic stability and functional exercises are performed. Numerous descriptive articles exist in the literature; however,

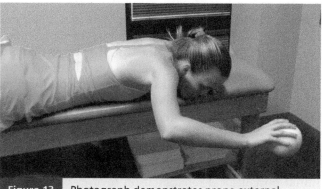

Figure 13 Photograph demonstrates prone external rotation with 90° of abduction with a handheld weight.

limited studies demonstrate the effectiveness of the programs in a prospective, systematic manner. Based on

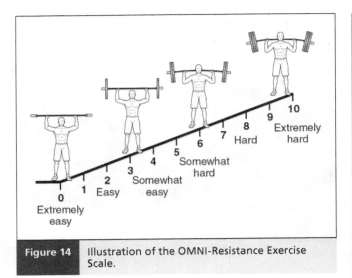

Figure 14 Illustration of the OMNI-Resistance Exercise Scale.

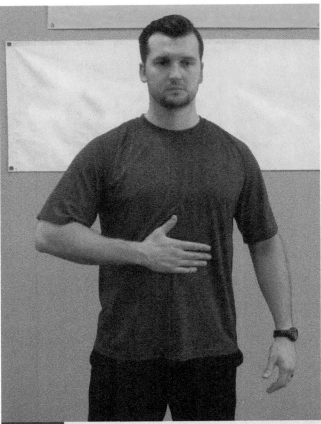

Figure 15 Photograph demonstrates the stomach rub exercise.

a 2009 systematic review, limited high-level evidence supports the effectiveness of some of these advanced interventions in rehabilitation with patients.[52] Plyometric exercises have been indicated in throwing athletes to increase throwing velocity and both concentric and eccentric strength.[53] A recent EMG study[54] quantified the muscular activity of plyometric shoulder exercises performed in 90° of abduction that are commonly used in high-level rehabilitation programs.[30] Finally, the use of isokinetic test results and training in shoulder rehabilitation is supported in the literature. An extensive review on this topic outlined evidence-based training paradigms, population-specific descriptive data, and exercise progressions.[55]

Postoperative Concepts

A 2012 research study compared the increase in rotator cuff repairs performed between 1996 and 2006 and identified national trends, including the increased number of total rotator cuff repairs as well as those that are performed arthroscopically (a 600% increase from 1996 to 2006).[56] Postoperative rehabilitation concepts (Figures 15 and 16) used by the authors of this chapter following arthroscopic rotator cuff repair are listed in Table 1.

ROM Concepts

Initial postsurgical rehabilitation focuses on ROM to prevent capsular adhesion while protecting the surgically repaired tissues. Some postsurgical protocols have specific ROM limitations that are applied during the first 6 weeks of rehabilitation. Several basic science studies provide a rationale for the safe application of glenohumeral joint ROM, specifically outlining the movement's joint excursions and capsular lengthening that provide safe inherent tensions in the repaired tendon. A 2001 cadaver model of repaired 1 × 2–cm supraspinatus tears studied the effects of humeral rotation ROM on the tension in the supraspinatus in 30° of elevation in the coronal, scapular, and sagittal planes.[57] Compared with tension in a position of neutral rotation, external rotation of 30° and 60° actually resulted in decreased tension within the supraspinatus musculotendinous unit. In contrast, 30° and 60° of internal rotation resulted in increased tension within the supraspinatus tendon. Because most patients are placed in positions of internal rotation following surgery during the immobilization period, internal shoulder rotation is performed despite the increased tension. In addition, the tensile load in the repaired supraspinatus tendon was compared in the coronal, scapular, and sagittal planes during humeral rotation simulation. Substantially higher loading was present in the supraspinatus tendon during humeral rotation in the sagittal plane compared with both the frontal and scapular planes. Therefore, early passive ROM should be performed in the directions of

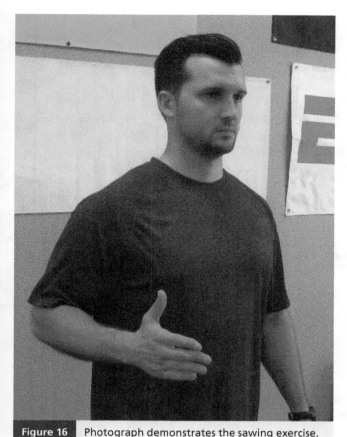

Figure 16 Photograph demonstrates the sawing exercise.

both external and internal humeral rotation using the scapular plane position to minimize tensile loading in the repaired tendon.

The effects of passive motion on tensile loading of the supraspinatus tendon were also studied in 2006.[58] No substantial increases in strain were found during the movement of cross-arm adduction in either the supraspinatus or infraspinatus tendons at 60° of elevation. However, internal rotation performed at 30° and 60° of elevation placed increased tension in the inferiormost portion of the infraspinatus tendon over the resting or neutral position. This study demonstrated the importance of knowing the degree of tendon involvement and repair because posteriorly based rotator cuff repairs (those involving the infraspinatus and teres minor) can be subjected to increased tensile loads if early internal rotation is applied during postoperative rehabilitation. Communication between the surgeon and treating therapist is of vital importance to ensure that optimal ROM is performed following repair.

Passive Versus Active-Assisted ROM

The progression from passive ROM applications to active-assisted and active ROM is important in the early stages of rehabilitation following arthroscopic rotator cuff repair. Some disagreement among clinicians exists regarding the amount of muscular activation occurring during activities commonly used for rehabilitation. A 1993 study clearly delineated the degree of muscular activation of the supraspinatus during supine assisted ROM and seated elevation with the use of a pulley.[59] Although both activities produce low levels of inherent muscular activation in the supraspinatus, the upright pulley activity produces substantially more muscular activity than the supine activities. The delay in upright pulley or active-assisted elevation exercises is present in several prominent rehabilitation protocols that inherently use only passive ROM in the initial 6-week period following surgery.[60] To truly minimize muscle activation, ROM performed by a physical therapist with the patient supine is indicated based on the results of the 1993 study.[59]

The levels of muscular activation during the Codman pendulum exercise have been quantified in a study that shows minimal levels of muscular activation in the rotator cuff musculature.[61] However, the exercise cannot be considered passive because the musculature is truly activated, especially in individuals with shoulder pathology. In addition, although many therapists do not recommend holding a weight in the hand during pendulum exercises to avoid potential anterior translation, activity in the rotator cuff musculature was not changed between performing the pendulum exercise with or without a handheld weight.

A more recent study measured supraspinatus and infraspinatus EMG activity in patients performing a series of early rehabilitation exercises following subacromial decompression and distal clavicular resection.[62] These exercises included therapist-assisted external rotation and elevation performed in the supine position, patient-assisted external rotation and elevation performed in the supine position, as well as pulleys, table flexion, and scapular retraction exercises. EMG activity during these early rehabilitation exercises was compared with baseline levels (standing at rest) in the infraspinatus and supraspinatus muscles. The findings showed no difference between therapist-assisted external rotation and elevation and baseline activity in the supraspinatus and infraspinatus. Pendulum exercises were also not different from baseline EMG levels in those muscles. This study supported therapist-assisted external rotation and elevation for patients following shoulder surgery because the level of muscular activity inherent in these maneuvers facilitates early joint motion and mobilization without musculotendinous unit activation above baseline (standing posture) levels.

Rehabilitation in the first 2 to 4 weeks following rotator cuff repair typically consists of truly passive and several minimally active or active-assisted exercises for the

Table 1

Postoperative Rehabilitation Protocol for Arthroscopic Rotator Cuff Repair of a Medium-Size Tear

General Guidelines

Progression of resistance exercise and ROM depends on patient tolerance.

Resistance exercise should not be performed with specific shoulder joint pain or pain over the incision site.

A sling is provided for support as needed with daily activities and to wear at night. The patient should be weaned from the sling as tolerated and under the direction of the referring surgeon.

Early home exercises given to the patient following surgery should include stomach rubs (Figure 15), sawing (Figure 16), and distal gripping activity.

Progression to assisted ROM against gravity and duration of sling use is determined by the size of the rotator cuff tear and the quality of the tissue and fixation.

Postoperative Weeks 1 and 2

Early postoperative ROM to patient tolerance during the first 4 to 6 weeks

  Flexion

  Scapular and coronal plane abduction

  IR/ER with 90° to 45° abduction as tolerated

Mobilization of the glenohumeral joint and scapulothoracic joint. Passive stretching of elbow, forearm, and wrist to terminal ranges.

Side-lying scapular protraction/retraction resistance to encourage early serratus anterior and lower trapezius activation and endurance.

Home exercise instruction:

  Postoperative and active-assisted ROM exercises with T-bar, pulleys, or opposite-arm assistance in supine position using ROM to patient tolerance.

  Weight-bearing (closed chain) Codman exercise over a ball or countertop/table

  Therapeutic putty for grip strength maintenance

Postoperative Week 3

Continue above-shoulder ROM and add isometric strength program (IR/ER in neutral) to patient tolerance.

Begin active scapular strengthening exercises and continue side-lying manual scapular stabilization exercise:

  Scapular retraction

  Scapular retraction with depression

Begin submaximal rhythmic stabilization using the balance point position (90° to 100° elevation) in supine position to initiate dynamic stabilization.

ER = external rotation, IR = internal rotation, ROM = range of motion.

rotator cuff such as active-assisted elevation and pendulum exercises. The balance point position (90° of shoulder elevation in the scapular plane) in the supine position is also used: the patient is queued to perform small active motions of flexion/extension from the 90° starting position to recruit rotator cuff and scapular muscular activity. These exercises, coupled with early scapular stabilization via manual resistance techniques emphasizing direct hand contact on the scapula to bypass force application to the rotator cuff and optimize trapezius, rhomboid, and serratus anterior muscular activation, are recommended.

Early scapular stabilization exercises have also been advocated using EMG quantification of low-level closed chain exercise such as weight shifting on a rocker board.[25,63] The low levels (< 10%) of activation of the rotator cuff and scapular musculature during application were highlighted as well as several exercises such as robbery and the low row, which produce low to moderate levels of scapular stabilizer activation while not placing the shoulder with a repaired rotator cuff in harmful positions.

Table 1 (continiued)

Postoperative Rehabilitation Protocol for Arthroscopic Rotator Cuff Repair of a Medium-Size Tear

Postoperative Weeks 5 and 6

Initiate isometric and isotonic resistance exercise focusing on the following movements:

 Standing IR/ER isometric step-outs with elastic resistance

 Sidelying ER

 Prone extension

 Prone horizontal abduction (range limited to 45°; 8 weeks postoperative)

 Side-lying flexion to 90°

A low-resistance/high-repetition (for example, 30 repetitions) format is recommended initially using no resistance (such as the weight of the arm).

Progression to full postoperative and assisted ROM in all planes including ER and IR in neutral adduction, progressing from the 90° abducted position used initially postoperatively.

ER oscillation (resisted ER with a towel roll under axilla and a body blade or flexion bar)

Home exercise program for strengthening the rotator cuff and scapular musculature with isotonic weights and/or elastic tubing.

Postoperative Week 10

Begin closed chain step-ups and quadruped rhythmic stabilization exercise.

Initiate upper extremity plyometric chest passes and functional two-hand rotation tennis groundstroke or golf swing simulation using small exercise ball progressing to light medicine ball as tolerated.

Postoperative Week 12

Initiation of submaximal isokinetic exercise for IR/ER in the modified neutral position.

Criterion for progression to isokinetic exercise:

 Patient has IR/ER ROM greater than that used during the isokinetic exercise.

 Patient can complete isotonic exercise program pain-free with a 2- to 3-lb weight or medium resistance surgical tubing or elastic band.

Progression to 90° abducted rotational training in patients returning to overhead work or sport.

 Prone ER

 Standing ER/IR with 90° abduction in the scapular plane

 Statue of Liberty (ER oscillation in the 90/90 position)

Reevaluation of strength with isometric IR/ER strength (at side), goniometric ROM (active and passive ROM), and functional outcome measures

Postoperative Week 16

Progression to maximal isokinetics in IR/ER and isokinetic test results to assess strength in modified base 30/30/30 position. Formal documentation of assisted ROM, postoperative ROM, and shoulder rating scales.

Begin interval return programs if following criteria have been met:

 IR/ER strength at minimum of 85% of contralateral extremity

 ER/IR ratio is 60% or higher

 Pain-free ROM

 Negative impingement and instability signs during clinical examination

Preparation for discharge from formal physical therapy to home program phase

ER = external rotation, IR = internal rotation, ROM = range of motion.

Resistance Exercise

The progression to resistance exercise for strengthening the rotator cuff and scapular musculature typically occurs in an interval of approximately 6 weeks following surgery. The time for initiation of resistance exercise varies substantially[64,65] and is based on several factors including, but not limited to, tear size, tear type, tendon retraction, tissue quality, fatty infiltration, concomitant surgical procedures, patient health status, and age. Communication between the referring surgeon and physical therapist is critical to ensure information is shared regarding fixation limitations, tissue challenges, and/or other concomitant relative factors that would limit the progression of postsurgical rehabilitation.

The clinical application of resistance exercise during this critical stage of rehabilitation should be guided by both the literature detailing the level of muscular activity within the individual muscles of the rotator cuff and scapular stabilizers and the patient's demonstrated exercise tolerance.[32,33,37,41,44,54] The application of low resistance levels used in a repetitive format are recommended both for safety and relative protection of the repaired tissues as well as to improve local muscular endurance. Multiple sets of 15 to 20 repetitions have been recommended and described in several training studies to improve muscular strength in the rotator cuff and scapular stabilizing musculature.[66-68] Exercise patterns that use shorter lever arms and maintain the glenohumeral joint in positions less than 90° of elevation and anterior to the coronal plane of the body (such as the scapular plane) are theorized to reduce the risks of both compressive irritation and capsular loading/attenuation.[65] In addition, early focus on the rotator cuff and scapular stabilizers without emphasis on larger, primary muscles such as the deltoid, pectorals, and upper trapezius are recommended to minimize joint shear and inappropriate arthrokinematics as well as optimizing external/internal rotation muscle balance.[69]

One specific exercise that has been described extensively in the literature is the empty can exercise: scapular plane elevation with an internally rotated (thumb pointed down) arm position. Although EMG studies have shown high levels of supraspinatus activation during the empty can exercise,[41,70,71] the combined movements of elevation and internal rotation have produced clinically disappointing results in practical application as well as common patterns of substitution and improper biomechanical execution. A 2006 study quantified these compensations objectively and showed increases in scapular internal rotation and anterior tilting when comparing the empty can and full can (scapular plane elevation with external rotation) exercises using motion analysis.[42] Movement patterns characterized by scapular internal rotation and anterior tilt theoretically decrease the subacromial space and could compromise the ability to perform repetitive movement patterns required to improve strength during shoulder rehabilitation.

Progression to Functional Activities

The patient evaluation used to determine return to functional and recreational activities requires reexamination of clinical test results, objective determination of ROM and muscular strength, and the ability to simulate functional movement patterns without symptoms or unwanted compensatory movement deviations. Progression to advanced strengthening exercises, including isokinetic training, emphasizes the movement of internal and external rotation, which prepares the patient for the increased loading and faster angular joint movements inherent in most functional activities.[55] The contralateral extremity is used as the baseline for most patients and allows a meaningful comparison of postsurgical ROM and muscular strength. Although the goal is a full return of both passive and active ROM as well as muscular strength and endurance, these indices cannot always be measured during the initial length of many rehabilitation programs. Formal rehabilitation should restore 85% to 90% of rotational strength compared with that of the contralateral uninjured extremity, as well as muscular balance represented via an external/internal rotation strength ratio of at least 60% (66% to 75% is the preferred ratio), before recommending the patient return to functional activities such as upper extremity sports and aggressive activities of daily living. In addition, clinical impingement and instability signs should also be eliminated before higher level activities can be recommended.

Short-term follow-up of patients for 12 weeks following both mini-open[65] and arthroscopic[72] rotator cuff repair shows the return of almost full active and passive ROM, with deficits in muscular strength ranging from 10% to 30% in internal and external rotation compared with the uninjured extremity. Greater deficits following both mini-open and arthroscopic rotator cuff repair have been reported in the posterior rotator cuff (external rotator muscles) despite emphasis placed on these structures during postsurgical rehabilitation.

Early Versus Delayed ROM: Effect on Outcome

Early versus delayed ROM is likely one of the areas of greatest controversy and variation in rehabilitation following rotator cuff repair. Given the increase in the numbers of arthroscopic rotator cuff repairs being performed, rehabilitation professionals and surgeons have been investigating this particular issue for some time. A systematic review in 2009[73] found insufficient evidence to provide an evidence-based conclusion or recommendation regarding immobilization versus early passive ROM for rotator cuff repair rehabilitation.[74]

Five randomized controlled trials (RCTs) have been published comparing early passive ROM to sling immobilization following arthroscopic rotator cuff repair.[74-78] A meta-analysis identified the important findings from these RCTs for clinical application.[79] Advocates of early passive ROM following surgery cite the most common complication following arthroscopic rotator cuff repair (postoperative stiffness) as the primary rationale for early mobilization and movement;[80,81] opponents cite the high incidence of re-tear.[82,83] The meta-analysis[79] shows that early postoperative passive ROM results in substantial increases in shoulder flexion at 3, 6, and 12 months after surgery compared with immobilization. External rotation ROM also increased across the early passive ROM groups; however, this increase was only significant at 3 months after surgery. Perhaps most important, early passive ROM did not result in increased rotator cuff re-tear rates at a minimum follow-up of 1 year. The studies included in this analysis excluded massive rotator cuff tears. A 2012 study also excluded retracted tears and those that extended beyond a single tendon.[74]

These results indicate that early passive ROM is not a risk factor for increased re-tear rates following arthroscopic rotator cuff repairs. The early motion performed in these studies included pendulum exercises and manual passive ROM performed by a physical therapist. A 2013 study showed that therapist-assisted passive ROM does not produce EMG activity in the supraspinatus and infraspinatus above baseline levels (postural standing at rest).[62] This finding, coupled with the results of increased ROM in elevation and external rotation in the meta-analysis,[79] supports the use of early passive ROM following rotator cuff repair.

A 2011 study applied a modified early ROM protocol in 79 patients with identified risk factors for stiffness following arthroscopic rotator cuff repair.[60] These risk factors included calcific tendinitis, partial articular supraspinatus tendon avulsion lesions, concomitant superior labrum anterior to posterior repairs, preoperative adhesive capsulitis, and single-tendon rotator cuff repairs. The protocol included patient-directed ROM with a polyvinyl chloride bar as well as the use of table slides performed in a seated position next to a table top. No patient experienced any postoperative stiffness with the modified treatment protocol following rotator cuff repair, and an early motion protocol is advocated for patients following rotator cuff repair.

Summary

It is important to review the current concepts and evidence regarding key elements of rehabilitation for rotator cuff pathology. The benefits and indications for ROM and rotator cuff and scapular strengthening form the primary focus of rehabilitation efforts presently recommended and supported in the current literature. Further research is always needed and is indeed forthcoming regarding greater delineation of the specific parameters and characteristics of exercise interventions as well as additional randomized clinical trials to develop optimal protocols for rehabilitation of the patient with rotator cuff pathology.

Key Study Points

- Rotator cuff rehabilitation involves specific application of exercise interventions that activate the rotator cuff and scapular musculature at high levels without placing the cuff in positions or movement patterns that promote impingement or instability.

- It is imperative that both nonsurgical and postoperative rotator cuff rehabilitation begin with a key foundation of scapular stabilization exercises. Weakness or dykinesis of the scapula is a common clinical finding in patients with rotator cuff disorders, and early rehabilitation and emphasis on the serratus anterior and lower trapezius force couple is recommended.

- Postoperative rotator cuff rehabilitation begins with early passive range of motion to protect the repair while preventing the development of postoperative stiffness, followed by scapular stabilization exercise and finally rotator cuff strengthening to restore full active motion, muscular strength, and endurance.

Annotated References

1. Picavet HS, Schouten JS: Musculoskeletal pain in the Netherlands: Prevalences, consequences and risk groups, the DMC(3)-study. *Pain* 2003;102(1-2):167-178.

2. Davies GJ, Gould J, Larson R: Functional examination of the shoulder girdle. *Phys Sportsmed* 1981;9(6):82-104.

3. Jobe FW, Kvitne RS, Giangarra CE: Shoulder pain in the overhand or throwing athlete. The relationship of anterior instability and rotator cuff impingement. *Orthop Rev* 1989;18(9):963-975.

4. Walch G, Boileau P, Noel E, Donell ST: Impingement of the deep surface of the supraspinatus tendon on the

posterosuperior glenoid rim: An arthroscopic study. *J Shoulder Elbow Surg* 1992;1(5):238-245.

5. Tate AR, McClure PW, Young IA, Salvatori R, Michener LA: Comprehensive impairment-based exercise and manual therapy intervention for patients with subacromial impingement syndrome: A case series. *J Orthop Sports Phys Ther* 2010;40(8):474-493.

   This case series reviewed the use of manual therapy, exercise, and thrust and nonthrust manipulations for patients with subacromial impingement. At 12 weeks, 80% of patients had a successful outcome (50% improvement in the Disabilities of the Arm, Shoulder and Hand score). This study supports the use of exercise and manual therapy for patients with subacromial impingement. Level of evidence: IV.

6. Ainsworth R, Lewis JS: Exercise therapy for the conservative management of full thickness tears of the rotator cuff: A systematic review. *Br J Sports Med* 2007;41(4):200-210.

7. Bang MD, Deyle GD: Comparison of supervised exercise with and without manual physical therapy for patients with shoulder impingement syndrome. *J Orthop Sports Phys Ther* 2000;30(3):126-137.

8. Haahr JP, Østergaard S, Dalsgaard J, et al: Exercises versus arthroscopic decompression in patients with subacromial impingement: A randomised, controlled study in 90 cases with a one year follow up. *Ann Rheum Dis* 2005;64(5):760-764.

9. Ketola S, Lehtinen J, Arnala I, et al: Does arthroscopic acromioplasty provide any additional value in the treatment of shoulder impingement syndrome?: A two-year randomised controlled trial. *J Bone Joint Surg Br* 2009;91-B(10):1326-1334.

   One hundred forty patients were randomized into groups undergoing either arthroscopic acromioplasty and postoperative exercise or exercise alone. Analysis of the visual analog scale pain ratings showed that arthroscopic acromioplasty did not provide an additional benefit over exercise rehabilitation alone in patients with subacromial impingement.

10. McClure PW, Bialker J, Neff N, Williams G, Karduna A: Shoulder function and 3-dimensional kinematics in people with shoulder impingement syndrome before and after a 6-week exercise program. *Phys Ther* 2004;84(9):832-848.

11. Senbursa G, Baltaci G, Atay A: Comparison of conservative treatment with and without manual physical therapy for patients with shoulder impingement syndrome: A prospective, randomized clinical trial. *Knee Surg Sports Traumatol Arthrosc* 2007;15(7):915-921.

12. Michener LA, Walsworth MK, Burnet EN: Effectiveness of rehabilitation for patients with subacromial impingement syndrome: A systematic review. *J Hand Ther* 2004;17(2):152-164.

13. Kuhn JE: Exercise in the treatment of rotator cuff impingement: A systematic review and a synthesized evidence-based rehabilitation protocol. *J Shoulder Elbow Surg* 2009;18(1):138-160.

   This review of 11 RCTs focused on the effect of exercise for patients with subacromial impingement. The results of the studies showed that exercise had a substantial effect on improving pain and function but not directly on ROM and increasing strength.

14. Desmeules F, Côté CH, Frémont P: Therapeutic exercise and orthopedic manual therapy for impingement syndrome: A systematic review. *Clin J Sport Med* 2003;13(3):176-182.

15. Grant HJ, Arthur A, Pichora DR: Evaluation of interventions for rotator cuff pathology: A systematic review. *J Hand Ther* 2004;17(2):274-299.

16. Green S, Buchbinder R, Hetrick S: Physiotherapy interventions for shoulder pain. *Cochrane Database Syst Rev* 2003;2:CD004258.

17. Brudvig TJ, Kulkarni H, Shah S: The effect of therapeutic exercise and mobilization on patients with shoulder dysfunction : A systematic review with meta-analysis. *J Orthop Sports Phys Ther* 2011;41(10):734-748.

   Seven RCTs were identified that used therapeutic exercise and manual therapy for patients with shoulder disorders. Manual therapy did not provide an additional benefit scientifically to exercise in patients with rotator cuff pathology. Level of evidence: 1a.

18. Marinko LN, Chacko JM, Dalton D, Chacko CC: The effectiveness of therapeutic exercise for painful shoulder conditions: A meta-analysis. *J Shoulder Elbow Surg* 2011;20(8):1351-1359.

   This meta-analysis of 19 articles specific to the use of exercise in shoulder rehabilitation concluded that exercise made a positive contribution to pain reduction and the improvement of function in patients with shoulder conditions. Level of evidence: 1a.

19. Ellenbecker TS, Davies GJ, Rowinski MJ: Concentric versus eccentric isokinetic strengthening of the rotator cuff. Objective data versus functional test. *Am J Sports Med* 1988;16(1):64-69.

20. Mont MA, Cohen DB, Campbell KR, Gravare K, Mathur SK: Isokinetic concentric versus eccentric training of shoulder rotators with functional evaluation of performance enhancement in elite tennis players. *Am J Sports Med* 1994;22(4):513-517.

21. Treiber FA, Lott J, Duncan J, Slavens G, Davis H: Effects of Theraband and lightweight dumbbell training on shoulder rotation torque and serve performance in college tennis players. *Am J Sports Med* 1998;26(4):510-515.

22. Byrnes E, Simpson L, Stephens G, Riemann BL, Davies GJ: Comparison of random vs blocked protocol design for

upper extremity rehabilitation: a prospective randomized controlled training study (Honorable mention financial award). Graduate Student Research Presentations, - AASU, Savannah, GA, April, 17, 2007 (MS Thesis, 2007).

23. Moseley JB Jr, Jobe FW, Pink M, Perry J, Tibone J: EMG analysis of the scapular muscles during a shoulder rehabilitation program. *Am J Sports Med* 1992;20(2):128-134.

24. Ekstrom RA, Donatelli RA, Soderberg GL: Surface electromyographic analysis of exercises for the trapezius and serratus anterior muscles. *J Orthop Sports Phys Ther* 2003;33(5):247-258.

25. Kibler WB, Sciascia AD, Uhl TL, Tambay N, Cunningham T: Electromyographic analysis of specific exercises for scapular control in early phases of shoulder rehabilitation. *Am J Sports Med* 2008;36(9):1789-1798.

26. Wilk KE, Yenchak AJ, Arrigo CA, Andrews JR: The Advanced Throwers Ten Exercise Program: A new exercise series for enhanced dynamic shoulder control in the overhead throwing athlete. *Phys Sportsmed* 2011;39(4):90-97.

   This commentary included advanced shoulder exercises focusing on bilateral upper extremity performance and use of a physio ball to improve shoulder activation and provide a training stimulus to progressively improve shoulder strength and endurance. The exercises provided can be incorporated into advanced rehabilitation programs for patients with shoulder pathology. Level of evidence: V.

27. Decker MJ, Hintermeister RA, Faber KJ, Hawkins RJ: Serratus anterior muscle activity during selected rehabilitation exercises. *Am J Sports Med* 1999;27(6):784-791.

28. Tsuruike M, Ellenbecker TS: Serratus anterior and lower trapezius muscle activities during multi-joint isotonic scapular exercises and isometric contractions. *J Athl Train* 2015;50(2):199-210.

   This study provided EMG analysis of several key scapular exercises used in rehabilitation of shoulder patients including a quadruped arm elevation, robbery, and lawnmower exercises. The interactions of exercise intensity with external loading and muscle activation of the serratus anterior and lower trapezius are provided in this clinically applicable study. Level of evidence: Cross-sectional laboratory study.

29. McCabe RA, Orishimo KF, McHugh MP, Nicholas SJ: Surface electromygraphic analysis of the lower trapezius muscle during exercises performed below ninety degrees of shoulder elevation in healthy subjects. *N Am J Sports Phys Ther* 2007;2(1):34-43.

30. Ellenbecker TS, Cools A: Rehabilitation of shoulder impingement syndrome and rotator cuff injuries: An evidence-based review. *Br J Sports Med* 2010;44(5):319-327.

   This paper reviews evidence for the treatment of rotator cuff pathology. Detailed reviews of therapeutic exercise, manual therapy including rotator cuff strengthening, and scapular stabilization are provided. Exercises that promote activation of the lower trapezius and serratus anterior in addition to rotator cuff activation are recommended and summarized. Level of evidence: V.

31. Andersen CH, Zebis MK, Saervoll C, et al: Scapular muscle activity from selected strengthening exercises performed at low and high intensities. *J Strength Cond Res* 2012;26(9):2408-2416.

   This study analyzed EMG activity between the upper and lower trapezius musculature under Borg scale 3 and 8 conditions. Increased lower trapezius activation and reduced upper trapezius activation was found with lower intensity exercises for scapular stabilization (Borg scale 3) compared with higher intensity exercise. This study has important clinical application for therapists designing optimal programs for patients with shoulder pathology. Level of evidence: Controlled laboratory study.

32. Reinold MM, Wilk KE, Fleisig GS, et al: Electromyographic analysis of the rotator cuff and deltoid musculature during common shoulder external rotation exercises. *J Orthop Sports Phys Ther* 2004;34(7):385-394.

33. Hintermeister RA, Lange GW, Schultheis JM, Bey MJ, Hawkins RJ: Electromyographic activity and applied load during shoulder rehabilitation exercises using elastic resistance. *Am J Sports Med* 1998;26(2):210-220.

34. Rathbun JB, Macnab I: The microvascular pattern of the rotator cuff. *J Bone Joint Surg Br* 1970;52(3):540-553.

35. Biberthaler P, Wiedemann E, Nerlich A, et al: Microcirculation associated with degenerative rotator cuff lesions. In vivo assessment with orthogonal polarization spectral imaging during arthroscopy of the shoulder. *J Bone Joint Surg Am* 2003;85-A(3):475-480.

36. Saha AK: The classic. Mechanism of shoulder movements and a plea for the recognition of "zero position" of glenohumeral joint. *Clin Orthop Relat Res* 1983;173:3-10.

37. Reinold MM, Macrina LC, Wilk KE, et al: Electromyographic analysis of the supraspinatus and deltoid muscles during 3 common rehabilitation exercises. *J Athl Train* 2007;42(4):464-469.

38. Graichen H, Hinterwimmer S, von Eisenhart-Rothe R, Vogl T, Englmeier KH, Eckstein F: Effect of abducting and adducting muscle activity on glenohumeral translation, scapular kinematics and subacromial space width in vivo. *J Biomech* 2005;38(4):755-760.

39. Hinterwimmer S, Von Eisenhart-Rothe R, Siebert M, et al: Influence of adducting and abducting muscle forces on the subacromial space width. *Med Sci Sports Exerc* 2003;35(12):2055-2059.

40. Jobe FW, Moynes DR: Delineation of diagnostic criteria and a rehabilitation program for rotator cuff injuries. *Am J Sports Med* 1982;10(6):336-339.

41. Townsend H, Jobe FW, Pink M, Perry J: Electromyographic analysis of the glenohumeral muscles during

a baseball rehabilitation program. *Am J Sports Med* 1991;19(3):264-272.

42. Thigpen CA, Padua DA, Morgan N, Kreps C, Karas SG: Scapular kinematics during supraspinatus rehabilitation exercise: A comparison of full-can versus empty-can techniques. *Am J Sports Med* 2006;34(4):644-652.

43. Takeda Y, Kashiwaguchi S, Endo K, Matsuura T, Sasa T: The most effective exercise for strengthening the supraspinatus muscle: Evaluation by magnetic resonance imaging. *Am J Sports Med* 2002;30(3):374-381.

44. Ballantyne BT, O'Hare SJ, Paschall JL, et al: Electromyographic activity of selected shoulder muscles in commonly used therapeutic exercises. *Phys Ther* 1993;73(10):668-677, discussion 677-682.

45. Alpert SW, Pink MM, Jobe FW, McMahon PJ, Mathiyakom W: Electromyographic analysis of deltoid and rotator cuff function under varying loads and speeds. *J Shoulder Elbow Surg* 2000;9(1):47-58.

46. Bitter NL, Clisby EF, Jones MA, Magarey ME, Jaberzadeh S, Sandow MJ: Relative contributions of infraspinatus and deltoid during external rotation in healthy shoulders. *J Shoulder Elbow Surg* 2007;16(5):563-568.

47. Carroll TJ, Abernethy PJ, Logan PA, Barber M, McEniery MT: Resistance training frequency: Strength and myosin heavy chain responses to two and three bouts per week. *Eur J Appl Physiol Occup Physiol* 1998;78(3):270-275.

48. Durrall C, Hermsen D, Demuth C: Systemic review of single-set versus multiple-set resistance- training randomized controlled trials: Implications for rehabilitation. *Crit Rev Phys Rehabil Med* 2006;18(2):107-116.

49. Lovering RM, Russ DW: Fiber type composition of cadaveric human rotator cuff muscles. *J Orthop Sports Phys Ther* 2008;38(11):674-680.

50. Colado JC, Garcia-Masso X, Triplett TN, Flandez J, Borreani S, Tella V: Concurrent validation of the OMNI-resistance exercise scale of perceived exertion with Thera-band resistance bands. *J Strength Cond Res* 2012;26(11):3018-3024.

This study validated using the OMNI-Resistance Exercise Scale to objectively evaluate exercise intensity using a visual scale. This allows clinicians to accurately understand the exercise intensity from the patient for optimal resistance exercise progression and strength development.

51. Colado JC, Garcia-Masso X, Triplett NT, et al: Construct and concurrent validation of a new resistance intensity scale for exercise with thera-band® elastic bands. *J Sports Sci Med* 2014;13(4):758-766.

This study focused on the use of elastic resistance using a validated progression of color-based elastic bands and concomitant exercise intensity.

52. Zech A, Hübscher M, Vogt L, Banzer W, Hänsel F, Pfeifer K: Neuromuscular training for rehabilitation of sports injuries: A systematic review. *Med Sci Sports Exerc* 2009;41(10):1831-1841.

This systematic review identified 20 RCTs that supported the use of balance training and proprioceptive training to improve neuromuscular control in patients with orthopaedic injuries. This study supports the current use of proprioceptive exercise interventions and provides key objective evidence for its inclusion in rehabilitation programs. Level of evidence: Systematic review.

53. Carter AB, Kaminski TW, Douex AT Jr, Knight CA, Richards JG: Effects of high volume upper extremity plyometric training on throwing velocity and functional strength ratios of the shoulder rotators in collegiate baseball players. *J Strength Cond Res* 2007;21(1):208-215.

54. Ellenbecker TS, Sueyoshi T, Bailie DS: Muscular activation during plyometric exercises in 90° of glenohumeral joint abduction. *Sports Health* 2015;7(1):75-79.

This study analyzed the EMG results of two plyometric exercises performed in 90° of glenohumeral joint abduction, which had high activation levels of the infraspinatus, lower trapezius, and serratus anterior. 0.5- and 1-kg exercise loads were used. These exercises are recommended for clinical use to increase rotator cuff and scapular strength. Level of evidence: Controlled laboratory study.

55. Ellenbecker TS, Davies GJ: The application of isokinetics in testing and rehabilitation of the shoulder complex. *J Athl Train* 2000;35(3):338-350.

56. Colvin AC, Egorova N, Harrison AK, Moskowitz A, Flatow EL: National trends in rotator cuff repair. *J Bone Joint Surg Am* 2012;94(3):227-233.

This study analyzed the number of rotator cuff repairs between 1996 and 2006. A 141% increase was found in the number of rotator cuff repairs and a 600% increase in the repairs performed arthroscopically were reported.

57. Hatakeyama Y, Itoi E, Urayama M, Pradhan RL, Sato K: Effect of superior capsule and coracohumeral ligament release on strain in the repaired rotator cuff tendon. A cadaveric study. *Am J Sports Med* 2001;29(5):633-640.

58. Muraki T, Aoki M, Uchiyama E, Murakami G, Miyamoto S: The effect of arm position on stretching of the supraspinatus, infraspinatus, and posterior portion of deltoid muscles: A cadaveric study. *Clin Biomech (Bristol, Avon)* 2006;21(5):474-480.

59. McCann PD, Wootten ME, Kadaba MP, Bigliani LU: A kinematic and electromyographic study of shoulder rehabilitation exercises. *Clin Orthop Relat Res* 1993;288:179-188.

60. Koo SS, Parsley BK, Burkhart SS, Schoolfield JD: Reduction of postoperative stiffness after arthroscopic rotator cuff repair: Results of a customized physical therapy regimen based on risk factors for stiffness. *Arthroscopy* 2011;27(2):155-160.

This case series studied 152 patients (152) who underwent rotator cuff repair; 79 were at high risk for stiffness. Patients in this subgroup were given a table slide exercise in addition to a standardized rehabilitation program. The patients in this group did not develop stiffness and the authors recommend this exercise for patients who are at risk for stiffness following rotator cuff repair.

61. Ellsworth AA, Mullaney M, Tyler TF, McHugh M, Nicholas S: Electromyography of selected shoulder musculature during un-weighted and weighted pendulum exercises. *N Am J Sports Phys Ther* 2006;1(2):73-79.

62. Murphy CA, McDermott WJ, Petersen RK, Johnson SE, Baxter SA: Electromyographic analysis of the rotator cuff in postoperative shoulder patients during passive rehabilitation exercises. *J Shoulder Elbow Surg* 2013;22(1):102-107.

This study examined 14 passive shoulder rehabilitation exercises and compared them with baseline activity in the shoulder 4 days following shoulder surgery using fine wire electrodes. Exercises such as therapist-assisted supine ROM and external rotation, pendulum exercises, and isometric internal rotation created supraspinatus activity level similar to baseline. Actual levels were not reported but were measured relative to baseline activity. This information provides key evidence for clinicians on early muscle activation during passive exercises used following rotator cuff repair. Level of evidence: EMG laboratory study.

63. Kibler WB, Livingston B, Bruce R: Current concepts in shoulder rehabilitation, in *Advances in Operative Orthopaedics* .St Louis, Mosby, 1995, pp 249-297, vol 3.

64. Wilk KE, Arrigo C: Current concepts in the rehabilitation of the athletic shoulder. *J Orthop Sports Phys Ther* 1993;18(1):365-378.

65. Ellenbecker TS, Elmore E, Bailie DS: Descriptive report of shoulder range of motion and rotational strength 6 and 12 weeks following rotator cuff repair using a mini-open deltoid splitting technique. *J Orthop Sports Phys Ther* 2006;36(5):326-335.

66. Moncrief SA, Lau JD, Gale JR, Scott SA: Effect of rotator cuff exercise on humeral rotation torque in healthy individuals. *J Strength Cond Res* 2002;16(2):262-270.

67. Wang CH, McClure P, Pratt NE, Nobilini R: Stretching and strengthening exercises: Their effect on three-dimensional scapular kinematics. *Arch Phys Med Rehabil* 1999;80(8):923-929.

68. Giannakopoulos K, Beneka A, Malliou P, Godolias G: Isolated vs. complex exercise in strengthening the rotator cuff muscle group. *J Strength Cond Res* 2004;18(1):144-148.

69. Lee SB, An KN: Dynamic glenohumeral stability provided by three heads of the deltoid muscle. *Clin Orthop Relat Res* 2002;400:40-47.

70. Malanga GA, Jenp YN, Growney ES, An KN: EMG analysis of shoulder positioning in testing and strengthening the supraspinatus. *Med Sci Sports Exerc* 1996;28(6):661-664.

71. Kelly BT, Kadrmas WR, Speer KP: The manual muscle examination for rotator cuff strength. An electromyographic investigation. *Am J Sports Med* 1996;24(5):581-588.

72. Ellenbecker TS, Fischer DJ, Zeman D: Glenohumeral joint range of motion, rotational isokinetic strength, and functional self-report measures following All-Arthroscopic rotator cuff repair.[Abstract]. *J Orthop Sports Phys Ther* 2006;36(1):A68.

73. Baumgarten KM, Vidal AF, Wright RW: Rotator cuff repair rehabilitation. A level I and II systematic review. *Sports Health* 2009;1(2):125-130.

This systematic review of rotator cuff repair rehabilitation studies noted a paucity of evidence identified in high-level studies. The use of continuous passive motion was not supported by the literature by one study included in this review. Level of evidence: I.

74. Arndt J, Clavert P, Mielcarek P, Bouchaib J, Meyer N, Kempf JF; French Society for Shoulder & Elbow (SOFEC): Immediate passive motion versus immobilization after endoscopic supraspinatus tendon repair: A prospective randomized study. *Orthop Traumatol Surg Res* 2012;98(6, Suppl):S131-S138.

This study analyzed the effects of immediate passive ROM following rotator cuff repair with complete immobilization for 6 weeks following surgery. Improved functional results were found in the early passive ROM group without decreases in healing. This study supports early passive ROM following rotator cuff repair. Level of evidence: I.

75. Cuff DJ, Pupello DR: Prospective randomized study of arthroscopic rotator cuff repair using an early versus delayed postoperative physical therapy protocol. *J Shoulder Elbow Surg* 2012;21(11):1450-1455.

This prospective, randomized controlled trial studied 68 patients who either started physical therapy on postoperative day 2 or were immobilized and had ROM initiated after 6 weeks. No significant difference was reported between groups in ROM, re-tear rates, and patient satisfaction at 1 year. Level of evidence: I.

76. Kim YS, Chung SW, Kim JY, Ok JH, Park I, Oh JH: Is early passive motion exercise necessary after arthroscopic rotator cuff repair? *Am J Sports Med* 2012;40(4):815-821.

In this study, 105 patients underwent arthroscopic rotator cuff repair (excluding large and massive tears) and were randomized into either an early ROM group with motion three to four times per day while wearing an immobilizer, or into a delayed motion group with no motion for 4 to 5 weeks. ROM and VAS pain ratings were compared at 1-year follow-up and several other intervals and no substantial differences were found between the two groups. Early passive postoperative ROM did not produce greater ROM but also did not increase re-tear rates.

77. Lee BG, Cho NS, Rhee YG: Effect of two rehabilitation protocols on range of motion and healing rates after arthroscopic rotator cuff repair: Aggressive versus limited early passive exercises. *Arthroscopy* 2012;28(1):34-42.

In this study, 64 patients were assigned to either an aggressive early motion and unlimited self-stretching group or a limited passive exercise group following arthroscopic rotator cuff repair. Patients in the early motion group showed an early increase in shoulder ROM over the limited passive motion group. No substantial difference was found in ROM at 1-year follow up. No substantial difference in re-tear rates was found between the two groups.

78. Keener JD, Galatz LM, Stobbs-Cucchi G, Patton R, Yamaguchi K: Rehabilitation following arthroscopic rotator cuff repair: A prospective randomized trial of immobilization compared with early motion. *J Bone Joint Surg Am* 2014;96(1):11-19.

In this study, 122 patients younger than 65 years underwent arthroscopic rotator cuff repair and either underwent a traditional rehabilitation program with early passive ROM or were immobilized for 6 weeks with no motion. No long-term differences were found in functional return, ROM, and strength between groups and no difference in rotator cuff healing was seen between the two groups. Level of evidence: I.

79. Riboh JC, Garrigues GE: Early passive motion versus immobilization after arthroscopic rotator cuff repair. *Arthroscopy* 2014;30(8):997-1005.

This meta-analysis identified five RCTs of early passive ROM following arthroscopic rotator cuff repair. Improved flexion ROM was noted at 3 months, 6 months, and 12 months postoperatively. External rotation was only identified as superior with early motion at 3 months. No difference was noted in re-tear rates between early and delayed passive ROM. Level of evidence: II.

80. Brislin KJ, Field LD, Savoie FH III: Complications after arthroscopic rotator cuff repair. *Arthroscopy* 2007;23(2):124-128.

81. Namdari S, Green A: Range of motion limitation after rotator cuff repair. *J Shoulder Elbow Surg* 2010;19(2):290-296.

In this review of 345 patients who underwent rotator cuff repair, mean active forward flexion was 90%, external rotation was 78%, and internal rotation was 80% of the contralateral side at 3-month follow-up. Patients with restricted preoperative ROM were more likely to have limited ROM postoperative that was significant. Only 3 of 47 patients who had stiffness at 1 year required capsular release.

82. Galatz LM, Ball CM, Teefey SA, Middleton WD, Yamaguchi K: The outcome and repair integrity of completely arthroscopically repaired large and massive rotator cuff tears. *J Bone Joint Surg Am* 2004;86-A(2):219-224.

83. Tashjian RZ, Hollins AM, Kim HM, et al: Factors affecting healing rates after arthroscopic double-row rotator cuff repair. *Am J Sports Med* 2010;38(12):2435-2442.

In this study, 49 shoulders with full-thickness rotator cuff tears underwent arthroscopic double-row repair and were evaluated for tendon healing at a minimum 6-month follow-up: at ultrasonographic evaluation, 51% of tendons were healed, 67% of single-tendon tears showed complete healing, and 36% of multiple-tendon tears showed healing. Increased age and longer follow-up time were significant factors for healing limitations in this study.

Chapter 24

Nonsurgical and Postoperative Rehabilitation for Injuries of the Overhead Athlete's Elbow

Kevin E. Wilk, PT, DPT, FAPTA   Todd R. Hooks, PT, ATC, OCS, SCS, NREMT-1, CSCS, CMTPT, FAAOMPT

Abstract

Overhead athletes are subject to injuries at the elbow joint as a result of high levels of forces imparted onto the elbow during the throwing motion. Injuries can be acute to the point of tissue failure, or chronic as a result of repetitive overuse. It is imperative that the restoration of elbow function is achieved to allow the elbow to return to its prior level of function. Systematic and progressive rehabilitation programs can help avoid overstressing healing tissues. The treatment programs are designed to restore full motion, muscular strength, and endurance, and restore neuromuscular control. Multiphased rehabilitation programs are designed to restore function in the overhead athlete's elbow and include both nonsurgical and specific postoperative pathologies of the overhead athlete.

Keywords: overhead athlete; ulnar collateral ligament; elbow; rehabilitation

Dr. Wilk or an immediate family member serves as a paid consultant to LiteCure Medical, IntelliSkin, and ZetrOz; serves as an unpaid consultant to AlterG; has received research or institutional support from IntelliSkin; and has received nonincome support (such as equipment or services), commercially derived honoraria, or other non–research-related funding (such as paid travel) from Educational Grant, Bauerfeind, and ERMI. Neither Mr. Hooks nor any immediate family member has received anything of value from or has stock or stock options held in a commercial company or institution related directly or indirectly to the subject of this chapter.

Introduction

Elbow injuries are common in the overhead athlete because of the repetitive nature of overhead sporting activities. Elbow injuries have been reported to represent approximately 22% to 26% of all injuries in Major League Baseball.[1,2] The elbow extends at more than 2300°/s during overhead throwing, which produces a medial shear force of 300 N and a compressive force of 900 N.[3] These forces impart a valgus stress of 64 N·m[3] during the acceleration phase of throwing, which exceeds the ultimate tensile strength of the ulnar collateral ligament (UCL).

Throughout the throwing motion, several forces converge at the elbow.[3] During the acceleration phase of throwing, valgus stresses at the elbow create tension across the medial elbow, whereas compression forces are applied to the lateral aspect of the elbow during this phase of throwing.[3] During the acceleration and deceleration phases of throwing, the posterior compartment is subject to valgus extension overload as a result of tensile, compressive, and torsional forces that can cause osteophyte formation, stress fractures of the olecranon, or physeal injury.[4,5]

The rehabilitation program described in this chapter uses a multiphased approach focused on returning the athlete to the prior level of function via a systematic process. This program is divided into four phases that are designed to follow a gradual progression of exercises and stresses applied methodically to restore strength, dynamic stability, and neuromuscular control. The key to a successful and effective treatment program is the identification of each athlete's causative factors, facilitating the design of a specific treatment program to address these factors. Guidelines for rehabilitation following elbow injury (Table 1) and elbow arthroscopy (Table 2) are presented. The postoperative rehabilitation programs for specific pathologies and for surgical intervention also are included.

Table 1

Nonsurgical Rehabilitation Program for Elbow Injuries

I. Acute Phase (Week 1)

Goals: To improve motion, diminish pain and inflammation, retard muscle atrophy

Exercises

1. Stretches for wrist, elbow, and shoulder joint

2. Strengthening exercises; isometrics for wrist, elbow, and shoulder musculature

3. Pain and inflammation control: cryotherapy, HVGS, ultrasound, and whirlpool

II. Intermediate Phase (Weeks 2-4)

Goals: To normalize motion; improve muscular strength, power, and endurance

Week 2

1. Initiate isotonic strengthening for wrist and elbow muscles.

2. Initiate exercise tubing exercises for shoulder.

3. Continue using cryotherapy and other pain-control modalities.

Week 3

1. Initiate rhythmic stabilization drills for elbow and shoulder joint.

2. Progress isotonic strengthening for entire upper extremity.

3. Initiate isokinetic strengthening exercises for elbow flexion/extension.

Week 4

1. Initiate Thrower's Ten Program.

2. Emphasize work on eccentric biceps, concentric triceps, and wrist flexor.

3. Progress endurance training.

4. Initiate light plyometric drills.

5. Initiate swinging drills.

III. Advanced Strengthening Phase (Weeks 4-8)

Goals: To prepare athlete for return to functional activities

Criteria: To progress to advanced phase

1. Full nonpainful ROM

2. No pain or tenderness

3. Satisfactory isokinetic test

4. Satisfactory clinical examination

Table 1 (continued)

Nonsurgical Rehabilitation Program for Elbow Injuries

Weeks 4-5

1. Continue daily strengthening exercises, endurance drills, and flexibility exercises.

2. Continue Thrower's Ten Program.

3. Progress plyometric drills.

4. Emphasize maintenance program based on pathology.

5. Progress swinging drills (for example, hitting).

Weeks 6-8

1. Initiate interval sport program as determined by physician.

2. Begin Phase I program.

IV. Return-to-Activity Phase (Weeks 6-9)

Return to play depends on the athlete's condition and progress; physician determines when it is safe.

1. Continue strengthening program and Thrower's Ten Program.

2. Continue flexibility program.

3. Progress functional drills to unrestricted play.

HGVS = high-voltage galvanic stimulation, ROM = range of motion.

Data from Wilk KE, Reinhold MM, Andrews JR: Rehabilitation of the thrower's elbow. *Tech Hand Up Extrem Surg* 2003;7(4):197-216.

Nonsurgical Rehabilitation

Phase I: Acute Phase

The first phase of the elbow rehabilitation program is designed to reduce pain and inflammation, normalize range of motion (ROM) and muscle balance, correct postural adaptations, and re-establish baseline dynamic joint stability. During this phase, the athlete may be prescribed NSAIDs and/or local injections. In addition, the clinician can use local therapeutic modalities such as ice, iontophoresis, phonophoresis, and electrical stimulation to reduce pain and inflammation. The athlete also is educated about activity avoidance and activity modification during throwing, exercise, and other strenuous activities. Following the initial acute inflammation phase, the clinician can use moist heat, a warm whirlpool, and/or ultrasound to increase local circulation and soft-tissue extensibility to increase the pliability of the joint capsule and musculotendinous tissues.

ROM activities are initiated in the acute phase of treatment to ensure the normalization of motion. All aspects of elbow mobility should be assessed, but it is common for the overhead athlete to display a loss of elbow extension

Table 2

Postoperative Rehabilitation Protocol for Elbow Arthroscopy

I. Initial Phase (Week 1)

Goals: Full wrist and elbow ROM, swelling and pain reduction, retardation of muscle atrophy

Day of surgery

Begin gently moving elbow in bulky dressing.

Postoperative days 1 and 2

Replace bulky dressing with elastic bandages.

Immediate postoperative hand, wrist, and elbow exercises

 Putty/grip strengthening

 Wrist flexor stretches

 Wrist extensor stretches

 Wrist curls

 Reverse wrist curls

 Neutral wrist curls

 Pronation/supination

 AROM elbow extension/flexion

Postoperative days 3 through 7

PROM elbow extension/flexion (motion to tolerance)

Begin PRE exercises with 1-lb weight.

 Wrist curls

 Reverse wrist curls

 Neutral wrist curls

 Pronation/supination

 Broomstick roll-up

II. Intermediate Phase (Weeks 2-4)

Goal: To improve muscular strength and endurance, normalize joint arthrokinematics

Week 2

 ROM exercises (overpressure into extension)

 Add biceps curl and triceps extension.

 Continue to progress PRE weight and repetitions as tolerable.

 Supraspinatus

 Scapulothoracic strengthening

Table 2 (*continued*)

Postoperative Rehabilitation Protocol for Elbow Arthroscopy

Week 3

 Initiate biceps eccentric exercise program.

 Initiate shoulder exercise program.

  External rotators

  Internal rotators

  Deltoid

  Supraspinatus

  Scapulothoracic strengthening

III. Advanced Phase (Weeks 4-8)

Goal: To prepare athlete for return to functional activities

Criteria to progress to advanced phase

 Full nonpainful ROM

 Absence of pain or tenderness

 Isokinetic test that fulfills criteria to throw

 Satisfactory clinical examination

Weeks 4 through 6

 Continue maintenance program, emphasizing muscular strength, endurance, flexibility.

 Initiate interval throwing program phase

ROM = range of motion, AROM = active range of motion, PROM = passive range of motion, PRE = progressive resistance exercise.

in particular. The authors of a 2006 study evaluated 33 professional baseball players during the preseason and determined a mean loss of elbow extension of 7° and a mean loss of elbow flexion of 5.5°, compared with the contralateral elbow.[6] The elbow is predisposed to flexion contractures because of the intimate congruency of the joint articulations, the tightness of the joint capsule, and the tendency of the anterior capsule to develop adhesions following injury.[7] Furthermore, the brachialis muscle attaches to the anterior joint capsule as it crosses the elbow joint, and injury to the elbow joint can create excessive scar tissue formation of the brachialis muscle, causing functional splinting of the elbow.[7] Therefore, ROM activities should be performed for all planes of elbow and wrist motions to prevent the formation of scar tissue and adhesions by providing nourishment to the articular cartilage and assisting in the synthesis, alignment, and organization of collagen tissue.[7-9,] Restoring full elbow extension or preinjury ROM is the primary goal of early ROM activities, to minimize the occurrence of elbow flexion contractures.[10] Determining the athlete's preinjury ROM helps to guide the clinician in restoring motion. The athlete also can be queried whether full elbow extension was present before injury.

Joint mobilization may be performed to minimize the occurrence of joint contractures and improve joint mobility. Grade I and II mobilizations are used initially and

4. Rehabilitation

are progressed to grade III and IV mobilizations during the later stages of rehabilitation, as symptoms subside. Grade I and II mobilization techniques also may be used to neuromodulate pain by stimulating type I and type II articular receptors. Posterior glides of the humeroulnar joint are performed at end range of joint mobility to assist in the regaining of full elbow extension (**Figure 1**). In addition, the clinician may perform mobilization for the radiocapitellar and radioulnar joints.

The aggressiveness of the stretching and mobilization techniques is determined by the healing constraints of the involved tissues, the specific pathology or surgery, and the amount of motion and end feel. If the patient presents with a reduction in motion and a hard end feel without pain, aggressive stretching and mobilization techniques may be used. Conversely, a patient who exhibits pain before resistance or an empty end feel should be progressed slowly with gentle stretching. In addition, it

is beneficial to be aggressive with glenohumeral rehabilitation to improve ROM through internal rotation and external rotation stretching.

Occasionally, patients may continue to have difficulty achieving full elbow extension. In such cases, the clinician can implement a low-load, long duration (LLLD) stretch to produce deformation or creep of the collagen tissue, which results in tissue elongation. Clinically, this stretch can be performed by having the patient lie supine with a towel roll placed under the distal humerus to act as a cushion and fulcrum. Light resistance exercise tubing is applied to the patient's wrist and secured to the table or to a dumbbell on the ground (**Figure 2, A**) as the patient is instructed to relax for the duration of 10 to 15 minutes of LLLD treatment. The amount of resistance applied should be of low magnitude to enable the patient to perform the stretch for the entire duration without pain or muscle spasm; this technique should impart a low-load but a long-duration stretch. Patients are instructed to perform the LLLD stretches several times per day, equaling at least 60 minutes of total end range time. This type of program has been referred to as the total end range time program.[11] The program has been extremely beneficial for patients with a stiff elbow. In some patients, it may be beneficial to use splinting and bracing to create the LLLD stretch (**Figure 2, B**).

The early phase of rehabilitation also focuses on the voluntary activation of muscle and the retardation of muscular atrophy. Pain-free submaximal isometrics are performed initially for the elbow flexors and extensors, wrist flexors and extensors, as well as the forearm pronators and supinators. Shoulder isometrics also may be

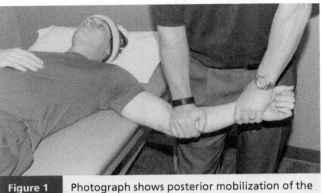

Figure 1 Photograph shows posterior mobilization of the ulna to improve elbow extension.

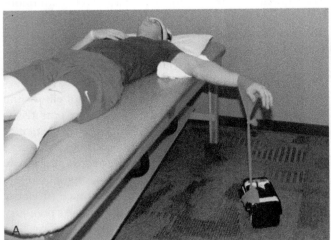

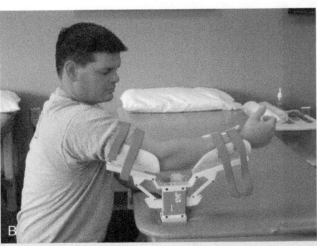

Figure 2 Photographs demonstrate the low-load, long duration (LLLD) stretch to increase elbow extension. **A,** The stretch is performed using light resistance while the shoulder is placed in internal rotation, with the forearm pronated to minimize compensation and best isolate the stretch on the elbow joint. **B,** Splinting and bracing using a commercial device also can be used to create the LLLD stretch and perform elbow extension range of motion as part of a home exercise program.

© 2016 American Academy of Orthopaedic Surgeons

performed during this phase, with caution against internal rotation and external rotation exercises if they are painful. Alternating rhythmic stabilization drills for shoulder flexion, extension, horizontal abduction, and adduction as well as shoulder internal rotation and external rotation are performed. Elbow flexion, extension, supination, and pronation also are performed to begin reestablishing proprioception and neuromuscular control of the upper extremity. Furthermore, the patient's shoulder joint ROM may be addressed during this phase using a stretching program to improve internal rotation and horizontal adduction.

Phase II: Intermediate Phase

Phase II is initiated when the patient has achieved full ROM, experiences minimal pain and tenderness, and has a good (4/5) score with manual muscle testing of the elbow flexor and extensor musculature. The goals of this phase of treatment are to progress the strengthening program, maintain normal physiologic flexibility, mobility, and ROM of the elbow, and enhance neuromuscular control.

Stretching and ROM exercises of the elbow, shoulder, and trunk are progressed throughout this phase of rehabilitation. Joint mobilization techniques may be progressed to grades III and IV to apply a stretch to the joint capsule and improve joint mobility. Flexibility exercises are continued for the wrist flexors, extensors, pronators, and supinators, with increased emphasis on improving elbow extension and forearm pronation flexibility.

Shoulder mobility and flexibility should be assessed, because it is common for the overhead athlete to lose internal rotation and horizontal adduction. The loss of internal rotation commonly is described as a glenohumeral internal rotation deficit (GIRD). An 18° loss of internal rotation in the throwing shoulder has been implicated in elbow injuries.[12] GIRD has been attributed to osseous adaptations, posterior rotator cuff tightness, posterior capsule tightness, and an anteriorly tilted scapula.[12-14] A proper clinical assessment to differentiate between altered scapula positioning, posterior capsule tightness, and/or posterior shoulder tightness is essential for the clinician to direct the appropriate treatment program. Shoulder external rotation also should be assessed, because a loss of motion can result in increased strain on the medial aspect of the elbow during the throwing motion. Shoulder flexibility exercises in all planes of movement also are continued during this phase. The clinician may assess for the total arc of motion and compare the motion to the contralateral shoulder.

Strengthening exercises are progressed to include isotonic exercises, beginning with concentric activities and progressing to eccentric activities. Although emphasis is

Table 3

Exercises for the Scapular Musculature

- Seated scapular neuromuscular control with manual resistance
- Sidelying scapular neuromuscular control with manual resistance
- Prone horizontal abduction (prone T's) on table or stability ball
- Prone full can (prone Y's) on table or stability ball
- Prone rowing into external rotation (prone W's) on table or stability ball
- Prone extensions (prone I's) on table or stability ball
- Seated modified robbery movement for lower trapezius
- Wall circles
- Corner stretch for pectoralis minor

placed on the entire elbow and forearm musculature, the clinician should incorporate strengthening exercises for the glenohumeral and scapulothoracic musculature as well. The Thrower's Ten Program,[15] which is based on electromyography (EMG) data to ensure the restoration of muscle balance in the treatment of the overhead athlete, can be used.[16,17] Because the external rotators are commonly weak, particular focus is placed on this muscle group by the inclusion of sidelying shoulder external rotation and prone rowing into shoulder external rotation exercises, because these movements have been shown to have high EMG activity of the posterior rotator cuff.[18]

The scapula is critical for optimal arm function, because it provides the proximal stability needed for efficient distal arm mobility. The importance of the scapular muscles in facilitating optimal shoulder function has been well described by numerous authors.[19,20] The scapular retractors, protractors, and depressors are emphasized because of their commonly noted weakness. Specific exercises (Table 3) have been developed, designed to normalize the force couples of the scapular musculature and enhance proprioceptive and kinesthetic awareness to facilitate neuromuscular control of the scapulothoracic joint.[21]

Closed kinetic chain exercises are advanced to include proprioceptive drills such as table push-ups on a tilt board or ball (Figure 3). These drills have been shown to generate increased upper and middle trapezius and serratus anterior activity compared with a standard push-up exercise.[22] Rhythmic stabilization drills can be performed by having the athlete place a hand on a small ball against a wall as the clinician performs perturbation drills to the athlete's arm (Figure 4). Additionally, neuromuscular

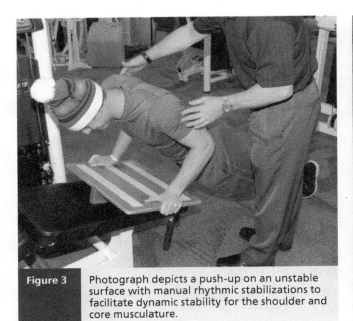

Figure 3   Photograph depicts a push-up on an unstable surface with manual rhythmic stabilizations to facilitate dynamic stability for the shoulder and core musculature.

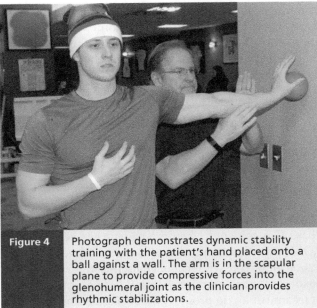

Figure 4   Photograph demonstrates dynamic stability training with the patient's hand placed onto a ball against a wall. The arm is in the scapular plane to provide compressive forces into the glenohumeral joint as the clinician provides rhythmic stabilizations.

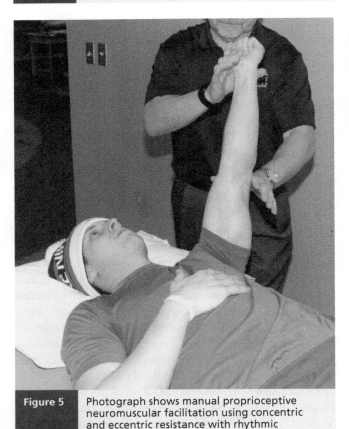

Figure 5   Photograph shows manual proprioceptive neuromuscular facilitation using concentric and eccentric resistance with rhythmic stabilizations.

control exercises can be performed for the upper extremity, including proprioceptive neuromuscular facilitation exercises with rhythmic stabilizations and manual resistance drills (Figure 5).

Phase III: Advanced Strengthening Phase

Phase III is designed to initiate aggressive strengthening exercises, progress functional drills, enhance power and endurance, and improve neuromuscular control to prepare for a gradual return to sport. Before advancing to this phase, the athlete should exhibit full nonpainful ROM, have no pain or tenderness, and demonstrate strength that is 70% of that of the contralateral extremity.

Muscle fatigue has been shown to decrease neuromuscular control and diminish proprioceptive sense.[23] Therefore, the athlete is progressed with strengthening activities using the Advanced Thrower's Ten Exercise Program, which incorporates high-level endurance and alternating movement patterns to further challenge neuromuscular control and restore muscle balance and symmetry in the throwing athlete.[24] The incorporation of sustained holds challenges the athlete to maintain a set position while the opposite extremity performs isotonic exercises. Three sets are incorporated into each exercise, each following a sequential progression that integrates bilateral isotonic movement and unilateral isotonic movement with a contralateral sustained hold and alternating isotonic/sustained-hold sequencing. The athlete can be instructed to perform these exercises on a stability ball to further challenge the core. Manual resistance drills can be added to increase muscle excitation and promote endurance. Manual resistance provided by the clinician is applied to seated stability ball exercises to augment muscle excitation and improve the endurance of the shoulder and core musculature (Figure 6).

Elbow flexion exercises are progressed to emphasize

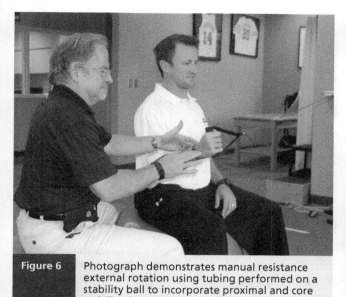

Figure 6 Photograph demonstrates manual resistance external rotation using tubing performed on a stability ball to incorporate proximal and core stabilization.

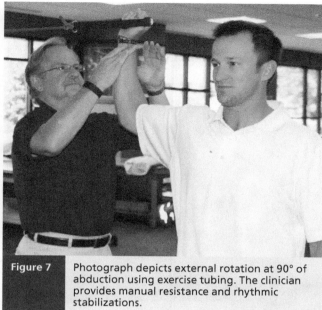

Figure 7 Photograph depicts external rotation at 90° of abduction using exercise tubing. The clinician provides manual resistance and rhythmic stabilizations.

eccentric control. The biceps muscle is an important stabilizer during the follow-through phase of overhead throwing, because it eccentrically controls the deceleration of the elbow and therefore prevents pathologic abutment of the olecranon within the fossa.[25] Elbow flexion can be performed with elastic tubing to emphasis slow- and fast-speed concentric and eccentric contractions. Manual resistance can be applied for concentric and eccentric contractions of the elbow flexors. The triceps are exercised primarily with a concentric contraction because of the acceleration (muscle shortening) activity of this muscle during the acceleration phase of throwing. Aggressive strengthening exercises with weight machines also are incorporated during this phase. These exercises most commonly begin with bench presses, seated rowing, and front latissimus dorsi pulldowns.

Neuromuscular control exercises are progressed to include sidelying external rotation with manual resistance. Concentric and eccentric external rotation are performed against the clinician's resistance, with the addition of rhythmic stabilization at end range. This manual resistance exercise may be progressed to standing external rotation with exercise tubing at 0° and finally at 90° (Figure 7).

Plyometric exercises are initiated to further enhance dynamic stability and proprioception and to introduce and gradually increase functional stresses to the shoulder joint. Enhanced joint position sense and kinesthesia as well as decreased time for peak torque generation were seen following 6 weeks of single-arm plyometric tosses performed at 90° of shoulder abduction as demonstrated with isokinetic testing.[26] In a comparison of 8 weeks of plyometric exercises with conventional isotonic training, an increase of shoulder internal rotation power and throwing distance was reported.[27] Plyometric exercises begin with a rapid prestretch eccentric contraction that stimulates the muscle spindle, followed by the amortization phase, which marks the time between the eccentric and concentric phase. To allow an effective transfer of energy and prevent the beneficial neurologic effects of the prestretch from being dissipated as heat, this phase should be as short as possible. The athlete is instructed to coordinate the trunk and lower extremity to most efficiently facilitate the transfer of energy into the upper extremity during the plyometric drills. A plyometric program has been described that systematically introduces stresses on the healing tissues, beginning with two-hand drills such as the chest pass, side-to-side throws, side throws, and overhead soccer throws.[28] On successful completion of these two-hand drills, the athlete can progress to one-hand drills, including standing one-hand throws, wall dribbles, and plyometric step-and-throw exercises. Specific plyometric drills for the forearm musculature include wrist flexion (Figure 8) and extension flips, which are important components of an elbow rehabilitation program that emphasize the forearm and hand musculature.

Muscle fatigue has been shown to diminish proprioceptive sense and alter biomechanics; therefore, muscle endurance training should be included in any rehabilitation program for overhead athletes.[29] Kinematic and kinetic motion analysis reported in a 2001 study showed that shoulder external rotation and ball velocity declined along with lead knee flexion and shoulder

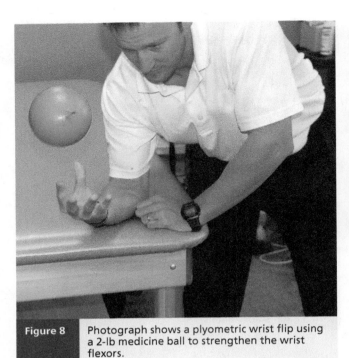

Figure 8 | Photograph shows a plyometric wrist flip using a 2-lb medicine ball to strengthen the wrist flexors.

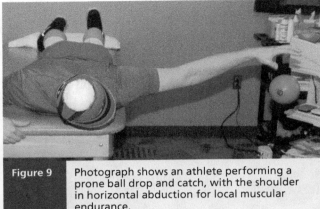

Figure 9 | Photograph shows an athlete performing a prone ball drop and catch, with the shoulder in horizontal abduction for local muscular endurance.

adduction torque after a thrower became fatigued.[30] Endurance training performed by the athlete includes wall dribbles with a medicine ball, prone ball drops (Figure 9) wall arm circles, the upper-body cycle, and Advanced Thrower's Ten Program exercises.

Phase IV: Return-to-Activity Phase

Phase IV of the rehabilitation program enables the athlete to continue progressing with activities that allow a return to full competition. This phase includes an interval throwing program (ITP). The criteria required to begin phase IV of treatment include the achievement of full ROM, the absence of pain or tenderness, a satisfactory isokinetic test result, and a satisfactory clinical examination. Isokinetic testing is performed at 180°/s and 300°/s. Data indicate that the bilateral comparison at 180°/s for the throwing arm's elbow flexion is 10% to 20% stronger and the dominant extensors are typically 5% to 15% stronger than those of the nonthrowing arm.[7]

The ITP was developed to gradually introduce the quantity, distance, intensity, and types of throws needed to facilitate the restoration of normal throwing motions. The ITP is divided into two phases. Phase I is a long-toss program (Table 4 and Table 5) that is initiated at 45 feet (15 m) and is progressed with increased distances and volume of throws. Phase II is a mound throwing program used for pitchers. During phase I, the athlete is instructed to use a crow-hop method of throwing, to incorporate synchronization of the trunk and lower extremities, while throwing with a slight arc for each prescribed distance. It is necessary to implement a slight arc (versus throwing on a line) in the long-toss program as a way to regulate the intensity of each throw and ensure that the athlete is not throwing harder than needed for each distance. During the long-toss program, as intensity and distance increase, the stresses also increase on the patient's medial elbow and anterior shoulder joint. A 2011 study reported that the longer throwing distances substantially increased these forces.[31] The long-toss program is designed to gradually introduce loads and strains and should be completed successfully before throwing from the mound is allowed. Position players additionally can begin a progressive hitting program that begins with swinging a light bat and progresses to hitting off a tee, soft-toss hitting, and finally, batting practice.

Following the completion of a long-toss program, pitchers progress to phase II of the throwing program, throwing off a mound (Table 6). In phase II, the number of throws, the intensity, and the type of pitch are progressed to gradually increase stress on the elbow and shoulder joints. Generally, the pitcher begins at 50% of intensity and gradually progresses to 75%, 90%, and 100% over a 4-week to 6-week period. Breaking balls are initiated after the pitcher can throw 40 to 50 pitches at least at 80% of intensity without symptoms. During this phase, position players will be progressed with position-specific fielding drills and functional drills.

The athlete is instructed to continue with all previously described exercises and drills to maintain and improve upper extremity, core, and lower extremity strength, power, and endurance during this phase of rehabilitation. It is also important to teach the athlete a year-round conditioning program, including the periodization of throwing and strength-training activities, to help prevent overtraining and throwing when poorly conditioned and also to prepare for the upcoming season. A 1992 study

Table 4

Interval Throwing Program for Baseball Positional Players

45-Feet Phase

Step 1

A) Warm-up throwing	D) Warm-up throwing
B) 45 feet (25 throws)	E) 45 feet (25 throws)
C) Rest 5-10 min	

Step 2

A) Warm-up throwing	E) 45 feet (25 throws)
B) 45 feet (25 throws)	F) Rest 5-10 min
C) Rest 5-10 min	G) Warm-up throwing
D) Warm-up throwing	H) 45 feet (25 throws)

60-Feet Phase

Step 3

A) Warm-up throwing	D) Warm-up throwing
B) 60 feet (25 throws)	E) 60 feet (25 throws)
C) Rest 5-10 min	

Step 4

A) Warm-up throwing	E) 60 feet (25 throws)
B) 60 feet (25 throws)	F) Rest 5-10 min
C) Rest 5-10 min	G) Warm-up throwing
D) Warm-up throwing	H) 60 feet (25 throws)

90-Feet Phase

Step 5

A) Warm-up throwing	D) Warm-up throwing
B) 90 feet (25 throws)	E) 90 feet (25 throws)
C) Rest 5-10 min	

Step 6

A) Warm-up throwing	E) 90 feet (25 throws)
B) 90 feet (25 throws)	F) Rest 5-10 min
C) Rest 5-10 min	G) Warm-up throwing
D) Warm-up throwing	H) 90 feet (25 throws)

120-Feet Phase

Step 7

A) Warm-up throwing	D) Warm-up throwing
B) 120 feet (25 throws)	E) 120 feet (25 throws)
C) Rest 5-10 min	

Step 8

A) Warm-up throwing	E) 120 feet (25 throws)
B) 120 feet (25 throws)	F) Rest 5-10 min
C) Rest 5-10 min	G) Warm-up throwing
D) Warm-up throwing	H) 120 feet (25 throws)

Table 4 (continued)

Interval Throwing Program for Baseball Positional Players

150-Feet Phase

Step 9

A) Warm-up throwing	D) Warm-up throwing
B) 150 feet (25 throws)	E) 150 feet (25 throws)
C) Rest 3-5 min	

Step 10

A) Warm-up throwing	E) 150 feet (25 throws)
B) 150 feet (25 throws)	F) Rest 3-5 min
C) Rest 3-5 min	G) Warm-up throwing
D) Warm-up throwing	H) 150 feet (25 throws)

180-Feet Phase

Step 11

A) Warm-up throwing	D) Warm-up throwing
B) 180 feet (25 throws)	E) 180 feet (25 throws)
C) Rest 3-5 min	

Step 12

A) Warm-up throwing	E) 180 feet (25 throws)
B) 180 feet (25 throws)	F) Rest 3-5 min
C) Rest 3-5 min	G) Warm-up throwing
D) Warm-up throwing	H) 180 feet (25 throws)

Step 13

A) Warm-up throwing	G) Warm-up throwing
B) 180 feet (25 throws)	H) 180 feet (20 throws)
C) Rest 3-5 min	I) Rest 3-5 min
D) Warm-up throwing	J) Warm-up throwing
E) 180 feet (25 throws)	K) 15 throws progressing from 120 feet to 90 feet to 60 feet
F) Rest 3-5 min	

Step 14: Return to field position

All throws should be on an arc with a crow-hop. Warm-up throws consist of 10 to 20 throws at approximately 30 feet. The throwing program should be performed every other day, 3 times per week, unless otherwise specified by the physician or rehabilitation specialist. Each step is performed ____ times before progressing to the next step.

Data adapted from Wilk KE, Reinhold MM, Andrews JR: Rehabilitation of the thrower's elbow. *Sports Med Arthrosc Rev* 2003;11(1):79-95, and Ellenbacker TS, Wilk KE, Reinhold MM, Murphy TM, Paine RM: Use of interval return programs for shoulder rehabilitation, in Ellenbecker TS: *Shoulder Rehabilitation: Non-Operative Treatment*. New York, NY, Thieme, 2006, pp 139-165.

showed that a dynamic variable resistance exercise program significantly increased throwing velocity.[32] Similarly, the throwing velocity in high school baseball players was increased using a program that includes a variety of resistance exercises, including plyometric training and a Thrower's Ten training program.[33]

Table 5

Interval Throwing Program for Baseball Pitchers: Phase I

45-Feet Phase

Step 1

A) Warm-up throwing
B) 45 feet (25 throws)
C) Rest 3-5 min

D) Warm-up throwing
E) 45 feet (25 throws)

Step 2

A) Warm-up throwing
B) 45 feet (25 throws)
C) Rest 3-5 min
D) Warm-up throwing

E) 45 feet (25 throws)
F) Rest 3-5 min
G) Warm-up throwing
H) 45 feet (25 throws)

60-Feet Phase

Step 3

A) Warm-up throwing
B) 60 feet (25 throws)
C) Rest 3-5 min

D) Warm-up throwing
E) 60 feet (25 throws)

Step 4

A) Warm-up throwing
B) 60 feet (25 throws)
C) Rest 3-5 min
D) Warm-up throwing

E) 60 feet (25 throws)
F) Rest 3-5 min
G) Warm-up throwing
H) 60 feet (25 throws)

90-Feet Phase

Step 5

A) 60 feet (10 throws)
B) 90 feet (20 throws)
C) Rest 3-5 min

D) 60 feet (10 throws)
E) 90 feet (20 throws)

Step 6

A) 60 feet (7 throws)
B) 90 feet (18 throws)
C) Rest 3-5 min
D) 60 feet (7 throws)

E) 90 feet (18 throws)
F) Rest 3-5 min
G) 60 feet (7 throws)
H) 90 feet (18 throws)

120-Feet Phase

Step 7

A) 60 feet (5-7 throws)
B) 90 feet (5-7 throws)
C) 120 feet (15 throws)
D) Rest 3-5 min

E) 60 feet (5-7 throws)
F) 90 feet (5-7 throws)
G) 120 feet (15 throws)

Step 8

A) 60 feet (5 throws)
B) 90 feet (10 throws)
C) 120 feet (15 throws)
D) Rest 3-5 min

E) 60 feet (5 throws)
F) 90 feet (10 throws)
G) 120 feet (15 throws)

Table 5 (continued)

Interval Throwing Program for Baseball Pitchers: Phase I

Flat Throwing

Step 9

A) Throw 60 feet (10-15 throws)
B) Throw 90 feet (10 throws)

C) Throw 120 feet (10 throws)
D) Throw 60 feet (flat ground) using pitching mechanics (20-30 throws)

Step 10

A) Throw 60 feet (10-15 throws)
B) Throw 90 feet (10 throws)
C) Throw 120 feet (10 throws)
D) Throw 60 feet (flat ground) using pitching mechanics (20-30 throws)

E) Rest 3-5 min
F) Throw 60-90 feet (10-15 throws)
G) Throw 60 feet (flat ground) using pitching mechanics (20 throws)

Throwing program should be performed every other day, with one day of rest between steps, unless otherwise specified by the physician. Each step is performed 2 times before progressing to the next step.

Data from Wilk KE, Reinhold MM, Andrews JR: Rehabilitation of the thrower's elbow. *Tech Hand Up Extrem Surg* 2003;7(4):197-216, and Wilk KE, Reinhold MM, Andrews JR: Rehabilitation of the thrower's elbow. *Sports Med Arthrosc Rev* 2003;11(1):79-95.

Specific Nonsurgical Rehabilitation Guidelines

UCL Injury

Nonsurgical treatment is attempted for partial tears and sprains of the UCL, although surgical reconstruction may be warranted for complete tears or if nonsurgical treatment is unsuccessful. A nonsurgical rehabilitation program is outlined in Table 7. Initially, a brace can be used to restrict ROM and prevent valgus stresses from limiting movement so additional adverse stresses on the UCL can be avoided. ROM usually is permitted, although in a nonpainful arc of motion, typically from 10° to 100°, to allow inflammation to subside and collagen tissue to align. Isometric exercises are performed for the shoulder, elbow, and wrist to prevent muscular atrophy. Ice and anti-inflammatory medications are prescribed to control pain and inflammation. Elbow flexion and extension ROM is increased gradually by 5° to 10° per week during the second phase of rehabilitation or as tolerated, with full ROM achieved by at least 3 to 4 weeks. The clinician should ensure the restoration of full shoulder ROM by incorporating manual stretches, ROM exercises, and

© 2016 American Academy of Orthopaedic Surgeons

Table 6

Interval Throwing Program: Phase II, Throwing Off the Mound

Stage I: Fastballs Only[a]

Step 1: Interval throwing
15 throws off mound at 50%[b]

Step 2: Interval throwing
30 throws off mound at 50%

Step 3: Interval throwing
45 throws off mound at 50%

Step 4: Interval throwing
60 throws off mound at 50%

Step 5: Interval throwing
70 throws off mound at 50%

Step 6: 45 throws off mound at 50%
30 throws off mound at 75%

Step 7: 30 throws off mound at 50%
45 throws off mound at 75%

Step 8: 10 throws off mound at 50%
65 throws off mound at 75%

Stage II: Fastballs Only

Step 9: 60 throws off mound at 75%
15 throws in batting practice

Step 10: 50-60 throws off mound at 75%
30 throws in batting practice

Step 11: 45-50 throws off mound at 5%
45 throws in batting practice

Stage III

Step 12: 30 throws off mound at 75% warm-up
15 throws off mound at 50%; begin breaking balls
45-60 throws in batting practice (fastball only)

Step 13: 30 throws off mound at 75%
30 breaking balls at 75%
30 throws in batting practice

Step 14: 30 throws off mound at 75%
60-90 throws in batting practice (gradually increase breaking balls)

Step 15: Simulated game; progress by 15 throws per workout (pitch count)

All throwing off the mound should be done in the presence of the pitching coach or sport biomechanist to stress proper throwing mechanics. Use speed gun to aid in effort control.

[a] For steps 1 through 5, use the interval throwing at 120 feet (36.6 m) phase as a warm-up.

[b] Percentage of effort.

Data from Azar M, Wilk KE: Nonoperative treatment of the elbow in throwers. *Oper Tech Sports Med* 1996;4(2):91-99.

mobilization techniques. Although all aspects of shoulder ROM should be addressed, glenohumeral internal rotation should be emphasized, because a loss of internal rotation ROM has been implemented in elbow injuries.[12]

Rhythmic stabilization exercises are initiated as tolerated in the acute stages of rehabilitation to develop dynamic stabilization and neuromuscular control of the upper extremity. As dynamic stability is advanced, isotonic exercises are incorporated for the entire upper extremity. The flexor carpi ulnaris and flexor digitorum superficialis overlay the UCL; therefore, strengthening exercises for these muscles can assist the UCL in resisting valgus stresses at the elbow.[34] In addition, posterior rotator cuff and scapular strengthening exercises are performed to restore proximal stabilization. The advanced strengthening phase usually is initiated at 6 to 7 weeks after injury, with valgus loading monitored throughout the rehabilitation program. An interval return-to-throwing program is initiated after the athlete regains full motion, adequate strength, and dynamic stability of the elbow. The athlete is allowed to return to competition following the asymptomatic completion of the interval sport program. If symptoms recur during the interval throwing program, they typically present when throwing at longer distances or with greater intensity or during throwing from the mound. If symptoms persist, the athlete is reassessed and surgical intervention is considered.

Medial Epicondylitis and Flexor-Pronator Tendinitis

Medial epicondylitis occurs because of changes within the musculotendinous flexor-pronator unit, characterized by microscopic or macroscopic tearing within the flexor carpi radialis or pronator teres near the origin on the medial epicondyle. Overhead throwers who exhibit flexor-pronator tendinitis also may have UCL pathology that creates this secondary pathology due to the underlying increased laxity. Furthermore, it may be beneficial to determine the number of episodes and the chronicity of medial epicondylar symptoms. Patients with long histories of medial epicondylitis may exhibit a chronic degeneration known as tendinosis or tendinopathy, not true tendinitis.

The treatment of tendinopathy is based on a careful examination to determine the exact pathology present. Often, patients in whom tendinitis has been diagnosed only later discover that the tendon had undergone a degenerative process referred to as tendinosis.[35,36] The differential diagnosis of tendinosis may be made using MRI, ultrasonography, or tissue biopsy.

The treatment of tendinitis typically focuses on reducing inflammation and pain. This goal is accomplished through the reduction of activities, steroid injections, anti-inflammatory medications, cryotherapy, iontophoresis,

Table 7

Nonsurgical Treatment Following Ulnar Collateral Ligament Sprains of the Elbow

Immediate Motion Phase	Intermediate Phase	Advanced Phase	Return-to-Activity Phase
Weeks 0 through 2	Weeks 3 through 6	Weeks 6 through 12	Weeks 12 through 14
NA	NA	Criteria to progress: Full ROM, no pain or tenderness, no increase in laxity, strength 4/5 of elbow flexion/extension	Criteria to progress to return to throwing: Full nonpainful ROM, no increase in laxity, fulfillment of isokinetic test criteria, successful clinical examination
Goals: To increase ROM, promote healing of UCL, retard muscular atrophy, reduce pain and inflammation	Goals: To increase ROM, improve strength and endurance, reduce pain and inflammation, promote stability	Goals: To increase strength, power and endurance; improve neuromuscular control; initiate high-speed exercise drills	Goals: Maintain strength, power, and endurance gains. Maintain ROM and flexibility.
ROM: Brace (optional) for nonpainful ROM (20°-90°), AAROM, PROM elbow and wrist (nonpainful ROM)	ROM: Gradually increase motion 0° to 135° increase 10 per week	ROM: Progress to full elbow ROM	Maintain full elbow ROM and elbow and forearm muscle flexibility
Exercises: Isometrics for wrist and elbow musculature; shoulder strengthening (no ER strengthening)	Exercises: Initiate isotonic exercises: wrist curls, wrist extensions, pronation/supination, biceps/triceps; dumbbells: glenohumeral ER and IR, deltoid, supraspinatus, rhomboids	Exercises: Initiate exercise tubing, shoulder program: Thrower's Ten program, biceps/triceps program, supination/pronation, wrist extension/flexion, plyometrics, throwing drills	Exercises: Initiate interval throwing, continue Thrower's Ten Program, continue plyometrics
Modalities: Ice, compression	Modalities: Ice, compression	Modalities: Moist hot pack pretreatment; ice posttreatment	Modalities: Moist hot pack pretreatment; ice posttreatment

ROM = range of motion, UCL = ulnar collateral ligament, AAROM = active-assisted range of motion, PROM = passive range of motion, ER = external rotation, IR = internal rotation, NA = not applicable.

Data from Wilk KE, Reinhold MM, Andrews JR: Rehabilitation of the thrower's elbow. *Sports Med Arthrosc Rev* 2003;11(1):79-95.

light exercise, and stretching. Conversely, the treatment of tendinosis focuses on increasing the circulation to promote collagen synthesis and collagen organization. Such treatment would include heat, stretching, eccentric exercises, laser therapy, transverse massage, and soft-tissue mobilization. These therapies are performed to increase the circulation and promote tissue healing. Dry needling has been advocated for this pathology to promote tendon healing.[37]

Platelet-rich plasma (PRP) therapy is a promising intervention in which a small sample of the patient's own blood is separated and the platelet-rich layer is injected into the site of injury. The proposed mechanism delivers humoral mediators and growth factors locally to induce a healing response. Other advantages of PRP therapy are

that it is minimally invasive, provokes a local response only, and avoids an inflammatory response. Disadvantages can include the cost of treatment, a lack of supporting evidence, and increased staff time to withdraw and centrifuge the blood, and then reinject it into the site of pathology. Early research on the clinical application of PRP to promote healing and an adaptive response is promising.[38,39] Substantial benefits of PRP were shown in patients with chronic lateral epicondylitis.[39] Basic science and controlled studies have yet to report the efficacy of such a treatment.

The nonsurgical approach (Table 8) for the treatment of epicondylitis (tendinitis and/or paratendinitis) focuses on diminishing the pain and inflammation and then gradually improving muscular strength. The primary

Table 8

Epicondylitis Rehabilitation Protocol

Phase I: Acute Phase	Phase II: Subacute Phase	Phase III: Chronic Phase
Goals: To reduce inflammation, promote tissue healing, retard muscular atrophy	Goals: To improve flexibility, increase muscular strength/endurance, increase functional activities, promote return to function	Goals: To improve muscular strength and endurance, maintain/enhance flexibility, gradually return to sport and high-level activities
Therapies and exercises: Cryotherapy Whirlpool Stretching to increase flexibility: wrist extension/flexion, elbow extension/flexion, forearm supination/pronation Isometrics: wrist extension/flexion, elbow extension/flexion, forearm supination/pronation High-voltage galvanic stimulation Phonophoresis Friction massage Iontophoresis (with anti-inflammatory drug, eg, dexamethasone) Avoidance of painful movements (eg, gripping)	Exercises: Emphasize concentric/eccentric strengthening Concentrate on involved muscle group Wrist extension/flexion Forearm pronation/supination Elbow flexion/extension Initiate shoulder strengthening (if deficiencies are noted) Continue flexibility exercises May use counterforce brace Continue using cryotherapy after exercise/function Gradually return to stressful activities Gradually reinitiate formerly painful movements	Exercises: Continue strengthening exercises (emphasize eccentric/concentric) Continue to emphasize deficiencies in shoulder and elbow strength Continue flexibility exercises Gradually decrease use of counterforce brace Use cryotherapy as needed Gradually return to sport activity Modify equipment (grip size, string tension, playing surface) Emphasize maintenance program

Data from Wilk KE, Macrina LC: Rehabilitation for elbow instability: Emphasis on the throwing athlete, in Skirven TM, Osterman AL, Fedorczyk J, Amadio PC: *Rehabilitation of the Hand and Upper Extremity*. Philadelphia, PA, Elsevier, 2011, pp 1143-1156.

goals of rehabilitation are to control the applied loads and create an environment for healing. The initial treatment consists of warm whirlpool baths, iontophoresis, stretching exercises, and light strengthening exercises to stimulate a repair response. Therapeutic modalities often are used by rehabilitation specialists to reduce inflammation and promote healing. Very limited evidence supports using these modalities in isolation. Common modalities can include massage, cold laser therapy, iontophoresis, ultrasound, nitric oxide, and extracorporeal shock wave therapy. When used in combination with exercise or with other modalities, however, studies have shown improved tissue quality and outcomes.[40-42] Conversely, patients with tendinosis are treated with transverse friction massage, forceful stretching, a focus on eccentric strengthening with gradually progressing loads, and warm modalities to promote tendon regeneration.

After the patient's symptoms have subsided, an aggressive stretching and strengthening program featuring high loads and low repetitions that emphasizes eccentric contractions is initiated. Wrist flexion and extension activities should be performed, initially with the elbow flexed 30° to 45°. A gradual progression through plyometric and throwing activities precedes the initiation of the ITP.

Ulnar Neuropathy

Ulnar nerve changes can result from tensile forces, compressive forces, or nerve instability. Ulnar neuropathy occurs in three stages.[43] The first stage is characterized by an acute onset of radicular symptoms. During the second stage, a recurrence of symptoms occurs as the athlete attempts to return to competition. The third stage is distinguished by persistent motor weakness and sensory changes. If the athlete presents in the third stage of injury, nonsurgical management may not be effective.

A leading mechanism for tensile force on the ulnar nerve is valgus stress. This mechanism may be coupled with an external rotation supination stress overload mechanism. The traction forces are magnified further when underlying valgus instability from UCL injury is present. Ulnar neuropathy is often a secondary pathology of UCL insufficiency. Compression of the ulnar nerve is often due to hypertrophy of the surrounding soft tissues or the presence of scar tissue. The nerve also may be trapped between the two heads of the flexor carpi ulnaris. Repetitive flexion and extension of the elbow with an unstable nerve can irritate or inflame the nerve. Additionally, the nerve may subluxate or rest on the medial epicondyle, rendering it vulnerable to direct trauma.

The nonsurgical treatment of ulnar neuropathy focuses on reducing ulnar nerve irritation, enhancing dynamic medial joint stability, and returning the athlete to competition gradually. Using a night splint with the elbow flexed to 45° can help to restrict movement and prevent ulnar nerve irritation. NSAIDs can be prescribed as well as an iontophoresis disposable patch and cryotherapy. Throwing athletes are instructed to discontinue throwing activities for at least 4 weeks, depending on the severity and chronicity of symptoms. They will be progressed through the immediate motion and intermediate phases over 4 to 6 weeks, with emphasis on eccentric and dynamic stabilization drills. Plyometric exercises are used to facilitate further dynamic stabilization of the medial elbow. The athlete is allowed to begin an ITP when full pain-free ROM and muscle performance are achieved without neurologic symptoms.

Osteochondritis Dissecans

Osteochondritis dissecans (OCD) of the elbow can develop as a result of the valgus strain on the elbow joint, which produces not only medial tension but also a lateral compressive force.[44] This is observed as the capitellum of the humerus is compressed against the radial head. Patients often report lateral elbow pain on palpation and valgus stress. Classification of the pathologic progression of OCD has been described in three stages.[45] Stage I describes patients without evidence of subchondral displacement or fracture, whereas stage II refers to lesions showing evidence of subchondral detachment or articular cartilage fracture. Stage III lesions involve detached osteochondral fragments, resulting in intra-articular loose bodies. Nonsurgical treatment is attempted for stage 1 patients only and consists of relative rest and immobilization until elbow symptoms have resolved.

Nonsurgical treatment includes 3 to 6 weeks of immobilization at 90° of elbow flexion. ROM activities for the shoulder, elbow, and wrist are performed three to four times a day. As symptoms resolve, a strengthening program is initiated with isometric exercises. Isotonic exercises are added after approximately 1 week of isometric exercise. Aggressive high-speed, eccentric, and plyometric exercises are included progressively to prepare the athlete for the start of an ITP.

If nonsurgical treatment fails or evidence of loose bodies exists, surgical intervention, including arthroscopic abrading and drilling of the lesion with fixation

or removal of the loose bodies, is indicated.[46] Long-term follow-up studies regarding the outcome of patients undergoing surgery to drill or reattach the lesions have not reported favorable results, suggesting that prevention and early detection of symptoms may be the best form of treatment.[46]

Little Leaguer's Elbow

During the arm-cocking and acceleration phases of throwing, the medial epicondyle physis is subject to repetitive tensile and valgus forces that can lead to a spectrum of injuries to the medial epicondylar apophysis, ranging from microtrauma to the physis to fracture and displacement of the medial epicondyle through the apophysis. Pain in the medial elbow is common is adolescent throwers. These forces can result in microtraumatic injury to the physis, with potential fragmentation, hypertrophy, separation of the epiphysis, or avulsion of the medial epicondyle.

In the absence of an avulsion, a nonsurgical rehabilitation program similar to that used for the UCL is initiated. Initial emphasis is placed on the reduction of pain and inflammation and the restoration of motion and strength. Strengthening exercises are performed in a gradual fashion. First, isometrics are performed, then, light isotonic strengthening exercises are initiated. Young throwing athletes often exhibit poor core and scapular control, along with weakness of the shoulder musculature; therefore, core, leg, and shoulder strengthening are emphasized. In addition, stretching exercises are performed to normalize shoulder ROM, especially into internal rotation and horizontal adduction. No heavy lifting is permitted for 12 to 14 weeks. An ITP is initiated as tolerated when symptoms subside.

In the presence of a nondisplaced or minimally displaced avulsion, a brief period of immobilization for approximately 7 days is encouraged, followed by a gradual progression of ROM, flexibility, and strength. An ITP usually is allowed at week 6 to 8. If the avulsion is displaced, open reduction and internal fixation may be required.

Specific Postoperative Rehabilitation Guidelines

UCL Reconstruction

Surgical reconstruction of the UCL attempts to restore the stabilizing functions of the anterior bundle of the UCL.[47] Several types of surgical procedures are available to reconstruct the UCL.[12,48,49] The modified Jobe procedure can be used, in which the palmaris longus or gracilis graft source is obtained and passed in a figure-of-8 pattern through drill holes in the sublime tubercle of the ulna and the medial epicondyle.[47] A subcutaneous ulnar nerve transposition is performed at the time of reconstruction.

Table 9

Postoperative Rehabilitation Protocol Following Ulnar Collateral Ligament Reconstruction Using Autogenous Palmaris Longus Graft (Accelerated ROM)

Immediate Postoperative Phase (0-3 Weeks)

Goals: To protect healing tissue, reduce pain and inflammation, retard muscular atrophy, protect graft site to allow healing

Week 1

Brace: Posterior splint at 90° elbow flexion

ROM: Wrist AROM extension/flexion immediately after surgery

Elbow: Postoperative compression dressing 5-7 days

Wrist (graft site) compression dressing 7-10 days as needed

Exercises: Gripping exercises, wrist ROM, shoulder isometrics (no shoulder ER), biceps isometrics

Cryotherapy to elbow joint and to graft site at wrist

Week 2

Brace: Elbow ROM 15°-105° or as tolerated

Motion to tolerance

Exercises: Continue all exercises listed above

Elbow ROM in brace 30°-105°

Initiate elbow extension isometrics

Continue wrist ROM exercises

Initiate light scar mobilization over distal incision (graft)

Cryotherapy: Continue ice to elbow and graft site

Week 3

Brace: Elbow ROM 5°/10° to 115°/120°, motion to tolerance

Exercises: Continue all exercises listed above

Elbow ROM in brace

Initiate AROM wrist and elbow (No resistance)

Initiate light wrist flexion stretching

Initiate AROM shoulder

Full can

Lateral raises

ER/IR tubing

Elbow flexion/extension

Initiate light scapular strengthening exercises

May incorporate bicycle for lower extremity strength, endurance

Table 9 (*continued*)

Postoperative Rehabilitation Protocol Following Ulnar Collateral Ligament Reconstruction Using Autogenous Palmaris Longus Graft (Accelerated ROM)

Intermediate Phase (Weeks 4-7)

Goals: Gradual increase to full ROM, promote healing of repaired tissue, regain and improve muscular strength, restore full function of graft site

Week 4

Brace: Elbow ROM 0°-135°, motion to tolerance

Exercises: Begin light resistance exercises for arm (1 lb); wrist curls, extension, pronation, supination; elbow extension/flexion

Progress shoulder program emphasize rotator cuff and scapular strengthening

Initiate shoulder strengthening with light dumbbells

Week 5

ROM: Elbow ROM 0°-135°

Discontinue brace

Maintain full ROM

Continue all exercises; progress all shoulder and upper extremity exercises (progress weight 1 lb)

Week 6

AROM: 0°-145° without brace or full ROM

Exercises: Initiate Thrower's Ten Program, progress elbow strengthening exercises, initiate shoulder ER strengthening, progress shoulder program

Week 7

Progress Thrower's Ten Program (progress weights)

Initiate PNF diagonal patterns (light)

Advanced Strengthening Phase (Week 8-14)

Goals: To increase strength, power, endurance; maintain full elbow ROM; gradually initiate sporting activities

Week 8

Exercises: Initiate eccentric elbow flexion/extension, continue isotonic program: forearm and wrist, continue shoulder program (Thrower's Ten Program), manual resistance diagonal patterns, initiate plyometric exercise program (two-hand plyometrics close to body only), chest pass, side throw close to body, continue stretching calf and hamstrings

Week 10

Exercises: Continue all exercises listed above; program plyometrics to two-hand drills away from body: side-to-side throws, soccer throws, side throws

Table 9 (*continued*)

Postoperative Rehabilitation Protocol Following Ulnar Collateral Ligament Reconstruction Using Autogenous Palmaris Longus Graft (Accelerated ROM)

Weeks 12-14

Continue all exercises; initiate isotonic machines strengthening exercises (if desired): bench press (seated), lat pull down; initiate golf, swimming; initiate interval hitting program

Return-to Activity Phase (Weeks 14-32)

Goals: Continue to increase strength, power, endurance of upper extremity musculature; gradually return to sport activities

Week 14

Exercises: Continue strengthening program; emphasize elbow and wrist strengthening and flexibility exercises; maintain full elbow ROM; initiate one-hand plyometric throwing (stationary throws); initiate one-hand wall dribble; initiate one-hand baseball throws into wall

Week 16

Exercises: Initiate interval throwing program (phase I, long-toss program); continue Thrower's Ten Program and plyometrics; continue stretching before and after throwing

Weeks 22-24

Exercises: Progress to phase II throwing (after phase I successfully completed).

Weeks 30-32

Exercises: Gradually progress to competitive throwing/sports.

ROM = range of motion, AROM = active range of motion, ER = external rotation, IR = internal rotation, PNF = proprioceptive neuromuscular facilitation.

Data from Wilk KE, Arrigo CA, Andrews JR, Azar FM: Rehabilitation following elbow surgery in the throwing athlete. *Oper Tech Sports Med* 1996;4(2):114-132.

The rehabilitation program in current use following UCL reconstruction is outlined in Table 9. The athlete's arm is placed in a posterior splint with the elbow immobilized at 90° of flexion for the first 7 days postoperatively to allow early healing of the UCL graft and fascial slings involved in the nerve transposition. The patient is allowed to perform wrist ROM and gripping and submaximal isometrics for the wrist and elbow. The patient is progressed from the posterior splint to a hinged elbow ROM brace to protect the healing tissues from valgus stresses that can be detrimental. The brace is discontinued at the beginning of week 5.

Passive ROM activities are initiated immediately to reduce pain and slowly stress the healing tissues. Initially, the focus of the rehabilitation is on obtaining full elbow extension while gradually progressing flexion. Elbow extension is encouraged early, to at least 15°, but full extension is allowed if the patient can comfortably achieve it as long as no discomfort is present. A recent study demonstrated that passive ROM of the elbow produced 3% or less strain in both bands of the reconstructed ligament and approximately 1% strain for the anterior band of the UCL.[50] Therefore, it has been determined that in the immediate postoperative period, full elbow extension is safe and does not place excessive stress on the healing graft. Conversely, elbow flexion to 100° is allowed and should be progressed at about 10° per week until full ROM is achieved by 4 to 6 weeks postoperatively.

Isometric exercises are progressed to include light resistance isotonic exercises at week 4 and the full Thrower's Ten Program by week 6. Progressive resistance exercises are incorporated at week 8 to 9. Again, focus is placed on developing dynamic stabilization of the medial elbow. Because of the anatomic orientation of the flexor carpi ulnaris and the flexor digitorum superficialis overlying the UCL, isotonic and stabilization activities for these muscles can assist the UCL in stabilizing valgus stress at the medial elbow.[34] Thus, concentric and eccentric strengthening of these muscles is performed.

Aggressive exercises involving eccentric and plyometric contractions are included in the advanced phase, usually weeks 12 through 16. The Advanced Thrower's Ten Exercise Program is initiated at week 12 after surgery. Two-hand plyometric drills are performed at week 12, and one-hand drills are executed at week 14. An ITP is allowed at postoperative week 16. Progression to throwing from a mound may occur within 4 to 6 weeks following the initiation of an ITP, and a return to competitive throwing may commence at approximately 9 months following surgery.

A 2010 study reported the outcomes of UCL reconstruction of the elbow in 743 athletes during a 2-year minimum follow-up.[51] The authors stated that UCL reconstruction with subcutaneous ulnar nerve transposition was found to be effective in correcting valgus elbow instability in the overhead athlete and that the procedure allowed most athletes (83%, 616 patients) to return to the previous or a higher level of competition in less than 1 year. Major complications were noted in only 4% (30 patients).

Ulnar Nerve Transposition

An ulnar nerve transposition can be performed in a subcutaneous fashion using fascial slings. The clinician should use caution to avoid overstressing the soft-tissue structures

© 2016 American Academy of Orthopaedic Surgeons

Table 10

Postoperative Rehabilitation Following Ulnar Nerve Transposition

Phase I: Immediate Postoperative Phase	Phase II: Intermediate Phase	Phase III: Advanced Strengthening Phase	Phase IV: Return-to-Activity Phase
Week 0-2	Weeks 3-7	Weeks 8-12	Weeks 12-16
Goals: To allow soft-tissue healing of relocated nerve, reduce pain and inflammation, retard muscular atrophy	Goals: To restore full pain-free ROM; improve strength, power, endurance of upper-extremity musculature; gradually increase functional demands	Goals: To increase strength, power, endurance; gradually initiate sporting activities	Goal: To gradually return to sporting activities
Week 1	Week 3	Week 8	Week 12
Posterior splint at 90° elbow flexion with wrist free for motion (sling for comfort); compression dressing; exercises such as gripping exercises, wrist ROM, shoulder isometrics	Discontinue posterior splint; progress elbow ROM and emphasize full extension; initiate flexibility exercise for wrist extension/flexion, forearm supination/pronation, and elbow extension/flexion; initiate strengthening exercises for wrist extension/flexion, forearm supination/pronation, elbow extensors/flexors, and a shoulder program	Initiate eccentric exercise program; begin plyometric exercise drills; continue shoulder and elbow strengthening and flexibility exercises; initiate interval throwing program	Return to competitive throwing; continue Thrower's Ten program
Week 2	Week 6	NA	NA
Remove posterior splint for exercise and bathing; progress elbow ROM (PROM 15° -120°); initiate elbow and wrist isometrics; continue shoulder isometrics	Continue all exercises listed above; initiate light sports activities		

ROM = range of motion, PROM = passive range of motion, NA = not applicable.

involved in relocating the nerve while soft-tissue healing occurs.[28] The rehabilitation guidelines following an ulnar nerve transposition are outlined in Table 10. A posterior splint at 90° of elbow flexion is used for the first postoperative week to prevent excessive extension ROM and tension on the nerve. The splint is discontinued at the beginning of week 2, and light ROM activities are initiated. Full ROM usually is restored by weeks 3 to 4. Gentle isotonic strengthening is begun during week 3 to 4 and progressed to the full Thrower's Ten Program by 4 to 6 weeks after surgery. Aggressive strengthening, including eccentric training, the Advanced Thrower's Ten Exercise Program, and plyometric training, is incorporated at week 8 and an ITP is begun at week 8 to 9 if all previously outlined criteria are met. A return to competition usually occurs between weeks 12 and 16 postoperatively.

Posterior Olecranon Osteophyte Excision

Surgical excision of posterior olecranon osteophytes is performed arthroscopically using an osteotome or motorized burr. Approximately 5 to 10 mm of the olecranon tip is removed, and a motorized burr is used to contour the coronoid, olecranon tip, and fossa to prevent further impingement during extreme flexion and extension.[52]

The rehabilitation program following arthroscopic posterior olecranon osteophyte excision is slightly more conservative in restoring full elbow extension secondary to postsurgical pain. ROM is progressed within the patient's tolerance, but by 10 days after surgery, the patient should exhibit at least 15° to 105°/110° of ROM, and 5°-10° to 115° by day 14. Full ROM (0° to 145°) typically is restored by day 20 to 25 after surgery. The rate of ROM progression most often is limited by osseous pain and synovial joint inflammation, usually located at the top of the olecranon.

The strengthening program is similar to the previously discussed progression. Isometric exercises are performed for the first 10 to 14 days, and isotonic strengthening is performed from weeks 2 to 6. During the first 2 weeks following surgery, forceful triceps contractions can produce posterior elbow pain; therefore, the clinician should avoid initiating or reducing the force produced by the triceps muscle. The full Thrower's Ten Program is initiated by week 6. An ITP is included by week 10 to week 12. Emphasis again is placed on eccentric control of the elbow flexors and dynamic stabilization of the medial elbow.

The outcomes of elbow surgery in 72 professional baseball players have been reported.[53] Of these athletes, 47 exhibited a posterior olecranon osteophyte, and 18 of the athletes who underwent an isolated olecranon excision later required a UCL reconstruction.[53] These findings suggest that subtle medial instability can accelerate osteophyte formation.

Summary

The elbow joint is a common site of injury in athletes, especially in the overhead athlete, because of the repetitive forces occurring at the elbow that create repetitive microtraumatic injuries. Conversely, in athletes playing in collision sports such as football, wrestling, soccer, and gymnastics, elbow injury often results from macrotraumatic forces to the elbow, leading to fractures, dislocations, and ligamentous injuries. Rehabilitation of the elbow, whether after injury or surgery, must follow a progressive and sequential order to ensure that the healing tissues are not overstressed. The rehabilitation program should limit immobilization and achieve full ROM early, especially elbow extension ROM. Furthermore, the rehabilitation program should restore strength and neuromuscular control progressively and should incorporate sport-specific activities gradually to successfully return the athlete to his or her previous level of competition as quickly and safely as possible. Additionally, the rehabilitation of the elbow must include the entire kinetic chain (the scapula, shoulder, hand, core/hips, and legs) to ensure the athlete's return to high-level sports participation.

Key Study Points

- Multiphased rehabilitation programs allow individualized progression of the athlete as determined by successful completion of each phase.
- A complete and thorough evaluation allows the rehabilitation specialist to properly design an effective treatment program for each athlete.
- The rehabilitation programs are designed to gradually introduce functional forces and stresses through functional and sport-specific drills to prepare for a return to prior level of function.

Annotated References

1. Conte S, Requa RK, Garrick JG: Disability days in major league baseball. *Am J Sports Med* 2001;29(4):431-436.

2. Posner M, Cameron KL, Wolf JM, Belmont PJ Jr, Owens BD: Epidemiology of Major League Baseball injuries. *Am J Sports Med* 2011;39(8):1676-1680.

   The authors analyzed the Major League Baseball disabled list from 2002 to 2008. They examined the differences in injuries between seasons and occurring on a monthly basis during the season. These injuries were categorized by anatomic regions. Injuries also were categorized for position and pitchers.

3. Fleisig GS, Escamilla RF: Biomechanics of the elbow in the throwing athlete. *Oper Tech Sports Med* 1996;4(2):62-68.

4. Andrews JR, Craven WM: Lesions of the posterior compartment of the elbow. *Clin Sports Med* 1991;10(3):637-652.

5. Wilson FD, Andrews JR, Blackburn TA, McCluskey G: Valgus extension overload in the pitching elbow. *Am J Sports Med* 1983;11(2):83-88.

6. Wright RW, Steger-May K, Wasserlauf BL, O'Neal ME, Weinberg BW, Paletta GA: Elbow range of motion in professional baseball pitchers. *Am J Sports Med* 2006;34(2):190-193.

7. Wilk KE, Arrigo C, Andrews JR: Rehabilitation of the elbow in the throwing athlete. *J Orthop Sports Phys Ther* 1993;17(6):305-317.

8. Salter RB, Hamilton HW, Wedge JH, et al: Clinical application of basic research on continuous passive motion for disorders and injuries of synovial joints: A preliminary report of a feasibility study. *J Orthop Res* 1984;1(3):325-342.

9. Salter RB, Simmonds DF, Malcolm BW, Rumble EJ, MacMichael D, Clements ND: The biological effect of continuous passive motion on the healing of full-thickness defects

in articular cartilage. An experimental investigation in the rabbit. *J Bone Joint Surg Am* 1980;62(8):1232-1251.

10. Green DP, McCoy H: Turnbuckle orthotic correction of elbow-flexion contractures after acute injuries. *J Bone Joint Surg Am* 1979;61(7):1092-1095.

11. McClure PW, Blackburn LG, Dusold C: The use of splints in the treatment of joint stiffness: Biologic rationale and an algorithm for making clinical decisions. *Phys Ther* 1994;74(12):1101-1107.

12. Dines JS, Frank JB, Akerman M, Yocum LA: Glenohumeral internal rotation deficits in baseball players with ulnar collateral ligament insufficiency. *Am J Sports Med* 2009;37(3):566-570.

    The authors demographically matched 29 baseball players with UCL insufficiency to a control group of baseball players with no history of shoulder, elbow, or cervical injuries and measure passive glenohumeral internal and external rotation, elbow flexion and extension, and forearm pronation and supination. The authors reported a significant difference between players with UCL injury versus control patients for dominant arm internal rotation, internal rotation deficit, and total ROM. The authors concluded that pathologic glenohumeral internal rotation deficit can be associated with elbow valgus instability. Level of evidence: III.

13. Crockett HC, Gross LB, Wilk KE, et al: Osseous adaptation and range of motion at the glenohumeral joint in professional baseball pitchers. *Am J Sports Med* 2002;30(1):20-26.

14. Thomas SJ, Swanik CB, Higginson JS, et al: A bilateral comparison of posterior capsule thickness and its correlation with glenohumeral range of motion and scapular upward rotation in collegiate baseball players. *J Shoulder Elbow Surg* 2011;20(5):708-716.

    The authors measured the posterior capsule thickness (PCT) using a 10-MHz transducer to determine the correlation with glenohumeral internal rotation, external rotation, and scapular upward rotation. The authors reported that PCT was greater on the dominant shoulder than on the nondominant shoulder. A negative correlation was noted between PCT and internal rotation. A positive correlation was found between PCT and external rotation and between PCT and scapular upward rotation at 60°, 90°, and 120° of glenohumeral abduction. Level of evidence: III.

15. Wilk KE, Andrews JR, Arrigo C: *Preventive and Rehabilitative Exercises for the Shoulder and Elbow* ,ed 6. Birmingham, AL, American Sports Medicine Institute, 2001.

16. Moseley JB Jr, Jobe FW, Pink M, Perry J, Tibone J: EMG analysis of the scapular muscles during a shoulder rehabilitation program. *Am J Sports Med* 1992;20(2):128-134.

17. Townsend H, Jobe FW, Pink M, Perry J: Electromyographic analysis of the glenohumeral muscles during

a baseball rehabilitation program. *Am J Sports Med* 1991;19(3):264-272.

18. Reinold MM, Wilk KE, Fleisig GS, et al: Electromyographic analysis of the rotator cuff and deltoid musculature during common shoulder external rotation exercises. *J Orthop Sports Phys Ther* 2004;34(7):385-394.

19. Kibler WB: The role of the scapula in athletic shoulder function. *Am J Sports Med* 1998;26(2):325-337.

20. Paine RM: The role of the scapula in the shoulder, in Andrews JR, Wilk KE, eds: *The Athlete's Shoulder* .New York, Churchill Livingstone, 1994, pp 495-512.

21. Wilk KE, Arrigo CA: An integrated approach to upper extremity exercises. *Orthop Phys Ther Clin North Am* 1992;1:337-360.

22. Tucker WS, Armstrong CW, Gribble PA, Timmons MK, Yeasting RA: Scapular muscle activity in overhead athletes with symptoms of secondary shoulder impingement during closed chain exercises. *Arch Phys Med Rehabil* 2010;91(4):550-556.

    Using EMG data, this controlled laboratory study was performed to compare the scapular muscle activation patterns in 15 overhead athletes having symptoms of shoulder impingement with the patterns of 15 overhead athletes with no shoulder pathology. The authors noted altered muscle activation of the middle trapezius, and the serratus anterior and upper trapezius had similar muscle activation.

23. Carpenter JE, Blasier RB, Pellizzon GG: The effects of muscle fatigue on shoulder joint position sense. *Am J Sports Med* 1998;26(2):262-265.

24. Wilk KE, Yenchak AJ, Arrigo CA, Andrews JR: The Advanced Throwers Ten Exercise Program: A new exercise series for enhanced dynamic shoulder control in the overhead throwing athlete. *Phys Sportsmed* 2011;39(4):90-97.

    The authors describe the Advanced Thrower's Ten Exercise Program.

25. Andrews JR, Jobe FW: Valgus extension overload in the pitching elbow, in Andrews JR, Zarins B, Carson WB, eds: *Injuries to the Throwing Arm* .Philadelphia, Saunders, 1985, pp 250-257.

26. Swanik KA, Lephart SM, Swanik CB, Lephart SP, Stone DA, Fu FH: The effects of shoulder plyometric training on proprioception and selected muscle performance characteristics. *J Shoulder Elbow Surg* 2002;11(6):579-586.

27. Fortun CM, Davies GJ, Kernozck TW: The effects of plyometric training on the shoulder internal rotators. *Phys Ther* 1998;78(51):S87.

28. Wilk KE, Voight ML, Keirns MA, Gambetta V, Andrews JR, Dillman CJ: Stretch-shortening drills for the upper extremities: Theory and clinical application. *J Orthop Sports Phys Ther* 1993;17(5):225-239.

29. Voight ML, Hardin JA, Blackburn TA, Tippett S, Canner GC: The effects of muscle fatigue on and the relationship of arm dominance to shoulder proprioception. *J Orthop Sports Phys Ther* 1996;23(6):348-352.

30. Murray TA, Cook TD, Werner SL, Schlegel TF, Hawkins RJ: The effects of extended play on professional baseball pitchers. *Am J Sports Med* 2001;29(2):137-142.

31. Fleisig GS, Bolt B, Fortenbaugh D, Wilk KE, Andrews JR: Biomechanical comparison of baseball pitching and long-toss: Implications for training and rehabilitation. *J Orthop Sports Phys Ther* 2011;41(5):296-303.

   This kinematic and kinetic analysis examined the differences between pitching from a mound and long-toss pitching in 17 healthy college pitchers. The results indicated that horizontal flat throws produced biomechanical patterns similar to pitching, whereas maximum-distance throws had increased torques compared with mound pitching.

32. Wooden MJ, Greenfield B, Johanson M, Litzelman L, Mundrane M, Donatelli RA: Effects of strength training on throwing velocity and shoulder muscle performance in teenage baseball players. *J Orthop Sports Phys Ther* 1992;15(5):223-228.

33. Escamilla RF, Ionno M, deMahy MS, et al: Comparison of three baseball-specific 6-week training programs on throwing velocity in high school baseball players. *J Strength Cond Res* 2012;26(7):1767-1781.

   The authors compared throwing velocity following a 6-week training program in 68 high school baseball players. The subjects were divided into three training groups (the Thrower's Ten, Keiser Pneumatic [Keiser], and Plyometric) and a control group. Compared with pretest throwing velocity values, posttest velocity values were significantly greater in the Thrower's Ten group (1.7%), the Keiser Pneumatic (1.2%), and the Plyometric (2.0%) groups than in the control group, with no significant difference in the control group. Level of evidence: II.

34. Davidson PA, Pink M, Perry J, Jobe FW: Functional anatomy of the flexor pronator muscle group in relation to the medial collateral ligament of the elbow. *Am J Sports Med* 1995;23(2):245-250.

35. Kraushaar BS, Nirschl RP: Tendinosis of the elbow (tennis elbow). Clinical features and findings of histological, immunohistochemical, and electron microscopy studies. *J Bone Joint Surg Am* 1999;81(2):259-278.

36. Nirschl RP, Ashman ES: Tennis elbow tendinosis (epicondylitis). *Instr Course Lect* 2004;53:587-598.

37. Suresh SP, Ali KE, Jones H, Connell DA: Medial epicondylitis: Is ultrasound guided autologous blood injection an effective treatment? *Br J Sports Med* 2006;40(11):935-939, discussion 939.

38. de Mos M, van der Windt AE, Jahr H, et al: Can platelet-rich plasma enhance tendon repair? A cell culture study. *Am J Sports Med* 2008;36(6):1171-1178.

39. Mishra A, Pavelko T: Treatment of chronic elbow tendinosis with buffered platelet-rich plasma. *Am J Sports Med* 2006;34(11):1774-1778.

40. Gum SL, Reddy GK, Stehno-Bittel L, Enwemeka CS: Combined ultrasound, electrical stimulation, and laser promote collagen synthesis with moderate changes in tendon biomechanics. *Am J Phys Med Rehabil* 1997;76(4):288-296.

41. Reddy GK, Gum S, Stehno-Bittel L, Enwemeka CS: Biochemistry and biomechanics of healing tendon: Part II. Effects of combined laser therapy and electrical stimulation. *Med Sci Sports Exerc* 1998;30(6):794-800.

42. Stergioulas A, Stergioula M, Aarskog R, Lopes-Martins RA, Bjordal JM: Effects of low-level laser therapy and eccentric exercises in the treatment of recreational athletes with chronic achilles tendinopathy. *Am J Sports Med* 2008;36(5):881-887.

43. Alley RM, Pappas AM: Acute and performance related injuries of the elbow, in Pappas AM, ed: *Upper Extremity Injuries in the Athlete* .New York, Churchill Livingstone, 1995, pp 339-364.

44. Andrews JR, Whiteside JA: Common elbow problems in the athlete. *J Orthop Sports Phys Ther* 1993;17(6):289-295.

45. Morrey BF: Osteochondritis Dessicans, in DeLee JC, Drez D, eds: *Orthopedic Sports Medicine* .Philadelphia, Saunders, 1994, pp 908-912.

46. Bauer M, Jonsson K, Josefsson PO, Lindén B: Osteochondritis dissecans of the elbow. A long-term follow-up study. *Clin Orthop Relat Res* 1992;284:156-160.

47. Andrews JR, Jelsma RD, Joyce ME, Timmerman LA: Open surgical procedures for injuries of the elbow in throwers. *Oper Tech Sports Med* 1996;4(2):109-113.

48. Dines JS, ElAttrache NS, Conway JE, Smith W, Ahmad CS: Clinical outcomes of the DANE TJ technique to treat ulnar collateral ligament insufficiency of the elbow. *Am J Sports Med* 2007;35(12):2039-2044.

49. Rohrbough JT, Altchek DW, Hyman J, Williams RJ III, Botts JD: Medial collateral ligament reconstruction of the elbow using the docking technique. *Am J Sports Med* 2002;30(4):541-548.

50. Bernas GA, Ruberte Thiele RA, Kinnaman KA, Hughes RE, Miller BS, Carpenter JE: Defining safe rehabilitation for ulnar collateral ligament reconstruction of the elbow: A biomechanical study. *Am J Sports Med* 2009;37(12):2392-2400.

   This controlled laboratory study evaluated the strain on the UCL in eight cadaver elbows following UCL reconstruction using a gracilis tendon graft. Strain was measured with elbow passive ROM, 22.2 N isometric flexion and extension contraction, and 3.34 N · m varus and valgus torque at 90° flexion. From 0° to 50° flexion, strain was less than 3%, and at 90° flexion, strain was 7%. No substantial strain with forearm rotation was noted.

51. Cain EL Jr, Andrews JR, Dugas JR, et al: Outcome of ulnar collateral ligament reconstruction of the elbow in 1281 athletes: Results in 743 athletes with minimum 2-year follow-up. *Am J Sports Med* 2010;38(12):2426-2434.

This retrospective outcome study reported the outcomes and the return to play in athletes following UCL reconstruction at a minimum of 2-year follow-up. Of all athletes, 83% were able to return to their previous level of competition or higher. The mean time for the initiation of throwing was 4.4 months, and the mean time for the return to full competition was 11.6 months. Level of evidence: IV.

52. Martin SD, Baumgarten TE: Elbow injuries in the throwing athlete: Diagnosis and arthroscopic treatment. *Oper Tech Sports Med* 1996;4(2):100-108.

53. Andrews JR, Timmerman LA: Outcome of elbow surgery in professional baseball players. *Am J Sports Med* 1995;23(4):407-413.

Chapter 25
Hip Rehabilitation

Keelan Enseki, MS, PT, OCS, SCS, ATC, CSCS   Dave Kohlrieser, DPT, PT, OCS, SCS, CSCS

Ashley Young, PT, DPT, CSCS

Abstract

Injuries to the hip joint in athletes have recently gained increased attention. Intra-articular conditions resulting from femoroacetabular impingement and hypermobility have been of particular interest. Because evidence to support both nonsurgical and postoperative rehabilitation protocols is relatively limited, intervention should be based on impairments and functional limitations identified using structured evaluation. The known characteristics of specific athletes related to hip injuries should be considered when developing treatment programs. Future emphasis should be placed on critical appraisal of nonsurgical treatment, postoperative rehabilitation protocols, and return-to-play considerations for athletes with hip injuries.

Keywords: hip; rehabilitation; femoroacetabular impingement; hypermobility

Introduction

Rehabilitation of hip injuries in the athletic population is a rapidly growing subject of interest in the field of sports medicine. Intra-articular pathology such as acetabular labral tears and associated underlying mechanisms such as femoroacetabular impingement (FAI) and joint hypermobility have prompted innovations in surgical and nonsurgical treatment. Nonsurgical and postoperative rehabilitation for these individuals must consider the mechanical factors of underlying injury (and associated surgery when applicable), the demands of the athlete, and most current available evidence.

None of the following authors or any immediate family member has received anything of value from or has stock or stock options held in a commercial company or institution related directly or indirectly to the subject of this chapter: Dr. Enseki, Dr. Kohlrieser, and Dr. Young.

Femoroacetabular Impingement

The treatment of symptomatic FAI has been debated recently. Although literature reporting generally positive results for the surgical treatment of FAI in athletes is increasing,[1] the current lack of definitive evidence justifies a trial of nonsurgical treatment of this population. Nonsurgical rehabilitation should focus on activity modification, treatment of physical impairments, and optimization of joint function.[2,3]

Reasonable training modifications should be the initial recommendation when treating symptomatic FAI. Activities that place the hip in a position of impingement should be minimized. Although impingement can occur in various positions, combined positions of flexion, adduction, and internal rotation are commonly associated with increased symptoms associated with FAI. Deep squatting, lunging, cycling, and hurdling are examples of activities that may require modification during rehabilitation. Effective training while modifying symptomatic activities can be difficult for competitive athletes participating in sports that require frequent performance of these activities.

Impaired strength has been noted in individuals with nonarthritic hip pain, including those with FAI. Particular deficits of the abductors and external rotators of the hip have been noted.[4] Uncontrolled pelvic motion in the frontal and transverse planes can contribute to the pain associated with FAI.[5] Strengthening exercises should be advanced to include weight-bearing activities that challenge the patient to control excessive adduction and internal rotation of the hip. Exercises that maximize gluteal recruitment and minimize use of the tensor fascia lata should be emphasized, including the resisted clam shell (Figure 1), the resisted sidestep (Figure 2), the unilateral bridge (Figure 3), and quadruped hip extension exercises.[6] Exercises to strengthen the lumbopelvic muscles should also be considered. Appropriate control can help to decrease the occurrence of excessive anterior pelvic tilt associated with impingement secondary to altered acetabular orientation.[7]

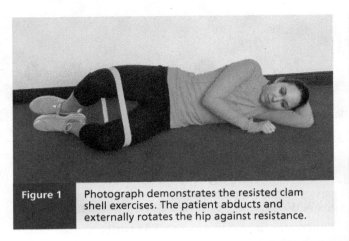

Figure 1 Photograph demonstrates the resisted clam shell exercises. The patient abducts and externally rotates the hip against resistance.

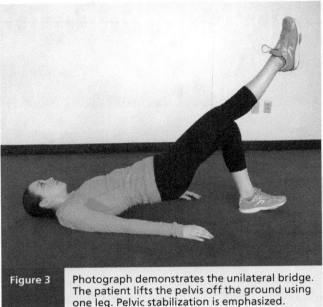

Figure 3 Photograph demonstrates the unilateral bridge. The patient lifts the pelvis off the ground using one leg. Pelvic stabilization is emphasized.

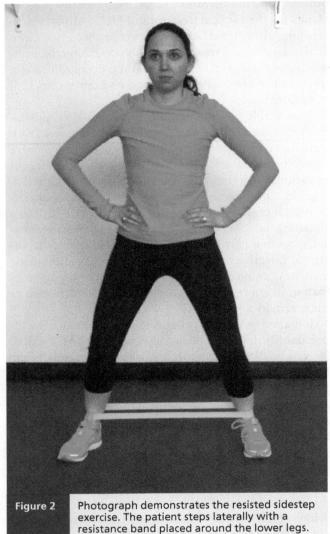

Figure 2 Photograph demonstrates the resisted sidestep exercise. The patient steps laterally with a resistance band placed around the lower legs.

the athlete to move the hip through the ranges of motion (ROMs) associated with symptomatic impingement. Treating hip flexor tightness should be a priority. Excessive tightness of this muscle group can be associated with anterior pelvic tilt. Anterior pelvic tilt has been correlated with the occurrence of FAI earlier in hip ROM.[7] When prescribing stretching activities, clinicians must be cautious to avoid placing the patient in positions associated with symptomatic impingement.[2]

Physical therapy techniques should be considered for patients with FAI. Joint mobilization may be indicated when the patient's examination suggests a loss of capsular mobility. Possible examination findings include loss of passive ROM, a capsular end-feel with passive ROM assessment, and a decrease of symptoms with manual distraction of the hip joint. Because FAI can be part of a spectrum of changes and a precursor to hip osteoarthritis in some individuals,[8] capsular changes should be considered. Soft-tissue mobilization can be useful when the tissue restricts joint mobility. A loss of motion associated with an elastic end-feel coupled with an immediate response to manual treatment of the target tissue indicates soft-tissue mobilization as a potentially useful intervention.[2]

Joint Hypermobility

Following a diagnosis of hypermobility or structural instability of the hip joint, patient education and counseling regarding activity modification is of primary concern to protect and/or avoid further injury in the region. It is recommended that the individuals avoid activities

Patients with symptomatic FAI may demonstrate impaired hip flexibility and pelvic musculature.[3] Flexibility activities should treat muscle tightness that can cause involving uncontrolled, forceful end-range extension and/or rotation that can place repetitive strain on the passive restraints of the hip.[2]

The correction of muscular imbalances of the hip and lumbopelvic region should be emphasized in athletes with hypermobility. An individualized program should be developed to treat impairments identified through evaluation. Flexibility exercises should be prescribed with caution only after end-feels have been assessed and are to be discouraged in those patients with excessive ROM.[2] ROM measurements should be recorded and compared with the contralateral limb. Individuals with rotational hip ROM imbalances demonstrate specific patterns of strength deficits. Individuals with excessive hip external rotation ROM have decreased strength of the hip internal rotators, and those with excessive internal rotation ROM have decreased strength of the hip external rotators.[9] The development and maintenance of sufficient strength to limit and/or control excessive hip ROM is essential in the nonsurgical management of this population.[2]

Strengthening programs designed for individuals with hip joint hypermobility should primarily focus on the hip abductor and external rotator muscle groups because of their role in controlling lower extremity alignment during functional activities. These specific muscle groups are responsible for maintaining a level pelvis and preventing adduction and internal rotation of the lower extremity while in single-leg stance.[10] Decreased hip rotational stability and/or strength has also been noted in individuals with symptomatic acetabular labral tears.[2]

In the presence of joint hypermobility, neuromuscular re-education including proprioceptive and perturbation training may be beneficial. Neuromuscular reeducation has had positive effects with other pathologies of the lower extremity. Individuals with labral pathology and compromised hip stability may benefit from the inclusion of dynamic stabilization and/or perturbation training (Figure 4) to increase the efficiency of the surrounding musculature, which can improve dynamic hip joint control during functional activities.[2]

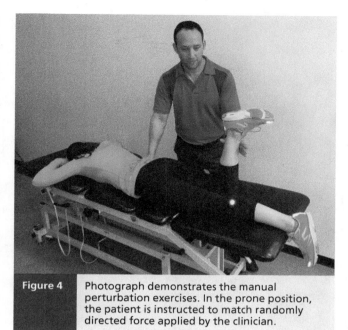

Figure 4 Photograph demonstrates the manual perturbation exercises. In the prone position, the patient is instructed to match randomly directed force applied by the clinician.

 Video 25.1: Manual Perturbation, Prone and Quaduped. Keelan Enseki, MS, PT, OCS (1 min)

Postoperative Concerns for Athletes Undergoing Hip Arthroscopy

In the patient who has undergone hip arthroscopy, postoperative goals are similar irrespective of the specific procedure performed. The main objectives are to reduce both the joint and postoperative inflammation quickly while protecting the repaired structures. Many complications in rehabilitation are preventable and can be avoided with deliberate patient education regarding the postoperative rehabilitation protocol, appropriate level of activity progression, and early activity modification strategies. Problems can occur during this period if the patient is not compliant with the prescribed period of limited weight bearing, participates in forceful ROM exercises, and/or is progressed too rapidly through the rehabilitation protocol.[11]

Procedure-specific considerations should be applied to the rehabilitation program. Prevention of postoperative joint stiffness and/or the formation of intra-articular adhesions should be emphasized immediately after hip arthroscopy. Circumduction ROM exercises (Figure 5) are used early in the rehabilitation program. Early application of circumduction exercises during the postoperative period has been associated with a lower rate of revision procedures.[12]

Acetabular labrum repair should be protected during the initial postoperative period by limiting hip flexion, extension, and external rotation ROM. The specific motion limitations depend on the location of the repair. Hip flexion is typically limited to 90° to protect posterior repairs, and hip extension and external rotation are often limited to neutral to protect anterior labral repairs. When the anterior joint capsule is involved (plication procedures), external rotation is often restricted for up to 4 weeks after surgery. ROM is typically progressed over the course of 2 months. Fewer precautions are used if labral débridement is performed.[11]

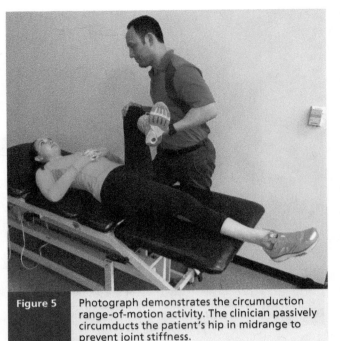

Figure 5 Photograph demonstrates the circumduction range-of-motion activity. The clinician passively circumducts the patient's hip in midrange to prevent joint stiffness.

Weight-bearing precautions vary depending on the surgical procedures performed. In less-invasive procedures such as isolated labral débridement, a short period of partial weight bearing (2 weeks or less) is often recommended.[13] For more involved procedures such as labral repair, protected weight bearing is maintained for an extended period. In such cases, patients typically bear weight as tolerated with an appropriate assistive device such as axial crutches for approximately 4 weeks.[11,14] When using crutches, patients should be encouraged to bear partial weight through the involved lower extremity while demonstrating a normal heel-to-toe gait pattern. This decreases the compression forces across the hip joint and can decrease potential iliopsoas irritation that can result from a sustained contraction while maintaining a toe-touch gait pattern.[11,13] Patients should continue to use crutches or an appropriate assistive device until the ability to ambulate without deviation can be demonstrated, even if crutch or device use persists beyond timeframes stated in postoperative guidelines. Weaning patients from crutches who are ambulating with compensatory patterns can delay recovery by contributing to continued intra-articular irritation and/or overuse of accessory musculature around the hip.[13,14]

Osteoplasty is often performed during hip arthroscopy to treat FAI. Up to 30% of the diameter of the anterolateral femoral neck can be resected to treat cam deformities without decreasing the load-bearing capacity of the femur.[15,16] Resection of 30% of the femoral neck diameter can significantly decrease the amount of energy required to produce a fracture.[16] Although rare, femoral neck fractures can occur following arthroscopic osteoplasty; therefore, weight bearing must be limited after procedures that include osteoplasty. Weight-bearing precautions specific to these procedures vary, but a period of partial weight bearing of up to 6 weeks is often recommended.[16]

When capsular modification procedures are performed to treat laxity, the rehabilitation program should be adjusted to protect the integrity of the repaired tissues. In these cases, ROM precautions specific to the procedure are recommended.[13] If capsulectomy was performed, often to visualize a cam lesion in the peripheral compartment, extension and external rotation ROM is avoided in the early postoperative period. With anterior capsular repair, avoiding external rotation greater than 20° is often recommended during the immediate postoperative period.[11]

Microfracture procedures can be performed in patients with focal full-thickness cartilage lesions of appropriate size.[17] The immature marrow clot should be protected during rehabilitation. Recommendations support extending the protected or limited weight bearing period to 6 to 8 weeks.[11,13,18] In conjunction with weight-bearing precautions, continuous passive motion can be recommended after microfracture to avoid intra-articular adhesions and scar formation. It is commonly recommended that continuous passive motion be used 4 hours per day during the first 2 to 4 weeks, with ROM set between 30° and 70°. ROM should be based on patient tolerance and progressed gradually during this period.[11,19]

Sport-Specific Rehabilitation Concerns for Athletes With Hip Injuries

Running

Hip musculature is often involved in various running-related injuries, including iliotibial band syndrome and gluteal muscle strain. Previous research has demonstrated that hip joint moments are greatest during the loading response phase of running, with the gluteus medius bearing the greatest load, followed by the gluteus minimus, gluteus maximus, and rectus femoris.[20] Increasing the step rate has been shown to increase loading of the hamstring and gluteal muscles in late swing phase. Conversely, increased step rate has been shown to decrease gluteal and piriformis muscle loading in stance phase.[21] For distance runners, the effect of step rate on specific muscles during various phases of gait should be considered.

Soccer

Most severe injuries in soccer players occur in the lower extremity. Although these injuries are more common in the knee and ankle, elite athletes often report unilateral or bilateral groin pain. Groin pain affects many different aspects of play, including kicking, accelerating, and changing direction. Athletes with groin pain have been found to produce notably less torque during hip adduction tasks than those without groin pain.[22] In uninjured players, a marginal difference exists between isometric measurements of hip adduction and abduction strength between the dominant and nondominant sides.[22] When determining return-to-play criteria for soccer players, a near-identical side-to-side measurement of isometric hip abduction and adduction strength indicates strength recovery. In cases of bilateral involvement, a ratio of 1.0 for ipsilateral hip abductors versus adductors may be considered ideal.

Golf

Most golf injuries occur at the lumbar spine; few occur at the hip joint. However, because of the close association of the lumbar spine and pelvis, issues with hip rotation ROM are thought to influence spinal injuries. During the swing of right-handed female golfers, the hip joint primarily rotates in the transverse plane, with the lead leg using 50% to 75% of available external rotation during the backswing and 84% to 131% of internal rotation during the downswing. The lag leg rotates substantially less during a full swing, creating an asymmetric movement pattern at the hip.[23] Because golf is a weight-bearing activity, it is recommended that ROM be clinically assessed during weight bearing, rather than in the traditional positions of sitting and prone. In addition, when treating hip injuries in golfers, obtaining full lead leg internal rotation through joint or soft tissue-mobilization techniques must be emphasized to minimize compensatory ROM through the lumbar spine.

Ballet

Ballet dancers require an extreme amount of motion at the hip, which often results in compensatory soft-tissue laxity. This pronounced amount of flexion, extension, abduction, and external rotation renders these athletes more susceptible to labral injuries, femoroacetabular subluxation, tendinopathies, and muscular imbalances. Generally, dancers exhibit increased external rotation at hip at the expense of internal rotation ROM.[24] External rotation strength in dancers has not been found to be greater than in nondancers; however, dancers generate a substantially greater angle-specific torque at extreme ranges of external rotation.[25] Rehabilitation should focus on establishing external rotation strength, particularly at the extreme ROMs commonly used by dancers.

Return-to-Play Considerations for Athletes With Hip Injuries

A relatively small body of literature describes functional testing and return-to-play considerations for athletes being treated nonsurgically or postoperatively following injuries in the hip region. Currently, clinicians must use the limited available evidence combined with established functional tests and protocols for other lower extremity injuries. Variations of deep squat test results have been described for individuals with FAI.[26] Hip abductor function has been correlated to performance on the single-leg squat and star excursion balance test. However, this association has only been studied in nonsymptomatic individuals.[26] Postoperative return-to-play criteria have often been adapted from protocols described following athletic knee injuries.[1]

Several patient-reported outcome measures have been validated for the younger, active population with hip injuries. The International Hip Outcome Tool (iHOT-33) has shown reliability and validity for assessing the quality of life in young, active patients.[27] The Hip Outcome Score has shown reliability and validity in patients undergoing hip arthroscopy. Additionally, the Hip Outcome Score contains a sports subscale.[28] Using patient-reported outcome measures may help the clinician assess perceived characteristics that affect an athlete's readiness for return to sports.

Summary

Hip and groin pain can become a chronic condition in athletes, potentially affecting performance and athletic participation. Recent advances in diagnostic imaging and improved understanding of pertinent examination findings should result in more rapid and accurate diagnosis of these pathologies. Many factors need to be considered by clinicians when implementing guidelines for nonsurgical management or a specific postoperative rehabilitation program. To achieve the most effective results and desired outcomes, the rehabilitation program should be based on the most current literature, individualized to treat impairments identified during clinical examination, and modified to consider athlete's diagnosis, history, and specific surgical procedure performed. A paucity of evidence exists detailing objective criterion-based progression through nonsurgical or postoperative rehabilitation. For this reason, decisions to advance exercise or activity level should be based on the individual's ability to demonstrate correct mechanics and appropriate dynamic control during functional activities versus advancing solely on time-based measures. Current evidence provides a theoretical foundation on which to base rehabilitation; however, future research should focus on comparisons between interventions and/or protocols to improve effectiveness of care.

Key Study Points

- Treatment techniques applicable to athletes with symptomatic FAI and hypermobility of the hip joint must be identified.

- The appropriate postoperative treatment progression to athletes undergoing hip arthroscopy should be applied.

- Sport-specific factors affect rehabilitation of athletes with hip injuries.

Annotated References

1. Tranovich MJ, Salzler MJ, Enseki KR, Wright VJ: A review of femoroacetabular impingement and hip arthroscopy in the athlete. *Phys Sportsmed* 2014;42(1):75-87.

   This clinical review explores recent evidence on the evaluation, recognition, and treatment of FAI, and discusses nonsurgical management, postoperative rehabilitation, and treatment in the pediatric and master athlete populations. Level of evidence: V.

2. Enseki K, Harris-Hayes M, White DM, et al; Orthopaedic Section of the American Physical Therapy Association: Nonarthritic hip joint pain. *J Orthop Sports Phys Ther* 2014;44(6):A1-A32.

   These guidelines developed by the Orthopaedic Section of the American Physical Therapy Association describe evidence-based physical therapy practice for treatment of nonarthritic hip pain. Level of evidence: I.

3. Yazbek PM, Ovanessian V, Martin RL, Fukuda TY: Nonsurgical treatment of acetabular labrum tears: A case series. *J Orthop Sports Phys Ther* 2011;41(5):346-353.

   This case series describes a nonsurgical program for those with clinical evidence of an acetabular labrum tear and found all patients demonstrated decreased pain, functional improvement, and correction of muscular imbalances. Level of evidence: IV.

4. Harris-Hayes M, Mueller MJ, Sahrmann SA, et al: Persons with chronic hip joint pain exhibit reduced hip muscle strength. *J Orthop Sports Phys Ther* 2014;44(11):890-898.

   This controlled laboratory cross-sectional study assessing hip abduction and rotator strength characteristics in individuals with chronic hip pain and control patients found substantial differences exist between experimental and control groups. Level of evidence: III.

5. Austin AB, Souza RB, Meyer JL, Powers CM: Identification of abnormal hip motion associated with acetabular labral pathology. *J Orthop Sports Phys Ther* 2008;38(9):558-565.

6. Selkowitz DM, Beneck GJ, Powers CM: Which exercises target the gluteal muscles while minimizing activation of the tensor fascia lata? Electromyographic assessment using fine-wire electrodes. *J Orthop Sports Phys Ther* 2013;43(2):54-64.

   This controlled laboratory study used electromyographic data to determine gluteal muscle activity during selected exercises and identified specific exercises that recruit the gluteal muscles while minimizing tensor fascia lata recruitment. Level of evidence: III.

7. Ross JR, Nepple JJ, Philippon MJ, Kelly BT, Larson CM, Bedi A: Effect of changes in pelvic tilt on range of motion to impingement and radiographic parameters of acetabular morphologic characteristics. *Am J Sports Med* 2014;42(10):2402-2409.

   This controlled laboratory study examining the effect of changes in pelvic tilt on terminal hip ROM and measurements of acetabular version found dynamic changes in pelvic tilt substantially influence the functional orientation of the acetabulum. Level of evidence: III.

8. Bedi A, Lynch EB, Sibilsky Enselman ER, et al: Elevation in circulating biomarkers of cartilage damage and inflammation in athletes with femoroacetabular impingement. *Am J Sports Med* 2013;41(11):2585-2590.

   This controlled laboratory study measured biomarkers of cartilage degradation and inflammation in athletes with FAI compared with control patients and found the results were substantially higher in the experimental group. Level of evidence: III.

9. Cibulka MT, Strube MJ, Meier D, et al: Symmetrical and asymmetrical hip rotation and its relationship to hip rotator muscle strength. *Clin Biomech (Bristol, Avon)* 2010;25(1):56-62.

10. Leetun DT, Ireland ML, Willson JD, Ballantyne BT, Davis IM: Core stability measures as risk factors for lower extremity injury in athletes. *Med Sci Sports Exerc* 2004;36(6):926-934.

    This study examined strength measurements in subjects with symmetrical and asymmetrical hip rotation ROM and found that strength values depended on the position that the hip rotator muscle is tested and the type of hip rotation symmetry or asymmetry present. Level of evidence: III.

11. Spencer-Gardner L, Eischen JJ, Levy BA, Sierra RJ, Engasser WM, Krych AJ: A comprehensive five-phase rehabilitation programme after hip arthroscopy for femoroacetabular impingement. *Knee Surg Sports Traumatol Arthrosc* 2014;22(4):848-859.

    This case series describes a nonsurgical program for patients with clinical evidence of an acetabular labrum tear that emphasizes hip and lumbopelvic stabilization, correction of hip muscle imbalances, biomechanical control, and sport-specific functional progression. Level of evidence: IV.

12. Willimon SC, Briggs KK, Philippon MJ: Intra-articular adhesions following hip arthroscopy: A risk factor analysis. *Knee Surg Sports Traumatol Arthrosc* 2014;22(4):822-825.

This case series was conducted to evaluate the possible risk factors for adhesions after hip arthroscopy and found adhesions following hip arthroscopy were reduced with modification of rehabilitation protocols. Level of evidence: IV.

13. Enseki KR, Kohlrieser D: Rehabilitation following hip arthroscopy: An evolving process. *Int J Sports Phys Ther* 2014;9(6):765-773.

14. Edelstein J, Ranawat A, Enseki KR, Yun RJ, Draovitch P: Post-operative guidelines following hip arthroscopy. *Curr Rev Musculoskelet Med* 2012;5(1):15-23.

This clinical commentary details a multiphase rehabilitation protocol following hip arthroscopy. Level of evidence: V.

15. Ayeni OR, Bedi A, Lorich DG, Kelly BT: Femoral neck fracture after arthroscopic management of femoroacetabular impingement: A case report. *J Bone Joint Surg Am* 2011;93(9):e47.

The authors reported a case description of a patient experiencing fracture of the femoral neck following arthroscopic osteoplasty for FAI. Level of evidence: V.

16. Mardones RM, Gonzalez C, Chen Q, Zobitz M, Kaufman KR, Trousdale RT: Surgical treatment of femoroacetabular impingement: Evaluation of the effect of the size of the resection. *J Bone Joint Surg Am* 2005;87(2):273-279.

17. Haughom BD, Erickson BJ, Rybalko D, Hellman M, Nho SJ: Arthroscopic acetabular microfracture with the use of flexible drills: A technique guide. *Arthrosc Tech* 2014;3(4):e459-e463.

The authors reported a technical description of an arthroscopic microfracture technique for the hip using a flexible microfracture drill. Level of evidence: V.

18. Yen YM, Kocher MS: Chondral lesions of the hip: Microfracture and chondroplasty. *Sports Med Arthrosc* 2010;18(2):83-89.

This clinical commentary describes chondral injuries that occur in the hip joint and arthroscopic procedures to treat such pathology. Level of evidence: V.

19. Enseki KR, Martin RL, Draovitch P, Kelly BT, Philippon MJ, Schenker ML: The hip joint: Arthroscopic procedures and postoperative rehabilitation. *J Orthop Sports Phys Ther* 2006;36(7):516-525.

20. Schache AG, Blanch PD, Dorn TW, Brown NA, Rosemond D, Pandy MG: Effect of running speed on lower limb joint kinetics. *Med Sci Sports Exerc* 2011;43(7):1260-1271.

This controlled laboratory study evaluated the effect of running speed on lower limb kinetics and found hip extensor and knee flexor muscles during terminal swing demonstrated the most dramatic increase in biomechanical load when running speed progressed toward sprinting. Level of evidence: III.

21. Lenhart R, Thelen D, Heiderscheit B: Hip muscle loads during running at various step rates. *J Orthop Sports Phys Ther* 2014;44(10):766-774, A1-A4.

This cross-sectional controlled study characterizing hip muscle forces and powers during running and how these measurements change with step-rate demonstrated increasing step rate and increased hamstring and gluteal muscle loading in late swing, but decreased loading of gluteal muscles and piriformis during stance-phase. Level of evidence: III.

22. Thorborg K, Serner A, Petersen J, Madsen TM, Magnusson P, Hölmich P: Hip adduction and abduction strength profiles in elite soccer players: Implications for clinical evaluation of hip adductor muscle recovery after injury. *Am J Sports Med* 2011;39(1):121-126.

This cross-sectional study comparing isometric hip adduction and abduction strength between dominant and nondominant sides demonstrated that a comparison between nondominant and dominant isometric hip adduction strength and ipsilateral hip adduction/abduction strength ratio should be used as a guideline for soccer players with groin pain. Level of evidence: III.

23. Gulgin H, Armstrong C, Gribble P: Weight-bearing hip rotation range of motion in female golfers. *N Am J Sports Phys Ther* 2010;5(2):55-62.

This controlled laboratory study measuring weight bearing hip rotation ROM in female golfers compared with actual hip rotation ROM occurring during a full swing demonstrated that weight-bearing ROM limits were not exceeded during swing, but the lead hip demonstrated decreased weight-bearing internal rotation. Level of evidence: III.

24. Weber AE, Bedi A, Tibor LM, Zaltz I, Larson CM: The hyperflexible hip: Managing hip pain in the dancer and gymnast. *Sports Health: A Multidisciplinary Approach.* 2014; April 23 [Epub ahead of print].

25. Gupta A, Fernihough B, Bailey G, Bombeck P, Clarke A, Hopper D: An evaluation of differences in hip external rotation strength and range of motion between female dancers and non-dancers. *Br J Sports Med* 2004;38(6):778-783.

26. Kivlan BR, Martin RL: Functional performance testing of the hip in athletes: A systematic review for reliability and validity. *Int J Sports Phys Ther* 2012;7(4):402-412.

This systematic review examining performance tests for the younger active population with hip pathology found the use of functional performance tests in the assessment of hip dysfunction has not been well established in the current literature. Level of evidence: IIb.

4: Rehabilitation

27. Mohtadi NG, Griffin DR, Pedersen ME, et al. Multicenter Arthroscopy of the Hip Outcomes Research Network: The development and validation of a self-administered quality-of-life outcome measure for young, active patients with symptomatic hip disease: the International Hip Outcome Tool (iHOT-33). *Arthroscopy* 2012;28(5):595-605.

This study describes the development of a self-administered evaluative tool to measure health-related quality of life in young, active patients with hip disorders that resulted in the development of a new quality-of-life patient-reported outcome measure, the 33-item International Hip Outcome Tool (iHOT-33). Level of evidence: IIa.

28. Martin RL, Philippon MJ: Evidence of reliability and responsiveness for the hip outcome score. *Arthroscopy* 2008;24(6):676-682.

Video Reference

25.1: Enseki K: Video. *Manual Perturbation, Prone and Quadruped.* Pittsburgh, PA, 2015.

Current Rehabilitation Concepts Following Anterior Cruciate Ligament Reconstruction

Penny Lauren Goldberg, PT, DPT, ATC   Giorgio Zeppieri Jr, PT, SCS, CSCS   Debi Jones, PT, DPT, SCS, OCS
Terese L. Chmielewski, PT, PhD, SCS

Abstract

Injuries to the anterior cruciate ligament (ACL) are common in sports. Patients usually are recommended to undergo ACL reconstruction to regain the knee stability that is necessary for resuming preinjury sports participation. Recent evidence indicates that ACL reconstruction outcomes include a low return-to-sport rate, a high incidence of second ACL injury, and the development of posttraumatic knee osteoarthritis, however; ACL reconstruction outcomes can be improved with a comprehensive preoperative and postoperative rehabilitation program that addresses knee impairments, patient expectations, psychosocial factors, and movement pattern deviations. Deciding when to allow a patient to return to sports participation or other high-demand activities is challenging and should be judicious, based on the results of a battery of objective tests.

Keywords: anterior cruciate ligament; rehabilitation; return to sports

Introduction

Knee ligament injuries are common musculoskeletal injuries that often occur during sports participation. The anterior cruciate ligament (ACL) is the knee ligament with the highest prevalence of injury.[1] ACL injury usually

None of the following authors or any immediate family member has received anything of value from or has stock or stock options held in a commercial company or institution related directly or indirectly to the subject of this chapter: Dr. Goldberg, Mr. Zeppieri, Dr. Jones, and Dr. Chmielewski.

results in knee instability that leads to reduced knee function and a lower activity level. Most patients require ACL reconstruction to regain knee stability and resume sports or other high-demand activities.[2] Consequently, ACL reconstruction rehabilitation receives substantial attention in clinical and research settings.

It is not surprising that most patients who undergo ACL reconstruction expect to return to sports participation.[3] Only approximately 60% of affected patients actually return to preinjury sports participation after ACL reconstruction.[4,5] Moreover, within 2 years after ACL reconstruction, as many as 20% sustain a second ACL injury to either the surgical or nonsurgical knee, with a slightly higher risk to the nonsurgical knee.[6,7] Within 10 years after ACL reconstruction, up to 80% show signs of posttraumatic knee osteoarthritis,[8] which can reduce knee function progressively. Clinicians should be mindful of these outcomes and should seek ways to improve ACL reconstruction rehabilitation to enhance return-to-sport (RTS) rates, guard against a second injury, and protect long-term joint health.

Patients undergoing ACL reconstruction ideally should undergo a brief period of rehabilitation before surgery and more extensive rehabilitation after surgery. Postsurgical ACL reconstruction rehabilitation can be divided broadly into early rehabilitation and late rehabilitation. Early rehabilitation focuses on resolving knee impairments and reintroducing low-level functional activity, whereas late rehabilitation focuses on preparing and transitioning the patient back to high-demand activity, including sports participation. Although general agreement about this approach to ACL reconstruction rehabilitation exists, consensus has not been reached on when to initiate certain exercises—especially those that impart high loads to the graft or knee articular surfaces—or what criteria to use when progressing patients between rehabilitation phases or back to sports participation.[9,10] In addition, altered psychosocial factors[11,12] and movement patterns[13] have been identified after ACL reconstruction, which can negatively influence rehabilitation outcomes. These impairments are not addressed routinely in most ACL reconstruction rehabilitation protocols.

This chapter describes the current concepts in ACL reconstruction rehabilitation. Although the focus is ACL reconstruction rehabilitation, many of the concepts are applicable to the rehabilitation of other knee ligament injuries.

Preoperative Rehabilitation

A primary goal of preoperative rehabilitation is to resolve knee impairments to the greatest extent possible. Acute knee impairments resulting from ACL injury, including pain, effusion, quadriceps inhibition, and loss of motion, should be addressed because they can contribute to the development of postoperative knee arthrofibrosis.[14] Quadriceps weakness occurs in almost all patients after ACL injury, likely because of effusion and pain.[15] Quadriceps muscle inhibition is common after ACL injury and can contribute to quadriceps weakness.[1] High-intensity neuromuscular electrical stimulation can be used to reduce quadriceps muscle inhibition and increase strength.[15,16] Additional exercises to improve quadriceps activation include the quad set and straight leg raise. Patients usually adopt an antalgic gait after injury and benefit from gait training to reestablish knee extension and symmetric weight bearing.

A subject not addressed routinely in preoperative rehabilitation that could influence postoperative outcomes is patient expectations. Patients should be educated about the course of ACL reconstruction rehabilitation and need to be engaged in a discussion about their expectations of postoperative outcomes to prevent postoperative dissatisfaction.[3] Practitioners should establish baseline expectations for rehabilitation milestones, create RTS criteria, and provide direction to prevent unrealistic patient expectations.[17] Practitioners also should be aware that the conventional criteria used to determine success following ACL reconstruction, such as knee laxity or functional testing, may fail to capture the patient's definition of a successful rehabilitation outcome. Excellent clinical and functional outcomes do not always equate to patient satisfaction.[17,18] Recent evidence has shown that patient expectations following ACL reconstruction are higher in younger, highly active patients without a history of previous knee surgery;[3] however, the influence of these factors on expectations may be unique to the individual and case.[17] Patient education aimed at managing expectations

is necessary, because failure to address expectations early in rehabilitation can lead to dissatisfaction and increased health care utilization and cost.[17]

Patients often have an elevated fear of reinjury following ACL injury,[19] and fear of reinjury is a key reason for not returning to sports participation after ACL reconstruction.[20] Fear of reinjury is high immediately after ACL injury but tends to decline substantially in the first month after ACL reconstruction and throughout early rehabilitation,[21] at the same time as knee impairments are improving. However, psychologic disturbances can follow a "U" pattern, in which disturbances are high immediately after ACL injury, improve through early rehabilitation, and increase again on RTS.[22] Preliminary work in this area suggests that the level of a patient's fear of reinjury immediately after ACL injury does not affect RTS.[11] During the preoperative period, however, it might be beneficial to assess the level of a patient's fear of reinjury. If a high fear of reinjury is present, the patient could be engaged in a discussion about the underlying reasons for the fear to begin reducing the anxiety about reinjury.[23] The Tampa Scale for Kinesiophobia is a questionnaire that could be used to assess levels of a patient's fear of reinjury.[24] A recent survey showed that 50% of physicians discuss the fear of reinjury with their patients; this type of discussion could be done more regularly.[25]

Early Postoperative Rehabilitation

Immediate Postoperative Phase

The goals of the immediate postoperative phase are to reduce knee effusion and pain, increase knee range of motion (ROM), obtain good quadriceps contraction, improve proprioception, and normalize gait. Weight bearing should begin immediately after surgery to restore proper gait sequencing. Patients should be transitioned from protected weight bearing with assistive devices to weight bearing without assistive devices when they can achieve full knee extension and can effectively control pain. The immediate postoperative phase continues to focus on resolving acute knee impairments, because surgery reactivates the inflammatory process.

Reducing postoperative knee effusion following ACL reconstruction is imperative because persistent effusion has been shown to negatively affect intra-articular structures, inhibit quadriceps contraction, interfere with the recovery of knee ROM, disrupt gait mechanics, and prolong rehabilitation.[14,26] A failure to reduce knee effusion can lead to patellofemoral pain, increased postoperative pain, posttraumatic osteoarthritis, and an increased risk of arthrofibrosis.[14,26-28] Strategies to reduce knee effusion include the use of compression wraps, limb elevation, modalities such as cryotherapy and high-voltage electrical stimulation, and knee ROM exercises.[29]

Initiating knee ROM exercises and restoring knee ROM in the immediate postoperative phase of rehabilitation are essential. Delaying knee motion can cause complications, including articular cartilage degradation, arthrofibrosis, impedance of graft remodeling, capsular contractures, patellofemoral pain, gait dysfunction, and scar tissue formation in the intercondylar notch.[14,26,28,30] Achieving knee extension that is symmetric to the contralateral knee is critical because extension deficit is a potential risk factor for the development of osteoarthritis and knee stiffness.[20] Therefore, rehabilitation should be directed first toward the achievement of symmetric full knee extension to the contralateral side, followed by full knee flexion.[28] Heel slides or active assisted ROM exercises performed while seated in a chair or on the edge of a bed can be used to improve extension and flexion ROM. If a patient has difficulty regaining full knee extension, passive interventions that use low-load long-duration stretching can be implemented, such as heel props (**Figure 1**) and prone hangs. Patellar mobilization in the superior direction can assist the recovery of knee extension by facilitating quadriceps activation and preventing infrapatellar fat pad contracture.[14,28] Soft-tissue mobilizations should be performed along the incision and portal sites to minimize the risk of adhesions, which can cause pain and interfere with knee ROM and patellar mobility.

Reestablishing proprioception is essential following ACL reconstruction to assist in muscle activation, dynamic joint stability, the reduction of joint forces, and the relearning of movement patterns.[13] Initially, weight shifts can be used to provide somatosensory input and promote weight bearing on the surgical limb. Weight shifts can be progressed to single-leg standing with 5° to 30° of knee flexion.

Intermediate Postoperative Phase

Before beginning the intermediate postoperative phase, the patient should have achieved full-extension ROM, nearly full-flexion ROM, a normalized gait pattern, and minimal to no effusion, with no joint line or patellofemoral pain.[15,29] The goals of this phase are to resolve any remaining acute knee impairments, increase muscle strength and endurance, restore neuromuscular control, and normalize movement patterns in low-demand functional activities. A factor that could delay progress during this phase is persistent knee effusion, which can limit knee ROM and inhibit quadriceps contraction. Functional activities should be progressed to gradually increase the load on the knee. In addition, the graft type will determine exercise progression so that the load on the healing

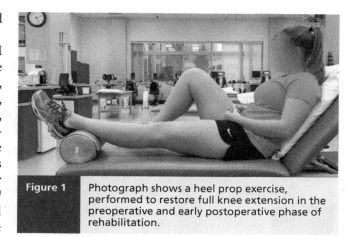

Figure 1 Photograph shows a heel prop exercise, performed to restore full knee extension in the preoperative and early postoperative phase of rehabilitation.

tissue is increased gradually.

Quadriceps strengthening is important during this phase, but it must not compromise the integrity of the graft. After the patient can elicit a visible quadriceps contraction and perform a straight leg raise without an extension lag, exercises to increase quadriceps strength and endurance can be implemented. Seated knee extension is an open kinetic chain exercise that isolates the quadriceps muscle; it should be performed from 90° to 40° of knee flexion to minimize anterior tibial translation in ranges that can be harmful to the healing graft.[14,31] Conversely, closed kinetic chain multijoint exercises should be performed in the range of 0° to 60° of knee flexion. Examples of closed kinetic chain exercises include the leg press (**Figure 2**), squats, lunges, and forward or lateral step-ups. Strengthening exercises should incorporate concentric and eccentric training of the lower extremity. Studies have shown that patients who include eccentric training have more quadriceps strength and perform better on hopping tasks than those who trained with traditional exercise alone.[32] High-intensity neuromuscular electrical stimulation may be continued in the intermediate phase if the patient continues to have difficulty producing a quadriceps contraction, has marked weakness, or experiences pain during open or closed kinetic chain exercises.

Movement pattern deviations during closed kinetic chain exercise or other functional activities are common after ACL reconstruction. One potential deviation is reduced weight bearing on the surgical side, which may result from quadriceps weakness and could be addressed with strengthening exercises. However, many patients continue to reduce weight bearing on the surgical side even after acquiring sufficient quadriceps strength. In such cases, patients may benefit from instruction from the rehabilitation specialist and feedback from a force measuring device (such as a force plate or scale), mirror, or video.

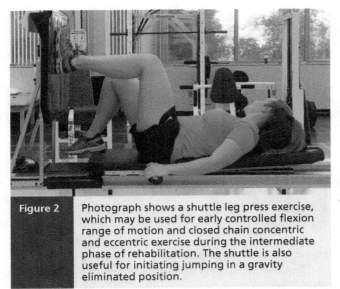

Figure 2 | Photograph shows a shuttle leg press exercise, which may be used for early controlled flexion range of motion and closed chain concentric and eccentric exercise during the intermediate phase of rehabilitation. The shuttle is also useful for initiating jumping in a gravity eliminated position.

Video 26.1: Perturbation Training for Neuromuscular Control and Dynamic Stability. Penny Goldberg, PT, DPT, ATC (0.13 min)

Video 26.2: Anticipatory Strategies to Enhance Neuromuscular Control and Proprioception. Penny Goldberg, PT, DPT, ATC (0.16 min)

Video 26.3: Reactive Strategies to Enhance Neuromuscular Control and Proprioception. Penny Goldberg, PT, DPT, ATC (0.17 min)

It is widely accepted that abnormal femoral motion has the potential to directly affect tibiofemoral joint mechanics and specifically the soft-tissue restraints that connect the distal femur to the tibia.[33] Another potential movement pattern deviation is medial deviation of the knee in the frontal plane secondary to hip adduction and internal rotation, resulting from hip muscle weakness. This deviation is addressed best with strengthening exercises such as resisted clam shells, side stepping with elastic resistance, the unilateral bridge, and quadruped hip extension with knee flexion.[34] This movement pattern, often referred to as dynamic knee valgus, has been associated with ACL injury[35] and may continue to be present even after ACL reconstruction if not addressed.[29] If sufficient hip strength is present, this medial deviation in the frontal plane may be a learned movement pattern that requires instruction and feedback.

A final consideration for the intermediate phase is trunk control and core stabilization, because reduced core proprioception has been linked to knee injuries.[36] Most high-level activities require core stabilization and trunk control to maintain the body's center of mass within the base of support in response to unexpected perturbations, so that potentially injurious forces are minimized. Potential beneficial exercises include bridges, planks, crunches, and double-leg and single-leg dead lifts. Perturbation training using stable and unstable surfaces (Video 26.1) as well as training anticipatory strategies (Video 26.2) and reactive balance strategies (Video 26.3) should be incorporated to enhance proprioception and neuromuscular control of the lower extremity (Figure 3).

Tasks that train anticipatory strategies include stepping onto unstable surfaces or moving the other extremity outside of the base of support. Reactive strategies can be taught using catching tasks with weighted balls; the patient must react to the ball and stabilize after the catch.

Completion of the intermediate phase is marked by full, pain-free knee ROM, adequate quadriceps and hamstring strength, good proprioception and balance, and minimal pain or effusion during activities of daily living.[15,16,29] The quadriceps index, a ratio between the strength of the involved side to that of the uninvolved side, is an important predictor of performance, emphasizing the role quadriceps strength plays in function and performance.[37] Quadriceps strength can be measured using an isokinetic or hand-held dynamometer or by isometric strength testing or one-repetition maximum testing. Values ranging from 65% to 90% have been reported as adequate to begin higher-level rehabilitation activities.[14,16,29,37-39]

Late Postoperative Rehabilitation

The goal of the late phase of ACL reconstruction rehabilitation is to initiate high-demand activities in preparation for RTS.[15,16,29] A combination of in-line running, agility, and sport-specific exercises are implemented progressively to appropriately challenge the patient's strength and endurance. Increasing levels of intensity should be used to ensure that the patient is physically fit enough to return to full, unrestricted participation in sports. Proper movement patterns are emphasized during these activities, and neuromuscular training should play a major role in late-phase rehabilitation to reinforce appropriate muscle firing patterns and a suitable reaction to external forces, which contribute to proper joint biomechanics and possibly help prevent knee osteoarthritis[40] and reduce the risk of reinjury.[41] Strengthening and flexibility exercises are

4: Rehabilitation

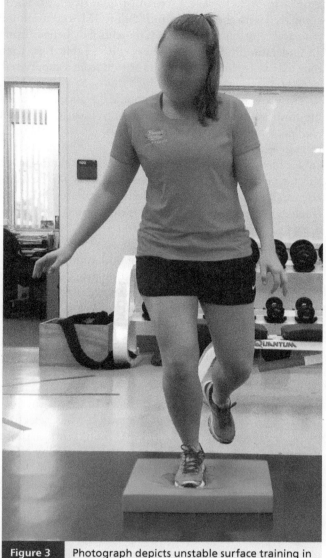

| Figure 3 | Photograph depicts unstable surface training in a single-leg stance to enhance neuromuscular control of the lower extremity. Adding perturbations or throwing and catching tasks can be used to increase the difficulty of the drill. |

| Figure 4 | Photograph shows a ladder drill, which can be used to incorporate lateral movements and ready the patient for a return to sport during the late phase of rehabilitation. |

continued and move to a maintenance or home exercise program as impairments resolve.

Straight-plane running for 4 to 6 weeks should be performed before the introduction of lateral movements into the rehabilitation program to allow the patient to build unilateral strength and force generation through the dynamic nature of running.[16] Activities that pose a high risk of ACL injury include landing a jump,[42] sidestepping, and cutting maneuvers.[43] Double-leg or single-leg landing tasks and ladder or cone drills should be incorporated during this phase (Figures 4 and 5). The chosen activities should mimic the movements most likely to be encountered by each individual athlete. Movement patterns should be assessed continually for the presence of dynamic valgus, weight-bearing asymmetries,[44] and decreased knee flexion to minimize the risk of ACL injury.[45] If weakness in the hip and quadriceps muscles has been addressed earlier in the early phase of rehabilitation, these movement pattern deviations are less likely to be present.

Although the specific criteria for the return to sport-specific activities vary, the protocols generally use a combination of the quadriceps strength index, ROM, knee laxity, episodes of instability, pain, effusion, and self-reporting of function to determine the achievement of each milestone to indicate readiness for the next milestone.[16] Common criteria used to assess readiness to begin running include a 65% to 90%[14,16,29,37-39] return of quadriceps strength compared with the healthy limb, full ROM, and minimal pain and effusion. Additionally, patients may benefit from an understanding of the soreness rules (Table 1) so that they may self-manage during transition from a supervised to an unsupervised progression.[16]

The progression of activities should advance from double-limb activities to single-limb activities. Tasks that challenge proximal control of the lower extremity should remain a focus of the program (Figure 6). Although critical for identifying limb and weight-bearing asymmetries, success in bilateral tasks alone has been shown to be inadequate in identifying other underlying unilateral deficits (such as strength, endurance, proprioception) even when activities are biased toward the affected limb.[46] Plyometric exercise to develop neuromuscular coordination during the explosive elements of running and athletic activities should be included in the rehabilitation program. Surface electromyography to the gluteus maximus and medius as well as the medial and lateral hamstrings of the dominant limb has been used to evaluate the activation of these muscles during common plyometric exercises.[47] Single-leg and double-leg sagittal plane hurdle hops consistently produced more muscle activity in the hamstrings and gluteal muscles, whereas jumping while rotating the body 180° during the flight phase produced the least activation of these muscles. This suggests that when selecting plyometric exercise, the practitioner should choose those performed in the sagittal plane, because they may effectively reduce load to the ACL and prevent dynamic knee valgus than those performed in the frontal plane.

A combination of visual, verbal, and tactile feedback may be beneficial when responding to athletes regarding gait deviations, limb asymmetries, and abnormal

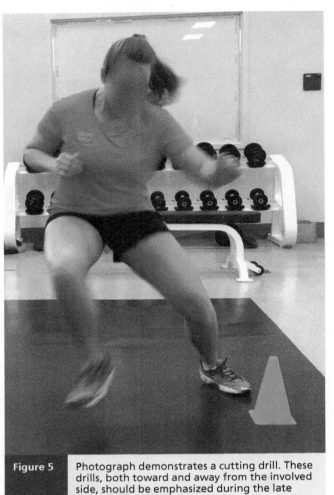

| Figure 5 | Photograph demonstrates a cutting drill. These drills, both toward and away from the involved side, should be emphasized during the late phase of rehabilitation. |

Table 1		
Soreness Rules		
Criterion	**Action**	
Soreness during warm-up that continues	2 days off, drop down 1 level	
Soreness during warm-up that goes away	Stay at level that led to soreness	
Soreness during warm-up that goes away but redevelops during the session	2 days off, drop down 1 level	
Soreness the day after lifting (not muscle soreness)	1 day off, do not advance program to the next level	
No soreness	Advance 1 level per week or as instructed by health care professional	

Reproduced with permission from Fees M, Decker T, Snyder-Mackler L, Axe MJ: Upper extremity weight-training modifications for the injured athlete: A clinical perspective. *Am J Sports Med* 1998;26(5):735.

© 2016 American Academy of Orthopaedic Surgeons

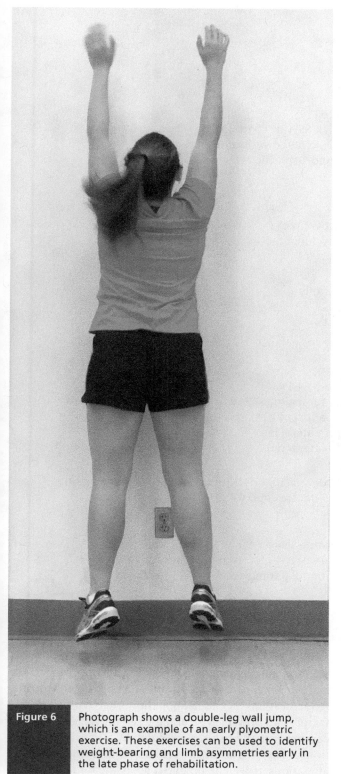

Figure 6 Photograph shows a double-leg wall jump, which is an example of an early plyometric exercise. These exercises can be used to identify weight-bearing and limb asymmetries early in the late phase of rehabilitation.

movement patterns compared with the healthy limb.[48] Programs that target individual biomechanical corrections have proved to be efficient in changing movement patterns,[49] potentially leading to improved postoperative outcomes. The incorporation of mirrors, video feedback, or force plates in addition to verbal cueing after visual assessment may improve performance. Multiple stable and unstable surfaces, which replicate sport-specific demands, should be used in jumping and landing tasks. Additionally, exercises that include anticipated and unanticipated movements will prepare the athlete to accept the various forces most likely to be encountered during sports participation. Depending on surgical protocol timelines, an athlete should complete agility and jump training for a period of several weeks to several months to ensure that adequate strength, endurance, and neuromuscular control are achieved before the initiation of RTS testing.

No single test can be performed to determine the readiness for RTS. Instead, a battery of tests should be used to create a complete picture of the athlete's strength and functional status.[15] Functional performance tests such as hop tests can identify limb asymmetries. The most common hop tests are the single hop for distance, the crossover hop for distance, the triple hop for distance, and the 6-meter timed hop.[16,37,38] The limb symmetry index is commonly used to determine when muscle strength and hop performance are normal. Generally, hop testing is included in the RTS testing, but it has been suggested that specific criteria to be achieved before initiating hop testing include full ROM, a quadriceps index greater than 80%, and no pain with single-leg hopping.[16] Similarly, a wide variety of criteria are used to determine if a patient is ready to begin the RTS progression (Table 2). The most common criteria are full, pain-free ROM,[9,14,15,29] 80% to 90% on the quadriceps index,[9,14-16,29,46] and limb symmetry index scores of 80% to 90% of the uninvolved side.[16,29,39]

At the time of RTS, the effect of quadriceps strength asymmetry on functional performance and self-reported function after ACL reconstruction has been established.[37] More quadriceps weakness is associated with lower self-reported knee function and poorer performance in all functional testing. Additionally, a quadriceps index score less than 85% negatively affected function, whereas patients with a quadriceps index score of 90% or greater performed in a manner similar to uninjured individuals.[37]

For many athletes, rehabilitation will end with RTS, but clinicians may choose to continue to monitor the patient after full RTS has occurred. Issues of strength or biomechanics that were not resolved completely during the late phase of rehabilitation can continue to be addressed both during and after RTS. Additionally, the

4: Rehabilitation

Table 2

Return-to-Sport Criteria From Published Protocols

Authors and Year	Criteria
van Grinsven et al (2010)[14]	• Full range of motion • Hop tests ≥ 85% of contralateral side • Hamstrings and quadriceps strength ≥ 85% of contralateral side • Hamstrings/quadriceps ratio < 15% compared with contralateral side • No increased pain or swelling with sport-specific activities
Adams et al (2012)[16]	• ≥ 12 wk postoperative • ≥ 90% on quadriceps index • ≥ 90% on all hop tests • ≥ 90% on Knee Outcome Survey Activities of Daily Living Scale • ≥ 90% on global rating score of knee function
Manske et al (2012)[15]	• Full pain-free range of motion • No patellofemoral irritation • 90% quadriceps and hamstring strength • Sufficient proprioception • Physician clearance for advanced activities
Wilk et al (2012)[29]	• Satisfactory clinical examination • Symmetric pain-free range of motion • Quadriceps bilateral comparison ≥ 80% • Quadriceps torque–body weight ratio ≥ 65% • Hamstrings-quadriceps ratio > 66% for males, > 75% for females • Acceleration rate at 0.2 s 80% of quadriceps peak torque • KT-2000 test within 2.5 mm of contralateral leg • Functional hop test ≥ 85% of contralateral side
Kyritsis and Witvrouw (2014)[38]	• No pain or swelling • Isokinetic test at 60°/s, 180°/s, and 300°/s > 10% deficit in quadriceps and hamstrings • Isokinetic test at 60°/s hamstring/quadriceps ratio 0.7–0.9 • Student • Limb symmetry index > 90% • Knee Injury and Osteoarthritis Outcome Score > 90 on each subscale • Patient-Specific Functional Scale score of 9–10 for each reported activity • On-field Sports-Specific Rehabilitation fully completed

athlete may demonstrate higher levels of kinesiophobia and may benefit from continued training to develop appropriate levels of confidence.

Summary

ACL reconstruction rehabilitation continually evolves and currently is being scrutinized for ways to improve RTS rates, reduce second ACL injury rates, and minimize the development of posttraumatic knee osteoarthritis. ACL reconstruction rehabilitation protocols commonly address acute knee impairments (pain, effusion, loss of motion and quadriceps weakness), which is important because these knee impairments can adversely affect ACL reconstruction outcomes. Clinicians should cautiously progress patients from early to late rehabilitation in the presence of persistent knee impairments because progression too quickly may impede RTS and contribute to the early development of posttraumatic knee osteoarthritis. Awareness has increased about how altered psychosocial factors can prevent RTS and altered movement patterns can increase the risk for a second ACL injury. Recognition of key psychosocial factors and movement pattern alterations as well as potential assessment methods and interventions is important. Even though standardized clinical guidelines for ACL reconstruction rehabilitation are not available, the concepts presented provide guidance during the decision-making process.

Key Study Points

- RTS rate, the second ACL injury rate, and the incidence of posttraumatic knee osteoarthritis are important ACL reconstruction rehabilitation outcomes that require improvement.

- Knee impairments (effusion, pain, loss of ROM, and quadriceps weakness) can negatively affect ACL reconstruction rehabilitation outcomes and are the focus of early rehabilitation.

- Movement patterns should be assessed for common deviations, particularly in late rehabilitation, when sport-specific tasks imparting high forces to the lower extremity are introduced.

- Psychosocial factors (such as patient expectations, the fear of reinjury, and self-efficacy) should be monitored throughout ACL reconstruction rehabilitation because they can negatively affect ACL reconstruction rehabilitation outcomes.

Annotated References

1. Nicolini AP, de Carvalho RT, Matsuda MM, Sayum JF, Cohen M: Common injuries in athletes' knee: Experience of a specialized center. *Acta Ortop Bras* 2014;22(3):127-131.

   In this cross-sectional comparison of common knee injuries in various sports, it was determined that ACL injuries were most common in football, basketball, and volleyball players. Level of evidence: IV.

2. Hurd WJ, Axe MJ, Snyder-Mackler LA: 10-year prospective trial of a patient management algorithm and screening examination for highly active individuals with ACL injury: Part II. Determinants of dynamic knee stability. *Am J Sports Med* 2008;36(1):48-56.

   This cohort study (diagnosis) found that neither knee laxity nor quadriceps strength differed in potential copers and noncopers. Additionally, quadriceps strength influenced hop test performance more than activity level or knee laxity. Level of evidence: I.

3. Feucht MJ, Cotic M, Saier T, et al: Patient expectations of primary and revision anterior cruciate ligament reconstruction. *Knee Surg Sports Traumatol Arthrosc* 2014. [Epub ahead of print]

   This prospective study demonstrated that younger patients, patients without a history of knee surgery, and highly active patients have high expectations for RTS following ACL reconstruction. Level of evidence: IV.

4. Ardern CL, Taylor NF, Feller JA, Webster KE: Fifty-five per cent return to competitive sport following anterior cruciate ligament reconstruction surgery: An updated systematic review and meta-analysis including aspects of physical functioning and contextual factors. *Br J Sports Med* 2014;48(21):1543-1552.

   This update of a previous systematic review discusses RTS rates following ACL reconstruction surgery. Level of evidence: III.

5. McCullough KA, Phelps KD, Spindler KP, et al.Return to High School and College Level Football Following ACL Reconstruction: A MOON Cohort Study.2012;40(11):2523-2529.

   This article is a retrospective analysis of RTS rates, self-report performance and reasons for RTS, and risk factors for not returning to the same level of play in football players. Level of evidence: III.

6. Kamath GV, Murphy T, Creighton RA, Viradia N, Taft TN, Spang JT: Anterior cruciate ligament injury, return to play, and reinjury in the elite collegiate athlete: Analysis of an NCAA Division I Cohort. *Am J Sports Med* 2014;42(7):1638-1643.

   This case series of athletes undergoing ACL reconstruction before or during collegiate competition presents data on graft survivorship, reoperation rates, and career length. Level of evidence: IV.

7. Paterno MV, Rauh MJ, Schmitt LC, Ford KR, Hewett TE: Incidence of second ACL injuries 2 years after primary ACL reconstruction and return to sport. *Am J Sports Med* 2014;42(7):1567-1573.

   This cohort study to determine the incidence of repeat ACL injury following ACL reconstruction and RTS showed that, following ACL reconstruction and RTS, patients have a higher risk of suffering a second ACL injury than those with healthy knees. Level of evidence: II.

8. Øiestad BE, Holm I, Aune AK, et al: Knee function and prevalence of knee osteoarthritis after anterior cruciate ligament reconstruction: A prospective study with 10 to 15 years of follow-up. *Am J Sports Med* 2010;38(11):2201-2210.

   This prospective cohort examination of long-term changes in knee function after ACL reconstruction and ACL reconstruction with concomitant injuries found a significantly higher prevalence of osteoarthritis in those who had undergone ACL reconstruction with concomitant injuries. Level of evidence: II.

9. Barber-Westin SD, Noyes FR: Factors used to determine return to unrestricted sports activities after anterior cruciate ligament reconstruction. *Arthroscopy* 2011;27(12):1697-1705.

   This article is a systematic review of published criteria to explore the factors used to determine when to allow athletes to return to unrestricted sports activities after ACL reconstruction.

10. Thomeé R, Kaplan Y, Kvist J, et al: Muscle strength and hop performance criteria prior to return to sports after ACL reconstruction. *Knee Surg Sports Traumatol Arthrosc* 2011;19(11):1798-1805.

This article uses relevant literature to present recommendations for new muscle strength and hop performance criteria to be used for RTS decisions following ACL reconstruction. Level of evidence: IV.

11. Ardern CL, Taylor NF, Feller JA, Whitehead TS, Webster KE: Psychological responses matter in returning to preinjury level of sport after anterior cruciate ligament reconstruction surgery. *Am J Sports Med* 2013;41(7):1549-1558.

    In this case-controlled study exploring whether psychologic factors predicted RTS at 12 months after ACL reconstruction, several psychologic factors were independent contributors to RTS. Level of evidence: III.

12. Czuppon S, Racette BA, Klein SE, Harris-Hayes M: Variables associated with return to sport following anterior cruciate ligament reconstruction: A systematic review. *Br J Sports Med* 2014;48(5):356-364.

    The authors present a systematic review of the variables proposed to be associated with RTS following ACL reconstruction, including knee impairments, function, and psychological status. Level of evidence: IV.

13. Risberg MA, Mørk M, Jenssen HK, Holm I: Design and implementation of a neuromuscular training program following anterior cruciate ligament reconstruction. *J Orthop Sports Phys Ther* 2001;31(11):620-631.

14. van Grinsven S, van Cingel RE, Holla CJ, van Loon CJ: Evidence-based rehabilitation following anterior cruciate ligament reconstruction. *Knee Surg Sports Traumatol Arthrosc* 2010;18(8):1128-1144.

    This systematic review creates an evidence-based postoperative rehabilitation protocol for ACL reconstruction.

15. Manske RC, Prohaska D, Lucas B: Recent advances following anterior cruciate ligament reconstruction: rehabilitation perspectives : Critical reviews in rehabilitation medicine. *Curr Rev Musculoskelet Med* 2012;5(1):59-71.

    The authors of this critical review discuss various phases of rehabilitation, using the current research on the early return of passive motion, early weight bearing, bracing, kinetic chain exercises, neuromuscular electrical stimulation, and accelerated rehabilitation.

16. Adams D, Logerstedt DS, Hunter-Giordano A, Axe MJ, Snyder-Mackler L: Current concepts for anterior cruciate ligament reconstruction: A criterion-based rehabilitation progression. *J Orthop Sports Phys Ther* 2012;42(7):601-614.

    This article presents an updated postoperative rehabilitation guideline for ACL reconstruction, including the timelines and criteria for various milestones throughout the rehabilitation process to reflect the most current available research. Level of evidence: V.

17. Bialosky JE, Bishop MD, Cleland JA: Individual expectation: An overlooked, but pertinent, factor in the treatment of individuals experiencing musculoskeletal pain. *Phys Ther* 2010;90(9):1345-1355.

    This clinical perspective paper describes the role of expectations in clinical outcomes in individuals with musculoskeletal pain.

18. Becker R, Döring C, Denecke A, Brosz M: Expectation, satisfaction and clinical outcome of patients after total knee arthroplasty. *Knee Surg Sports Traumatol Arthrosc* 2011;19(9):1433-1441.

    This prospective study determined that patient satisfaction correlates with Knee Society Score, Western Ontario & McMaster Universities Osteoarthritis Index, and Short Form-36 Health Survey outcomes in a patient's status after total knee arthroplasty. Level of evidence: II.

19. Hartigan EH, Lynch AD, Logerstedt DS, Chmielewski TL, Snyder-Mackler L: Kinesiophobia after anterior cruciate ligament rupture and reconstruction: Noncopers versus potential copers. *J Orthop Sports Phys Ther* 2013;43(11):821-832.

    This secondary analysis, longitudinal cohort study examining kinesiophobia in noncopers and potential copers before and after ACL reconstruction found that preoperative kinesiophobia was high in noncopers and potential copers and that noncopers had greater reductions in fear after surgery.

20. Ardern CL, Webster KE, Taylor NF, Feller JA: Return to sport following anterior cruciate ligament reconstruction surgery: A systematic review and meta-analysis of the state of play. *Br J Sports Med* 2011;45(7):596-606.

    This article is a systematic review of postoperative RTS outcomes after ACL reconstruction.

21. Chmielewski TL, Zeppieri G Jr, Lentz TA, et al: Longitudinal changes in psychosocial factors and their association with knee pain and function after anterior cruciate ligament reconstruction. *Phys Ther* 2011;91(9):1355-1366.

    This prospective, longitudinal, observational compares the changes in psychosocial factors and their associations with knee pain and function following ACL reconstruction. All factors changed across a 12-week period and early scores were not predictive of pain or function.

22. Morrey MA, Stuart MJ, Smith AM, Wiese-Bjornstal DM: A longitudinal examination of athletes' emotional and cognitive responses to anterior cruciate ligament injury. *Clin J Sport Med* 1999;9(2):63-69.

23. Nicholas MK, George SZ: Psychologically informed interventions for low back pain: An update for physical therapists. *Phys Ther* 2011;91(5):765-776.

    This article discusses the application of empirically based psychological principles and clinical reasoning to assist physical therapists in managing the psychological obstacles that arise with activity-based interventions in patients with low back pain.

24. Woby SR, Roach NK, Urmston M, Watson PJ: Psychometric properties of the TSK-11: A shortened version of the Tampa Scale for Kinesiophobia. *Pain* 2005;117(1-2):137-144.

25. Mann BJ, Grana WA, Indelicato PA, O'Neill DF, George SZ: A survey of sports medicine physicians regarding psychological issues in patient-athletes. *Am J Sports Med* 2007;35(12):2140-2147.

26. Saka T: Principles of postoperative anterior cruciate ligament rehabilitation. *World J Orthop* 2014;5(4):450-459.

This article is a review of postoperative brace use, early ROM, electrical stimulation, proprioception, and open chain and closed chain strengthening in ACL reconstruction rehabilitation.

27. Shelbourne KD, Urch SE, Gray T, Freeman H: Loss of normal knee motion after anterior cruciate ligament reconstruction is associated with radiographic arthritic changes after surgery. *Am J Sports Med* 2012;40(1):108-113.

This prospective cohort study found that radiographic osteoarthritis is lower in patients who achieve normal ROM regardless of meniscal condition at 5-year follow-up after ACL reconstruction. Level of evidence: III.

28. Shelbourne KD, Freeman H, Gray T: Osteoarthritis after anterior cruciate ligament reconstruction: The importance of regaining and maintaining full range of motion. *Sports Health* 2012;4(1):79-85.

This literature review discusses the association between ROM and osteoarthritis following ACL reconstruction.

29. Wilk KE, Macrina LC, Cain EL, Dugas JR, Andrews JR: Recent advances in the rehabilitation of anterior cruciate ligament injuries. *J Orthop Sports Phys Ther* 2012;42(3):153-171.

This evidence-based commentary describes an accelerated rehabilitation program following ACL reconstruction with additional considerations for special populations, including female athletes and patients with concomitant knee injuries.

30. Shelbourne KD, Gray T: Minimum 10-year results after anterior cruciate ligament reconstruction: How the loss of normal knee motion compounds other factors related to the development of osteoarthritis after surgery. *Am J Sports Med* 2009;37(3):471-480.

This prospective cohort study examining ROM losses found that patients with a loss of knee extension of 3° to 5° including hyperextension had lower subjective and objective International Knee Documentation Committee scores at 10-year follow-up from ACL reconstruction. Level of evidence: II.

31. Escamilla RF, Macleod TD, Wilk KE, Paulos L, Andrews JR: Anterior cruciate ligament strain and tensile forces for weight-bearing and non-weight-bearing exercises: A guide to exercise selection. *J Orthop Sports Phys Ther* 2012;42(3):208-220.

This article is a descriptive laboratory investigation of the tensile and strain forces to the ACL during several common weight-bearing and non–weight-bearing rehabilitation exercises. It includes a review of similar studies and makes recommendations for the clinical utility of the findings.

32. Gerber JP, Marcus RL, Dibble LE, Greis PE, Burks RT, LaStayo PC: Effects of early progressive eccentric exercise on muscle size and function after anterior cruciate ligament reconstruction: A 1-year follow-up study of a randomized clinical trial. *Phys Ther* 2009;89(1):51-59.

This article presents 1-year follow-up data to a randomized clinical trial that investigated the effect of early eccentric resistance training after ACL reconstruction. Eccentric exercise led to increased quadriceps and gluteus maximus volume as well as quadriceps strength and hopping distance.

33. Powers CM: The influence of abnormal hip mechanics on knee injury: A biomechanical perspective. *J Orthop Sports Phys Ther* 2010;40(2):42-51.

This clinical commentary focuses primarily on the potentially detrimental effects that altered hip biomechanics produce at the knee joint. Level of evidence: V.

34. Selkowitz DM, Beneck GJ, Powers CM: Which exercises target the gluteal muscles while minimizing activation of the tensor fascia lata? Electromyographic assessment using fine-wire electrodes. *J Orthop Sports Phys Ther* 2013;43(2):54-64.

This controlled laboratory study used a repeated-measures design to determine which exercises activate gluteal muscles while simultaneously minimizing tensor fascia lata (TFL) activity. Five exercises scored greater than or equal to 50 on the gluteal-to-TFL index, a ratio of gluteal activity to TFL activation.

35. Hewett TE, Myer GD, Ford KR, et al: Biomechanical measures of neuromuscular control and valgus loading of the knee predict anterior cruciate ligament injury risk in female athletes: A prospective study. *Am J Sports Med* 2005;33(4):492-501.

36. Zazulak BT, Hewett TE, Reeves NP, Goldberg B, Cholewicki J: The effects of core proprioception on knee injury: A prospective biomechanical-epidemiological study. *Am J Sports Med* 2007;35(3):368-373.

37. Schmitt LC, Paterno MV, Hewett TE: The impact of quadriceps femoris strength asymmetry on functional performance at return to sport following anterior cruciate ligament reconstruction. *J Orthop Sports Phys Ther* 2012;42(9):750-759.

This article is a cross-sectional examination of the effect of quadriceps asymmetry on RTS using self-reported function and functional performance following ACL reconstruction. Those with weaker quadriceps had reduced function, whereas those with better strength performed similarly to uninjured individuals.

38. Kyritsis P, Witvrouw E: Return to sport after anterior cruciate ligament reconstruction: A literature review. *J Nov Physiother* 2014;4(1):1-6.

This literature review examines RTS criteria following ACL reconstruction.

39. Munro AG, Herrington LC: Between-session reliability of four hop tests and the agility T-test. *J Strength Cond Res* 2011;25(5):1470-1477.

This article is an evaluation of the reliability and learning effects of hop tests and agility tests used after ACL reconstruction. Participants achieved greater than or equal to 90% symmetry on hop tests, leading to a recommendation that this threshold be used in RTS decision making.

40. Culvenor AG, Schache AG, Vicenzino B, et al: Are knee biomechanics different in those with and without patellofemoral osteoarthritis after anterior cruciate ligament reconstruction? *Arthritis Care Res (Hoboken)* 2014;66(10):1566-1570.

This article is a cross-sectional investigation of knee rotational angles during running and walking after ACL reconstruction in subjects with and without patellofemoral osteoarthritis. Less internal knee rotation was found in subjects with patellofemoral osteoarthritis and valgus alignment.

41. Paterno MV, Schmitt LC, Ford KR, et al: Biomechanical measures during landing and postural stability predict second anterior cruciate ligament injury after anterior cruciate ligament reconstruction and return to sport. *Am J Sports Med* 2010;38(10):1968-1978.

This prospective cohort study of three-dimensional biomechanical factors associated with ACL graft failure reported that altered neuromuscular control of the hip and knee predicted secondary injury after primary ACL reconstruction. Level of evidence: II.

42. Ferretti A, Papandrea P, Conteduca F, Mariani PP: Knee ligament injuries in volleyball players. *Am J Sports Med* 1992;20(2):203-207.

43. Cochrane JL, Lloyd DG, Buttfield A, Seward H, McGivern J: Characteristics of anterior cruciate ligament injuries in Australian football. *J Sci Med Sport* 2007;10(2):96-104.

44. Gardinier ES, Di Stasi S, Manal K, Buchanan TS, Snyder-Mackler L: Knee contact force asymmetries in patients who failed return-to-sport readiness criteria 6 months after anterior cruciate ligament reconstruction. *Am J Sports Med* 2014;42(12):2917-2925.

This descriptive laboratory study of contact force symmetries in patients who underwent RTS readiness testing 6 months after ACL reconstruction reported that patients in whom testing failed demonstrated significant and meaningful contact force asymmetries.

45. Myer GD, Ford KR, Khoury J, Succop P, Hewett TE: Development and validation of a clinic-based prediction tool to identify female athletes at high risk for anterior cruciate ligament injury. *Am J Sports Med* 2010;38(10):2025-2033.

This article is a cross-sectional cohort study of the clinical predictors of increased knee abduction moment during landing tasks. Increased valgus, knee flexion ROM, body mass, tibia length, and quadriceps-to-hamstrings ratio correlated with increased knee abduction moment in a female population. Level of evidence: II.

46. Myer GD, Schmitt LC, Brent JL, et al: Utilization of modified NFL combine testing to identify functional deficits in athletes following ACL reconstruction. *J Orthop Sports Phys Ther* 2011;41(6):377-387.

This case-controlled study of modified National Football League Combine drills attempted to determine whether bilateral tasks adequately identified unilateral deficits when biased toward the involved side. The modified tests failed to identify deficits found with hop testing.

47. Struminger AH, Lewek MD, Goto S, Hibberd E, Blackburn JT: Comparison of gluteal and hamstring activation during five commonly used plyometric exercises. *Clin Biomech (Bristol, Avon)* 2013;28(7):783-789.

This descriptive laboratory study used electromyography to investigate gluteal and hamstring muscle activity during common plyometric exercises. Sagittal plane plyometric exercises produced greater levels of muscle activation than those in the frontal plane.

48. Barrett DS: Proprioception and function after anterior cruciate reconstruction. *J Bone Joint Surg Br* 1991;73(5):833-837.

49. Pappas E, Nightingale EJ, Simic M, Ford KR, Hewett TE, Myer GD: Do exercises used in injury prevention programmes modify cutting task biomechanics? A systematic review with meta-analysis. *Br J Sports Med* 2015;49(10):673-680.

This article is a systematic review of the effect of injury prevention programs on biomechanical changes during cutting tasks. Injury prevention programs have the potential to improve biomechanics during cutting tasks, particularly when they target technique correction in postpubertal female athletes.

Video References

26.1: Goldberg P: Video. *Pertubation Training for Neuromuscular Control and Dynamic Stability.* Gainesville, FL, 2015.

26.2: Goldberg P: Video. *Anticipatory Strategies to Enhance Neuromuscular Control and Proprioception.* Gainesville, FL, 2015.

26.3: Goldberg P. Video. *Reactive Strategies to Enhance Neuromuscular Control and Proprioception.* Gainesville, FL, 2015.

Chapter 27

Patellofemoral Pain Syndrome: Current Concepts in Rehabilitation

Mark V. Paterno, PT, PhD, MBA, SCS, ATC   Jeffery A. Taylor-Haas, PT, DPT, OCS, CSCS

Abstract

Patellofemoral pain is the most prevalent condition involving the knee that is referred to physical therapy, and it results from a diverse range of pathomechanics and pathoanatomic lesions. Despite the condition's prevalence, only limited evidence concerning the etiology, risk factors, and optimal management of this condition exists in the literature. An evidence-based approach for the evaluation and nonsurgical management of patellofemoral pain is suggested. The interventions are classified by proximal factors related to the hip and trunk, local factors specific to the knee joint, and distal factors focused on the distal shank and foot. Successful management is rooted in the detection of underlying impairments and functional limitations found during a thorough evaluation and in the appropriate application of interventions designed to target individually identified deficits.

Keywords: rehabilitation; patellofemoral pain syndrome; proximal factors; local factors; distal factors

Introduction

Patellofemoral pain syndrome (PFPS) is the most prevalent disorder involving the knee[1] and is the second most common musculoskeletal symptom presenting to physical therapists.[1] Despite this high prevalence, the etiology of and risk factors for developing PFPS remain unclear,[2] and a variety of theories about its etiology and rehabilitation exist. The most common etiologic theories describe alterations and/or impairments in anatomic morphology[3] and dynamic neuromuscular function.[4] Rehabilitative and etiologic investigations have focused on three areas of dynamic neuromuscular function and their associated effect on PFPS: the proximal area at the trunk and pelvis, the distal area at the foot and ankle, and the local area at the quadriceps and the patellofemoral joint (PFJ) itself.

Before implementing a course of rehabilitation for a patient with PFPS, it is critical to complete an accurate and thorough history and physical evaluation to determine the underlying mechanism. The identification of specific impairments and dysfunctions associated with the patient's reports of pain should drive the treatment planning and specific interventions. The authors of a 2000 study linked intrinsic risk factors to the development of PFPS.[5] They outlined local factors—including a reduction in quadriceps flexibility, altered neuromuscular coordination between the vastus medialis oblique (VMO) and the vastus lateralis, decreased quadriceps strength, and patellar hypermobility—to the development of PFPS. More recently, other authors examining multimodal factors have identified the interaction of local and proximal variables such as hip rotation weakness as being related to the presence of PFPS.[6] Another study relates more distal factors such as foot mechanics to PFPS.[7] This lack of consensus underscores the theory that no single mechanism for the development of PFPS exists. Therefore, a thorough evaluation of the potential underlying factors that may contribute to the development of PFPS must be undertaken by the physical therapist before developing an evidence-based intervention program. Specific interventions exist to address the proximal, local, and distal factors that may contribute to PFPS. An ideal rehabilitation program should incorporate components of each of these areas, as deemed necessary by the initial evaluation.

Dr. Paterno or an immediate family member serves as a board member, owner, officer, or committee member of Pediatric and Adolescent Research in Sports Medicine and serves as a consultant for DJO Global. Neither Dr. Taylor-Haas nor any immediate family member has received anything of value from or has stock or stock options held in a commercial company or institution related directly or indirectly to the subject of this chapter.

Proximal Interventions

Of all the etiologic and rehabilitative theories, none has received more recent attention than that focusing on the proximal factors that may contribute to the development of PFPS. A 2003 study theorized that biomechanical deviations of the femur into excessive adduction and/or internal rotation might result in a relative lateralization of the patella with respect to the trochlear groove.[4] These abnormal mechanics were believed to result in increased infrapatellar compression, pain, and dysfunction.[4] A 2010 study provided preliminary theoretical support when reporting that, compared with an uninjured cohort, adult females with PFPS demonstrate greater femoral internal rotation during the closed chain single-leg squat.[8] Accordingly, enhancing strength and/or neuromuscular activation to the muscles of the pelvic girdle may have a clinically relevant role.[4] Over the past decade, many studies have advocated assessing the role of hip muscle strength, hip neuromuscular activation, and dynamic lower extremity biomechanics on PFPS.[1,9,10] Emerging research highlights the contribution of dynamic trunk mechanics to altered PFJ stress.[11]

Recent prospective research has been conducted on the risk factors that contribute to PFPS. In a military population performing a jump landing task, prospective risk factors for the development of PFPS included decreased knee flexion angle, decreased vertical ground-reaction force, and increased hip internal rotation angle.[9] In adolescent girls, a large knee abduction moment incurred during a drop vertical jump task was linked prospectively with the later development of PFPS.[12] In adult female runners, greater hip adduction, but not hip internal rotation, has been linked prospectively with the development of PFPS.[13] This finding agrees, in part, with several cross-sectional studies that have identified excessive hip adduction and/or hip internal rotation in women with PFPS compared with age- and sex-matched controls.[14-16] These altered mechanics are not reported consistently in male runners,[14] indicating the differing role that sex may play in the development and treatment of PFPS in adults. Recent evidence suggests that, compared with women with PFPS, men with PFPS squat and run with less hip adduction and increased knee adduction or varus.[17] Further prospective studies in males are needed to delineate the relative risk of proximal biomechanical abnormalities on the development of PFPS.

Reductions in hip strength have been cited consistently in adolescent girls and women with PFPS, compared with age- and sex-matched controls.[18-20] In a systematic review of five cross-sectional studies, the authors of a 2009 study summarized strong evidence suggesting that females with

PFPS have weaker hip external rotators, hip abductors, and hip extensors than controls.[19] Moderate evidence indicates that females with PFPS have weaker hip internal rotators and hip flexors compared with controls, whereas no evidence indicates differences in hip adductor strength between cohorts.[19] In two separate cross-sectional studies, male and female runners with PFPS demonstrated increased hip adduction and hip internal rotation range of motion, compared with controls, and these deficits correlated with endurance deficits to the hip abductor and hip extensor musculature, respectively.[21,22] Future longitudinal work is needed to validate a casual relationship between these variables.

Rehabilitation efforts that focus on hip abductor and hip external rotator strength have resulted in positive outcomes, including short-term reductions in pain and improvements in function, in patients with PFPS.[10,23] A recent randomized controlled trial demonstrated that, compared with quadriceps strengthening alone, posterolateral hip strengthening resulted in superior outcomes in terms of pain reduction and functional improvement.[24] Although it is theorized that improvements in hip muscle strength may reduce stress on the PFJ through kinematic alterations to the hip joint and the knee joint in the frontal and transverse planes,[4] several authors have found no changes in hip and knee kinematics after implementing a variety of hip-strengthening protocols.[10,23] Thus, further investigations are required to understand the association between hip muscle strengthening, hip and knee kinematics, pain, and functional outcomes.

Recent investigations have focused on the association between PFPS, alterations in hip neuromuscular activation, and lower extremity kinematics. Compared with control subjects, adults with PFPS demonstrate a delayed and shorter duration of gluteus medius muscle activation during stair negotiation.[25] Furthermore, preliminary evidence indicates that gluteus medius activity is delayed and of shorter duration during running, whereas gluteus maximus activity is increased during stair descent in those with PFPS.[25] In women with PFPS, increased hip adduction and hip internal rotation excursion were correlated with later onset in the gluteus medius and gluteus maximus, respectively.[26] Because of the cross-sectional nature of the studies, however, cause and effect cannot be established, and further prospective studies are warranted.

Dynamic trunk mechanics may influence stress on the PFJ. A 2014 study demonstrated that, in a cohort of healthy adult male runners, increased sagittal-plane trunk flexion was associated with reduced peak PFJ stress.[11] In a cohort of adolescent girls with PFPS, a reduction in sagittal-plane trunk flexion during a single-leg squat was one of several variables—along with altered hip and

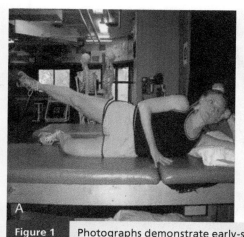
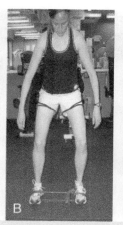
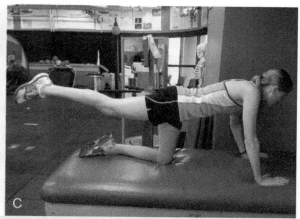

Figure 1 Photographs demonstrate early-stage interventions to address impaired hip strength. **A**, A hip abduction straight leg raise is shown. **B**, Lateral side stepping with band resistance facilitates gluteus medius muscle activity. **C**, Quadruped hip extension is shown with the knee straight.

knee kinematics—differentiating injured from uninjured patients.[27] From a kinetics standpoint, increasing trunk flexion reduces the external flexor moment acting upon the PFJ and therefore may reduce the internal knee extensor moment. The net effect is a reduction in compressive forces acting upon the PFJ. Altered dynamic trunk mechanics in the frontal plane also may influence motion and thus stress to the PFJ. Compared with controls, men and women with PFPS demonstrate increased ipsilateral trunk lean and contralateral pelvic drop.[28] An increased ipsilateral trunk lean may result in an increased external knee abduction moment acting upon the PFJ, which, in turn, may result in altered frontal-plane knee positioning and thus stress to the PFJ.[12,29,30] Therefore, rehabilitative efforts centered on altering the abnormal frontal-plane and sagittal-plane trunk mechanics in patients presenting with PFPS may have a clinically relevant role.

A rehabilitation plan of care designed to target proximal impairments often will focus on hip strength and muscle activation and can be staged into early interventions and return-to-function interventions. Early interventions focus on improving gluteal muscle recruitment while limiting pain reproduction, whereas return-to-function interventions focus primarily on closed-chain neuromuscular reeducation that targets the specific movement dysfunctions and participation limitations unique to the patient.

Early interventions to address impaired hip strength may be staged into exercises that gradually progress the neuromuscular activation of the gluteal musculature from low to high. Exercises in the low category, which recruit less than or equal to 40% of the muscle's maximal voluntary isometric contraction (MVIC), frequently begin with non–weight-bearing open kinetic chain activities such as side-lying leg lifts (**Figure 1, A**) and side-lying hip external rotation with band resistance.[31] These foundational exercises target the isolated hip muscle weakness often seen in patients with PFPS. Other early-stage intervention options to activate the gluteal musculature while minimizing activation of the tensor fascia latae include sidestepping with bands (**Figure 1, B**), single-leg bridging, and quadruped hip extension with the knee straight and bent[32] (**Figure 1, C**).

Interventions in the intermediate stage of therapy encompass open kinematic chain and closed kinematic chain interventions designed to increase gluteal and trunk muscle recruitment and to address altered neuromuscular movement patterns. Open kinetic chain interventions with moderate gluteal recruitment (40% to 60% of MVIC) include alternating arm and leg (for the gluteus maximus) elevation in quadruped and single-leg bridges[33] (for the gluteus medius, **Figure 2, A**). Closed kinetic chain interventions with similar gluteal recruitment levels include a variety of lunges and step-ups onto a box, including a retro step up.[34] Interventions targeted to improve trunk muscle recruitment and stability include a mix of exercises on stable surfaces such as anterior/front planks (**Figure 2, B**) and side planks (**Figure 2, C**) and exercises that introduce instability such as those conducted using a therapeutic ball.

Return-to-activity interventions are designed to maximally recruit and strengthen the proximal musculature and to normalize faulty movement patterns to prepare for the return to activity. Strengthening exercises that maximally recruit the gluteal musculature (greater than 60% of MVIC) include resisted lateral sidestepping, single-limb deadlifts (**Figure 3, A**), and single-limb squats[31] (**Figure 3, B**).

© 2016 American Academy of Orthopaedic Surgeons

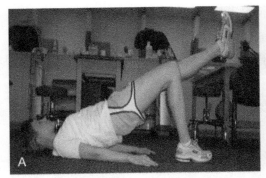
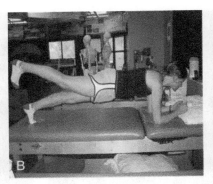
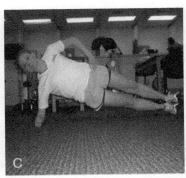
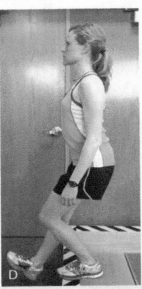
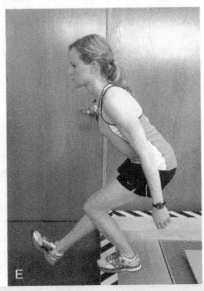

Figure 2 Photographs show interventions from the intermediate stage of rehabilitation, including single-leg bridging (**A**), a prone plank (**B**), a side plank (**C**), single-leg step down focusing on quadriceps femoris recruitment (**D**), and single-leg step down focusing on gluteus maximus recruitment (**E**).

In addition to strengthening, optimizing the technique and muscle activation are critical. Modifications to technique can result in a more targeted approach to certain interventions. For example, a single-leg step down can focus more on quadriceps recruitment (Figure 2, D) if executed with a more erect posture. Conversely, if executed with an increase in hip and trunk flexion, additional gluteal muscle recruitment is required to successfully accomplish the task (Figure 2, E). Modifications to the technique can influence the desired outcome of an intervention. Finally, proximal muscle recruitment is necessary to optimally align the lower extremity during dynamic movement. Prior research has identified hip adduction moment as a potential risk factor for the development of PFP in young athletes.[12] Interventions that target neuromuscular recruitment during dynamic tasks may facilitate optimal muscle activity and, ultimately, more normal movement patterns in this population.

Local Interventions

Local interventions, specific to the knee joint, long have been advocated in the rehabilitation of patients with PFPS. This philosophy was driven by the theory that PFPS was rooted in deficits in local factors, such as patellar tracking, limited muscle flexibility, or altered balance of quadriceps muscle function.[4,35] These local contributing factors could be the result of pathoanatomic or structural factors, such as patellar apprehension, tibial tubercle deviations, patellar alta, the presence of patellofemoral articular cartilage injury, and abnormal trochlea morphology.[36,37] In addition, biomechanical and neuromuscular factors related to the quadriceps femoris muscle such as VMO response time and the total cross-sectional area of the quadriceps have been linked to outcomes in this population.[36] A 2005 study described a clinical classification scheme focused on local factors that guided treatment

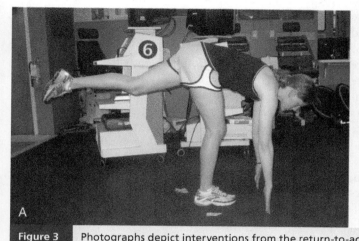
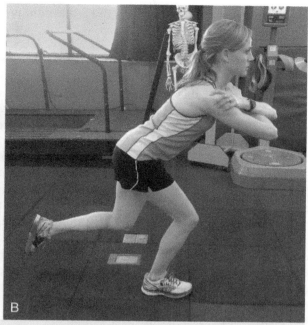
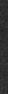

Figure 3 Photographs depict interventions from the return-to-activity stage of rehabilitation, including single-leg deadlifting (**A**) and single-leg squatting (**B**).

based on malalignment and muscular dysfunction, inclusive of strength deficits, neuromuscular dysfunction, and flexibility deficits.[38] These muscular deficits provide a template for addressing local modifiable impairments in patients with PFPS.

A primary modifiable local impairment often associated with PFPS is altered quadriceps femoris function. Reduction in quadriceps femoris strength limits the knee's ability to provide dynamic stability to the PFJ. Coupled with potential pathoanatomic factors, this reduction in strength may result in pain, instability, or loss of function. Interventions to target isolated quadriceps femoris weakness can use closed kinetic chain activities such as those described previously. Although these activities may successfully strengthen the lower kinetic chain, they may fail to address isolated weaknesses if compensatory patterns of movement develop. As a result, if the presence of isolated quadriceps weakness is appreciated at the evaluation, open kinetic chain quadriceps strengthening may be indicated. This intervention must be approached with caution, however, because open kinetic chain knee extension has the potential to increase shear forces on the PFJ. Recent research has identified safe ranges of motion in which to execute this task.[39] Specifically, the authors recommend a range of extension from 90° to 45°. Conversely, a closed kinetic chain squat is safest when performed from full extension to 45° of knee flexion.

Other local interventions have been reported in the literature with varying efficacy. Deficits in quadriceps, hamstring, and gastrocnemius-soleus complex flexibility have been identified in patients with PFPS[40]; however, the efficacy of targeted interventions to address these impairments has not been reported. Patellar taping to improve alignment and muscle activation also has been reported in the literature as a way to reduce PFPS and increase self-reported function in a period of less than 1 year.[1,41,42] Interestingly, a systematic review performed in 2008 showed that limited evidence in lower quality studies supported using patellar bracing as an effective means to manage PFPS. In summary, local interventions having the strongest evidence to improve short-term outcomes in patients with PFPS are focused on therapeutic exercises.[41]

Distal Interventions

Abnormalities in distal lower extremity biomechanics may be related to PFPS.[4] During dynamic activity, the foot and ankle provide the initial shock absorption and affect the proximal lower extremity motion. Because of the tight articulation of the talus within the distal tibial-fibular joint, pronation at the foot and ankle is coupled proximally with tibial internal rotation and knee internal rotation.[43] Thus, a theoretical construct exists, in which abnormalities in arch structure and dynamic function may lead to abnormal mechanics, stress, and ultimately pain and dysfunction at the PFJ.[4,44]

Evidence supporting this theoretical construct is mixed, with several authors finding no differences in pronation excursion between subjects with PFPS and uninjured cohorts during walking[45,46] and running.[13,15,46-48] Others have found increases in pronation variables in walkers.[49,50] A recent investigation using an altered definition of excessive pronation found that runners with PFPS used more of their available rear foot range of motion than did controls.[47] Additional prospective investigations are warranted to appreciate the association between altered distal lower extremity mechanics and the risk for PFPS.

Many clinicians assess foot posture as a static measure in an attempt to infer dynamic motion. Limited evidence links reduced medial longitudinal arch height and increased dynamic foot pronation in asymptomatic adults during walking[50,51] and running.[51,52] Limited evidence also links reduced medial longitudinal arch height and increased dynamic foot pronation in adults with PFPS.[49] Because of the nature of the cross-sectional study design, caution must be used in interpreting the results. Prospective findings are needed to better establish a cause-and-effect relationship between static arch height, dynamic foot pronation, and the risk of incurring PFPS. In a prospective study of novice recreational adult runners, no association was found between static arch structure and the future development of PFPS.[7] Additional prospective studies in subjects of different ages and activity levels are warranted to better understand the relationship between static arch structure and the risk of developing PFPS.

Because of the coupling between foot pronation and internal rotation of the tibia and knee, clinicians often prescribe over-the-counter (OTC) or custom foot orthoses in an attempt to modify distal biomechanics that may affect PFJ stress and dynamic function. The biomechanical evidence of the effect of OTC or custom foot orthoses on walking and running biomechanics is mixed. Several authors, using a heterogeneous approach to foot orthoses fabrication, have found no effect in healthy runners of a custom foot orthosis on such biomechanical variables as rearfoot eversion pronation,[53-55] tibial internal rotation,[55,56] or knee kinematics.[57] Others have found that custom foot orthoses do significantly reduce pronation-related variables at the rearfoot,[56,58] tibia,[53,54,59] and knee, however.[55,60] Differences in study results may be explained partially by heterogeneity in study design, subject populations, and outcome variable selection.

Biomechanics aside, individuals provided orthotic devices as part of a treatment program for PFPS frequently report reductions in pain[61-63] and improvement in the quality of life.[62] Limited evidence suggests that, compared with a flat insert, OTC foot orthoses reduce knee internal rotation and improve the short-term quality of life in individuals with PFPS.[64] Furthermore, limited evidence suggests that a combination of physical therapy (PT) and an OTC foot orthosis is better at reducing pain and improving quality of life than an OTC foot orthosis alone.[61,64] Compared with individuals receiving only PT, those receiving PT combined with an OTC foot orthosis have mixed outcomes, with some reports detailing improved subject outcomes[65] and others finding no difference.[61] Further randomized controlled trials are needed to better understand the added value, if any, of foot orthoses in enhancing patient outcomes.

Although rehabilitation frequently has focused on improving dynamic lower extremity alignment by enhancing hip and quadriceps muscle strength and neuromuscular activation, emerging evidence suggests that gait retraining may play a role in modifying stress to the PFJ. In runners, two key areas have been studied: step rate manipulation and visual gait retraining.

An increased stride length in runners results in increased PFJ stress.[66] An increased step rate has an inverse relationship with stride length[67] and PFJ forces.[68] The proposed mechanisms for reductions in PFJ stress may include alterations to hip kinematics,[67] knee kinematics,[67] hip neuromuscular activation,[69] and the external ground reaction force vector acting upon the PFJ.[66] Additional studies with long-term follow-up in injured patients are warranted to better understand the role that step rate manipulation may have on the improvement of functional outcomes in runners with PFPS.

Although step rate manipulation seeks to alter stride length as a means of influencing key kinematic and kinetic variables associated with PFPS, visual gait retraining primarily focuses on the alteration of frontal plane kinematic variables at the knee, pelvis, and trunk. Limited evidence suggests that real-time visual gait retraining using a computer[70] or a mirror[71] alters pelvic kinematics,[70,71] hip kinematics,[70,71] loading rate variables,[70] and external knee moments[71] and leads to short-term improvements in pain[70,71] and function.[70,71] The effect of running visual gait retraining on an untrained task of single-leg squat mechanics is mixed, with one study reporting a significant alteration in squat mechanics[71] and another finding no significant effect.[70] Limitations in these studies include their retrospective nature, homogenous subject populations, and short-term follow-up periods. Further randomized controlled trials with long-term follow-up are warranted to better understand the role that visual gait retraining may have on the reduction of pain and the improvement of function in subjects with PFPS.

Summary

Despite the current high prevalence of PFPS, optimal nonsurgical management has yet to be outlined in the literature. Success in rehabilitation is dependent on a thorough history and physical examination to identify the underlying mechanism. After the syndrome is identified, the development of a targeted intervention program addressing appropriate proximal, local, and distal factors is necessary to ensure the best outcome in this population.

Key Study Points

- Successful conservative management of PFPS is dependent on a thorough history and physical examination.

- Following identification of the unique mechanism underlying an individual's PFPS, it is imperative to apply targeted proximal, local, and distal interventions as appropriate to meet the patient's needs.

- A targeted plan of care is often unique to the specific impairments and functional limitations of each patient.

Annotated References

1. Davis IS, Powers CM: Patellofemoral pain syndrome: Proximal, distal, and local factors, an international retreat, April 30-May 2, 2009, Fells Point, Baltimore, MD. *J Orthop Sports Phys Ther* 2010;40(3):A1-A16.

   This article is a summary statement of the 2009 Patellofemoral Pain Retreat. Level of evidence: V.

2. Wilson T, Carter N, Thomas G: A multicenter, single-masked study of medial, neutral, and lateral patellar taping in individuals with patellofemoral pain syndrome. *J Orthop Sports Phys Ther* 2003;33(8):437-443, discussion 444-448.

3. McConnell J: The management of chondromalacia patellae: A long term solution. *Aust J Physiother* 1986;32(4):215-223.

4. Powers CM: The influence of altered lower-extremity kinematics on patellofemoral joint dysfunction: A theoretical perspective. *J Orthop Sports Phys Ther* 2003;33(11):639-646.

5. Witvrouw E, Lysens R, Bellemans J, Cambier D, Vanderstraeten G: Intrinsic risk factors for the development of anterior knee pain in an athletic population. A two-year prospective study. *Am J Sports Med* 2000;28(4):480-489.

6. Lankhorst NE, Bierma-Zeinstra SM, van Middelkoop M: Factors associated with patellofemoral pain syndrome: A systematic review. *Br J Sports Med* 2013;47(4):193-206.

   This review systematically summarized factors associated with PFPS. Factors noted were a larger Q-angle, sulcus angle, and patellar tilt angle; less hip abduction strength; a lower knee extension peak torque; and less hip external rotation strength in PFPS patients than in controls. Level of evidence: IA.

7. Thijs Y, De Clercq D, Roosen P, Witvrouw E: Gait-related intrinsic risk factors for patellofemoral pain in novice recreational runners. *Br J Sports Med* 2008;42(6):466-471.

8. Souza RB, Draper CE, Fredericson M, Powers CM: Femur rotation and patellofemoral joint kinematics: A weight-bearing magnetic resonance imaging analysis. *J Orthop Sports Phys Ther* 2010;40(5):277-285.

   Altered PFJ kinematics in females with patellofemoral pain appear to be related to excessive medial femoral rotation, as opposed to lateral patella rotation. Control of femoral rotation may be important in restoring normal PFJ kinematics. Level of evidence: IV.

9. Boling MC, Padua DA, Marshall SW, Guskiewicz K, Pyne S, Beutler A: A prospective investigation of biomechanical risk factors for patellofemoral pain syndrome: The Joint Undertaking to Monitor and Prevent ACL Injury (JUMP-ACL) cohort. *Am J Sports Med* 2009;37(11):2108-2116.

   This study suggested risk factors for the development of PFPS included decreased knee flexion angle, decreased vertical ground-reaction force, and increased hip internal rotation angle during the jump-landing task. In addition, decreased quadriceps and hamstring strength, increased hip external rotator strength, and increased navicular drop were risk factors for the development of patellofemoral pain syndrome. Level of evidence: III.

10. Earl JE, Hoch AZ: A proximal strengthening program improves pain, function, and biomechanics in women with patellofemoral pain syndrome. *Am J Sports Med* 2011;39(1):154-163.

    In this study, hip-focused and core-focused rehabilitation improved symptoms and patient-reported outcomes in female patients with PFP. Level of evidence: IV.

11. Teng HL, Powers CM: Sagittal plane trunk posture influences patellofemoral joint stress during running. *J Orthop Sports Phys Ther* 2014;44(10):785-792.

    This study suggests that increased forward trunk lean may be a strategy to reduce PFJ stress. Level of evidence: IV.

12. Myer GD, Ford KR, Di Stasi SL, Foss KD, Micheli LJ, Hewett TE: High knee abduction moments are common risk factors for patellofemoral pain (PFP) and anterior cruciate ligament (ACL) injury in girls: Is PFP itself a predictor for subsequent ACL injury? *Br J Sports Med* 2015;49(2):118-122.

    This study suggests that in girls age 13.3 years and older than 16.1 years, greater than 15 Nm and greater than 25 Nm of knee abduction load during landing, respectively, are associated with a greater likelihood of the development of PFP. Level of evidence: III.

13. Noehren B, Hamill J, Davis I: Prospective evidence for a hip etiology in patellofemoral pain. *Med Sci Sports Exerc* 2013;45(6):1120-1124.

    This study showed that adult female runners in whom PFP developed exhibited significantly greater hip adduction. No differences were found for the hip internal rotation angle or rearfoot eversion. Level of evidence: III.

14. Nakagawa TH, Moriya ET, Maciel CD, Serrão AF: Frontal plane biomechanics in males and females with and without patellofemoral pain. *Med Sci Sports Exerc* 2012;44(9):1747-1755.

    In this study, females presented with altered frontal plane biomechanics, which may predispose them to knee injury. Individuals with PFPS showed frontal-plane biomechanics that could increase the lateral PFJ stress. Level of evidence: IV.

15. Noehren B, Pohl MB, Sanchez Z, Cunningham T, Lattermann C: Proximal and distal kinematics in female runners with patellofemoral pain. *Clin Biomech (Bristol, Avon)* 2012;27(4):366-371.

    In this study, greater hip adduction, hip internal rotation, and shank internal rotation were seen in female runners with PFP. Less contralateral trunk lean in the PFP group also was noted. Level of evidence: IV.

16. Willson JD, Petrowitz I, Butler RJ, Kernozek TW: Male and female gluteal muscle activity and lower extremity kinematics during running. *Clin Biomech (Bristol, Avon)* 2012;27(10):1052-1057.

    This study showed that females run with a greater peak gluteus maximus activation level and a greater average activation level than do males. Female runners also displayed greater hip adduction and knee abduction angles at initial contact, greater hip adduction at peak vertical ground-reaction force, and less knee internal rotation excursion than did males. Level of evidence: IV.

17. Willy RW, Manal KT, Witvrouw EE, Davis IS: Are mechanics different between male and female runners with patellofemoral pain? *Med Sci Sports Exerc* 2012;44(11):2165-2171.

    In this study, males with PFP ran and squatted in greater peak knee adduction and demonstrated greater peak knee external adduction moment compared with healthy male controls. Males with PFP ran and squatted with less peak hip adduction and greater peak knee adduction than did females with PFP. Level of evidence: IV.

18. Cichanowski HR, Schmitt JS, Johnson RJ, Niemuth PE: Hip strength in collegiate female athletes with patellofemoral pain. *Med Sci Sports Exerc* 2007;39(8):1227-1232.

19. Prins MR, van der Wurff P: Females with patellofemoral pain syndrome have weak hip muscles: A systematic review. *Aust J Physiother* 2009;55(1):9-15.

    This systematic review suggests that females with PFPS demonstrate decreased abduction, external rotation, and extension strength in the affected limb compared to healthy controls. Level of evidence: II.

20. Souza RB, Powers CM: Differences in hip kinematics, muscle strength, and muscle activation between subjects with and without patellofemoral pain. *J Orthop Sports Phys Ther* 2009;39(1):12-19.

    This study suggested that females with PFP presented with greater hip internal rotation and decreased hip abduction and extension torque production compared with control subjects without PFPS. Greater gluteus maximus recruitment was present in patients with PFPS during running and step down tasks. Level of evidence: IV.

21. Souza RB, Powers CM: Predictors of hip internal rotation during running: An evaluation of hip strength and femoral structure in women with and without patellofemoral pain. *Am J Sports Med* 2009;37(3):579-587.

    Patients with PFP had less hip internal rotation, reduced hip muscle strength, and greater femoral inclination compared with control patients. Isotonic hip extension endurance predicted hip internal rotation motion. Level of evidence: IV.

22. Dierks TA, Manal KT, Hamill J, Davis I: Lower extremity kinematics in runners with patellofemoral pain during a prolonged run. *Med Sci Sports Exerc* 2011;43(4):693-700.

    In this study, the PFP group displayed less overall motion than did controls. Three distinct PFP subgroups were noted: a knee valgus group, a hip abduction group, and a hip and knee transverse plane group. Level of evidence: IV.

23. Ferber R, Kendall KD, Farr L: Changes in knee biomechanics after a hip-abductor strengthening protocol for runners with patellofemoral pain syndrome. *J Athl Train* 2011;46(2):142-149.

    This research showed that hip abductor muscle strengthening was effective in increasing muscle strength and reducing pain and improving knee kinematics in individuals with PFPS. Level of evidence: IV.

24. Khayambashi K, Fallah A, Movahedi A, Bagwell J, Powers C: Posterolateral hip muscle strengthening versus quadriceps strengthening for patellofemoral pain: A comparative control trial. *Arch Phys Med Rehabil* 2014;95(5):900-907.

    In this study, outcomes in the posterolateral hip exercise group were superior to those in the quadriceps exercise group. The superior outcomes obtained in the posterolateral hip exercise group were maintained for 6 months after intervention. Level of evidence: III.

25. Barton CJ, Lack S, Malliaras P, Morrissey D: Gluteal muscle activity and patellofemoral pain syndrome: A systematic review. *Br J Sports Med* 2013;47(4):207-214.

    This study presented current evidence indicating that gluteus medius activity is delayed and of shorter duration during stair negotiation in patients with PFPS. In addition, limited evidence indicates that gluteus medius activity is delayed and of shorter duration during running and gluteus maximus activity is increased during stair descent. Level of evidence: I.

26. Willson JD, Kernozek TW, Arndt RL, Reznichek DA, Scott Straker J: Gluteal muscle activation during running in females with and without patellofemoral pain syndrome. *Clin Biomech (Bristol, Avon)* 2011;26(7):735-740.

   In this study, females with PFP demonstrated delayed and shorter gluteus medius activation than females without knee pain during running. The magnitude and timing of gluteus maximus activation was not different between groups. Greater hip adduction and internal rotation excursion were correlated with later onset in the gluteus medius and gluteus maximus, respectively. Level of evidence: IV.

27. Scattone Silva R, Serrão FV: Sex differences in trunk, pelvis, hip and knee kinematics and eccentric hip torque in adolescents. *Clin Biomech (Bristol, Avon)* 2014;29(9):1063-1069.

   In this study, adolescent females presented with greater hip adduction, hip external rotation, and knee abduction and smaller trunk flexion during the single-leg squat than did males. Additionally, adolescent females showed smaller isokinetic eccentric hip torque normalized by body mass in all planes than did males. Level of evidence: IV.

28. Nakagawa TH, Moriya ET, Maciel CD, Serrão FV: Trunk, pelvis, hip, and knee kinematics, hip strength, and gluteal muscle activation during a single-leg squat in males and females with and without patellofemoral pain syndrome. *J Orthop Sports Phys Ther* 2012;42(6):491-501.

   In this study, individuals with PFPS had greater ipsilateral trunk lean, contralateral pelvic drop, hip adduction, and knee abduction when performing a single-leg squat than did controls. Individuals with PFPS also had 18% less hip abduction and 17% less hip external rotation strength. Compared with female controls, females with PFPS had more hip internal rotation and less muscle activation of the gluteus medius during the single-leg squat. Level of evidence: IV.

29. Powers CM, Ward SR, Fredericson M, Guillet M, Shellock FG: Patellofemoral kinematics during weight-bearing and non-weight-bearing knee extension in persons with lateral subluxation of the patella: A preliminary study. *J Orthop Sports Phys Ther* 2003;33(11):677-685.

30. Myer GD, Ford KR, Barber Foss KD, et al: The incidence and potential pathomechanics of patellofemoral pain in female athletes. *Clin Biomech (Bristol, Avon)* 2010;25(7):700-707.

   The authors prospectively evaluated measures of frontal-plane knee loading during landing to determine their relationship to the development of PFP. The new PFP group demonstrated increased knee abduction moment at initial contact on the most symptomatic limb and maximum knee abduction moment on the least symptomatic limb or the asymptomatic limb relative to the matched control limbs. Level of evidence: III.

31. Distefano LJ, Blackburn JT, Marshall SW, Padua DA: Gluteal muscle activation during common therapeutic exercises. *J Orthop Sports Phys Ther* 2009;39(7):532-540.

   This study describes the relative gluteal muscle activation during several common therapeutic exercises. Side-lying hip abduction resulted in the greatest gluteus medius activity while single limb squatting and single-limb dead-lifting led to the greatest gluteus maximus activity. Level of evidence: IV.

32. Selkowitz DM, Beneck GJ, Powers CM: Which exercises target the gluteal muscles while minimizing activation of the tensor fascia lata? Electromyographic assessment using fine-wire electrodes. *J Orthop Sports Phys Ther* 2013;43(2):54-64.

   This study showed that the clamshell, side step, unilateral bridge, and both quadruped hip extension exercises would appear to be the most appropriate to preferentially activate the gluteal muscles while minimizing tensor fascia latae activation. Level of evidence: IV.

33. Ekstrom RA, Donatelli RA, Carp KC: Electromyographic analysis of core trunk, hip, and thigh muscles during 9 rehabilitation exercises. *J Orthop Sports Phys Ther* 2007;37(12):754-762.

34. Ayotte NW, Stetts DM, Keenan G, Greenway EH: Electromyographical analysis of selected lower extremity muscles during 5 unilateral weight-bearing exercises. *J Orthop Sports Phys Ther* 2007;37(2):48-55.

35. Werner S: Anterior knee pain: An update of physical therapy. *Knee Surg Sports Traumatol Arthrosc* 2014;22(10):2286-2294.

   This clinical commentary provides a general update on phsycial therapy management of anterior knee pain. Level of evidence: V.

36. Lack S, Barton C, Vicenzino B, Morrissey D: Outcome predictors for conservative patellofemoral pain management: A systematic review and meta-analysis. *Sports Med* 2014;44(12):1703-1716.

   This systematic review and meta-analysis sought to evaluate the efficacy of proximal rehabilitation of PFP, compare various rehabilitation protocols and identify biomechanical mechanisms to optimize proximal rehabilitation. The review suggests proximal rehabilitation of PFPF should be included in conservative management. Level of evidence: II.

37. Witvrouw E, Crossley K, Davis I, McConnell J, Powers CM: The 3rd International Patellofemoral Research Retreat: An international expert consensus meeting to improve the scientific understanding and clinical management of patellofemoral pain. *Br J Sports Med* 2014;48(6):408.

   The authors discussed the consensus statement from the 3rd International Patellofemoral Research Retreat, which attempts to summarize current trends and research priorities in the area of patellofemoral pain. Level of evidence: V.

38. Witvrouw E, Werner S, Mikkelsen C, Van Tiggelen D, Vanden Berghe L, Cerulli G: Clinical classification of patellofemoral pain syndrome: Guidelines for non-operative treatment. *Knee Surg Sports Traumatol Arthrosc* 2005;13(2):122-130.

39. Powers CM, Ho KY, Chen YJ, Souza RB, Farrokhi S: Patellofemoral joint stress during weight-bearing and non-weight-bearing quadriceps exercises. *J Orthop Sports Phys Ther* 2014;44(5):320-327.

    This study suggests that, to minimize PFJ stress while performing quadriceps exercises, the squat exercise should be performed from 45° to 0° of knee flexion and the knee-extension-with-variable-resistance exercise should be performed from 90° to 45° of knee flexion. Level of evidence: IV.

40. Piva SR, Goodnite EA, Childs JD: Strength around the hip and flexibility of soft tissues in individuals with and without patellofemoral pain syndrome. *J Orthop Sports Phys Ther* 2005;35(12):793-801.

41. Witvrouw E, Callaghan MJ, Stefanik JJ, et al: Patellofemoral pain: Consensus statement from the 3rd International Patellofemoral Pain Research Retreat held in Vancouver, September 2013. *Br J Sports Med* 2014;48(6):411-414.

    A consensus statement from the 2013 Patellofemoral Pain Retreat is discussed. Level of evidence: V.

42. Warden SJ, Hinman RS, Watson MA Jr, Avin KG, Bialocerkowski AE, Crossley KM: Patellar taping and bracing for the treatment of chronic knee pain: A systematic review and meta-analysis. *Arthritis Rheum* 2008;59(1):73-83.

43. McClay I, Manal K: A comparison of three-dimensional lower extremity kinematics during running between excessive pronators and normals. *Clin Biomech (Bristol, Avon)* 1998;13(3):195-203.

44. Tiberio D: The effect of excessive subtalar joint pronation on patellofemoral mechanics: A theoretical model. *J Orthop Sports Phys Ther* 1987;9(4):160-165.

45. Powers CM, Chen PY, Reischl SF, Perry J: Comparison of foot pronation and lower extremity rotation in persons with and without patellofemoral pain. *Foot Ankle Int* 2002;23(7):634-640.

46. Hetsroni I, Finestone A, Milgrom C, et al: A prospective biomechanical study of the association between foot pronation and the incidence of anterior knee pain among military recruits. *J Bone Joint Surg Br* 2006;88(7):905-908.

47. Rodrigues P, TenBroek T, Hamill J: Runners with anterior knee pain use a greater percentage of their available pronation range of motion. *J Appl Biomech* 2013;29(2):141-146.

    In this study, no differences in traditional pronation variables were noted between healthy and injured runners. In contrast, injured runners used significantly more of their available range of motion than did healthy runners. Level of evidence: IV.

48. Rodrigues P, Chang R, TenBroek T, Hamill J: Medially posted insoles consistently influence foot pronation in runners with and without anterior knee pain. *Gait Posture* 2013;37(4):526-531.

    In this study, insoles, on average, reduced peak eversion, peak eversion velocity, and eversion range of motion. Although insoles reduced eversion variables, however, they had small influences on the transverse-plane kinematics of the tibia or knee. Level of evidence: IV.

49. Barton CJ, Levinger P, Crossley KM, Webster KE, Menz HB: Relationships between the Foot Posture Index and foot kinematics during gait in individuals with and without patellofemoral pain syndrome. *J Foot Ankle Res* 2011;4:10.

    In individuals with and without PFPS, a fair to moderate association was found between the foot posture index and some parameters of dynamic foot function. Inconsistent findings between the PFPS group and the control group indicate that pathology may play a role in the relationship between static foot posture and dynamic function. Level of evidence: IV.

50. Barton CJ, Levinger P, Crossley KM, Webster KE, Menz HB: The relationship between rearfoot, tibial and hip kinematics in individuals with patellofemoral pain syndrome. *Clin Biomech (Bristol, Avon)* 2012;27(7):702-705.

    In this study, greater peak rearfoot eversion was associated with greater peak tibial internal rotation in the PFPS group. Greater rearfoot eversion range of motion was associated with greater hip adduction range of motion in the PFPS and control groups and greater peak hip adduction in the control group. Level of evidence: IV.

51. McPoil TG, Cornwall MW: Prediction of dynamic foot posture during running using the longitudinal arch angle. *J Am Podiatr Med Assoc* 2007;97(2):102-107.

52. Franettovich MM, McPoil TG, Russell T, Skardoon G, Vicenzino B: The ability to predict dynamic foot posture from static measurements. *J Am Podiatr Med Assoc* 2007;97(2):115-120.

53. Mündermann A, Nigg BM, Humble RN, Stefanyshyn DJ: Foot orthotics affect lower extremity kinematics and kinetics during running. *Clin Biomech (Bristol, Avon)* 2003;18(3):254-262.

54. Stacoff A, Reinschmidt C, Nigg BM, et al: Effects of foot orthoses on skeletal motion during running. *Clin Biomech (Bristol, Avon)* 2000;15(1):54-64.

55. Williams DS III, McClay Davis I, Baitch SP: Effect of inverted orthoses on lower-extremity mechanics in runners. *Med Sci Sports Exerc* 2003;35(12):2060-2068.

56. Eslami M, Begon M, Hinse S, Sadeghi H, Popov P, Allard P: Effect of foot orthoses on magnitude and timing of rearfoot and tibial motions, ground reaction force and knee moment during running. *J Sci Med Sport* 2009;12(6):679-684.

The authors reported foot orthoses could reduce rearfoot eversion so that this can be associated with a reduction of knee adduction moment during the first 60% stance phase of running. These findings imply that modifying rearfoot and tibial motions during running could not be related to a reduction of the ground reaction force. Level of evidence: IV.

57. Boldt AR, Willson JD, Barrios JA, Kernozek TW: Effects of medially wedged foot orthoses on knee and hip joint running mechanics in females with and without patellofemoral pain syndrome. *J Appl Biomech* 2013;29(1):68-77.

In this research, no significant group × condition or calcaneal angle × condition effects were observed. The addition of medially wedged foot orthoses to standardized running shoes during running had a minimal effect on knee and hip joint mechanics thought to be associated with PFPS symptoms. These effects did not appear to depend on injury status or standing calcaneal posture. Level of evidence: IV.

58. MacLean C, Davis IM, Hamill J: Influence of a custom foot orthotic intervention on lower extremity dynamics in healthy runners. *Clin Biomech (Bristol, Avon)* 2006;21(6):623-630.

59. Nawoczenski DA, Cook TM, Saltzman CL: The effect of foot orthotics on three-dimensional kinematics of the leg and rearfoot during running. *J Orthop Sports Phys Ther* 1995;21(6):317-327.

60. Stackhouse CL, Davis IM, Hamill J: Orthotic intervention in forefoot and rearfoot strike running patterns. *Clin Biomech (Bristol, Avon)* 2004;19(1):64-70.

61. Collins N, Crossley K, Beller E, Darnell R, McPoil T, Vicenzino B: Foot orthoses and physiotherapy in the treatment of patellofemoral pain syndrome: Randomised clinical trial. *Br J Sports Med* 2009;43(3):169-171.

This randomized controlled trial investigating the efficacy of foot orthoses and physical therapy in patients with PFPS noted that foot orthoses were superior to flat inserts but similar to physiotherapy and do not improve outcome when added to physiotherapy. Level of evidence: II.

62. Johnston LB, Gross MT: Effects of foot orthoses on quality of life for individuals with patellofemoral pain syndrome. *J Orthop Sports Phys Ther* 2004;34(8):440-448.

63. McPoil TG, Vicenzino B, Cornwall MW: Effect of foot orthoses contour on pain perception in individuals with patellofemoral pain. *J Am Podiatr Med Assoc* 2011;101(1):7-16.

In this study, all participants perceived greater support with contoured orthoses in the heel and arch regions. All of the participants rated cushioning as equivalent, despite differences in material hardness. In the patellofemoral pain group, six individuals reported a clinically significant reduction in knee pain as a result of wearing foot orthoses. Level of evidence: III.

64. Barton CJ, Munteanu SE, Menz HB, Crossley KM: The efficacy of foot orthoses in the treatment of individuals with patellofemoral pain syndrome: A systematic review. *Sports Med* 2010;40(5):377-395.

Limited evidence shows that prefabricated foot orthoses better reduce the range of transverse-plane knee rotation and provide greater short-term improvements in individuals with PFPS than do flat inserts. Findings also indicate that combining physical therapy with prefabricated foot orthoses may be superior to prefabricated foot orthoses alone. Level of evidence: I.

65. Eng JJ, Pierrynowski MR: Evaluation of soft foot orthotics in the treatment of patellofemoral pain syndrome. *Phys Ther* 1993;73(2):62-68, discussion 68-70.

66. Willson JD, Sharpee R, Meardon SA, Kernozek TW: Effects of step length on patellofemoral joint stress in female runners with and without patellofemoral pain. *Clin Biomech (Bristol, Avon)* 2014;29(3):243-247.

In this study, PFJ stress per step increased in the long step-length condition and decreased in the short step-length condition. Total stress per mile experienced at the PFJ declined with a short step length despite the greater number of steps necessary to cover the distance. Level of evidence: IV.

67. Heiderscheit BC, Chumanov ES, Michalski MP, Wille CM, Ryan MB: Effects of step rate manipulation on joint mechanics during running. *Med Sci Sports Exerc* 2011;43(2):296-302.

This study showed that increased step rate results in an altered peak hip adduction angle as well as a reduction in peak hip adduction and internal rotation moments. Level of evidence: IV.

68. Lenhart RL, Thelen DG, Wille CM, Chumanov ES, Heiderscheit BC: Increasing running step rate reduces patellofemoral joint forces. *Med Sci Sports Exerc* 2014;46(3):557-564.

In this study, increasing the step rate reduced peak PFJ force. Peak muscle forces were altered as a result of the increased step rate, with hip, knee, and ankle extensor forces and hip abductor forces all reduced in midstance. Level of evidence: IV.

69. Chumanov ES, Wille CM, Michalski MP, Heiderscheit BC: Changes in muscle activation patterns when running step rate is increased. *Gait Posture* 2012;36(2):231-235.

An increase in late swing phase muscle activity occurs when the step rate is increased, suggesting an anticipatory preactivation for the foot-ground contact. Muscle activities during the loading response were not reduced as the step rate increased. Level of evidence: IV.

70. Noehren B, Scholz J, Davis I: The effect of real-time gait retraining on hip kinematics, pain and function in subjects with patellofemoral pain syndrome. *Br J Sports Med* 2011;45(9):691-696.

In this study, a reduction in hip adduction and contralateral pelvic drop while running was seen following gait retraining. Improvements in pain and function also were seen. Subjects were able to maintain their improvements in running mechanics, pain, and function at 1-month follow-up. Level of evidence: IV.

71. Willy RW, Scholz JP, Davis IS: Mirror gait retraining for the treatment of patellofemoral pain in female runners. *Clin Biomech (Bristol, Avon)* 2012;27(10):1045-1051.

This study found decreased peaks of hip adduction, contralateral pelvic drop, and hip abduction moment during running with gait retraining. Skill transfer to single-leg squatting and step descent was noted. Subjects reported improvements in pain and function and maintained them throughout the 3 months after retraining. Level of evidence: IV.

© 2016 American Academy of Orthopaedic Surgeons

Chapter 28

Foot and Ankle Rehabilitation

RobRoy L. Martin, PhD, PT

Abstract

Manual therapy, taping, and exercise are commonly included in a comprehensive foot and ankle rehabilitation program. These interventions typically are performed to decrease pain and restore normal motion, muscle function, proprioception, and biomechanics. Manual therapy procedures can have biomechanical, neurophysiologic, and psychologic effects. Taping techniques are typically used to reinforce normal protective support structures, improve proprioception, enhance neuromuscular activation, and/or alter biomechanics whereas exercise typically is directed toward improving range of motion, recruitment pattern, strength, and/or endurance. Eccentric exercise can also be used to promote tendon remodeling. It is important to review the literature related to the potential effectiveness of manual therapy procedures, taping techniques, and exercise in foot and ankle rehabilitation, and review specific evidence to support the use of these interventions for individuals with heel pain, plantar fasciitis, Achilles tendinopathy, and lateral ankle sprain.

Keywords: manual therapy; taping; exercise; evidence-based practice

Introduction

Manual therapy, taping, and exercise are commonly included in comprehensive foot and ankle rehabilitation programs. These interventions typically decrease pain and restore normal motion, muscle function, proprioception, and biomechanics. The potential effectiveness of manual therapy procedures, taping techniques, and exercise in foot and ankle rehabilitation has been reviewed, and

Neither Dr. Martin nor any immediate family member has received anything of value from or has stock or stock options held in a commercial company or institution related directly or indirectly to the subject of this chapter.

specific evidence outlined to support the use of these interventions for individuals with heel pain, plantar fasciitis, Achilles tendinopathy, and lateral ankle sprain.

Manual Therapy

Manual therapy can include joint and soft-tissue mobilization techniques. The effects of these techniques can be biomechanical, neurophysiologic, and psychologic and have been outlined in a comprehensive model.[1] A literature review supported using manual therapy as an intervention to treat lower extremity conditions.[2] From a biomechanical perspective, joint and soft-tissue mobilization techniques theoretically address restrictions in capsular, ligamentous, tendinous, muscular, and/or fascial structures. Another potential biomechanical effect of joint mobilization is the realignment of bony structures. Generally positive biomechanical effects can be associated with improved range of motion. Soft-tissue mobilization can be directed toward increasing circulation, improving venous and lymphatic flow, and promoting collagen realignment. The neurophysiologic effects of manual therapy can include altering central pain processing, muscle recruitment, and reflex activity patterns, which can result in improved force production and decreased pain perception. The psychologic effects of manual therapy may be placebo in nature and associated with "a feeling of being helped;" however, these effects should not be underestimated and can change an individual's pain perception, stress levels, and overall emotional state.[1]

Taping

Taping techniques can reinforce normal protective support structures, improve proprioception, enhance neuromuscular activation, and/or alter biomechanics. Taping techniques that correct lower extremity kinematics and muscle activation in individuals with abnormal pronation are generally categorized as antipronation. A review of the literature showed that antipronation taping can increase medial longitudinal arch height, reduce calcaneal eversion, reduce tibial internal rotation, and reduce tibialis posterior muscle activity.[3] The treatment-directed test uses antipronation taping techniques to guide orthotic prescription.[4] Research has disproved many theories[5] traditionally used in foot assessment and orthotic fabrication.[6-8] Because clinical examination may not be able to predict dynamic foot function, clinical findings may not be as helpful as previously assumed in orthotic prescription. However, the individualized approach to orthotic fabrication based on response to taping through the treatment-directed test has reduced pain and improved function.[9]

Exercise

Typically, active exercise is directed toward changing the characteristics of a muscle contraction by improving recruitment pattern, strength, and/or endurance. Stretching exercises are typically used to improve range of motion and flexibility. Because muscles do not work in isolation, active exercises should target not only muscles in the foot and ankle but also include proximal muscle groups in functional activities. Exercises often attempt to correct abnormal pronation by improving the function of muscles that support the medial longitudinal arch, particularly the posterior tibialis. Because hindfoot pronation has been coupled with hip internal rotation,[10] exercises that target hip musculature can be beneficial. One study found that individuals with overuse injuries had strength deficits in the hip musculature.[11] It is also theorized that exercise should include muscle groups of the lumbopelvic region to facilitate a stable platform for lower extremity movement.

In addition to exercise being directed toward correcting abnormal pronation and improving functional stability, exercise also can be directed at tendon remodeling using an eccentric exercise program. A program developed for individuals with tendinopathies consists of progressive eccentric loading with resistance high enough to cause moderate but not disabling pain.[12] The exact mechanisms behind the success of eccentric training can involve altering tendon blood flow, collagen synthesis, and production of growth factors. A 2013 study suggested that eccentric exercise that loads the tendon in a lengthened position can cause "squeezing out" and resolution of abnormal neovascularity.[13]

Evidence-Based Practice

Evidence-based clinical practice guidelines for the orthopaedic physical therapy management of individuals with common foot and ankle-related musculoskeletal impairments have been published. These guidelines outline evidence for the use of manual therapy, taping, and exercise in individuals with heel pain/plantar fasciitis,[14] Achilles tendinopathy,[15] and lateral ankle sprain.[16]

Plantar Fasciitis

Plantar fasciitis usually presents as a chronic condition in both nonathletic and athletic populations.[14] Limited ankle dorsiflexion range of motion, high body mass index in nonathletic individuals, running, and work-related weight-bearing activities under conditions with poor shock absorption have been identified as risk factors for the development of plantar fasciitis. Strong evidence indicates that plantar fasciitis can be diagnosed based on plantarmedial heel pain that is most noticeable with initial steps following a period of inactivity but also may be worsened following prolonged weight bearing; the onset of pain associated with a recent increase in weight-bearing activity; pain with palpation of the proximal insertion of the plantar fascia; a positive windlass test result; and negative tarsal tunnel test results.[14] The treatment of plantar fasciitis of the heel is summarized in Table 1 and includes strong evidence for manual therapy, taping, and exercise.[14]

Manual Therapy

A 2014 review[14] recommended that manual therapy consisting of joint and soft-tissue mobilization procedures be used to treat relevant lower extremity joint mobility and calf flexibility deficits and to decrease pain and improve function in individuals with heel pain/plantar fasciitis. Level I research studies supported this recommendation. Authors of a 2009 study[17] found that patients who underwent exercise and manual therapy had better function and global self-reported outcomes at both 4 weeks and 6 months when compared with patients in the group treated with exercise and iontophoresis. Manual therapy consisted of soft-tissue mobilization directed toward the calf and plantar fascia and joint mobilization directed toward identified range of motion restrictions of the hip, knee, ankle, and foot. Because limited ankle dorsiflexion is often identified in those with plantar fasciitis, anterior to posterior talar glides (Figure 1) are commonly performed. Authors of a 2011 study[18] found that patients who underwent the addition of soft-tissue mobilization techniques directed at gastrocnemius and soleus myofascial trigger points had better pain reduction at 4 weeks when compared with patients who underwent self-stretching only.

Taping

The authors of the 2014 review also recommended that clinicians should use antipronation taping for immediate (up to 3 weeks) pain reduction and improved function for individuals with plantar fasciitis.[14] Systematic reviews have

Table 1

Summary of Evidence in the Treatment of Plantar Fasciitis

Strong Evidence

Treatment	Intervention
Manual therapy	Lower extremity joint mobilization
	Plantar fascia, gastrocnemius, and soleus soft-tissue mobilization
Taping	Antipronation technique
Exercise	Plantar fascia stretching
	Gastrocnemius and soleus stretching
Foot orthoses	Over-the-counter/prefabricated or a custom foot orthoses that supports the medial arch and/or provides cushion to the heel region
Night splints	

Weak Evidence

Treatment	Intervention
Physical agents	Iontophoresis with dexamethasone or acetic acid
	Low-level laser
	Phonophoresis with ketoprofen gel

(Data from Martin RL, Davenport TE, Reischl SF, et al: Heel pain-plantar fasciitis: Revision 2014. *J Orthop Sports Phys Ther* 2014;44[11]:A1-A33. http://dx.doi.org/10.2519/jospt.2014.0303.)

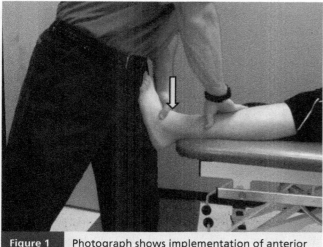

Figure 1 Photograph shows implementation of anterior to posterior talar glides (arrow) to increase ankle dorsiflexion range of motion.

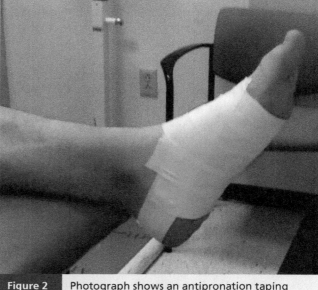

Figure 2 Photograph shows an antipronation taping technique.

found antipronation taping to be effective in reducing pain at 1-week follow-up in subjects with plantar fasciitis.[19,20] An example of antipronation tape is demonstrated in Figure 2. A level I study not included in these reviews found therapeutic elastic tape applied to the gastrocnemius and plantar fascia improved pain scores and reduced plantar fascia thickness when compared with ultrasound and electrotherapy treatments at 1-week follow-up.[21] Additionally, a level II study found that antipronation taping reduced pain and improved function over a 3-week period in individuals with plantar fasciitis.[22]

Exercise

Clinicians should use plantar fascia–specific and gastrocnemius/soleus stretching to provide short-term (1 week to 4 months) pain relief for individuals with plantar fasciitis.[14] Two systematic reviews concluded that stretching exercises for the ankle and foot can provide short-term (2 weeks to 4 months) improvements,[20,23] with plantar fascia–specific stretching being more beneficial than Achilles

4: Rehabilitation

Table 2

Summary of Evidence in the Treatment of Individuals With Achilles Tendinopathy

	Strong Evidence	
Treatment	**Intervention**	
Exercises	Eccentric loading of the Achilles tendon	
Physical agents	Low-level laser	
	Iontophoresis with dexamethasone	
	Weak Evidence	
Treatment	**Intervention**	
Exercise	Plantar flexor stretching	
Foot orthoses	Custom semirigid inserts	
Manual therapy	Achilles tendon soft-tissue mobilization	
	Expert Opinion	
Treatment	**Intervention**	
Taping	Directed toward decreased strain on the Achilles tendon	

(Data from Carcia CR, Martin RL, Houck J, Wukich DK; Orthopaedic Section of the American Physical Therapy Association: Achilles pain, stiffness, and muscle power deficits: Achilles tendinitis. *J Orthop Sports Phys Ther* 2010;40[9]:A1-A26. http://dx.doi.org/10.2519/jospt.2010.0305.)

stretching.[20] A study not included in these reviews found improved self-reported outcome scores when comparing plantar fascia–specific stretching with shockwave therapy at 2- and 4-month follow-up.[24]

Achilles Tendinopathy

Achilles tendinopathy is a common pathology in active individuals. Intrinsic risk factors associated with Achilles tendinopathy include abnormal dorsiflexion range of motion, abnormal subtalar joint range of motion, decreased ankle plantar flexion strength, increased foot pronation, and abnormal tendon structure.[15] A recent study suggested that high body mass index may also be a risk factor for developing Achilles pathology.[25] A 2010 review[15] found that Achilles tendinopathy can be diagnosed by the following findings: local tenderness of the Achilles tendon 2 to 6 cm proximal to its insertion; a positive arc sign where the area of palpated swelling moves with dorsiflexion and plantar flexion; and a positive Royal London Hospital Test result where Achilles tenderness in slight plantar flexion decreases as the ankle dorsiflexes. Evidence supporting interventions in the treatment of Achilles tendinopathy is summarized in Table 2 and include weak evidence for manual therapy, expert opinion for taping, and strong evidence for exercise.

Manual Therapy

For individuals with Achilles tendinopathy, soft-tissue mobilization can be used to reduce pain, increase mobility,

and improve function. This recommendation was further supported by a recent systematic review in 2012[26] that outlined low-level evidence for soft-tissue mobilization in individuals with Achilles tendinopathy. One soft-tissue mobilization technique consisted of gliding a hypomobile Achilles tendon in conjunction with stretching and muscular contraction.[27] Although not extensively studied, joint and soft-tissue mobilization could be justified for increasing ankle dorsiflexion range of motion.

Taping

Taping can also be used to decrease tendon strain in patients with Achilles tendinopathy.[15] According to a systematic review,[26] there is low-level evidence to support antipronation taping. Given that abnormal pronation is a risk factor for developing Achilles tendinopathy, the use of antipronation taping techniques could be justified as an appropriate intervention. A case study of an individual with Achilles tendinopathy reported that antipronation taping reduced symptoms and produced a tenfold increase in pain-free jogging distance.[28] Other taping techniques include "off-loading" and "equinus-constraint," which decrease strain on the Achilles tendon and limit dorsiflexion range of motion.[29] Figure 3 demonstrates the 'off-loading' taping technique.

Exercise

Clinicians should implement an eccentric loading program to decrease pain and improve function in individuals with Achilles tendinopathy.[15] This recommendation

© 2016 American Academy of Orthopaedic Surgeons

was further supported in other literature reviews.[26,30] One study not included in these reviews found eccentric strengthening was more effective than concentric strengthening in reducing pain and improving function in individuals with Achilles tendinopathy.[31] Additionally, a 5-year follow-up study noted that although long-term improvement in symptoms can be expected, mild pain may persist.[32]

Ankle Sprain

The incidence of ankle sprain was found to be highest in young, active individuals, especially those who participate in court sports such as basketball.[16] The following risk factors have been identified for an acute lateral ankle sprain: previous ankle sprain; not using external support; not properly warming up with static stretching and dynamic movement before activity; abnormal ankle dorsiflexion range of motion; and not participating in balance and proprioceptive prevention programs after a lateral ligament injury. Clinicians should use the clinical findings of decreased function, ligamentous laxity, hemorrhage, point tenderness, total ankle motion, swelling, and pain to classify a patient with acute ankle ligament sprain. Tests to assess lateral ligament stability have not shown desirable diagnostic accuracy when performed in isolation. Additional research has shown medial ankle joint pain with palpation and dorsiflexion at 4 weeks as the most valuable prognostic indicators of function 4 months after injury.[33] Recurrent lateral ankle sprains are not uncommon, with reinjury occurring in 3% to 34% of

individuals between 2 weeks and 96 months after initial injury.[16] Individuals with long-term symptoms following lateral ankle sprain are commonly characterized as having either chronic mechanical or functional ankle instability. The treatment of acute lateral ankle sprain and chronic ankle instability is summarized in Tables 3 and 4, respectively. Strong evidence has been found for manual therapy, weight bearing with support, and exercise for those with an acute lateral ankle injury. Moderate and weak evidence were identified for manual therapy and exercise, respectively, for those with chronic ankle instability.

Manual Therapy

Clinicians should use manual therapy procedures such as lymphatic drainage, active and passive soft-tissue and

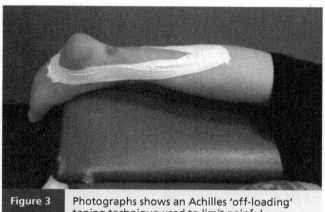

| Figure 3 | Photographs shows an Achilles 'off-loading' taping technique used to limit painful dorsiflexion range of motion. |

4. Rehabilitation

Table 3

Summary of Evidence in the Treatment of Acute Lateral Ankle Sprain

Strong Evidence	
Treatment	**Intervention**
Exercise	Structured rehabilitation program including progressive active range of motion and resistance exercises incorporating weight bearing with support
Physical agents	Cyrotherapy
Moderate Evidence	
Treatment	**Intervention**
Manual therapy	Anterior-to-posterior talar mobilization, lymphatic drainage, active and passive soft-tissue and joint mobilization procedures
Weak Evidence	
Treatment	**Intervention**
Physical agents	Diathermy

(Data from Martin RL, Davenport TE, Paulseth S, Wukich DK, Godges JJ, Orthopaedic Section American Physical Therapy Association: Ankle stability and movement coordination impairments: Ankle ligament sprains. *J Orthop Sports Phys Ther* 2013;43[9]:A1-A40. http://dx.doi.org/10.2519/jospt.2013.0305.)

Table 4	
Summary of Evidence in the Treatment of Chronic Ankle Instability	
Strong Evidence	
Treatment	**Intervention**
Manual therapy	Non–weight-bearing and weight-bearing joint mobilization
Weak Evidence	
Treatment	**Intervention**
Exercise	Weight-bearing functional/sports-related exercises and single-limb balance activities using unstable surfaces

(Data from Martin RL, Davenport TE, Paulseth S, Wukich DK, Godges JJ, Orthopaedic Section American Physical Therapy Association: Ankle stability and movement coordination impairments: Ankle ligament sprains. *J Orthop Sports Phys Ther* 2013;43[9]:A1-A40. http://dx.doi.org/10.2519/jospt.2013.0305.)

joint mobilization, and anterior-to-posterior talar mobilization (Figure 1) procedures to reduce swelling, improve pain-free ankle and foot mobility, and normalize gait parameters in individuals with acute lateral ankle sprain.[16] According to a level II study, a single session of manual therapy in the emergency department was associated with decreased edema and pain in individuals presenting with acute ankle sprain.[34] Soft-tissue mobilization, joint mobilization, isometric mobilization, contract/relax, positional release, and lymphatic drainage procedures directed toward identified impairments are examples of manual therapy. A separate level II study found individuals with acute ankle sprains who received pain-free posterior talar joint mobilizations had better outcomes, achieving full range of motion and symmetric step length within the first two to three treatments.[35] The use of manual therapy was further supported by a recent systematic review.[36] Recent evidence also exists that the addition of myofascial therapy to thrust and nonthrust manipulation and exercise can further improve outcomes in those with acute lateral ankle sprain.[37]

In individuals with nonacute lateral ankle injuries, clinicians should include nonweight-bearing and weight-bearing joint mobilization to improve ankle dorsiflexion range of motion, proprioception, and weight-bearing tolerance.[16] A weight-bearing joint mobilization that can be used to improve ankle dorsiflexion is demonstrated in Figure 4. In addition, a systematic review concluded that manual therapy techniques improve ankle range of motion, decrease pain, and improve function for those with signs and symptoms consistent with a subacute/chronic lateral ankle sprain.[36] A study not included in that review found that posterior talar mobilizations were associated with improved measures of function for at least 1 week in individuals with chronic ankle instability.[38]

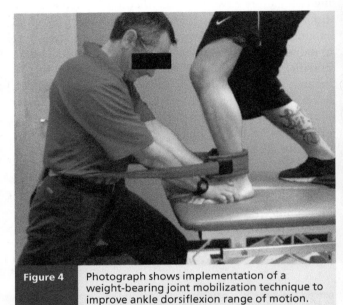

Figure 4 Photograph shows implementation of a weight-bearing joint mobilization technique to improve ankle dorsiflexion range of motion.

Taping

Clinicians should strongly encourage use of external support and progressive weight bearing on the affected extremity in patients with acute lateral ankle sprain. The type of external support (which can include tape) and gait-assistance device recommended should be based on the severity of the injury, phase of tissue healing, level of protection indicated, extent of pain, and patient preference. In patients with more severe injuries, immobilization ranging from semirigid bracing to casting below the knee may be indicated.[16] The authors of a systematic review[39] found that using a semirigid ankle support rather than an elastic wrap was associated with substantially shorter return to work and sports, as well as decreased reports of instability. External support from tape was most frequently associated with complications, such as skin irritation. Although some studies have noted a positive effect of taping and bracing on proprioception, a recent meta-analysis noted the use of an ankle brace or tape had no overall effect on proprioceptive acuity in those with recurrent ankle sprain or functional ankle instability.[40] Conflicting evidence exists that fibular reposition taping[41,42] and therapeutic elastic tape[43,44] can improve postural control and proprioception.

Exercise

Clinicians should implement a rehabilitation program that includes therapeutic exercises for patients with acute lateral ankle sprain, along with active range of motion and progressive resistance exercises for the ankle and foot. A study that supports this recommendation found functional improvement in individuals with a severe ankle sprain who underwent physical therapy intervention and conventional medical treatment compared with those who underwent conventional medical treatment alone.[45]

For chronic ankle instability, clinicians should include weight-bearing sport-specific exercises and single-limb balance activities using unstable surfaces to improve mobility, strength, coordination, and postural control. This recommendation is supported by a systematic review that concludes functional exercises and activities, especially using unstable surfaces, promote improvement in dynamic postural control.[46]

Summary

Foot and ankle rehabilitation programs can include manual therapy, taping, and exercise. Manual therapy procedures can have biomechanical, neurophysiologic, and psychologic effects. Taping techniques are typically used to reinforce normal protective support structures, improve proprioception, enhance neuromuscular activation, and/or alter biomechanics; exercise typically is directed toward improving range of motion, recruitment pattern, strength, and/or endurance. Eccentric exercise can also be used to promote tendon remodeling. Strong evidence supports manual therapy used in individuals with plantar fasciitis and chronic ankle instability, moderate evidence in those with acute lateral ankle sprain, and weak evidence in those with Achilles tendinopathy. Strong evidence exists for taping in those with plantar fasciitis and expert opinion in those with Achilles tendinopathy. Strong evidence exists for using exercise in those with plantar fasciitis, Achilles tendinopathy, and acute lateral ankle sprain but weak evidence for those with chronic ankle instability.

Key Study Points

- The potential effectiveness of manual therapy procedures, taping techniques, and exercise in foot and ankle rehabilitation is described according to the current literature.
- There is specific evidence to support the use of manual therapy, taping, and exercise for individuals with heel pain/plantar fasciitis, Achilles tendinopathy, and lateral ankle sprain.

Annotated References

1. Bialosky JE, Bishop MD, Price DD, Robinson ME, George SZ: The mechanisms of manual therapy in the treatment of musculoskeletal pain: A comprehensive model. *Man Ther* 2009;14(5):531-538.

   The authors present a model of potential mechanisms for manual therapy.

2. Brantingham JW, Bonnefin D, Perle SM, et al: Manipulative therapy for lower extremity conditions: Update of a literature review. *J Manipulative Physiol Ther* 2012;35(2):127-166.

   This systematic review outlines the evidence for manipulative therapy in the management of various lower extremity conditions, including plantar fasciitis. Level of evidence: II.

3. Franettovich M, Chapman A, Blanch P, Vicenzino B: A physiological and psychological basis for anti-pronation taping from a critical review of the literature. *Sports Med* 2008;38(8):617-631.

4. Vicenzino B: Foot orthotics in the treatment of lower limb conditions: A musculoskeletal physiotherapy perspective. *Man Ther* 2004;9(4):185-196.

5. Root M, Orien WP, Weed JH: *Normal And Abnormal Function of the Foot: Clinical Biomechanics.* Los Angeles, CA, Clincial Biomechanics, 1977, vol 2.

6. Cornwall MW, McPoil TG: Motion of the calcaneus, navicular, and first metatarsal during the stance phase of walking. *J Am Podiatr Med Assoc* 2002;92(2):67-76.

7. McPoil T, Cornwall MW: Relationship between neutral subtalar joint position and pattern of rearfoot motion during walking. *Foot Ankle Int* 1994;15(3):141-145.

8. McPoil TG, Cornwall MW: Relationship between three static angles of the rearfoot and the pattern of rearfoot motion during walking. *J Orthop Sports Phys Ther* 1996;23(6):370-375.

9. Meier K, McPoil TG, Cornwall MW, Lyle T: Use of anti-pronation taping to determine foot orthoses prescription: A case series. *Res Sports Med* 2008;16(4):257-271.

10. Souza TR, Pinto RZ, Trede RG, Kirkwood RN, Fonseca ST: Temporal couplings between rearfoot-shank complex and hip joint during walking. *Clin Biomech (Bristol, Avon)* 2010;25(7):745-748.

    The study found evidence to support a temporal coupling of rearfoot pronation with hip internal rotation and rearfoot supination with hip external rotation during walking. Level of evidence: IV.

11. Kulig K, Popovich JM Jr, Noceti-Dewit LM, Reischl SF, Kim D: Women with posterior tibial tendon dysfunction have diminished ankle and hip muscle performance. *J Orthop Sports Phys Ther* 2011;41(9):687-694.

    The authors found women with posterior tibial tendon dysfunction had decreased ankle and hip muscle performance. Level of evidence: III.

12. Alfredson H, Pietilä T, Jonsson P, Lorentzon R: Heavy-load eccentric calf muscle training for the treatment of chronic Achilles tendinosis. *Am J Sports Med* 1998;26(3):360-366.

13. McCreesh KM, Riley SJ, Crotty JM: Neovascularity in patellar tendinopathy and the response to eccentric training: A case report using Power Doppler ultrasound. *Man Ther* 2013;18(6):602-605.

    This case report describes complete resolution of abnormal neovascularity, using ultrasound imaging, after 8 weeks of eccentric exercise in a subject with chronic patellar tendinopathy. Level of evidence: IV.

14. Martin RL, Davenport TE, Reischl SF, et al: Heel pain-plantar fasciitis: Revision 2014. *J Orthop Sports Phys Ther* 2014;44(11):A1-A33.

    The authors summarize the evidence related to the diagnosis, examination, and intervention for those with heel pain/plantar fasciitis.

15. Carcia CR, Martin RL, Houck J, Wukich DK; Orthopaedic Section of the American Physical Therapy Association: Achilles pain, stiffness, and muscle power deficits: Achilles tendinitis. *J Orthop Sports Phys Ther* 2010;40(9):A1-A26.

    The authors summarize the evidence related to the diagnosis, examination, and intervention for those with Achilles tendinopathy.

16. Martin RL, Davenport TE, Paulseth S, Wukich DK, Godges JJ, Orthopaedic Section American Physical Therapy Association: Ankle stability and movement coordination impairments: Ankle ligament sprains. *J Orthop Sports Phys Ther* 2013;43(9):A1-A40.

    The authors summarize the evidence related to the diagnosis, examination, and intervention for those with acute and chronic lateral ankle injuries.

17. Cleland JA, Abbott JH, Kidd MO, et al: Manual physical therapy and exercise versus electrophysical agents and exercise in the management of plantar heel pain: A multicenter randomized clinical trial. *J Orthop Sports Phys Ther* 2009;39(8):573-585.

    This study found patients who underwent exercise and manual therapy had better function and global self-reported outcomes at both 4 weeks and 6 months when compared with patients in the group treated with exercise and iontophoresis. Level of evidence: I.

18. Renan-Ordine R, Alburquerque-Sendín F, de Souza DP, Cleland JA, Fernández-de-Las-Peñas C: Effectiveness of myofascial trigger point manual therapy combined with a self-stretching protocol for the management of plantar heel pain: A randomized controlled trial. *J Orthop Sports Phys Ther* 2011;41(2):43-50.

    The authors found patients who underwent the addition of soft-tissue mobilization techniques directed at gastrocnemius and soleus myofascial trigger points had better pain reduction at 4 weeks when compared with patients who underwent self-stretching only. Level of evidence: I.

19. van de Water AT, Speksnijder CM: Efficacy of taping for the treatment of plantar fasciosis: A systematic review of controlled trials. *J Am Podiatr Med Assoc* 2010;100(1):41-51.

    The authors reviewed controlled trials and found limited evidence indicating the effectiveness of taping to reduce pain in patients with plantar fasciosis.

20. Landorf KB, Menz HB: Plantar heel pain and fasciitis. *BMJ Clin Evid* 2008;2008:1111.

21. Tsai CT, Chang WD, Lee JP: Effects of short-term treatment with kinesiotaping for plantar fasciitis. *J Musculoskelet Pain* 2010;18:71-80.

    This study found therapeutic elastic tape applied to the gastrocnemius and plantar fascia improved pain scores and reduced plantar fascia thickness when compared with ultrasound and electrotherapy treatments at 1-week follow-up in patients with plantar fasciitis. Level of evidence: I.

22. Abd El Salam MS, Abd Elhafz YN: Low-dye taping versus medial arch support in managing pain and pain-related disability in patients with plantar fasciitis. *Foot Ankle Spec* 2011;4(2):86-91.

    These authors found that antipronation taping reduced pain and improved function over a 3-week period in patients with plantar fasciitis. Level of evidence: II.

23. Sweeting D, Parish B, Hooper L, Chester R: The effectiveness of manual stretching in the treatment of plantar heel pain: A systematic review. *J Foot Ankle Res* 2011;4:19.

    This systematic review concluded the main pain-relieving benefits of stretching appear to occur within the first 2 weeks to 4 months after the initiation of treatment. Level of evidence: I.

© 2016 American Academy of Orthopaedic Surgeons

24. Rompe JD, Cacchio A, Weil L Jr, et al: Plantar fascia-specific stretching versus radial shock-wave therapy as initial treatment of plantar fasciopathy. *J Bone Joint Surg Am* 2010;92(15):2514-2522.

The authors concluded that manual stretching is more effective than shock-wave therapy in the treatment of plantar fasciopathy. Level of evidence: I.

25. Scott RT, Hyer CF, Granata A: The correlation of Achilles tendinopathy and body mass index. *Foot Ankle Spec* 2013;6(4):283-285.

Statistical analysis was performed to determine the correlation between body mass index and Achilles tendon pathology. Patients with Achilles tendon pathology had a greater body mass index than those without. Level of evidence: II.

26. Rowe V, Hemmings S, Barton C, Malliaras P, Maffulli N, Morrissey D: Conservative management of midportion Achilles tendinopathy: A mixed methods study, integrating systematic review and clinical reasoning. *Sports Med* 2012;42(11):941-967.

This systematic review found case-study evidence to support the use of soft-tissue mobilization for those with Achilles tendinopathy. Level of evidence: IV.

27. Christenson RE: Effectiveness of specific soft tissue mobilizations for the management of Achilles tendinosis: Single case study—experimental design. *Man Ther* 2007;12(1):63-71.

28. Smith M, Brooker S, Vicenzino B, McPoil T: Use of anti-pronation taping to assess suitability of orthotic prescription: Case report. *Aust J Physiother* 2004;50(2):111-113.

29. Martin RL, Paulseth S, Carcia CR: Taping techniques for achilles tendinopathy. *Orthopaedic Physical Therapy Practice*. 2009;20:106-107.

This clinical commentary describes two taping techniques that can be used to decrease pain for patients with Achilles tendinopathy. Level of evidence: V.

30. Sussmilch-Leitch SP, Collins NJ, Bialocerkowski AE, Warden SJ, Crossley KM: Physical therapies for Achilles tendinopathy: Systematic review and meta-analysis. *J Foot Ankle Res* 2012;5(1):15.

The findings of this systematic review supported the use of eccentric exercise as an initial intervention for patients with Achilles tendinopathy. Level of evidence: I.

31. Yu J, Park D, Lee G: Effect of eccentric strengthening on pain, muscle strength, endurance, and functional fitness factors in male patients with achilles tendinopathy. *Am J Phys Med Rehabil* 2013;92(1):68-76.

The authors found eccentric strengthening to be more effective than concentric strengthening in reducing pain and improving function in patients with Achilles tendinopathy. Level of evidence: I.

32. van der Plas A, de Jonge S, de Vos RJ, et al: A 5-year follow-up study of Alfredson's heel-drop exercise programme in chronic midportion Achilles tendinopathy. *Br J Sports Med* 2012;46(3):214-218.

This study found a significant increase in VISA-A scores at 5 years following an intervention that included an eccentric exercise. The authors noted that although improvement of symptoms can be expected with eccentric exercises, mild pain may remain long term. Level of evidence: I.

33. O'Connor SR, Bleakley CM, Tully MA, McDonough SM: Predicting functional recovery after acute ankle sprain. *PLoS One* 2013;8(8):e72124.

The authors found clinical assessment variables at 4 weeks were the strongest predictors of recovery, explaining 50% of the variance in ankle function at 4 months.

34. Eisenhart AW, Gaeta TJ, Yens DP: Osteopathic manipulative treatment in the emergency department for patients with acute ankle injuries. *J Am Osteopath Assoc* 2003;103(9):417-421.

35. Green T, Refshauge K, Crosbie J, Adams R: A randomized controlled trial of a passive accessory joint mobilization on acute ankle inversion sprains. *Phys Ther* 2001;81(4):984-994.

36. Loudon JK, Reiman MP, Sylvain J: The efficacy of manual joint mobilisation/manipulation in treatment of lateral ankle sprains: A systematic review. *Br J Sports Med* 2014;48(5):365-370.

This systematic review found manual joint mobilization diminished pain and increased dorsiflexion range of motion in those with acute ankle sprains and improved ankle range of motion, decreased pain, and improved function in those with subacute/chronic lateral ankle sprains. Level of evidence: I.

37. Truyols-Domí Nguez S, Salom-Moreno J, Abian-Vicen J, Cleland JA, Fernández-de-Las-Peñas C: Efficacy of thrust and nonthrust manipulation and exercise with or without the addition of myofascial therapy for the management of acute inversion ankle sprain: A randomized clinical trial. *J Orthop Sports Phys Ther* 2013;43(5):300-309.

These authors found the addition of myofascial therapy to thrust and nonthrust manipulation and exercise can further improve outcomes in those with acute lateral ankle sprain. Level of evidence: I.

38. Hoch MC, Andreatta RD, Mullineaux DR, et al: Two-week joint mobilization intervention improves self-reported function, range of motion, and dynamic balance in those with chronic ankle instability. *J Orthop Res* 2012;30(11):1798-1804.

This study found posterior talar mobilizations were associated with improved measures of function for at least 1 week in individuals with chronic ankle instability. Level of evidence: II.

39. Kerkhoffs GM, Rowe BH, Assendelft WJ, Kelly KD, Struijs PA, van Dijk CN: Immobilisation for acute ankle

sprain. A systematic review. *Arch Orthop Trauma Surg* 2001;121(8):462-471.

40. Raymond J, Nicholson LL, Hiller CE, Refshauge KM: The effect of ankle taping or bracing on proprioception in functional ankle instability: A systematic review and meta-analysis. *J Sci Med Sport* 2012;15(5):386-392.

    The authors wanted to determine if wearing an ankle brace or taping the ankle, compared with no brace or tape, improves proprioceptive acuity in individuals with a history of ankle sprain or functional ankle instability. The pooled evidence found that using an ankle brace or ankle tape had no effect on proprioceptive acuity in participants with recurrent ankle sprain or who have functional ankle instability.

41. Someeh M, Norasteh AA, Daneshmandi H, Asadi A: Immediate effects of Mulligan's fibular repositioning taping on postural control in athletes with and without chronic ankle instability. *Phys Ther Sport* 2015;16(2):135-139.

    This study found that fibular repositioning taping significantly improved postural control in athletes with chronic ankle instability. Level of evidence: III.

42. Wheeler TJ, Basnett CR, Hanish MJ, et al: Fibular taping does not influence ankle dorsiflexion range of motion or balance measures in individuals with chronic ankle instability. *J Sci Med Sport* 2013;16(6):488-492.

    The authors did not find a significant change in ankle dorsiflexion range of motion or dynamic balance when comparing fibular taping to sham taping in patients with chronic ankle instability. Level of evidence: III.

43. Simon J, Garcia W, Docherty CL: The effect of kinesio tape on force sense in people with functional ankle instability. *Clin J Sport Med* 2014;24(4):289-294.

    This study noted that in patients with functional ankle instability, proprioceptive deficits were not improved immediately after application of kinesio tape, however, but did improve after wearing the tape for 72 hours. Level of evidence: III.

44. Shields CA, Needle AR, Rose WC, Swanik CB, Kaminski TW: Effect of elastic taping on postural control deficits in subjects with healthy ankles, copers, and individuals with functional ankle instability. *Foot Ankle Int* 2013;34(10):1427-1435.

    The results of this study did not support the use of kinesio tape for improving postural control deficits in those with ankle instability. Level of evidence: III.

45. van Rijn RM, van Heest JA, van der Wees P, Koes BW, Bierma-Zeinstra SM: Some benefit from physiotherapy intervention in the subgroup of patients with severe ankle sprain as determined by the ankle function score: A randomised trial. *Aust J Physiother* 2009;55(2):107-113.

    The authors found functional improvement in individuals with a severe ankle sprain who underwent physical therapy intervention and conventional medical treatment compared with those who underwent conventional medical treatment alone. Level of evidence: I.

46. Webster KA, Gribble PA: Functional rehabilitation interventions for chronic ankle instability: A systematic review. *J Sport Rehabil* 2010;19(1):98-114.

    This systematic review concluded that functional exercises and activities promote improvement in dynamic postural control for those with chronic ankle instability. Level of evidence: II.

Chapter 29

Core Stabilization

Rafael F. Escamilla, PhD, PT, CSCS, FACSM

Abstract

Muscle recruitment patterns of lumbopelvic-hip musculature, which is commonly referred to as the core, and loading of the lumbar spine during core exercises common used during core strengthening programs are described in the literature. The orthopaedic surgeon should be knowledgeable about why the core is important, what muscles comprise the core and which ones contribute the most to core stability, the benefits and risks of core stabilization exercises, biomechanical differences between abdominal hollowing (drawing-in maneuver) and abdominal bracing techniques, traditional and nontraditional exercises used for core stability, biomechanical differences between abdominal exercises that cause active hip or trunk flexion or control hip or trunk extension, biomechanical differences between the crunch and the bent-knee sit-up, and abdominal and oblique recruitment between the crunch and reverse crunch.

Keywords: stability; abdominal hollowing; abdominal bracing; electromyography; EMG; low back pain

Introduction

It is important for the orthopaedic surgeon to understand muscle recruitment patterns of lumbopelvic-hip musculature (commonly referred to as the core) and loading of the lumbar spine during core exercises commonly used during core strengthening programs. In addition, the importance of the core, which core muscles are most important for core stability, the benefits and risks of traditional and nontraditional core stabilization exercises, lumbar spinal

Neither Dr. Escamilla nor any immediate family member has received anything of value from or has stock or stock options held in a commercial company or institution related directly or indirectly to the subject of this chapter.

loading and injury risk during exercises commonly used to enhance core stability, and biomechanical differences between abdominal hollowing and bracing exercises, trunk flexion and extension exercises, and crunch and bent-knee sit-up exercises are important concepts to therapists and other health care or fitness specialists who develop specific core exercises for rehabilitation or training.

Why is the Core Important?

In functional and athletic events, the core provides proximal stability for distal mobility.[1] Trunk musculature helps stabilize the core by compressing and stiffening the spine, which is important because the osteoligamentous lumbar spine buckles under compressive loads of only 90 N (approximately 20 lb).[2] Core muscles act as guy wires around the human spine to prevent spinal buckling. In addition, intra-abdominal pressure increases as core muscles contract,[3] which further increases spinal stiffness and enhances core stability.[4]

Core Muscles and Stability

Considerable debate exists regarding which core muscles are the most important in optimizing core stability (spinal stabilization). Some studies suggest that the transversus abdominis and multifidi muscles are key to enhancing spinal stability,[5,6] but others have questioned the importance of these muscles as major spine stabilizers.[2,7] Therefore, the effectiveness of the transversus abdominis and multifidi on lumbar stability is not clear. Isolated contractions from the transversus abdominis have not been demonstrated during functional higher demand activities that require all abdominal muscles to become active.[8]

In healthy individuals without lumbar pathology, the transversus abdominis contracts before upper extremity motion irrespective of the direction of the motion.[9] However, a 2012 study reported that transversus abdominis activation is direction-specific and that symmetric, bilateral preactivation of the transversus abdominis does not normally occur in healthy individuals without lumbar pathology during rapid, unilateral arm movements.[7]

This is important because bilaterally, preactivation of the transversus abdominis theoretically provides lumbar spine stability in anticipation of perturbations of posture.[9] In contrast, transversus abdominis activation is substantially delayed in patients with low back pain with all movements, indicating a motor control deficit that can result in inefficient muscular stabilization of the spine. However, select low-intensity exercises such as abdominal hollowing (drawing in) have been shown to preferentially activate the transversus abdominis in patients with chronic low back pain during exercise.[10] Moreover, evidence exists that the deep abdominal muscles (transversus abdominis and internal oblique muscles) can be preferentially trained in individuals with chronic low back pain using targeted exercises such as abdominal hollowing.[11]

To optimize core stabilization, numerous muscles, including smaller, deeper core muscles (such as the transversospinales, transversus abdominis, internal oblique, and quadratus lumborum) and larger superficial core muscles (such as the erector spinae, external oblique, and rectus abdominis), must be activated in sequence, with appropriate timing and tension.[2] A 2002 study reported that no single core muscle can be identified as the most important for lumbar spine stability, that the relative contribution of each core muscle to lumbar spine stability depends on trunk loading direction (spinal instability was greatest during trunk flexion) and magnitude, and that no single muscle contributed more than 30% to overall spine stability.[12] Therefore, lumbar stabilization exercises may be most effective when they involve the entire spinal musculature and its motor control under various loading conditions of the spine.[12]

Benefits and Risks of Core Stabilization Exercises

Core strengthening of the lumbopelvic region can decrease the risk of injury to the thoracolumbar spine by enhancing spinal stability[13] and has been shown to decrease the risk of injury to lower extremities and to enhance performance;[14] however, no strong relationship exists between core stability and performance and the results are inconclusive.[15,16] Appropriate spinal loading enhances spinal stability, whereas excessive spinal loading can increase the risk of injury to the lumbar spine.[13] Therefore, adequate spinal loading is required to maximize core stability; excessive loading can cause injury to the lumbar spine. For example, lifting extremely heavy weights during the deadlift exercise has resulted in estimated lumbar compression forces between 18,000 to 36,000 N.[17,18] These extremely high lumbar compression forces, which result from both the heavy external load being lifted and the high muscle forces that are generated during heavy lifting, can result in injury to the lumbar spine.[17,18]

The literature is scarce regarding the effectiveness of lumbar stabilization exercises on lumbar pathology, and more research is needed.[19] Although lumbar stabilization exercise programs have been effective in treating individuals with chronic low back pain,[20] these programs have not conclusively demonstrated that lumbar stabilization programs are more effective in treating individuals with chronic low back pain compared with a generalized, less-specific exercise program.[19]

Biomechanical Differences Between Abdominal Hollowing and Bracing

Abdominal hollowing is often performed supine with the hips flexed 45° and the knees flexed 90° (hook lying position); individuals are instructed to take a deep breath and exhale while pulling their navels up and in toward the spine.[21] In abdominal bracing, individuals are instructed to globally activate all abdominal and low back muscles by tensing all core musculature, without drawing in or pushing out the abdominal cavity.[8,22]

Abdominal hollowing is effective in the preferential recruitment of the deeper abdominal (transversus abdominis and internal oblique muscles) and lumbar (multifidi) muscles.[23,24] A 2006 study[24] demonstrated that the transversus abdominis and internal oblique contract bilaterally to form a musculofascial corset that appears to tighten during abdominal hollowing, enhancing lumbar spine stability and decreasing the risk of injury to the lumbar spine. Transversus abdominis and internal oblique activity is thought to enhance lumbar stability by increasing intra-abdominal pressure[3] and placing tension on the thoracolumbar fascia, but the multifidi provides additional spinal stability by directly controlling lumbar intersegmental movement.[6,25] Moreover, contraction of the transversus abdominis has been shown to substantially decrease sacroiliac joint laxity to a greater extent in abdominal hollowing compared with abdominal bracing.[25] These data provide some evidence that abdominal hollowing can enhance spinal stability and be beneficial for individuals with select lumbar pathologies.

Using biomechanical models, abdominal hollowing has been compared with abdominal bracing with respect to spinal stability and muscle activity.[8,21,25] A 2007 study reported that abdominal hollowing was not as effective as abdominal bracing for increasing lumbar spine stability, reporting that abdominal bracing improved lumbar spine stability by 32% with only a 15% increase in lumbar spine compression (higher benefit of lumbar stability with decreased risk of lumbar injury).[8] Moreover, the transversus abdominis alone had little effect on lumbar spine stability. However, when the effects of internal oblique and intra-abdominal pressure are combined with the effects of the transversus abdominis, core stability improved as more core muscles were activated, which occurs during abdominal bracing.

The authors of a 2007 study investigated the effectiveness of abdominal hollowing and bracing techniques in controlling spinal mobility and stability against rapid perturbations and reported that abdominal bracing performed better.[22] During rapid perturbations, abdominal bracing actively stabilized the spine and reduced lumbar spine displacement, whereas abdominal hollowing was not effective in spinal stabilization. Using these data, it can be inferred that abdominal bracing is more effective during functional activities such as lifting, jumping, pushing, and pressing activities in sports or activities of daily living. However, core muscle co-contraction during abdominal bracing substantially increases lumbar compression loads compared with abdominal hollowing, which can be problematic in those with lumbar pain and pathology. External oblique and rectus abdominis activity was substantially greater in abdominal bracing than abdominal hollowing. Moreover, abdominal hollowing demonstrated a higher spinal compression loading–to–spine stability (cost-benefit) ratio, which implies that hollowing resulted in higher spinal compression loads (increased injury risk) with less spinal stability. During abdominal hollowing, individuals were not able to activate the deep abdominal muscles in isolation, but always included substantial activity from both the external and internal oblique muscles.[22]

The effect of abdominal stabilization contractions during abdominal hollowing and bracing on posteroanterior spinal stiffness was investigated in a 2008 study; it was reported that stiffness was substantially greater in abdominal bracing.[26] More work is needed to assess the long-term effects of abdominal hollowing and bracing on posteroanterior spinal stiffness in individuals with lumbar pain and pathologies.

Abdominal hollowing or bracing techniques have been performed immediately before core-strengthening exercises.[21,23,27] Compared with the curl-up (crunch) without abdominal hollowing or bracing, the curl-up with abdominal hollowing or bracing resulted in the deep abdominal muscles (the transversus abdominis and internal oblique) being recruited earlier than the superficial abdominal muscles (the rectus abdominis and external oblique).[23]

Using ultrasonography, deep abdominal recruitment patterns were examined during numerous abdominal exercises (crunch, sit-back, leg lowering, side plank) and low back exercises (quadruped opposite arm–and–leg lift) performed immediately after abdominal hollowing.[21]

The highest recruitment of the transversus abdominis and internal oblique muscles occurred during the side plank. High activity from several important core muscles (the quadratus lumborum, internal oblique, external oblique) was reported during the side plank (resulting in enhanced spinal stability) with moderate spinal compressive loading.[2,28] A 2008 study reported high recruitment of the transversus abdominis and internal oblique muscles and low compressive spinal loading during the crunch performed after abdominal hollowing,[21] which is similar to the results of a 1997 study.[13] Performing the quadruped opposite arm–and–leg lift after abdominal hollowing preferentially recruited the transversus abdominis muscle with minimal recruitment of the internal oblique muscle, which provides evidence for its use in the early phases of motor control exercise programs that emphasize the firing of the transversus abdominis without concomitant high recruitment from other abdominal muscles.[21] Performing abdominal hollowing before abdominal exercises is beneficial to improving core muscle recruitment and spinal stability.

The effects of prone hip extension exercises on hip and back muscle activity and anterior pelvic tilt performed with and without abdominal hollowing were investigated.[27] Hip extension performed with abdominal hollowing resulted in significantly less erector spinae activity (17% ± 12% versus 49 ± 14% maximum voluntary isometric contraction [MVIC]) and significantly greater activity in the gluteus maximus (52% ± 15% versus 24% ± 8% MVIC) and medial hamstring (58% ± 20% versus 47% ± 14% MVIC) muscles. Moreover, anterior pelvic tilt was significantly greater without abdominal hollowing (10° ± 2°) than with hollowing (3° ± 1°). Performing abdominal hollowing with hip extension can be an effective strategy when the goal is to minimize anterior pelvic tilt, lumbar motion, and erector spinae activity, and to maximize hip extensor activity.

Traditional and Nontraditional Exercises for Core Stability

Traditional and nontraditional exercises (Figures 1 through 6) are used to enhance core stability. Although these exercises are primarily used to strengthen the abdominal musculature, they also recruit additional core muscles such as the latissimus dorsi and lumbar paraspinal muscles.

The abdominal musculature helps stabilize the trunk and unload the lumbar spine,[13] and is commonly activated by concentric muscle action during trunk flexion such as during the bent-knee sit-up (Figure 2, A) or crunch (Figure 2, B). During the crunch, the hips remain at a

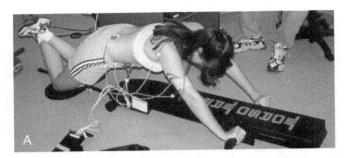

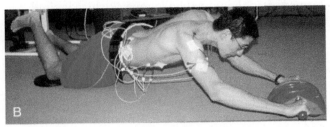

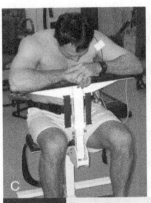

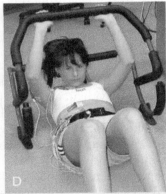

Figure 1 Photographs depict the Torso Track (Torso Track Inc.) (**A**), Ab Slide (Skyway Intertrade) (**B**), Super Abdominal Machine (Wayne Connor, Super Ab Machine) (**C**), and Ab Roller (Tristar Products, Inc.) (**D**). (Reproduced with permission from Escamilla RF, McTaggart MS, Fricklas EJ, et al: An electromyographic analysis of commercial and common abdominal exercises: Implications for rehabilitation and training. *J Orthop Sports Phys Ther* 2006;36[2]:45-57.)

(EMG) to report core muscle activity during these and similar exercises.[29-31] One study examined core muscle activity among the crunch, bent-knee sit-up, prone plank on toes, and side plank on toes[30] (Table 1). Several important differences were found: (1) upper rectus abdominis activity was greater in the crunch than in both the prone and side planks on toes, and greater in the bent-knee sit-up than in the side plank on toes; (2) lower rectus abdominis activity was less in the side plank on toes than in the remaining three exercises; (3) external oblique activity was greater in the side plank on toes than in the other three exercises; (4) latissimus dorsi activity was greater in the prone plank on toes than in the crunch and bent-knee sit-up; (5) lumbar paraspinal activity was greater in the side plank on toes than in the other three exercises; and (6) rectus femoris activity was greater in the bent-knee sit-up than in the side plank on toes and crunch, and greater in the prone plank on toes than in the crunch.

During the prone and side planks on toes, similar activity in the rectus abdominis and external oblique has been reported, along with moderate to high activity in the longissimus thoracis, lumbar multifidi, gluteus medius, and gluteus maximus during the side plank on toes. [32] In addition, the internal oblique and quadratus lumborum have demonstrated moderate to high activity during the side plank on toes.[32] Therefore, the side plank on toes effectively recruits core muscles that are important for core stability. However, the lumbar compression force is relatively high in the side plank on toes,[33] which can be problematic for individuals with lumbar pathologies. The prone plank on toes and crunch produce similar amounts of activity in the rectus abdominis, internal oblique, and external oblique muscles, but the prone plank on toes was more effective than the crunch in recruiting the latissimus dorsi and rectus femoris muscles.

Abdominal musculature is activated in a different manner during nontraditional core exercises than with the traditional crunch and bent-knee sit-up. One example is the reverse crunch (performing the traditional crunch in reverse), which involves flexing the trunk by posteriorly rotating the pelvis (Figure 4). Nontraditional core exercises can also involve controlling trunk extension (against an external force such as gravity) using isometric or eccentric muscle contractions, such as when performing the Swiss ball decline push-up (Figure 5, D) while keeping a neutral pelvis and spine.

The Swiss Ball (Figure 5) or commercial devices or machines (Figures 1 and 6) can also be used during nontraditional core exercises. Some devices or machines allow only uniplanar motion such as trunk flexion; others allow multiplanar motions such as trunk flexion and rotation or trunk extension and rotation.[29-31,34] Adding rotational

constant angle and the pelvis does not rotate; during the bent-knee sit-up, the hips flex and the pelvis rotates anteriorly. Although the bent-knee sit-up has been effective in activating the rectus abdominis and internal and external oblique musculature, the crunch has been recommended instead of the bent-knee sit-up.[29-31] Although the abdominal musculature is activated similarly between the crunch and bent-knee sit-up, the relatively high hip flexor activity that occurs during the bent-knee sit-up can increase lumbar spine stress.[13,29-31]

Other traditional abdominal exercises include the prone plank on toes (Figure 3, A) and side plank on toes (Figure 3, B), and several studies have used electromyography

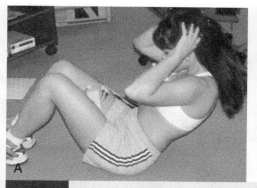
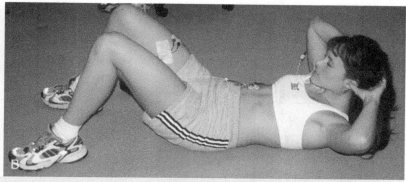

Figure 2 Photographs depict bent-knee sit-up (**A**) and the crunch (**B**). (Reproduced with permission from Escamilla RF, McTaggart MS, Fricklas EJ, et al: An electromyographic analysis of commercial and common abdominal exercises: Implications for rehabilitation and training. *J Orthop Sports Phys Ther* 2006;36[2]:45-57.)

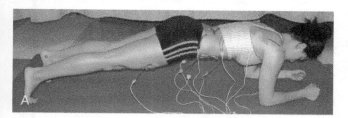

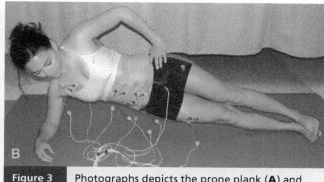

Figure 3 Photographs depicts the prone plank (**A**) and side plank (**B**) plank.

components to trunk flexion can be advantageous in internal or external oblique recruitment. The crunch combined with the Ab Roller with rotation results in simultaneous trunk flexion and rotation. Performing these exercises with left rotation (the oblique crunch and Ab Roller oblique) results in greater right external oblique activity compared with performing the crunch and ab roller with trunk flexion with no rotation (normal crunch and Ab Roller crunch)[31] (Table 2). EMG data on performing nontraditional abdominal exercises with or without abdominal devices are limited.[29-31,35-39] Core muscle activity has been quantified while performing abdominal exercises using commercial machines or devices, such as the Torso Track (Torso Track Inc.), Power Wheel (Jon H. Hindes, Lifeline USA), hanging strap, Super Abdominal Machine, Ab Revolutionizer, Ab Slide (Skyway Intertrade), Ab

Doer, Ab Shaper, Ab-Flex, Ab-Roller (Tristar Products), Ab Rocker, Ab Vice, and Ab Twister.[29-31,34-39] Several abdominal devices do not appear to offer any advantage in recruiting abdominal musculature compared with the crunch, reverse crunch, and bent-knee sit-up.[29,31] However, one advantage of the Ab Revolutionizer is that external weight can be added, thereby varying exercise intensity. The reverse crunch flat and Ab Revolutionizer reverse crunch are almost identical, only differing in that the former was performed without using an abdominal device. In addition, the crunch and Ab Roller, which are also almost identical, produced similar amounts of abdominal activity (Table 2). One advantage of the Ab Roller is that the head is supported (**Figure 1, D**), which may be more comfortable; therefore, many individuals may prefer it over the crunch. Exercises performed with abdominal devices reportedly do not appear to offer any advantage in recruiting abdominal musculature compared with performing similar exercises without devices.[34]

Some commercial devices exhibited substantially less abdominal muscle activity than the traditional crunch, reverse crunch, and bent-knee sit-up, and substantially less abdominal activity compared with other commercial abdominal devices studied.[31] Moreover, the devices tend to generate relatively high rectus femoris or lumbar paraspinal activity, which may be contraindicated in individuals with lumbar spine pathologies.

Core muscle activity was quantified in 27 traditional and nontraditional core exercises with and without various commercial abdominal devices and machines.[29,31] Twelve of the exercises are illustrated in **Figures 1, 2, 4,** and **6**); EMG data are shown in **Tables 2** and **3**. Among these exercises, upper rectus abdominis activity was highest for the Power Wheel roll-out, hanging knee-up with straps, reverse crunch inclined 30°, Ab Slide, Torso Track, crunch, and Ab Roller; and lowest for the Ab Revolutionizer, reverse crunch, Ab Twister, Ab Rocker, and Ab

Table 1

Prone and Side Plank Exercises Compared With Traditional Abdominal Crunch and Sit-Up Exercises

Exercise	Upper Rectus Abdominis	Lower Rectus Abdominis	Internal Oblique	External Oblique	Latissimus Dorsi	Lumbar Paraspinal	Rectus Femoris
Prone plank on toes	34 ± 15[c]	40 ± 10	29 ± 12	40 ± 21[b]	18 ± 12	5 ± 2[b]	20 ± 7
Side plank on toes	26 ± 15[c,d]	21 ± 9[a,c,d]	28 ± 12	62 ± 37	12 ± 10	29 ± 16	14 ± 4[d]
Crunch	53 ± 19	39 ± 16	33 ± 13	28 ± 17[b]	8 ± 3[a]	5 ± 2[b]	6 ± 4[a,d]
Bent-knee sit-up	40 ± 13	35 ± 14	31 ± 11	36 ± 14[b]	8 ± 3[a]	6 ± 2[b]	23 ± 12

Average electromyographic (EMG) (± SD) activity for each muscle and exercise expressed as a percentage of each muscle's maximum isometric voluntary contraction. A significant difference ($P < 0.001$) in EMG activity among abdominal exercises was reported for all muscles.

Pairwise comparisons ($P < 0.01$):

[a]Significantly less EMG activity compared with the prone plank on toes;

[b]Significantly less EMG activity compared with the side plank on toes;

[c]Significantly less EMG activity compared with the crunch;

[d]Significantly less EMG activity compared with the bent-knee sit-up.

Data from Escamilla RF, Lewis C, Bell D, et al: Core muscle activation during Swiss ball and traditional abdominal exercises. *J Orthop Sports Phys Ther* 2010;40[5]:265-276. Medline http://dx.doi.org/10.2519/jospt.2010.3073; and Escamilla RF, Lewis C, Pecson A, Imamura R, Andrews JR. Electromyographic comparison among supine, prone and side position exercises with and without a Swiss Ball. *Sports Health J*; in press.

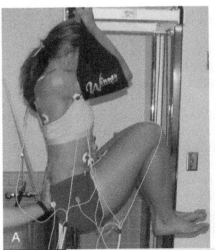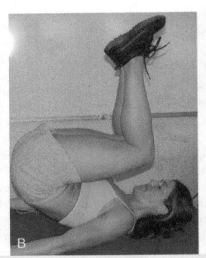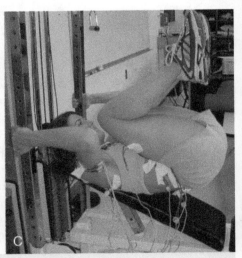

Figure 4 Photographs depict the hanging knee-ups with straps (**A**), reverse crunch flat (**B**), and reverse crunch incline 30° (**C**). (Reproduced with permission from Escamilla RF, Babb E, DeWitt R, et al: Electromyographic analysis of traditional and nontraditional abdominal exercises: Implications for rehabilitation and training. *Phys Ther* 2006;86[5]:656-671.)

Doer. Lower rectus abdominis activity was highest for the Power Wheel roll-out, hanging knee-up with straps, Ab Slide, and Torso Track; and lowest for the Ab Twister, Ab Rocker, and Ab Doer. External oblique activity was highest for the Power Wheel pike, Power Wheel knee-up, hanging knee-up with straps, Ab Slide, and bent-knee sit-up; and lowest for the crunch, Ab Roller, and Ab Doer. Internal oblique activity was highest for the Power Wheel

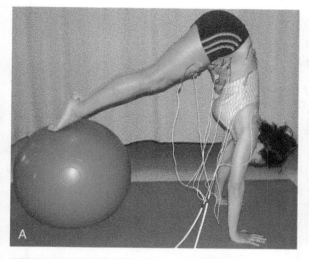
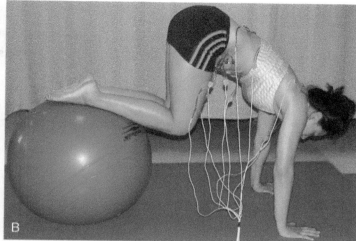
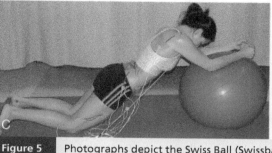
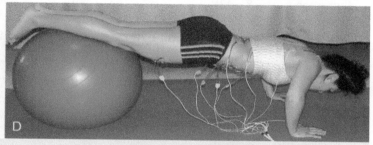

Figure 5 Photographs depict the Swiss Ball (Swissball, TheraGear) pike (**A**), knee-up (**B**), roll-out (**C**), and decline push-up (**D**). (Reproduced with permission from Escamilla RF, Lewis C, Bell D, et al: Core muscle activation during Swiss ball and traditional abdominal exercises. *J Orthop Sports Phys Ther* 2010;40[5]:265-276.)

roll-out, Power Wheel pike, Power Wheel knee-up, hanging knee-up with straps, reverse crunch inclined 30°, Ab Slide, Torso Track, bent-knee sit-up, and crunch; and lowest for the Ab Roller, Ab Twister, Ab Rocker, and Ab Doer. Although the traditional crunch and bent-knee sit-up are effective in recruiting abdominal musculature, abdominal recruitment was higher in the Power Wheel roll-out, Power Wheel pike, Power Wheel knee-up, hanging knee-up with straps, reverse crunch inclined 30°, Ab Slide, and Torso Track.

Many exercises performed with commercial abdominal devices or machines can also be performed using a Swiss ball, and many studies have quantified core muscle activity during various Swiss Ball exercises.[30,37,40-49] A 2010 study quantified core muscle activity (Table 4) between several Swiss Ball exercises (Figure 5) and the traditional crunch and bent-knee sit-up[30] (Figure 2). Rectus abdominis activity was greatest in the Swiss ball roll-out, Swiss Ball pike, and crunch, whereas external and internal oblique activity was greatest in the Swiss Ball roll-out, Swiss Ball pike, and Swiss Ball knee-up. Latissimus dorsi activity was greatest in the Swiss Ball pike, Swiss Ball knee-up, and Swiss Ball decline push-up, whereas rectus femoris activity was greatest in the Swiss Ball pike, Swiss

Ball knee-up, and bent-knee sit-up. Lumbar paraspinal activity was relativity low in all exercises. Although rectus abdominis recruitment is similar among the crunch, bent-knee sit-up, and Swiss Ball exercises, internal and external oblique activities were generally greater in Swiss ball exercises than in the crunch and bent-knee sit-up.

Many abdominal exercises traditionally performed on a flat surface can also be performed on a Swiss Ball, such as the push-up, bench press, and crunch. Several studies have reported an increase in abdominal muscle activity when the push-up is performed on an unstable surface (such as a Swiss Ball) compared with a stable surface.[44,50-52] Abdominal muscle activity is greater when a bench press is performed on a Swiss ball compared with a flat stable surface.[52,53] Other studies have demonstrated an increase in abdominal muscle activity when performing the crunch on a Swiss Ball compared with a flat surface.[41,48,49] Bridging using an unstable surface (Swiss Ball and BOSU ball) has also demonstrated greater abdominal activity compared with bridging on a flat surface.[42]

One study reported that compared with a nonlabile surface, the use of a labile surface Swiss Ball enhanced lumbar multifidus activity in individuals with chronic low back pain.[46] However, another study reported that the

Table 2

Abdominal Exercises Performed With Machine Devices Compared With Traditional Abdominal Crunch and Sit-Up Exercises

Exercise or Machine	Upper Rectus Abdominis	Lower Rectus Abdominis	Internal Oblique	External Oblique	Latissimus Dorsi	Lumbar Paraspinal Muscles	Rectus Femoris
Ab Slide	67 ± 26	72 ± 19	53 ± 15	40 ± 16	10 ± 4	3 ± 2	5 ± 3[d]
Torso Track	67 ± 25	72 ± 17	58 ± 14	32 ± 18	10 ± 5	2 ± 2	6 ± 5[d]
Crunch (normal)	51 ± 9	50 ± 8[ab]	41 ± 9	16 ± 11[ac]	5 ± 1[d]	2 ± 1	3 ± 2[d]
Crunch (oblique)	50 ± 15	39 ± 14[ab]	40 ± 11	32 ± 22	8 ± 5	5 ± 3	3 ± 2[d]
Bent-knee sit-up	38 ± 12[ab]	44 ± 13[ab]	49 ± 21	41 ± 16	6 ± 3[d]	4 ± 2	36 ± 16
Super Abdominal Machine	42 ± 17[ab]	50 ± 20[ab]	36 ± 13[b]	31 ± 21	12 ± 6	4 ± 2	20 ± 15
Ab Roller (crunch)	46 ± 17	42 ± 12[ab]	38 ± 9[b]	13 ± 8[ac]	5 ± 2[d]	3 ± 2	1 ± 1[d]
Ab Roller (oblique)	49 ± 12	36 ± 16[ab]	25 ± 11[abc]	20 ± 9	6 ± 2[d]	3 ± 2	2 ± 2[d]

Average electromyographic (EMG) (± SD) activity for each muscle and exercise expressed as a percentage of maximum isometric voluntary contraction. A significant difference ($P < 0.001$) in EMG activity among abdominal exercises was reported for all muscles.

Pairwise comparisons ($P < 0.01$):

[a]Significantly less EMG activity compared with the Ab Slide (straight and curved);

[b]Significantly less EMG activity compared with the Torso Track;

[c]Significantly less EMG activity compared with the bent-knee sit-up;

[d]Significantly less EMG activity compared with the Super Abdominal Machine.

Data from Escamilla RF, McTaggart MS, Fricklas EJ, et al: An electromyographic analysis of commercial and common abdominal exercises: Implications for rehabilitation and training. *J Orthop Sports Phys Ther* 2006;36[2]:45-57. http://dx.doi.org/10.2519/jospt.2006.36.2.45.

Swiss Ball may not provide a potential effect on erector spinae activity during Pilates isometric exercises with similar posture when compared with stable surfaces.[54]

In addition to being effective in activating abdominal musculature, the 12 exercises evaluated in this chapter are also effective in activating the latissimus dorsi[29-31] (Tables 1 through 4), which tenses the thoracolumbar fascia when it contracts and helps stabilize the trunk. Moreover, tension in thoracolumbar fascia resulting from contractions of the internal oblique (and presumably the transversus abdominis) muscle can further enhance lumbar stability, and most of these exercises produce high activity in the internal oblique muscle. However, except for the Power Wheel roll-out, Swiss Ball roll-out, Ab Slide, and Torso Track, these exercises also exhibited significant rectus femoris activity (and to a lesser extent lumbar paraspinal activity), which can be problematic for some individuals with low back pathologies because of the tendency of the hip flexors and lumbar extensors to accentuate lumbar lordosis, lumbar compression, and intradiscal pressure.[3,13] Therefore, the Power Wheel roll-out, Swiss Ball roll-out, Ab Slide, and Torso Track may be the most effective methods of recruiting abdominal and latissimus dorsi musculature while minimizing rectus femoris and lumbar paraspinal activity. During these roll-out exercises, the latissimus dorsi contract eccentrically during the initial roll-out phase to control the rate of shoulder flexion, and concentrically in the return phase as the shoulders extend. Moreover, although it is logical to assume that the rectus femoris contracts eccentrically

Table 3

Power Wheel and Reverse Crunch Exercises Compared With Traditional Abdominal Crunch and Sit-Up Exercises

Exercise or Machine	Upper Rectus Abdominis	Lower Rectus Abdominis	Internal Oblique	External Oblique	Latissimus Dorsi	Lumbar Paraspinal Muscles	Rectus Femoris
Power Wheel roll-out	76 ± 26	81 ± 29	66 ± 25	64 ± 27[b]	15 ± 7[bcf]	5 ± 2[bcde]	6 ± 4[bcdeh]
Power Wheel pike	41 ± 11[adeg]	53 ± 16[ad]	83 ± 31	96 ± 32	27 ± 16	8 ± 3	26 ± 11[c]
Power Wheel knee-up	41 ± 18[adeg]	45 ± 12[ad]	72 ± 32	80 ± 30	25 ± 12	8 ± 4	43 ± 18
Hanging knee-up with straps	69 ± 21	75 ± 16	85 ± 40	79 ± 25	21 ± 12	7 ± 3	15 ± 8[bc]
Reverse crunch inclined 30°	77 ± 27	53 ± 13[ad]	86 ± 37	50 ± 19[bcd]	14 ± 8[bcf]	8 ± 4	22 ± 12[c]
Reverse crunch flat	41 ± 20[adeg]	30 ± 13[abcdeg]	52 ± 24[bcde]	39 ± 16[abcd]	23 ± 14	6 ± 3[bce]	11 ± 5[bceh]
Crunch	56 ± 17[ae]	48 ± 13[ad]	42 ± 10[bcde]	27 ± 16[abcdeh]	5 ± 3[abcdef]	3 ± 1[bcdefh]	3 ± 3[bcdeh]
Bent-knee sit-up	39 ± 9[adeg]	38 ± 11[abde]	49 ± 22[bcde]	50 ± 16[bcd]	6 ± 3[abcdf]	6 ± 3[bce]	22 ± 12[c]

Average electromyographic (EMG) (± SD) activity for each muscle and exercise expressed as a percentage of maximum isometric voluntary contraction. A significant difference ($P < 0.001$) in EMG activity among abdominal exercises was reported for all muscles.

Pairwise comparisons ($P < 0.01$):

[a]Significantly less EMG activity compared with the Power Wheel roll-out;

[b]Significantly less EMG activity compared with the Power Wheel pike;

[c]Significantly less EMG activity compared with the Power Wheel knee-up;

[d]Significantly less EMG activity compared with the hanging knee-up with straps;

[e]Significantly less EMG activity compared with the reverse crunch inclined 30°;

[f]Significantly less EMG activity compared with the reverse crunch flat;

[g]Significantly less EMG activity compared with the crunch;

[h]Significantly less EMG activity compared with the bent-knee sit-up.

Data from Escamilla RF, Babb E, DeWitt R, et al: Electromyographic analysis of traditional and nontraditional abdominal exercises: Implications for rehabilitation and training. *Phys Ther* 2006;86[5]:656-671.

during the initial rollout phase (to control the rate of hip extension) and concentrically during the return phase (to cause hip flexion), rectus femoris activity was low during these four exercises. This may partially be explained by the neutral pelvic and spine positions that are maintained while performing these exercises. It has been reported that abdominal activity tends to increase and rectus femoris activity tends to decrease when the pelvis is maintained in neutral or posteriorly tilted positions compared with an anteriorly tilted position.[55] Therefore, the latissimus dorsi (and upper extremity muscles in general) may play a greater role in both controlling and causing the roll-out and rollback movements during these exercises than the hip flexors.

Exercises that recruit the rectus femoris and lumbar paraspinal muscles may be contraindicated for those with weak abdominal muscles or lumbar instability. The forces generated when the hip flexors and lumbar extensors contract cause anterior pelvis rotation and increase the lordotic curve of the lumbar spine, as well as increase L4-L5

Table 4

Prone Position Swiss Ball Exercises Compared With Traditional Supine Position Abdominal Crunch and Sit-Up Exercises

Exercise or Machine	Upper Rectus Abdominis	Lower Rectus Abdominis	Internal Oblique	External Oblique	Latissimus Dorsi	Lumbar Paraspinal	Rectus Femoris
Swiss Ball rollout	63 ± 30	53 ± 23	46 ± 21	46 ± 18[b]	12 ± 9[b,c]	6 ± 2	8 ± 5[b,c,e]
Swiss Ball pike	47 ± 18	55 ± 16	56 ± 22	84 ± 37	25 ± 11	8 ± 3	24 ± 6
Swiss Ball Knee-up	32 ± 15[a,d]	35 ± 14	41 ± 16	64 ± 39	22 ± 13	6 ± 3	23 ± 8
Crunch	53 ± 19	39 ± 16	33 ± 13[b]	28 ± 17[b,c]	8 ± 3[b,c,f]	5 ± 2	6 ± 4[b,c,e]
Bent-knee Sit-up	40 ± 13[a]	35 ± 14	31 ± 11[b]	36 ± 14[b,c]	8 ± 3[b,c,f]	6 ± 2	23 ± 12
Swiss ball decline pushup	38 ± 20[a]	37 ± 16	33 ± 18[b]	36 ± 24[b,c]	18 ± 12	6 ± 2	10 ± 6[b,c,e]

Average electromyographic (EMG) (± SD) activity for each muscle and exercise expressed as a percentage of each muscle's maximum isometric voluntary contraction. A significant difference ($P < 0.001$) in EMG activity among abdominal exercises was reported for all muscles.

Pairwise comparisons ($P < 0.01$):

[a]Significantly less EMG activity compared with the Swiss ball roll-out;

[b]Significantly less EMG activity compared with the Swiss ball pike;

[c]Significantly less EMG activity compared with the Swiss ball knee-up;

[d]Significantly less EMG activity compared with the crunch;

[e]Significantly less EMG activity compared with the bent-knee sit-up;

[f]Significantly less EMG activity compared with the Swiss ball decline push-up.

Data from Escamilla RF, Lewis C, Bell D, et al: Core muscle activation during Swiss ball and traditional abdominal exercises. *J Orthop Sports Phys Ther* 2010;40[5]:265-276. http://dx.doi.org/10.2519/jospt.2010.3073.

compression and intradiscal pressure;[3] when coupled with weak abdominal musculature, the risk of low back pathologies increases during these conditions.[13] Exercises such as the bent-knee sit-up, Power Wheel pike, Power Wheel knee-up, reverse crunch inclined 30°, and reverse crunch flat, which have relatively high rectus femoris or lumbar paraspinal activity compared with the crunch, Ab Roller, Ab Slide, Torso Track, and Power Wheel roll-out, may be contraindicated in individuals with weak abdominal muscles or lumbar instability.[13,29,30] Moreover, during abdominal exercises, the EMG magnitude and recruitment pattern of the psoas and iliacus is similar (within 10%) to that of the rectus femoris,[56] which implies that the psoas, iliacus, and rectus femoris may exhibit similar EMG recruitment patterns and magnitudes when performing the aforementioned abdominal exercises. The psoas muscle, because of its attachments to the lumbar spine, attempts to hyperextend the spine as it flexes the hip, and this action may be detrimental to some individuals with lumbar instability. The psoas muscle can also generate lumbar compression and anterior shear force at L5-S1,[13,57] which can be problematic for those with lumbar disk pathologies. Although muscle force from the lumbar paraspinal muscles can also increase lumbar spine compression, the aforementioned abdominal exercises generated relatively low muscle activity (< 10% of MVIC) from the lumbar paraspinal muscles[29,31] (Tables 1 and 2).

Biomechanical Differences Between Abdominal Exercises That Cause Active Hip or Trunk Flexion and Control Hip or Trunk Extension

Some core exercises may be appropriate for some individuals but not others. Some core exercises (for example, the bent-knee sit-up) cause hip and trunk flexion; other core exercises (for example, the Power Wheel roll-out or

Swiss Ball roll-out) control hip and trunk extension. Core exercises that actively flex the trunk can be problematic for some individuals with lumbar disk pathologies because of increased intradiscal pressure and lumbar spine compression,[3,13] as well as individuals with osteoporosis because of the risk of vertebral compression fractures.[58] In these individuals, it may be more beneficial to maintain a neutral pelvis and spine (such as when performing the Power Wheel or Swiss Ball roll-out) rather than forceful flexion of the lumbar spine (such as when performing the bent-knee sit-up). Lumbar stabilization exercises using a Swiss Ball have been demonstrated as effective interventional therapy to alleviate chronic low back pain and to increase bone mineral density.[59]

Some individuals with facet joint syndrome, spondylolisthesis, and vertebral or intervertebral foramen stenosis may not tolerate exercises in which the trunk is maintained in extension, but may better tolerate trunk flexion exercises such as the crunch. In these individuals, trunk flexion exercises can decrease facet joint stress and pain and increase vertebral or intervertebral foramina openings, decreasing the risk of spinal cord impingement, nerve root impingement, or facet joint syndrome.

Although rollout exercises (such as the Swiss Ball roll-out) and reverse crunch–type exercises (such as the hanging knee-up with straps) are effective in activating abdominal musculature, the exercises are performed in a different manner. During rollout exercises, the abdominal musculature contracts eccentrically or isometrically to resist gravity and extend the trunk and rotate the pelvis. During the return motion, the abdominal musculature contracts concentrically or isometrically. If the pelvis and spine are stabilized and maintained in a neutral position throughout the rollout and return movements, the abdominal musculature primarily contracts isometrically. A relatively neutral pelvis and spine are maintained while performing rollout exercises. In contrast, in reverse crunch–type exercises (such as the hanging knee-up), the abdominal musculature initially contracts concentrically as the hips flex, the pelvis rotates posteriorly, and the lumbar spine flexes. As the knees are lowered and the hips extend, the reverse movements occur, and the abdominal musculature contracts eccentrically to control the rate of return to the starting position.

The hanging knee-up with straps, Swiss Ball pike, Power Wheel pike, Swiss Ball knee-up, and Power Wheel knee-up are all performed similarly by flexing the hips, posteriorly rotating the pelvis, and flattening the lumbar spine, which is basically the reverse action of what occurs during the bent-knee sit-up, which involves trunk flexion followed by hip flexion (bent-knee sit-up only).[29-31] One limitation to the hanging knee-up with straps is a

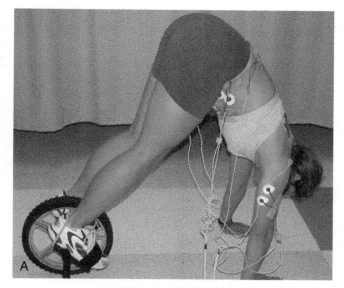

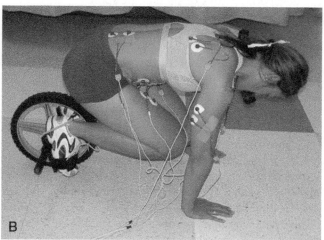

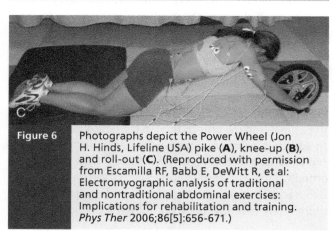

Figure 6   Photographs depict the Power Wheel (Jon H. Hinds, Lifeline USA) pike (**A**), knee-up (**B**), and roll-out (**C**). (Reproduced with permission from Escamilla RF, Babb E, DeWitt R, et al: Electromyographic analysis of traditional and nontraditional abdominal exercises: Implications for rehabilitation and training. *Phys Ther* 2006;86[5]:656-671.)

relatively high L4-L5 disk compression that occurs; however, compression has been shown to be slightly higher in the bent-knee sit-up.[13] Furthermore, EMG from the upper and lower rectus abdominis and internal and external oblique muscles are all substantially greater in the hanging knee-up with straps compared with the bent-knee sit-up.[29] Therefore, the hanging knee-up with straps may be preferred over the bent-knee sit-up for higher level individuals who want to elicit a greater challenge to the abdominal musculature; however, neither exercise may be appropriate for some individuals with lumbar pathologies because of relatively high L4-L5 compression.

When the lumbar spine is forcefully flexed, which can occur when using commercial abdominal machines such as the Ab Twister, Ab Rocker, and Ab Doer, the anterior fibers of the intervertebral disk are compressed and the posterior fibers are in tension. In addition, in extreme lumbar flexion, intradiscal pressure can increase several times above normal from a resting supine position.[3] Although the stresses on the disk may not be problematic for the normal healthy disk, they can be detrimental to the degenerative disk or pathologic spine.

Biomechanical Differences Between the Crunch and Bent-Knee Sit-Up

Not all abdominal exercises involve the same degree of lumbar spine flexion. One study demonstrated that lumbar spine flexion was only 3° during the crunch but approximately 30° during the bent-knee sit-up.[60] In addition, the bent-knee sit-up has been shown to generate greater lumbar intradiscal pressure[3] and compression[13] compared with exercises similar to the crunch, largely because of increased lumbar flexion.[57] This finding implies that the crunch may be safer than the bent-knee sit-up for some individuals who need minimize lumbar spinal flexion or compressive forces because of lumbar pathology.[13]

Although the crunch and bent-knee sit-up are both effective in recruiting abdominal musculature (Tables 2 through 4), some differences exist. Several studies have shown that external oblique activity and, to a lesser extent, internal oblique activity, are substantially greater in the bent-knee sit-up compared with the crunch.[13,29-31,57] However, upper rectus abdominis activity has been shown to be greater in the crunch than in the bent-knee sit-up.[29-31] In addition, rectus femoris and psoas activity have been reported as greater in the bent-knee sit-up than in the crunch.[28-31,57] Increased muscle activity from the rectus femoris and psoas can exacerbate low back pain in some individuals with low back pathologies.

Abdominal and Oblique Recruitment Between the Crunch and Reverse Crunch

Performing the reverse crunch flat activates the lower abdominals and external oblique to a greater extent than the crunch.[61] In contrast, several studies reported substantially greater upper and lower rectus abdominis activities in the crunch than in the reverse crunch flat, and external and internal oblique activity was not substantially different between the exercises.[29,31,36] These discrepancies may be the result of methodologic differences among studies. In one study, the reverse crunch flat was performed by having subjects raise the lower half of the body off the table as far as possible;[61] in two other studies, the subjects were instructed to posteriorly tilt the pelvis and flex the hips to maximal extent.[29,31] However, during the reverse crunch inclined 30°, which involved a higher degree of difficulty compared with both the crunch and reverse crunch flat, activity in the upper rectus abdominis, internal oblique, and external oblique muscles was significantly greater than in the crunch and reverse crunch flat, but no significant difference was reported in lower rectus abdominis activity between the reverse crunch inclined 30° and the crunch[29] (Table 2). These data show that the increasing difficulty of the reverse crunch inclined 30° results in proportional increases in muscle activity.

Summary

Understanding how different exercises elicit core muscle activity and load the lumbar spine is useful to therapists and other health care or fitness specialists who develop specific core exercises for the rehabilitation or training needs of their patients or clients. It is important to be knowledgeable about the relevant literature regarding core stability, core muscle activity during common abdominal exercises, and lumbar spinal loading and injury risk during exercises commonly used to enhance core stability. The core exercises discussed in this chapter activated abdominal muscles and loaded the lumbar spine in various ways such as actively flexing the trunk, controlling trunk extension, flexing the hips with posterior pelvis rotation, or a combination of flexing the trunk and flexing the hips with spinal and pelvis rotation. Several nontraditional abdominal exercises generated substantially greater rectus abdominis, internal oblique, and external oblique activity compared with traditional abdominal exercises such as the crunch and bent-knee sit-up. Although both the crunch and bent-knee sit-up demonstrated similar amounts of abdominal activity, the crunch may be a safer exercise for individuals with low back pathologies because of relatively high rectus femoris activity and lumbar intradiscal pressure generated during the bent-knee sit-up. Roll-out exercises (for example, Power Wheel roll-out, Swiss Ball roll-out, Ab Slide, and Torso Track) were shown to be the most effective exercises in activating rectus abdominis, internal oblique, external oblique, and latissimus dorsi muscles while minimizing lumbar paraspinal and rectus femoris muscle activity. The Power Wheel pike, Swiss Ball pike, Power Wheel knee-up, Swiss Ball knee-up, hanging knee-up with straps, and reverse crunch inclined 30° were all shown to be effective exercises in activating rectus abdominis, internal oblique, external oblique, and latissimus dorsi muscles, but at a cost of also producing relatively high rectus femoris or lumbar paraspinal activity (which can be problematic for individuals with lumbar pathologies). Many exercises that generated high activity from multiple core muscles, such as abdominal bracing, also produced the greatest core stability as well as relatively high lumbar compressive loads (which can increase injury risk to the lumbar spine). Exercises that activated only a few muscles, such as abdominal hollowing, may not be effective in producing the level of core stability needed for many functional activities, such as lifting, running, and jumping. However, these types of exercises may be appropriate early in a core stabilization program, as well as for individuals who cannot tolerate high lumbar compression loading. Many individuals, such as athletes who are training, use a wide array of sport-specific functional exercises to develop core muscles and enhance core stability. However, research involving the effectiveness of performing higher level functional exercises on core stability are needed, and this should be the focus of future research.

Key Study Points

- An understand of the importance of the core, the muscles that comprise the core, and which muscles contribute the most to core stability is important to provide effective rehabilitation or training programs.
- Biomechanical differences exist between abdominal hollowing (drawing-in maneuver) and abdominal bracing techniques.
- Biomechanical differences exist between abdominal exercises that cause active hip or trunk flexion or control hip or trunk extension.

Annotated References

1. Kibler WB, Press J, Sciascia A: The role of core stability in athletic function. *Sports Med* 2006;36(3):189-198.

2. McGill SM: Low back stability: From formal description to issues for performance and rehabilitation. *Exerc Sport Sci Rev* 2001;29(1):26-31.

3. Nachemson AL: Disc pressure measurements. *Spine (Phila Pa 1976)* 1981;6(1):93-97.

4. Essendrop M, Andersen TB, Schibye B: Increase in spinal stability obtained at levels of intra-abdominal pressure and back muscle activity realistic to work situations. *Appl Ergon* 2002;33(5):471-476.

5. Hodges PW: Is there a role for transversus abdominis in lumbo-pelvic stability? *Man Ther* 1999;4(2):74-86.

6. Wilke HJ, Wolf S, Claes LE, Arand M, Wiesend A: Stability increase of the lumbar spine with different muscle groups. A biomechanical in vitro study. *Spine (Phila Pa 1976)* 1995;20(2):192-198.

7. Morris SL, Lay B, Allison GT: Corset hypothesis rebutted—transversus abdominis does not co-contract in unison prior to rapid arm movements. *Clin Biomech (Bristol, Avon)* 2012;27(3):249-254.

   The authors tested the "corset" model of spinal stability, specifically the hypothesis that feed forward transversus abdominis activity is bilaterally symmetric and independent of the direction of perturbation to posture because of arm movements. This study assessed transversus abdominis EMG activity bilaterally. Level of evidence: I.

8. Grenier SG, McGill SM: Quantification of lumbar stability by using 2 different abdominal activation strategies. *Arch Phys Med Rehabil* 2007;88(1):54-62.

9. Hodges PW, Richardson CA: Inefficient muscular stabilization of the lumbar spine associated with low back pain. A motor control evaluation of transversus abdominis. *Spine (Phila Pa 1976)* 1996;21(22):2640-2650.

10. Teyhen DS, Miltenberger CE, Deiters HM, et al: The use of ultrasound imaging of the abdominal drawing-in maneuver in subjects with low back pain. *J Orthop Sports Phys Ther* 2005;35(6):346-355.

11. O'Sullivan PB, Twomey L, Allison GT: Altered abdominal muscle recruitment in patients with chronic back pain following a specific exercise intervention. *J Orthop Sports Phys Ther* 1998;27(2):114-124.

12. Cholewicki J, VanVliet JJ IV: Relative contribution of trunk muscles to the stability of the lumbar spine during isometric exertions. *Clin Biomech (Bristol, Avon)* 2002;17(2):99-105.

13. Axler CT, McGill SM: Low back loads over a variety of abdominal exercises: Searching for the safest abdominal challenge. *Med Sci Sports Exerc* 1997;29(6):804-811.

14. Willson JD, Dougherty CP, Ireland ML, Davis IM: Core stability and its relationship to lower extremity function and injury. *J Am Acad Orthop Surg* 2005;13(5):316-325.

15. Okada T, Huxel KC, Nesser TW: Relationship between core stability, functional movement, and performance. *J Strength Cond Res* 2011;25(1):252-261.

The authors determined the relationship between core stability, functional movement, and performance. Level of evidence: II.

16. Reed CA, Ford KR, Myer GD, Hewett TE: The effects of isolated and integrated 'core stability' training on athletic performance measures: A systematic review. *Sports Med* 2012;42(8):697-706.

    The authors provided a systematic review that focuses on identification of the association between core stability and sports-related performance measures. A secondary objective was to identify difficulties encountered when training core stability to improve athletic performance. Level of evidence: II.

17. Cholewicki J, McGill SM, Norman RW: Lumbar spine loads during the lifting of extremely heavy weights. *Med Sci Sports Exerc* 1991;23(10):1179-1186.

18. Granhed H, Jonson R, Hansson T: The loads on the lumbar spine during extreme weight lifting. *Spine (Phila Pa 1976)* 1987;12(2):146-149.

19. Standaert CJ, Weinstein SM, Rumpeltes J: Evidence-informed management of chronic low back pain with lumbar stabilization exercises. *Spine J* 2008;8(1):114-120.

20. Wang XQ, Zheng JJ, Yu ZW, et al: A meta-analysis of core stability exercise versus general exercise for chronic low back pain. *PLoS One* 2012;7(12):e52082.

    The authors reviewed the effects of core stability exercise or general exercise for patients with chronic low back pain. Level of evidence: II.

21. Teyhen DS, Rieger JL, Westrick RB, Miller AC, Molloy JM, Childs JD: Changes in deep abdominal muscle thickness during common trunk-strengthening exercises using ultrasound imaging. *J Orthop Sports Phys Ther* 2008;38(10):596-605.

22. Vera-Garcia FJ, Elvira JL, Brown SH, McGill SM: Effects of abdominal stabilization maneuvers on the control of spine motion and stability against sudden trunk perturbations. *J Electromyogr Kinesiol* 2007;17(5):556-567.

23. Barnett F, Gilleard W: The use of lumbar spinal stabilization techniques during the performance of abdominal strengthening exercise variations. *J Sports Med Phys Fitness* 2005;45(1):38-43.

24. Hides J, Wilson S, Stanton W, et al: An MRI investigation into the function of the transversus abdominis muscle during "drawing-in" of the abdominal wall. *Spine (Phila Pa 1976)* 2006;31(6):E175-E178.

25. Richardson CA, Snijders CJ, Hides JA, Damen L, Pas MS, Storm J: The relation between the transversus abdominis muscles, sacroiliac joint mechanics, and low back pain. *Spine (Phila Pa 1976)* 2002;27(4):399-405.

26. Stanton T, Kawchuk G: The effect of abdominal stabilization contractions on posteroanterior spinal stiffness. *Spine (Phila Pa 1976)* 2008;33(6):694-701.

27. Oh JS, Cynn HS, Won JH, Kwon OY, Yi CH: Effects of performing an abdominal drawing-in maneuver during prone hip extension exercises on hip and back extensor muscle activity and amount of anterior pelvic tilt. *J Orthop Sports Phys Ther* 2007;37(6):320-324.

28. McGill S, Juker D, Kropf P: Quantitative intramuscular myoelectric activity of quadratus lumborum during a wide variety of tasks. *Clin Biomech (Bristol, Avon)* 1996;11(3):170-172.

29. Escamilla RF, Babb E, DeWitt R, et al: Electromyographic analysis of traditional and nontraditional abdominal exercises: Implications for rehabilitation and training. *Phys Ther* 2006;86(5):656-671.

30. Escamilla RF, Lewis C, Bell D, et al: Core muscle activation during Swiss ball and traditional abdominal exercises. *J Orthop Sports Phys Ther* 2010;40(5):265-276.

    The authors tested the ability of eight Swiss ball exercises (roll-out, pike, knee-up, skier, hip extension right, hip extension left, decline push-up, and sitting march right) and two traditional abdominal exercises (crunch and bent-knee sit-up) on activating core musculature (lumbopelvic hip complex). Level of evidence: II.

31. Escamilla RF, McTaggart MS, Fricklas EJ, et al: An electromyographic analysis of commercial and common abdominal exercises: Implications for rehabilitation and training. *J Orthop Sports Phys Ther* 2006;36(2):45-57.

32. Ekstrom RA, Donatelli RA, Carp KC: Electromyographic analysis of core trunk, hip, and thigh muscles during 9 rehabilitation exercises. *J Orthop Sports Phys Ther* 2007;37(12):754-762.

33. Kavcic N, Grenier S, McGill SM: Quantifying tissue loads and spine stability while performing commonly prescribed low back stabilization exercises. *Spine (Phila Pa 1976)* 2004;29(20):2319-2329.

34. Schoffstall JE, Titcomb DA, Kilbourne BF: Electromyographic response of the abdominal musculature to varying abdominal exercises. *J Strength Cond Res* 2010;24(12):3422-3426.

    The authors examined the EMG response of the upper rectus abdominis, lower rectus abdominis, internal oblique, external oblique, and rectus femoris muscles during various abdominal exercises (crunch, supine V-up, prone V-up on ball, prone V-up on slide board, prone V-up on TRX, and prone V-up on Power Wheel). Level of evidence: II.

35. Avedisian L, Kowalsky DS, Albro RC, Goldner D, Gill RC: Abdominal strengthening using the AbVice machine as measured by surface electromyographic activation levels. *J Strength Cond Res* 2005;19(3):709-712.

36. Clark KM, Holt LE, Sinyard J: Electromyographic comparison of the upper and lower rectus abdominis during abdominal exercises. *J Strength Cond Res* 2003;17(3):475-483.

37. Hildenbrand K, Noble L: Abdominal Muscle Activity While Performing Trunk-Flexion Exercises Using the Ab Roller, ABslide, FitBall, and Conventionally Performed Trunk Curls. *J Athl Train* 2004;39(1):37-43.

38. Sternlicht E, Rugg S: Electromyographic analysis of abdominal muscle activity using portable abdominal exercise devices and a traditional crunch. *J Strength Cond Res* 2003;17(3):463-468.

39. Warden SJ, Wajswelner H, Bennell KL: Comparison of Abshaper and conventionally performed abdominal exercises using surface electromyography. *Med Sci Sports Exerc* 1999;31(11):1656-1664.

40. Behm DG, Leonard AM, Young WB, Bonsey WA, MacKinnon SN: Trunk muscle electromyographic activity with unstable and unilateral exercises. *J Strength Cond Res* 2005;19(1):193-201.

41. Cosio-Lima LM, Reynolds KL, Winter C, Paolone V, Jones MT: Effects of physioball and conventional floor exercises on early phase adaptations in back and abdominal core stability and balance in women. *J Strength Cond Res* 2003;17(4):721-725.

42. Czaprowski D, Afeltowicz A, Gębicka A, et al: Abdominal muscle EMG-activity during bridge exercises on stable and unstable surfaces. *Phys Ther Sport* 2014;15(3):162-168.

    The authors assessed abdominal muscle activity during prone, side, and supine bridge on stable and unstable surfaces (BOSU, Swiss ball). Level of evidence: II.

43. Imai A, Kaneoka K, Okubo Y, et al: Trunk muscle activity during lumbar stabilization exercises on both a stable and unstable surface. *J Orthop Sports Phys Ther* 2010;40(6):369-375.

    The authors examined whether differences in surface stability influence trunk muscle activity. Level of evidence: II.

44. Marshall PW, Murphy BA: Core stability exercises on and off a Swiss ball. *Arch Phys Med Rehabil* 2005;86(2):242-249.

45. Mori A: Electromyographic activity of selected trunk muscles during stabilization exercises using a gym ball. *Electromyogr Clin Neurophysiol* 2004;44(1):57-64.

46. Scott IR, Vaughan AR, Hall J: Swiss ball enhances lumbar multifidus activity in chronic low back pain. *Phys Ther Sport* 2015;16(1):40-44.

    The authors examined the effects of sitting surfaces on the cross-sectional area of the lumbar multifidus in patients with chronic low back pain and healthy control patients. Level of evidence: II.

47. Stanton R, Reaburn PR, Humphries B: The effect of short-term Swiss ball training on core stability and running economy. *J Strength Cond Res* 2004;18(3):522-528.

48. Sternlicht E, Rugg S, Fujii LL, Tomomitsu KF, Seki MM: Electromyographic comparison of a stability ball crunch with a traditional crunch. *J Strength Cond Res* 2007;21(2):506-509.

49. Vera-Garcia FJ, Grenier SG, McGill SM: Abdominal muscle response during curl-ups on both stable and labile surfaces. *Phys Ther* 2000;80(6):564-569.

50. Calatayud J, Borreani S, Colado JC, Martin F, Rogers ME: Muscle activity levels in upper-body push exercises with different loads and stability conditions. *Phys Sportsmed* 2014;42(4):106-119.

    The authors compared the muscle activation levels during push-up variations (such as suspended push-ups with/without visual input on different suspension systems, and push-ups on the floor with/without additional elastic resistance) with the bench press exercise and the standing cable press exercise both performed at 50%, 70%, and 85% of the one-repetition maximum. Level of evidence: II.

51. Lehman GJ, MacMillan B, MacIntyre I, Chivers M, Fluter M: Shoulder muscle EMG activity during push up variations on and off a Swiss ball. *Dyn Med* 2006;5:7.

52. Marshall PW, Murphy BA: Increased deltoid and abdominal muscle activity during Swiss ball bench press. *J Strength Cond Res* 2006;20(4):745-750.

53. Norwood JT, Anderson GS, Gaetz MB, Twist PW: Electromyographic activity of the trunk stabilizers during stable and unstable bench press. *J Strength Cond Res* 2007;21(2):343-347.

54. Paz G, Maia M, Santiago F, Lima V, Miranda H: Muscle activity of the erector spinae during Pilates isometric exercises on and off Swiss Ball. *J Sports Med Phys Fitness* 2014;54(5):575-580.

    The authors investigated the muscle activity of the erector spinae during Pilates isometric exercises performed on and off a Swiss ball. Level of evidence: II.

55. Workman JC, Docherty D, Parfrey KC, Behm DG: Influence of pelvis position on the activation of abdominal and hip flexor muscles. *J Strength Cond Res* 2008;22(5):1563-1569.

56. McGill S, Juker D, Kropf P: Appropriately placed surface EMG electrodes reflect deep muscle activity (psoas, quadratus lumborum, abdominal wall) in the lumbar spine. *J Biomech* 1996;29(11):1503-1507.

57. Juker D, McGill S, Kropf P, Steffen T: Quantitative intramuscular myoelectric activity of lumbar portions of psoas and the abdominal wall during a wide variety of tasks. *Med Sci Sports Exerc* 1998;30(2):301-310.

58. Sinaki M: Exercise for patients with osteoporosis: Management of vertebral compression fractures and trunk strengthening for fall prevention. *PM R* 2012;4(11):882-888.

   The authors examined the effects of exercise for patients with osteoporosis and the management of vertebral compression fractures and trunk strengthening for fall prevention. Level of evidence: II.

59. Yoon JS, Lee JH, Kim JS: The effect of swiss ball stabilization exercise on pain and bone mineral density of patients with chronic low back pain. *J Phys Ther Sci* 2013;25(8):953-956.

   The authors examined the effects of a 16-week lumbar stabilization exercise program using a Swiss ball targeting patients with chronic low back pain on alleviating the pain and increasing bone mineral density. Level of evidence: II.

60. Halpern AA, Bleck EE: Sit-up exercises: An electromyographic study. *Clin Orthop Relat Res* 1979;145:172-178.

61. Willett GM, Hyde JE, Uhrlaub MB, Wendel CL, Karst GM: Relative activity of abdominal muscles during commonly prescribed strengthening exercises. *J Strength Cond Res* 2001;15(4):480-485.

Head and Spine

SECTION EDITOR

Francis H. Shen, MD

Chapter 30
Concussion

Siobhan M. Statuta, MD, CAQSM   John M. MacKnight, MD, FACSM   Jeremy B Kent, MD, CAQSM

Jeremy L. Riehm, DO

Abstract

Concussion is, undoubtedly, one of the most prevalent topics within the sports medicine arena. New discoveries are improving understanding of what exactly occurs on the subcellular and cellular levels, and how they manifest certain clinical features displayed by the athlete. Despite these advances in knowledge, each concussion presents and plays out in a unique fashion that depends on variables such as sport played, position of the athlete, and age of the athlete. Several tests are available to help diagnose concussion and track symptoms. Using these data, medical providers can help guide the athlete back into sports in a safe, stepwise pattern. Concussion complications such as postconcussive syndrome and second-impact syndrome are real entities that could have lasting effects and devastating results. Education and early identification of these conditions is crucial.

Keywords: concussions; sports-related concussion

Introduction

Concussion is currently one of the most frequently discussed topics in sports medicine. Concerted efforts have been made on the national and local levels to improve education regarding concussions in an attempt to better diagnose and manage this condition. Special attention is being directed to improve understanding of what specifically occurs both acutely and over time within the brain, and to answer some important questions: What transpires on the cellular level? Can this cellular activity explain the subsequent alterations observed in athlete behavior and function? What are the long-term effects of concussion?

Concussions can result from simple falls, motor vehicle accidents, assaults, or any similar motion causing sudden acceleration or deceleration to the brain. The annual incidence of recreational or sports-related concussion (SRC) is estimated to be 3.8 million,[1,2] although these values are considered low because of underreporting.

Certain behaviors place an individual at increased risk for sustaining a concussion. In athletic activities, certain sports and athlete positions produce more concussion events than others. Contact sports confer the greatest risk, particularly American football, ice hockey, soccer, boxing, and rugby. Athletes with a previous history of SRC are at increased risk of sustaining another concussive event. The accumulation of concussion episodes, severity of the concussion, and growing symptom duration correlate with prolonged recovery. Female athletes are more likely than male athletes to sustain SRC in similar sports. Children and adolescent athletes appear to have a higher risk of concussive events, with prolonged recovery courses or a subsequent catastrophic event.[1]

Definition

The term "concussion" is derived from the Latin word concutere, meaning "to shake violently" and often is referred to as commotio cerebri in countries outside the United States. No single, agreed-on definition for concussion exists. Concussion can be categorized as a mild, diffuse brain injury resulting in clinical symptoms but not necessarily attributed to a pathologic injury. When a concussive head injury occurs, the brain sustains a contusion. If the head is stationary and is struck by a moving object, a coup injury ensues, resulting in a focal injury of the brain under the site of skull impact. A contrecoup injury—or bruise to the opposite side of the brain—likely results when the moving head strikes an immobile object.

Dr. MacKnight or an immediate family member serves as a board member, owner, officer, or committee member of the American College of Sports Medicine. None of the following authors or any immediate family member has received anything of value from or has stock or stock options held in a commercial company or institution related directly or indirectly to the subject of this chapter: Dr. Statuta, Dr. Kent, and Dr. Riehm.

Although often used interchangeably with the term "mild traumatic brain injury" (mTBI), concussion refers to a specific, less severe subset of the traumatic brain injury (TBI) spectrum.[2] Symptoms are generally limited, with resolution within a few weeks.[1,2]

When the head is jolted, the biomechanical forces imparted to the brain trigger a complex neuronal pathophysiologic cascade, resulting in changes to personality, emotional and physical status, and rate and precision of cognition. Each concussion is unique in its presentation, yet according to the consensus statement released at the 4th International Conference on Concussion in Sport,[2] the following generalities appear to hold true:

1. Concussion may be caused by a direct blow to the head, face, neck, or other part of the body, with an impulsive force transmitted to the head.

2. Concussion typically results in the rapid onset of a short-lived impairment of neurologic function that resolves spontaneously. In some cases, symptoms and signs may evolve over several minutes to hours.

3. Concussion may result in neuropathologic changes, but these acute clinical symptoms largely reflect a functional disturbance rather than a structural injury; therefore, no abnormality is seen on standard structural neuroimaging studies.

4. Concussion results in a graded set of clinical symptoms that may or may not involve the loss of consciousness. Resolution of the clinical and cognitive symptoms typically follows a sequential course. It is important to note that symptoms may be prolonged in some cases.

The diagnosis can include a single impairment or more in one or several clinical domains, including physical symptoms or signs, behavioral changes, cognitive impairment, or sleep disturbances.

Pathophysiology

Questions have been raised regarding what occurs on the microscopic level that effects such behavioral and emotional changes. Studies reveal that, following a concussive force to the brain, neurologic changes result without macroscopic neural damage.[3] As each individual concussion differs, the threshold needed to sustain a clinical concussion also differs among athletes. At the neural cellular level, an alteration occurs to the mechanoporation of the membranes, which triggers an abnormal exchange of substances into and out of the neurons—the neurometabolic cascade. The neurotransmitter glutamate is leaked, followed by an ionic flux. Potassium exits the cells while an influx of sodium and calcium occurs. This ion fluctuation can result in a cellular depolarization, which in turn affects the reactivity of voltage or ligand-gated ion

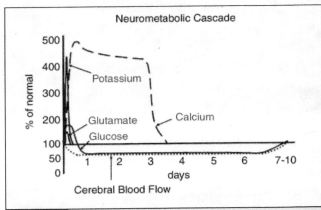

Figure 1 Diagram shows the acute cellular biologic processes occurring after concussion or mild traumatic brain injury. (Reproduced with permission from Giza CC, Hovda DA: The new metabolic cascade of concussion. *Neurosurgery* 2014;75(4):S35.)

channels, resulting in a state of sluggishness (Figure 1).

The brain is left in a state of ionic disarray. Adenosine triphosphate (ATP)-dependent pumps go into action to attempt to restore homeostasis. This process requires energy obtained via hyperglycolysis, which rapidly leaves the brain in a state of energy depletion and with a surplus of adenosine diphosphate (ADP). Consequently, a demand for an increase in energy reserves occurs at the same time as a paradoxical drop in cerebral perfusion. An energy crisis ensues because of this mismatch of supply and demand.[3]

This disarray continues on the mitochondrial level as well as the cellular level. The cells receive an overwhelming influx of calcium. To manage this influx, mitochondria attempt to sequester the excess, but doing so leads to mitochondrial dysfunction. Mitochondria play a crucial role in oxidative metabolism, responsible for the formation of ATP. If they are malfunctioning, the mitochondria exacerbate the energy crisis by slowing down the recycling of ATP. In addition to the mitochondrial malfunction, shifts in subcellular metabolic pathways occur, resulting in the production of damaging free radicals. This process leaves the brain even more vulnerable to reinjury. After the initial insult and neurometabolic cascade, glucose metabolism rates slow paradoxically. This slowness can last up to 7 to 10 days and has been observed to result in behavioral and learning impairments in animal models.[3]

The structure, or cytoskeleton, of the brain also can be affected by these traumatic biomechanical forces. The delicate axons, dendrites, and astrocytic processes are thought to undergo a loss of structural integrity, subsequently leading to an interference of normal neurotransmission. On a more severe level, axonal stretch is postulated to lead to atrophy and shrinkage of neurons without necessarily resulting in cell death. The damaged cell is likely incapable of normal function, as demonstrated in different animal models.

Classification of Concussion

TBI is a spectrum of pathology ranging from mild to severe, with SRC representing a subset of mild TBI.[4] The Glasgow Coma Scale (GCS) helps assess the level of consciousness following head trauma using an objective scoring scale that is reliable and reproducible. GCS scores for moderate head trauma range from 9 to 12; in severe trauma, scores drop to a range of 3 to 8. For concussions, the GCS is typically normal, and any alterations of consciousness or amnesia are relatively brief. Grading systems for concussions have been proposed in the past but are no longer used because of their inability to reliably predict severity or patient outcomes.[2]

The most recent concussion management guidelines use a more generalized scheme of predicting severity instead of grading scales[2] (Table 1). In this revised system, each predictor is not necessarily cumulative. The provided list of symptoms is not all-inclusive, but can be used as a management tool on an individualized basis when attempting to predict intractable symptoms. Loss of consciousness (LOC) is no longer considered an important prognosticator of SRC. Most LOC events during concussions last only seconds and thus are not predictive of severity. Consensus guidelines recommend considering LOC that lasts longer than 1 minute as a possible predictor of greater severity.[2]

Evaluation and Assessment Tools

The evaluation for SRC ideally begins in the preseason with the preparticipation physical examination. This in-depth, detailed examination offers the provider time to uncover any preexisting conditions that are potential concussion modifiers as listed in Table 1. Additionally, the athlete also can complete baseline neurocognitive and balance tests at this time to assist with management and treatment plans. These tests will be discussed later in this chapter.

During sideline coverage, the astute physician must be aware of what is occurring on the playing field as well as along the sideline. The outward, objective signs of a concussion may be very subtle. A concussed athlete may simply wobble upon standing or have a vacant stare. When the physician does not personally know the affected athlete, he or she should rely on athletic trainers and assistants, who prove invaluable in providing input on possible emotional or personality changes.

Table 1

Concussion Modifiers

Factors	Modifier
Symptoms	Number
	Duration (>10 days)
	Severity
Signs	Prolonged LOC (>1 min), amnesia
Sequelae	Concussive convulsions
Temporal factors	Frequency – repeated concussions over time
	Timing – injuries close together in time
	Recency – recent concussion or TBI
Threshold	Repeated concussions occurring with progressively less impact force or slower recovery after each successive concussion
Age	Child and adolescent (<18 years)
Comorbidities and premorbidities	Migraine, depression or other mental health disorders, ADHD, LD, sleep disorders
Medication	Psychoactive drugs, anticoagulants
Behavior	Dangerous style of play
Sport	High-risk activity, contact and collision sport, high athletic level

LOC = loss of consciousness, min = minute, TBI = traumatic brain injury, ADHD = attention deficit hyperactivity disorder, LD = learning disability

Reproduced with permission from McCrory P, Meeuwisse W, Aubry M, et al: Consensus statement on concussion in sport–the 4th international conference on concussion in sport held in Zurich, November 2012. *Clin J Sports Med* 2013;23(2):89-117.

If the sports medicine provider suspects an SRC, the coaches should be made aware that the athlete is being assessed by the medical staff and is not available for participation. Evaluation of the athlete begins with basic life support. After the athlete is deemed stable, the secondary survey can commence, specifically focusing on the athlete's mental status, any neurologic deficit, and possible cervical spine injuries. Findings such as focal neural deficits, progressively worsening symptoms, or prolonged LOC as well as suspicion of a skull or cervical spine fracture warrant further evaluation with conventional neuroimaging.

If and when the athlete is deemed stable following the secondary survey, the provider should proceed with a more detailed sideline evaluation for concussion. During

Table 2

Symptom Evaluation
How do you feel? Score yourself on the following symptoms, based on how you feel now.

Symptom	None	Mild		Moderate		Severe	
Headache	0	1	2	3	4	5	6
Pressure in head	0	1	2	3	4	5	6
Neck pain	0	1	2	3	4	5	6
Nausea or vomiting	0	1	2	3	4	5	6
Dizziness	0	1	2	3	4	5	6
Blurred vision	0	1	2	3	4	5	6
Balance problems	0	1	2	3	4	5	6
Sensitivity to light	0	1	2	3	4	5	6
Sensitivity to noise	0	1	2	3	4	5	6
Feeling slowed down	0	1	2	3	4	5	6
Feeling like "in a fog"	0	1	2	3	4	5	6
"Don't feel right"	0	1	2	3	4	5	6
Difficulty concentrating	0	1	2	3	4	5	6
Difficulty remembering	0	1	2	3	4	5	6
Fatigue or low energy	0	1	2	3	4	5	6
Confusion	0	1	2	3	4	5	6
Drowsiness	0	1	2	3	4	5	6
Trouble falling asleep	0	1	2	3	4	5	6
Feeling more emotional	0	1	2	3	4	5	6
Irritability	0	1	2	3	4	5	6
Sadness	0	1	2	3	4	5	6
Nervousness or anxiety	0	1	2	3	4	5	6

Reproduced with permission from McCrory P, Meeuwisse W, Aubry M, et al: Consensus statement on concussion in sport–the 4th international conference on concussion in sport held in Zurich, November 2012. *Clin J Sports Med* 2013;23(2):89-117.

this time, the player is removed from play for sideline testing. Removing a vital piece of equipment, such as a helmet, can assist in preventing the athlete from returning to play prematurely without approval by the physician.

Several commonly used sideline concussion assessment tools are available, including the Sport Concussion Assessment Tool 3rd edition (SCAT3), the Centers for Disease Control and Prevention Acute Concussion Evaluation, and the National Football League Sideline Concussion Assessment Tool. The SCAT3 is the most widely used sideline tool and has been validated in athletes older than 13 years. The Child-SCAT3 is a variation that has been validated in athletes age 5 to 12 years.[2] Included in each of these assessments is a symptom checklist, a questionnaire assessing neurocognition, and a balance test.

The sideline assessment begins with a symptom checklist such as the one contained in the SCAT3[2,5] (Table 2).

This checklist is associated with a Likert scale allowing for the assessment of symptom severity and has proved to be a reliable and valid predictor of concussions. The sports medicine provider also can use the symptom checklist in the continued management of SRC through ongoing, serial assessments.[6]

The Standardized Assessment of Concussion (SAC) is the tool classically used for neurocognitive testing on the sidelines. It evaluates four categories: orientation, immediate memory, concentration, and delayed recall. The SAC takes approximately 5 minutes to complete and can be administered by physicians or nonmedical personnel. It is scored on a scale in which the normal scores average 26.5 to 30. Concussed athletes average 23 to 30, or a 3.5-point drop below baseline. The SAC is most successful in identifying concussion early in the injury process and is therefore valuable for the acute sideline situation.[7,8]

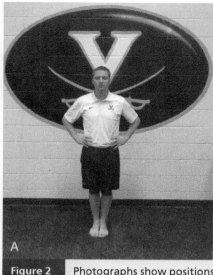
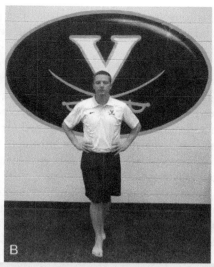
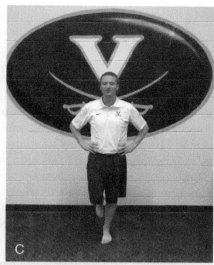

Figure 2 Photographs show positions from the modified Balance Error Scoring System. **A**, Double-leg stance. **B**, Heel-to-toe stance. **C**, Single-leg stance on nondominant foot. The athlete should maintain hands on hips, and eyes closed for each position for a period of 20 seconds on a firm surface. Any position changes, eye opening, or hands coming off hips are recorded as errors.

Balance dysfunction is a hallmark of SRC. Balance, or postural stability, demands a complex coordination between the brain and the musculoskeletal system. A concussed brain demonstrates disturbances in the neural pathways governing balance, and concussed athletes display balance deficits for 3 to 5 days after injury.[7] The Balance Error Scoring System (BESS) is a brief intervention to assess for such a balance dysfunction. The BESS uses three stances on two surfaces, firm and soft. The athlete's goal is to maintain balance in each stance with the eyes closed for a 20-second interval.[9] The test supervisor keeps a record of the number of errors, such as eyes opening or loss of balance. The modified BESS is a scaled-down version using a firm surface (Figure 2) and is most applicable for sideline evaluation. Yet another option is the tandem gait test (Figure 3) as described in the SCAT3, which can substitute for the modified BESS test. With this test, the subject is asked to walk heel-to-toe back and forth over the length of a 3-m line of athletic tape. Grading for this test assesses errors such as stepping off the line as well as completion time. The average time of completion for a nonconcussed individual is approximately 11 seconds. Although simple to complete, the tandem gait test is limited because of a lack of evidence and validity in the concussed individual.[8]

Technologic advances have prompted the development of more precise, increasingly objective methods to measure subtle physical deficits. One such application is demonstrated with the Sensory Organization Test (SOT), another method of testing balance. This system is more sophisticated, using force plates to measure minute

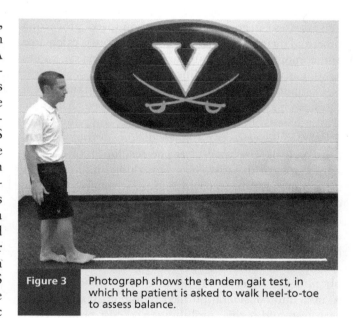

Figure 3 Photograph shows the tandem gait test, in which the patient is asked to walk heel-to-toe to assess balance.

impairments via vertical ground reactive forces, allowing assessment of the somatosensory, visual, and vestibular systems. The SOT is sensitive to tiny changes in postural stability, thus it is superior to the BESS test for detecting balance disturbances. Although the SOT is more accurate than the BESS, its limitation is the cost of the machine.[9] Other examples include the increasingly popular software programs designed to use an accelerometer in smartphones to measure balance. These programs have shown some promising results. The software uses the BESS test as a framework and detects errors while the subject holds the smartphone. These smartphone applications are commonplace and easy to use but are limited by the type of data that are collected.[10]

Apart from the sideline evaluation, formal neuropsychologic evaluation is an effective tool to evaluate SRC. Two forms of neuropsychologic testing are available: paper and pencil questionnaires or computer-based testing. Computer-based testing has become the predominant method because of its ease of administration and interpretation. The computer testing allows a broader spectrum of health care providers such as team physicians or athletic trainers to use the testing results than do paper-and-pencil tests, which require interpretation by neuropsychologists. Various computer-based neuropsychologic tests are available, including Immediate Post-Concussion Assessment and Cognitive Testing (ImPACT, ImPACT Applications), Computerized Cognitive Assessment Tool (CCAT, Cogstate Sports), Computerized neurocognitive test battery (CNS Vital Signs), and Automated Neuropsychological Assessment Metrics (ANAM, Vista LifeSciences). Each test takes approximately 25 to 30 minutes to complete and assesses categories such as reaction speed, processing time, and memory. A final performance score is calculated and compared with population-based normative values as well as individual baseline results.[11,12]

Computer-based tests are best used as management tools after a concussion has been diagnosed. Although they can assist in the diagnosis of SRC, computer-based tests are far less effective as a sole diagnostic tool. Instead, they typically are used after the resolution of concussive symptoms to assist decision making on the athlete's readiness to return to participation. Obtaining baseline computer-based neuropsychologic testing has become the norm, because it accounts for individual variability inherent in the test and gives the provider another data point to help in the diagnosis and management in the concussed athlete. Some uncertainty remains about the usefulness of obtaining baseline testing because it lacks evidence, fails to take into consideration the random error inherent in each test, and is time prohibitive and cost prohibitive.[12] Speculation regarding poor athlete effort or intentional poor performance has been a further concern about the validity of this test.

Additional tools are available that the sports medicine provider can use to assist with the diagnosis of concussion. One such instrument is the King-Devick test (**Figure 4**). The King-Devick test originally was developed to study abnormalities in the saccadic eye movements of children with reading difficulties but was later shown to be effective in diagnosing SRC. The King-Devick test specifically evaluates processing speed, saccadic eye movements, and visual tracking using single-digit numbers displayed on three cards. The patient reads the numbers aloud from left to right as accurately and quickly as possible. The test administrator records the time to completion and the number of errors, which are compared with baseline testing or normative data. The King-Devick test has good reliability and has shown results equivalent to those of computer-based neurocognitive testing.[13,14] Overall, studies are limited for the King-Devick test, but it appears to be a promising tool that is quick, inexpensive, and readily administered by a layperson in the setting of a suspected concussion.

Concussions are not discriminating injuries, and they have far-reaching neurophysiologic effects. One area of the brain that SRC alters is the vestibular system, evidenced by the postural instability uncovered in the BESS, the SOT, and other balance tests. Balance is controlled through the vestibular-spinal system. SRC also affects the vestibular-ocular system. Recent studies have looked to the eyes as "a window to concussion." SRC affects saccadic eye movements, near convergence, and smooth pursuit. Concussed athletes have more pronounced saccadic movements as well as distorted near-convergence and smooth pursuits. Administering these eye tests also will provoke concussion symptoms. Ongoing studies are exploring vestibular-ocular screening tests for concussion diagnostic purposes. At this point, additional data are needed to determine the reliability and validity.

In the ideal setting, the athlete with a suspected SRC would be forthright in declaring his or her symptoms, but this rarely happens in reality. Athletes have been notoriously unreliable in reporting, thus rendering the subjective symptom score invalid. Subsequently, the diagnosis of SRC becomes exponentially more challenging. The search continues for more objective measures to add to the available diagnostic approaches. Biomarkers and advanced neuroimaging are two promising modalities gaining increasing research attention. The ideal biomarker would be a quick and reliable substance that is easily acquired on the sideline or in the locker room. Blood, saliva, urine, and cerebrospinal fluid are all potential sources for biomarkers, although to date, no single biomarker has met the previously described criteria. Certain substances show promise, but none are without substantial flaws. The most studied biomarker is the S100B protein, which is found within astrocytes. Other biomarkers include neuron-specific enolase, glial fibrillary acidic protein, and myelin basic protein, among others. Given the relatively early stages of research, more data are essential before application on the sideline or in the clinical setting is feasible.[15]

Although concussion is a clinical diagnosis, neuroimaging such as CT or MRI are beneficial to rule out a possible secondary process such as a hemorrhage. Research

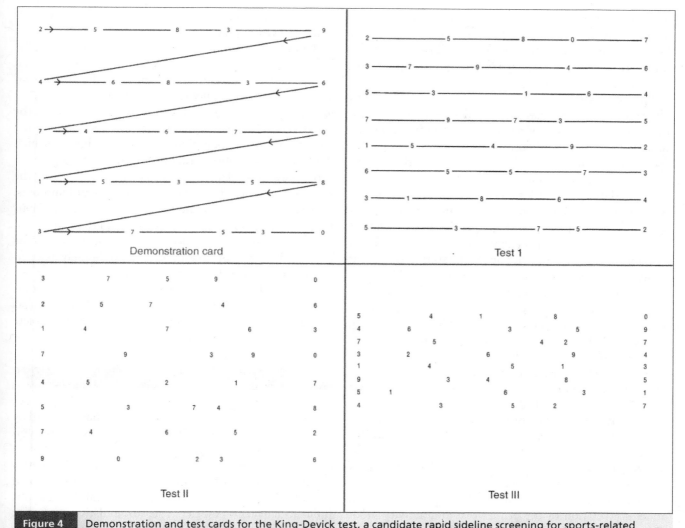

Figure 4 Demonstration and test cards for the King-Devick test, a candidate rapid sideline screening for sports-related concussion based on the time to perform rapid number naming. (Reproduced with permission from Galetta KM, Brandes LE, Maki K, et al: The King-Devick test and sports-related concussion: Study of a rapid visual screening tool in a collegiate cohort. *J Neurol Sci* 2011;309:34-39.)

is underway to explore using other more advanced imaging modalities to assist with the actual diagnosis and evaluation of concussion. Specifically, functional MRI, diffusion tensor imaging, magnetic resonance spectroscopy, and positron emission tomography have shown potential, because findings in these images appear to correlate with symptom severity and concussion resolution. Although these modalities are promising, uncertainties remain about how to interpret or incorporate them into the evaluation and management process of SRC.[15]

Management

If the sideline assessments reveal no worrisome signs, plans for the athlete's departure home may begin. It is advisable to provide the athlete and caregiver with written informational guidelines as a reliable resource to which they can refer. This handout should include a list of specific red-flag signs and symptoms that necessitate immediate medical attention. Such concerning findings include focal weakness, seizure, or increasing confusion. Additionally, an explanation detailing the definition of "appropriate physical, mental, and emotional rest" should be included, covering commonly overlooked exertions such as video games, watching complex television shows, or texting. Athletes with SRC must be reminded to avoid substances that can impair judgment and cognitive function, such as benzodiazepines, alcohol, or even common over-the-counter products such as cough medicines. Extra caution should be taken with certain masking medications, which can treat symptoms and give a false sense of recovery. Acetaminophen is permitted for simple headaches; however, antiplatelet drugs such as aspirin or ibuprofen should be avoided, given the acute concerns for latent intracranial bleeding. The athlete must be closely followed to ensure a pattern of improvement, particularly during the first several days after injury.

Sports activities are restricted to maximize the body's ability to resume normal cerebral perfusion and ensure the greatest likelihood of resuming normal function. Although the athlete should continue physically resting from sports until asymptomatic, low to moderate activity levels are reasonable to maintain daily activities.

Beyond limiting physical activity, cognitive rest also is recommended. This can prove challenging, particularly in middle school, high school, and collegiate arenas, where it is expected that the athletes maintain academic standards. Prompt communication with academic staff is important to facilitate a reasonable modification to the student athlete curriculum without unnecessary delay. Interventions to minimize symptom aggravation should be considered such as limiting continuous hours of reading or restricting screen time. Allowance of additional testing time or due date adjustments also may be warranted as the concussed athlete recovers. The creation of an individualized "return-to-learn" plan allows reintegration into the normal curriculum with as little disruption as possible.

Throughout this entire process, anticipatory guidance for family members, teachers, and coaching staff is critical, particularly given the individual nuances of the recovery process. Often, no outward, objective signs of injury are present with concussions, so the individuals surrounding an affected athlete naturally may have an underappreciation of the proper rest and activity modifications required for recovery. Most athletes become asymptomatic by the end of the first week,[16] but reminding all involved that some cases can take longer will help manage expectations.

Return to Play

Under no circumstances should the athlete be allowed a same-day return to any physical play.[1,2,17] This is a relatively recent yet paramount difference to the way concussions were managed just a few years ago. Although a player suffering an insult capable of resulting in a concussion ideally should be examined by a medical professional, such a professional may not always be available. This is particularly true in the younger or more rural athletic populations. Consequently, mounting efforts to educate parents, coaches, and referees regarding better recognition of concussion have arisen. This heightened awareness reduces the risk of returning to play after such an injury. Assessment by a health professional in the aftermath is

recommended and is now required by law in most states before return to play.

A gradual return to normal social and academic activity precedes a return to sport. A health care professional should make note of this when clearing the athlete and approving initiation into a graduated return-to-play program. A commonly used protocol is that offered by the consensus statement presented at the 4th International Conference on Concussion in Sport[2] (Table 3), which delineates a stepwise return. Advancing through each progressive stage depends on successfully completing the related level of activity without a recurrence of symptoms. Typically, each level should take advantage of a 24-hour time frame to allow for the exertion and for the monitoring of symptoms. If no exacerbation of symptoms occurs, the entire protocol takes approximately 1 week. If symptom recurrence occurs at any point, however, the athlete should revert to the level at which no symptoms occurred to allow further recovery. When the athlete has no symptoms, the progression may resume until complete reintegration into full play occurs.

Postconcussion Syndrome

Postconcussion syndrome (PCS) is a relatively rare but well-described concussion complication characterized by persistent symptoms that may last weeks or, more typically, months or even years. Most concussions follow a characteristic period of resolution. Although 80% to 90% of concussions resolve within 2 weeks,[2,18] the accepted period for recovery is not scientifically established and is influenced by factors such as age, sex, and history of prior concussions.[19] The World Health Organization defines PCS as "a syndrome that occurs following head trauma (usually sufficiently severe to result in loss of consciousness) and includes a number of disparate symptoms such as headache, dizziness, fatigue, irritability, difficulty in concentration and performing mental tasks, impairment of memory, insomnia, and reduced tolerance to stress, emotional excitement, or alcohol."[20] Headache is the most common clinical feature and is often the symptom that prompts medical attention. Athletes also may report vision disturbance, light and sound sensitivity, restlessness, cognitive intolerance, executive dysfunction, vestibular dysfunction, provocation of symptoms with exercise, and concurrent depression.

The progression of a concussion to PCS is poorly defined and understood. Predictors of PCS are not known with certainty, but some clinical variables appear to increase the risk. They include a history of prior concussions, male sex, younger age, a history of cognitive dysfunction, and affective disorders such as anxiety and

Table 3

Protocol for a Graduated Return to Play

Rehabilitation Stage	Functional Exercise	Objective
1. No activity	Symptom-limited physical and cognitive rest	Recovery
2. Light aerobic exercise	Walking, swimming, or stationary cycling, keeping intensity <70% maximum permitted heart rate	Increase heart rate
3. Sport-specific exercise	Skating drills in ice hockey, running drills in soccer; no head impact activities	Add movement
4. Noncontact training drills	Progression to more complex training drills, eg, passing drills in football and ice hockey; may start resistance training	Exercise, coordination, and cognitive load
5. Full-contact practice	Following medical clearance, participation in normal training activities	Restore confidence and assess functional skills by coaching staff
6. Return to play	Normal game play	—

Reproduced with permission from McCrory P, Meeuwisse W, Aubry M, et al: Consensus statement on concussion in sport–the 4th international conference on concussion in sport held in Zurich, November 2012. *Clin J Sports Med* 2013;23(2):89-117.

depression.[19,21] It has been shown that high school and college athletes with LOC, posttraumatic and retrograde amnesia, and greater symptom severity within the first 24 hours following concussion experience longer recoveries.[18] Youth with a history of multiple concussions also have been found to be at greater risk for prolonged recovery and PCS.[19,22] No study has yet identified injury severity as a factor contributing to the development of PCS.

Formal evaluations should be performed by a neurologist and/or neuropsychologist experienced in caring for individuals with head injury to make a definitive diagnosis of PCS. Important alternative diagnoses to consider include cervical injury, migraine headaches, depression, chronic pain, vestibular dysfunction, visual dysfunction, or a combination of these conditions. A battery of neuropsychologic studies may be necessary to fully understand the degree of impairment experienced by the PCS patient. Whenever possible, some measure of baseline neurocognitive testing should be performed before contact sport exposure to allow postinjury comparisons. Conventional neuroimaging can be used to rule out structural pathology, but currently, insufficient data exist to recommend its routine use or the use of advanced neuroimaging techniques.[2] As described previously, several biomarkers also are being investigated for potential use in the diagnosis of PCS. None to date have been shown to consistently predict the development of PCS after concussion, and further research is required to determine their potential clinical utility.

The management of PCS is provided ideally by a health care team that works with concussion on a regular basis. The basic management for PCS focuses on the same general principles as those used for acute concussion. Physical and cognitive rest are the primary interventions, although several complementary therapies are becoming increasingly accepted. PCS patients may derive benefit from cognitive, vestibular, physical, and psychologic therapies.[2] Low-level subsymptom threshold exercise also should be a core component of treatment for those slow to recover from PCS. Athletes with persistent dizziness may derive functional and symptomatic benefit from neuromotor retraining, sensorimotor retraining, and vestibular physiotherapy.

The most common medications prescribed for PCS are antidepressants. Selective serotonin reuptake inhibitors have become the primary treatment of the depression that is associated with head injury and also can improve the cognitive deficits associated with concussion. Tricyclic antidepressants such as low-dose amitriptyline often are used clinically to aid sleep and headaches in patients with PCS, but no controlled trials exist that show their efficacy in restoring normal function. Amantadine is an accepted therapy for the management of moderate to severe traumatic brain injury and can be a valuable therapy in modifying the effects of PCS.

For competitive athletes at all levels, the development of PCS should stimulate discussion about the appropriateness of returning to competitive athletics. These individuals, even after symptoms eventually resolve, maintain a higher risk for reinjury than their nonconcussed peers, and PCS symptoms are more likely to develop again if the affected athletes experience additional concussions.

Second-Impact Syndrome

Second-impact syndrome (SIS), or malignant cerebral edema, is a rare but often fatal complication of multiple concurrent concussive injuries.[23] Although several cases have been described in the literature, the existence of SIS remains controversial, and the underlying triggering mechanisms are still unclear.[24] Classically, SIS arises rapidly after an athlete suffers head trauma while still symptomatic from a prior unresolved concussion.[25] Although this second impact often occurs relatively soon after the initial concussion, SIS can occur up to 2 weeks after the initial head trauma. This second injury may initially appear mild but can rapidly lead to collapse, LOC, respiratory failure, and death.[26]

The exact pathophysiology of SIS is poorly understood. Reinjury to neuronal cells during a vulnerable period following previous injury is postulated to be the most likely mechanism for SIS.[27] This reinjury then sets in motion a cascade of processes, including a loss of cerebral autoregulation, vascular engorgement, and a resulting massive cerebral edema.[23,28] These changes, often coupled with local hemorrhage, then result in a rapid, marked increase in intracranial pressure and ultimately to cerebral herniation and death if unrecognized or untreated.

Except in cases associated with boxing, nearly all cases of SIS have been described in children and adolescents younger than 21 years, with a strong male predominance. Research to date has identified no definitive risk factors for this complication, although increased relative fragility of the younger brain is commonly postulated. Football is the primary sport resulting in described SIS cases, but any sport with contact or collision risk may be implicated.

The prevention of SIS focuses on a timely and accurate diagnosis of the initial concussion and appropriate management, including disqualification from sport, to prevent the risk of "second impact" exposure. When a concussion is suspected, the athlete should be removed immediately from all activity, and a concussion screening evaluation (SCAT3 or an equivalent) should be administered. Every potential concussive injury must be evaluated in a systematic manner to ensure an accurate diagnosis and to determine whether the athlete may return to sport safely. Any dysfunction on such assessment mandates a disqualification from ongoing sport exposure on the same day, at a minimum. If inadvertently allowed to return to sport in the face of an active concussion, the athlete is at risk for SIS.

After a concussion is diagnosed, it is crucial that the athlete be monitored closely during the initial minutes after injury. Athletes with SIS very rapidly deteriorate clinically as their intracranial pressure increases. The level of consciousness may decline precipitously, along with marked declines in cognitive status. Affected athletes can may present with focal neurologic deficits relating to edema and cerebral bleeding. Edema and herniation

develop so rapidly that a favorable outcome is likely only in settings in which medical care is immediately available. Development of any of the clinical features described previously is an indication for immediate transport for urgent brain imaging via CT or MRI and neurologic or neurosurgical consultation. Imaging findings of marked cerebral edema and impending herniation mandate emergent neurosurgical measures to rapidly lower central nervous system pressure and prevent frank brain damage or even death. Additionally, a recent review of death caused by blunt trauma found subdural hematoma to be the cause of all 17 cases of SIS.[29] It is unclear whether concussion increased the risk of bleeding or if the initial injuries were occult subdural injuries diagnosed as concussions.

Health care providers must always be aware that SIS is inherently preventable. As such, it is critical that a concussed athlete never return to sport until a return-to-play protocol following the current standard of care guidelines has been completed, and the athlete has been formally released to resume full contact activities.

Summary

The understanding of exactly what occurs during a concussive injury has advanced greatly, and sports medicine physicians now comprehend that each and every concussion is unique to the individual. Education is imperative for those involved at all levels, beginning with the coaching and athletic staff and incorporating athletes and their parents. Research continues to achieve a greater understanding of head injury and to find more expedient, accurate methods of diagnosis to better treat those who are affected.

Key Study Points

- The presence of certain risk factors, including participation in a contact sport, the position played within the sport, previous athlete history of concussion, female sex, and adolescent or child athletes, increases the likelihood that a concussion will result from an insult.

- A concussion results from a force that causes the brain to sustain a contusion. A collision or fall is not necessary for this to occur.

- Concussion can result in long-term neuropathologic changes, but acutely, clinical symptoms reflect a functional disturbance.

- Under no circumstances should the athlete be allowed a same-day return to any physical play following concussion.

Annotated References

1. Harmon KG, Drezner J, Gammons M, et al; American Medical Society for Sports Medicine: American Medical Society for Sports Medicine position statement: Concussion in sport. *Clin J Sport Med* 2013;23(1):1-18.

   This position statement released by the American Medical Society for Sports Medicine provides an evidence-based approach to the evaluation and management of sports concussion.

2. McCrory P, Meeuwisse W, Aubry M, et al; Kathryn Schneider, PT, PhD, Charles H. Tator, MD, PHD: Consensus statement on concussion in sport—the 4th International Conference on Concussion in Sport held in Zurich, November 2012. *Clin J Sports Med* 2013;23(2):89-117.

   The authors present a revision and update of the recommendations developed following deliberations at the 4th International Conference on Concussion in Sport held in Zurich, November 2012.

3. Giza CC, Hovda DA: The new neurometabolic cascade of concussion. *Neurosurgery* 2014;75(Suppl 4):S24-S33.

   The authors attempt to further explain the postconcussive pathophysiology on the cellular and subcellular levels. These physiologic changes can be linked to the displayed concussive symptoms, which help in understanding what happens during concussive insults.

4. Bailes JE, Hudson V: Classification of sport-related head trauma: A spectrum of mild to severe injury. *J Athl Train* 2001;36(3):236-243.

5. 2013 Concussion in Sport Group. Sport concussion assessment tool - 3rd edition. http://bjsm.bmj.com/. Updated 2014. Accessed November 11, 2014.

   The authors have developed this SCAT3 as a standardized tool for evaluating injured athletes for concussion and may be used in athletes age 13 years or older. It is a modification from the original SCAT and SCAT2.

6. Lovell MR, Iverson GL, Collins MW, et al: Measurement of symptoms following sports-related concussion: Reliability and normative data for the post-concussion scale. *Appl Neuropsychol* 2006;13(3):166-174. .

7. McCrea M, Kelly JP, Randolph C, et al: Standardized assessment of concussion (SAC): On-site mental status evaluation of the athlete. *J Head Trauma Rehabil* 1998;13(2):27-35.

8. Guskiewicz KM, Register-Mihalik J, McCrory P, et al: Evidence-based approach to revising the SCAT2: Introducing the SCAT3. *Br J Sports Med* 2013;47(5):289-293.

   The authors review the evidence for making changes to the SCAT2. They offer specific recommendations to make the SCAT3 a more reliable concussion tool.

9. Ruhe A, Fejer R, Gänsslen A, Klein W: Assessing postural stability in the concussed athlete: What to do, what to expect, and when. *Sports Health* 2014;6(5):427-433.

   The authors investigate the reliability and validity of the BESS and the SOT. They conclude that both tests have limitations, but both can serve as adequate tools for assessing postural stability.

10. Patterson JA, Amick RZ, Thummar T, Rogers ME: Validation of measures from the smartphone sway balance application: A pilot study. *Int J Sports Phys Ther* 2014;9(2):135-139.

    The authors investigate the validity of a smartphone application to assess postural stability. The application's results were no different than previously validated postural stability tests, and the authors concluded that the smartphone application may be a promising objective measure to assess balance.

11. Giza CC, Kutcher JS, Ashwal S, et al: Summary of evidence-based guideline update: Evaluation and management of concussion in sports: Report of the Guideline Development Subcommittee of the American Academy of Neurology. *Neurology* 2013;80(24):2250-2257.

    The authors provide practice guidelines and seek to update previous recommendations based on the most recent evidence. They focus on four areas, including risk factors for concussion, diagnostic concussion tools, risk factors for postconcussive symptoms, and concussion interventions.

12. Resch JE, McCrea MA, Cullum CM: Computerized neurocognitive testing in the management of sport-related concussion: An update. *Neuropsychol Rev* 2013;23(4):335-349.

    The authors review the most recent evidence on computer-based neurocognitive testing. They compare the validity and reliability of the most commonly used computer-based examinations.

13. Galetta KM, Brandes LE, Maki K, et al: The King-Devick test and sports-related concussion: Study of a rapid visual screening tool in a collegiate cohort. *J Neurol Sci* 2011;309(1-2):34-39.

    The authors compared the King-Devick test to the SAC test in collegiate athletes. Their results show evidence for the King-Devick as a sideline assessment tool for concussion.

14. Tjarks BJ, Dorman JC, Valentine VD, et al: Comparison and utility of King-Devick and ImPACT® composite scores in adolescent concussion patients. *J Neurol Sci* 2013;334(1-2):148-153.

    The authors compared the King-Devick test with ImPACT and found similar score improvements in both tests during postconcussive recovery.

15. Cook GA, Hawley JS: A review of mild traumatic brain injury diagnostics: Current perspectives, limitations, and emerging technology. *Mil Med* 2014;179(10):1083-1089.

    The authors evaluate the most recent evidence on emerging technologies in the diagnosis of mild traumatic brain

5: Head and Spine

injury, including biomarkers, advanced neuroimaging, and quantitative electroencephalography.

16. McCrea M, Guskiewicz KM, Marshall SW, et al: Acute effects and recovery time following concussion in collegiate football players: The NCAA Concussion Study. *JAMA* 2003;290(19):2556-2563.

17. Herring SA, Cantu RC, Guskiewicz KM, et al; American College of Sports Medicine: Concussion (mild traumatic brain injury) and the team physician: A consensus statement—2011 update. *Med Sci Sports Exerc* 2011;43(12):2412-2422.

    This article presents a revised consensus statement from the 2006 document. The update focuses on the key revisions, in topics ranging from changes in return-to-play guidelines to emerging technologies and their role in concussion research.

18. McCrea M, Guskiewicz K, Randolph C, et al: Incidence, clinical course, and predictors of prolonged recovery time following sport-related concussion in high school and college athletes. *J Int Neuropsychol Soc* 2013;19(1):22-33.

    The authors investigate the incidence of prolonged recovery in a cohort of athlete seasons over 10 years. Prolonged recovery was associated with unconsciousness, posttraumatic amnesia, and more severe acute symptoms.

19. Guskiewicz KM, McCrea M, Marshall SW, et al: Cumulative effects associated with recurrent concussion in collegiate football players: The NCAA Concussion Study. *JAMA* 2003;290(19):2549-2555.

20. World Health Organization: International statistical classification of diseases and related health problems, 10th revision. Available at: http://apps.who.int/classifications. Updated 2010. Accessed August 6, 2015.

    This volume of the ICD-10 (International Statistical Classification of Diseases and Related Health Problems 10th Revision) contains guidelines for recording and coding, along with much new material on the practical aspects of the classification's use, as well as an outline of the historical background of the classification.

21. Guskiewicz KM, Marshall SW, Bailes J, et al: Recurrent concussion and risk of depression in retired professional football players. *Med Sci Sports Exerc* 2007;39(6):903-909.

22. Kerr ZY, Marshall SW, Harding HP Jr, Guskiewicz KM: Nine-year risk of depression diagnosis increases with increasing self-reported concussions in retired professional football players. *Am J Sports Med* 2012;40(10):2206-2212.

    The authors used survey data obtained over 9 years to prospectively study the effects of recurrent concussions on the clinical diagnosis of depression in a group of retired National Football League players. The risk of depression increased as the numbers of self-reported concussions rose.

23. Wetjen NM, Pichelmann MA, Atkinson JL: Second impact syndrome: Concussion and second injury brain complications. *J Am Coll Surg* 2010;211(4):553-557.

    The authors provide a review of the pathophysiology of second impact syndrome and the several mechanisms postulated to play a role in this condition. They review animal research data and include illustrative case summaries.

24. McCrory P, Davis G, Makdissi M: Second impact syndrome or cerebral swelling after sporting head injury. *Curr Sports Med Rep* 2012;11(1):21-23.

    The authors reviewed scientific data regarding the existence of second-impact syndrome, its pathophysiology, the risk factors for its development, and issues relating to prevention in athletes.

25. Weinstein E, Turner M, Kuzma BB, Feuer H: Second impact syndrome in football: New imaging and insights into a rare and devastating condition. *J Neurosurg Pediatr* 2013;11(3):331-334.

    The authors reviewed a case of second impact syndrome in which neuroimaging was obtained between the first and second impacts. This review offers new insights into the pathophysiology of this process and the potential risk factors.

26. Cantu RC: Second-impact syndrome. *Clin Sports Med* 1998;17(1):37-44.

27. Cantu RC: Recurrent athletic head injury: Risks and when to retire. *Clin Sports Med* 2003;22(3):593-603, x.

28. Longhi L, Saatman KE, Fujimoto S, et al: Temporal window of vulnerability to repetitive experimental concussive brain injury. *Neurosurgery* 2005;56(2):364-374, discussion 364-374.

29. Thomas M, Haas TS, Doerer JJ, et al: Epidemiology of sudden death in young, competitive athletes due to blunt trauma. *Pediatrics* 2011;128(1):e1-e8.

    The authors analyzed the US National Registry of Sudden Death in Young Athletes and found that deaths caused by blunt trauma in athletes were uncommon. Of the total, a large number occurred after head blows sustained after a recent symptomatic concussion.

© 2016 American Academy of Orthopaedic Surgeons

Chapter 31

Traumatic Spine Injuries in the Athlete

Sophia A. Strike, MD   Hamid Hassanzadeh, MD

Abstract

As the fourth most common cause of spinal cord injury, sports participation remains an important area of focus in the study of head and neck injuries. Spinal cord injury in the athlete is an important and potentially catastrophic occurrence. Historical developments have led to improved safety; however, these injuries continue to occur. Understanding the pathophysiology as well as keys to initial, on-field, and in-hospital management allows for complete care of these patients. Controversial topics include removal of protective equipment, use of steroids, and hypothermia.

Keywords: spine injuries; athlete; management of spine injuries; spinal cord injuries; transient quadriparesis; neurapraxia

Introduction and Epidemiology

As of 2013, the incidence of spinal cord injury (SCI) in the United States was estimated at 12,500 cases per year.[1,2] According to the National Spinal Cord Injury Statistical Center, the fourth most common cause of SCI is sports participation, with more substantial damage occurring from injuries to the cervical spine than to the lower segments.[3,4] Motor vehicle collisions and violence, most commonly from gunshot wounds, continue to be the first and second most common causes of traumatic SCI, whereas the proportion of SCI from sporting events is declining, and the proportion from falls has been rising since 2005.[1-3] Between 1991 and 1995, 35.9% of SCIs resulted from

motor vehicles collisions, 29.5% from violent acts, 20.3% from falls, and 7.3% from sporting activities, with more recent rates reported as 38% from motor vehicle collisions, 30% from falls, 14.3% from violence and 9% from sporting activities between 2010 and 2014.[1,2,5] First-year costs per mechanism of injury were highest for sports-related SCI, at $295,643 in 1995, and lower for the other three most common mechanisms of SCI.[5] Patients with sports-related injuries comprised the youngest group, at a mean age of 24 years.[5] For 1995, the aggregate overall cost of traumatic SCI from all causes was estimated to be $7.736 billion.[5]

Sports-related injuries to the spinal cord are associated with football, ice hockey, gymnastics, wrestling, rugby, and trampolining.[6] Gymnastics and ice hockey have higher rates of severe head and spine injury, but football is associated with the largest total number of catastrophic cervical spine injuries, based on the popularity of the sport.[3] According to the National Center for Catastrophic Sport Injury Research, an estimated 4.2 million people participate in football at various levels in the United States annually. Most of these players participate in sandlot or unorganized games, with 1.1 million participants at the high school level and approximately 100,000 participants in college or more competitive levels.[1] Between 1945 and 2000, 16% of deaths in all levels of football were attributable to cervical spine injuries.[4] Between 1945 and 1994, only 1 year (1990) saw no recorded fatality in football from head or cervical spine injury.[7] Throughout this time, 684 fatalities in football occurred, with 85% due to head injuries (465 patients, 68%) or cervical spine injuries (116 patients, 17%).[7] The highest percentage of football fatalities due to head and/or cervical spine injury occurred in the decade from 1965 to 1974.[7] Most of the fatalities from cervical spine injury were fractures and/or dislocations.[7] Involvement in an offensive or defensive tackle was the most common activity at the time of fatal cervical spine injury.[7]

The development of improved football helmets reduced the incidence of football-related deaths from intracranial

Neither of the following authors nor any immediate family member has received anything of value from or has stock or stock options held in a commercial company or institution related directly or indirectly to the subject of this chapter: Dr. Strike and Dr. Hassanzadeh.

hemorrhages. A coincident increase in cervical spine injuries, including fractures and dislocations with resultant quadriplegia, occurred because of the players' newfound ability to hit opponents headfirst, producing an axial load along the cervical spine.[3,4] The elimination of dangerous methods of tackling subsequently reduced the incidence of these injuries.[4] Similarly, changes in checking practices in ice hockey were implemented in an attempt to reduce the occurrence of cervical spine injuries.[3] Multiple national organizations have used epidemiologic data to effect a reduction in head and neck injuries related to sports activities through improvements in the design and manufacturing of safety equipment, the elimination of dangerous sports practices, and increased public awareness of the risks of such injuries.[4]

The National Football Head and Neck Injury Registry was established in 1975 to evaluate national trends in catastrophic football-related injuries.[6,7] In 1975, 12 players sustained head or neck injuries while performing a headfirst tackle or block, in Pennsylvania and New Jersey.[6] In an analysis of head and neck injuries from 1959 to 1963, in comparison with the period 1971 to 1975, the authors found that the number of intracranial hemorrhages and deaths had declined, by 66% and 42%, respectively.[6] Over this same comparison period, a 204% increase in cervical spine fractures and/or dislocations and a 116% increase in cervical quadriplegia occurred.[6] The authors concluded that a concomitant increase in cervical spine injuries occurred because of improved head protection, resulting in an increase in the headfirst tackling technique, which subjected the cervical spine to axial loading.[6] After the presentation of these results in 1976, rule changes rendered headfirst tackling or "spearing" of opponents as well as butt blocking illegal in an attempt to mitigate this upward trend of cervical spine injuries.[6,7] From 1976 to 1987, the number of cervical spine fractures, subluxations, and dislocations declined at the high school and college levels by 70% and 60%, respectively. Complete quadriplegia from cervical spine injury followed a similar trend.[6] Between 1969 and 1998, 51 rules changes were made by the National Collegiate Athletic Association to prevent head and cervical spine injury in football.[7] All helmets now must be certified by the National Operating Committee on Standards for Athletic Equipment prior to use by a high school or collegiate football player.[7] Proper helmet fitting, education about and enforcement of safe tackling techniques, improved physical conditioning of athletes, and an increased presence of medical providers on the sidelines all are factors thought to have reduced the occurrence of death from head and cervical spine injury in football.[7]

Pathophysiology

Spinal Cord Injuries

The bony structures of the spine protect the spinal cord from injury during loading. Anterior structures, including the intervertebral disks and vertebral bodies, resist compression, whereas posterior structures, including the ligamentum flavum, interspinous ligament, and paraspinal muscles, resist distraction. The facet joints prevent the translation of vertebrae.[3] The space for the spinal cord is narrowest at the C4-7 levels.[3] For most contact sports, the mechanism of injury is compression of the cervical spine.[3] Hyperextension of the cervical spine and direct impact to the lower cervical spine from the posterior rim of the football helmet were discredited as major mechanisms of injury in the 1980s.[7] Compression forces can lead to SCI through two major mechanisms. First, a flexion posture with compressive load shortens the anterior column of the spine while distracting the posterior column, leading to overall instability.[3] Second, flexion of the neck during sports activity moves the cervical spine into straight alignment and removes the paraspinal musculature as a supportive shock absorber, and force is no longer appropriately transferred distally to the thorax.[6,8,9] Initially, the energy of the axial load is absorbed by the intervertebral disks, but with the continued application of force, failure of the disks and/or surrounding ligamentous and osseous structures eventually occurs, resulting in fractures and/or dislocations of the cervical spine.[8] Neck flexion to 30° is described as the straightest position of the cervical spine when it is most susceptible to injury from axial loading.[6,8] A pure axial load on the anterior and posterior columns leads to a burst fracture, with SCI resulting from the retropulsion of bony fragments from the vertebral body into the spinal canal.[3] Bilateral facet joint dislocations and burst fractures are associated with SCI.[3,10] A herniated nucleus pulposus, with the characteristic symptoms of acute posterior neck pain with or without radicular symptoms, can lead to transient or permanent cord injury.[3] Klippel-Feil syndrome, odontoid hypoplasia, and os odontoideum are important congenital cervical spine abnormalities, and they must be considered to be conditions that predispose a player to a traumatic cervical spine injury.[3]

Secondary mechanisms of SCI include ischemia, edema, and hemorrhage.[9] Vascular trauma also must be considered in the evaluation of the injured patient with a neurologic deficit. Dissection, thrombus or embolism, and occlusion from direct trauma or secondary compression can occur. Above C6, the vertebral artery may be damaged. Symptoms indicating dysfunction of a cerebral hemisphere or a spinal cord syndrome can appear acutely or develop over time.[9] Magnetic resonance angiography or CT angiography should be performed emergently if vascular trauma is a concern.[9]

Patients with neurologic deficit after a cervical spine fracture or dislocation are more likely to have sustained an injury to the lower cervical spine.[11] Mean sagittal canal diameters decrease proximally to distally within the cervical spine, with a nadir at C6, averaging 23.9 mm at C1 to 17.9 mm at C7.[11] In a review of 98 patients with cervical spine fractures and/or dislocations, the authors found substantially smaller sagittal cervical spine canal diameters in those patients with complete SCI than in those with no neurologic deficits or incomplete deficits, suggesting that a large spinal canal is a protective factor for SCI.[11]

Studies of squid axons suggest that the mechanical deformation of axons alters membrane permeability and thus the cytosolic calcium concentration, as well as local vasospasm and the resulting incoming blood flow.[8] These changes affect the ability of the axon to conduct signals, to a reversible, partially reversible, or irreversible degree, based on the applied amount of tension.[8] In a transient neurapraxia of the spinal cord, as discussed later, an elastic deformation of axons is thought to occur, leading to a change in membrane permeability that causes a minimal increase in intracellular calcium and thus only a temporary alteration in function with no residual deficit.[8] Injuries rendering the cervical spine more unstable (such as unilateral or bilateral facet dislocations, severe fractures) can lead to spinal cord deformation causing the maximal elastic or plastic deformation of axons and thus longer periods of anoxia and cytosolic calcium build-up.[8] These intracellular changes result in incompletely reversible or irreversible SCI.[8]

Transient Quadriparesis

Transient SCI, or transient quadriparesis, manifests as weakness with or without sensory changes, most commonly in all four extremities but occasionally only hemiparetically.[9] The pathophysiology of transient quadriparesis is described as a physiologic—as opposed to an anatomic—disruption in normal spinal cord signaling.[3] A neurapraxia results from "contusion" of the spinal cord after dynamic narrowing of the spinal canal.[3] As in peripheral neurapraxia, symptoms last from minutes to 2 days and resolve completely.[3,8,9] Symptoms include bilateral upper-extremity or lower-extremity pain, paresthesias, and/or tingling, with possible motor weakness as severe as that seen in complete quadriplegia.[3,8] As described previously, transient quadriparesis typically is not associated with cervical spine pain and, with resolution of symptoms, full painless range of motion of the cervical

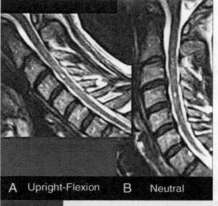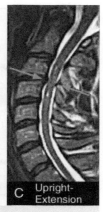

| | | |
| A Upright-Flexion | B Neutral | C Upright-Extension |

Figure 1 Images show transient quadriparesis. The upright flexion (**A**) and extension (**C**) images show spinal cord contusions at the C3-4 level that resulted in the acute transient paralysis. This was not visible on the neutral upright scan (**B**). (Courtesy of Jean Pierre J. Elsig, MD, Zurich, Switzerland.)

spine is noted.[8] Radiographs of the cervical spine are negative for fractures and/or dislocations.[8]

The pathophysiology of these "spinal cord concussions" had been postulated to be a temporary loss of signal transmission from an acute and transient impingement of the spinal cord.[9] Permanent damage is not thought to occur, and thus persistent radiologic changes are not observed.[9] A smaller anteroposterior sagittal canal diameter in an athlete has been thought to predispose to cervical spine neurapraxia. The etiology is thought to be mechanical and to be related to an acute compression of the spinal cord between the posteroinferior aspect of the supradjacent vertebral body and the subjacent anterosuperior aspect of the spinal laminar line or vice versa, with hyperflexion or hyperextension but without fracture or dislocation[8](Figure 1).

Neurapraxia (Stingers and Burners)

Stingers is a term used to describe a transient sensation of burning, pain, numbness or tingling in a unilateral upper extremity. This sensation may be accompanied by motor weakness.[12] Symptoms in bilateral upper extremities or in either lower extremity should alert the clinician to the possibility of a spinal cord injury, rather than to peripheral nerve injury.[12] Stingers are thought to result from traction on the brachial plexus or compression of a cervical spine root at the level of the neuroforamen[3,12,13](Figure 2). A dermatomal distribution of radiating pain with possible weakness in the corresponding nerve root distribution is indicative of an injury at the cervical nerve root level. The mechanism of injury of cervical root impingement is a compression loading on the neck through an axial

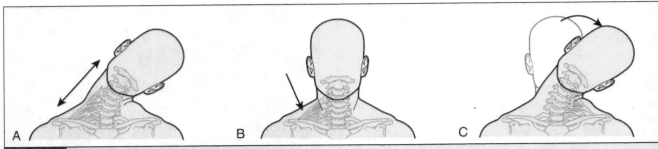

Figure 2 Drawings show the mechanisms of injury for burners. **A,** Traction to the brachial plexus from the ipsilateral shoulder depression and contralateral lateral neck flexion are shown. **B,** A direct blow occurs to the supraclavicular fossa at the Erb point. **C,** Compression of the cervical roots or brachial plexus from ipsilateral lateral flexion and hyperextension is shown.

blow to the head or extension and ipsilateral rotation of the neck.[3,12,13] Burners or stingers involving the brachial plexus are more likely to affect multiple muscle groups and a wider sensory area.[9] Brachial plexus stretch occurs after a direct blow to the head or shoulder, causing extension and traction in the region of the plexus.[12,13]

In scholastic athletes, the Torg-Pavlov ratio (the spinal canal AP width to the vertebral body AP width) and the foramen/vertebral body ratio (the height ratio of the neuroforamen to the subjacent vertebra at the largest points) were found to be substantially different in players who had sustained burners than in control group players who had not. This finding suggests that an increased risk of cervical canal stenosis and foraminal stenosis is present in players who have sustained a burner-type injury. No stratification of players based on mechanism was performed, however. It has been proposed that extension-compression mechanisms are more likely to be associated with root-level injuries. Further subgroup analysis may have provided an even stronger association with cervical canal stenosis and foraminal stenosis in this subset.[13]

For most patients, pain will resolve within minutes, and full sensorimotor symptoms will resolve within 1 to 2 days.[3] Persistence or recurrence of symptoms, an abnormal physical examination, or symptoms concerning for a more central process preclude a player from returning to the game and require further imaging such as cervical spine MRI.[12] Symptoms that continue longer than 2 weeks should be evaluated with electromyography (EMG).[12] Although EMG will differentiate the level of peripheral nerve injury, it typically is not useful until 3 weeks after injury.[9]

Management

Advanced Trauma Life Support
A primary survey of airway, breathing, and circulation always must be performed in an injured player.[9,14] A neurologic evaluation and determination of consciousness follows if the primary survey is negative for abnormality.[9] Unconscious patients or those with neurologic symptoms including burning, numbness, tingling, and weakness should be managed as if a cervical spine injury is present.[9,15] Cervical spine injuries during sporting events are unique in the need to accommodate protective gear and on-field conditions when evaluating and immobilizing the potentially injured player.[3]

Accessibility of the airway is necessary for the management of injured players. In contrast to the prior recommendation to leave a helmet in place for the player with a cervical spine injury, the most current recommendation from the National Athletic Trainers' Association (NATA) is that the provider with the highest level of training remove all athletic equipment prior to transport to the hospital including the helmet and shoulder pads, although this recommendation remains controversial.[16] According to the National Athletic Trainers' Association (NATA), exposure of the airway must be completed urgently. The jaw-thrust maneuver for airway patency is preferred over a head-tilt to protect the cervical spine from potentially damaging motion.[15] For all sports, on-field personnel should become familiar with the related protective equipment and make all attempts to keep the cervical spine in neutral alignment.[15,16] Recognizing less severe but more common soft-tissue injuries such as ligament and muscle strains is important for the complete evaluation of the athlete.[4]

Boarding and Transferring Patients
In a 2007 review of the literature on positioning of the cervical spine when boarding an injured player, the authors concluded that the shoulder pads and helmet should be left in place in football and in ice hockey to keep the cervical spine at zero elevation and allow maximal space for the spinal cord within the canal, however, the updated recommendation is to remove all protective equipment

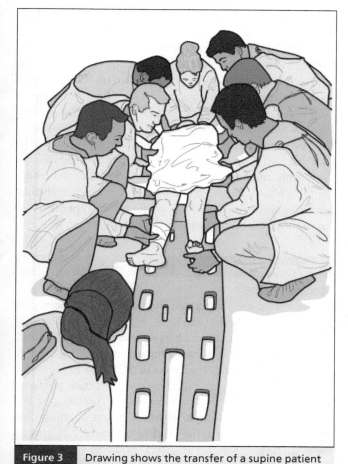

Figure 3 Drawing shows the transfer of a supine patient to a spine board using the 6 + lift and slide technique.

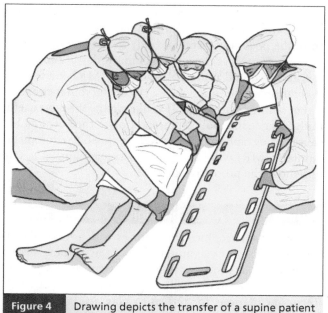

Figure 4 Drawing depicts the transfer of a supine patient to a spine board using the log-roll technique.

to the board.[9] An additional form of immobilization of the head also should be used.[9] A cervical collar provides the best immobilization of the cervical spine.[9] The spine of the prone player should be examined prior to the log roll.[15] Repositioning movements on the long board should be performed in a longitudinal direction rather than perpendicular to the axis of the spine.[15]

Imaging

Evaluation begins with a thorough examination and cervical spine radiographs, including flexion and extension views. Radiographic evaluation is necessary in any patient with symptoms or clinical signs of neurologic injury.[9] Transient bilateral sensory and/or motor deficits occurring after a head or neck injury are suggestive of an SCI.[12] Cervical spine radiographs serve as the initial modality.[9] CT or MRI of the spine may be necessary to detect bony or ligamentous injury as well as spinal cord injury or nerve root compression.[12] MRI is the optimal imaging study for the evaluation of a traumatic intervertebral disk herniation, hematoma, or local swelling in the cervical spine.[9] MRI also allows evaluation of possible spinal stenosis because it provides optimal visualization of the vertebral bodies, the intervertebral disks, the spinal cord, and the canal.[9,17]

In a review of cervical spine imaging in football players, it was proposed that athletes with neurologic symptoms have flexion and extension radiographs of the cervical spine performed for the evaluation of stability.[17]

prior to transport to the hospital.[9,16] The least ideal positioning is extension of the cervical spine; therefore, leaving shoulder pads in place and allowing the head to rest on the backboard is not recommended.[9] NATA recommends immediate stabilization of the cervical spine in a neutral position when injury is suspected.[15] Immobilization of the cervical spine and head should be maintained with external devices (cervical collar, blocks, towel rolls) and manual stabilization, if possible.[15]

Full-body immobilization in the form of a long board or vacuum splint is also necessary for transfer.[15] The head should be secured at the forehead and chin for optimal immobilization of the spine.[15] Two techniques for transferring patients to the rigid board are currently used. The six-person lift technique involves lifting the patient approximately 6 inches off the ground and sliding a board below (Figure 3). Alternatively, the patient can be log rolled onto a board placed beneath the patient to support the cervical spine[15] (Figure 4). NATA recommends the lift-and-slide technique, citing less motion at the cervical spine.[15] At least three straps should secure the patient

Furthermore, it was proposed that any athlete with neurologic symptoms and a sagittal canal diameter (measured from the posterior vertebral body to the anterior aspect of the lamina) less than two standard deviations below the mean should undergo functional MRI for further evaluation of the function reserve of the spinal canal.[17]

For helmeted athletes, CT is likely to be the most useful initial diagnostic tool on presentation to the hospital, because radiographs will be limited by sporting equipment. Similarly, MRI will have to be postponed until it is safe to remove the protective gear.[15]

Return to Play After Spine Injury

Although catastrophic spine injuries with a residual neurologic deficit or concomitant head injury clearly necessitate future abstinence from contact sports, less severe injuries may allow the player to resume such activities. Recommendations for return to play are largely experience based and are tailored to the player.[9,14,18] As an overall guideline, return to play requires the absence of neurologic symptoms and pain as well as full range of motion of the cervical spine.[18] For stingers or burners, the immediate resolution of symptoms with no recurrence and a normal examination may allow same-day return to sports activity.[3] A neck roll to prevent hyperextension and a neck and shoulder muscular training program also should be considered to prevent future injury in these players.[18]

A 2007 study cites evidence that prodromal symptoms are unlikely to occur prior to catastrophic SCI.[9] Furthermore, no evidence shows that stenosis alone predicts a future catastrophic injury.[9] Players with transient SCI—and thus no permanent neurologic sequelae—as well as preserved cerebrospinal fluid on MRI can be allowed to return to contact sport.[9] Radiologic evidence of disk herniation, cord contusion or impingement from osteophytes or surrounding ligaments, or instability should preclude players from contact sports in the future.[9] Repetitive episodes of transient quadriparesis warrant further consideration for discontinuing participation in contact sports.[9,18] Congenital conditions involving the odontoid (hypoplasia, os odontoideum), atlanto-occipital fusion, and Klippel-Feil anomaly involving fusion of the cervical spine to the upper thoracic spine are absolute contraindications to return to play.[18] Players with spear tackler spine or the clinical combination of cervical spine stenosis, persistent loss of cervical lordosis, posttraumatic radiographic changes, and a history of spear tackling should not return to play at any time.[18] Players with stable spine fractures, such as spinous process fractures and compression and endplate vertebral body fractures with no sagittal changes or concomitant ligamentous injury and without neurologic symptoms may be considered for return to play.[18] Stability must be confirmed with flexion-extension cervical spine radiographs.[9] Players must not have any neurologic symptoms or cervical spine pain.[14] Players with spinal fractures requiring surgical stabilization or spinal cord injuries are advised against return to contact sports.[9] Players who have previously undergone spine surgery specifically for disk herniation may return to play after bony fusion is complete.[9] In the absence of neurologic symptoms and pain, fusion of one vertebral level does not prohibit play, whereas the fusion of two to three levels is a relative contraindication. Having four or more levels of fusion is an absolute contraindication to return to play.[18]

Controversies

Steroid Protocol

The systemic use of steroids in acute SCI has been proposed as a method to reduce the effect of secondary mechanisms of damage such as edema and inflammation. A Cochrane review of randomized trials using methylprednisolone sodium succinate in SCI patients revealed only eight adequate studies; however, practice guidance has been based on these outcomes.[19] Treatment of SCI with methylprednisolone within 8 hours of injury has become standard practice and is supported by the reviewed trials.[19] The dosing and duration of treatment are based on the time from injury. Patients given methylprednisolone within 3 hours of injury should receive a bolus of 30 mg/kg intravenously for 15 minutes followed by a maintenance infusion of 5.4 mg/kg starting 45 minutes later for the next 23 hours; no benefit is gained by continuing therapy longer than 24 hours. Patients given methylprednisolone between 3 and 8 hours from the time of injury should receive the same initial bolus but should receive 48 hours of total therapy, because motor and functional outcomes are improved with an increased length of therapy in this group of patients.[19] Furthermore, the reviewed trials showed no evidence of an increase in medical complications or mortality from changing to the 48-hour regimen of dosing from the 24-hour regimen.[19] Since the publication of that review, the Congress of Neurological Surgeons has recommended against using methylprednisolone, citing the off-label use and the lack of well-designed studies.[20] In a survey of the members of the Cervical Spine Research Society, researchers found a significant reduction from 89% to 56% of members using methylprednisolone in acute SCI in 2013 versus in 2006. Members cited sepsis, gastrointestinal bleeding, and SCI occurring more than 8 hours prior to the possible administration of steroids as the most common contraindications.[21] Similarly, according to recommendations by NATA, treatment of acute SCI with methylprednisolone remains a controversial technique. Its use in the injured athlete requires a discussion of the risks and benefits with the patient and the family.[15] In contrast, peripheral neurapraxias, including stingers and brachial plexopathies, are a contraindication to steroid use.[22]

Hypothermia

The benefits of additional interventions in the setting of an acute SCI include mitigating the secondary injury and increasing the patient's chances for improved future function.[23] Moderate systemic hypothermia has been proposed as a mechanism for reducing potentially irreversible histopathologic changes within the spinal cord.[23] Well-defined protocols for using hypothermia in the acute management of SCIs are not available, however.[9,23,24]

A National Football League player who sustained a C3-4 fracture/dislocation and an SCI graded A on the American Spinal Injury Association (ASIA) impairment scale was treated with surgical decompression, intravenous methylprednisolone, and early moderate hypothermia. The player's neurologic function improved within weeks, and at the time of the report, his neurologic status was graded as ASIA D.[25] Based on this single report, the improvement in neurologic status could not be attributed entirely to systemic hypothermic treatment; however, the case highlights the need and potential clinical utility of further studies on its use in SCI.[25] In a case series of 20 patients with a complete SCI treated with surgical decompression, glucocorticoids, and local spinal cord cooling, overall improvements in neurologic status were observed. With confounding treatments and no controls, clinical application is limited, but the authors suggest that, based on this experience, well-designed clinical trials using local hypothermia are worth undertaking.[26]

The American Association of Neurological Surgeons (AANS)/Congress of Neurological Surgeons (CNS) Joint Section on Disorders of the Spine and Peripheral Nerves and Joint Section on Trauma released an update to their initial 2007 position statement on using hypothermia in SCI, noting the lack of comparative studies available on which to base recommendations.[27] The authors cite insufficient evidence for or against using hypothermia in acute SCI and note promising level IV evidence that hypothermia is a potentially safe intervention requiring further study.[27]

Hypothermia was used originally as a local treatment performed by surrounding the exposed spinal cord with cold saline during decompression procedures, with occasional beneficial results. This technique was confounded by the surgery itself as well as by the use of steroids in the acute setting, thus precluding its standard adoption.[23]

Local cooling was advantageous because systemic responses to hypothermia, such as arrythmias, hypotension, venous thromboembolic events, acute respiratory distress syndrome (ARDS) and/or infection, are avoided.[23,24] Surface cooling using blankets and water baths help facilitate hypothermic treatment, given its noninvasive nature; however, the process is variable, and depending on patient size can be inefficient in producing hypothermic changes.[24] Intravascular cooling allows more controlled hypothermia but is associated with the previously described risks.[23] In one study of 14 patients receiving moderate hypothermia for the prevention of SCI, most complications were respiratory (pneumonia, atelectasis, ARDS, pulmonary edema). It was unclear whether this result could be attributed directly to the hypothermic protocol, however, because no significant difference, except pulmonary edema, was seen when compared with complications in a matched control group.[24,28] Importantly, 6 patients (42.8%) improved in neurologic status from ASIA/International Medical Society of Paraplegia impairment scale grade A at initial presentation and maintained this improvement after discharge, with a greater number of patients converting to a better ASIA status than in the control group.[28] None of the patients demonstrated an ascending neurologic level.[28] In a rat model of spinal cord contusion treated with post-SCI hypothermia, the treatment group was noted to have increased gray and white matter volumes, increased neuron cell preservation near the site of injury, and maintenance of long-tract reticulospinal axons.[29] Clinically, the rats showed increased rates of locomotor recovery and increased limb strength.[29]

Multiple pathophysiologic mechanisms are thought to provide protection in moderate hypothermia. Reduced cerebral metabolic demands provide an increased energy source for the area of damage.[23] Hypothermia is thought further to decrease the release of glutamate, an excitatory neurotransmitter. The expression of relevant neurotransmitter receptors, including N-methyl-D-aspartic acid also seems to be altered by temperature changes.[23] An overall change in the excitatory state of the brain is thought to protect neuronal vulnerability.[13,29] Hypothermic states reduce vascular permeability and thus prevent the loss of the blood-brain barrier.[23] Intracellularly, multiple signaling pathways affecting calcium concentration and the cytoskeletal infrastructure also seem to be sensitive to temperature alterations.[23] Inflammatory responses, via cytokines such as tumor necrosis factor–α and interleukin-1, are thought to be blunted by therapeutic hypothermia, protecting neurons from secondary insult.[23] An overall change in the ability to retard tissue damage after traumatic insult to the spinal cord underlies the mechanisms of protection produced by mild to moderate hypothermia.[29]

© 2016 American Academy of Orthopaedic Surgeons

Summary

Cervical spine trauma in the athlete is a significant occurrence, with potentially catastrophic results. Football remains one of the most common and most well-studied sports activities associated with spine injuries. Transient spinal cord and peripheral nerve injuries may manifest as quadriparesis or burners/stingers with symptoms that resolve completely. More severe spinal cord injuries, typically from axial loading on the cervical spine, cause bilateral symptoms with residual neurologic deficit. Advanced Trauma Life Support principles always must be applied to the player with a potential spine injury. Reducing the movement of the cervical spine through immobilization and accessing the airway, either through removal of all protective equipment or just removal of the facemask while leaving appropriate padding in place remains controversial, but is key to managing and transferring SCI players off the field. The use of steroids in acute SCI remains controversial. Moderate systemic hypothermia provides theoretical benefits for reducing spinal cord damage in the setting of an acute injury. Although this technique has been studied in the laboratory, only a few clinical trials have been performed, and further research is necessary before routine implementation of hypothermia protocols can be recommended.

Key Study Points

- Sports participation has consistently been the fourth leading cause of spinal cord injury, with the most injuries occurring in football players. Although deaths from intracranial hemorrhage decreased with use of helmets, an initial increase in cervical spine injuries was halted by rules changes forbidding head-first tackling and other dangerous maneuvers.

- Initial management of players with a potential spinal cord injury includes applying the principles of Advanced Trauma Life Support, especially securing an airway. Removal of protective athletic equipment continues to be a controversial topic with recent recommendations by the National Athletic Trainers' Association to do so on the field. Boarding and transfer require stabilization of the cervical spine to prevent additional injury.

- Controversial treatments for spinal cord injury include steroid protocols and use of acute hypothermia. Although laboratory data suggest a theoretical benefit, clinical use is not yet prevalent.

Annotated References

1. Injury SC: (SCI) Facts and Figures at a Glance. National Spinal Cord Injury Statistical Center. August 2014. Available at: https://www.nscisc.uab.edu/PublicDocuments/fact_figures_docs/Facts%202014.pdf Accessed on August 18, 2015.

   The up-to-date demographics of spinal cord injury patients are summarized and reviewed. Lifetime costs, life expectancy, and cause of death are also discussed.

2. Annual Survey of Football Injury Research: 1931-2013. National Center for Catastrophic Sport Injury Research. Available at: http://nccsir.unc.edu/files/2014/06/Annual-Football-2013-Fatalities-Final.pdf Accessed on August 18, 2015.

   A summary of survey results from the American Football Coaches Association is presented regarding fatalities related to football participation, with the goal to prevent future fatalities and improve the safety of the sport.

3. Banerjee R, Palumbo MA, Fadale PD: Catastrophic cervical spine injuries in the collision sport athlete, part 1: Epidemiology, functional anatomy, and diagnosis. *Am J Sports Med* 2004;32(4):1077-1087.

4. Cooper MT, McGee KM, Anderson DG: Epidemiology of athletic head and neck injuries. *Clin Sports Med* 2003;22(3):427-443, vii.

5. DeVivo MJ: Causes and costs of spinal cord injury in the United States. *Spinal Cord* 1997;35(12):809-813.

6. Torg JS, Vegso JJ, O'Neill MJ, Sennett B: The epidemiologic, pathologic, biomechanical, and cinematographic analysis of football-induced cervical spine trauma. *Am J Sports Med* 1990;18(1):50-57.

7. Mueller FO: Fatalities from head and cervical spine injuries occurring in tackle football: 50 years' experience. *Clin Sports Med* 1998;17(1):169-182.

8. Torg JS, Thibault L, Sennett B, Pavlov H: The Nicolas Andry Award. The pathomechanics and pathophysiology of cervical spinal cord injury. *Clin Orthop Relat Res* 1995;321:259-269.

9. Bailes JE, Petschauer M, Guskiewicz KM, Marano G: Management of cervical spine injuries in athletes. *J Athl Train* 2007;42(1):126-134.

10. Coelho DG, Brasil AV, Ferreira NP: Risk factors of neurological lesions in low cervical spine fractures and dislocations. *Arq Neuropsiquiatr* 2000;58(4):1030-1034.

11. Eismont FJ, Clifford S, Goldberg M, Green B: Cervical sagittal spinal canal size in spine injury. *Spine (Phila Pa 1976)* 1984;9(7):663-666.

12. Cantu RC: Stingers, transient quadriplegia, and cervical spinal stenosis: Return to play criteria. *Med Sci Sports Exerc* 1997;29(7, Suppl)S233-S235.

13. Kelly JD IV, Aliquo D, Sitler MR, Odgers C, Moyer RA: Association of burners with cervical canal and foraminal stenosis. *Am J Sports Med* 2000;28(2):214-217.

14. Ghiselli G, Schaadt G, McAllister DR: On-the-field evaluation of an athlete with a head or neck injury. *Clin Sports Med* 2003;22(3):445-465.

15. Swartz EE, Boden BP, Courson RW, et al: National athletic trainers' association position statement: Acute management of the cervical spine-injured athlete. *J Athl Train* 2009;44(3):306-331.

    Recommendations on the acute management of players with possible cervical spine injury are made by the National Athletic Trainers Association. This includes airway management, transfer, and the controversial topic of removal of athletic protective equipment.

16. National Athletic Trainers' Association: Appropriate Care of the Spine Injured Athlete: Updated From 1998 document, 2015. Available at: http://www.nata.org/sites/default/files/Executive-Summary-Spine-Injury.pdf Accessed on October 20, 2015.

    The executive summary update of the 1998 document provides revised recommendations regarding management of athletes with cervical spine injuries.

17. Herzog RJ, Wiens JJ, Dillingham MF, Sontag MJ: Normal cervical spine morphometry and cervical spinal stenosis in asymptomatic professional football players. Plain film radiography, multiplanar computed tomography, and magnetic resonance imaging. *Spine (Phila Pa 1976)* 1991;16(6, Suppl):S178-S186.

18. Torg JS: Cervical spine injuries and the return to football. *Sports Health* 2009;1(5):376-383.

    A systematic review of the National Football Head and Neck Registry as well as relevant literature was performed to provide recommendations on return to football play after cervical spine injury. The major recommendation is that any player returning to football should be pain free, without neurological deficit, and with intact range of cervical spine motion.

19. Bracken MB: Steroids for acute spinal cord injury. *Cochrane Database Syst Rev* 2012;1:CD001046.

    Randomized controlled trials of steroid treatment in acute spinal cord injury are reviewed. Methylprednisolone is identified as the only pharmacologic therapy shown to have any benefit, and a call for more research is made.

20. Hurlbert RJ, Hadley MN, Walters BC, et al: Pharmacological therapy for acute spinal cord injury. *Neurosurgery* 2013;72(Suppl 2):93-105.

    The authors recommend against use of methylprednisolone or GM-1 ganglioside in the acute management of spinal cord injury based on a literature review. They cite the limited number of pharmacologic agents studied and the need for more research.

21. Schroeder GD, Kwon BK, Eck JC, Savage JW, Hsu WK, Patel AA: Survey of Cervical Spine Research Society members on the use of high-dose steroids for acute spinal cord injuries. *Spine (Phila Pa 1976)* 2014;39(12):971-977.

    Data from a questionnaire survey of the members of the Cervical Spine Research Society regarding use of methylprednisolone and trends over time are presented. The number of surgeons using high-dose steroids has decreased over time. Side effects including gastrointestinal bleeding, sepsis, and late presentation are reported as reasons for the decrease in use.

22. Castro FP Jr: Stingers, cervical cord neurapraxia, and stenosis. *Clin Sports Med* 2003;22(3):483-492.

23. Dietrich WD, Levi AD, Wang M, Green BA: Hypothermic treatment for acute spinal cord injury. *Neurotherapeutics* 2011;8(2):229-239.

    A review of the historical use, clinical studies, and pathophysiology of induced hypothermia in the treatment of spinal cord injury is presented. Additional research on detailed clinical protocols is needed.

24. Levi AD, Green BA, Wang MY, et al: Clinical application of modest hypothermia after spinal cord injury. *J Neurotrauma* 2009;26(3):407-415.

    A case series of 14 patients with spinal cord injury treated with hypothermia is presented. The authors detail their protocol and report an effective system for maintaining a consistent body temperature with the goal to provide background information for future studies.

25. Cappuccino A, Bisson LJ, Carpenter B, Marzo J, Dietrich WD III, Cappuccino H: The use of systemic hypothermia for the treatment of an acute cervical spinal cord injury in a professional football player. *Spine (Phila Pa 1976)* 2010;35(2):E57-E62.

    The authors discuss the case of an NFL football player who sustained a spinal cord injury and was treated with hypothermia. The patient rapidly recovered neurologic function.

26. Hansebout RR, Hansebout CR: Local cooling for traumatic spinal cord injury: Outcomes in 20 patients and review of the literature. *J Neurosurg Spine* 2014;20(5):550-561.

    Twenty patients with spinal cord injury undergoing a combination of surgical decompression, glucocorticoid administration, and hypothermia are discussed. The authors report improved results over standard treatments and call for more research in these areas of acute management.

27. Position statement: Otoole J, Wang M, Kaiser M. Hypothermia and human spinal cord injury: Position statement and evidence based recommendations from the AANS/CNS Joint Section on Disorders of the Spine and the AANS/CNS Joint Section on Trauma. Available at: http://www.spinesection.org/hypothermia.php.

This position statement reports insufficient evidence to recommend for the use of regional or systemic hypothermia in the management of spinal cord injury.

28. Levi AD, Casella G, Green BA, et al: Clinical outcomes using modest intravascular hypothermia after acute cervical spinal cord injury. *Neurosurgery* 2010;66(4):670-677.

A retrospective review of 14 patients with spinal cord injury managed with intravascular hypothermia was performed. Complication rates were comparable to those of patients with normothermia.

29. Lo TP Jr, Cho KS, Garg MS, et al: Systemic hypothermia improves histological and functional outcome after cervical spinal cord contusion in rats. *J Comp Neurol* 2009;514(5):433-448.

A rat model of spinal cord injury was used to study the effects of transient hypothermia. Histologic and functional results suggest that mild systemic hypothermia may slow tissue damage and reduce neurologic deficits.

Chapter 32

The Cervical Spine

William R. Miele, MD   Brian J. Neuman, MD   A. Jay Khanna, MD, MBA

Abstract

Injuries to the cervical spine constitute a range of conditions from acute traumatic injuries to chronic overuse and degenerative conditions. In addition to trauma to the cervical spine, several degenerative conditions present in athletes, and may be of substantial consequence to long-term function and career longevity. The sports physician will benefit from being familiar with examination of the neck and cervical spine, the neurologic examination, and presenting histories of common conditions, and imaging modalities and findings.

Keywords: spine; sports medicine; spinal injuries

Introduction

Of the approximately 10,000 cervical spinal cord injuries in the United States each year, 10% are sports related, with most of these injuries occurring in unsupervised or informal sporting events and activities.[1] More than 11,000 cervical spine injuries resulting from football injuries alone are evaluated in emergency departments

Dr. Khanna or an immediate family member serves as a paid consultant to Orthofix; has stock or stock options held in New Era Orthopaedics, Cortical Concepts, and Avitus Orthopaedics; has received nonincome support (such as equipment or services), commercially derived honoraria, or other non–research-related funding (such as paid travel) from Siemens Healthcare and Thieme Medical Publishers; and serves as a board member, owner, officer, or committee member of the American Academy of Orthopaedic Surgeons, the Johns Hopkins Center for Bioengineering, Innovation, and Design, and the North American Spine Society. Neither of the following authors nor any immediate family member has received anything of value from or has stock or stock options held in a commercial company or institution related directly or indirectly to the subject of this chapter: Dr. Miele and Dr. Neuman.

yearly.[2] Cervical spine injuries in the athlete can range from minor cervical strain to permanent quadriplegia.

Contact and collision sports are of the most concern for cervical spine injury. Of football players, 10% to 15% sustain a cervical spine injury at least once in their careers,[3] and injuries are seen at all levels of play. One study found that up to 32% of college football recruits had radiographs demonstrating prior cervical spinal injury or degenerative changes.[4] Even at the highest level of play, injuries are not infrequent. A study of spine injuries in professional football players demonstrated that spine injuries comprise 7% of all football injuries, with 44% of spine injuries occurring in the cervical spine.[5]

The occurrence of cervical spine injury in the contact athlete is of particular concern; one study of professional football players demonstrated that incurring a cervical disk herniation resulted in a 28% chance of the athlete never returning to play.[6] Another study demonstrated a substantial negative effect on the careers of athletes with cervical spine pathology. Football players who underwent preexisting cervical spinal surgery or conditions were less likely to be selected in a draft pick and had shorter careers.[7]

Despite the focus on cervical spine injuries in collision contact sports, such injuries occur across sporting events, including hockey, skiing, diving, track and field, cheerleading, baseball, lacrosse, and wrestling.[8] A review of the clinical features of some sports-related cervical spine conditions is important for the physician to make a clinical diagnosis. The potential for catastrophic cervical spinal cord injury or substantial time lost from participation threatens with any cervical spine injury.

History and Physical Examination

Acute Injuries

Prior to any contact sport event, preparations should be made to ensure that the basic equipment needed to support the evaluation, on-field treatment, and transport of injured players is on hand. Necessary supplies include tools for the removal of protective equipment, an emergency cervical collar, a spine board, and sandbags or another cervical immobilization system for helmeted players. First-aid supplies and airway access instruments should be readily available, and trained personnel should be present and able to properly coordinate an emergency situation and provide on-field evaluation and emergency treatment. Recent recommendations are available for the management of the cervical spine-injured athlete.[8]

Unstable or unconscious patients should be treated according to American Heart Association Basic Life Support guidelines. Attention should be given to maintaining immobilization of the cervical spine. Any player with a suspected cervical spine injury should undergo a physical and neurologic evaluation on the field before being moved or before the neck is manipulated. Following neurologic assessment, examination of the neck can include palpation of the posterior bony elements, palpation for muscular spasm, and assessment of pain with axial compression or isometric resistance. Active range of motion may be assessed if the player is able to move the neck without pain. Players with findings indicative of cervical spine injuries should not be moved, and the neck must be immobilized.

If the helmet of a player with a suspected cervical spine injury cannot be removed without moving the cervical spine, the helmet and shoulder pads should not be removed.[8,9] The facemask may need to be removed for airway access, and the helmet also may need to be removed if the facemask alone cannot be removed. Prompt transfer to a medical facility must be arranged for players who are unconscious or who have persistently altered mentation, neurologic symptoms in two or more extremities, substantial neck pain, or cervical spine bony tenderness with a concerning injury mechanism.

Players with acute injuries must be immobilized in a rigid cervical collar. The patient's neck is immobilized in the midline and neutral in flexion-extension. The collar must fit snugly, so that one or two fingers can be placed beneath the patient's closed jaw and the collar chin-piece. The neck should be fit into the collar via gentle straightening and distraction if necessary, but any deformity or malangulation of the neck should not be forcibly straightened. Players with normal mentation, no bony tenderness, full active range of motion, and no neurologic symptoms or substantial distracting injuries typically may be deemed free of cervical spine injury.

Determining the mechanism of injury and the amount of force sustained by the neck are ways of rapidly ascribing a level of risk. Most spinal cord injuries in sports result from axial loading injuries incurred during spear tackling in football, head collision into boards in hockey, and diving injuries. Important components of the patient's account include pain or neurologic symptoms at the time of injury and the duration or persistence of symptoms (Table 1). The history and physical examination must

Table 1

Key Patient History Factors in Evaluation of Spinal Cord Injury

Location and quality of pain in the neck

Location and quality of pain in the arms

Presence of numbness and/or paresthesia

Presence of limb weakness or functional disability

Pattern and timeline of the progression of symptoms

include a detailed neurologic assessment. Neurologic injuries follow reproducible patterns and typically can be differentiated on the basis of the history and physical examination.

Stingers and Burners

Stingers and burners are a form of cervical nerve root or brachial plexus injury. A football tackle conducted with the shoulder while the neck is laterally flexed is part of the typical history. This position places the brachial plexus contralateral to neck lateral flexion in maximal tension and maximally narrows the cervical neuroforamina ipsilateral to neck lateral flexion on impact. The result is brachial plexus stretch or cervical nerve root compression injury. A blow to the supraclavicular region also can result in brachial plexus injury. Stinging or burning pain in the shoulder radiates to the arm and hand. Sensory symptoms are transient and typically resolve after several minutes, although they can remit and recur in an episodic fashion. The sensory symptoms may precede weakness of the shoulder, arm, or hand that occurs up to 1 week later.[10] Stingers occur frequently in football, with more than 50% of college-level players reporting at least one occurrence.[11]

Nerve Root Injury

Cervical nerve root injuries are most often the result of root compression by intervertebral disk herniation, although any compressive lesion, including fracture fragments or dislocation, may result in radiculopathy. The most constant features of nerve root injury are radicular pain, paresthesia, and sensory loss. Motor examination in cervical nerve root injury may be normal or can demonstrate weakness in a myotomal distribution. The loss of a deep tendon reflex can reflect nerve root injury, and reflex loss may be noted even if full motor strength is present.

Transient Quadriplegia or Quadriparesis

Transient quadriplegia/paresis (transient cervical cord neuropraxia) is diagnosed when no acute fracture or ligamentous injury occurs and neurologic symptoms completely resolve. Symptoms may last from a few minutes to 36 hours, with the player demonstrating motor deficit in two or more extremities. Extremity heaviness, functional limitation, and paresthesia also can occur. Neurologic examination initially may demonstrate weakness, sensory deficit, and limb apraxia that improve to normal. One study demonstrated that more than 90% of players experiencing a single episode of transient quadriparesis had abnormal radiographs or MRI despite the complete resolution of symptoms,[12] and the probability of substantial structural pathology in players with this presentation must be considered. The syndrome is associated with cervical spinal stenosis.[13]

Spinal Cord Injury

Spinal cord injury most typically presents in one of three patterns: complete spinal cord injury, incomplete spinal cord injury, and central spinal cord injury. The level of injury is determined in reference to the most caudal spinal level with completely normal function. Complete spinal cord injury indicates no spinal cord function below the level of the injury. Incomplete spinal cord injury can be sensory incomplete or motor incomplete.

Central spinal cord injury is a form of incomplete injury that most often presents with neurologic deficit in the distal cervical levels (wrist and hand function), dysesthetic upper extremity pain, and sometimes a deficit in the lower extremities. Lower extremity deficit is present to a lesser degree than in the upper extremities. The mildest form of central cord syndrome presents with bilateral burning pain and tingling in the hands and is sometimes referred to as burning hand syndrome. It is important to clinically differentiate this condition from a stinger or burner. Central spinal cord injury is most often the result of hyperextension injuries.

The American Spinal Injury Association (ASIA) Impairment Scale worksheet is useful in determining the level and classification of spinal cord injury.[14] In complete spinal cord injury, reflexive movement may be present. The ability to withdraw to deep pain or pressure in the absence of voluntary movement commonly is not seen in spinal cord injury. Lower limb flexion to pain may have the appearance of limb withdrawal, and attention must be given to differentiating withdrawal from reflexive flexion. Spontaneous flexion movements can be seen in complete spinal cord injury and should not be mistaken for voluntary movement.

A deficit of sensation below a spinal level can help determine the level of injury. Somatic sensation is tested best with light touch and pin sensation. Touching the skin with an open safety pin is the easiest method of testing somatic sensation via the spinothalamic tracts. Sensory function of the dorsal column-medial lemniscus pathway is tested via joint position sense at the distal interphalangeal joints of the hand and the interphalangeal joint of the great toe, as well as via deep pressure and vibratory sense.

Although not generally part of an on-field examination, detailed reflex testing should be conducted after a patient with a suspected spinal cord injury arrives at the hospital. Involuntary reflexes to be tested include deep tendon reflexes, the abdominal cutaneous reflex, and the anal sphincter and bulbocavernosus reflexes. Myelopathy most classically results in deep tendon hyperreflexia below the level of injury. This is typically a late finding, however, and may be hypoactive or absent in acute spinal cord injury reflexes.

Subacute Presentations

The duration, severity, time and setting of onset, exacerbating or alleviating factors, functional impairment, and history of prior problems are all important factors. Any musculoskeletal and neurologic symptoms should be solicited.

Many comprehensive resources are available for reviewing the clinical examination and anatomy.[15,16] The surface anatomy is examined with the patient in a neutral position, seated or supine. Simple inspection will allow assessment of the neutral head position, the symmetry of the posture, and the gross appearance of the neck. With the patient in a neutral sitting or standing position, lateral viewing of the cervical spine should evidence a gentle lordosis, with the head centered over the trunk. Viewed anteriorly, the chin should be centered over the sternal notch, and symmetry of the sternocleidomastoid muscles should be apparent.

Active range of motion in the cervical spine is observed with the patient seated and should be full and pain free. Full flexion results in contact of the chin and chest, and full extension allows the patient to bring the face parallel to the horizontal. Normal rotation allows 60° to 90° of axial rotation in either direction. Lateral bending should allow the ear to touch the shrugged shoulder.

The posterior spinous elements from the inion to the upper thoracic spinous processes should be palpated, and any point tenderness, step-off deformities, malalignment of spinous processes, or spasm of the paraspinal musculature should be noted. The inion and C2 spinous process are easily palpable, C3-5 are small bifid processes that may not be individually palpable, and C6, C7, and T1 are typically prominent. The lateral masses and facet joints are not palpable individually, although tenderness lateral to the adjacent spinous process can corroborate facet pathology at that level. Anteriorly, the midline structures

5: Head and Spine

Table 2	
Clinical Signs in Evaluation of the Cervical Spinal Cord and Nerve Roots	
Spurling sign	The head is extended slightly and axially rotated to the affected side, and gentle axial compression is applied. The reproduction of radicular symptoms suggests neuroforaminal stenosis.
Lhermitte sign	The patient performs maximal active flexion of the neck and trunk. The resulting electrical, shooting, or other paresthesia symptoms down the spine or into the bilateral arms suggest cervical spinal stenosis.
Romberg sign	The patient is asked to stand with the feet together and the arms outstretched, with palms up. The patient then closes the eyes. An inability to maintain balance suggests dorsal column dysfunction. This test can help to identify myelopathy in patients with gait or balance problems.
Hoffman sign	The distal phalanx of the third digit is flicked at the distal interphalangeal joint. Thumb flexion in response is considered a positive sign and may indicate cervical myelopathy. The Hoffman sign demonstrates a hyperactive C8 deep tendon reflex, not a pathologic reflex.

that can be palpated are the hyoid bone, trachea, thyroid and cricoid cartilage, sternocleidomastoid muscles, carotid tubercle of C6, and carotid arteries. Neck strength can be tested in flexion, extension, lateral bending, and axial rotation. The sternocleidomastoid muscle rotates the neck in a contralateral direction.

Neurologic examination is conducted as described previously. Special maneuvers include the Spurling, Lhermitte, Romberg, and Hoffman tests (Table 2). Dermatomal sensation is tested via pin tip and light touch. Deep tendon reflexes may be tested at the C5, C6, C7, and C8 roots. Deep tendon reflexes in the lower extremities, plantar stimulation (the Babinski maneuver), and distal joint position sense in the lower extremities are mandatory tests in patients with symptoms that suggest cervical spinal stenosis. Symptoms of spinal cord injury may be apparent by patient history before physical signs of myelopathy appear. Subjective numbness, paresthesia, hand weakness, dyscoordination or functional limitation in the extremities, poor coordination, gait problems, or imbalance all can be seen with myelopathy. Unilateral or bilateral cervical radicular symptoms may be present.

Imaging

Plain Radiography

CT has virtually supplanted plain radiography for emergency assessment. When CT cannot be performed expediently, cross-table lateral radiographs are useful for assessing for cervical dislocations in unconscious patients or in those who cannot be examined for other reasons. Plain radiography can be useful as an initial study before the removal of protective equipment.

When plain radiographs are obtained as a primary radiographic evaluation, images should include AP, lateral, and AP open-mouth odontoid views. The swimmer view is used to assess the cervicothoracic junction. Oblique views are useful in assessing for foraminal stenosis or osteophytes. Cervical alignment is assessed best with neutral upright AP and lateral radiographs. Lateral projections are used to assess alignment; the anterior spinous line, posterior spinous line, spinolaminar line, and spinous process line are evaluated. Fracture, listhesis, segmental angulation, loss of lordosis, splaying of the spinous processes, or widened prevertebral soft tissue all can be signs of cervical spine injury. Lateral and open-mouth odontoid views allow assessment of the occiput-C1-C2 junction.

Lateral flexion-extension radiographs are the basis for excluding instability of the cervical spine. If confirmed to have normal static radiographs, no neck pain, no neurologic symptoms, and full active range of motion, the patient may have flexion-extension radiography. Patients with substantial distraction injuries should not have flexion-extension radiographs obtained and instead may need to remain in the cervical collar and/or undergo MRI. Full excursion in range of motion must be evident on radiographs for the examination to be valid.

Computed Tomography

Most CT protocols now include multiplanar reconstruction in the coronal and sagittal planes that readily allow the identification of fractures, malalignment, and dislocations. CT should be performed for any patient with abnormal plain radiographs following injury or when adequate plain radiographs cannot be obtained.

Magnetic Resonance Imaging

MRI can be performed to assess for injury to the nonosseous structures in the cervical spine. Image sequences to be reviewed include T2-weighted, short tau inversion

---

recovery (STIR), T1-weighted, and axial gradient echo/fast field echo (GRE/FFE) sequences. T2-weighted images offer the best contrast of cervical spinal structures and are the easiest to interpret. STIR sequences are the next most useful. STIR is optimized to highlight tissue edema and makes possible the identification of acute fractures, ligamentous disruption, or acute spinal cord contusions. T1-weighted images are of limited usefulness in emergency cervical spine imaging but have the best spatial resolution and can help to distinguish abnormal signal in areas that are equivocal on other imaging sequences. GRE/FFE axial images are high-contrast sequences allowing imaging of the spinal canal and neural elements in a manner comparable to CT myelography and are a useful adjunct.

Imaging in Cervical Collar Management

Acute cervical spine injuries are managed initially by immobilization in a rigid cervical collar. Patients with a radiographic injury, normal radiographs but substantial pain, or distracting injury are maintained in a cervical collar. In patients with no apparent injury who have been placed in a cervical collar, some broadly accepted criteria are available for determining which patients need imaging. The Canadian C-Spine Rule and (National Emergency X-Radiography Utilization Study) Low-Risk Criteria are two commonly used sets of guidelines.[17]

Collar clearance protocols for patients undergoing imaging vary by practice, and some controversy exists. In general, patients with normal plain radiographs or CT, no neck pain, full active range of motion, and no distracting injury can have the cervical collar removed. Patients with substantial distracting injury need to have either flexion-extension lateral radiographs or MRI confirmed as normal before the cervical collar is removed. In patients with normal plain radiographs or CT and neck pain without neurologic deficit, some protocols recommend immobilization in a collar followed by repeat clinical evaluation and flexion-extension radiographs after pain subsides and full and pain-free range of motion is achieved. Other protocols recommend MRI. MRI should be performed in all players with neurologic deficit or symptoms following a cervical spine injury.

Types of Cervical Spine Injuries

Occiput, C1, and C2 Injuries

Occipitocervical C1 and C2 injuries often present without neurologic injury. Axial loading injuries, high-energy blows to the head, or acceleration-deceleration injuries are the most common mechanisms of injury. Imaging for high-energy cervical injuries should include multiplanar

reconstruction CT and MRI. Some practitioners recommend vascular imaging for all players presenting with C1 or C2 fractures. Treatment algorithms for C2 fractures may involve immobilization in a cervical collar, capital fixation via halo vest, or surgical fixation.

Occipital condyle fractures occur via axial loading of the skull onto the C1 lateral mass, with a resulting fracture of the condyle. They also can occur from lateral hyperflexion. Occipito-atlantal dissociation typically is seen only in the setting of high-energy injuries and results from disruption of the alar ligaments and tectorial membrane. These injuries can be fatal in adults; nonfatal iterations need to be considered highly unstable. Two methods are available for assessing for occipitoatlantal dissociation on radiographs: the Powers ratio, which identifies only anterior subluxation, and the basion-axial interval/basion-dens interval (BAI/BDI) method.

Atlantoaxial instability may be demonstrated by a widened atlanto-dens interval (ADI) or dynamic changes to ADI on flexion-extension radiographs. ADI is less than 3 mm in the healthy adult male, less than 2.5 mm in the healthy adult female, and less than 5 mm in children age 15 years or younger.

C1 fractures most typically result from axial loading injuries, resulting in a burst fracture (Jefferson fracture), with fragments moving outward and away from the spinal canal (Figure 1, A). Axial T2-weighted images on MRI assess the integrity of the transverse/cruciate ligament. Rupture of the transverse ligament is suggested by overhang of the C1 lateral masses on C2 totaling more than 7 mm on AP radiographs (Figure 1, B).

Odontoid fractures are the most common type of C2 fractures, accounting for one-half of all C2 fractures. The mechanism of injury is hyperflexion or hyperextension (Figure 1, C through E). Hangman fracture is a hyperextension and axial loading injury resulting in bilateral C2 pars fractures (traumatic spondylolisthesis). It is most commonly seen in diving injuries in the sports setting.

Subaxial Cervical Spine Injuries

More than one-half of subaxial cervical spine injuries are hyperflexion injuries. The force is greatest at C4-7 in hyperflexion, and injury most commonly occurs at C5-6. Hyperflexion injuries can result in end plate or compression fractures, burst fractures, facet dislocation, and injury to the posterior ligaments.

A compression fracture is an anterior wedge fracture of the vertebral body. It is considered to be a stable injury if no evidence exists of severe kyphotic angulation, canal compromise, or associated severe ligamentous disruption. Flexion teardrop fracture is a fracture through the anterior vertebral body, with an anterior-superior fracture

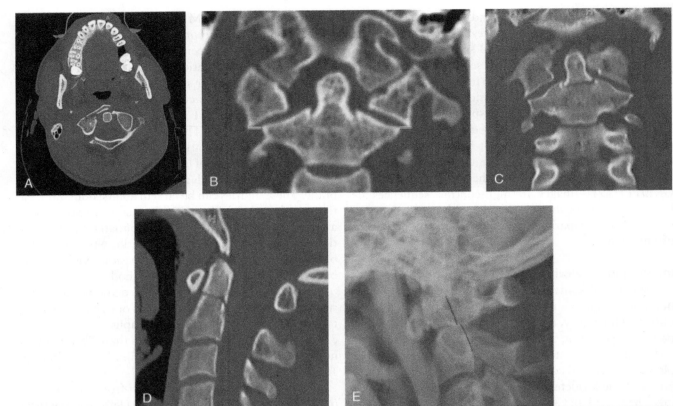

Figure 1 Images show fractures of C1 and C2. **A**, An axial CT scan displays a Jefferson fracture of C1 in a 22-year-old man following an axial loading injury during a helmeted fall. Because of the ring structure of the C1 vertebra, fracture is obligatory at two or more sites. **B**, Coronal CT reconstruction of a Jefferson fracture. Combined lateral mass overhang (red lines) of greater than 7 mm is thought to indicate rupture of the transverse ligament. Coronal (**C**) and sagittal CT reconstruction (**D**) show a type II fracture of the dens. **E**, Follow-up lateral radiograph shows slight anterior displacement that was not evident on the initial CT. The patient was treated with odontoid fixation via an anteriorly placed cannulated lag screw and postoperative immobilization in a cervical collar for treatment of an associated Jefferson fracture. (Panel **B** reproduced with permission from Radcliffe KE, Sonagli MA, Rodrigues LM, Sidhu ES, Albert TJ, Vaccaro R: Does C1 fracture displacement correlate with transverse ligament integrity? *Orthop Surg* 2013;5:94-99.)

fragment, often associated with posterior displacement of the posterior aspect of the vertebral body into the spinal canal and an interspinous ligament tear (Figure 2, **A** and **B**). A facet capsule injury can be unilateral or bilateral. On lateral radiographs, the facet joint should be no more than 2 mm wide and should align evenly with the remaining facet joints. Distraction of a facet, or perched facet, is indicative of joint dislocation (Figure 2, **C**) and can be associated with fractures or discoligamentous injury. Locked facet dislocation, or jumped facet, occurs when the inferior articular process is pulled anteriorly and ventrally over the superior articulating process of the level below. It can be unilateral or bilateral. A high rate of cervical spinal cord injury occurs in bilateral locked facet dislocation, with 30% of patients presenting with complete spinal cord injury[18] (Figure 2, **D**).

Extension injuries can occur with direct facial trauma.

Ligamentous injury of the anterior longitudinal ligament, intervertebral disk injury, pedicle/pillar fractures, spinous process fractures, or facet fractures all can be seen in hyperextension injuries. Clay shoveler's fracture is a fracture of the spinous process tip. It most commonly occurs in the cervical spine at spinous process C6 or C7 and can occur in the upper thoracic spine (Figure 2, **E**). Spinous process apophysitis is seen at prominent spinous processes C6 or C7 that can appear as calcifications of supraspinatus ligaments or small fracture fragments of the spinous process tip, and indicates repetitive microtrauma (Figure 2, **F** and **G**).

Axial loading injuries most typically result in subaxial cervical injury in combination with another force vector. Flexion-compression injury is seen in diving injuries, spear tackling, or other instances of uncontrolled impact to the top of the head. Dislocations in the subaxial

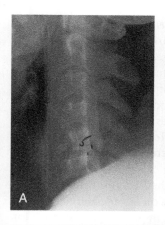
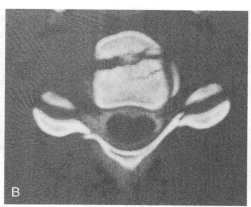
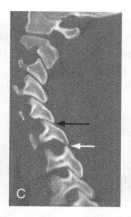
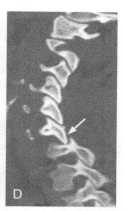

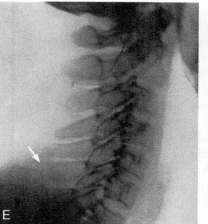
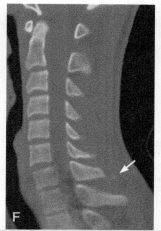
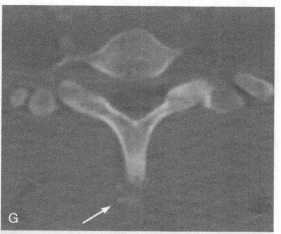

Figure 2 Images show subaxial cervical spine injuries. **A,** Lateral cervical radiograph demonstrates a flexion teardrop fracture of C5. A coronally oriented fracture is seen through the vertebral body, and posterior displacement of the dorsal fracture fragment also is seen. **B,** Axial CT scan demonstrates the same vertebral body fracture and shows widened facet joints. **C,** Sagittal CT reconstruction shows a facet capsule injury resulting in uncovering of the C6 articular surface secondary to anterior subluxation of the C5 facet (black arrow) and dislocation at C6-7 resulting in a perched facet (white arrow). **D,** Sagittal CT reconstruction depicts anterior translation of a dislocated facet, resulting in a locked dislocation or jumped facet (arrow). **E,** A lateral radiograph shows a fracture of the C6 spinous process, or clay shoveler's fracture (arrow), which was first described as a result of avulsion by violent paraspinal muscle contraction. Fractures of this type are seen in hyperextension injury. Sagittal reconstruction CT (**F**) and axial CT (**G**) demonstrate calcifications superficial to the C7 spinous process tip (arrows) in an 18-year-old man with a cervical strain injury. (Panels **A** and **B** reproduced with permission from Fisher CG, Dvorak MFS, Leith J, Wing P: Comparison of outcomes for lower cervical flexion teardrop fractures managed with halo thoracic vest versus anterior corpectomy and plating. *Spine (Phila Pa 1976)* 2002;27:160-166. Panels **C** and **D** reproduced with permission from Raniga SB, Menon V, Al Muzahmi KS, Butt S: MDCT of acute subaxial cervical spine trauma: A mechanism based approach. *Insights Imaging* 2014;5:321-338. Panel **E** reproduced with permission from McKellar Hall RD: Clay-shoveler's fracture. *J Bone Joint Surg Am* 1940;22[1]:63-75.)

cervical spine are most commonly the result of flexion combined with axial loading; diving injury is a classic mechanism of injury.

Ligamentous Injury

The anterior and posterior longitudinal ligaments, interspinous ligaments, and facet capsules provide flexibility and structural integrity to the subaxial cervical spine, and injury to one or more of these structures can compromise the stability of the cervical spine. Ligamentous injury is diagnosed when radiographs or CT demonstrates signs of ligamentous instability, or when direct imaging of ligamentous disruption or edema is evident on MRI (**Figure 3**). Injuries of this type vary in severity from minor (associated with no serious risk of late spinal instability or neurologic injury) to highly unstable (requiring surgical fixation). For this reason, the injured player with normal static plain radiographs or CT should not be presumed to be without a destabilizing injury.

Spinal Stenosis

Spinal stenosis can take the form of congenital stenosis or developmental (degenerative) spinal stenosis in the athlete. The relationship between spinal stenosis and cervical spinal cord injury has been a topic of study because an increased incidence of spinal stenosis has been observed in players with transient quadriparesis or neurologic injury.[12]

On lateral radiographs, the ratio of the spinal canal to the AP diameter of the vertebral body can be used as an indicator of congenital spinal stenosis (Figure 4, A). A Torg ratio less than 0.8 indicates congenital spinal stenosis.[19] Problems arise in using the Torg ratio to define spinal stenosis because a Torg ratio less than 0.8 has been shown to have low predictive value for future spinal cord injury.[13] Another study demonstrated that 49% of professional football players had a Torg ratio less than 0.8, but only 13% had stenosis on advanced imaging.[20] A diagnosis of spinal stenosis has important implications for return to play following neurologic injuries or transient quadriparesis.[12,13,21-23] MRI is the test of choice to evaluate for true spinal stenosis because spinal canal diameter with respect to the spinal cord is the true determinant of spinal stenosis. Contact of the structural spinal tissues with the surface of the spinal cord is thought to be the best indicator of functional spinal stenosis (Figure 4, B and C).

Congenital Anomalies

Congenital anomalies of the cervical spine may be of interest to the sports physician in screening for clearance or return to play, or can be seen as incidental findings. Some types of Klippel-Feil anomalies, os odontoideum,

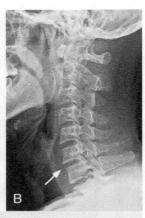

Figure 3 Images show cervical ligamentous injury and traumatic subluxation. **A**, Short T1 inversion recovery T2-weighted sagittal MRI demonstrates hyperintensity of the interspinous ligaments of C4-5, C5-6, and C6-7 (arrow) in a 20-year-old man following an injury sustained during downhill skiing. **B**, Lateral radiograph shows a C7 superior articular process fracture and anterolisthesis of C6 on C7 (arrow).

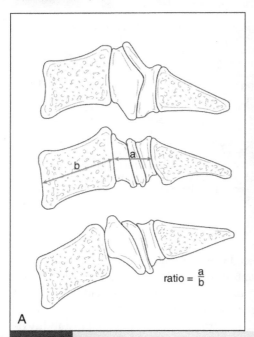
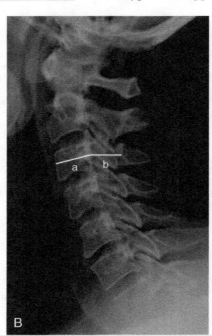
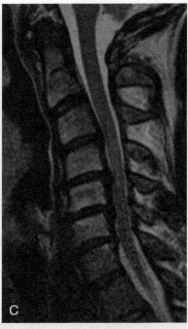

ratio = $\frac{a}{b}$

Figure 4 Images of the Torg ratio. **A**, Illustration depicts the Torg ratio, defined as the ratio of the spinal canal AP diameter (a) to the vertebral body AP diameter (b). A Torg ratio less than 0.8 is considered radiographic evidence of congenital or developmental spinal stenosis. **B**, Lateral radiograph demonstrates the measurements of the vertebral body and the spinal canal AP diameter at C3. **C**, Sagittal T2-weighted magnetic resonance image demonstrates a congenitally narrow spinal canal, hypertrophy of the posterior longitudinal ligament, and a central disk bulge at C3-4 to C6-7.

congenital assimilation of the atlas, and other conditions can be associated with an increased risk of spinal cord injury to contact athletes, and these players may be advised against engaging in contact sports. A full discussion of congenital anomalies of the cervical spine and recommendations on suitability for sports participation were proposed in 1997 and reviewed in 2002.[21,23]

Cervical Strain and Sprain

Sports-related cervical sprain and strain account for a substantial portion of all neck injuries. A review of epidemiologic data found that 24% of all cervical sprain or strain injuries seen in the emergency department, excluding those from automobile accidents, resulted from sports injuries.[24] Sprain and strain injuries are soft-tissue injuries, and the presenting history is of axial neck pain, stiffness, or painful range of motion following neck injury.

Cervical strain is defined as a stretch injury to the muscles and tendons of the neck without injury to the vertebrae or ligaments. CT and MRI are normal in cervical strain. Plain radiographs may demonstrate a loss of cervical lordosis, which indicates muscular spasm. The treatment of acute cervical strain consists of immobilization in a cervical collar. Patients typically are immobilized for 2 weeks or until they are pain free. Removal of the cervical collar is considered when the patient has no neck pain and has pain-free, full, active range of motion. Lateral flexion-extension radiographs need to be obtained to ensure that no instability is present before discontinuing the cervical collar.

Cervical sprain is a term describing nondestabilizing cervical ligamentous injury. Minor ligamentous injuries can manifest clinically only as axial neck pain, with MRI demonstrating minor tears or edema of one or more ligaments. Acute ligamentous injury is demonstrated best by focal STIR sequence hyperintensity on MRI. MRI with STIR sequences can be performed within 72 hours of injury to evaluate for ligamentous injury. After 72 hours, MRI loses sensitivity for ligamentous edema.

For cervical strain injuries, cervical sprains should be managed initially via immobilization in a cervical collar. The cervical collar can be removed when axial neck pain is resolved and the patient has pain-free, full, active range of motion. Lateral flexion-extension radiographs are obtained at that time. Dynamic instability may warrant continued rigid immobilization or surgical stabilization.

Severe ligamentous injuries also may be symptomatic only as axial neck pain, but imaging may show signs of substantial ligamentous disruption, listhesis, malangulation, or injury to multiple ligaments. Severe cervical spinal ligamentous injury typically is treated via immobilization in a rigid cervical collar for 6 or more weeks, and destabilizing injuries may require surgical stabilization. Severe or destabilizing ligamentous injury generally is not considered a cervical sprain.

Because athletes with cervical strains and sprains may not present acutely, management of the athlete presenting with a subacute injury suggestive of cervical strain or sprain typically should be the same as for those presenting acutely. If the player has pain that prevents normal active flexion and extension, then immobilization in a rigid cervical collar is indicated. Plain radiographs should be obtained, and for mild instances without limitation of full active range of motion, lateral flexion-extension radiographs are obtained to exclude instability. Athletes with spinal instability or abnormal imaging or those unable to undergo radiographic assessment for instability are immobilized in a cervical collar. Lateral flexion-extension radiographs can be performed after pain has resolved and the patient can participate in full, active range of motion.

In the absence of instability, no cervical collar is needed, although immobilization may provide symptomatic relief. Treatment consists of withdrawal from play, NSAIDs, and ice application.

Cervical Disk Herniation

Athletes may be at increased risk for cervical disk degeneration, and the implication of this diagnosis for the athlete is important.[25] One review demonstrated that cervical disk herniation resulted in an average of 85 days lost from play in professional football players, a figure superseded only by fractures of the cervical or thoracic spine.[5] Although the surgical management of cervical disk herniation demonstrates excellent functional results in the general population, the diagnosis can result in career limitation for elite athletes.

Symptomatic disk herniation results in one of several manifestations: neck pain, radiculopathy, or myelopathy. Often, the initial, or only, reports are axial neck pain and interscapular pain, which may precede the development of radicular symptoms. Two common patterns of injury can result in symptomatic disk herniation: acute disk herniation and chronic "hard disk" or disk-osteophyte complex. Acute disk herniation may result in a herniated nucleus pulposus fragment compressing the exiting cervical nerve root or spinal canal stenosis. Chronic or repetitive injury may result in the development of osteophytes and disk-osteophyte complex, which leads to neuroforaminal stenosis and chronic or recurrent radicular symptoms (Figure 5, A through C). Patients with radicular or myelopathic symptoms are evaluated best with MRI. Large or central disk herniation can result in stenosis of the spinal canal,

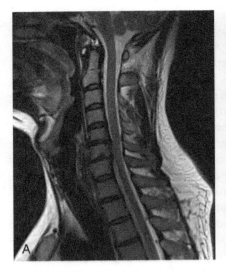
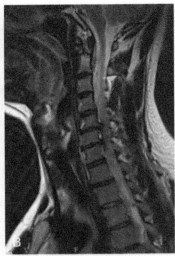
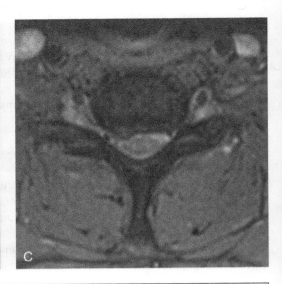

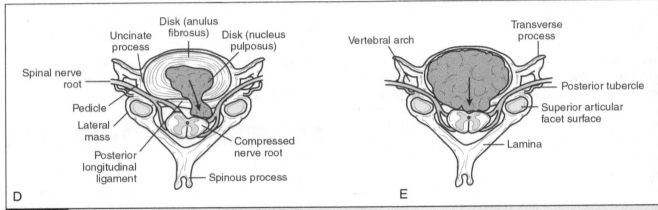

Figure 5 Images show cervical disk herniation. **A,** Midline T2-weighted magnetic resonance image demonstrates C5-6 and C6-7 disk herniations in a 29-year-old man who plays basketball. **B,** Paramedian image shows prominent foraminal disk bulges. **C,** Axial T2-weighted image at C6-7 demonstrates a right paramedian disk herniation abutting the spinal cord and narrowing the right C6-7 neuroforamen. Axial illustrations (**D** and **E**) show the difference between paramedian disc herniation abutting a nerve root, and central disk herniation compressing the spinal cord. A left posterolateral disk protrusion (**D,** arrow) results in mild deformity of the cord and compression of the exiting nerve root. Central canal stenosis and cord impingement secondary to a large central disk protrusion (**E,** arrow) is shown.

compression of the spinal cord, and symptoms of myelopathy. In the most extreme instances, a large traumatic cervical disk herniation can result in acute spinal cord injury (Figure 5, D and E).

The management of cervical disk herniation varies according to its presentation. Patients with radicular symptoms alone and all motor functional groups greater than 3/5 in strength can initially be treated nonsurgically. Oral corticosteroids, NSAIDs, and oral analgesics can help relieve radicular pain. Most cases of acute cervical radiculopathy resolve with nonsurgical management. Epidural or transforaminal steroid injections may provide relief of radicular pain if oral medications are ineffective. For intractable symptoms, surgery may be recommended.

In patients with a severe motor deficit on presentation, immediate surgery can facilitate motor recovery. Patients with motor power of 2/5 or less in the distribution of the affected nerve should undergo urgent surgery. The surgical treatment of paramedian cervical disk herniation resulting in radiculopathy consists only of posterior cervical laminoforaminotomy, anterior cervical diskectomy and fusion (ACDF), or total disk arthroplasty (TDA). Currently, TDA is not considered a treatment option for athletes planning a return to contact sports.

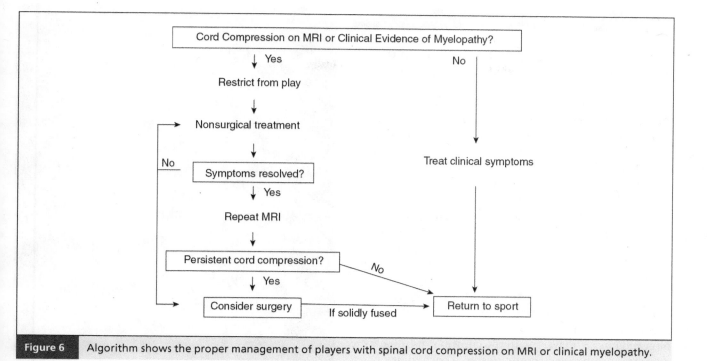

Figure 6 Algorithm shows the proper management of players with spinal cord compression on MRI or clinical myelopathy.

Video 32.1: Anterior Interbody Fusion in Cervical Disc Herniation. Cesare Faldini, MD; Alessandro Gasbarrini, MD; Mohammadreza Chehrassan, MD; Maria Teresa Miscione, MD; Francesco Arci, MD; Michele d'Amato, MD; Luca Boriani, MD; Stefano Boriani, MD; and Sandro Giannini, MD (18 min)

Some controversy exists in the current management of cervical radiculopathy in professional athletes over non-surgical versus surgical treatment of players with chronic or recurrent cervical radicular symptoms. In one study, National Football League (NFL) players returning to play after undergoing surgery for one-level disk herniation did not have a shortened career or reduction in performance level.[6] Furthermore, 72% of players undergoing surgery returned to play, compared with 46% of players treated nonsurgically. A subsequent study of 15 professional football players and wrestlers undergoing ACDF for radicular and myelopathic symptoms demonstrated that all players were approved for return to play following surgery, with 13 players eventually returning to professional play at an average of 6 months following surgery.[26] In a study of 16 NFL players treated for cervical disk herniation, all players treated nonsurgically for radiculopathy returned to play.[27] Return to play should be considered after neck pain has resolved and pain-free, full, active range of motion is present. Players with persistent neck pain, limited range of motion, radicular symptoms, myelopathy, or radiographic spinal cord compression should not return to play. Decisions regarding return to play following surgery are controversial, but it is generally believed that players with one-level or two-level cervical fusions can return to play after demonstrating a solid arthrodesis on CT.

Cervical disk herniation can have a substantial effect on athletes in noncontact sports. A review of cervical disk herniation in 11 Major League Baseball pitchers demonstrated substantial morbidity.[25] Seven players underwent ACDF and one player underwent TDA. Of eight players undergoing surgery, seven returned to play, and one of the three treated nonsurgically returned to play. The mean time for return to play for the eight players who did so was 11.6 months. Career longevity extended to a mean of 63 games pitched over a mean of 3.7 years, figures interpreted as successful management.

Players presenting with spinal cord compression may require urgent or emergent surgery. Acute disk herniation with myelopathy is managed surgically for decompression of the spinal cord. Substantial radiographic cord impingement or T2-weighted/STIR signal change within the spinal cord on MRI may warrant surgical treatment even in asymptomatic patients. An algorithm has been proposed for the management of myelopathy from cervical disk herniation in NFL athletes[27] (Figure 6).

Spear Tackler Spine

Spear tackling (or spearing) refers to the use of the helmet to make initial contact while tackling in American football. Spear tackling was made illegal by a rule change in 1976 after the recognition of a substantially higher incidence of cervical spine injuries in players initiating a tackle with the helmet. The incidence of cervical spine fractures and quadriplegia dropped appreciably in high school and college football between 1976 and 1978.[28,29]

The natural flexibility of the cervical spine protects the structural components from fracture or dislocation through dissipation of force. Strong supporting cervical paraspinal muscles and the intervertebral disks allow controlled movement and help to absorb and dissipate applied forces. The mechanism of spear tackling places the cervical spine in slight flexion, and the nonlordotic cervical spine is unprotected from failure during the application of axial loading forces. A 1993 study popularized the term "spear tackler spine" to describe the clinical entity and its biomechanics.[22] Players with the clinical syndrome were considered to be predisposed to spinal cord injury when subjected to axial loading forces. The recommendation that players meeting the criteria for spear tackler spine be precluded from further participation in contact sports is widely accepted.[22,23]

Three radiographic features define spear tackler spine: cervical spinal stenosis, the loss of lordosis or kyphosis, and imaging findings consistent with prior cervical spine injury. All three findings in conjunction with a prior history of engaging in spear tackling qualify a player for this diagnosis (Figure 7).

Cervical Spinal Stenosis

Congenital or posttraumatic developmental spinal stenosis was present in all players in the initial series.[22] In one study of 23 players experiencing an episode of transient quadriparesis, all were shown to have a Torg ratio of less than 0.8.[19] A normal Torg ratio does not exclude spinal stenosis. MRI is the imaging modality of choice for the diagnosis of spinal stenosis and is more useful than plain radiographs in players presenting with neurologic symptoms.

Loss of Lordosis or Kyphosis

Players in the study on spear tackler spine all demonstrated persistent abnormal straightening of the cervical spine on neutral upright lateral cervical radiographs.[22] Players with an abnormal loss of lordosis were categorized as having permanent loss of lordosis, presumably secondary to repetitive trauma, or reversible loss of lordosis. Either finding was considered reason to preclude

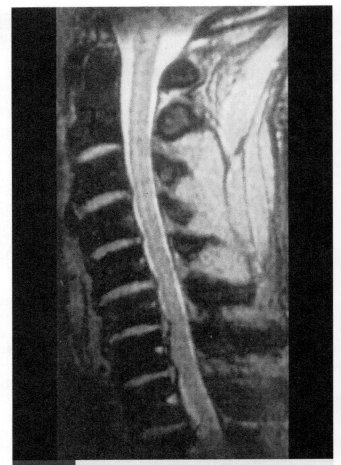

Figure 7 Sagittal MRI demonstrates the features of spear tackler spine in a 25-year-old man who plays professional football following an episode of transient quadriparesis. Congenital or developmental cervical stenosis, the loss of cervical lordosis, and findings of prior cervical spinal injury are the three characteristic radiographic findings in spear tackler spine. Having the three radiographic features precludes play in contact sports by current guidelines. (Reproduced with permission from Torg JS, Ramsey-Mermen JA: Suggested management guidelines for participation in collision activities with congenital, developmental, or postinjury lesions involving the cervical spine. *Med Sci Sports Exercise* 1997;29:256-272.)

involvement in contact sports, although a return of lordotic alignment in reversible cases was thought to warrant reassessment.

Posttraumatic Findings on Radiographic Studies

Prior compression fractures, limbus vertebrae, intervertebral disk herniation, ligamentous laxity, subluxation, and other radiographic findings consistent with prior cervical spine trauma were present on imaging studies. The

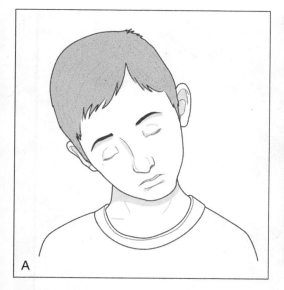

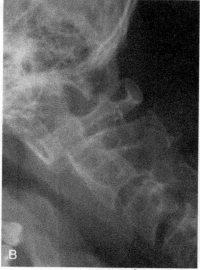

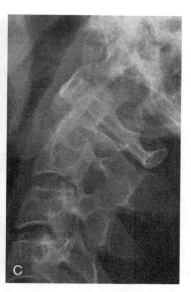

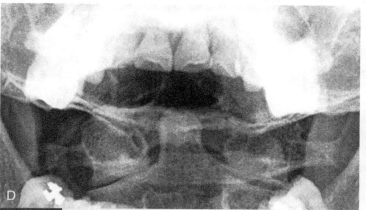

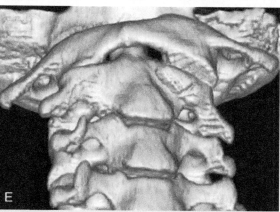

Figure 8 Images depict atlanto axial rotatory subluxation. **A,** Illustration shows the cock robin torticollis position. The head is held in approximately 20° of lateral flexion and 20° of contralateral rotation. The patient can actively correct the deformity to neutral but cannot turn the head beyond neutral to the contralateral direction. **B** and **C,** Lateral flexion and extension radiographs, respectively, demonstrate a fixed widened atlanto-dens interval in a 34-year-old man after a fall. **D,** AP open-mouth odontoid view demonstrates a skewed dens-C2 lateral mass relationship, a finding that can be easily missed on the AP open-mouth view. **E,** Three-dimensional CT reformat demonstrates rotation of C1 about the right C1-2 articulation, with fixed subluxation of the C1 lateral mass anterior to the C2 lateral mass. A fracture of the left C2 superior articular surface is seen. (Panels **B, C, D,** and **E** reproduced with permission from Kim YS, Lee JK, Moon SJ, Kim SH: et al: Posttraumatic atlantoaxial rotatory fixation in an adult. *Spine (Phila PA 1976)* 2007;32:E682-E687.)

clinical presentation of players in the original description of injury was in all 15 cases, either for "neck injury" or for neurapraxia localizing to the cervical spinal cord, cervical nerve roots, or brachial plexus.[22]

Atlantoaxial Rotatory Subluxation

Atlantoaxial rotatory subluxation (AARS), also called atlantoaxial rotatory dislocation or atlantoaxial rotatory fixation, is an uncommon injury following cervical spine trauma. The condition occurs most commonly in children. A recent review of isolated AARS in adults identified the condition as case reportable, with only 14 cases

appearing in the literature.[30,31] Few data in the sports literature address the condition. Several reports describe AARS occurring following rugby injuries and one following a diving injury.[31] Current guidelines denote the condition as an absolute contraindication to return to contact sports.[21,23]

People with syndromes of ligamentous or connective tissue laxity are thought to be at increased risk. In children, AARS can occur after minor trauma. In one series, patients had a mean age of 20 years and presented most often following upper respiratory infection or major or minor trauma.[32] The classic presentation is torticollis, with the head held approximately 20° in lateral bending

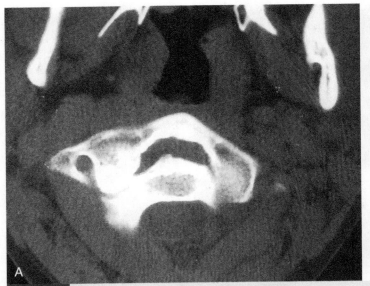
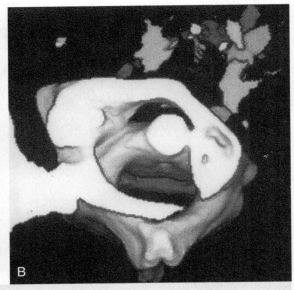

Figure 9 **A,** Axial CT image shows axial rotation and greater than 5 mm anterior subluxation of C1 on C2 in a 9-year-old boy with neck pain and torticollis. **B,** Three-dimensional CT reconstruction shows rotatory displacement of C1 on C2 and in situ fusion in the rotated position. This CT was obtained 14 months following the onset of symptoms, highlighting the likelihood of delay in the diagnosis of children with atlantoaxial rotatory subluxation. (Reproduced with permission from Roche CJ, O'Malley M, Dorgan JC, Larty HM: A pictorial review of atlanto-axial rotatory fixation: Key points for the radiologist. *Clin Radiol* 2001;56:947-958.)

and 20° in contralateral axial rotation with slight flexion, the "cock robin" position (Figure 8, A). Sternocleidomastoid muscle spasm may be present, and patients are able to voluntarily correct their deformity but cannot move their head beyond neutral. In one series, the average delay in diagnosis was 11.6 months. Plain radiographs detected only six of eight cases in another series of patients with radiographs followed by CT.[33] The wide availability of multiplanar reconstruction CT may improve the sensitivity (Figure 8, B through E and Figure 9).

The treatment algorithms for AARS are controversial, and it should be considered that pediatric AARS following only minor trauma and AARS in skeletally mature athletes from higher energy injuries are different entities. In unilateral anterior subluxation without injury to the transverse ligament or another associated fracture or ligament injury, traction reduction and immobilization in a cervical collar comprise a commonly recommended treatment.[31,32,34-36] Controversy exists over whether reduction is necessary in pediatric cases, and current evidence is limited to small case series and expert opinion.[34] Immobilization in a halo vest or surgical fixation may be indicated in recurrent cases. In one series of seven pediatric patients, six patients with recurrent AARS eventually required surgical fixation.[35] Recurrence was seen only in patients first presenting with symptoms of 3 weeks' duration.

In the athlete presenting acutely with neck injury and AARS, the management is the same as that for an unstable cervical spine injury. Halter traction or Gardner-Wells traction can be applied to help reduce the subluxation in the context of any associated fractures or ligamentous injury. Immobilization in a halo vest or surgical fixation may be necessary. Neurologic deficit, transverse ligament rupture, and fractures are indications for surgical reduction and fixation. Substantial spinal canal stenosis or neural element compression may require emergent surgical reduction or decompression and surgical fixation. C1-2 fusion is considered an absolute contraindication to return to sports in commonly used guidelines.[23]

Summary

Cervical spine injuries in the athlete range in severity from minor transient injuries to catastrophic injuries with permanent neurologic disability. A thorough understanding of the types of injuries, presenting history and examination findings, and radiographic findings is vital for the sports physician to treat and counsel players with injuries and disorders of the cervical spine. Minor injuries and chronic conditions can result in substantial time away from play, and can be associated with the risk of further injury to the sports participant. Differentiating injuries and conditions that are self-limiting from those necessitating referral to a spine specialist is important in the management of both injuries and chronic conditions.

Available evidence for the management of spine injuries as relevant to professional and high-performing athletes is mostly limited to observational studies.

Key Study Points

- A complete neurologic examination is mandatory in players with suspected cervical spine injuries. Players with abnormal neurologic examination results or histories that suggest neurologic involvement are evaluated best with MRI.

- Understanding the differential diagnosis of cervical spinal injuries and the localization of neurologic injury via history taking and physical examination is paramount for the sports medicine provider.

- Axial loading and hyperflexion injuries are the most common causes of sports-related catastrophic cervical spine injuries. Uncontrolled impact to the top of the head in recreational sports accounts for most sports-related spinal cord injuries.

- Cervical sprains and strains are stretch injuries to the musculotendinous units or ligaments of the cervical spine. Sprains and strains typically do not have major late consequences, but players should be withdrawn from play until the resolution of neck pain and the return of full, active, pain-free range of motion.

- Patients with cervical disk herniation can present with neck pain, radiculopathy, or myelopathy. The diagnosis has a substantial effect on players and results in a mean time away from play of 85 days. Radiculopathy may be managed symptomatically or surgically. Myelopathy or radiographic spinal cord compression may require surgical treatment.

- Spear tackler spine is defined as the concomitant occurrence of cervical spinal stenosis, the loss of cervical spinal lordosis or development of cervical kyphosis, and radiographic findings consistent with prior cervical spinal trauma. Players with this condition are at increased risk of spinal cord injury and may not participate in contact sports.

- AARS is an uncommon injury in adults and can present in children following seemingly minor trauma. Children with spontaneous torticollis or players with acute torticollis following sports injury should be evaluated for AARS.

Annotated References

1. Maroon JC, Bailes JE: Athletes with cervical spine injury. *Spine (Phila Pa 1976)* 1996;21(19):2294-2299.

2. Rihn JA, Anderson DT, Lamb K, et al: Cervical spine injuries in American football. *Sports Med* 2009;39(9):697-708.

   This review discusses root/brachial plexus neuropraxia, cervical cord neurapraxia, catastrophic neurologic injury, early evaluation and management, and return to play in the context of American football.

3. Thomas BE, McCullen GM, Yuan HA: Cervical spine injuries in football players. *J Am Acad Orthop Surg* 1999;7(5):338-347.

4. Albright JP, Moses JM, Feldick HG, Dolan KD, Burmeister LF: Nonfatal cervical spine injuries in interscholastic football. *JAMA* 1976;236(11):1243-1245.   5. Mall NA, Buchowski J, Zebala L, Brophy RH, Wright RW, Matava MJ: Spine and axial skeleton injuries in the National Football League. *Am J Sports Med* 2012;40(8):1755-1761.

   This epidemiologic study reviews 11 years of data on injuries to the spinal and axial skeleton sustained by NFL players. Spine injuries resulted in a mean of 25.7 days lost from play per injury, and cervical disk herniation resulted in a mean of 85 days lost per injury. Level of evidence: II-C.

5. Mall NA, Buchowski J, Zebala L, Brophy RH, Wright RW, Matava MJ: Spine and axial skeleton injuries in the National Football League. *Am J Sports Med* 2012;40(8):1755-1761.

   This epidemiologic study reviews 11 years of data on injuries to the spinal and axial skeleton sustained by NFL players. Spine injuries resulted in a mean of 25.7 days lost from play per injury, and cervical disk herniation resulted in a mean of 85 days lost per injury. Level of evidence: II-C.

6. Hsu WK: Outcomes following nonoperative and operative treatment for cervical disc herniations in National Football League athletes. *Spine (Phila Pa 1976)* 2011;36(10):800-805.

   This retrospective cohort study used newspaper archives and team databases to identify NFL players in whom cervical disk herniations had been diagnosed. Of all players, 72% returned to play following surgery for disc herniation compared with 46% of those managed nonsurgically. Level of evidence: IV.

7. Schroeder GD, Lynch TS, Gibbs DB, et al: The impact of a cervical spine diagnosis on the careers of National Football League athletes. *Spine (Phila Pa 1976)* 2014;39(12):947-952. chttp://dx.doi.ocg/10.1097/BRS.0000000000000321

   This case-controlled cohort study compared the careers of entering NFL players with a diagnosis of prior cervical spinal injury or pathology with matched controls. Players with the cervical spine diagnosis were less likely to be drafted onto a team and had shorter careers. Level of evidence: III-B.

8. Swartz EE, Boden BP, Courson RW, et al: National athletic trainers' association position statement: Acute management of the cervical spine-injured athlete. *J Athl Train* 2009;44(3):306-331.

This position statement from the NATA outlines preparation for events, necessary training for personnel, and on-field evaluation and management algorithms. This is an in-depth review and treatment of available evidence for the early management of sports players with cervical spine injuries.

9. Waninger KN: Management of the helmeted athlete with suspected cervical spine injury. *Am J Sports Med* 2004;32(5):1331-1350.

10. Robertson WC Jr, Eichman PL, Clancy WG: Upper trunk brachial plexopathy in football players. *JAMA* 1979;241(14):1480-1482.

11. Sallis RE, Jones K, Knopp W: Burners: Offensive strategy for an underreported injury. *Phys Sportsmed* 1992;20:47-55.

12. Torg JS, Corcoran TA, Thibault LE, et al: Cervical cord neurapraxia: Classification, pathomechanics, morbidity, and management guidelines. *J Neurosurg* 1997b;87(6):843-850.

13. Torg JS, Naranja RJ Jr, Pavlov H, Galinat BJ, Warren R, Stine RA: The relationship of developmental narrowing of the cervical spinal canal to reversible and irreversible injury of the cervical spinal cord in football players. *J Bone Joint Surg Am* 1996;78(9):1308-1314.

14. ASIA Learning Center Materials - International Standards for Neurological Classification of SCI (ISNCSCI) Exam Worksheet. Available at: http://www.asia-spinalinjury.org/elearning/ISNCSCI.php. . Accessed August 12, 2015.

15. Hoppenfeld S: *Physical examination of the cervical spine and temporomandibular joint. Physical examination of the spine & extremities.* Upper Saddle River, NJ, Prentice Hall, 1976, pp 105-132.

16. Wetzel FT, Reider B: Cervical and thoracic spine, in Reider B, ed: The Orthopaedic Physical Examination, ed 2. Philadelphia, PA, Elsevier Saunders, 2005, pp 297-334.

17. Stiell IG, Clement CM, McKnight RD, et al: The Canadian C-spine rule versus the NEXUS low-risk criteria in patients with trauma. *N Engl J Med* 2003;349(26):2510-2518.

18. Grant GA, Mirza SK, Chapman JR, et al: Risk of early closed reduction in cervical spine subluxation injuries. *J Neurosurg* 1999;90(Suppl 1):13-18.

19. Pavlov H, Torg JS, Robie B, Jahre C: Cervical spinal stenosis: Determination with vertebral body ratio method. *Radiology* 1987;164(3):771-775.

20. Herzog RJ, Wiens JJ, Dillingham MF, Sontag MJ: Normal cervical spine morphometry and cervical spinal stenosis in asymptomatic professional football players. Plain film radiography, multiplanar computed tomography, and magnetic resonance imaging. *Spine (Phila Pa 1976)* 1991;16(6, Suppl)S178-S186.

21. Torg JS, Ramsey-Emrhein JA: Suggested management guidelines for participation in collision activities with congenital, developmental, or postinjury lesions involving the cervical spine. *Med Sci Sports Exerc* 1997;29(7, Suppl)S256-S272.

22. Torg JS, Sennett B, Pavlov H, Leventhal MR, Glasgow SG: Spear tackler's spine. An entity precluding participation in tackle football and collision activities that expose the cervical spine to axial energy inputs. *Am J Sports Med* 1993;21(5):640-649.

23. Vaccaro AR, Klein GR, Ciccoti M, et al: Return to play criteria for the athlete with cervical spine injuries resulting in stinger and transient quadriplegia/paresis. *Spine J* 2002;2(5):351-356.

24. Versteegen GJ, Kingma J, Meijler WJ, ten Duis HJ: Neck sprain not arising from car accidents: A retrospective study covering 25 years. *Eur Spine J* 1998;7(3):201-205.

25. Roberts DW, Roc GJ, Hsu WK: Outcomes of cervical and lumbar disk herniations in Major League Baseball pitchers. *Orthopedics* 2011;34(8):602-609.

Eleven Major League Baseball pitchers with a diagnosis of cervical disc herniation were identified. At an average of 1.6 months following diagnosis, eight returned to play. Eight underwent surgical treatment. Management controversies are also discussed. Level of evidence: IV.

26. Maroon JC, Bost JW, Petraglia AL, et al: Outcomes after anterior cervical discectomy and fusion in professional athletes. *Neurosurgery* 2013;73(1):103-112, discussion 112.

A series of 15 professional football players or wrestlers who underwent anterior cervical diskectomy and fusion was retrospectively studied. All players were eventually cleared for return to play, with 13 actually returning a mean of 6 months postoperatively. Level of evidence: IV.

27. Meredith DS, Jones KJ, Barnes R, Rodeo SA, Cammisa FP, Warren RF: Operative and nonoperative treatment of cervical disc herniation in National Football League athletes. *Am J Sports Med* 2013;41(9):2054-2058.

Sixteen NFL players with a diagnosis of cervical disk herniation were identified. Of the players, three were treated surgically, one of whom returned to play. In the nonsurgical group, 8 of 13 returned to play. Management strategies are reviewed. Level of evidence: IV.

© 2016 American Academy of Orthopaedic Surgeons

28. Torg JS, Truex R Jr, Quedenfeld TC, Burstein A, Spealman A, Nichols C III: The National Football Head and Neck Injury Registry. Report and conclusions 1978. *JAMA* 1979;241(14):1477-1479.

29. Torg JS, Vegso JJ, Sennett B, Das M: The National Football Head and Neck Injury Registry. 14-year report on cervical quadriplegia, 1971 through 1984. *JAMA* 1985;254(24):3439-3443.

30. Crook TB, Eynon CA: Traumatic atlantoaxial rotatory subluxation. *Emerg Med J* 2005;22(9):671-672.

31. Venkatesan M, Bhatt R, Newey ML: Traumatic atlantoaxial rotatory subluxation (TAARS) in adults: A report of two cases and literature review. *Injury* 2012;43(7):1212-1215.

   The authors discuss a case presentation and review of 12 papers presenting cases of traumatic atlantoaxial rotatory subluxation in adult patients. The report describes traumatic AARS and the management as applicable to sports and other injuries in skeletally mature patients. Level of evidence: IV.

32. Fielding JW, Hawkins RJ: Atlanto-axial rotatory fixation. (Fixed rotatory subluxation of the atlanto-axial joint). *J Bone Joint Surg Am* 1977;59(1):37-44.

33. Woodring JH, Lee C: The role and limitations of computed tomographic scanning in the evaluation of cervical trauma. *J Trauma* 1992;33(5):698-708.

34. Pang D: Atlantoaxial rotatory fixation. *Neurosurgery* 2010;66(3, Suppl)161-183.

   The biomechanics of the C1-2 joint in AARS is described extensively, and the pathophysiology of AARS in children is hypothesized and a clinical grading system is presented. A management algorithm based on the grading system is proposed. Level of evidence: IV.

35. Subach BR, McLaughlin MR, Albright AL, Pollack IF: Current management of pediatric atlantoaxial rotatory subluxation. *Spine (Phila Pa 1976)* 1998;23(20):2174-2179.

36. Kim YS, Lee JK, Moon SJ, Kim SH: Post-traumatic atlantoaxial rotatory fixation in an adult: A case report. *Spine (Phila Pa 1976)* 2007;32(23):E682-E687.

Video Reference

32.1: Faldini C, Gasbarrini A, Chehrassan M, et al: Video. *Anterior Interbody Fusion in Cervical Disc Herniation*. Bologna, Italy, University of Bologna Istituto Ortopedico Rizzoli, 2012.

Chapter 33

Thoracolumbar Spine

Anuj Singla, MD   Christopher A. Burks, MD

Abstract

Low back pain and related symptoms are common reasons for clinical visits to spine surgeons. The incidence of back pain continues to increase, which is attributed to lifestyle changes and increased involvement in sporting activities. Careful attention should be paid to the inciting event while eliciting history and neurologic examination as well as radiologic evaluation. Some of the most common reasons for nonremitting and recurring back pain include disk degeneration, disk herniation, spinal stenosis, spondylolysis, and spondylolisthesis. The management of spinal problems is highly individualized, based on pathology, symptomatic involvement, and the activity/physical demands of the patient. Conservative treatment is usually the first line of treatment for most of these disorders. Return to activity (including sports) is a big challenge and often requires aggressive and prolonged rehabilitation.

Keywords: thoracic spine; lumbar spine; degeneration; spondylosis; disk herniation; spondylolisthesis

Introduction

Low back pain is one of the most common symptoms for which patients seek medical care. The lifetime incidence ranges between 60% and 90%, with 26% of people reporting an episode of low back pain within the previous 3 months.[1] Direct medical expenditures for the treatment of low back pain is more than $100 billion annually and is increasing.[2] Low back pain is a significant source of short-term and long-term disability, lost productivity, and work absenteeism. Up to 25% of all missed work days in the United States are attributed to low back pain.[3] The condition is also common in the adolescent population, with more than 75% of episodes having no clear diagnosis.[4] The common nontraumatic spinal pathologies affecting the thoracolumbar spine include disk degeneration, disk herniation, spinal stenosis, spondylolysis, and spondylolisthesis. The management of thoracolumbar and lumbosacral spine-related pain differs, depending on the exact etiology of the patient's symptoms.

History and Physical Examination

The approach to the active patient with low back pain with or without leg pain begins with a thorough history and physical examination. It is important to establish a timeline for the patient's symptoms and to identify the nature, duration, onset, and characterization of the symptoms. When eliciting the history, the physician must focus on any inciting event and the presence or absence of certain red flags. Red flag signs indicate the potential for an underlying pathology that warrants a timely and focused workup. Evaluation of a patient presenting with low back or leg pain and a history of fevers, chills, weight loss, cancer, immunosuppression, and/or intravenous drug abuse should prompt the clinician to consider infection or malignancy as a possible etiology. Evaluation of a patient presenting with back pain and reports of clumsiness, gait instability, or bowel, bladder, or sexual dysfunction should prompt the physician to carefully assess for causes of spinal cord dysfunction, such as cervical or thoracic myelopathy.

Asking the patient to describe the pain in relation to certain activities can help identify a possible etiology. Discogenic pain related to disk degeneration or disk herniation may be worse in flexion, while sitting, or with prolonged axial loading and often is described in a diffuse, band-like distribution. Facet-mediated pain related to facet arthrosis or spondylolysis may be worse in extension and is often activity related and well localized.

A thorough examination should begin by observing the patient walk, which allows an assessment of coordination,

Dr. Burks or an immediate family member has stock or stock options held in Smith & Nephew. Neither Dr. Singla nor any immediate family member has received anything of value from or has stock or stock options held in a commercial company or institution related directly or indirectly to the subject of this chapter.

Table 1			
Common Physical Examination Findings			
Level	**Motor**	**Sensory**	**Reflex**
L1	None	Inguinal crease	None
L2	Hip flexion	Anterior upper/inner thigh	None
L3	Hip flexion/adduction	Anterior/inner thigh	None
L4	Knee extension	Lateral thigh, anterior knee, medial leg	Patellar
L5	Ankle/toe dorsiflexion, hip abduction	Lateral leg, dorsum of foot	None
S1	Ankle plantar flexion, foot eversion	Posterior leg, lateral foot	Achilles
S2	Toe plantar flexion	Plantar foot	None
S3-4	Bowel/bladder	Perianal	Cremasteric

strength, and symmetry of motion. Palpation of the back should assess for any points of maximal tenderness such as in the facets, the paraspinal musculature, or the sacroiliac joints. Assessing the range of motion of the hips can help to rule out referred pain due to hip arthrosis. A thorough sensorimotor examination should follow (Table 1).

Provocative tests can be performed to elicit responses that corroborate physical examination or imaging findings. These tests may include testing for nerve root tension signs such as a straight leg raise, contralateral straight leg raise, or femoral nerve stretch test. For the purpose of detecting lumbar disk herniation, the straight leg raise test is more sensitive but less specific than the contralateral straight leg raise test in patients with single-leg radicular pain.[5]

The provider must be aware of possible indications of nonorganic or psychologic pain etiology. The five categories of signs for such an etiology, as described by Waddell,[6] are tenderness, simulation, distraction, regional disturbances, and overreaction. The presence of three or more Waddell signs should prompt the physician to evaluate for other etiologies of the symptoms such as depression, hypochondriasis, or secondary gain issues. The presence of three or more Waddell signs does not discount the possibility of a spine problem but is associated with higher pain scores and poorer treatment outcomes overall.

Thoracic Herniated Disk

Epidemiology

Symptomatic thoracic disk herniation has an incidence of approximately 0.5% in the population and occurs most commonly in males between the ages of 40 and 50 years.[7] It can occur at any level in the thoracic spine, but 75% occur below T8, with most occurring at T11-12 because of increased relative mobility at this level. In a study of MRIs of asymptomatic individuals, 73% had disk degeneration, and 29% were found to have thoracic disk herniation with a resultant spinal cord deformation.[8]

Clinical Presentation

Thoracic disk herniation may present in a variety of ways. Approximately half of patients will identify a specific traumatic event that led to the onset of symptoms; many will report insidious onset consistent with chronic degenerative changes, however. The most common presentation is axial pain in the mid to low thoracic spine that may extend into the lumbar spine. The second most common presentation is radiating pain in a dermatomal pattern that may be unilateral or bilateral. Common dermatomal reference levels are the nipple line corresponding to T4, the xiphoid process corresponding to T7, the umbilicus corresponding to T10, and the inguinal crease corresponding to T12. Percussion of the posterior elements of the thoracic spine may reproduce or exacerbate axial and/or radicular pain. Lower thoracic disk herniations may even present with an isolated unilateral footdrop associated with upper motor neuron signs.[9]

The least common presentation, but one that must be readily identified, is that of progressive myelopathy. Because of the chronic degenerative process associated with disk herniations, patients often will present with a myriad of symptoms consistent with more common lumbar spine etiologies. A thorough assessment of root level sensorimotor function and upper motor neuron function should occur. In a review of 427 patients with symptomatic thoracic stenosis due to disk herniation or ossified ligamentum flavum, 81% had lower extremity weakness, and 64% reported lower extremity sensory deficits.[10] Bowel, bladder, and sexual dysfunction may be noted in 15% to 20% of patients.[11] Sustained clonus, a positive Babinski sign, hyperreflexia, and altered gait should prompt the physician to consider cervical level or thoracic level disk spinal cord compression in the diagnosis. A positive Romberg test is highly sensitive for early myelopathy due to dorsal column dysfunction, resulting in decreased proprioception. Although most often considered part of the routine evaluation of idiopathic scoliosis, abdominal reflexes also may be asymmetric in patients with thoracic myelopathy.

Diagnostic Imaging

Diagnosis of a symptomatic thoracic disk herniation requires confirmatory imaging. The most common imaging modality for the detection of thoracic disk herniation is MRI, which is highly sensitive and therefore associated with a high rate of false-positive results. One potential drawback to MRI is its limitations with respect to evaluating for calcified disk fragments or ossified ligamentum flavum. In patients in whom a high suspicion exists for disk or ligamentum ossification or in those with an inability to undergo MRI, CT myelography provides a viable option. Like MRI, CT myelography identifies a high rate of asymptomatic herniations. Plain radiography is of little utility in the diagnosis of thoracic disk herniation but is useful in assessing for transitional anatomy or the presence of any instability or malalignment and to compare with intraoperative localization in the surgical patient.

Treatment

Symptomatic thoracic disk herniations have a variety of presentations varying from mild pain to frank paraparesis. Therefore, the treatment timeline and treatment strategy can vary significantly. Most symptomatic thoracic disk herniations may be treated with nonsurgical measures similar to those used for lumbar disk herniations. These treatments include NSAIDs, muscle relaxants, short-term narcotics, antineuropathic medications, and physical therapy. For the patient with acute pain, physical therapy initially should be restricted to passive treatment modalities such as heat, ultrasound, and massage, but as symptoms diminish, more active therapy such as extension-based exercises, core strengthening, and range-of-motion exercises can be introduced. For patients with substantial radicular pain, an intercostal nerve block may be an effective adjunct treatment option.[12] Except in the case of acutely progressive myelopathy, nonsurgical treatment should be undertaken for a minimum of 4 to 6 weeks before surgery is considered.

Thoracic disk herniations are associated with more lost time from games and practice than are lumbar disk herniations. In a retrospective review[13] of the National Football League's (NFL) surveillance database, players with thoracic disk herniations missed significantly more practices and games (72 and 17, respectively) on average than those with lumbar disk herniations (39 and 11, respectively).

Surgical treatment is appropriate for patients with radicular pain recalcitrant to prolonged nonsurgical management, weakness, and acute myelopathy. Approximately 4% of thoracic disk herniations present with acute myelopathy with severe functional limitations (**Figure 1**). Some authors have advocated a more aggressive, urgent approach to surgical decompression and stabilization in these patients.[14] One of the most challenging aspects of the surgical treatment of thoracic disk herniation is the appropriate localization of the correct level intraoperatively.[15] Proper localization is paramount to successful surgical treatment and the avoidance of litigation.

The thoracic spinal cord is not as amenable to manipulation as is the thecal sac in the lumbar spine. Multiple surgical approaches are used to decompress the thoracic spine—the anterior approach through a thoracotomy or combined thoracoabdominal approach, the direct lateral retropleural approach, the posterolateral approach via a costotransversectomy, and the transpedicular approach, as well as posterior thoracic laminectomy—although no strategy has been shown to be consistently superior, and each is associated with its own risks and complications. Regardless of the approach taken, the decision to perform instrumentation and fusion is dependent on the degree of instability imparted by the approach.[15] Recently, minimally invasive endoscopic techniques have been described with promising results in small case series.[16,17] In appropriately selected patients, these newer techniques may result in less morbidity and allow an earlier return to play for athletes.

Lumbar Disk Herniation

Lumbar disk herniation is a common finding on MRI of the lumbar spine. Although often an asymptomatic, incidental finding, it can be associated with significant back and extremity pain, as well as sensory and motor deficits. Although lumbar disk herniation can occur in children and young adults, it is most common in people older than 50 years, representing a single point in the degenerative cascade of the intervertebral disk, much like a degenerative meniscus tear. The herniation occurs as a result of tensile failure of the anulus fibrosus following internal disk disruption.

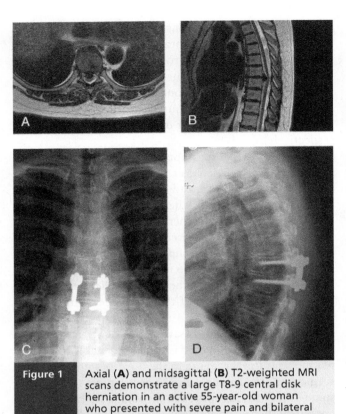

Figure 1 Axial (**A**) and midsagittal (**B**) T2-weighted MRI scans demonstrate a large T8-9 central disk herniation in an active 55-year-old woman who presented with severe pain and bilateral lower-extremity weakness. She underwent T8-9 diskectomy and T8-T9 instrumented fusion via a posterior extracavitary approach. AP (**C**) and lateral (**D**) radiographs show postoperative views. The patient experienced immediate improvement in pain and lower extremity weakness.

Lumbar disk herniations can be characterized by their location and the integrity of the annulus and posterior longitudinal ligament. With regard to location, disk herniations may be central, paracentral, foraminal, or extraforaminal; paracentral herniations are most common because of the relatively reduced strength of the posterior longitudinal ligament. A disk herniation also may be described as a bulge or protrusion when the anulus fibrosus is intact; conversely, it may be extruded through an annular or ligamentous defect or sequestered without attachment to the native disk. Obesity, occupations that involve heavy lifting, exposure to persistent vibration, smoking, and genetics have been identified as risk factors for lumbar disk herniation.[18]

Clinical Presentation

The clinical presentation of symptomatic herniated disks may include isolated back pain, single-leg radicular pain, weakness, or numbness, or cauda equina syndrome. Often, a prodromal history of low back pain is noted by the patient when describing the symptoms. Most patients are unable to pinpoint a specific inciting event but relate that it began spontaneously. As always when presented with a patient with low back pain and/or leg pain, it is imperative to rule out potentially serious etiologies by inquiring about bowel and bladder dysfunction, the presence of fever, or progressive neurologic deterioration.

A thorough physical examination can help to elicit weakness and sensory deficits, but most commonly, the patient's description of radicular symptoms can give a clue or provide further information to confirm a diagnosis. Observing the patient's gait can be useful in detecting subtle weakness. Nerve root tension signs such as the straight leg raise and femoral stretch test are more specific for lumbar disk herniation than is dermatomal distribution, because significant overlap exists. Straight leg raises are considered positive when pain is reproduced between 35° and 75°, which is the point at which stretch is applied to the sciatic nerve. An assessment of reflexes should be performed, because hyporeflexia would be expected to be present in cases of nerve root compression from a herniated disk.

Diagnostic Imaging

The most common imaging study used to identify a lumbar disk herniation is MRI. T2-weighted axial and sagittal images best delineate the space-occupying nature of the disk in relation to the thecal sac, given the contrast provided by the cerebrospinal fluid. T1-weighted sagittal images provide the best view of the exiting nerve root and the overall foraminal space because of the fat surrounding the nerve root (Figure 2). Plain radiographs cannot show disk herniations, but they may demonstrate disk space narrowing, spondylolisthesis, or spasm-induced scoliosis, although these findings may be nonspecific and may not indicate a specific spinal level. In patients with contraindications to MRI or those having lumbar instrumentation from prior surgery, CT myelography can provide similar information regarding space-occupying lesions. In patients with prior surgical decompression, MRI enhanced with gadolinium can help to delineate recurrent herniation from postoperative scar tissue.

The location of the disk herniation dictates which nerve root is affected. The most common location is paracentral, because of the relative weakness of the posterior longitudinal ligament. This type will cause stenosis within the lateral recess, impinging on the traversing nerve root exiting under the caudal pedicle. A disk herniation within or lateral to the foramen will impinge on the root exiting through that foramen. For example, a left-side L4-5 paracentral disk herniation most likely will impinge on the left L5 nerve root, whereas a foraminal herniation

© 2016 American Academy of Orthopaedic Surgeons

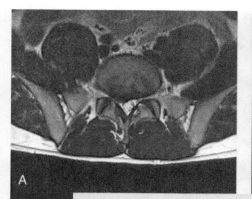
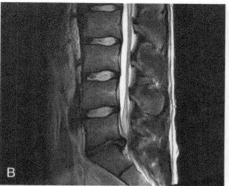
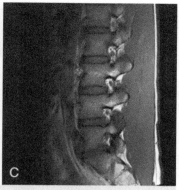

Figure 2 Axial (**A**) and parasagittal (**B**) T2-weighted MRI scans demonstrate a left-side paracentral disk herniation at L5-S1 impinging on the traversing S1 nerve root and show the loss of disk height and signal changes within the disk at L5-S1. Sagittal T1-weighted MRI scan (**C**) demonstrates nerve roots (dark) surrounded by fat (white) within the intervertebral foramen. Note the decrease in fat signal around the nerve root at L5-S1 as a result of disk height loss.

will impinge on the L4 nerve root as it travels under the left L4 pedicle in the intervertebral foramen.

Although the condition is rare, care must be taken to appropriately identify patients with cauda equina syndrome caused by a large central disk herniation. Cauda equina syndrome is a clinical diagnosis confirmed with correlating imaging. It is associated with progressive bilateral sensorimotor changes, bowel or bladder dysfunction such as retention or incontinence, and perianal sensory deficits as the result of a centrally based space-occupying lesion compressing the lumbosacral nerve roots distal to the conus medullaris. Quick identification and urgent surgical decompression is imperative in these patients to mitigate the risk of permanent neurologic dysfunction.

Treatment

Lumbar radiculopathy resulting from a disk herniation often responds to a course of nonsurgical management. Multiple modalities, including NSAIDs, muscle relaxants, short-term narcotics, antineuropathic medications, physical therapy, and epidural or transforaminal steroid injections may be used. No consensus exists about the optimum nonsurgical treatment strategy for lumbar radiculopathy secondary to disk herniation. Steroid injections have provided short-term improvement of symptoms of lumbar radiculopathy. A prospective randomized controlled trial demonstrated a greater than 50% reduction in pain at 1 month in 54% of patients who received a transforaminal steroid injection, which was significantly better than the results in those receiving normal saline or local anesthetic injections.[19] Repeat injections were noted to be less likely to provide substantial relief.

In a study of 27 NFL players treated with epidural steroid injections for lumbar radiculopathy secondary to lumbar disk herniation, 89% (24 patients) returned to play with an average loss of 2.8 practices and 0.6 games.[20] Three players eventually required surgery, and all were noted to have sequestered disk herniations along with weakness. In an analysis of 342 professional athletes with lumbar disk herniations, 82% (280 of 342) were able to return to play; of those who underwent surgical decompression, 81% (184 of 226) returned to play.[21] Major League Baseball players had a higher rate of return to play than did NFL players. No consensus exists on the return-to-play criteria; however, the resolution of preinjury symptoms and the completion of a structured rehabilitation program have been advocated.[22] A recent review article summarized the available case series and expert opinion regarding return-to-play criteria following lumbar microdiskectomy, demonstrating wide variability. The time to return to play was reported as 1 to 2 months for golf, 6 to 8 weeks for noncontact sports, and 2 to 6 months for contact sports.[23]

Patients in whom nonsurgical management has failed as previously described and with good correlation between imaging and physical examination may benefit from surgical decompression. In a recent prospective study on the cost effectiveness of continued medical management of lumbar disk herniation in surgical candidates, it was shown that continued nonsurgical treatment strategies were not cost effective.[24] After 6 weeks of nonsurgical treatment, outcome measures failed to improve with continued nonsurgical care in patients with imaging-confirmed spine pathology. In an analysis of 137 NFL players with lumbar disk herniations, those who underwent surgery experienced greater career longevity (36 games played) compared with those treated nonsurgically (20 games played).[25]

The gold standard for the surgical treatment of lumbar disk herniation is diskectomy. Considerable debate exists about the best surgical technique. Multiple systematic reviews have failed to demonstrate a consistent benefit of any single technique, including open discectomy, microdiskectomy, tubular microdiskectomy, percutaneous or endoscopic discectomy, over any other.[26-28]

The Spine Patients Outcomes Research Trial was a multicenter trial that followed patients with multiple lumbar spine diagnoses. Although initially designed as a randomized controlled trial with a secondary observational group, significant crossover in the randomized patients has led to the data being evaluated "as treated." The observational arm of the study has provided substantial data on lumbar disk herniation and the effect of multiple treatments. Despite demographic differences between those who underwent surgery and those who did not, those who underwent surgery demonstrated improvements in all primary outcome measures at 2, 4, and 8 years.[29,30] Those with symptoms lasting longer than 6 months, sequestered fragments, and increased back pain, and those who were not working experienced greater benefits from surgery.[30] Subgroup analysis of the data showed that preoperative epidural steroid injection did not influence surgical outcome and that obesity is associated with a lower clinical benefit from surgical or nonsurgical treatment.[31-33]

Total Disk Replacement

Total disk replacement (TDR) is an appealing option for younger patients in whom nonsurgical management has failed, with the theoretical advantage of saving motion segments and minimizing adjacent segment disease when compared with fusion. TDR typically is not indicated for the treatment of lumbar disk herniation but instead for the treatment of degenerative disk disease and discogenic back pain. The mainstay treatment for degenerative disk disease and discogenic back pain continues to be nonsurgical. Multiple clinical trials have determined lumbar TDR to be "not inferior" to circumferential lumbar fusion; concern for bias exists with many of these studies.[34,35] One study examined lumbar TDR in a cohort of 39 young, athletic individuals. The athletes were allowed to return to noncontact sports at 3 months and to contact sports at 4 to 6 months. Of the total, 95% (37 of 39) returned to sports activity, with 85% (33 of 39) reporting improved performance from the preoperative status.[36] High-quality clinical studies are needed to determine the efficacy of total lumbar disk replacement compared with current conventional treatment in the athletic population.

Spondylolysis

Spondylolysis is commonly associated with young athletes and is a stress reaction leading to osteolysis or fracture

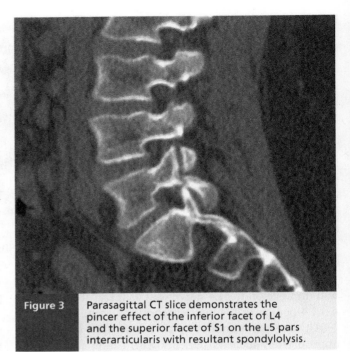

Figure 3 Parasagittal CT slice demonstrates the pincer effect of the inferior facet of L4 and the superior facet of S1 on the L5 pars interarticularis with resultant spondylolysis.

of the pars interarticularis, a narrow isthmus of bone connecting the superior and inferior facets of the lumbar vertebra. It is most common at L5 because of the decreased distance between the L4 inferior facet and the S1 superior facet, which leads to excessive repetitive loading of the pars interarticularis of L5[37] (Figure 3). This condition particularly affects athletes involved in sports that require repetitive hyperextension of the lumbar spine, such as gymnasts, football linemen, rowers, and soccer players. The condition once was thought to be congenital; however, multiple studies have shown it to be an acquired defect.[38]

Epidemiology

The exact incidence of spondylolysis is unknown, because it often may be asymptomatic. The overall prevalence was found to be 4.2% in a cadaver study of approximately 4,200 specimens.[39] It occurs predominantly at L5 (85%) and less often at L4 (10% to 15%) in a 2:1 male-to-female ratio; however, female athletes may be at a higher risk than males because of the female athlete triad.[40,41] It is bilateral in 80% of cases and rarely (4%) found at more than one level.[42]

Clinical Presentation

Spondylolysis most often is asymptomatic and may be an incidental finding on radiography; back pain frequently develops in active youth with spondylolysis, which leads to a physician visit. The onset of pain may occur after a specific inciting event, but often symptom onset will not be readily definable. Initially, patients may have back pain only with activity that improves with rest, but chronic, low-level pain may be present at all times. The most common report is of back pain that increases with high-intensity activity; however, radicular pain into the buttocks or posterior thigh may be present rarely in isolated spondylolysis. In spondylolytic spondylolisthesis, foraminal stenosis may cause radicular symptoms.

On physical examination, focal tenderness to palpation often is noted adjacent to the midline and in the paraspinal musculature at the level of spondylolysis. Forward flexion does not elicit any pain (in contrast to extension, which may be limited). Extension/hyperextension of the spine may be painful. Other physical examination findings may be hamstring tightness, antalgic gait, functional scoliosis due to muscle spasm, palpable step-off of the spinous process in cases of spondylolysis with spondylolisthesis, and increased lumbar lordosis. A single-leg lumbar hyperextension test can be used to assess for unilateral versus bilateral spondylolysis, but it has poor specificity for spondylolysis because it may be positive in multiple lumbar spine disorders. A thorough neurologic examination should be performed but is often normal.

Diagnostic Imaging

Patients with persistent activity-related back pain without neurologic symptoms should be evaluated with standing AP and lateral lumbar radiographs. Historically, oblique views also were obtained to evaluate for spondylolysis, but they have not been shown to increase diagnostic accuracy, and they increase cost and radiation exposure.[43] Plain radiographs were shown to be diagnostic in 86% of patients who had spondylolysis.[44] The lateral view demonstrates a lucency or lytic defect in the pars interarticularis and allows assessment of any spondylolisthesis. This view also assesses lumbopelvic parameters such as slip angle, pelvic incidence, and sacral slope, which help to predict the risk of slip development or progression.

In cases of suspected spondylolysis with negative radiographs, other imaging modalities can be used, although the most appropriate study to use is a topic of debate. Radionuclide bone scans and single photon emission CT (SPECT) can be used and are based on the metabolic activity of the region. "Hot" bone scans indicate increased radionuclide uptake as a result of increased metabolic activity in areas of active spondylolysis. They may be "cold" or normal in chronic cases that have ceased the attempted reparative process. SPECT has improved sensitivity and specificity than radionuclide bone scans and allows better delineation of bony anatomy but has higher costs and radiation exposure.[44]

CT has high sensitivity and specificity for detecting bony defects of the pars interarticularis and is the gold standard for characterizing fractures because of its excellent visualization of bony anatomy. Care must be taken when evaluating both the axial and sagittal images to avoid mistaking facets for pars interarticularis defects. CT also can be used to evaluate the healing process. The drawback to CT is its high radiation exposure, poor evaluation of soft-tissue structures, and inability to evaluate prelysis conditions.

Recently, MRI has been used in the assessment of the young patient with back pain in whom spondylolysis is a concern. MRI is better than CT at characterizing the soft tissues of the lumbar spine and detecting early stress-related changes in the pars interarticularis. A classification system was developed for using MRI in the diagnosis of stress reactions through complete fractures of the pars interarticularis.[45] A recent study showed that MRI was equivalent to bone scans in ability to detect stress reactions of the pars interarticularis without overt fracture and equivalent to CT in ability to detect complete injuries.[46] Because of its ability to assess active versus inactive stress reactions, MRI largely has supplanted bone scan and SPECT in the diagnosis of spondylolysis. A role for CT remains in the diagnosis and assessment of the treatment for spondylolysis.

Treatment

Spondylolysis is most often treated nonsurgically, which may include cessation of sports participation, activity modification, physical therapy, and bracing. The key to successful treatment begins with the early diagnosis of an acute pars interarticularis fracture. In a study of 32 young athletes with radiographically negative, bone scan-positive spondylolysis for an average of 9 years, 91% (29 of 32 athletes) reported good to excellent low back functional outcomes at final follow-up, despite the absence of healing on radiographs.[47]

In a recent retrospective review,[48] the effect of sports cessation compliance on long-term results was studied in 132 pediatric patients with spondylolysis without spondylolisthesis. Although no nonsurgical treatment strategy was uniformly applied, all patients were advised to cease sporting activities for a minimum of 3 months. Sixty-five percent of patients (86 of 132) stopped their sports activity for at least 3 months and 35% (46 of 132) stopped for a variable period of time. Patients who stopped sports activity for 3 months were 16 times more likely to experience excellent resolution of their symptoms. Bony fusion did not have an association with a better outcome; however, it was more likely to occur with cessation of sports activity.

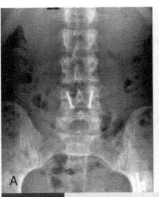
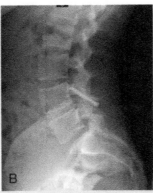

Figure 4 AP (**A**) and lateral (**B**) radiographs show direct pars repair with interlaminar screw fixation of bilateral L4 spondylolysis.

There is a lack of high-quality studies examining the effectiveness of nonsurgical modalities such as bracing, functional rehabilitation, and electric stimulation because most studies are small case series. Studies indicate that athletes should be asymptomatic before being allowed to return to sports, and nonunion or fibrous union is not associated with a failure to return to play or good functional outcome.[48-50]

The indications for surgical treatment of spondylolysis without spondylolisthesis are failure of 6 months of nonsurgical treatment or 9 to 12 months of persistent back pain with nonunion.[51] The goals of surgical treatment are débridement of any fibrous nonunion and stabilization of the pars interarticularis. Many surgical techniques are available, including single-level fusion using screw-rod constructs, transverse process wiring, and noninstrumented posterolateral arthrodesis. More recently, direct pars interarticularis repair with débridement and interlaminar screw fixation has gained favor following failed nonsurgical treatment but requires a healthy intervertebral disk[52] (Figure 4).

The choice of bone graft or bone graft substitutes for the augmentation of bony healing remains controversial. The authors of a 2014 study reported on 31 patients treated with direct interlaminar screw repair with iliac crest autograft for spondylolysis.[53] Of the total, 90% reported successful outcomes with reduced postoperative visual analog scale scores, and 76% of the competitive athletes in the series returned to their respective sports. Another study[54] reported on 29 pars interarticularis defects in competitive athletes treated with direct screw repair and recombinant human bone morphogenetic protein; bony fusion was achieved in all but one defect, and 100% return to play was seen. Conversely, a prospective outcomes study was conducted on 47 military members who underwent pars screw repair following

failure of nonsurgical management.[55] Fifty-five percent achieved union, with 53% of patients satisfied with their outcome. Oswestry Disability Index and 12-Item Short Form Health Survey scores were significantly improved from baseline at 6 months but had a tendency to decline after 12 months. Return to high-intensity sports activity following surgical stabilization is possible if the patient is asymptomatic, has a demonstrated fusion, and has fully rehabilitated to prior playing status.[51] As in lumbar disk herniation, return-to-play criteria following surgery are based on expert opinion and vary widely. For patients who have undergone single-level lumbar or lumbosacral fusion for spondylolysis or spondylolisthesis, various authors have advocated waiting a range of times before allowing a return to sports participation, including 6 to 12 months for noncontact sports, 1 year for contact sports, or never for contact or collision sports.[51,56,57]

Spondylolisthesis

Spondylolisthesis refers to the translation of one vertebral body in relation to an adjacent body. The Wiltse classification of spondylolisthesis has five types[58] (Table 2). The most common are types I and II, which will be the focus of this section. Type III, degenerative spondylolisthesis, occurs as a continuation of the degenerative cascade of disk degeneration, with progressive facet capsule incompetence leading to instability and subsequent translation without structural changes in the vertebrae. Type IV is a result of traumatic or iatrogenic defects of the posterior elements. Type V results from a pathologic process. Despite the Wiltse classification's widespread use, it does not provide any prognostic value, but it does allow communication between providers for these distinct processes.

Dysplastic spondylolisthesis, type I, occurs secondary to a developmental defect in the facet complex, resulting in poorly restrained motion, most commonly at the L5-S1 complex. The superior S1 facet or inferior L5 facet may be missing, underdeveloped, or oriented in the sagittal plane. Spina bifida occulta often is seen in conjunction with dysplastic spondylolisthesis. Compared with spondylolysis, which is more prevalent in males, dysplastic spondylolisthesis is twice as common in females and accounts for 15% to 20% of pediatric spondylolisthesis.[59]

Isthmic spondylolisthesis, type II, can be divided into three subtypes, based on the integrity of the pars interarticularis. Type IIA is defined as a defect of the pars interarticularis secondary to a stress fracture as described previously in the section on spondylolysis. Type IIB, isthmic spondylolisthesis, is defined as an elongation of the pars interarticularis without a defect, caused by repetitive microtrauma and bony remodeling of the pars

Table 2

Classification of Spondylolisthesis

Type	Description	Key Notes
I	Dysplastic	Developmental anomalies of the facet complex or posterior elements
II	Isthmic	Defect in pars interarticularis
IIA	Spondylolytic	Stress fracture of the pars interarticularis
IIB	Elongated pars	Elongation of the pars interarticularis from bony remodeling
IIC	Traumatic	Acute fractures of the pars interarticularis
III	Degenerative	Secondary to chronic facet complex instability
IV	Posttraumatic	Prior posterior element fracture or iatrogenic instability
V	Pathologic	Secondary to generalized disease process with destruction of posterior elements

interarticularis. Type IIC is a traumatic pars interarticularis fracture and is the least common isthmic subtype.

Clinical Presentation

Spondylolisthesis in the young active patient presents most commonly with back pain of insidious onset, except in the case of acute pars interarticularis fractures. Radiculopathy is uncommon but when present, is most often bilateral. The most common level of isthmic and dysplastic spondylolisthesis is L5-S1, with the L5 nerve root the most commonly affected root. The nerve root may be irritated as a result of two different mechanisms. In higher grade slips, traction on the nerve root may cause irritation. In the spondylolytic and isthmic types, repeated attempts at healing the defect may lead to a proliferation of fibrous tissue, which impinges on the exiting nerve root and in some cases also may irritate the traversing nerve root.

A thorough physical examination may indicate subtle weakness in the extensor hallucis longus or a slight Trendelenburg gait due to hip external rotator weakness; pain with lumbar extension is the most common finding. One of the most common signs associated with spondylolisthesis is a decreased popliteal femoral angle due to hamstring tightness. No neurologic basis exists for the tightness; it is likely a manifestation of chronic postural changes made in an attempt to maintain normal sagittal balance.[60] Palpation of the lumbar spine may demonstrate a step-off at the L4-L5 spinous process in isthmic spondylolisthesis and, conversely, at the L5-S1 junction in the dysplastic type.

Diagnostic Imaging

Plain radiography of the lumbar spine is sufficient to demonstrate most cases of spondylolisthesis. As described previously, oblique views were historically obtained to evaluate for isthmic spondylolisthesis, but this practice has been shown to be associated with a higher rate of radiation exposure without any increased diagnostic utility. The lateral standing radiograph can be used to calculate multiple spinal alignment parameters, the most useful of which is the slip angle. The slip angle is the angle formed by a line perpendicular to the posterior cortex of the sacrum and a line parallel to the inferior end plate of L5. Slip angles greater than 55° are associated with an increased risk of slip progression.[61]

CT can be useful in evaluating for subtle pars interarticularis fractures or spina bifida occulta. Detection of spina bifida occulta is important when surgical correction is planned, to reduce the risk of inadvertent durotomy or neurologic injury. MRI should be used in patients with neurologic symptoms to evaluate the site or sites of compression for preoperative planning.

Treatment

Asymptomatic or minimally symptomatic spondylolisthesis in the young, active patient can be successfully treated nonsurgically. Surgical treatment is reserved for patients with symptomatic spondylolisthesis in whom nonsurgical management has failed and for those with significant functional limitations, high-grade slips with a high slip angle, and altered sagittal alignment. Multiple surgical techniques can be used, including instrumented and noninstrumented in situ arthrodesis or reduction of the slip with instrumented fusion. The addition of interbody grafts, performed via an anterior, lateral, or posterior approach, has been shown to increase the rate of fusion in spondylolisthesis and result in greater restoration of lordosis and disk space height, compared with instrumented posterolateral fusion alone in the treatment of spondylolisthesis.[62,63] One systematic review of the evidence for in situ arthrodesis versus spondylolisthesis reduction[64] found a higher rate of pseudarthrosis in the

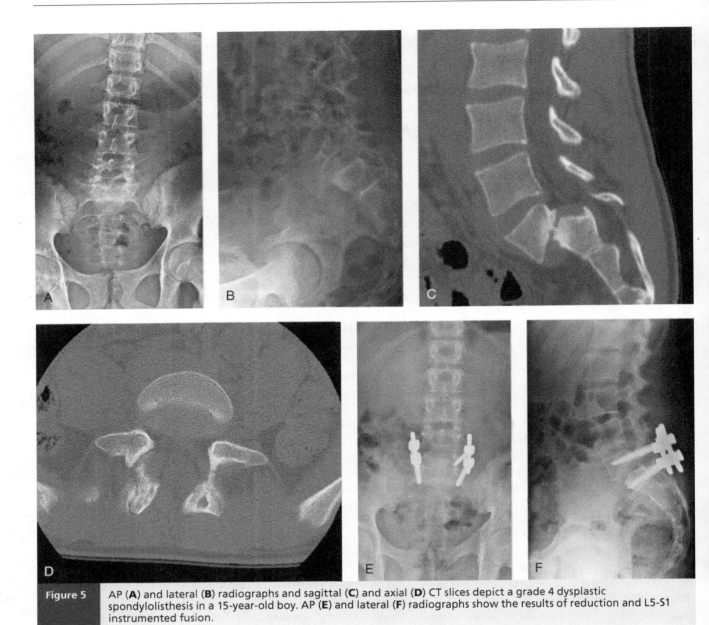

Figure 5 AP (**A**) and lateral (**B**) radiographs and sagittal (**C**) and axial (**D**) CT slices depict a grade 4 dysplastic spondylolisthesis in a 15-year-old boy. AP (**E**) and lateral (**F**) radiographs show the results of reduction and L5-S1 instrumented fusion.

in situ group (17.8% versus 5.5%), greater improvement in slip angle and percent slip in the reduction group, and no difference in the incidence of postoperative neurologic deficit between the groups. The reduction of high-grade slips has been shown to lead to an overall improvement in global sagittal alignment, providing optimal spinal biomechanics to mitigate the risk of adjacent segment disease[65] (Figure 5).

A recent retrospective review of 53 adolescents with high-grade spondylolisthesis demonstrated that those who were asymptomatic or minimally symptomatic could be treated nonsurgically without risk of neurologic problems.[66] In addition, those who were treated surgically

because their symptoms progressed had long-term results similar to those who did not have surgery. Those with higher slip angles had worse long-term outcomes, as measured by the Scoliosis Research Society (SRS) 30 questionnaire, independent of surgical or nonsurgical treatment. Another study examined the improvements in health-related quality of life (HRQOL) as measured by the SRS 22 questionnaire in 28 patients with high-grade slips[67] and reported a significant improvement in HRQOL in surgically treated patients, with patients having lower baseline scores experiencing the most improvement. Return-to-play criteria for surgically treated spondylolisthesis are described in the section on spondylolysis.

Summary

Low back pain is a common report of the young, active patient and most often is a self-limiting episode without underlying etiology. Careful attention to the history and a diligent physical examination can help diagnose those cases of underlying spinal pathology. Nonsurgical treatment is often successful in cases of thoracic and lumbar disk herniation, spondylolysis, and spondylolisthesis. In patients who require surgery, a return to sports or activity is certainly possible following successful rehabilitation.

No standardized return-to-play guidelines are available for any of the previously discussed conditions and treatments. The surgeon must make an individualized plan for each athlete that takes into account the athlete's participation level, individual sport requirements, and overall treatment outcome.

Key Study Points

- Low back pain and thoracolumbar spine-related issues continue to increase in adolescent and young adults. Careful attention should be paid to any inciting trauma, history, and related symptoms.
- Lumbar/thoracic disk pathology and herniation, spinal stenosis, spondylolysis, and spondylolisthesis are some of the common diagnoses associated with chronic back pain, and require detailed clinical and radiologic evaluation.
- Nonsurgical treatment is usually first, unless substantial or worsening neurologic involvement, infection, or spine instability are present.
- Return to sports or high-demand activity is often possible with either surgical or nonsurgical treatment, after successful rehabilitation.

Annotated References

1. Deyo RA, Mirza SK, Martin BI: Back pain prevalence and visit rates: Estimates from U.S. national surveys, 2002. *Spine (Phila Pa 1976)* 2006;31(23):2724-2727.

2. Martin BI, Deyo RA, Mirza SK, et al: Expenditures and health status among adults with back and neck problems. *JAMA* 2008;299(6):656-664.

3. Devereaux M: Low back pain. *Med Clin North Am* 2009;93(2):477-501, x.

   This article provides a detailed overview of low back pain and is especially targeted at general practitioners and family physicians. The important points of history taking and clinical and radiological examination to be considered when managing low back pain and related issues are discussed.

4. Bhatia NN, Chow G, Timon SJ, Watts HG: Diagnostic modalities for the evaluation of pediatric back pain: A prospective study. *J Pediatr Orthop* 2008;28(2):230-233.

5. Andersson GB, Deyo RA: History and physical examination in patients with herniated lumbar discs. *Spine (Phila Pa 1976)* 1996;21(24, Suppl)10S-18S.

6. Waddell G, McCulloch JA, Kummel E, Venner RM: Nonorganic physical signs in low-back pain. *Spine (Phila Pa 1976)* 1980;5(2):117-125.

7. Arce CA, Dohrmann GJ: Herniated thoracic disks. *Neurol Clin* 1985;3(2):383-392.

8. Wood KB, Garvey TA, Gundry C, Heithoff KB: Magnetic resonance imaging of the thoracic spine. Evaluation of asymptomatic individuals. *J Bone Joint Surg Am* 1995;77(11):1631-1638.

9. Zhang C, Xue Y, Wang P, Yang Z, Dai Q, Zhou HF: Foot drop caused by single-level disc protrusion between T10 and L1. *Spine (Phila Pa 1976)* 2013;38(26):2295-2301.

   The authors present their experience in this case series of 25 cases of unilateral foot drop in patients with a single disk herniation between T10 and L1. Level of evidence: IV.

10. Hou X, Sun C, Liu X, et al: Clinical features of thoracic spinal stenosis-associated myelopathy: A retrospective analysis of 427 cases. *J Spinal Disord Tech* 2014 [Epub ahead of print].

    The authors report on the epidemiology of thoracic stenosis and on the constellation of symptoms at presentation in 427 consecutive patients treated surgically at a single institution. Level of evidence: III.

11. Vanichkachorn JS, Vaccaro AR: Thoracic disk disease: Diagnosis and treatment. *J Am Acad Orthop Surg* 2000;8(3):159-169.

12. Eckel TS, Bartynski WS: Epidural steroid injections and selective nerve root blocks. *Tech Vasc Interv Radiol* 2009;12(1):11-21.

    This review article discusses the indications and technique of epidural and selective nerve root injections in the cervical, thoracic, and lumbar spine.

13. Gray BL, Buchowski JM, Bumpass DB, Lehman RA Jr, Mall NA, Matava MJ: Disc herniations in the national football league. *Spine* 2013;38:1934-1938.

    The authors use the National Football League players' injury database to describe the incidence and characteristics of disk herniations in professional football players and the impact they have on playing status.

5: Head and Spine

14. Cornips EM, Janssen ML, Beuls EA: Thoracic disc herniation and acute myelopathy: Clinical presentation, neuroimaging findings, surgical considerations, and outcome. *J Neurosurg Spine* 2011;14(4):520-528.

    The authors report their experience with the surgical treatment of thoracic disk herniations presenting with acute myelopathy in a series of eight patients.

15. Yoshihara H: Surgical treatment for thoracic disc herniation: An update. *Spine (Phila Pa 1976)* 2014;39(6):E406-E412.

    The author provides an updated look at the outcomes and techniques for the surgical treatment of thoracic disk herniations.

16. Choi KY, Eun SS, Lee SH, Lee HY: Percutaneous endoscopic thoracic discectomy; transforaminal approach. *Minim Invasive Neurosurg* 2010;53(1):25-28.

    In this case series, the authors describe their technique and the outcomes of 14 patients treated with percutaneous endoscopic thoracic diskectomy for soft disk herniations. Level of evidence: IV.

17. Smith JS, Eichholz KM, Shafizadeh S, Ogden AT, O'Toole JE, Fessler RG: Minimally invasive thoracic microendoscopic diskectomy: Surgical technique and case series. *World Neurosurg* 2013;80(3-4):421-427.

    In this case series, the authors present their results of minimally invasive thoracic diskectomy for soft disk herniations. Level of evidence: IV.

18. Hadjipavlou AG, Tzermiadianos MN, Bogduk N, Zindrick MR: The pathophysiology of disc degeneration: A critical review. *J Bone Joint Surg Br* 2008;90(10):1261-1270.

19. Ghahreman A, Ferch R, Bogduk N: The efficacy of transforaminal injection of steroids for the treatment of lumbar radicular pain. *Pain Med* 2010;11(8):1149-1168.

    In this randomized controlled study, the authors sought to evaluate the route of steroid injection—transforaminal versus intramuscular—for the treatment of lumbar radicular pain. Level of evidence: I.

20. Krych AJ, Richman D, Drakos M, et al: Epidural steroid injection for lumbar disc herniation in NFL athletes. *Med Sci Sports Exerc* 2012;44(2):193-198.

    In this retrospective case series, the authors discuss the utility of epidural steroid injections in improving return-to-play time in professional football players with symptomatic lumbar disk herniations. Level of evidence: IV.

21. Hsu WK, McCarthy KJ, Savage JW, et al: The Professional Athlete Spine Initiative: Outcomes after lumbar disc herniation in 342 elite professional athletes. *Spine J* 2011;11(3):180-186.

    In this retrospective cohort study, the authors present the results and 2-year outcomes data of the surgical and nonsurgical treatment of lumbar disk herniation in 342 professional athletes. Level of evidence: III.

22. Burgmeier RJ, Hsu WK: Spine surgery in athletes with low back pain-considerations for management and treatment. *Asian J Sports Med* 2014;5(4):e24284.

    This review article summarizes the current evidence and treatment thoughts for athletes with a spectrum of spinal disorders.

23. Li Y, Hresko MT: Lumbar spine surgery in athletes: Outcomes and return-to-play criteria. *Clin Sports Med* 2012;31(3):487-498.

    This review article discusses the implications of lumbar spine surgery in pediatric athletes. Treatment variation, functional outcomes, and return-to-play criteria are discussed.

24. Parker SL, Godil SS, Mendenhall SK, Zuckerman SL, Shau DN, McGirt MJ: Two-year comprehensive medical management of degenerative lumbar spine disease (lumbar spondylolisthesis, stenosis, or disc herniation): A value analysis of cost, pain, disability, and quality of life: Clinical article. *J Neurosurg Spine* 2014;21(2):143-149.

    The authors used a prospective quality-of-life spine registry to perform a cost-benefit analysis of nonsurgical treatment options after 6 weeks in patients with identifiable surgical lesions. They found no benefit to continued nonsurgical therapy.

25. Hsu WK: Performance-based outcomes following lumbar discectomy in professional athletes in the National Football League. *Spine (Phila Pa 1976)* 2010;35(12):1247-1251.

    The author presents the results of 137 NFL players treated for lumbar disk herniation. Surgically treated herniations resulted in improved career longevity.

26. Kamper SJ, Ostelo RW, Rubinstein SM, et al: Minimally invasive surgery for lumbar disc herniation: A systematic review and meta-analysis. *Eur Spine J* 2014;23(5):1021-1043.

    The results of a systematic review and meta-analysis of available clinical trials comparing conventional open discectomy with minimally invasive diskectomy are presented.

27. Rasouli MR, Rahimi-Movaghar V, Shokraneh F, Moradi-Lakeh M, Chou R: Minimally invasive discectomy versus microdiscectomy/open discectomy for symptomatic lumbar disc herniation. *Cochrane Database Syst Rev* 2014;9:CD010328.

    Cochrane review data of available clinical trials comparing conventional open discectomy versus minimally invasive diskectomy are presented. Level of evidence: II.

28. Jacobs WC, van Tulder M, Arts M, et al: Surgery versus conservative management of sciatica due to a lumbar herniated disc: A systematic review. *Eur Spine J* 2011;20(4):513-522.

    This systematic review discusses the effectiveness of surgery versus the nonsurgical management of sciatica due to lumbar disk herniation. It found that early surgery

5: Head and Spine

demonstrated earlier pain relief than did nonsurgical management. Level of evidence: IV.

29. Lurie JD, Tosteson TD, Tosteson AN, et al: Surgical versus nonoperative treatment for lumbar disc herniation: Eight-year results for the spine patient outcomes research trial. *Spine (Phila Pa 1976)* 2014;39(1):3-16.

    This article presents the 8-year outcomes data from the Spine Patient Outcomes Research Trial (SPORT) in patients who underwent treatment of lumbar disk herniation. No degradation in outcomes was seen in the surgical or nonsurgical group. Level of evidence: II.

30. Kerr D, Zhao W, Lurie JD: What are long-term predictors of outcomes for lumbar disc herniation? A randomized and observational study. *Clin Orthop Relat Res* 2015;473(6):1920-1930.

    Evaluation of the 8-year SPORT data for lumbar disk herniations demonstrated the following factors as associated with better outcomes with surgery: higher levels of baseline back pain accompanying radiculopathy, a longer duration of symptoms, and patients who were neither working nor disabled at baseline. Level of evidence: II.

31. Lurie JD, Faucett SC, Hanscom B, et al: Lumbar discectomy outcomes vary by herniation level in the Spine Patient Outcomes Research Trial. *J Bone Joint Surg Am* 2008;90(9):1811-1819.

32. Rihn JA, Radcliff K, Hilibrand AS, et al: Does obesity affect outcomes of treatment for lumbar stenosis and degenerative spondylolisthesis? Analysis of the Spine Patient Outcomes Research Trial (SPORT). *Spine (Phila Pa 1976)* 2012;37(23):1933-1946.

    This subgroup analysis of the SPORT data showed that obese patients improved with surgery for lumbar stenosis and spondylolisthesis, but the gains were lower than in patients who were not obese. Level of evidence: II.

33. Rihn JA, Kurd M, Hilibrand AS, et al: The influence of obesity on the outcome of treatment of lumbar disc herniation: Analysis of the Spine Patient Outcomes Research Trial (SPORT). *J Bone Joint Surg Am* 2013;95(1):1-8.

    This subgroup analysis of the SPORT data showed that obese patients improved with surgery for lumbar disk herniation but the gains were lower than in patients who were not obese. Level of evidence: II.

34. van den Eerenbeemt KD, Ostelo RW, van Royen BJ, Peul WC, van Tulder MW: Total disc replacement surgery for symptomatic degenerative lumbar disc disease: A systematic review of the literature. *Eur Spine J* 2010;19(8):1262-1280.

    This article is a systematic review of available clinical trials evaluating lumbar disk arthroplasty for the treatment of degenerative disk disease. Level of evidence: III.

35. Jacobs W, Van der Gaag NA, Tuschel A, et al: Total disc replacement for chronic back pain in the presence of disc degeneration. *Cochrane Database Syst Rev* 2012;9:CD008326.

    This article is a Cochrane Review of available clinical trials evaluating lumbar disk arthroplasty for the treatment of degenerative disk disease. Level of evidenve: III.

36. Siepe CJ, Wiechert K, Khattab MF, Korge A, Mayer HM: Total lumbar disc replacement in athletes: Clinical results, return to sport and athletic performance. *Eur Spine J* 2007;16(7):1001-1013.

37. Zehnder SW, Ward CV, Crow AJ, Alander D, Latimer B: Radiographic assessment of lumbar facet distance spacing and pediatric spondylolysis. *Spine (Phila Pa 1976)* 2009;34(3):285-290.

    This retrospective radiographic review describes narrowed intrafacet distance as a possible etiology of lumbar pars defects. Level of evidence: III.

38. Reitman CA, Gertzbein SD, Francis WR Jr: Lumbar isthmic defects in teenagers resulting from stress fractures. *Spine J* 2002;2(4):303-306.

39. Roche MB, Rowe GG: The incidence of separate neural arch and coincident bone variations; A summary. *J Bone Joint Surg Am* 1952;34-A(2):491-494.

40. Takemitsu M, El Rassi G, Woratanarat P, Shah SA: Low back pain in pediatric athletes with unilateral tracer uptake at the pars interarticularis on single photon emission computed tomography. *Spine (Phila Pa 1976)* 2006;31(8):909-914.

41. Kim HJ, Green DW: Spondylolysis in the adolescent athlete. *Curr Opin Pediatr* 2011;23(1):68-72.

    This review article discusses the presentation, diagnostic workup, and treatment of spondylolysis in the pediatric athlete.

42. Gurd DP: Back pain in the young athlete. *Sports Med Arthrosc* 2011;19(1):7-16.

    This review article discusses the presentation, diagnostic workup, and treatment of back pain in the pediatric athlete.

43. Beck NA, Miller R, Baldwin K, et al: Do oblique views add value in the diagnosis of spondylolysis in adolescents? *J Bone Joint Surg Am* 2013;95(10):e65. I

    This radiographic study evaluates the utility of oblique lumbar views for the detection of spondylolysis. The authors conclude that the views are not necessary nor worth the cost of radiation exposure. Level of evidence: III.

44. Miller R, Beck NA, Sampson NR, Zhu X, Flynn JM, Drummond D: Imaging modalities for low back pain in children: A review of spondyloysis and undiagnosed mechanical back pain. *J Pediatr Orthop* 2013;33(3):282-288.

    This retrospective study evaluates the epidemiology of mechanical back pain in the adolescent, the utility of imaging studies, and the common causes of back pain. Level of evidence: III.

45. Hollenberg GM, Beattie PF, Meyers SP, Weinberg EP, Adams MJ: Stress reactions of the lumbar pars interarticularis: The development of a new MRI classification system. *Spine (Phila Pa 1976)* 2002;27(2):181-186.

46. Rush JK, Astur N, Scott S, Kelly DM, Sawyer JR, Warner WC Jr: The use of magnetic resonance imaging in the evaluation of spondylolysis. *J Pediatr Orthop* 2015;35(3):271-275.

    The authors explore the efficacy of MRI in the diagnosis and evaluation of spondylolysis compared with CT in the management of spondylolysis. Level of evidence: III.

47. Miller SF, Congeni J, Swanson K: Long-term functional and anatomical follow-up of early detected spondylolysis in young athletes. *Am J Sports Med* 2004;32(4):928-933.

48. El Rassi G, Takemitsu M, Glutting J, Shah SA: Effect of sports modification on clinical outcome in children and adolescent athletes with symptomatic lumbar spondylolysis. *Am J Phys Med Rehabil* 2013;92(12):1070-1074.

    The authors evaluated the impact of sports cessation on long-term outcomes in the treatment of symptomatic lumbar spondylolysis. Sports cessation for a period of 3 months was associated with the improved possibility of an excellent long-term outcome. Level of evidence: III.

49. Standaert CJ, Herring SA: Expert opinion and controversies in sports and musculoskeletal medicine: The diagnosis and treatment of spondylolysis in adolescent athletes. *Arch Phys Med Rehabil* 2007;88(4):537-540.

50. Bouras T, Korovessis P: Management of spondylolysis and low-grade spondylolisthesis in fine athletes. A comprehensive review. *Eur J Orthop Surg Traumatol* 2015;25(Suppl 1):167-175.

    The authors present an excellent review of the management of spondylolysis and spondylolisthesis in athletes, with a focus on surgical treatment modalities.

51. Radcliff KE, Kalantar SB, Reitman CA: Surgical management of spondylolysis and spondylolisthesis in athletes: Indications and return to play. *Curr Sports Med Rep* 2009;8(1):35-40.

    In this review article, the authors discuss the surgical management of type 2 spondylolisthesis and the clinical criteria for return to play.

52. Drazin D, Shirzadi A, Jeswani S, et al: Direct surgical repair of spondylolysis in athletes: Indications, techniques, and outcomes. *Neurosurg Focus* 2011;31(5):E9.

    This article is a systematic review of the available literature on the surgical management of spondylolysis in athletes. The authors conclude that the ideal candidate is younger than 20 years and without degenerative disk changes.

53. Menga EN, Kebaish KM, Jain A, Carrino JA, Sponseller PD: Clinical results and functional outcomes after direct intralaminar screw repair of spondylolysis. *Spine (Phila Pa 1976)* 2014;39(1):104-110.

    This study describes the results of a cohort of patients with spondylolysis treated with direct repair via interlaminar screw fixation. Level of evidence: IV.

54. Snyder LA, Shufflebarger H, O'Brien MF, Thind H, Theodore N, Kakarla UK: Spondylolysis outcomes in adolescents after direct screw repair of the pars interarticularis. *J Neurosurg Spine* 2014;21(3):329-333.

    This meta-analysis looks at the relevant surgical literature on the outcomes of pars repair with direct fixation. Level of evidence: III.

55. Lee GW, Lee SM, Suh BG: Direct repair surgery with screw fixation for young patients with lumbar spondylolysis: Patient-reported outcomes and fusion rate in a prospective interventional study. *Spine (Phila Pa 1976)* 2015;40(4):E234-E241.

    This study discussed the results of direct repair to treat lumbar spondylolysis, and it was concluded that this surgery in young patients with lumbar spondylolysis may lead to suboptimal results 1 year postoperatively. Level of evidence: II.

56. Eck JC, Riley LH III: Return to play after lumbar spine conditions and surgeries. *Clin Sports Med* 2004;23(3):367-379, viii.

    In this review article, the authors discuss return-to-play criteria for spine conditions following surgical and nonsurgical management.

57. Rubery PT, Bradford DS: Athletic activity after spine surgery in children and adolescents: Results of a survey. *Spine (Phila Pa 1976)* 2002;27(4):423-427.

    In this study, the authors polled spine surgeons on their return-to-play criteria for a variety of lumbar spine conditions. Significant variability was noted among responses. Level of evidence: V.

58. Wiltse LL, Newman PH, Macnab I: Classification of spondylolisis and spondylolisthesis. *Clin Orthop Relat Res* 1976;117:23-29.

59. Newman PH: Surgical treatment for spondylolisthesis in the adult. *Clin Orthop Relat Res* 1976;117:106-111.

60. Barash HL, Galante JO, Lambert CN, Ray RD: Spondylolisthesis and tight hamstrings. *J Bone Joint Surg Am* 1970;52(7):1319-1328.

61. Min WK, Lee CH: Comparison and correlation of pelvic parameters between low-grade and high-grade spondylolisthesis. *J Spinal Disord Tech* 2014;27(3):162-165.

    This radiographic study looks at the differences in various spinopelvic parameters in patients with low-grade versus high-grade spondylolisthesis.

62. Liu X, Wang Y, Qiu G, Weng X, Yu B: A systematic review with meta-analysis of posterior interbody fusion versus posterolateral fusion in lumbar spondylolisthesis. *Eur Spine J* 2014;23(1):43-56.

The authors perform a systematic review of the surgical outcomes of degenerative lumbar spondylolisthesis based on surgical technique. Level of evidence: III.

63. Mummaneni PV, Dhall SS, Eck JC, et al: Guideline update for the performance of fusion procedures for degenerative disease of the lumbar spine. Part 11: Interbody techniques for lumbar fusion. *J Neurosurg Spine* 2014;21(1):67-74.

This article is a guidelines update regarding the best new evidence for the use of interbody devices in the treatment of lumbar spondylolisthesis.

64. Longo UG, Loppini M, Romeo G, Maffulli N, Denaro V: Evidence-based surgical management of spondylolisthesis: Reduction or arthrodesis in situ. *J Bone Joint Surg Am* 2014;96(1):53-58.

This systematic review shows that reduction of spondylolisthesis is associated with improvements in spinal biomechanics but not with an increased risk of neurologic deficits. Level of evidence: III.

65. Thomas D, Bachy M, Courvoisier A, Dubory A, Bouloussa H, Vialle R: Progressive restoration of spinal sagittal balance after surgical correction of lumbosacral spondylolisthesis before skeletal maturity. *J Neurosurg Spine* 2015;22(3):294-300.

In this radiographic study, the authors evaluate the preoperative and postoperative radiographic spinopelvic parameters in patients managed with surgical reduction of high-grade dysplastic spondylolisthesis.

66. Lundine KM, Lewis SJ, Al-Aubaidi Z, Alman B, Howard AW: Patient outcomes in the operative and nonoperative management of high-grade spondylolisthesis in children. *J Pediatr Orthop* 2014;34(5):483-489.

The authors performed a retrospective review of patients with high-grade spondylolisthesis. They found that delayed surgical intervention does not lead to worse outcomes in patients who are minimally symptomatic. Level of evidence: III.

67. Bourassa-Moreau É, Mac-Thiong JM, Joncas J, Parent S, Labelle H: Quality of life of patients with high-grade spondylolisthesis: Minimum 2-year follow-up after surgical and nonsurgical treatments. *Spine J* 2013;13(7):770-774.

The authors followed 28 patients for 2 years following treatment of high-grade spondylolisthesis. They found improved health-related quality-of-life scores with surgical treatment. Level of evidence: II.

Miscellaneous Topics

SECTION EDITOR

Stephen R. Thompson, MD, Med, FRCSC

Chapter 34

The Team Physician and the Ethics of Sports Medicine

Andrew M. Watson, MD, MS   Warren R. Dunn, MD, MPH

Abstract

Team physicians are confronted with a wide range of unique ethical dilemmas in providing care to athletes. The primary goals of medicine and athletic competition are not always aligned and the considerable internal and external pressures to prioritize short-term benefit and athletic success can potentially influence medical decision-making. As the media exposure and economic effect of sports increase in modern society, team physicians and athletes alike are presented with a number of potential conflicts of interest that threaten the principles of traditional medical practice. It is recommended that the team physician properly recognize these pressures and conflicts of interest to adopt a shared decision-making model that engenders trust, promotes patient autonomy and prioritizes long-term health outcomes for the athletes in his or her care.

Keywords: ethics; team physician

Introduction

Sports and medicine have had opposing objectives ever since organized athletics and rational medicine emerged in ancient Greece.[1] The goal of athletic competition is victory, and that of medicine is health. These goals come into conflict if the pursuit of athletic success threatens the health of the athlete. The rigorous training regimens, dietary habits, obsessive commitment, and personal sacrifice characteristic of an athlete's lifestyle stand in contrast

---

Dr. Dunn or an immediate family member serves as a paid consultant to or is an employee of CONMED Linvatec and serves as a board member, owner, officer, or committee member of the American Academy of Orthopaedic Surgeons, the American Orthopaedic Society for Sports Medicine, and the American Shoulder and Elbow Surgeons.

to the moderation promoted by rational medicine. As a result, medicine and sports historically have had an adversarial relationship. The relationship evolved during the course of the 20th century with the emergence of sports medicine as a specialty dedicated to facilitating athletic achievement by improving both performance and health. The role of medicine in athletic culture shifted from observation and even disapproval to recognition of the value of sports and active involvement that is intended to improve the health of athletes, who are a vulnerable population. Sports medicine has become integrated into athletic culture, and the role of the team physician increasingly is integrated into organized athletics.[1]

The new relationship of medicine and sports presents unique ethical challenges. The divergent objectives remain and can threaten the ethical foundations of medical practice.[2] Beneficence, a fundamental principle of medicine, obligates physicians to give first priority to their patients' well-being, even at a potential cost to themselves. Physicians and patients traditionally work cooperatively toward a common goal of improving patient health, but physicians and athletes may not have the same goals.[3] For example, some athletes are willing to risk health damage and violate the law by taking a drug to improve athletic success.[4] This divergence of goals presents a greater challenge to the classic physician-patient dyad than is found in other medical specialties.

The demands of a team sport can exert external pressures on the athlete and physician and can lead to the emergence of an ethically challenging physician-patient-team triad.[2] The financial and employment relationships of players, physicians, and teams vary considerably by levels of competition. The physician may be acting as a volunteer with a local recreational or scholastic team, the medical director of a large-scale single event, a general practitioner caring for athletes, an employee of a university athletic department, or a specialist who has paid for the right to treat the players on a professional team.[5] These relationships are different from those in a typical office-based medical practice. Potential conflicts of interest and threats to confidentiality and patient autonomy are inevitable, and in modern sports they are exaggerated by the increasing influence of prestige, market power, advertising, media coverage, and interested third parties.[2,3,6,7] In an attempt to guide physicians confronted with ethical dilemmas, several organizations and governing bodies have developed codes of conduct.[8-10] Nonetheless, no widely accepted code of ethics has fully dealt with the varied situations in sports medicine. As the sports landscape continues to rapidly change, new and challenging scenarios are likely to appear.

Conflicts of Interest

For the practicing sports medicine physician, the greatest threat to the principle of beneficence arises from divergent opposing goals within the physician-patient-team triad.[2] An athlete's decision making can be significantly influenced by real or perceived external pressures unrelated to her or his overall or long-term health, and the pressures are exacerbated by media presence and the economic effect of sports.[7] The most obvious conflict occurs if an athlete's health and athletic success require different interventions. For example, an athlete with a repairable meniscus tear incurred near the end of the competitive season could be treated with a meniscus repair or a meniscectomy. The meniscectomy could allow a more rapid return to play, with participation in postseason competition, and thus would further the goal of team success. However, the meniscus repair could decrease the long-term risk of degenerative joint disease and thus further the goal of improving the athlete's long-term health. The physician may believe that the long-term benefits of meniscus repair outweigh the short-term benefits of a rapid return to play, but the patient and/or the team may hold the opposite opinion. For the high school player in competition for an athletic scholarship, an early end to the season could jeopardize the only opportunity for college acceptance.

Athletes are under considerable internal pressure because of the real or perceived financial effect of injury and time lost from play. In high-level sports, players increasingly are motivated by financial considerations such as salary and advertising revenue, and early return to play is likely to become a higher priority than long-term health. The loss of a partial or entire season of play can have a considerable financial impact on an athlete as well as family and friends who stand to benefit from the athlete's success.[11] An athlete may attempt to hide past injuries from a new physician, team, or athletic organization for fear of being prevented from further participation. The perceived threat to the athlete's financial success can create a dysfunctional relationship with medical staff.[7]

The perception that the public prizes athletic toughness and teamwork can create great pressure to play through injury or sacrifice individual health to benefit the team or achieve individual success. The iconic image of an injured athlete fighting to compete and struggling through pain to glory represents an extremely strong influence on athletes. Such athletes are almost deified in television, movies, advertisements, and the public eye. Many athletes have a strong desire to please a coach or another authority figure, and their decision-making process may be strongly influenced by a belief that a certain decision will displease the coach. A research study found that minimizing the severity of pain and playing through pain are learned behaviors that develop in young players at least partly in response to athletic coaching.[12] Sports participation often is an important part of an athlete's identity. Athletes may fear that injury-caused loss of playing time will undermine their position on a team as well as their standing with teammates and in the community.[13] On a professional level, the financial consequences of lost time can cause an athlete to fear inability to satisfy obligations to family members and friends. Actions resulting from such motivations can significantly conflict with actions designed to ensure the athlete's health.[5,6]

Team physicians are exposed to psychosocial pressures that can influence their decision making. As a member of a team, the team physician naturally has an emotional attachment to the team's success, and typically it is accepted, if not expected, that the team physician is an active supporter of the team. This factor can consciously or unconsciously influence the physician's decision making in the care of an individual athlete. A physician also may be responsible for covering the care of players on an opposing team, and this factor opens a further possibility for conflict with the beneficence principle. Although it is clearly unethical to promote a team's chance of success at the expense of an athlete's health, the potential for unconscious influence must be recognized. This conflict is unique to sports medicine.[6]

High-level sports decisions can be complicated by the influence of media exposure. The physician may be subject to public scrutiny of his or her medical decisions and interventions. For example, the physician's choice of treatment for an athlete with a torn meniscus could become publicly controversial.[2] A decision to pursue meniscus repair rather than meniscectomy might be in the best long-term interest of the patient but could be negatively perceived by the public. The community may revere a physician who is able to quickly return athletes to play, but there is little acclaim for a physician who enables a player to retire years later with a nonarthritic joint. This sort of decision making can have considerable personal and professional consequences for a high-level team physician, and the potential influence of the media should not be minimized.

In general, ethical questions surround team physicians affiliated with a professional sports organization. Affiliation with a professional sports organization can be so financially beneficial that physician groups and hospitals are willing to pay a considerable sum to obtain the affiliation.[2] The public may believe that a team physician's affiliation with a professional team is a function only of clinical experience or skill, although in fact it may have resulted from a bidding competition. Paying to become a team medical provider is not recommended, but the current reality is that the position of team physician is directly linked to marketing contracts, particularly in professional sports. Team physicians should attempt to minimize the inherent conflict.[2] The American Academy of Orthopaedic Surgeons Committee on Ethics recommends that publicity should not be used in an untruthful, misleading, or deceptive manner.[14] Team physicians should disclose relevant financial arrangements in an attempt to ensure that the patients who seek their care are motivated by their ability to manage medical conditions rather than their relationship with a sports organization.

Athletic teams have an obvious interest in players' and physicians' medical decision making, and the role of the team within the physician-patient-team triad should not be minimized. At all levels of athletic competition, team administrators, coaches, and teammates of an injured player feel pressure to succeed. Desire for short-term success may outweigh concern for the long-term health of the athlete with an injury. Particularly during the competitive season, emotions are strong, and the desire to return an athlete to play despite the risk can be overwhelming. In addition, the team may have a substantial financial investment in the player, and the pressure for on-field success may be in conflict with medical decision making based on long-term patient health.[7] The result is real or perceived pressure on the athlete and team physician to return the athlete to play as quickly as possible. The pressure can be particularly intense if the team physician is employed by or otherwise formally affiliated with the athletic organization; the physician may feel torn between an obligation to the athlete's health and the priorities, demands, or expectations of the employer. Failure to ensure an athlete's rapid return to play can jeopardize the relationship between a team physician and the professional sports organization and may threaten the benefits of the affiliation for the physician.[2] Such a situation is similar to that of a company-employed physician who must make a medical decision affecting the speed of an employee's return to work after a workplace injury, with a substantial effect on the financial success of the company.

These conflicts can create complex and unique concerns for the team physician.[15] In no other medical specialty are practitioners so often confronted with disparate goals and motivations, with substantial financial and public relations ramifications. In successfully counseling and caring for athletes, team physicians should actively work to understand the internal and external pressures affecting an athlete's priorities and health decisions. Failure to recognize these influences threatens the physician-patient relationship and can lead to adversarial interactions, often at the expense of an athlete's health and performance. The ethical team physician must resist such influences and be guided solely by the best interests of the individual athlete.

Three Principles of Modern Medical Practice

Patient Autonomy

The practice of medicine traditionally has been predicated on the principle of beneficence; in modern medical practice, beneficence has been superseded by patient autonomy. Medical practice fundamentally was paternalistic until the second half of the 20th century. Physicians were thought to be better able than patients to understand the risks and benefits of treatment options and therefore were capable of making the appropriate decision for the patient. This model failed to account for the values and priorities of the individual patient, however. As society increasingly emphasized individuality and personal values, a shared decision-making model came to dominate modern medicine. The process of medical decision making now is expected to incorporate not only the experience and knowledge of the medical practitioner but also the experiences and values of the individual patient.

The evolution from a paternalistic to a shared decision-making model may be contributing to resolution of some of the conflicts between medicine and athletics. Recognition of patient autonomy as a principle of medical ethics can improve the functional relationship of the physician and athlete. In a paternalistic environment, the physician's recommendations based on the patient's long-term health might be ignored in the interest of short-term athletic success. Recognizing and incorporating the athlete's goals and values enables physicians to develop and present treatment options that do not necessarily require the sacrifice of athletic success. Although the goals of athletes and physicians still differ, the shared decision-making model has facilitated an improved working relationship between the physician and the athlete.

In modern medicine, the patient's freedom to choose is paramount, even if the patient's choice is believed to be poor.[16] Athletes should enjoy the same ability to make their own health care decisions as patients in other medical settings. True autonomy may require an individual to be free of any outside influence, however. Athletes may not be capable of true autonomy because of the considerable internal and external pressure they experience.[17] During a game, the internal and external pressure for an athlete to return to play is extremely strong, and the athlete may be willing to risk her or his individual health in the interest of short-term personal or team success. Some retired athletes were found to regret their decisions when they looked back with a long-term perspective and experience of the consequences.[7] Some researchers argue that sports medicine practitioners have an obligation to protect players from the risk of dangerous injury and should consider a paternalistic intervention to counter undue pressure to risk injury.[17] Others argue for a shared decision-making model in which the physician protects the patient's autonomy through an unbiased presentation of treatment options that include the implications for long-term health outcomes.[2,3,6]

Informed Consent

The principle of informed consent is designed to satisfy the need for patient autonomy. Through the presentation of all relevant treatment options, the patient is able to make a truly autonomous decision based on a full understanding of the implications of each treatment option.[16,17] The American Medical Association Code of Medical Ethics subsection on sports medicine states that "physicians should assist athletes to make informed decisions about their participation in amateur and professional contact sports which entail risks of bodily injury."[9] The International Federation of Sports Medicine Code of Ethics makes an even stronger statement: "Never impose your authority in a way that impinges on the individual right of the athlete to make his/her own decisions....A basic ethical principle in health care is that of respect for autonomy. An essential component of autonomy is knowledge. Failure to obtain informed consent is to undermine an athlete's autonomy."[10]

Adherence to the principle of patient autonomy can be interpreted as requiring the team physician to depend entirely on informed consent to satisfy the duty to beneficence. Unable to exert paternalistic influence, a physician in any setting must rely on being able to convey information sufficient for the patient to make a decision that truly is in the patient's best interest, and the information must be conveyed without deliberately influencing the patient toward any particular intervention. It is obvious that an attempt to deceive or mislead the patient threatens autonomy, but autonomy is similarly undermined by the physician's failure to fully identify and disclose the available options in a way that is understandable to the patient. Because of the increasing volume and complexity of available treatment options as well as the difficulty of conveying sufficient information to a patient who has no medical background, some researchers have suggested that this goal is not truly attainable.[16] In fact, it has been suggested that physicians' attempts to fully inform and educate athletes during game situations are meaningless.[27]

To some extent, the team physician is relieved of the necessity of obtaining informed consent by the obligation to maintain the safety and well-being of the athlete. The American Medical Association Code of Medical Ethics includes this statement: "The professional responsibility of the physician who serves in a medical capacity at an athletic contest or sporting event is to protect the health and safety of the contestants. The desire of spectators, promoters of the event, or even the injured athlete that he or she should not be removed from the contest should not be controlling. The physician's judgment should be governed only by medical considerations."[9] The International Federation of Sports Medicine Code of Ethics includes a similar statement: "It is the responsibility of the sports medicine physician to determine whether the injured athletes should continue training or participate in competition. The outcome of the competition or the coaches should not influence the decision, but solely the possible risks and consequences to the health of the athlete."[10]

Despite the difficulties inherent in truly informed consent and the potential for external influence on the athlete's decision-making process, team physicians are constrained by the ethics of the medical profession. If the safety of an athlete or another participant is in jeopardy, the team physician is always required to protect individual safety without regard to individual or team athletic success. In other situations, however, modern medicine relies on patient autonomy, and athletes have the right to make decisions for themselves. This principle can relieve the physician of the burden of decision making but replaces it with the necessity of presenting a large amount of information in an easily understandable form. This ability should be developed as one of the most important clinical skills of the team physician because it can have a substantial impact on the ability of athletes to actively participate in their own care.

Confidentiality

In a traditional medical setting, physicians are obligated to maintain confidentiality regarding a patient's medical condition. Confidentiality is considered inviolable by most health care codes of ethics. Health care providers are legally bound to maintain patient confidentiality unless withholding information might harm the patient or another person. In sports medicine, the right to confidentiality may be challenged if a medical condition threatens the patient's ability to participate in the sport. For example, an athlete who has sustained a concussion is required to be removed from the game and not be returned to play.[18] The athlete may wish to keep the team physician's diagnosis of concussion confidential so as to be allowed to return to play. Because a return to play would directly threaten the athlete's health, the physician would need to violate patient confidentiality by informing the coaches of the diagnosis, thereby precluding the athlete's return to play and ensuring his or her safety. In high-level sports, extensive media attention can undermine patient confidentiality. The team physician should disclose to the media only the information clearly authorized by the athlete.

There may be an ethical and practical distinction based on whether a physician is acting as a team physician or an athlete's personal physician.[3] A physician hired by a team is an agent for the team and is obligated to give priority to the goals of the team. The team physician should inform the patient that the physician has an obligation to disclose relevant medical information to team officials, even if the patient has specifically requested that the information remain confidential. An athlete's personal physician has no obligation to the team and must honor the athlete's confidentiality. This distinction has been applied to the US Health Insurance Portability and Accountability Act of 1996 (HIPAA).[19] Team physicians can disclose a professional athlete's medical information to coaches and team officials because the information is part of the athlete's employment record and therefore is not protected under HIPAA. However, a physician who independently cares for a professional athlete in the physician's medical office is obligated by HIPAA to maintain confidentiality and cannot disclose information to team officials. Care provided to athletes through a university health service is regulated by the Federal Educational Rights and Privacy Act, which allows health care information to be disclosed only to educational entities unless the patient has given consent. Both the Federal Educational Rights and Privacy Act and HIPAA allow health information to be provided to other health care providers without patient consent. Although athletic trainers have not been fully defined as health care providers, this status typically is assumed, particularly in the context of emergency evaluation and treatment during a game.[19]

The unique context of medical care during sports events and within an athletic organization should be clarified for athletes, team physicians, coaches, and staff. Athletes should be informed that the team physician may need to disclose personal or private information to other providers in the interest of providing optimal care.[20] For example, the coaching staff and athletic trainers in the rehabilitation program may need to know an athlete's prognosis after an injury or illness. It is possible, however, that fear of repercussions may lead the athlete to avoid disclosing the information.[6] This is an important consideration, and the physician should seek to promote a common understanding of the nature of proper care in a team environment. A breach of confidentiality is the greatest threat to a successful physician-patient-team relationship, and establishing appropriate expectations is a required part of professional conduct.[6] Athletes should be advised that health care providers will be careful to avoid inadvertently revealing information to anyone not involved in the athlete's care and that aspects of the athlete's care that are not immediately relevant to sports participation or the safety of others will be kept strictly confidential.

Concussion

Sports-related concussion has received considerable media attention in recent years and has become a major public health concern.[18] Concussion is common in many sports and can have both short-term and long-term effects on an athlete's cognitive function and quality of life. Recurrent concussions appear to be associated with an even higher risk for dementia and other long-term deleterious effects on behavior and neurocognitive function.[21] In response to the emerging body of evidence, all 50 states and the District of Columbia have adopted legislation governing concussion management.[21] These laws generally cover removal from play if an athlete has a suspected concussion, return to play after a concussion diagnosis, and education on concussion for coaches, athletes, and parents. State laws differ substantially, and there is no federal concussion legislation. Team physicians must be familiar with their responsibilities under the laws of their state.

There is a universal recommendation that an athlete with a concussion should be immediately be removed from play for the remainder of the day. A team physician can encounter difficulty in identifying concussion during competition, however. Athletes often are motivated to hide concussion symptoms to avoid being removed from play.[22] Because of the subjective nature of many concussion symptoms, such as nausea, headache, and dizziness, the team physician may be unable to reach a definitive diagnosis within a brief period of time on the sideline. A gradual return to play, typically over 5 days, is required after a concussion diagnosis, and a concussion diagnosis during a busy season may preclude an athlete from participation in multiple events.[18] This situation is difficult for the team physician. An underdiagnosis places an athlete at risk of subsequent injury, but an overdiagnosis may unnecessarily preclude an athlete from participating in multiple events, to the detriment of the athlete and the team.

Because of the significant potential for harm, guidelines typically recommend withholding an athlete with any evidence of a concussion for the remainder of the competitive event. There should be a forthright discussion of the risks to ensure that the athlete understands that the decision to withhold from competition was not made lightly.[21] Nonetheless, the athlete may disagree with the diagnosis and resist medical advice. An athlete with a concussion may have impaired capacity for decision making. Despite the physician's obligation to respect patient autonomy, in this situation the athlete's immediate well-being is more important than the desire to resume participation. The team physician, trainers, and coaches must agree if they are to prevent a player from returning to play against medical advice, and a breach of confidentiality therefore is justified. One common means of preventing a football player with a concussion from immediately reentering the game is to take away the helmet.

The recommended process of recovery from concussion incorporates a stepwise return to play that is contingent on resolution of initial symptoms and continuing absence of symptoms.[18] Neurocognitive testing sometimes is necessary. Most concussion symptoms are resolved within days of the injury and allow a relatively quick return to play over the next several days. Occasionally, the symptoms of concussion persist for weeks or months, however, and the athlete is precluded from competing for an extended period of time. There may be external pressure from multiple directions to prematurely return the athlete to play, possibly to the benefit of the team but at great risk to the athlete's well-being. The team physician must openly discuss expectations and milestones for return to play with the athlete, coaches, and team administrators as soon as possible after the injury. Premature return to play after concussion should be understood as unacceptable under any circumstance. If all members of the team understand the reasons for a progressive return-to-play process (Table 1), external pressure to violate the standard of care is likely to diminish in importance.

Performance-Enhancing Drugs

The team physician may be approached by athletes about the use of performance-enhancing substances, or the physician may inadvertently learn about the use of such substances when an athlete's use is exposed. Athletes are strongly motivated to seek a competitive advantage, and scandals involving the use of banned substances are not

Table 1

Graduated Return to Play Protocol

Step 1: No activity (symptom limited physical and cognitive rest)

Step 2: Light aerobic exercises (walking, swimming or stationary bike keeping intensity < 70% maximum permitted heart rate. No resistance training)

Step 3: Sport-specific exercise (such as running drills in soccer. No head-impact activities)

Step 4: Noncontact training drills (progression to more complex training drills based on sport)

Medical clearance required prior to proceeding with step 5

Step 5: Full-contact training

Step 6: Return to competition

Adapted with permission from McCrory P, Meeuwisse WH, Aubry M, et al: Consensus statement on concussion in sport: The 4th International Conference on Concussion in Sport held in Zurich, November 2012. *Br J Sports Med* 2013;47(5):250-258.

uncommon. Modern ethical guidelines are unequivocal in condemning the use of banned substances. The International Federation of Sports Medicine Code of Ethics specifically forbids the use of certain substances as having adverse effects and providing an unfair advantage to the athlete.[10] Governing bodies such as the National Collegiate Athletic Association, the American College of Sports Medicine, and the International Olympic Committee also condemn nontherapeutic drug use.[2] Athletes sometimes disclose the use of such substances to the team physician, however, and as a result the physician must reconcile a conflict between the principles of beneficence and confidentiality. Under no circumstances should a team physician prescribe a banned substance, and the physician has an obligation to denounce the use of banned substances. However, if there is no immediate threat of significant harm to the athlete, the physician can honor patient confidentiality and need not disclose the use of a banned substance to coaches or team officials. The physician need not terminate the relationship with an athlete if the athlete chooses to ignore the advice to discontinue the use of a banned substance. The athlete probably will benefit from continuing information on the risks of use as well as the physician's surveillance and management of any adverse effects.

Although an athlete's use of a legal, accepted performance-enhancing drug may not be unethical, the team physician nonetheless should be cautious. Over-the-counter analgesics, for example, may be performance enhancing if they facilitate a return to play while the athlete has injury symptoms, with the risk of worsening the injury.[2]

If a legal substance is not universally available, its use by those with access has the potential to violate the spirit of competition.[3] In general, team physicians should discourage the use of any substances that are associated with a health risk for the athlete or unfairly benefit the athlete through a performance advantage. The physician should establish a trusting relationship with the athlete that promotes the disclosure of information and allows the dissemination of information, so that patient autonomy is preserved and the risk to the patient's health is minimized.

Genomics

The development of different types of genetic testing and their widespread availability have created new ethical dilemmas in sports medicine. Genetic testing can be used to determine an individual's health risks related to sports participation. For example, testing is useful in a patient who may have Marfan syndrome or long QT syndrome or who has a family history of hypertrophic cardiomyopathy or certain types of arrhythmias.[23,24] Genetic testing has been used in an attempt to identify genes predicting athletic performance; such testing could lead to discrimination if used to direct young athletes toward or away from certain activities.[7] The US Genetic Information Nondiscrimination Act prohibits the use of genetic information in employment decisions, and the use of genetic testing for athlete selection could be considered a violation of this act.[25]

Certain genetic tests can yield information on increased risk affecting participants in a specific sport. For example, the development of a test for apolipoprotein E4 could have important ramifications for athletes in contact sports such as football because adults with apolipoprotein E4 on even a single allele are at significantly increased risk of a poor long-term neurocognitive outcome after traumatic brain injury.[7] Screening could result in athletes with a positive genotype being restricted from play. In general, there is no consensus regarding the question of how much risk a fully informed player should be allowed to accept.

When genetic information is available to the team physician, the acceptability of using the information is not always clear. For example, if a team physician forbids participation based on a genetic test, the decision could be considered discriminatory and in violation of the Genetic Information Nondiscrimination Act.[25] However, ignoring the information and allowing an athlete to play could have catastrophic consequences, such as sudden cardiac death in an athlete known to be at risk for dysrhythmia. If an athlete ignores the advice to withdraw from play, disclosing information to team officials or coaches could represent a breach of confidentiality, depending on the severity of the risk. It is not always clear whether genetic testing information is useful. For example, the value of commercial genetic tests that purport to identify an individual's athletic abilities has not been proved. The extent of the risk associated with apolipoprotein E4 in athletes participating in contact sports also is unknown. Team physicians should be knowledgeable about the accuracy and usefulness of such tests in estimating the risk to individual athletes. This information is essential to allow the team physician to properly advise an athlete, while maintaining both autonomy and confidentiality.

Medical Innovations

Innovations in sports medicine–related drugs, supplements, surgical techniques, and rehabilitation are plentiful and rapidly advancing, but many medications or procedures lack a sufficient evidence base to guide their use.[2,7] Athletes, teams, and the public often believe that "newer is better," even if evidence is lacking. In professional sports, the media attention and financial considerations associated with medical and surgical interventions can place the team physician in a difficult position. The rapid pace of development and the relatively small number of athletes available for research studies often precludes the collection of sound evidence on the use of new procedures or medications. Paradoxically, the evidence remains scant until the modality is used on a large scale.[2]

The deliberate pursuit of truly informed consent is paramount whenever a new treatment is being considered. The physician is obligated to honestly and thoroughly evaluate the available evidence related to the proposed treatment. If a treatment has not been investigated or if only minimal, anecdotal evidence exists, the physician must fully inform the athlete of the experimental nature of the treatment. If a physician has participated in the development of a treatment as an inventor, industry consultant, or researcher, this information also must be disclosed. The physician may need to seek the informal advice of physician colleagues before considering an unproved or experimental treatment. The team physician should fully convey the risks and benefits associated with a treatment so the physician and the athlete can cooperatively arrive at an informed decision.[2]

Summary

The sports medicine clinical environment is unique in that medical decision making often involves conflicts of interest related to the physician-patient-team triad. Athletes, teams, and physicians are subject to real and perceived pressures that are exacerbated by the increasing media visibility and economic impact of sports in modern society. Team physicians are required to deal with situations in which the long-term health interests of an athlete are in conflict with short-term individual or team success. The medical treatment of athletes sometimes requires following legal and ethical guidelines that reflect a delicate balance among beneficence, autonomy, and confidentiality to achieve optimal care of an athlete. Physicians should actively identify the pressures that can motivate athletes and teams and should treat an athlete within a shared decision-making model that engenders trust. Informed consent always should be sought to preserve the athlete's autonomous decision-making ability. An athlete's informed decision that opposes the advice of the team physician should be respected, and an ongoing cooperative relationship should be pursued. Patient autonomy may need to be sacrificed, however, if there is a significant risk of harm to the athlete or others. In a rapidly changing environment, team physicians are obligated to remain aware of national organization recommendations as well as state and federal legislation related to the ethical care of the athlete.

Key Study Points

- The practice of sports medicine is confronted with a wide range of ethical dilemmas because of the considerable external pressures and potential conflicts of interest that may promote the sacrifice of long-term health outcomes for short-term benefit and athletic success.

- The physician-patient-team triad is a unique health care model with important implications for patient confidentiality, autonomy, and beneficence.

- As a health care provider, the team physician is obligated to identify and minimize conflicts of interest (for both himself/herself and the patient) in pursuit of a shared decision-making model that facilitates truly informed consent and protects patient autonomy.

- Team physicians are obligated to remain up to date on emerging therapeutic modalities, sport science, and the relevant legislation to ensure that athletes are truly informed before participating in unproven or experimental modalities.

Annotated References

1. Mathias MB: The competing demands of sport and health: An essay on the history of ethics in sports medicine. *Clin Sports Med* 2004;23(2):195-214, vi.

2. Dunn WR, George MS, Churchill L, Spindler KP: Ethics in sports medicine. *Am J Sports Med* 2007;35(5):840-844.

3. Bernstein J, Perlis C, Bartolozzi AR: Normative ethics in sports medicine. *Clin Orthop Relat Res* 2004;420:309-318.

4. Goldman B, Bush PJ, Klatz R: *Death in the Locker Room: Steroids and Sports.* South Bend, IN, Icarus Press, 1984.

5. Holm S, McNamee MJ, Pigozzi F: Ethical practice and sports physician protection: A proposal. *Br J Sports Med* 2011;45(15):1170-1173.

   The authors present a proposal for the navigation of the ethical dilemmas that confront the sports medicine physician. They argue that the contexts are varied, but not unique, and can be approached by drawing on the ethics of public health.

6. Stovitz SD, Satin DJ: Ethics and the athlete: Why sports are more than a game but less than a war. *Clin Sports Med* 2004;23(2):215-225, vi.

7. Testoni D, Hornik CP, Smith PB, Benjamin DK Jr, McKinney RE Jr: Sports medicine and ethics. *Am J Bioeth* 2013;13(10):4-12.

   The authors provide a thorough evaluation of the ethical principles that should guide sports medicine physicians in their approach to the care of athletes. They specifically address the implications of paternalistic versus shared decision-making models.

8. American College of Sports Medicine: Code of Ethics. Available at http://www.acsm.org/join-acsm/membership-resources/code-of-ethics. Accessed November 14, 2014.

   The code of ethics from the American College of Sports Medicine provides the practicing team physician with guidance to deal with the unique ethical dilemmas confronted in clinical practice.

9. American Medical Association: Code of Medical Ethics. http://www.ama-assn.org/ama/pub/physician-resources/medical-ethics/code-medical-ethics/opinion306.page? Accessed November 10, 2014.

   This code from the American Medical Association provides guidelines for clinical practice in the care of athletes. It identifies potential conflicts of interest for both athletes and physicians and makes recommendations for how to approach them ethically.

10. International Federation of Sports Medicine: Code of Ethics. Available at http://www.fims.org/en/general/code-of-ethics/. Accessed November 10, 2014.

The guidelines provided by this governing body attempt help the practicing team physician identify and manage ethical dilemmas in the care of athletes.

11. Greenfield BH, West CR: Ethical issues in sports medicine: A review and justification for ethical decision making and reasoning. *Sports Health* 2012;4(6):475-479.

    The authors present the inherent difficulty for healthcare providers in making return-to-play decisions for athletes, and the ethical principles that should guide proper decision-making.

12. Malcom NL: "Shaking it off" and "toughing it out": Socialization to pain and injury in girls' softball. *J Contemp Ethnogr* 2006;35(5):495-525.

13. Nixon HL: Social network analysis of sport: Emphasizing social-structure in sport sociology. *Sociol Sport J* 1993;10(3):315-321.

14. Hensinger RN: The principles of medical ethics in orthopaedic surgery. *J Bone Joint Surg Am* 1992;74(10):1439-1440.

15. Johnson R: The unique ethics of sports medicine. *Clin Sports Med* 2004;23(2):175-182.

16. Bunch WH, Dvonch VM: Informed consent in sports medicine. *Clin Sports Med* 2004;23(2):183-193, v.

17. Sim J: Sports medicine: Some ethical issues. *Br J Sports Med* 1993;27(2):95-100.

18. McCrory P, Meeuwisse WH, Aubry M, et al: Consensus statement on concussion in sport: The 4th International Conference on Concussion in Sport, Zurich, November 2012. *J Athl Train* 2013;48(4):554-575.

    This consensus statement uses the best available evidence to provide guidelines in the identification and management of sport-related concussion.

19. Magee JT, Almekinders LC, Taft TN: HIPAA and the team physician. *Sports Med Update* 2003:March-April;4-8.

20. Waddington I, Roderick M: Management of medical confidentiality in English professional football clubs: Some ethical problems and issues. *Br J Sports Med* 2002;36(2):118-123, discussion 123.

21. Kirschen MP, Tsou A, Nelson SB, Russell JA, Larriviere D; Ethics, Law, and Humanities Committee, a Joint Committee of the American Academy of Neurology, American Neurological Association, and Child Neurology Society: Legal and ethical implications in the evaluation and management of sports-related concussion. *Neurology* 2014;83(4):352-358.

    The authors present the ethical dilemma that faces the team physician in the context of identifying and managing sport-related concussion, and draw on a number of ethical principles to guide decision making.

22. Torres DM, Galetta KM, Phillips HW, et al: Sports-related concussion: Anonymous survey of a collegiate cohort. *Neurol Clin Pract* 2013;3(4):279-287.

    The authors present the results of a survey of collegiate athletes that suggests that although most are aware of the signs and symptoms of concussion, a large percentage reportedly knowingly withheld symptoms to continue participation.

23. Pelliccia A, Fagard R, Bjørnstad HH, et al; Study Group of Sports Cardiology of the Working Group of Cardiac Rehabilitation and Exercise Physiology; Working Group of Myocardial and Pericardial Diseases of the European Society of Cardiology: Recommendations for competitive sports participation in athletes with cardiovascular disease: A consensus document from the Study Group of Sports Cardiology of the Working Group of Cardiac Rehabilitation and Exercise Physiology and the Working Group of Myocardial and Pericardial Diseases of the European Society of Cardiology. *Eur Heart J* 2005;26(14):1422-1445.

24. Trusty JM, Beinborn DS, Jahangir A: Dysrhythmias and the athlete. *AACN Clin Issues* 2004;15(3):432-448.

25. Nemeth P, Bonnette TW: Genetic discrimination in employment. *Michigan Bar J* 2009: January; 42-45.

26. No pain, no gain: The dilemma of a team physician. *Br J Sports Med* 2001;35(3):141-142.

    This article outlines the Genetic Information Non-Discrimination Act and the prohibition against making employment decisions based on known genetic information.

6: Miscellaneous Topics

Chapter 35

Research Studies and Registries in Sports Medicine

Robert H. Brophy, MD   Matthew V. Smith, MD

Abstract

Prospective multicenter studies are an increasingly important component of medical research, including research related to orthopaedic surgery and sports medicine. Several recent publications related to rotator cuff disease, anterior cruciate ligament primary and revision reconstruction, and meniscus tears have resulted from prospective cohort studies and registries related to the shoulder and knee.

Keywords: anterior cruciate ligament reconstruction; meniscus tear; registry; rotator cuff tear

Introduction

The increasing emphasis on evidence-based medicine has led to a need for high-quality clinical research in orthopaedic surgery that is designed to improve patient care and identify risk factors for poor outcomes. For the purpose of conducting research or critically evaluating a published study to determine whether the conclusions are relevant to their clinical practice, orthopaedic surgeons must understand the fundamental principles of study design and statistical analysis.

Collaborative multicenter studies are increasingly important to orthopaedic surgery and sports medicine research. The importance of such studies cannot be overstated. By studying large cohorts from multiple sites, researchers are able to substantially increase the power

Dr. Brophy or an immediate family member has stock or stock options held in Ostesys; and serves as a board member, owner, officer, or committee member of the American Orthopaedic Society for Sports Medicine. Dr. Smith or an immediate family member serves as a paid consultant to ISTO Technologies.

and generalizability of research.[1] Multicenter studies are less common in orthopaedic surgery and sports medicine than in other medical specialties, although the gap is narrowing.[2]

There is an important distinction between prospective multicenter studies and registries. A prospective multicenter study is designed to collect data for the purpose of answering a specific question or set of questions. In contrast, a registry simply collects data on one or more types of surgical procedures. A research question can be investigated retrospectively in the context of a prospective multicenter study, but by design the research questions are retrospective in a registry-based study. The quality of a registry's data often is lower than that of a prospective cohort study's data. Although registry-based studies are useful, prospective multicenter studies generally provide a higher level of evidence and better-quality research.

Study Design

Research Question

Many important clinical questions cannot be answered completely with a single study. Instead, a series of studies, using different study designs, may be required to characterize the distribution of a disease or injury in a population (a descriptive study), investigate the risk factors for the disease or injury in the population (an analytic study), and evaluate the efficacy of treatment (an experimental study). The choice of a study design depends on an assessment of the accessibility of information, the prevalence of the disease in the population, and the findings of earlier research.

Several factors must be considered as a research protocol is developed. The starting point is identification of an important clinical question that is not adequately answered in the available literature. The research question is developed using the FINER criteria[3] (Feasible, Interesting, Novel, Ethical, Relevant) (Table 1). The study should be focused to answer a specific question. The research design also may provide insight into secondary

Table 1	
The FINER Criteria for Developing an Orthopaedic Research Question	
Criterion	**Defining Questions**
Feasible	Is the number of research subjects adequate?
	Does the research team have adequate technical expertise?
	Can the research be completed with the available time and money?
	Is the research manageable in scope?
Interesting	Is the research topic of interest to the investigator?
	Is the research topic of interest to orthopaedic surgeons?
Novel	Will the research results confirm or refute previous knowledge?
	Will the research provide new insight into what is already known?
	Will the research add to the body of knowledge?
Ethical	Will the research violate or uphold ethical principles?
Relevant	Will the research add to scientific knowledge?
	Will the research results lead to future additional research?

questions, but the primary outcome of interest should the main focus of the research design. When the primary research question has been formulated and the FINER criteria have been met, each component of the research protocol should be carefully considered. Fully vetting a study protocol before starting a research project is useful for identifying pitfalls that could impede the progress of the study or make it impossible to complete. Completing a research template helps to focus the research plan and ensure that key components of the study are thought out in advance (Table 2).

Research Hypothesis

With the exception of a purely descriptive study, most clinical research should be hypothesis driven. The null hypothesis (H_0) proposes that no difference exists between two variables. In contrast, the alternative hypothesis (H_A) proposes that a difference exists between two variables. The hypothesis should be specific to the primary outcome variable and should reflect the expected change in the primary outcome variable. For example, the following hypothesis statement is not sufficiently specific because the primary outcome variable is not clearly defined: "Patients with a full-thickness rotator cuff tear will have better outcomes after undergoing surgical treatment than nonsurgical treatment." This hypothesis must be refined to provide a precise statement of the expected outcome of the study, as in the following statement: "Patients with a full-thickness rotator cuff tear will have an average American Shoulder and Elbow Surgeons shoulder score 10 points higher after undergoing surgical treatment than after undergoing nonsurgical treatment."

Types of Studies

Studies can be observational or experimental. In an observational study, a population of interest is observed for a disease at a single point in time (a cross-sectional study), observed for exposure and resulting disease prospectively or retrospectively (a cohort study), or observed to determine the exposure history of those with and without a specific disease (a case-control study).[4] Observational studies can be descriptive or analytic. Analytic observational studies examine associations between exposure and disease. Descriptive studies examine the features of the study population such as the number of patients with a particular disease. Descriptive studies may establish the incidence or prevalence of a problem in a given population. Experimental studies evaluate an outcome of an intervention by assigning participants to a treatment and following them over time. Often an experimental study includes control subjects for comparison. The interventions may or may not be randomly assigned or blinded to participants and observers.

Case Report and Case Study

Case reports and case studies are observational studies that explore outcomes in a limited group of patients with a similar disease or with similar treatment of a disease. There are no control subjects, so the ability to make comparisons regarding treatment efficacy is limited, and it is difficult to critically evaluate causation. Such studies produce low-level evidence, but they are beneficial for describing treatment outcomes in uncommon diseases and can generate ideas for higher level controlled studies.

Table 2

Template for a Research Protocol

Component	Description
Study question	State the primary question the research aims to answer. The question should be focused and specific.
Significance	Describe why the research is important: • What is known? • What is unknown? • How will the study results be beneficial?
Hypothesis	State what you think the answer to the study question will be in specific terms.
Primary outcome	State the main outcome variable of interest.
Secondary outcome(s)	State other included outcome variables that may be important.
Study design	Describe the specific study design you intend to use to answer the study question.
Setting	Describe where the study will take place: • Who will be involved in subject recruitment? • Where will data be collected? • Will other institutions be included in the study?
Subjects	Describe the population you intend to study to answer the study question: • How many subjects will be enrolled? • How will subjects be recruited? • What are the inclusion and exclusion criteria?
Statistical approach	Describe the statistical methods you plan to use to analyze the data: • What criteria will be included in the power analysis? • What statistical tests will be used? • How do you plan to deal with missing or incomplete data?
Anticipated outcome	Describe how you think the findings from the study will add to the current literature

Case-Control Study

A case-control study is an observational study that analyzes the relationship between disease and exposure. The disease of interest already has occurred in the population of interest. The researcher selects an appropriately matched group of individuals who do not have the disease (control subjects) from the same source population as individuals with the disease (patients or cases). The exposure history of individuals in both groups is evaluated to identify risk factors for disease. The odds of an exposure in the control subjects compared with the patients provides an odds ratio (OR) for the disease related to the identified exposure.

Case-control studies provide evidence of causality between an exposure and the disease of interest. Conclusions regarding causality are limited by recall and sampling biases. This study design is useful for identifying possible causes of a relatively uncommon disease or little-known causes of a common disease. Case-control studies typically are less expensive and less time consuming than other studies that analyze causality, but they provide a lower level of evidence because of the inherent bias in the study design.

Cross-sectional Study

A cross-sectional study measures the prevalence of a disease. Prevalence is defined as the total number of incidences at a single point in time. Because a cross-sectional study identifies disease and exposure at the same time, it is helpful for identifying multiple possible risk factors for a disease in a specified population. Possible exposures can be identified for consideration in a cohort study. This type of study cannot provide a good assessment of the relationship between exposure and disease, and it is not suitable for identifying rare outcomes. A cross-sectional study is relatively quick and inexpensive to perform.

Cohort Study

Cohort studies are observational studies that can be descriptive by defining new incidences of disease or analytic by identifying risk factors for the development of disease. In cohort studies, an exposed study population is assessed over time for disease development. A cohort study can be prospective or retrospective. In a prospective cohort study, the exposed population is selected and followed for a period of time to identify the outcome of interest. For example, patients who undergo a partial meniscectomy (the exposure) are followed into the future to assess their risk for the development of osteoarthritis (the disease). Any additional factor that may influence the outcome, such as patient weight, sex, occupation, activity level, or trauma, is controlled for in the statistical analysis. The cohort study design provides a powerful assessment of the factors associated with the development of disease. Prospective cohort studies are advantageous because they reliably assess exposure without relying on recall of events by the study participants. The resulting evidence is relatively strong for cause and effect in the development of disease. The disadvantage of a prospective cohort study is that it is time consuming and often expensive to conduct.

In a retrospective cohort study, the exposure is in the past and the researcher is looking forward from the time of exposure to identify risk factors for the development of disease. For example, patients who underwent CT 10 years earlier can be followed during the subsequent study period to evaluate their risk for cancer. A retrospective cohort study provides a reasonable assessment of the risk factors associated with a disease, but its disadvantage is the limited reliability of information gathered from charts and information recall by study participants.

A retrospective case study looks backward in time to determine what exposure individuals with the disease of interest had. In contrast, a retrospective cohort study looks backward in time at individuals with a particular exposure to determine whether the disease developed. A retrospective cohort design provides the higher level of evidence for causality.

Often two cohorts from a given population, one group with exposure and the other without exposure, are followed for the same period of time (Figure 1). In such a dual cohort study, comparisons can be made about the risk of disease in those who were exposed or not exposed. Case-control studies provide an OR for a disease after an exposure. In contrast, cohort studies provide a relative risk (RR) of disease in individuals who were exposed or not exposed. The RR is defined as the incidence of the disease in individuals who were exposed divided by the incidence of the disease in individuals who were not exposed. The OR and the RR are not the same, although the figures calculated for them may be similar if the incidence of the disease is low. As the disease incidence increases, the discrepancy between the OR and the RR

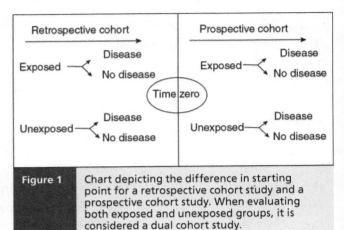

Figure 1   Chart depicting the difference in starting point for a retrospective cohort study and a prospective cohort study. When evaluating both exposed and unexposed groups, it is considered a dual cohort study.

also increases.

A nested case-control study can be performed from cohort study data. Cohort study data on participants who develop the disease can be analyzed with detailed exposure information. Exposure frequency in these participants can be compared with that of control subjects in the same cohort.

Cohort studies also provide disease incidence data. The incidence is defined as the number of new occurrences of the disease in the population during a specific time period. The disease incidence can be derived from a cohort study in which a population is evaluated repeatedly over time. Disease incidence is distinctly different from disease prevalence. The duration of the disease affects both the incidence and the prevalence. For example, if shoulder pain in a baseball pitcher typically is resolved when the pitcher stops throwing, the prevalence of shoulder pain in baseball pitchers may be high during the baseball season and low during the off-season, regardless of the incidence over the entire year. However, the incidence of osteoarthritis may be low during a specific year but the prevalence of osteoarthritis still will be high because osteoarthritis is a chronic, permanent disease.

Clinical Study

Clinical studies are experimental studies that evaluate the outcome in patients who undergo an intervention compared with control subjects. Clinical studies can be randomized or nonrandomized. Blinding observers and participants to treatment-arm assignments further reduces inherent bias. Blinded outcomes observation is difficult to achieve in surgical studies. Randomization reduces the inherent bias in the study by balancing the variables across the study groups. Randomization may not be possible if it would violate the need for clinical equipoise, however. Although randomized studies are considered the gold standard of clinical evidence for therapeutic studies, many clinical questions involve surgical intervention and are not amenable to a randomized control study. Randomized controlled studies are expensive, complex, and time consuming to conduct.

Systematic Review

A systematic review is a summary of the available published studies with an evaluation of their quality. The strength of the evidence in a systematic review is only as good as the study with the lowest level of evidence that is included in the analysis. A systematic review of high-level evidence that combines the information from several well-done studies provides the highest level of evidence. If the outcome measures used in the studies are similar, a meta-analysis of the data can provide strength to the conclusions by adding power to the studies. Both systematic reviews and meta-analyses can identify areas of weakness that future studies can build on. The challenges in conducting a systematic review lie in identifying a focused question, using strict inclusion and exclusion criteria, and dealing with the heterogeneity of the included studies.

Statistics

Type I and Type II Errors

The use of probabilities in hypothesis testing carries a risk of falsely rejecting or accepting the null hypothesis.[5] A false rejection of the null hypothesis, also called a type I or α error, consists of a decision that a difference exists between groups, when in fact there is no difference. The α value is a standard set before the statistical analysis is conducted and is used to determine how extreme an observed result must be to allow the null hypothesis to be rejected; the purpose is to minimize the risk of a type I error. The α value typically is set at 0.05 but can be adjusted if the research question requires tighter control for false-positive results. An α value of 0.05 simply means that, under the null hypothesis, a result at least this extreme will occur by chance 5% of the time.

A false acceptance of the null hypothesis, also called a type II or β error, consists of a decision that that there is no difference between groups when in fact there is a difference. Stated differently, it is the failure to detect a difference when a difference is present. To minimize the risk of a type II error, the sample size must be adequate to detect the magnitude of difference between the comparison groups. To detect a small change, the sample size needs to be larger. The generally accepted chance of a type II error in a study is 20%, but this percentage can be adjusted if it is important to minimize the number of false-negative results in the research outcomes.

Power Analysis

Power in a study is defined as the likelihood of detecting a true positive result. Usually studies are powered to an 80% likelihood of detecting a true positive result. Power analysis takes into consideration type II (or β) error. If the accepted type II error is 20%, the power is 1- β or 80%. If the chance of false negative results needs to be decreased for the study question to 10% or 5%, the power can be changed to 90% or 95% (1-β). Increasing the power increases the number of subjects needed for the study. A power analysis is needed for comparison studies so that an adequate sample size is available to avoid a type II error.[5] A power analysis includes the α value, the β value, the variability of the data, and the expected change in the outcome of interest (the effect size).

Variables

A variable is a measurable trait that has a changing value. A variable is either categorical; or continuous. Statistical tests are chosen based on the type of outcome variable. When designing or critically analyzing a research study, it is important to understand which statistical tests are appropriate for use with a particular type of variable. A categorical variable is assigned a specific rank (ordinal) or name (nominal). For example, the tumor stage in a patient with cancer is an ordinal variable, and the patient's sex is a nominal variable. A continuous variable changes along a continuum of values. Continuous variables can be nondiscrete or discrete. A nondiscrete variable can take on any value along a continuum; weight, temperature, and amount of surgical blood loss are examples. Nondiscrete values can be fractionated. A discrete variable is a specific value, such as the number of hospital admissions or surgical procedures per year. Discrete values cannot be fractionated. For example, a patient can weigh 150.2 lb (a nondiscrete value), but an individual surgeon cannot perform 35.2 surgical procedures in 1 month (a discrete value).

Descriptive statistics often are used to describe continuous data (Figure 2). Descriptive statistics help to find the central tendency of the data and determine its distribution.[6] The mean (average), median (middle number in the dataset), and mode (most common number in the dataset) are examples of descriptive statistics. Mean, median, and mode do not describe the dispersion of the data. Variance and standard deviation (SD) define the dispersion of the data from the mean.[6] The dispersion of the data is closer to the mean as variance and SD values become closer.

Descriptive statistics are used to determine whether the data are normally distributed in the study population. Normally distributed data should appear as a bell-shaped curve when plotted with a histogram. Many statistical

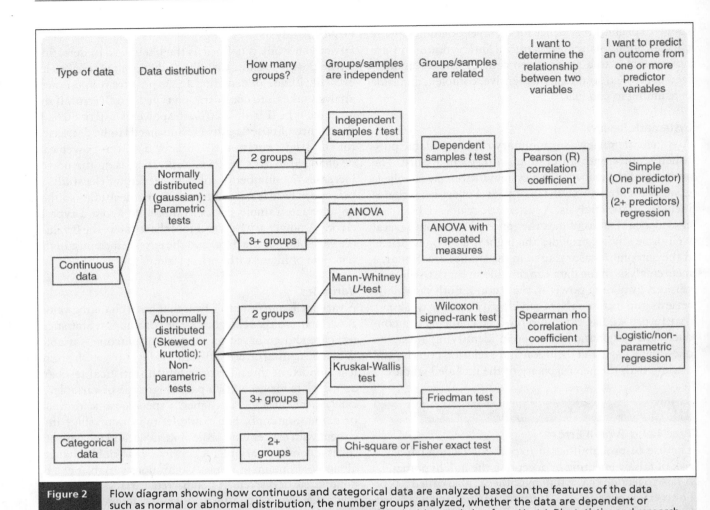

Figure 2 Flow diagram showing how continuous and categorical data are analyzed based on the features of the data such as normal or abnormal distribution, the number groups analyzed, whether the data are dependent or independent, and whether correlations exist. (Reproduced with permission from Hart J: Biostatistics and research design, in Miller M, Thompson S, eds: *Review of Orthopaedics*, ed 7. Philadelphia, PA, Elsevier, 2015, figure 13-6.)

(parametric) tests used to analyze continuous data assume a normal distribution of the data to estimate probability. Given a normal distribution, there is a 34% probability that a randomly selected data point from the sample population falls between the mean and 1 SD above or below the mean. Therefore, there is an approximately 68% chance that a randomly selected data point from the sample population will be within 1 SD from the mean. Similarly, there is a 95% probability that a randomly selected data point from the population is within 2 SDs from the mean.

In hypothesis testing using normally distributed continuous variables, probabilities are used to compare outcomes across the study population. For example, if a researcher wants to compare the effects of Treatment A and Treatment B in the study population, statistical tests will provide a probability (a *P* value) that a difference between the treatment effects exists or not. Given an α set at 0.05, if the mean and SD distribution of Treatment

A does not fall within the value 95% probability distribution of Treatment B, there is a statistically significant difference between the two variables. Because hypothesis testing deals with probability, it is inaccurate to say the null hypothesis or the alternative hypothesis is absolutely correct or incorrect. Rather, we reject the null hypothesis in favor of the alternative hypothesis.

Means Comparison

The Student *t* test is a statistical test used to compare the means of continuous variables between two groups. The Student *t* test assumes that the variables are independent and the data are normally distributed. An unpaired Student *t* test compares means from unrelated groups. A paired Student *t* test compares means from the same subject taken on separate occasions.[7,8] This test is not useful for comparing more than two means. Analysis of variance (ANOVA) is used to compare three or more means.

Comparing means with data that are not normally distributed requires a nonparametric statistical test. Non-parametric tests do not rely on the inferences of probability based on normal distribution of the data.[8] Ordinal variables are not normally distributed and, therefore, they require a nonparametric test. The sign test can be used when two observations from the study population are not independent, as in a paired Student t test. The difference between the observations is labeled as positive or negative depending on whether an increase or decrease occurred between the observations.[8] The number of positive and negative changes is used in the statistical analysis. The Wilcoxon signed-rank test is more commonly used than the sign test for two independent, nonnormally distributed groups.[8] As in the sign test, a positive or negative sign is applied, but the magnitude of difference is ranked and included in the analysis.

Categorical Data Analysis

The analysis of nominal data or other categorical data is different from that of continuous data. Continuous data sometimes also are categorical. To measure the association between categorical variables, the chi-square (χ^2) test is used to examine the proportion (frequency) of events. A chi-square test compares the observed frequency of events to the expected frequency of events.[9] This test does not provide a measure of the magnitude of the association, but it does provide a P value indicating whether there is an association. If the study is small, a chi-square analysis is not accurate, and a Fisher exact test should be used.

Correlation and Regression Analysis

Correlation establishes whether a relationship exists between two continuous, nondependent variables. Both correlation and regression analysis quantify the extent of the linear relationship between variables. The Pearson correlation coefficient, called r, is the interdependent association between two variables. An r equal to 1 indicates a perfect positive correlation. An r equal to −1 indicates a perfect negative correlation. An r equal to 0 indicates no correlation. A correlation coefficient does not imply causality, and it assumes that the data are normally distributed. If the data are not normally distributed a Spearman rank coefficient can be used.

Linear regression analysis seeks to use one or more variables (simple or multiple regression) to predict another variable.[8] To use linear regression, the outcome variable must be continuous. Linear regression assumes there is a linear relationship between variables. Logistic regression is used if the outcome of interest is categoric. For logistic regression, the data are logarithmically transformed to obtain the logarithmic odds. Logistic regression is then used to identify variables that are predictors for the outcome of interest, estimate the OR of the outcome for each one-unit change in the predictor, and estimate the absolute risk of the outcome of interest.[8] Multiple regression analysis, which is performed in linear and logistic regression, allows modeling of several variables while controlling for others. In addition, multiple regression analysis identifies potential interaction between predictor variables that affect the outcome variable.

Survival Analysis

Survival analysis is a nonparametric test that evaluates the probability of an event over a period of time, and it is used if one variable explains the time to an event such as death or hospital readmission. The Kaplan-Meier method of survival analysis calculates the cumulative probability of an event (and survival) based on conditional probabilities at each event time.[8] A Kaplan-Meier curve is most commonly used for a graphic display of survival probability. Cox proportional hazard modeling can assess the effect of multiple covariables on survival.

Multicenter and Registry-Based Research in Sports Medicine

Shoulder Research

The Multicenter Orthopaedic Outcomes Network (MOON) Shoulder Group was formed to conduct large multicenter studies on conditions of the shoulder.[10] The MOON Shoulder Group is made up of 16 fellowship-trained orthopaedic surgeons and research personnel from nine academic and private practice sites in the United States. The group initially was formed to identify research questions related to treatment of rotator cuff disease but has expanded its scope to include other shoulder pathology. To study rotator cuff disease, the group developed and standardized imaging protocols, assembled validated patient-oriented outcome forms, and conducted validation studies on the classification of rotator cuff tears based on MRI and arthroscopy videotapes as well as radiographic findings associated with rotator cuff disease.[11-13] After a systematic review to determine the effectiveness of physical therapy for treatment of rotator cuff disease, a standard physical therapy protocol was developed based on the evidence.[14] This process led to a prospective study of nonsurgical treatment of atraumatic full-thickness rotator cuff tears in a population of patients with symptoms, fewer than 25% of whom underwent surgery within the next 2 years.[10] Subsequent studies found that duration of symptoms, pain, and activity level were not correlated with the severity of rotator cuff disease in this population.[15-17]

6: Miscellaneous Topics

Knee Research
MOON Knee Group

The MOON Knee Group was formed in 1993 and evolved into a network consisting of seven institutions (Cleveland Clinic Foundation, OH; Hospital for Special Surgery, NY; The Ohio State University, OH; University of Colorado, CO; University of Iowa, IA; Vanderbilt Orthopaedic Institute, TN; Washington University, MO) and 17 surgeons. To establish a model for prospective, longitudinal, hypothesis-driven research, the MOON Knee Group began with interrater agreement among surgeons and focused on patient-reported outcomes.[18] Within 10 years, this group generated more than 40 publications. More than 4,400 patients were enrolled in a prospective study of anterior cruciate ligament (ACL) reconstruction. Recent publications included predictors of activity level and subsequent surgery after ACL reconstruction.[19,20] A significant interaction was found between activity level and graft choice with respect to the success or failure of ACL reconstruction.[21] Outcomes and return to play data were reported after ACL reconstruction in football and soccer players, and reconstruction was found to be a cost-effective treatment of ACL tears based on the MOON data.[22-24]

Multicenter ACL Revision Study

The finding of MOON and other studies that revision ACL reconstruction was associated with worse outcomes than primary ACL reconstruction provided the impetus for formation of the Multicenter ACL Revision Study (MARS).[25-27] This prospective longitudinal cohort study was developed through the American Orthopaedic Society for Sports Medicine (AOSSM), which has more than 2,000 members from private practice and academic settings predominantly in the United States and Canada. MARS was designed with multiple sites and multiple surgeons to determine modifiable predictors of outcome after revision ACL reconstruction.[28] All AOSSM members were invited to participate in MARS, and four training sessions were provided. Participating surgeons were required to read the final manual of operating procedures, obtain institutional review board approval, complete a trial data form, and sign an agreement to follow the manual of operating procedures. A total of 83 surgeons from 52 US and Canadian sites have enrolled patients in the study.[28]

Initial MARS cohort reports were on the epidemiology of the revision ACL reconstructions and reflected slightly more allograft use than autograft use (54% and 45%, respectively), with just over 1% using combined autograft and allograft.[28] Only 10% of patients had intact menisci and articular cartilage at the time of revision ACL reconstruction.[28] A comparison of knees at the time of revision ACL reconstruction and primary ACL reconstruction found that knees undergoing revision ACL reconstruction were less likely to have new lateral meniscus tears but more likely to have lateral compartment and patellar-trochlear chondral damage.[29] Previous partial meniscectomy but not previous meniscus repair was significantly associated with chondrosis at the time of revision ACL reconstruction.[30] Patients undergoing initial revision ACL reconstruction had higher activity levels, were less likely to have chondral damage in the medial and patellofemoral compartments, and had a higher rate of traumatic, recurrent injury of their graft compared to patients undergoing a multiple revision.[31]

Early Arthritis Therapies Study

The Early Arthritis Therapies (EARTH) study of patients with ACL is being developed by AOSSM. A feasibility study found that 93% of healthy adults age 18 to 30 years who had an ACL tear without earlier joint injury would be willing to participate in a randomized controlled study of early interventions to prevent osteoarthritis.[32]

ACL Registries

Several studies recently have been published from ACL registries in Denmark, Sweden, Norway, and the United States. The initial reports focused on epidemiology and early results.[33,34] The Norwegian registry study found that the risk of cartilage injury increased with the length of time between ACL injury and reconstruction.[35] This finding was reinforced by the findings of the US-based Kaiser Permanente ACL Registry.[36] In comparison with patients in the MOON cohort, the patients in the Norwegian registry were more likely to be men, were older, and were less likely to have an allograft.[37] The Kaiser Permanente ACL Registry was more similar to the Norwegian registry than the MOON Knee cohort in terms of patient age and sex.[38] Bone–patellar tendon–bone autografts were found to be used more often in relatively young male patients and by surgeons and centers with a high volume of such procedures.[39] A study that combined the Norwegian and Kaiser registries reported a higher incidence of concomitant medial collateral ligament injuries with ACL tears among American football players than basketball players; basketball players were more likely to have cartilage and lateral meniscus injuries.[40] In the Kaiser registry, patients who underwent primary and subsequent revision ACL reconstruction were more likely to have chondral injury and less likely to have a meniscus injury at the time of revision than at the primary surgery.[41]

As longitudinal studies from these registries are reported, the difficulty of patient follow-up has become apparent; follow-up percentages of 41%, 40% to 64%, and 54% of patients have been reported.[42-44] However, the completeness of registration (the percentage of ACL reconstructions captured in the registry) in the Danish registry increased from 60% in 2005 to 86% in 2011.[45]

Despite these challenges, interesting findings have been reported. The short-term reoperation rate after ACL reconstruction was low in the Kaiser registry, and approximately half of reoperations were related to the meniscus.[46] Another study from the Kaiser registry reported that hamstring autografts were associated with a higher rate of deep infection after ACL reconstruction than other types of grafts.[47] Studies from the Danish and Norwegian registries and a pooled analysis of the Scandinavian registries found a higher rate of revision ACL reconstruction when hamstring rather than bone–patellar tendon–bone autograft was used in the primary ACL reconstruction.[48-50] In the Swedish registry study, the risk of contralateral ACL injury was almost three times greater in patients younger than 20 years than in older patients.[51]

Meniscal Tear in Osteoarthritis Research Study

The Meniscal Tear in Osteoarthritis Research (METEOR) study was designed to compare the efficacy of arthroscopic partial meniscectomy with that of a standardized physical therapy regimen for patients with a symptomatic meniscus tear and concomitant mild to moderate osteoarthritis.[52] This US National Institutes of Health–funded prospective, randomized controlled study was conducted at seven academic medical centers (Brigham and Women's Hospital, MA; Cleveland Clinic, OH; Hospital for Special Surgery, NY; Mayo Clinic, MN; Rush University Medical Center, IL; Vanderbilt University, TN; Washington University, MO). In this study, 351 patients age 45 years or older with a meniscus tear and imaging evidence of mild to moderate osteoarthritis were randomly assigned to surgery and postoperative physical therapy or to a standardized physical therapy regimen (with the option to cross over to surgery at the discretion of the patient and surgeon).[53] In an intention-to-treat analysis, functional improvement based on the Western Ontario and McMaster Universities Osteoarthritis Index physical function score did not differ significantly after 6 months, although there was a 30% crossover to surgery in patients assigned to physical therapy alone.

Summary

An understanding of fundamental principles is required for successful sports medicine research. Multicenter cohort and research registry studies are becoming more common in orthopaedic sports medicine. Despite the challenges of designing and implementing such complex research efforts, the potential rewards are significant. Recent publications from such studies provided important information on the treatment of rotator cuff disease, ACL reconstruction, revision ACL reconstruction, and meniscus tears. To elevate the level of evidence and the generalizability of future research, orthopaedic sports medicine organizations should continue to invest in these studies.

Key Study Points

- An understanding of the fundamental principles and terminology of research and the potential benefits of prospective multicenter research cohort studies and registry-based studies will lead to improved patient care.

- An understanding of the primary published findings of such studies as related to the shoulder and knee in orthopaedic sports medicine can help improve outcomes.

Annotated References

1. Sprague S, Matta JM, Bhandari M, et al; Anterior Total Hip Arthroplasty Collaborative (ATHAC) Investigators: Multicenter collaboration in observational research: Improving generalizability and efficiency. *J Bone Joint Surg Am* 2009;91(Suppl 3):80-86.

   The successful conduct of multicenter studies requires careful study organization, a dedicated and experienced methods center, and motivated participating surgeons and study staff at the clinical sites as illustrated by a total hip arthroplasty collaborative.

2. Brophy RH, Smith MV, Latterman C, et al: Multi-investigator collaboration in orthopaedic surgery research compared to other medical fields. *J Orthop Res* 2012;30(10):1523-1528.

   Orthopaedic surgery has fewer publications from collaborative research and contributing authors and institutions than other medical specialties. There is an opportunity to stimulate this type of research in orthopaedic surgery. Level of evidence: IV.

3. Farrugia P, Petrisor BA, Farrokhyar F, Phil M, Bhandari M: Research questions, hypotheses and objectives. *Can J Surg* . 2010;53(4):278-281.

4. Kuhn JE, Greenfield ML, Wojtys EM: A statistics primer: Types of studies in the medical literature. *Am J Sports Med* 1997;25(2):272-274.

5. Kuhn JE, Greenfield ML, Wojtys EM: A statistics primer: Hypothesis testing. *Am J Sports Med* 1996;24(5):702-703.

6. Greenfield ML, Kuhn JE, Wojtys EM: A statistics primer: Descriptive measures for continuous data. *Am J Sports Med* 1997;25:720-723.

7. Greenfield ML, Wojtys EM, Kuhn JE: A statistics primer: Tests for continuous data. *Am J Sports Med* 1997;25(6):882-884.

8. Pagano M, Gauvreau K: *Principles of Biostatistics,* ed 2. Independence, KY, Cengage Learning, 2000.

9. Kuhn JE, Greenfield ML, Wojtys EM: A statistics primer: Statistical tests for discrete data. *Am J Sports Med* 1997;25(4):585-586.

10. Kuhn JE, Dunn WR, Sanders R, et al; MOON Shoulder Group: Effectiveness of physical therapy in treating atraumatic full-thickness rotator cuff tears: A multicenter prospective cohort study. *J Shoulder Elbow Surg* 2013;22(10):1371-1379.

    Nonsurgical treatment using physical therapy is effective for treating atraumatic full-thickness rotator cuff tears in approximately 75% of patients followed up for 2 years. Level of evidence: IV.

11. Baumgarten KM, Carey JL, Abboud JA, et al: Reliability of determining and measuring acromial enthesophytes. *HSS J* 2011;7(3):218-222.

    There is fair to moderate reliability among fellowship-trained shoulder surgeons in determining the presence of an acromial enthesophyte but poor reliability among observers in measuring the size of the enthesophyte. Level of evidence: IV.

12. Kuhn JE, Dunn WR, Ma B, et al; Multicenter Orthopaedic Outcomes Network-Shoulder (MOON Shoulder Group): Interobserver agreement in the classification of rotator cuff tears. *Am J Sports Med* 2007;35(3):437-441.

13. Spencer EE Jr, Dunn WR, Wright RW, et al; Shoulder Multicenter Orthopaedic Outcomes Network: Interobserver agreement in the classification of rotator cuff tears using magnetic resonance imaging. *Am J Sports Med* 2008;36(1):99-103.

14. Kuhn JE: Exercise in the treatment of rotator cuff impingement: A systematic review and a synthesized evidence-based rehabilitation protocol. *J Shoulder Elbow Surg* 2009;18(1):138-160.

    This systematic review demonstrated that exercise has statistically and clinically significant effects on pain reduction and improving function, but not on range of motion or strength for patients with rotator cuff impingement. Level of evidence: II.

15. Unruh KP, Kuhn JE, Sanders R, et al; MOON Shoulder Group: The duration of symptoms does not correlate with rotator cuff tear severity or other patient-related features: A cross-sectional study of patients with atraumatic, full-thickness rotator cuff tears. *J Shoulder Elbow Surg* 2014;23(7):1052-1058.

    In patients with atraumatic, full-thickness rotator cuff tears, duration of symptoms does not correlate with more severe rotator cuff disease, weakness, limited range of motion, tear size, fatty atrophy, or validated patient-reported outcome measures. Level of evidence: III.

16. Dunn WR, Kuhn JE, Sanders R, et al: Symptoms of pain do not correlate with rotator cuff tear severity: A cross-sectional study of 393 patients with a symptomatic atraumatic full-thickness rotator cuff tear. *J Bone Joint Surg Am* 2014;96(10):793-800.

    In patients with atraumatic, full-thickness rotator cuff tears, anatomic features defining the severity of atraumatic rotator cuff tears are not associated with pain level, whereas comorbidities, lower education level, and race are associated with pain level. Level of evidence: III.

17. Brophy RH, Dunn WR, Kuhn JE; MOON Shoulder Group: Shoulder activity level is not associated with the severity of symptomatic, atraumatic rotator cuff tears in patients electing nonoperative treatment. *Am J Sports Med* 2014;42(5):1150-1154.

    In patients with atraumatic, full-thickness rotator cuff tears, shoulder activity level is not associated with severity of the tear but is associated with patient age, sex, and occupation. Level of evidence: III.

18. Lynch TS, Parker RD, Patel RM, Andrish JT, Spindler KP; MOON Group: The impact of the Multicenter Orthopaedic Outcomes Network (MOON) research on anterior cruciate ligament reconstruction and orthopaedic practice. *J Am Acad Orthop Surg* 2015;23(3):154-163.

    The Multicenter Orthopaedic Outcomes Network consortium has enrolled more than 4,400 ACL reconstructions to establish a large level I prospective cohort. Studies from this cohort support the use of autograft for competitive athletes in their primary ACL reconstructions.

19. Dunn WR, Spindler KP; MOON Consortium: Predictors of activity level 2 years after anterior cruciate ligament reconstruction (ACLR): A Multicenter Orthopaedic Outcomes Network (MOON) ACLR cohort study. *Am J Sports Med* 2010;38(10):2040-2050.

    Higher baseline activity and lower body mass index predicted higher activity levels 2 years after ACL reconstruction while revision ACL reconstruction, smoking within 6 months of surgery, and female sex predicted lower activity levels. Level of evidence: II.

20. Hettrich CM, Dunn WR, Reinke EK, Spindler KP; MOON Group: The rate of subsequent surgery and predictors after anterior cruciate ligament reconstruction: Two- and 6-year follow-up results from a multicenter cohort. *Am J Sports Med* 2013;41(7):1534-1540.

    The rate of subsequent surgery is 18.9% on the ipsilateral knee within 6 years of ACL reconstruction, higher in younger patients and allograft reconstructions. There is a similar rate of ipsilateral graft tears (7.7%) and contralateral ACL tears (6.4%). Level of evidence: III.

© 2016 American Academy of Orthopaedic Surgeons

21. Kaeding CC, Aros B, Pedroza A, et al: Allograft versus autograft anterior cruciate ligament reconstruction: Predictors of failure from a MOON prospective longitudinal cohort. *Sports Health* 2011;3(1):73-81.

Patient age and ACL graft type predict graft failure following ACL reconstruction. Highest percentages of failures occurred in patients 10 to 19 years of age. Odds of graft rupture are four times higher with allograft than with autograft reconstructions.

22. McCullough KA, Phelps KD, Spindler KP, et al; MOON Group: Return to high school- and college-level football after anterior cruciate ligament reconstruction: A Multicenter Orthopaedic Outcomes Network (MOON) cohort study. *Am J Sports Med* 2012;40(11):2523-2529.

Return to football after ACL reconstruction was 63% in high school athletes and 69% in collegiate athletes. Only 43% reported getting back to the same self-described level of performance. Level of evidence: III.

23. Brophy RH, Schmitz L, Wright RW, et al: Return to play and future ACL injury risk after ACL reconstruction in soccer athletes from the Multicenter Orthopaedic Outcomes Network (MOON) group. *Am J Sports Med* 2012;40(11):2517-2522.

Return to soccer after ACL reconstruction was 72%, higher in younger and male athletes. There was a 3% risk of graft re-tear and a 9% risk of contralateral ACL tear. Level of evidence: III.

24. Mather RC III, Koenig L, Kocher MS, et al; MOON Knee Group: Societal and economic impact of anterior cruciate ligament tears. *J Bone Joint Surg Am* 2013;95(19):1751-1759.

ACL reconstruction is the preferred cost-effective treatment strategy for ACL tears compared to rehabilitation, reducing societal costs once indirect cost factors, such as work status and earnings, are considered.

25. Wright R, Spindler K, Huston L, et al: Revision ACL reconstruction outcomes: MOON cohort. *J Knee Surg* 2011;24(4):289-294.

Revision ACL reconstruction resulted in a significantly worse outcome as measured by Knee Injury and Osteoarthritis Outcome Scores, Knee Related Quality of Life, Sports and Recreation and Pain subscales, International Knee Documentation Committee, and Marx activity level at 2 years compared to primary ACL reconstruction.

26. Wright RW, Gill CS, Chen L, et al: Outcome of revision anterior cruciate ligament reconstruction: A systematic review. *J Bone Joint Surg Am* 2012;94(6):531-536.

Revision ACL reconstruction has nearly three to four times the failure rate of primary ACL reconstructions. Patient-reported outcome scores were inferior compared to previously published results of primary ACL reconstruction, but these differences may not be clinically important.

27. Lind M, Menhert F, Pedersen AB: Incidence and outcome after revision anterior cruciate ligament reconstruction: Results from the Danish registry for knee ligament reconstructions. *Am J Sports Med* 2012;40(7):1551-1557.

The rate of revision following primary ACL reconstruction was 4.1% compared to 5.4% following revision ACL reconstruction after 5 years in the Danish knee registry. Age younger than 20 years was associated with a higher revision rate following primary ACL reconstruction. Level of evidence: II.

28. Wright RW, Huston LJ, Spindler KP, et al; MARS Group: Descriptive epidemiology of the Multicenter ACL Revision Study (MARS) cohort. *Am J Sports Med* 2010;38(10):1979-1986.

Surgeons deemed traumatic reinjury to be the most common single mode of failure for knees undergoing revision ACL reconstruction. A combination of factors represented the most common mode of failure. Over 90% of knees had meniscal and/or cartilage injury. Level of evidence: II.

29. Borchers JR, Kaeding CC, Pedroza AD, Huston LJ, Spindler KP, Wright RW; MOON Consortium and the MARS Group: Intra-articular findings in primary and revision anterior cruciate ligament reconstruction surgery: A comparison of the MOON and MARS study groups. *Am J Sports Med* 2011;39(9):1889-1893.

Meniscal tears are common in primary and revision ACL reconstruction. Previous medial or lateral meniscectomy increases the OR of articular cartilage damage in the corresponding compartment. Revisions are more likely to have significant lateral compartment and patellar-trochlear chondral damage. Level of evidence: II.

30. Brophy RH, Wright RW, David TS, et al; Multicenter ACL Revision Study (MARS) Group: Association between previous meniscal surgery and the incidence of chondral lesions at revision anterior cruciate ligament reconstruction. *Am J Sports Med* 2012;40(4):808-814.

The status of articular cartilage at revision ACL reconstruction relates to previous meniscal surgery. Previous partial meniscectomy is associated with a higher incidence of articular cartilage damage, whereas previous meniscal repair is not. Level of evidence: II.

31. Chen JL, Allen CR, Stephens TE, et al; Multicenter ACL Revision Study (MARS) Group: Differences in mechanisms of failure, intraoperative findings, and surgical characteristics between single- and multiple-revision ACL reconstructions: A MARS cohort study. *Am J Sports Med* 2013;41(7):1571-1578.

Compared to initial revisions, multiple-revision ACL reconstructions have lower activity levels, more chondral injuries in the medial and patellofemoral compartments, and higher rate of nontraumatic, recurrent graft injury. Level of evidence: III.

32. Chu CR, Beynnon BD, Dragoo JL, et al; EARTH Group: The feasibility of randomized controlled trials for early arthritis therapies (EARTH) involving acute anterior cruciate ligament tear cohorts. *Am J Sports Med* 2012;40(11):2648-2652.

Adequate sample sizes to perform randomized controlled trials of early intervention strategies in ACL-injured cohorts comprising healthy young adults ages 18 to 30 years without prior joint injuries can be achieved.

33. Granan LP, Forssblad M, Lind M, Engebretsen L: The Scandinavian ACL registries 2004-2007: Baseline epidemiology. *Acta Orthop* 2009;80(5):563-567.

   The annual incidence of primary ACL reconstructions is higher in Denmark than Norway, except in young females. Despite a similar approach among Scandinavian surgeons, differences exist regarding graft and implant choice and treatment of simultaneous meniscal and cartilage injuries.

34. Lind M, Menhert F, Pedersen AB: The first results from the Danish ACL reconstruction registry: Epidemiologic and 2 year follow-up results from 5,818 knee ligament reconstructions. *Knee Surg Sports Traumatol Arthrosc* 2009;17(2):117-124.

   The initial 2-year follow-up study from the Danish ACL registry reported on 5,872 knees. Most were reconstructed with hamstring autograft (71%) and the overall revision rate was 3%. Follow up Knee Injury and Osteoarthritis Outcome Scores subscores were lower for revision and multiligament reconstructions.

35. Granan LP, Bahr R, Lie SA, Engebretsen L: Timing of anterior cruciate ligament reconstructive surgery and risk of cartilage lesions and meniscal tears: A cohort study based on the Norwegian National Knee Ligament Registry. *Am J Sports Med* 2009;37(5):955-961.

   Odds of cartilage injury increase by ~1% per month from the date of ACL injury until the date of ACL reconstruction surgery. Odds of cartilage injury were nearly twice as frequent if a meniscus tear is present, and vice versa. Level of evidence: II.

36. Chhadia AM, Inacio MC, Maletis GB, Csintalan RP, Davis BR, Funahashi TT: Are meniscus and cartilage injuries related to time to anterior cruciate ligament reconstruction? *Am J Sports Med* 2011;39(9):1894-1899.

   Increased time from ACL injury to ACL reconstruction surgery is associated with increased risk of medial meniscus injury, decreased meniscus repair rate, and increased risk of cartilage injury. Level of evidence: III.

37. Magnussen RA, Granan LP, Dunn WR, et al: Cross-cultural comparison of patients undergoing ACL reconstruction in the United States and Norway. *Knee Surg Traumatol Arthrosc* 2010;18(1):98-105.

   Patients were more likely to be male and older in the Norwegian cohort. There was less time between injury and surgery in the MOON cohort but more meniscus and articular cartilage injury and greater use of allograft.

38. Maletis GB, Granan LP, Inacio MC, Funahashi TT, Engebretsen L: Comparison of community-based ACL reconstruction registries in the U.S. and Norway. *J Bone Joint Surg Am* 2011;93(Suppl 3):31-36.

   The age of the Kaiser Permanent and Norwegian ACL reconstruction cohorts were similar. The Kaiser Permanente cohort had more males and a greater prevalence of meniscus tears.

39. Inacio MC, Paxton EW, Maletis GB, et al: Patient and surgeon characteristics associated with primary anterior cruciate ligament reconstruction graft selection. *Am J Sports Med* 2012;40(2):339-345.

   Bone-patellar tendon-bone autografts were used more often in younger and male patients. Non–fellowship-trained surgeons, lower volume sites, and/or lower volume surgeons were more likely to use allografts or hamstring autografts than bone-patellar tendon-bone autografts. Level of evidence: III.

40. Granan LP, Inacio MC, Maletis GB, Funahashi TT, Engebretsen L: Sport-specific injury pattern recorded during anterior cruciate ligament reconstruction. *Am J Sports Med* 2013;41(12):2814-2818.

   Knee ligament injury patterns were associated with certain sports. Skiing was associated with multiligament knee injuries while American football was associated with medial collateral ligament injuries and basketball was associated with concomitant meniscus and cartilage injuries. Level of evidence: III.

41. Wyatt RW, Inacio MC, Liddle KD, Maletis GB: Prevalence and incidence of cartilage injuries and meniscus tears in patients who underwent both primary and revision anterior cruciate ligament reconstructions. *Am J Sports Med* 2014;42(8):1841-1846.

   There was a higher prevalence of articular cartilage damage at revision ACL reconstruction compared to primary ACL reconstruction. The prevalence of medial meniscus tears was the same but the prevalence of lateral meniscus tears was lower at revision ACL reconstruction. Level of evidence: IV.

42. Ahldén M, Samuelsson K, Sernert N, Forssblad M, Karlsson J, Kartus J: The Swedish National Anterior Cruciate Ligament Register: A report on baseline variables and outcomes of surgery for almost 18,000 patients. *Am J Sports Med* 2012;40(10):2230-2235.

   In the Swedish national registry, all subscales of the Knee Injury and Osteoarthritis Outcome Score improved after primary ACL reconstruction. Revision ACL reconstructions and smokers have worse outcomes. There is a significant risk of subsequent ipsilateral and contralateral ACL injury in young female soccer players. Level of evidence: IV.

43. Barenius B, Forssblad M, Engström B, Eriksson K: Functional recovery after anterior cruciate ligament reconstruction: A study of health-related quality of life based on the Swedish National Knee Ligament Register. *Knee Surg Sports Traumatol Arthrosc* 2013;21(4):914-927.

   Male patients were more likely to have functional recovery after ACL reconstruction than female patients. Surgical treatment of the medial meniscus at ACL reconstruction,

6: Miscellaneous Topics Topics

previous meniscal surgery, and patellar tendon autograft predicted poor functional outcome. Level of evidence: II.

44. Røtterud JH, Sivertsen EA, Forssblad M, Engebretsen L, Arøen A: Effect of meniscal and focal cartilage lesions on patient-reported outcome after anterior cruciate ligament reconstruction: A nationwide cohort study from Norway and Sweden of 8476 patients with 2-year follow-up. *Am J Sports Med* 2013;41(3):535-543.

    Full-thickness cartilage lesions were associated with worse outcome in all of the Knee Injury and Osteoarthritis Outcome Score subscales compared with patients without cartilage lesions 2 years after ACL reconstruction whereas meniscal lesions and partial-thickness cartilage lesions were not. Level of evidence: II.

45. Rahr-Wagner L, Thillemann TM, Lind MC, Pedersen AB: Validation of 14,500 operated knees registered in the Danish Knee Ligament Reconstruction Register: Registration completeness and validity of key variables. *Clin Epidemiol* 2013;5:219-228.

    The completeness of the registration of patients in the Danish Knee Ligament Reconstruction Registry increased from 60% in 2005 to 86% in 2011. Large-volume hospitals had higher rates of completeness than small-volume hospitals.

46. Csintalan RP, Inacio MC, Funahashi TT, Maletis GB: Risk factors of subsequent operations after primary anterior cruciate ligament reconstruction. *Am J Sports Med* 2014;42(3):619-625.

    Short-term reoperation rates after ACL reconstruction are low, with median time to reoperation of 301 days. Risk factors include previous meniscal repair, female sex, allografts, prior surgery, older patient age, and having a sports medicine fellowship–trained surgeon. Level of evidence: III.

47. Maletis GB, Inacio MC, Reynolds S, Desmond JL, Maletis MM, Funahashi TT: Incidence of postoperative anterior cruciate ligament reconstruction infections: Graft choice makes a difference. *Am J Sports Med* 2013;41(8):1780-1785.

    The overall infection rate after ACL reconstruction was 0.48% (0.32% deep infections, 0.16% superficial infections). Hamstring tendon autografts had an 8.2 times higher risk compared with bone–patellar tendon–bone autografts. No difference in infection risk was identified between allografts and bone–patellar tendon–bone autografts. Level of evidence: II.

48. Gifstad T, Foss OA, Engebretsen L, et al: Lower risk of revision with patellar tendon autografts compared with hamstring autografts: A registry study based on 45,998 primary ACL reconstructions in Scandinavia. *Am J Sports Med* 2014;42(10):2319-2328.

    Although most ACL reconstructions in Scandinavia use hamstring autografts, there was a significantly lower risk

of revision using patellar tendon autografts compared to hamstrings (OR 0.63). Level of evidence: II.

49. Persson A, Fjeldsgaard K, Gjertsen JE, et al: Increased risk of revision with hamstring tendon grafts compared with patellar tendon grafts after anterior cruciate ligament reconstruction: A study of 12,643 patients from the Norwegian Cruciate Ligament Registry, 2004-2012. *Am J Sports Med* 2014;42(2):285-291.

    The failure rate of ACL reconstruction using hamstring autograft was twice that when using bone-patellar tendon-bone autograft. Younger age was the most important risk factor for failure. Level of evidence: II.

50. Rahr-Wagner L, Thillemann TM, Pedersen AB, Lind M: Comparison of hamstring tendon and patellar tendon grafts in anterior cruciate ligament reconstruction in a nationwide population-based cohort study: Results from the Danish registry of knee ligament reconstruction. *Am J Sports Med* 2014;42(2):278-284.

    Hamstring autografts had a higher failure rate than bone–patellar tendon–bone autografts at 1 and 5 years after ACL reconstruction. Level of evidence: II.

51. Andernord D, Desai N, Björnsson H, Gillén S, Karlsson J, Samuelsson K: Predictors of contralateral anterior cruciate ligament reconstruction: A cohort study of 9061 patients with 5-year follow-up. *Am J Sports Med* 2015;43(2):295-302.

    Male and female patients younger than 20 years had an almost three times higher 5-year risk of contralateral ACL reconstruction. Females undergoing reconstruction with contralateral autograft hamstring had more than three times higher 5-year risk of contralateral ACL reconstruction. Level of evidence: II.

52. Katz JN, Chaisson CE, Cole B, et al: The MeTeOR trial (Meniscal Tear in Osteoarthritis Research): Rationale and design features. *Contemp Clin Trials* 2012;33(6):1189-1196.

    This study explained the Meniscal Tear in Osteoarthritis Research Trial, a prospective randomized controlled trial of arthroscopic partial meniscectomy with standardized physical therapy versus standardized physical therapy alone to treat symptomatic meniscal tears in knees with mild to moderate osteoarthritis.

53. Katz JN, Brophy RH, Chaisson CE, et al: Surgery versus physical therapy for a meniscal tear and osteoarthritis. *N Engl J Med* 2013;368(18):1675-1684.

    Intention-to-treat analysis demonstrated no significant differences in functional improvement at 6 months between standardized physical therapy alone compared to arthroscopic partial meniscectomy and physical therapy; however, 30% of patients assigned to physical therapy alone underwent surgery within 6 months. Level of evidence: I.

Chapter 36

Current Concepts in Tendinopathy

Trevor Wilkes, MD   W. Benjamin Kibler, MD

Abstract

Tendinopathy is a common yet difficult-to-treat condition. The orthopaedic surgeon should examine the etiology and pathoanatomy of tendinopathy while acknowledging the large gaps in knowledge about this condition. It is important to be knowledgeable about treatment of commonly involved anatomic regions, including information on and physical therapy techniques, platelet-rich plasma, and novel molecular and genetic therapies.

Keywords: tendinopathy; tendon changes; tendon injury

Introduction

The scope and spectrum of tendinopathy are broad. Osteoarthritis probably is the only orthopaedic disease that rivals tendinopathy in prevalence, health care costs, and resulting loss of productivity. The etiology and treatment of tendinopathy continue to be extensively researched. Since 2009 approximately 400 peer-reviewed articles on tendinopathy have been published per year, and there have been approximately 176 clinical studies. Tendinopathy continues to be an area of both basic science and therapeutic interest.

The term tendinopathy is used clinically to describe a persistently painful and poorly functioning tendon. The model for understanding the etiology of tendinopathy is often divided into intrinsic (cellular) and extrinsic (overload) components. This model has limited usefulness, however, because the factors in the development of

Dr. Wilkes or an immediate family member is a member of a speakers' bureau or has made paid presentations on behalf of Arthrex. Dr. Kibler or an immediate family member serves as an unpaid consultant to Alignmed; has stock or stock options held in Alignmed; and serves as a board member, owner, officer, or committee member of the Arthroscopy Association of North America.

tendinopathy are numerous and interrelated. For example, the magnitude and repetition of load on the tendon of an assembly line worker cannot be precisely measured. In addition, a proxy such as age or nicotine use may not accurately define the physiology of an involved tendon.

The classic description of tendinopathy is that of a failed healing response. Five primary histologic features have been defined: collagen disruption, increased proteoglycan content, abnormal tenocytes, altered cell populations, and an increased number of microvessels and micronerves. Recent evidence has challenged and enhanced the understanding of this pathologic process. Research into gene therapy, the manipulation of cytokines and matrix metalloproteinases (MMPs), and the induction of collagen cross-linking may improve the arsenal of treatments.

Tendon Structure

The healthy tendon transmits the forces generated by muscles to their osseous insertions (entheses). Thus, the tendon acts as a tensile load-bearing structure that is essential to joint motion. Tendons are composed of a primary cell population, called tenocytes, and a carefully organized collagen network whose structure reflects its function (**Figure 1**) Type I collagen fibers are tightly packed and highly cross-linked for stiffness. Only small amounts of type II collagen exist in the normal tendon. In addition, glycosaminoglycans (GAGs) promote hydration of the extracellular matrix, fibril sliding, and collagen fiber assembly.

Tenocytes, which exist throughout the tendon, are derived from the fibroblast cell line. They are joined by gap junctions into longitudinal and lateral arrays. The tenocytes are spindle-shaped cells encapsulated by a pericellular sheath composed of versican, fibrillin, and type VI collagen that is believed to protect them from their environment. It is important to note that tenocytes are responsive to load. Mechanical stimulation activates metabolic pathways, and calcium-based signaling regulates collagen synthesis along the vectors of tension and stimulates extracellular matrix gene expression. These pathways are critical for maintenance of tendon structure, and their presence helps explain the manner in which exercise promotes the health of tendons.

Tendon structure begins at the level of collagen fibrils, which are encapsulated by epitenon and divided into fascicles by endotenon. The endotenon is a loose, fibrous sheath with intrinsic vascular, lymphatic, and nerve supply. More superficially, the tendon is surrounded in its entirety by the paratenon. The paratenon contains a similar fibrous sheath as well as a synovial lining with types I and II synoviocytes. The vascular supply to tendons varies widely by location. Arteries and arterioles course along the epitenon, and capillaries penetrate along the endotenon. However, it is well established that the blood supply to tendons is poor in certain regions such as the Codman zone of the supraspinatus tendon or the watershed zone of the Achilles tendon.

Acute Tendon Injury

The biology of tendons dictates that an acute injury requires more time to resolve than is needed in more vascular tissues. In addition, the anatomic location of the tendon defines its healing potential. The phases of the healing process include inflammation, repair, and remodeling. During the first 24 to 48 hours after injury, monocytes and macrophages migrate to the involved area to devour necrotic material. After the first 48 hours, fibroblasts and vascular cells facilitate the production of reparative tissue such as type III collagen and GAGs.

Regions within a tendon respond differently to injury. The paratenon and endotenon are metabolically active and produce more cellular signaling, proliferation, and vascularity than the tendon itself. Remodeling extends over a period of months as cell activity decreases and collagen matures. The tissue usually remains hypercellular and hypervascular, however. The histologic characteristics of the healed tendon reflect permanent disorganization, and its mechanical quality is poor. Regrown semitendinosus and gracilis tendons harvested for anterior cruciate ligament reconstruction were found to have less extracellular matrix, less collagen, and more cellularity than the native tendon.[1]

Chronic Tendon Injury

The traditional belief is that a chronic tendon injury represents a failed healing response. All components of the tendon including the epitenon, endotenon, and paratenon can be involved in a chronic tendon injury, as can locations within the macrostructure of the tendon, ranging from the musculotendinous junction to the tendon proper and osseous insertion. Enthesopathy is the pathologic

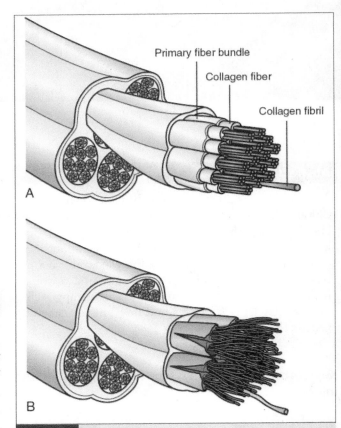

Figure 1 Schematic drawings showing the structure of a tendon. **A,** Normal architecture of the tendon. Primary fiber bundles, collagen fibers, and collagen fibrils are shown. **B,** Tendinopathic loss of organized architecture is shown.

cascade that occurs at the bone-tendon interface where the tendon is biomechanically weak. Typical histologic changes are noted in enthesopathy including irregularity of the tidemark, narrowing of the cortical bone, local bone marrow edema, and the development of bone spurs. However, the underlying pathology appears to lie within the tendon itself.

The Cellular Response to Injury

Knowledge of the tendon's response to injury and load at the cellular level is expanding. Repetitive loading in the setting of insufficient adaptation to such loading and insufficient repair appears to lead to collagen breakdown and dysregulated fibril assembly, as has been confirmed in animal models of tendon overload. When rat rotator cuffs were examined after induced treadmill running, increased cellularity and disorganized collagen were found.[2] Similarly, rats trained to perform repetitive reaching maneuvers with one limb had fibril fraying and increased

Table 1

Underlying Morphologic and Cellular Changes in Tendinosis

Tendon Component	Morphologic Changes	Cellular Changes
Collagen	Separation Disorganization Fibril breaks or tears Decreasing fibril diameter	Increasing matrix metalloproteinase activity Increasing collagen synthesis Increasing expression of collagen types I, II, III
Proteoglycan	Microvessel thickening Fibrocartilage metaplasia Scarring	Increasing versican Increasing aggrecan Increasing biglycan
Tenocytes	Abnormal distribution Mitotic figures Pyknotic nuclei	Increasing proliferation Increasing apoptosis Increasing migration
Abnormal cell populations	Mononuclear cells Granulocytes Mast cells Chondroid cells Fatty degeneration	Increasing CD3 Increasing CD68 Increasing mast cell tryptase
Vessels and nerves	Vascular hyperplasia Neural sprouting Edema Increased blood flow	Increasing vascular endothelial growth factor Increasing substance P

Adapted from Scott A, Khan K: Tendon overuse pathology: Implications for clinical management, in Kibler WB, ed: *Orthopaedic Knowledge Update: Sports Medicine*, ed 4. Rosemont, IL, American Academy of Orthopaedic Surgeons, 2009, p 308.

macrophages in comparison with the contralateral limb.[2] Increased levels of MMPs involved in collagen remodeling and repair were found with varying levels and isoforms in models of tendinopathy.[2] In this pathologic setting, collagen synthesis was mechanically inferior to that of a normal tendon and had less cross-linking. Collagen production predominantly was of type III rather than type I collagen, perhaps because an endotenon phenotype is assumed. The clinical implication is that regulation of MMPs and induction of type I collagen production can improve tendon integrity. Pilot studies found that the use of aprotinin, a serine proteinase inhibitor that can reduce collagenase activity, had positive results.[1] However, a randomized placebo-controlled study of peritendinous injection in Achilles tendinopathy found no significant benefit.[1]

The relationship between load intensity and tendon response has been a recent focus of research. A rat fatigue cyclic-loading model was used to investigate the relationship of MMP-13 and interleukin-1β (IL-1β) to osteoarthritis and general inflammation.[1] Low strain (0.6%) produced isolated collagen kinking as well as a striking 70% level of MMP-13 and IL-1β suppression. In contrast, moderate strain (1.7%) produced evidence of fiber separation, tearing, and a fivefold to sixfold increase in MMP-13 and IL-1β messenger RNA production. Thus, it appears that a low load has a suppressive effect but a moderate load leads to dramatically increased inflammatory signaling and tendon damage. In addition, real-time polymerase chain reaction of lacerated tendons revealed uniform collagen type I (*COL-1*) gene expression; fatigue-loaded tendons had diverse *COL-1* and *COL-3* subtype expression depending on the loading pattern[2,3] (Table 1).

Structural Changes in Tendinopathy

An increase in GAGs is found in pathologic tendons. The hydrophilic nature of GAGs is believed to be responsible for the increase in the tendon's water content to 75%, compared with the normal 65%.[1] GAGs are responsible for the increased T2-weighted MRI signal and ultrasonographic hypoechogenicity of tendons with tendinosis. An increase in vascular remodeling and cellular proliferation leads to increased GAG content.

Adipose and mast cells are examples of abnormal cell populations found in tendinopathy. The relationship of mast cells to nerves suggests a role in pain generation. Histologic specimens show chondroid metaplasia as another type of dysregulated cell proliferation. These abnormal cell foci negatively affect the integrity and function of the tendon. Therapeutic interventions targeted at inhibiting the vascular response and abnormal cell proliferation can help reduce proteoglycan levels and promote a more normal tendon architecture.

Perhaps the most notable histopathologic finding in tendinopathy is angiofibroblastic dysplasia. Microscopic slides reveal proliferation of endothelial and smooth muscle cells consistent with microvessel formation at a rate as much as 300% above that of normal tendons.[1] In addition, there is substantial proliferation of both autonomic and sensory nerves, which may be related to the development of chronic pain and central nervous system hypersensitivity.

Nonsurgical Therapeutic Interventions

Exercise Protocols

A patient-specific exercise prescription is considered the first-line, most evidence-based therapeutic treatment for tendinopathy. Loading the tendon has myriad cellular, structural, and possibly other autonomic effects. Research on the effects of exercise can be difficult to interpret because numerous parameters such as contraction type and speed, load, repetitions, and volume (number of sets) must be controlled.

Basic science research on the response of tendons to exercise-induced load found that the balance of the anabolic changes stimulated by load versus the catabolic effects of age and disuse is critical. Vascular flow can increase threefold, and oxygen levels can rise twofold to fivefold with exercise.[4] Tenocytes are stimulated to increase protein and specifically type I collagen production after a single session of load. With repetition and over time, load fundamentally improves the mechanical properties of tendons by increasing stiffness and decreasing strain. This improvement can be accomplished without an increase in the cross-sectional area of the tendon.

Eccentric rehabilitation protocols were first proposed in 1984 and have proved to be the workhorse intervention for tendinopathy. The therapeutic mechanism is not entirely understood, but it is believed that muscle-tendon lengthening alters the length-tension curve of the tendon unit. Evidence supports eccentric exercise as preferable to stretching in patients with lateral epicondylitis.[5] In addition, ballistic stretching was found to outperform a static exercise program in altering tendon stiffness.[5] In managing tendinopathy in an athlete during his or her sport season, it is crucial to consider the frequency and intensity of training sessions and games as related to the cumulative load on the involved tendon. Programs known to be beneficial during the off-season often are not advantageous in season. It can be challenging to control the pain level of an athlete in the setting of persistent intense load. Some data suggest that rehabilitation can be successful if the subjective pain score remains lower than 5 on a 10-point scale and diminishes to 0 by the following morning.[4]

Tendon-specific rehabilitation programs are unlikely to treat all of the underlying factors that led to the tendinopathy.[6] Carefully assessing and treating the entirety of the kinetic chain is required. Athletic or work-related gait, posture, and technique should be examined. Muscle imbalances and the flexibility of both the involved joint and the joints above and below it should be investigated.[5] Evidence shows that a full functional recovery allowing the athlete's sports demands to be accomplished can decrease the number of future episodes.[4]

In general, research has shown eccentric exercise programs to be effective in lower limb tendinopathy. Specifically, Achilles and patellar tendinopathies have been extensively studied.[5-8] Heel-drop eccentric exercises were found to be successful in 90% of patients with Achilles tendinopathy; this percentage can be used to encourage patients who become frustrated with their rehabilitation[7] (Figure 2). Controlled studies of eccentric exercise compared with ultrasound and massage found that eccentric exercise had better outcomes.[5] Not all studies have had positive findings for eccentric exercise, but histologic investigation found that eccentric exercise led to improved Achilles tendon structure and decreased vascularity.[8]

In the setting of patellar tendinopathy, the therapeutic response elicited by single-leg eccentric squats performed on a 25° decline board was superior to that of other nonsurgical treatments[5] (Figure 3). Improvement in tendon structure and excellent quadriceps activation was observed on electromyography after the use of this exercise. The addition of ultrasound has not been proved beneficial.[5] In-season programs have not had outcomes as positive as out-of-season programs.[4]

Exercise programs for upper extremity tendinopathy have had equivocal results, perhaps in part because of the intrinsic differences between a weight-bearing and a non–weight-bearing tendon. Exercise appears to be useful for patients with lateral epicondylitis, but it is questionable whether eccentric exercise adds value. Exercise was found to have better results than ultrasound, and improved forearm strength can reduce the risk of a recurrence.[9] Exercise protocols led to greater long-term patient satisfaction than corticosteroid injection.[9] In the rotator cuff, eccentric exercise has not been well studied. A program of rotator cuff isotonic exercise was as effective as arthroscopic subacromial decompression for treating tendinopathy.[2]

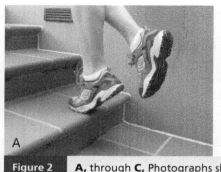
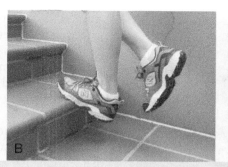
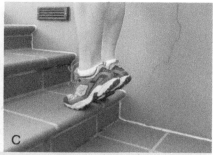

Figure 2   **A,** through **C,** Photographs show eccentric heel drop exercises for the treatment of Achilles tendinopathy. (Reproduced with permission from Andres BM, Murrell GA: Treatment of tendinopathy: What works, what does not, and what is on the horizon. *Clin Orthop Relat Res* 2008;466:1539-1554.)

Other Nonsurgical Interventions

Numerous interventions in addition to exercise have been used in an attempt to affect the imbalance of regenerative and degenerative changes in the tendon. The best means of intervening in the process is still poorly understood, however. Traditional treatment algorithms often incorporate the use of NSAIDs and corticosteroid injections. The lack of success of these treatments may reflect the complexity of tendinopathy and the absence of acute inflammation.

NSAIDs treat tendinopathy by interrupting inflammatory signals through the cyclooxygenase cascade, and they are effective only in the short term. In a recent review, 14 of 17 placebo-controlled studies of patients with Achilles tendinopathy found that NSAIDs provided substantial pain relief.[10] Success has been limited in patients with chronic conditions, and there is concern about the effect of NSAIDs on tendon healing. Any potential benefit must be carefully balanced against patient-specific risks to the gastrointestinal, cardiovascular, and renal systems. Data on local administration delivery systems such as gels and patches may be forthcoming. The use of these methods is increasing.

Like NSAIDs, corticosteroid injections are used to interrupt the local cycle of inflammatory signals. Several studies found short-term but not long-term benefit.[11] The exact mechanism of action is unclear, and there is concern about the effect on the structural integrity of the tendon. Short-term success has been documented, particularly in the lateral elbow and rotator cuff, but recurrence remains a concern.[12,13] The risk of using corticosteroid injections in the lower extremity and especially in the Achilles tendon should be carefully considered.

Only limited evidence supports the use of other modalities in tendinopathy. Some modalities were found to be successful when used in combination with a therapeutic exercise program but not in isolation. Ultrasound, the most studied modality, had beneficial effects in patients with lateral epicondylitis or calcific tendinitis of the supraspinatus,

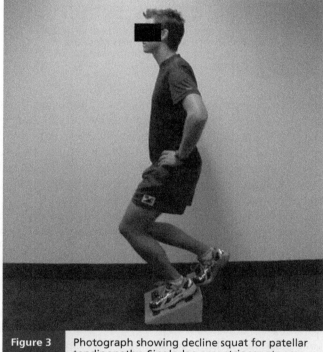

Figure 3   Photograph showing decline squat for patellar tendinopathy. Single-leg eccentric squats are performed on a decline board for treatment of patellar tendinopathy. (Reproduced with permission from Young MA, Cook JL, Purdam CR, Kiss ZS, Alfredson H: Eccentric decline squat protocol offers superior results at 12 months compared with traditional eccentric protocol for patellar tendinopathy in volleyball players. *Br J Sports Med* 2005;35:102-105.)

but the effect size was estimated at 15%.[1] Ultrasonography was not effective in Achilles tendinopathy or noncalcific rotator cuff tendinopathy.[4] Low-level laser treatment has had little or no benefit. Limited evidence supports iontophoresis or deep friction massage. Patients were found to have a positive response to hyperthermia.[4]

The use of blood, blood products, and stem cells has been investigated for the treatment of tendinopathy, and

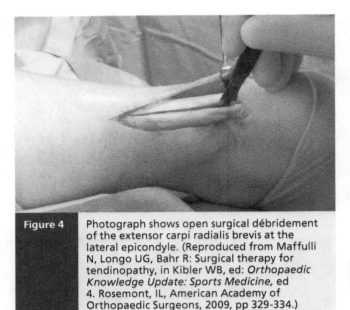

Figure 4 Photograph shows open surgical débridement of the extensor carpi radialis brevis at the lateral epicondyle. (Reproduced from Maffulli N, Longo UG, Bahr R: Surgical therapy for tendinopathy, in Kibler WB, ed: *Orthopaedic Knowledge Update: Sports Medicine*, ed 4. Rosemont, IL, American Academy of Orthopaedic Surgeons, 2009, pp 329-334.)

initial findings from animal studies were promising. Some techniques require bone marrow biopsy and cell line expansion, but these have not been widely incorporated into practice. A recent study of autologous tenocyte injection found encouraging outcomes in patients with lateral epicondylitis.[14] Patients with Achilles tendinopathy who received injection with skin-derived fibroblasts were found to have better results than control subjects.[15] The use of autogenous blood products such as platelet-rich plasma (PRP) has been readily accepted. Early studies suggested that growth factors such as vascular endothelial growth factor (VEGF) and insulin-like growth factor 1 stimulate tendon healing.[16] Small case control studies found benefit to using these growth factors, but high-quality evidence is scant.[17-19] A level I study of PRP for the treatment of midsubstance Achilles tendinopathy did not find it substantially beneficial.[20] Studies of PRP are difficult to interpret because concentrations, preparations, and injection protocols vary widely.[21] Research is continuing, and the indications for using PRP remain to be determined.[22-25]

Nitric oxide is a soluble molecule that acts as a cellular messenger. Glyceryl trinitrate has been used as a delivery system in attempt to induce healing responses in the tendon. In a rat model, a decrease in nitric oxide was found to be correlated with poor histologic findings and a low load to failure. Three randomized controlled studies found an approximately 20% positive treatment effect when nitric oxide or glyceryl trinitrate was used to treat elbow, shoulder, or Achilles tendinopathy.[26]

Extracorporeal shock wave therapy (ESWT) uses low-energy shock waves to treat tendinopathy. The mechanism of action is unclear. ESWT treatment protocols vary with respect to timing and intensity.[27] Randomized controlled studies found that ESWT had efficacy in patients with calcific tendinitis of the rotator cuff but not in patients with noncalcified tendinitis.[28,29] No substantial benefit was found in patients with lateral elbow tendinitis.

Sclerotherapy involves the injection of polidocanol or dextrose into blood vessels, often under ultrasound guidance.[30,31] The induced sclerosis may inhibit the proliferation of vascular cells and nerves, thus limiting pain generation. The effects of sclerotherapy on tendon structure have not been elucidated, but available data appear to support the safety and pain relief efficacy of sclerotherapy for use in the Achilles tendon.[32] Additional research from diverse sources is needed.

Surgical Management of Tendinopathy

Surgical intervention may be indicated for the treatment of tendinopathy after extensive unsuccessful nonsurgical treatment. There is a striking lack of evidence-based guidance for surgical treatment, however. Few double-blinded placebo-controlled studies have been conducted, and few accepted indications and techniques are available to guide the surgical management of tendinopathy. The literature is diverse and not based on universal outcome tools. Three studies with a total of more than 40 patients found that 70% to 90% had a successful outcome, and a review of research into surgery for tendinopathy found that studies with poor methodology reported better outcomes than studies with acceptable methodology.[4]

Surgical outcomes are known to be unpredictable, and complication rates are high. After clinically successful surgery, the tendon may not become normal and may remain biomechanically weak. The purposes of the surgical procedure are to excise pathologic tissue and promote repair, but there is controversy as to the most successful technique. The common techniques expose the involved tendon, strip the paratenon, create longitudinal tenotomies, and remove abnormal tissue. Insertional tendinopathies may require bursectomy, debridement, excision of calcific deposits, and sometimes release and repair of the tendon (Figure 4).

Achilles tendinopathy is associated with painful neovascularization on the ventral aspect of the tendon, which can be treated with several ultrasonographically guided and percutaneous techniques. The treatment may be most successful in the absence of substantial paratenon involvement. Little information is available for comparing these techniques to open surgery. Resection of more than 50% of the tendon may require reconstruction in an open procedure. Several techniques can be used to treat patellar tendinopathy, but research is limited. The primary procedures involve arthroscopically assisted or open drilling and excision. Ultrasonographically guided percutaneous techniques increasingly are used based on limited evidence.[33]

Recent Research on Tendinopathy

Research is revealing the limitations of current beliefs regarding the etiology of tendinopathy. Inflammatory cells such as macrophages and lymphocytes have been encountered in chronic tendinopathies, particularly in the paratenon and bursa. The predominant view of tendinopathy may be shifting toward a paradigm consistent with that of osteoarthritis. In osteoarthritis as well as the evolving understanding of tendinopathy, mechanical overload is the fundamental cause but ongoing active inflammation contributes to the cellular pathology. This view of tendinopathy has been clearly defined and is supported by the presence of elevated levels of inflammatory mediators such as substance P, the MMPs, VEGF, and cyclooxygenase. The classic cyclooxygenase pathway leads to elevated levels of prostaglandin E_1 and E_2, which have been found in models of tendinopathy.[1] Increased concentrations of MMPs are linked to tendinopathy and are upregulated in rotator cuff pathology. Injections of substance P into the peritenon stimulated vascularity and tenocyte proliferation with the altered ratios of type III collagen found in tendinopathy.[32] Novel interventions to attack these inflammatory signals may lead to treatments that will be more successful than the traditional treatments.[1,4]

Tumor necrosis factor-α (TNF-α) is a proinflammatory cytokine that stimulates IL-1, IL-6, MMPs, VEGF, and prostaglandin E_2. Higher-than-normal levels of TNF-α are associated with cellular apoptosis. Synthetic monoclonal biologic agents to inhibit TNF-α have been effective in controlling inflammatory conditions such as rheumatoid arthritis and ankylosing spondylitis.[1] The use of a diminished anti-TNF agent in tendinopathy has been recommended.[1] An investigation of adalimumab for use in Achilles tendinopathy found pain improvement and decreased blood flow at 12 weeks.[2] Important questions remain related to adalimumab dosage, cost, and immunosuppression, and further study is necessary.

Tissue inhibitor of matrix metalloproteases and MMPs are normal products of tenocytes for regulation of the extracellular matrix of proteoglycans. Therefore, the normal state of tendons involves a balance of synthesis and degradation. Disruption of this balance was found in messenger RNA profiles of chronically painful and ruptured tendons.[2] The MMP ADAMTS-5 (A disintegrin and metalloproteinase with thrombospondin motifs 5) is being investigated as a target of inhibition in osteoarthritis,

and it may have value for the treatment of tendinopathy.[2]

Substance P is known to be involved in nociception and upregulated in tendinopathy. A rabbit model of Achilles tendon overload found increased levels of substance P as well as hypercellularity and angiogenesis.[1] Substance P may become a viable target for intervention. Glutamate, a central nervous system signaling molecule, was found in increased levels in pathologic Achilles tendon tissue.[1] A histologic study of patellar tendinopathy found a tenfold increase in glutamate and a ninefold increase in N-methyl-D-aspartate receptor 1 (NMDAR1), a glutamate receptor, compared with control tissue.[1] These molecules also may become therapeutic targets. Specific inhibition of neovascularization and neoinnervation has generated interest. Inhibition of VEGF may reduce vascularity. Nerve growth factor is involved in the maintenance of sensory and sympathetic nerves and is believed to have a role in neuropathic pain. Tanezumab was found to be a monoclonal antibody against nerve growth factor in clinical studies, and this finding may have clinical application in treating chronic tendon pain.[1] The scleraxis gene in tenocytes is upregulated in repair and remodeling and also may become a target for gene therapy.

Summary

Therapeutic interventions for tendinopathy are evolving with increasing understanding of the condition. Some basic information on the incidence, prevalence, and prevention of tendinopathy remains to be determined, but progress is being made. Biochemical research is elucidating novel treatments and furthering the model of tissue pathology as well as its interactions with the central nervous system. It is critical to consider the tendon within its place in the kinetic chain and the patient's overall physiology. Continuing basic research and research into methodology and outcome measures should translate into improved clinical results.

Key Study Points

- Treatment of tendinopathy must take into account the patient-specific pathology of the tendon as well as its place in the kinetic chain.
- Tendinopathy represents a disruption in the anabolic/catabolic metabolic balance of the tendon.
- Scant high-level evidence is available to guide treatment protocols.
- Current research is targeting molecular and gene therapies for tendinopathy.

Annotated References

1. Rees JD, Stride M, Scott A: Tendons: Time to revisit inflammation. *Br J Sports Med* 2014;48(21):1553-1557.

   A review article examined historic and recent evidence that chronic tendinopathy incorporates elements of the inflammatory process and that this factor may offer potential therapeutic targets.

2. Neviaser A, Andarawis-Puri N, Flatow E: Basic mechanisms of tendon fatigue damage. *J Shoulder Elbow Surg* 2012;21(2):158-163.

   Molecular and mechanical changes and animal model research pertaining to rotator cuff tendon disease and treatment were reviewed.

3. September AV, Nell EM, O'Connell K, et al: A pathway-based approach investigating the genes encoding interleukin-1β, interleukin-6 and the interleukin-1 receptor antagonist provides new insight into the genetic susceptibility of Achilles tendinopathy. *Br J Sports Med* 2011;45(13):1040-1047.

   Variations in the IL genes and the COL5A1 BstUI CC genotypes were found to be collectively significantly associated with the risk of Achilles tendinopathy.

4. Scott A, Docking S, Vicenzino B, et al: Sports and exercise-related tendinopathies: A review of selected topical issues by participants of the second International Scientific Tendinopathy Symposium (ISTS) Vancouver 2012. *Br J Sports Med* 2013;47(9):536-544.

   Research and clinical practice issues were updated in a summary of a 2012 conference.

5. Dimitrios S, Pantelis M, Kalliopi S: Comparing the effects of eccentric training with eccentric training and static stretching exercises in the treatment of patellar tendinopathy: A controlled clinical trial. *Clin Rehabil* 2012;26(5):423-430.

   The addition of static stretching to a program of eccentric training for patellar tendinopathy significantly reduced pain and improved function. Level of evidence: II.

6. Ram R, Meeuwisse W, Patel C, Wiseman DA, Wiley JP: The limited effectiveness of a home-based eccentric training for treatment of Achilles tendinopathy. *Clin Invest Med* 2013;36(4):E197-E206.

   Home-based eccentric training was found not to meet patients' expectations for treatment of Achilles tendinopathy. Level of evidence: IV.

7. van der Plas A, de Jonge S, de Vos RJ, et al: A 5-year follow-up study of Alfredson's heel-drop exercise programme in chronic midportion Achilles tendinopathy. *Br J Sports Med* 2012;46(3):214-218.

   At long-term follow-up of a heel-drop exercise program for Achilles tendinopathy, patients had significant increases in outcome scores, but mild pain persisted and one-half of patients received other therapies after the conclusion of the 3-month program. Level of evidence: IV.

8. Horstmann T, Jud HM, Fröhlich V, Mündermann A, Grau S: Whole-body vibration versus eccentric training or a wait-and-see approach for chronic Achilles tendinopathy: A randomized clinical trial. *J Orthop Sports Phys Ther* 2013;43(11):794-803.

   Vibration training was a successful complement or alternative to eccentric training for chronic Achilles tendinopathy, especially for patients with insertional pain. Level of evidence: I.

9. Stasinopoulos D, Stasinopoulos I, Pantelis M, Stasinopoulou K: Comparison of effects of a home exercise programme and a supervised exercise programme for the management of lateral elbow tendinopathy. *Br J Sports Med* 2010;44(8):579-583.

   In 70 patients who underwent a home or supervised exercise program program for lateral elbow tendinopathy, the supervised program had significantly better results at 12- and 24-week follow-up. Level of evidence: II.

10. Maquirriain J, Kokalj A: Acute Achilles tendinopathy: Effect of pain control on leg stiffness. *J Musculoskelet Neuronal Interact* 2014;14(1):131-136.

    Athletes with unilateral Achilles tendinopathy had increased leg stiffness after receiving oral anti-inflammatory therapy. Level of evidence: III.

11. Karthikeyan S, Kwong HT, Upahyay PK, Parsons N, Drew SJ, Griffin D: A double-blind randomised controlled study comparing subacromial injection of tenoxicam or methylprednisolone in patients with subacromial impingement. *J Bone Joint Surg Br* 2010;92(1):77-82.

    Corticosteroid injection was found to have significantly better results than NSAID injection for shoulder function after 6 weeks in 58 randomly assigned patients. Level of evidence: I.

12. de Witte PB, Selten JW, Navas A, et al: Calcific tendinitis of the rotator cuff: A randomized controlled trial of ultrasound-guided needling and lavage versus subacromial corticosteroids. *Am J Sports Med* 2013;41(7):1665-1673.

    At 1-year follow-up, patients with calcific tendinitis of the rotator cuff who received ultrasound-guided needling and lavage combined with a subacromial bursa injection had better clinical and radiographic results than those who received the injection alone. Level of evidence: I.

13. Merolla G, Bianchi P, Porcellini G: Ultrasound-guided subacromial injections of sodium hyaluronate for the management of rotator cuff tendinopathy: A prospective comparative study with rehabilitation therapy. *Musculoskelet Surg* 2013;97(Suppl 1):49-56.

    Hyaluronic acid injection was found to provide better pain relief and outcome scores than rehabilitation therapy at weeks 4 and 12 but not at week 24. Level of evidence: II.

© 2016 American Academy of Orthopaedic Surgeons

14. Wang A, Breidahl W, Mackie KE, et al: Autologous tenocyte injection for the treatment of severe, chronic resistant lateral epicondylitis: A pilot study. *Am J Sports Med* 2013;41(12):2925-2932.

Twenty patients with lateral epicondylitis who were treated with autologous tenocyte injection had significant functional improvement and structural repair on MRI. Level of evidence: IV.

15. Obaid H, Clarke A, Rosenfeld P, Leach C, Connell D: Skin-derived fibroblasts for the treatment of refractory Achilles tendinosis: Preliminary short-term results. *J Bone Joint Surg Am* 2012;94(3):193-200.

A randomized double-blind study of 32 patients (40 Achilles tendons) found significant differences in outcome and pain scores and safety 6 weeks, 12 weeks, and 6 months after injection of skin-derived fibroblasts. Level of evidence: I.

16. Creaney L, Wallace A, Curtis M, Connell D: Growth factor-based therapies provide additional benefit beyond physical therapy in resistant elbow tendinopathy: A prospective, single-blind, randomised trial of autologous blood injections versus platelet-rich plasma injections. *Br J Sports Med* 2011;45(12):966-971.

PRP injections were found to be superior to autologous blood in the treatment of lateral epicondylitis. Level of evidence: II.

17. Mishra AK, Skrepnik NV, Edwards SG, et al: Efficacy of platelet-rich plasma for chronic tennis elbow: A double-blind, prospective, multicenter, randomized controlled trial of 230 patients. *Am J Sports Med* 2014;42(2):463-471.

No significant difference was found at 12-week follow-up based on whether patients with chronic tennis elbow had received leukocyte-rich PRP injection, but there was significant improvement at 24-week follow-up. Level of evidence: I.

18. Bell KJ, Fulcher ML, Rowlands DS, Kerse N: Impact of autologous blood injections in treatment of mid-portion Achilles tendinopathy: Double blind randomized controlled trial. *BMJ* 2013;346:f2310.

No additional benefit was found when two unguided peritendinous injections were added to a standard eccentric exercise program in patients with Achilles tendinopathy. Level of evidence: I.

19. Rha DW, Park GY, Kim YK, Kim MT, Lee SC: Comparison of the therapeutic effects of ultrasound-guided platelet-rich plasma injection and dry needling in rotator cuff disease: A randomized controlled trial. *Clin Rehabil* 2013;27(2):113-122.

In patients with tendinopathy or a partial tendon tear, PRP injection was found to be more effective than dry needling from 6-week to 6-month follow-up. Level of evidence: II.

20. de Jonge S, de Vos RJ, Weir A, et al: One-year follow-up of platelet-rich plasma treatment in chronic Achilles tendinopathy: A double-blind randomized placebo-controlled trial. *Am J Sports Med* 2011;39(8):1623-1629.

A study of 54 patients did not find PRP injection to be superior to placebo in combination with an eccentric exercise program at 1-year follow-up, as determined by outcome measures or ultrasound. Level of evidence: I.

21. Kesikburun S, Tan AK, Yilmaz B, Yaşar E, Yazicioğlu K: Platelet-rich plasma injections in the treatment of chronic rotator cuff tendinopathy: A randomized controlled trial with 1-year follow-up. *Am J Sports Med* 2013;41(11):2609-2616.

In patients with chronic rotator cuff tendinopathy, PRP injection was not found to be more effective than placebo in combination with an exercise program. Level of evidence: I.

22. Dragoo JL, Wasterlain AS, Braun HJ, Nead KT: Platelet-rich plasma as a treatment for patellar tendinopathy: A double-blind, randomized controlled trial. *Am J Sports Med* 2014;42(3):610-618.

Twenty-three patients with patellar tendinopathy who were randomly assigned to standard eccentric exercises with ultrasound-guided leukocyte rich PRP injection had accelerated recovery compared with patients who received exercises alone, but the results dissipated with time. Level of evidence: I.

23. Vetrano M, Castorina A, Vulpiani MC, Baldini R, Pavan A, Ferretti A: Platelet-rich plasma versus focused shock waves in the treatment of jumper's knee in athletes. *Am J Sports Med* 2013;41(4):795-803.

Two PRP injections were found to be more effective than ESWT at midterm clinical follow-up of patients with patellar tendinopathy. Level of evidence: II.

24. Gosens T, Den Oudsten BL, Fievez E, van 't Spijker P, Fievez A: Pain and activity levels before and after platelet-rich plasma injection treatment of patellar tendinopathy: A prospective cohort study and the influence of previous treatments. *Int Orthop* 2012;36(9):1941-1946.

PRP was significantly beneficial in the treatment of patellar tendinopathy, but patients who had undergone earlier surgical or injection treatments did not have a response to the treatment. Level of evidence: III.

25. Moraes VY, Lenza M, Tamaoki MJ, Faloppa F, Belloti JC: Platelet-rich therapies for musculoskeletal soft tissue injuries. *Cochrane Database Syst Rev* 2014;4:CD010071.

There was insufficient evidence to support the use of platelet-rich therapies in patients with musculoskeletal soft-tissue injury. Standardization of PRP preparation methods was recommended.

26. Steunebrink M, Zwerver J, Brandsema R, Groenenboom P, van den Akker-Scheek I, Weir A: Topical glyceryl trinitrate treatment of chronic patellar tendinopathy: A randomised, double-blind, placebo-controlled clinical trial. *Br J Sports Med* 2013;47(1):34-39.

© 2016 American Academy of Orthopaedic Surgeons

6: Miscellaneous Topics

Topical glyceryl trinitrate in addition to an eccentric exercise program did not lead to a superior clinical outcome compared with placebo patches in patients with chronic patellar tendinopathy. Level of evidence: I.

27. Zwerver J, Hartgens F, Verhagen E, van der Worp H, van den Akker-Scheek I, Diercks RL: No effect of extracorporeal shockwave therapy on patellar tendinopathy in jumping athletes during the competitive season: A randomized clinical trial. *Am J Sports Med* 2011;39(6):1191-1199.

   In 62 randomly assigned athletes with patellar tendinopathy symptoms of less than 12 months' duration, ESWT had no significant benefit over placebo. Level of evidence: II.

28. Kolk A, Yang KG, Tamminga R, van der Hoeven H: Radial extracorporeal shock-wave therapy in patients with chronic rotator cuff tendinitis: A prospective randomised double-blind placebo-controlled multicentre trial. *Bone Joint J* 2013;95-B(11):1521-1526.

   Treatment with radial ESWT did not reduce pain or improve function in patients with chronic rotator cuff tendinitis. Level of evidence: I.

29. Galasso O, Amelio E, Riccelli DA, Gasparini G: Short-term outcomes of extracorporeal shock wave therapy for the treatment of chronic non-calcific tendinopathy of the supraspinatus: A double-blind, randomized, placebo-controlled trial. *BMC Musculoskelet Disord* 2012;13:86.

   ESWT led to better pain scores and range of motion than placebo in 20 patients with chronic noncalcific tendinopathy of the supraspinatus at 12-week follow-up. Level of evidence: I.

30. Yelland MJ, Sweeting KR, Lyftogt JA, Ng SK, Scuffham PA, Evans KA: Prolotherapy injections and eccentric loading exercises for painful Achilles tendinosis: A randomised trial. *Br J Sports Med* 2011;45(5):421-428.

Prolotherapy injections with eccentric-loading exercises led to more rapid improvement in patients with Achilles tendinosis than eccentric-loading exercises along, but long-term results were similar. Level of evidence: II.

31. Hoksrud A, Torgalsen T, Harstad H, et al: Ultrasound-guided sclerosis of neovessels in patellar tendinopathy: A prospective study of 101 patients. *Am J Sports Med* 2012;40(3):542-547.

   Sclerosing treatment with polidocanol resulted in moderate improvement in patients with patellar tendinopathy, but most patients still were symptomatic at 24-month follow-up. Level of evidence: IV.

32. Gross CE, Hsu AR, Chahal J, Holmes GB Jr: Injectable treatments for noninsertional Achilles tendinosis: A systematic review. *Foot Ankle Int* 2013;34(5):619-628.

   A literature review found that injectable therapies had highly variable results in patients with noninsertional Achilles tendinosis. The evidence was inconclusive.

33. Koh JS, Mohan PC, Howe TS, et al: Fasciotomy and surgical tenotomy for recalcitrant lateral elbow tendinopathy: Early clinical experience with a novel device for minimally invasive percutaneous microresection. *Am J Sports Med* 2013;41(3):636-644.

   A proprietary device was used for minimally invasive ultrasonic tissue resection. Nineteen of 20 patients with recalcitrant lateral elbow tendinopathy had a good clinical result at 1-year follow-up. Level of evidence: IV.

Chapter 37

Current Applications of Orthobiologic Agents

Ryan M. Degen, MD, MSc, FRCSC   Scott A. Rodeo, MD

Abstract

The effectiveness of orthobiologic agents, such as autograft, allograft, and xenograft, in facilitating healing is currently being studied. An understanding of the science behind tissue healing is important to establish clinical indications for orthobiologic agents.

Keywords: orthobiologic agents; platelet-rich plasma; stem cells; growth factors; scaffolds; vitamin D deficiency; matrix metalloproteinase inhibitors

Introduction

Despite recent important innovations in orthopaedic surgical techniques, implants, and devices, the time required for healing remains a limiting factor in restoring function after injury. Heightened attention to understanding the basic biology of tissue healing has led to a concomitant interest in tissue regeneration. So-called orthobiologic agents have the potential to improve local biology and expedite or otherwise improve the healing process. Available orthobiologic agents include autograft, allograft, and xenograft biologic substances that can be further classified as having growth factor, cellular, or tissue therapeutic action. An increasingly large number of studies have been published on the available agents, but it can be difficult to use the literature to determine the efficacy and clinical usefulness of these agents.

Dr. Rodeo or an immediate family member serves as a paid consultant to Cytori, Pluristem, and Rotation Medical and has stock or stock options held in The Cayenne Company. Neither Dr. Degen nor any immediate family member has received anything of value from or has stock or stock options held in a commercial company or institution related directly or indirectly to the subject of this chapter.

Growth Factor Therapy

Platelet-Rich Plasma

The first treatments using platelet-rich plasma (PRP) were in maxillofacial surgery.[1] Positive results led to widespread interest and use in cardiovascular and plastic surgery, with more recent application in orthopaedic surgery.[2,3] Several preclinical and clinical studies have investigated the efficacy of PRP in treating orthopaedic conditions including fracture nonunion, diabetic fracture, tendinopathy, tendon-bone and ligament-bone healing, healing after spinal fusion, and cartilage repair.[2-5] Currently, there is no consensus on the use of PRP in the treatment of sport-related pathology.

PRP is a concentrate of autologous blood with a higher concentration of platelets than whole blood. Reported studies have used variable platelet concentrations. Clinical efficacy has been found at values as low as 200,000 platelets per μL, whereas other studies have defined PRP as having a concentration of at least 1 million platelets per μL in 5 mL of plasma.[1,3] Other identified differences in PRP formulations include variability in leukocyte concentration, the presence of fibrin architecture, and the need for an exogenous activating agent such as calcium chloride or thrombin.[6] Each of these factors affects the activity of PRP. The interpretation of clinical data is limited by an inability to determine the contribution of each component to the overall efficacy of PRP.

Preparation and Composition

More than 15 commercial preparation systems are currently available for creating PRP. Each system has its own whole blood volume requirement, centrifugation rate and time, platelet capture rate, and end volume (Table 1). As a result, PRP samples have substantial qualitative differences in platelet, growth factor, leukocyte, and neutrophil concentrations.[5]

The preparation of PRP involves drawing whole blood, mixing it with an anticoagulant, and centrifuging to separate the specimen into a red blood cell fraction

© 2016 American Academy of Orthopaedic Surgeons

Table 1

Characteristics of Commercial Platelet-Rich Plasma Separation Systems

Separation System	Whole Blood Volume (mL)	Anti-coagulant	Steps	Centrifuge Time / Speed	Final Volume of PRP (mL)	Activator	Final Platelet Concentration	Level of Growth Factor (compared with average)
Autologous Conditioned Plasma – Double Syringe (ACP-DS), Arthrex	9	ACD-A, 1.5 mL	Single spin	5 min / 1500 rpm	3	None	2-3x	PDGF (25x) EGF (5x) VEGF (11x) TGF-β1 (4x)
Cascade, MTF	9-18	Sodium citrate, 2 mL	Single spin for PRP, Double spin for platelet –rich fibrin matrix (PRFM)	6 min / 1100 g (PRP) +15 min /1450 g (PRFM)	4-9	Calcium chloride	1-1.5x	PDGF (N/A) EGF (5-10x) VEGF (5-10x) TGF-β1 (5-10x)
Gravitational Platelet Separation (GPS) III, Biomet	27-110	ACD-A, 6 mL	Single spin	15 min / 1900 g	3-12	Calcium chloride / autologous thrombin	3-8x	PDGF (N/A) EGF (3.9x) VEGF (6.2x) TGF-β1 (3.6x)
Magellan, Medtronic	30-60	ACD-A, 4 to 8 mL	Double spin	4-6 min / 1200 g	6	Calcium chloride	3-7x	—
Plasma Rich in Growth Factors – Endoret (PDGF-Endoret), BTI Biotechnology	9-72	Sodium citrate	Single spin	8 min / 580 g	4-32	Calcium chloride	2-3x	—
SmartPrep 2, Harvest Technologies	20-120	ACDA, 8 mL	Double spin	14 min / 1000 g	3-20 ml	Calcium chloride/ bovine thrombin	4-6x	PDGF (4.4x) EGF (4.4x) VEGF (4.4x) TGF-β1 (4.4x)

ACD-A = anticoagulant citrate dextrose solution A, PRP = platelet-rich plasma, EGF = epidermal growth factor, PDGF = platelet-derived growth factor, TGF-β1 = transforming growth factor β1, VEGF = vascular endothelial growth factor.

Table 2

Functions of Selected Growth Factors Released From Platelet α-Granules

Growth Factor	Function
Platelet-derived growth factor	Stimulates cell replication Stimulates angiogenesis Stimulates mitogen for fibroblasts
Vascular endothelial growth factor	Angiogenesis
Transforming growth factor-β1	Balances fibrosis and myocyte regeneration
Fibroblast growth factor	Stimulates myoblasts Stimulates angiogenesis
Epidermal growth factor	Stimulates proliferation of mesenchymal and epithelial cells Potentiates other growth factors
Insulin-like growth factor-1	Stimulates chondrogenic proliferation of mesenchymal stem cells Stimulates extra-cellular matrix production Downregulates catabolic effects of MMPs and interleukin-1

and a plasma fraction containing platelets, white blood cells (WBCs), and clotting factors. The plasma is further divided into platelet-poor plasma and PRP. The PRP can be mixed with an activator to stimulate the clotting and degranulation processes; if an activator is not added, clotting and degranulation occur more gradually after exposure to tissue-derived collagen.[5] PRP should be kept in an anticoagulated state until it is to be used because as much as 90% of the growth factors are released within the first 10 minutes after clotting, and more than 95% is released within the first hour.[1] Platelets can remain viable in the anticoagulated state for as long as 8 hours.[1] A second centrifugation of the plasma with calcium chloride converts the fibrinogen to fibrin and traps the platelets in a dense fibrin matrix (platelet-rich fibrin) to allow a gradual release of growth factors over 5 to 7 days.[6]

Platelets contain α-granules, in which proteins, cytokines, and growth factors help regulate the healing process.[2-4] Among the commonly recognized growth factors, each of which has a different function, are platelet-derived growth factor (PDGF), vascular endothelial growth factor, transforming growth factor β1 (TGF-β1), fibroblast growth factor (FGF), epidermal growth factor, and insulin-like growth factor 1 (**Table 2**). Platelets release these substances during degranulation, and they aid in the healing process by stimulating cell proliferation, chemotaxis, angiogenesis, matrix production, and cell differentiation.[2] In addition to growth factors, platelets release histamine and serotonin, which increase local capillary permeability and thereby improve access for inflammatory cells to start the reparative process.[3]

Platelet concentration and the subsequent release of growth factors initially were believed to represent the primary mechanism of action of PRP. What appeared to be a dose-response relationship was found between the concentration of platelets and the production of a cellular response in treated tissues, although this relationship was not always correlated with a measurable clinical effect.[1] More recently, other important constituents were identified as contributing to the healing activity of PRP; these include red blood cells, neutrophils, and WBCs (leukocytes), which are believed to propagate the local inflammatory response.[4] The benefit of WBCs in PRP is controversial. Several studies supported the use of WBCs, arguing that they potentiate the release of cytokines from platelets to improve healing and that, in vitro, they confer antimicrobial properties to reduce infection rates.[7,8] Other studies argued that the release of these cytokines causes a highly inflammatory reaction that creates a predisposition to fibrosis and structurally weaker tissue, without confirmed in vitro antimicrobial effects.[9,10] The clinical effect of WBCs and the other constituents of PRP remains unclear, and further study is warranted to quantify each substance and determine its specific clinical effects.

Uncertainty exists not only about the effects of individual PRP components but also about between-sample disparities in the concentration of the components. Concern over the heterogeneity of available PRP preparations and the generalizability of reported results led to a recent study of the cellular composition of PRP produced from several commercially available separation systems.[11] Marked differences in cellular composition were identified. In addition, variable platelet capture and WBC concentration

6. Miscellaneous Topics

were found when a single separation system was used to process sequential blood draws from individual patients. These findings should alert researchers and clinicians to carefully quantify the individual PRP preparation characteristics used in clinical studies, for the purpose of determining the true clinical efficacy of PRP and improving the applicability of reported results.

PRP in Tendinopathy

Tendon injuries can lead to substantial morbidity, interfering both with sports participation and activities of daily living. Healing tends to be slow because the injury often is in a relatively avascular region, and a complex, gradual process of inflammation, proliferation, and remodeling is required to restore structural integrity.[12] The interaction of several growth factors is important for generating the inflammatory phase that initiates repair. There has been significant interest in the potential ability of PRP to accelerate and improve healing by providing several requisite growth factors to the injury site early in the process. In addition, PRP may stimulate neovascularization to facilitate regeneration of the injured tissue.[4]

The use of PRP in treating various forms of tendinopathy as well as tendon rupture has been widely studied in recent years (Table 3). Rehabilitation coupled with PRP has been studied in acute and chronic Achilles tendon injuries, partial hamstring tears, lateral epicondylitis, and patellar tendinitis. A randomized controlled investigation of chronic Achilles tendinopathy treated with eccentric exercises and PRP or saline injection found no benefit to the use of PRP.[13] A retrospective cohort review of acute Achilles tendon rupture treated with functional rehabilitation and PRP also found no benefit to the use of PRP.[14] In contrast, partial hamstring tears were found to respond to ultrasound-guided PRP injection added to eccentric exercises; patients in the treatment group had better subjective pain scores and return-to-play timelines than those in the control group.[15] In two separate randomized controlled investigations, the use of PRP led to better pain scores and functional outcomes in patients with lateral epicondylitis, compared with dry needling or corticosteroid injection and physical therapy.[16,17] The utility of PRP in treating patellar tendinopathy is less clear, as two separate studies yielded mixed results.[18,19]

The success of PRP injections for tendinopathy is highly variable and depends in part on the pathology. Further study is warranted on the treatment of tendinopathy with PRP to more accurately quantify the administered PRP concentrate. Because some studies found that the treatment effect dissipated over time,[19,20] long-term follow-up is needed to determine whether the treatment effect is maintained.

PRP in Rotator Cuff Repair

The rotator cuff insertion consists of a specialized area of organized tissue that makes a gradual transition from tendon to unmineralized fibrocartilage, then to mineralized fibrocartilage, and finally to bone.[12] Tendon-bone healing typically proceeds in a stepwise fashion from an initial inflammatory phase to a repair phase and a remodeling phase. The inflammatory and repair phases occur within the first 14 days after injury; both rely heavily on platelet aggregation, fibrin deposition, and release of cytokines. These cytokines include growth factors that attract inflammatory cells as well as progenitor cells that rely on other signaling molecules for differentiation and proliferation and contribute to extracellular matrix synthesis.[21] Typically, the healing response after rupture or surgical repair does not lead to replication of the original organized structure but instead results in formation of significant fibrosis and scar tissue with weaker mechanical properties. PRP has been investigated in rotator cuff repair for its potential to stimulate cellular proliferation and differentiation leading to improved collagen orientation and structural integrity (Table 4). A randomized study of single-row repair of small rotator cuff tears found no significant differences in patient-reported outcomes (UCLA Shoulder Rating Scale, Constant shoulder score) or retear rates based on whether PRP was administered.[22] A retrospective cohort review found no measurable differences in patient-reported outcomes (UCLA, Constant, Simple Shoulder Test scores) based on whether PRP was used in double-row repair of large to massive rotator cuff tears.[23] A randomized controlled study of a platelet-rich fibrin matrix in the surgical repair construct of small to large rotator cuff tears found no benefit in any treatment group.[24] Results were evaluated using a combination of ultrasound-determined radiographic healing, dynamometer strength testing, and validated outcome measures (American Shoulder and Elbow Surgeons Shoulder Scale and L'Insalata Shoulder Questionnaire). In contrast, another study found improvement in radiographic outcomes (retearing rates and cross-sectional area) when PRP was added to a double-row suture bridge repair construct for treatment of large to massive tears; these findings were not correlated with improved clinical outcome scores, however.[25]

The currently available evidence appears to be insufficient to warrant the routine use of PRP in rotator cuff repairs. Many early studies were flawed by poor methodology and varying definitions of PRP composition.[26] Further study is warranted to determine whether there is a role for PRP in rotator cuff repair.

Table 3

Best Available Evidence for the Use of Platelet-Rich Plasma in Tendinopathy

Study (Year)	Disease	Treatment	Patient Number	Follow-up	Outcome Measures	Findings
Kaniki (2014)	Acute Achilles rupture	2 PRP injections and functional rehab versus rehab alone	73 patients in PRP group versus 72 in control	2 years	Calf circumference, Leppilahti scale, AOFAS hindfoot scale	No statistically significant differences in isokinetic strength or patient reported outcome measures to support use of PRP
de Vos (2010)	Chronic Achilles tendinopathy	Eccentric PT and PRP versus PT and placebo	54 pts (27 per group)	24 weeks	Primary: VISA-A Secondary: patient satisfaction; return to sports; adherence to PT	No differences between groups, with both improving on VISA-A scores No differences in secondary outcomes
A Hamid (2014)	Partial hamstring tear	Single PRP injection and rehab versus rehab alone	14 patients in each	N/A	Primary: return-to-play; time to full recovery Secondary: change in pain severity and intensity	Significantly faster return to play (27 days versus 48 days) and full recovery (26 weeks versus 39 weeks) in PRP group Substantially lower pain severity scores in PRP group
Mishra (2014)	Chronic lateral epicondylitis	Needling + PRP versus needling alone	116 pts in treatment; 114 pts in control	24 weeks	Primary: VAS with resisted wrist extension (25% improvement deemed a success) Secondary: PRTEE and extended wrist examination	At 12 weeks (192 available pts), no significant differences between groups. At 24 weeks (119 available pts), 84% success rate in PRP group versus 68% in control group (P = 0.037), despite 24% in PRP group reporting significant elbow tenderness
Peerbooms (2010)	Lateral epicondylitis	Corticosteroid versus PRP injection	100 pts; 51 in PRP, 49 in steroid	1 year	Primary: VAS (25% improvement deemed a success); DASH	Significantly better outcome on VAS and DASH following injection of PRP Effect of PRP maintained, transient effect of corticosteroid
Charousset (2014)	Patellar tendinopathy	PRP + eccentric strengthening PT	28 patients; no control	2 year (min.)	Primary: VISA-P, VAS, Lysholm Secondary: MRI for tendon healing	All outcome measures significantly improved with treatment MRI showed improved tendon structural integrity with return of normal architecture
Dragoo (2014)	Patellar tendinopathy	Dry needling + rehab versus PRP + rehab	23 pts (13 DN versus 10 PRP)	26 weeks	Primary: VISA-P Secondary: Tegner, Lysholm, VAS, SF-12	At 12 weeks, significantly better VISA-P scores in PRP group versus DN At 26 weeks, no significant differences between groups

AOFAS = American Orthopaedic Foot and Ankle Society, DASH = Disabilities of the Arm, Shoulder, and Hand questionnaire, PRP = platelet-rich plasma, PRTEE = Patient-rated Tennis Elbow Evaluation, SF-12 = Medical Outcomes Study 12-Item Short Form, VAS = Visual analog scale, VISA-A = Victorian Institute of Sports Assessment Achilles tendinopathy questionnaire, VISA-P = Victorian Institute of Sports Assessment patellar tendinopathy questionnaire.

8: Miscellaneous Topics

Table 4

Best Available Evidence for the Use of Platelet-Rich Plasma in Rotator Cuff Repair

Study (Year)	Disease	Treatment	Patient Number	Follow-up	Outcome Measures	Findings
Malavolta (2014)	Rotator cuff tear Small tear <3 cm retraction	Single-row repair PRP versus control	54 (27 per group)	2 years	Primary: UCLA Secondary: Constant; VAS; MRI	Similar improvements in UCLA, Constant and VAS scores noted in both groups No difference in re-tear rates on MRI
Charousset (2014)	Rotator cuff tear Large to massive tears	Double-row suture bridge L-PRP versus control	70 (35 per group)	2 years	Primary: MRI for healing Secondary: Constant; Simple Shoulder Test score; UCLA score; strength	No significant differences in any outcome measure
Jo (2013)	Rotator cuff tear Large to massive tears	Double-row suture bridge PRP versus control	48 (24 per group)	1 year	Primary: MRI or CTA for re-tear Secondary: Clinical outcome (pain, function, ROM, strength) and cross-sectional area	Significantly lower re-tear rate in the PRP group and increased cross-sectional area of supraspinatus; No difference in clinical outcomes
Rodeo (2012)	Rotator cuff tear Small to large	Platelet rich fibrin matrix versus control	79 (40 PRFM, 39 control)	1 year	Primary: U/S for tendon healing Secondary: ASES score, L'insalata score	No significant effects in healing or patient outcome measures
Chahal (2012)	Rotator cuff tear	PRP versus control	5 RCT studies selected	—	Primary: Re-tear rates Secondary: Constant, SST score, ASES score, UCLA score, SANE score	No significant differences in any of the identified studies

ASES = American Shoulder and Elbow Surgeons Shoulder Scale, PRP = platelet-rich plasma, RCT = randomized controlled trial, SANE = Single Assessment Numeric Evaluation, SST = Simple Shoulder Test, UCLA = UCLA Shoulder Rating Scale , VAS = visual analog scale.

PRP in Chondral Resurfacing

PRP has been studied for the treatment of chondral defects because some of the released growth factors have demonstrated anabolic effects in vitro by stimulating chondrocyte proliferation. TGF-β has been found to enhance matrix production, cell proliferation, and osteochondrogenic differentiation while it upregulates type II collagen and aggrecan gene expression.[27] PRP also has been found to have a chemotactic effect, stimulating both the migration of bone marrow stromal cells to the site of injury and subsequent chondrogenic differentiation.[27] In addition, PRP specifically increases the activity of TGF-β1, which can stimulate extracellular matrix synthesis, while downregulating the catabolic effects of interleukin 1 (IL-1) and matrix metalloproteinases (MMPs), which are known to degrade articular cartilage.[28] Insulin-like growth factor 1 has been found to have similar anabolic effects; it increases production of extracellular matrix, stimulates chondrogenic differentiation of mesenchymal stem cells (MSCs), downregulates the catabolic effects of IL-1 and MMPs, and has a synergistic effect when administered with TGF-β1.[28]

In the treatment of chondral defects, PRP can be injected locally to supply growth factors meant to stimulate an inflammatory response and neovascularization (to attract stem cells and fibroblasts), stimulate chondrocyte differentiation and proliferation, and downregulate catabolic enzyme activity (to allow articular cartilage regeneration).[27-29] A direct, intra-articular injection can be administered, or a scaffold can be used to deliver PRP to the intended site. The available polymer scaffolds are protein based (fibrin, collagen), carbohydrate based (hyaluronic acid, alginate), or synthetic (polylactic acid, polyglycolic acid).[29]

Animal studies found mixed results when osteochondral defects were treated with PRP, and few clinical studies exist. The effects of intra-articular PRP and hyaluronic acid injections were compared in treating talar osteochondral defects.[30] No scaffold was used. The PRP was activated with calcium chloride to allow a fibrin clot to form within the joint. Patients in both treatment groups had a decrease in visual analog scale (VAS) pain scores and improvement in American Orthopaedic Foot and Ankle Society ankle-hindfoot scores, but the outcomes were substantially better in the patients treated with PRP.[30] In the treatment of knee osteochondral defects, the use of a synthetic scaffold, in which PRP was combined with a poly-gamma glutamic acid (PGA)–hyaluronan scaffold, led to significant improvement in patient-reported outcomes on the Knee Injury and Osteoarthritis Outcome Score (KOOS) and to histologic evidence of hyaline-like repair tissue at the defect site at 1-year follow-up.[31] Five

patients treated for a patellar osteochondral defect using autologous matrix-induced chondrogenesis with added PRP had improved clinical outcome scores (KOOS, Kujala patellofemoral score, Tegner activity scale, VAS), despite lack of lesional filling on MRI at 1-year follow-up.[32] These studies suggest that PRP can be useful in treating osteochondral lesions, but further study is warranted to determine the best method of delivery and provide results.

PRP in Osteoarthritis

The progress of osteoarthritis is largely driven by proteolytic enzymes, with MMPs contributing to degradation of type II collagen and proteoglycan. PRP is thought to allow cartilage restoration by downregulating the effects of these enzymes while stimulating chondrocyte proliferation and extracellular matrix production.[28] Preclinical in vitro studies found a positive effect of PRP on chondrocyte metabolism and led to clinical studies.[33] A randomized clinical study comparing PRP with hyaluronic acid injections in the treatment of knee gonarthrosis found significantly better outcomes at 24-week follow-up in the patients who had PRP injections, as indicated by lower, maintained scores on the Western Ontario and McMaster Universities Osteoarthritis Index (WOMAC).[34] Another comparison of PRP with hyaluronic acid for treating osteoarthritis found improved International Knee Documentation Committee (IKDC) Subjective Knee Evaluation Form and VAS scores in both groups at 2-month follow-up, but at 6-month follow-up only the patients treated with PRP had maintained the improvement in outcome scores.[35] A double-blind, prospective randomized controlled study compared the effects of WBC-filtered PRP and normal saline injections in patients with osteoarthritis. Patients treated with one or two PRP injections had better scores on the WOMAC than those who received a saline injection, but the effect dissipated after 6 months.[20] Although these studies show a positive effect of single or multiple PRP injections for knee osteoarthritis, most of the results were limited to 6-month follow-up. Longer follow-up times are necessary to determine whether the effect is maintained.

PRP in Meniscal Repair

The inner two-thirds of the meniscus is a relatively avascular area with limited intrinsic healing capacity. Growth factor augmentation has the potential to stimulate neovascularization and improve healing in this region. An early study found that an exogenous clot could stimulate healing, but more recent clinical studies are lacking.[36] Animal studies found improved meniscal healing in rabbits after an introduced tear was repaired using PRP delivered with a gelatin hydrogel or hyaluronic acid–collagen composite

6: Miscellaneous Topics

matrix.[37,38] A clinical study of meniscal healing after open repair of a horizontal tear found excellent healing regardless of whether PRP had been injected into the repair site, but patients who received PRP had slightly better clinical outcomes (IKDC, KOOS scores) and radiographic meniscal appearance on postsurgical MRI.[39] Ongoing study is required to determine the usefulness of PRP and the optimal delivery method in meniscal injuries.

Isolated Growth Factors

Several active agents within PRP may be responsible for its clinical effects. Platelet aggregation and degranulation releases several different growth factors or cytokines that may contribute to the overall effect. The most commonly studied factors are PDGF, TGF-β, FGF, and bone morphogenetic protein (BMP), which have been shown to contribute to fibrosis and improved structural properties at the repair site.[21] The activity of several of these growth factors was upregulated during normal healing in an animal rotator cuff repair model.[40] It is not entirely clear which factors are most active in stimulating or contributing to soft-tissue or tendon-bone healing or whether their effects are synergistic.

PDGF exists as two subunits (A, B) and three isoforms (AA, BB, AB). PDGF-BB has been found to contribute to tendon-bone healing by stimulating cell chemotaxis and division as well as type I collagen synthesis.[21] Preclinical studies found that application of PDGF-BB in rabbit medial collateral ligament injuries and in rat and sheep rotator cuff injuries led to improvement in the histologic appearance of the healing ligaments and tendons, with increased tendon-bone interdigitation and increased biomechanical strength at the bone-ligament and bone-tendon interfaces.[21,40] Delivery of PDGF-BB in a collagen scaffold improved the histologic appearance of the bone-tendon interface in a rat rotator cuff repair model, although it appeared to have a detrimental effect on biomechanical properties, as shown by increased retearing rates and poor results on ultimate load-to-failure tests.[41] In addition to tendon-bone or ligament-bone healing, PDGF has been used in cartilage regeneration because it is a potent chemotactic and mitogenic factor that attracts MSCs, stimulates proliferation and differentiation (resulting in increased proteoglycan synthesis), and antagonizes interleukin 1β–mediated cartilage degradation.[29]

TGF-β is secreted after platelet degranulation. Its three isoforms (TGF-β1, TGF-β2, TGF-β3) have different functions. For example, TGF-β1 activity is greatest with scar tissue formation during wound healing, and TGF-β3 is active during fetal tendon formation. Experimental studies that manipulated these growth factors with exogenous application of TGF-β1 and TGF-β3 in a rat rotator cuff repair model found that administration of TGF-β3 improved the mechanical properties and histologic appearance of the healing rotator cuff better than TGF-β1.[42] After TGF-β1 was administered, with suppression of TGF-β2 and TGF-β3, the cross-sectional thickness of the rotator cuff increased. This thickness predominantly represented mechanically inferior scar tissue, however. In the same rat rotator cuff model, application of TGF-β3 and an osteoconductive calcium-phosphate matrix led to significant improvement in the strength of the repair at 4 weeks, with favorable histologic appearance and an improved ratio of type I to type III collagen.[43]

The FGF family of polypeptides has an affinity for heparin-binding sites. The role of FGFs in soft-tissue healing is primarily related to their contribution to angiogenesis, in which they stimulate division of capillary endothelial cells.[21,40] FGF-1 and FGF-2 are prevalent in adult tissue. Two studies of the effect of exogenous application of FGF-2 in a rat rotator cuff model found better repair strength in the treatment group than in the control group, although in one study the effect was maintained for only 6 weeks.[44,45] Similar results were found with the application of basic FGF for the treatment of patellar tendon defects in rats and flexor tendon injuries in chickens.[46,47] FGF-2 also has been used in cartilage regeneration. Exogenous administration in a mouse model led to a reduction in osteoarthritis, but administration in a mouse knockout model led to accelerated osteoarthritis.[29] Caution was recommended because large doses of exogenous FGF-2 upregulated MMP activity and accelerated the progress of arthritis.

The BMPs are a group of proteins constituting part of the TGF superfamily that regulates bone, tendon, and cartilage formation. The many BMP subtypes have been widely studied because of their distinctly different regulatory effects. BMP-12 and BMP-13 have a regulatory effect on new tendon formation. A study of the effects of BMP-12 applied in a sheep rotator cuff repair model found that treatment led to improved mechanical strength and an improved histologic appearance at the tendon-bone interface, with organized collagen fibrils. An investigation of the effect of BMP-13 in a rat rotator cuff model found no notable differences in histologic appearance or biomechanical testing.[48] A more recent study, again using a rat rotator cuff repair model, tested BMP-13 used in isolation and with PRP. On histologic analysis, BMP-13 was found to increase the ultimate load to failure as well as the amount of type III collagen.[49]

Despite preclinical evidence suggesting clinical efficacy of growth factors in the treatment of various conditions, clinical evidence is lacking, largely because of regulatory restrictions. Further preclinical studies are necessary to irrefutably demonstrate the efficacy of growth factors and establish a basis for approval of clinical studies.

Cellular Therapy

In addition to the gradual process of inflammation, repair, and remodeling, soft-tissue healing is often limited by the inadequate availability of native differentiated cells and tissues. The result can be an inflammatory process that leaves reactive scar tissue at the site of injury. MSC therapy is thought to have potential for improving the process. MSCs are regenerative cells capable of reparative healing; local paracrine activity, secretion of necessary growth factors, and attraction of additional cells lead to improved healing and restoration of native tissue organization. MSCs can be isolated from bone marrow, adipose tissue, synovial tissue, or periosteum. MSCs are useful in a multitude of areas; they maintain their multipotent status and, depending on their environmental cues, are able to differentiate into phenotypes including osteocytes, adipocytes, and chondrocytes. Despite tremendous interest and in vitro research activity, there is limited clinical evidence to support the use of MSCs in sports medicine.

Information is lacking on the number of cells required for a positive treatment effect. One study found that a relatively high concentration of progenitor cells produced a correspondingly greater clinical effect, as shown by improved healing rates when tibial nonunion was treated with a relatively high concentration of MSCs.[50] The yield of true pluripotent MSCs isolated from bone marrow aspirate is low, although it varies depending on the site from which the aspirate was drawn. A higher concentration was identified in iliac crest aspirates than in tibial or calcaneal aspirates.[51] Commercial systems can produce a bone marrow aspirate concentrate, but further study is necessary to determine the cell concentrations required to obtain a beneficial treatment effect in different tissues before widespread use can be recommended.

Stem cell use is limited not only by the lack of clinical evidence but also by the regulatory activity of the US FDA. Despite significant interest in the possible usefulness of stem cells in sports medicine, the US FDA allows only homologous use and limits the physical manipulation of stem cells. For example, isolated bone marrow–derived cells cannot be expanded in culture before use. Cell preconditioning is not allowed by the US FDA, despite evidence from in vitro studies that preconditioned cells confer a greater benefit than aspirate-concentrated cells.[37]

Stem Cells in Tendinopathy

Several preclinical studies found positive effects when MSCs derived from multiple sources were used in the treatment of tendinopathies in animal models. The relatively few clinical studies were done in Europe and involved isolation and amplification of skin-derived tenocytes, which are restricted in the United States.[52-54] These studies found positive effects in pain reduction and functional improvement when skin-derived fibroblast cells were used for treating patellar tendinopathy, lateral epicondylitis, or Achilles tendinosis. The stem cells were administered in conjunction with a plasma centrifugate, which may have affected interpretation of the clinical results. The clinical evidence is insufficient to support the routine use of stem cells in the treatment of tendinopathy.

Stem Cells in Rotator Cuff Repair

There is little clinical evidence to support the use of MSCs in rotator cuff repairs. Stem cells can be aspirated from the iliac crest or from the proximal humerus during arthroscopic rotator cuff repair, but only a few small studies have found a beneficial effect from their use. One study investigated the effect of adding autologous bone marrow–derived MSCs obtained from an iliac crest aspirate to a standard rotator cuff repair involving one to three tendons.[55] All 14 patients had MRI-demonstrated tendon integrity at 12-month follow-up, with satisfactory clinical outcomes (UCLA score); there was no control group. The researchers concluded that the use of bone marrow–derived MSCs offered a potential beneficial effect. In another study, all patients who received an iliac crest aspirate concentrate of bone marrow–derived MSCs with a standard repair of an isolated supraspinatus tear had healing on ultrasound and MRI at 6-month follow-up, compared with two-thirds of patients who received the standard repair alone.[56] The treatment effect was maintained at 2-year follow-up, when 87% of patients in the treatment group and only 44% of patients in the control group had an intact rotator cuff on ultrasound and MRI. A relationship was identified between tendon healing and the number of MSCs in the aspirate concentrate; higher failure rates were correlated with lower concentrations of MSCs.[56] This study did not report clinical outcome measures but did provide radiographic evidence to support the use of MSCs in rotator cuff repair. Further study is necessary to determine the associated clinical outcome.

Stem Cells in Chondral Resurfacing

It remains difficult to stimulate healing with appropriate tissue regeneration in chondral injuries. Attention has focused on the use of stem cells to allow regenerative cartilaginous healing as an expansion of the microfracture theory first proposed by Steadman, in which local growth factors and MSCs form a "super clot" that allows regenerative healing.[57] Early preclinical studies and case reports found improvement in healing when stem cells were used in chondral defects of rabbit knees and human patellae.[58,59] A clinical study investigated the use of MSCs in treating chondral injuries of the medial compartment of the knee, in conjunction with a high tibial osteotomy.[60] Stem cells were obtained from bone marrow aspirate, cultured, and embedded in a collagen gel that was delivered into the defect and secured with a periosteal patch. At 42-week follow-up, arthroscopic and histologic grading of the medial compartment in patients who received an MSC injection showed complete filling of the defects with metachromasia present. However, the clinical outcomes showed no statistically significant differences based on treatment with MSC injection.[60] A clinical study of the treatment of osteochondral defects of the distal femur compared the use of MSCs with the use of autologous chondrocyte implantation, both of which were inserted in a cell sheet secured under a periosteal patch. Patients in both groups had improvement, with no statistically significant differences. The researchers concluded that the use of MSCs was efficacious for treating chondral injuries, and that in comparison with autologous chondrocyte implantation MSCs offered lower surgical morbidity and a single-stage procedure.[61] Clinical and radiographic results were reported 3 years after focal osteochondral defects were treated with a single-stage knee arthroscopy with the use of iliac crest aspirate and the subsequent concentration, preparation, and delivery of a bone marrow–derived MSC-laden collagen membrane.[62] Improved IKDC scores and regenerative healing on imaging studies led the researchers to conclude that this procedure represented a viable option for treating osteochondral lesions of the knee.

Although these preliminary results show potential for using MSCs in the treatment of chondral injuries, further studies are required to determine the optimal delivery method, and long-term clinical follow-up is needed to ensure that the treatment effect is maintained.

Stem Cells in Osteoarthritis

Only limited clinical evidence is available to support stem cell use in the treatment of osteoarthritis. The use of infrapatellar fat pad–derived MSCs was investigated in the treatment of knee osteoarthritis.[63] The fat pad sample was harvested during knee arthroscopy, and the MSCs were concentrated, combined with 3.0 mL of PRP, and injected into the knee on the same day. Lysholm, VAS, and WOMAC scores improved, as did the global MRI rating for the knee. The study did not include a control group, and the earlier arthroscopic débridement of the patients' knees could have clouded the treatment effect. In addition, the administration of the MSCs with PRP creates

difficulty in discerning which agent led to the improvement. A second study by the same researchers reported on the second-look characteristics of isolated chondral defects in arthritic knees treated with MSC injection using a different delivery method.[64] Adipose-derived MSCs from buttock tissue were delivered in a synovial MSC suspension, which was injected onto the defect and allowed to adhere for 10 minutes before the knee was moved. The patients who underwent second-look arthroscopy had significant improvement in outcome measures (IKDC, Tegner scores), but extensive irregularity remained in the appearance of the regenerated cartilage, as determined using the International Cartilage Repair Society classification. A subsequent study by the same researchers added a group of patients treated using adipose-derived MSCs with fibrin glue as a carrier. During subsequent second-look arthroscopy, this method of delivery was found to improve the intra-articular appearance of the defect, compared with the earlier method.[65] Although these results are encouraging, ongoing study of the method of delivery and long-term clinical outcomes is needed.

Stem Cells in Meniscal Repair

Despite an abundance of preclinical evidence showing the positive effect of stem cells in the treatment of meniscal lesions, there is minimal evidence to support its clinical use. A novel clinical technique for meniscal repair used a collagen matrix incorporated into a suture repair of the meniscus, followed by injection of bone marrow–derived stem cells; effectively, the collagen matrix was used as a scaffold for delivering the stem cells to the site of injury.[66] This technique was used in 30 patients and, based on symptoms at 2.5-year follow-up, was considered successful in 27 (90%). There was no imaging to assess meniscal healing. Materials other than a collagen matrix could be used as scaffolds for stem cells in the treatment of meniscal lesions, but further study is necessary.

Tissue Therapy: Scaffolds

Scaffolds are collagen-rich extracellular matrixes derived from human or animal dermis or submucosal intestine.[76] A scaffold often is required for delivery of PRP or stem cells to the intended area of treatment. Scaffolds also can be used independently to augment soft-tissue healing, with the extracellular matrix providing immediate mechanical strength in the transient period of weakness during the healing phase after tendon or ligament repair. The use of scaffolds is limited by the immune response they can induce, their rate of degradation, and the overall biomechanical strength they confer to the local tissue.[67]

© 2016 American Academy of Orthopaedic Surgeons

Scaffolds are broadly classified as biologic or synthetic. Biologic scaffolds are thought to offer greater benefit than synthetic scaffolds because their natural composition allows better remodeling.[67] Animal-derived products are regulated by the US FDA. The cellular response and host response to the scaffold depends on its composition and the extent of chemical cross-linking; non–cross-linked scaffolds are rapidly remodeled, whereas cross-linked scaffolds undergo slower remodeling and incorporation into the host tissue.[68] Degradation of the scaffold is optimally balanced by local tissue regeneration to prevent any transient periods of weakened structural integrity during the healing process. Synthetic scaffolds are composed of chemical compounds, and they attempt to simulate native extracellular matrices to provide immediate mechanical strength to the adjacent local tissue while allowing cellular adhesion, differentiation, and proliferation.[67] The advantages of using a synthetic scaffold rather than a biologic scaffold are a potentially lower infection rate, a lower immunogenic response, a more consistent manufacturing process, and greater availability. The rate of degradation depends on the chemical composition of the scaffold, as it does with a biologic scaffold. Poly-L-lactic acid and polylactide-co-glycolide are among the more commonly used synthetic scaffolds.

The two most common uses for scaffolds in sports medicine are supported by preclinical and clinical evidence. In rotator cuff repair augmentation, the scaffold itself contributes mechanical strength during the healing process. In cartilage regeneration with cellular engineering, the scaffold essentially is a carrier for chondrocytes, MSCs, PRP, or other growth factors. Early clinical studies of rotator cuff augmentation using porcine small intestine mucosal patches had mixed results ranging from high failure rates and inflammatory reactions to improved outcomes on Constant and patient satisfaction scores with correlated MRI findings.[69,70] More recent studies found that the use of an acellular human dermal matrix allograft to augment a two-tendon rotator cuff tear (larger than 3 cm) led to statistically significant improvements in Constant and UCLA scores. There was a marked difference in tendon continuity between patients in the treated and control groups (85% or 40%, respectively).[71] A synthetic scaffold (polycarbonate polyurethane patch) used to augment rotator cuff repairs led to significant improvements in range of motion and patient-reported outcomes (American Shoulder and Elbow Surgeons, UCLA, Simple Shoulder Test scores). The retear rate was only 10%.[72]

Synthetic biomimetic scaffolds with three layers simulating the chondral, tidemark, and subchondral layers were used in the treatment of large defects in the knee.[73] Patients had improved outcomes (IKDC, Tegner, VAS

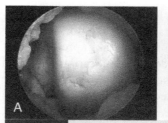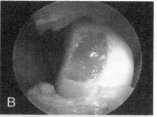

Figure 1 **A,** Chondral lesion of the medial femoral condyle. **B,** Medial femoral condyle lesion after débridement and application of Neocart scaffold. (Photos courtesy of Dr. Riley Williams.)

pain scores), with radiographically confirmed lesional filling in 70% of patients and an intact articular surface in 63%.

Scaffolds also are used to carry regenerative cells in cellular engineering. NeoCart (Histogenics) is one such product that is administered as a collagen matrix scaffold with autologous chondrocytes (**Figure 1**). A randomized clinical study found that the use of NeoCart led to excellent results in the treatment of osteochondral defects of the distal femur, in comparison with microfracture. Patients treated with NeoCart had significantly better outcomes (IKDC, KOOS, VAS scores) than those who were not treated with NeoCart.[74]

Although the studies appear to provide support for the use of scaffolds in the treatment of rotator cuff injuries and osteochondral defects, most are case control or case studies. Larger, randomized prospective clinical studies are necessary, with an appropriate-length follow-up.

Systemic Factors

Several systemic factors have been identified as contributing to the injury healing process, in addition to the cellular response to injury and its contribution to healing. The primary focus in recent years has been on the role of vitamin D in soft-tissue and tendon-bone healing, the role of MMP inhibitors in the treatment of osteoarthritis, and the effect of diabetes on soft-tissue and tendon-bone healing.

Vitamin D Deficiency

Vitamin D is a fat-soluble secosteroid that plays an integral part in the homeostasis of calcium and phosphate by affecting absorption and secretion in the intestine, kidneys, and skeletal system.[67,75] The primary source of vitamin D is ultraviolet light exposure of the skin, where 7-dehydrocholesterol is converted to previtamin D3. Previtamin D3 is slowly isomerized into vitamin D3, which travels to the liver and is metabolized into 25-hydroxyvitamin D, which travels to the kidney and is metabolized into 1,25-dihydroxyvitamin D; this represents the biologically active form. Dietary vitamin D is a minor, secondary component of the daily requirement. Skin production of vitamin D is affected by geographic location, age, and skin pigmentation. The process of hydroxylation in the liver and kidney is regulated by a complex interaction among calcium, phosphate, and parathyroid hormone. In addition to regulation of calcium and phosphate homeostasis, vitamin D affects neuromuscular junctions, inflammatory and immune responses, and gene expression and regulation of apoptosis.[67]

Most experts define vitamin D deficiency as a 1,25-dihydroxyvitamin D level of less than 20 ng per mL.[75] Vitamin D deficiency, or hypovitaminosis D, has been associated with cardiovascular disease, cancer, diabetes, and bone fragility. In sports medicine, it has been associated with decreased athletic performance and muscle function. Vitamin D is capable of stimulating muscle metabolism and growth through vitamin D receptors within muscle. The decrease in the number of these receptors with natural aging, in conjunction with decreasing muscular function, suggests that a vitamin D deficiency can contribute to decreasing muscle function and subsequent athletic performance.[75] In addition, vitamin D deficiency is correlated with increasing muscular atrophy, fatty infiltration, and muscle fibrosis, although most of these effects are reversible with vitamin D supplementation. Results from an observational study suggested that vitamin D deficiency may contribute to the progression of osteoarthritis, although the causal relationship has not been well defined.[76]

A recent study using a rat model investigated the effect of vitamin D deficiency on rotator cuff healing.[77] Compared with control rats, vitamin D–deficient rats had lower load-to-failure rates in early biomechanical testing and less structural integrity at the bone-tendon interface on histologic analysis. These results suggest that low vitamin D levels may adversely affect soft-tissue healing. This study represents the only preclinical evidence suggesting a deleterious effect of vitamin D deficiency on tendon-bone healing, but it should lead to increased attention to the effects of vitamin D on soft-tissue healing.

Matrix Metalloproteinases

The MMPs are a complex set of zinc-dependent enzymes that are responsible for maintenance and remodeling of the extracellular matrix. The MMPs are involved in normal activities including embryonal development, soft-tissue healing after injury, and remodeling after surgery. MMPs also are involved in pathologic activities including tumor growth and development of vascular aneurysmal disease. In sports medicine, excessive MMP activity has been related to osteoarthritis, tendinopathy, and rotator cuff disease.[29,78]

In native tissue, the activity of MMPs is primarily regulated by tissue inhibitors that control the balance between degradative and reparative processes. Evidence exists that in certain pathologic processes, such as rotator cuff degeneration or tearing, this balance is lost, with a resulting increase in MMP activity and decrease in levels of tissue inhibitors of MMPs.[78] Agents that act as MMP inhibitors may be able to reverse some of these effects or slow the degradative processes driven by the MMPs. PRP and BMP-7 are some of the substances that have been shown to inhibit MMP activity in the treatment of osteoarthritis or chondral defects.[29] In two separate rat-model studies, local administration of the MMP inhibitors α-2-macroglobulin and doxycycline after surgical rotator cuff detachment and repair led to significant improvement in collagen organization at the tendon-bone interface. However, biomechanical testing did not detect a significant maintained effect on failure strength at 4 weeks.[79,80]

The use of MMP inhibitors represents a potential means of restoring the native inhibitory processes to prevent ongoing degradative changes, but further study is necessary to determine the benefits beyond histologic improvement in the healing response. Preclinical and clinical studies are needed to define the indications for MMP inhibitors in the treatment of sports medicine pathology.

Diabetes Mellitus

Diabetes mellitus causes metabolic changes including glycosylation of proteins, microvascular abnormalities, and abnormal collagen accumulation, and it is strongly associated with vascular and neuropathic disease. In addition, the disease is related to musculoskeletal conditions such as adhesive capsulitis, tendinopathy, and rotator cuff tearing.[67] An observational study of rotator cuff characteristics and injury patterns in patients with diabetes and age-matched control subjects found that those with diabetes had significant tendon thickening as well as significantly higher rates of degenerative change in the rotator cuff (43% compared with 20%) and biceps tendon (27% compared with 8%).[81]

A review of outcomes of arthroscopic rotator cuff repair in patients with and without diabetes found less Constant score improvement in those with diabetes (from 49.2 to 60.8) than in those without diabetes (from 46.4 to 65.2).[82] Further analysis of the Constant score revealed that the patients with diabetes had more limitation in postsurgical range of motion, specifically forward flexion (150° compared with 157°) and external rotation (40° compared with 51°), than those without diabetes.

A rat study found that a persistent state of hyperglycemia has a negative effect on tendon-bone healing in rotator cuff repairs.[83] Diabetes was induced with an intraperitoneal injection of streptozotocin and confirmed by two glucose tolerance tests and hemoglobin A1c levels. In comparison with the control animals, those with diabetes were found to have less fibrocartilage and less well-organized collagen at the repair site, and they had a significantly reduced ultimate load to failure at 1 and 2 weeks.

These studies show the adverse effect that diabetes has on soft-tissue healing and surgical outcomes, particularly for tendon-bone healing. Patients should be encouraged to achieve appropriate glycemic control both as a preventive health measure and a potential factor in postsurgical recovery. Clinical study is necessary to determine whether glycemic control can improve outcomes after treatment of sports-related injuries.

Summary

Orthobiologic agents offer the potential to improve or expedite healing and improve outcomes after nonsurgical or surgical treatment of a variety of musculoskeletal injuries. A significant amount of preclinical research has been conducted, but clinical research with improved methodology, including standardization of biologic adjuvant preparation and method of delivery, is required before appropriate clinical indications can be established.

Key Study Points

- Orthobiologics, including PRP, mesenchymal stem cells, and tissue scaffolds, represent an exciting potential adjunct to traditional treatment of musculoskeletal injuries and sport-related pathology, although clinical data are currently lacking.
- Careful review of available literature, with ongoing clinical studies to further assess the efficacy of these agents should be performed prior to widespread utilization.

Annotated References

1. Marx RE: Platelet-rich plasma: Evidence to support its use. *J Oral Maxillofac Surg* 2004;62(4):489-496.

2. Sheth U, Simunovic N, Klein G, et al: Efficacy of autologous platelet-rich plasma use for orthopaedic indications: A meta-analysis. *J Bone Joint Surg Am* 2012;94(4):298-307.

This meta-analysis reviewed the usefulness of autologous blood concentrates in the treatment of orthopaedic bone and soft-tissue injuries. There are no clear indications for use because of variability in study protocols and concentrate preparation. Level of evidence: II.

3. Foster TE, Puskas BL, Mandelbaum BR, Gerhardt MB, Rodeo SA: Platelet-rich plasma: From basic science to clinical applications. *Am J Sports Med* 2009;37(11):2259-2272.

The basic science of PRP was reviewed, with clinical applications in orthopaedic sports medicine, human studies using PRP, the use of PRP in sports, and its regulation by antidoping agencies.

4. Hsu WK, Mishra A, Rodeo SR, et al: Platelet-rich plasma in orthopaedic applications: Evidence-based recommendations for treatment. *J Am Acad Orthop Surg* 2013;21(12):739-748.

The preparation and composition of PRP was reviewed with its current clinical applications and supporting evidence.

5. Hall MP, Band PA, Meislin RJ, Jazrawi LM, Cardone DA: Platelet-rich plasma: Current concepts and application in sports medicine. *J Am Acad Orthop Surg* 2009;17(10):602-608.

The composition and clinical applications of PRP with available evidence were reviewed.

6. Derwin KA, Kovacevic D, Kim M-S, Ricchetti ET: Biologic augmentation of rotator cuff healing, in Nicholson GP, ed: *OKU: Shoulder and Elbow* 4. Rosemont, IL, American Academy of Orthopaedic Surgeons, 2013, pp 31–44.

Available tissue-engineering strategies were reviewed as applied in the treatment of rotator cuff injuries. PRP, growth factors, and scaffolds were discussed with relevant clinical evidence.

7. Li G-Y, Yin J-M, Ding H, Jia W-T, Zhang C-Q: Efficacy of leukocyte- and platelet-rich plasma gel (L-PRP gel) in treating osteomyelitis in a rabbit model. *J Orthop Res* 2013;31(6):949-956.

The usefulness of leukocyte-rich PRP was reviewed in the treatment of osteomyelitis using an animal model.

8. Moojen DJ, Everts PA, Schure R-M, et al: Antimicrobial activity of platelet-leukocyte gel against Staphylococcus aureus. *J Orthop Res* 2008;26(3):404-410.

9. Lopez-Vidriero E, Goulding KA, Simon DA, Sanchez M, Johnson DH: The use of platelet-rich plasma in arthroscopy and sports medicine: Optimizing the healing environment. *Arthroscopy* 2010;26(2):269-278.

The composition, contribution to healing, and clinical application of PRP were reviewed.

10. Anitua E, Zalduendo MM, Prado R, Alkhraisat MH, Orive G: Morphogen and proinflammatory cytokine release kinetics from PRGF-Endoret fibrin scaffolds:

Evaluation of the effect of leukocyte inclusion. *J Biomed Mater Res A* 2015;103(3):1011-1020.

An in vitro study analyzed growth factor–release kinematics from leukocyte-free and leukocyte-rich PRP fibrin scaffolds. An increased release of growth factors and proinflammatory cytokines was identified with inclusion of leukocytes.

11. Mazzocca AD, McCarthy MB, Chowaniec DM, et al: Platelet-rich plasma differs according to preparation method and human variability. *J Bone Joint Surg Am* 2012;94(4):308-316.

The differences in qualitative composition of PRP derived from commercially available separation systems were reviewed, with identification of significant differences in component concentrations between samples.

12. Atesok K, Fu FH, Wolf MR, et al: Augmentation of tendon-to-bone healing. *J Bone Joint Surg Am* 2014;96(6):513-521.

This review covers challenges in achieving tendon-bone healing and related basic science research strategies.

13. de Vos RJ, Weir A, van Schie HT, et al: Platelet-rich plasma injection for chronic Achilles tendinopathy: A randomized controlled trial. *JAMA* 2010;303(2):144-149.

A randomized controlled study compared PRP injection and saline injection in patients who also performed eccentric exercises for the treatment of chronic Achilles tendinopathy. No significant improvement in pain and function was identified after PRP injection. Level of evidence: I.

14. Kaniki N, Willits K, Mohtadi NG, Fung V, Bryant D: A retrospective comparative study with historical control to determine the effectiveness of platelet-rich plasma as part of nonoperative treatment of acute Achilles tendon rupture. *Arthroscopy* 2014;30(9):1139-1145.

A retrospective study compared the effectiveness of PRP in the treatment of nonsurgically managed acute Achilles tendon ruptures. No significant benefit of PRP injection was identified. Level of evidence: III.

15. A Hamid MS, Mohamed Ali MR, Yusof A, George J, Lee LP: Platelet-rich plasma injections for the treatment of hamstring injuries: A randomized controlled trial. *Am J Sports Med* 2014;42(10):2410-2418.

A randomized controlled study investigated the effect of a single PRP injection coupled with rehabilitation for the treatment of grade 2 hamstring injuries, compared with rehabilitation alone. The addition of PRP injection led to significantly lower pain scores and earlier return to play. Level of evidence: II.

16. Mishra AK, Skrepnik NV, Edwards SG, et al: Efficacy of platelet-rich plasma for chronic tennis elbow: A double-blind, prospective, multicenter, randomized controlled trial of 230 patients. *Am J Sports Med* 2014;42(2):463-471.

A randomized controlled study evaluated the efficacy of PRP combined with dry needling for the treatment of lateral epicondylitis. There was significant improvement on the outcomes measure in patients treated with PRP at 24-week follow-up. Level of evidence: II.

17. Peerbooms JC, Sluimer J, Bruijn DJ, Gosens T: Positive effect of an autologous platelet concentrate in lateral epicondylitis in a double-blind randomized controlled trial: Platelet-rich plasma versus corticosteroid injection with a 1-year follow-up. *Am J Sports Med* 2010;38(2):255-262.

A randomized controlled study compared the effectiveness of PRP and corticosteroid injection in the treatment of chronic lateral epicondylitis. Patients in the PRP group had significantly better pain scores and function than those in the corticosteroid group. Level of evidence: I.

18. Charousset C, Zaoui A, Bellaiche L, Bouyer B: Are multiple platelet-rich plasma injections useful for treatment of chronic patellar tendinopathy in athletes? A prospective study. *Am J Sports Med* 2014;42(4):906-911.

A case study of PRP in the nonsurgical treatment of chronic patellar tendinopathy found that patients had significant improvement in symptoms and function after three ultrasound-guided injections of PRP, in comparison with those who received only rehabilitation. Level of evidence: IV.

19. Dragoo JL, Wasterlain AS, Braun HJ, Nead KT: Platelet-rich plasma as a treatment for patellar tendinopathy: A double-blind, randomized controlled trial. *Am J Sports Med* 2014;42(3):610-618.

A randomized controlled study of outcomes when patellar tendinopathy was treated with dry needling, with or without PRP injection found improvement in outcomes with dry needling but no apparent benefit of PRP injection. Level of evidence: I.

20. Patel S, Dhillon MS, Aggarwal S, Marwaha N, Jain A: Treatment with platelet-rich plasma is more effective than placebo for knee osteoarthritis: A prospective, double-blind, randomized trial. *Am J Sports Med* 2013;41(2):356-364.

A randomized controlled study evaluated the effect of PRP in the treatment of osteoarthritis. A single dose of WBC-filtered PRP provided transient improvement in pain and outcome scores, with dissipation of the treatment effect at 6 months. Level of evidence: I.

21. Weeks KD III, Dines JS, Rodeo SA, Bedi A: The basic science behind biologic augmentation of tendon-bone healing: A scientific review. *Instr Course Lect* 2014;63:443-450.

A review of the basic science behind tendon-bone healing included the relevant growth factors, bioengineering strategies used to augment rotator cuff repair, and supporting evidence.

22. Malavolta EA, Gracitelli ME, Ferreira Neto AA, Assunção JH, Bordalo-Rodrigues M, de Camargo OP: Platelet-rich plasma in rotator cuff repair: A prospective randomized study. *Am J Sports Med* 2014;42(10):2446-2454.

© 2016 American Academy of Orthopaedic Surgeons

A randomized controlled study investigated the effect of PRP in rotator cuff repair. No demonstrable benefit was found when PRP was added to the existing cuff repair construct. Level of evidence: I.

23. Charousset C, Zaoui A, Bellaïche L, Piterman M: Does autologous leukocyte-platelet-rich plasma improve tendon healing in arthroscopic repair of large or massive rotator cuff tears? *Arthroscopy* 2014;30(4):428-435.

   A case control study reviewed the effect of leukocyte-rich PRP injections in the treatment of rotator cuff repairs, compared with rehabilitation alone. No benefit was found in quality of tendon repair, retearing rates, or functional outcome. Level of evidence: III.

24. Rodeo SA, Delos D, Williams RJ, Adler RS, Pearle A, Warren RF: The effect of platelet-rich fibrin matrix on rotator cuff tendon healing: A prospective, randomized clinical study. *Am J Sports Med* 2012;40(6):1234-1241.

   A randomized clinical study assessed the efficacy of platelet-rich fibrin matrix on rotator cuff repair, compared with rehabilitation alone. No demonstrable effect of PRF application was found on tendon healing, vascularity, or function. Level of evidence: II.

25. Jo CH, Shin JS, Lee YG, et al: Platelet-rich plasma for arthroscopic repair of large to massive rotator cuff tears: A randomized, single-blind, parallel-group trial. *Am J Sports Med* 2013;41(10):2240-2248.

   A randomized controlled study assessed the efficacy of PRP in the treatment of rotator cuff repairs. PRP application was found to significantly improve structural properties, with lower retearing rates and a larger cross-sectional area, although no clinical improvement was noted. Level of evidence: I.

26. Chahal J, Van Thiel GS, Mall N, et al: The role of platelet-rich plasma in arthroscopic rotator cuff repair: A systematic review with quantitative synthesis. *Arthroscopy* 2012;28(11):1718-1727.

   A systematic review of the efficacy of PRP in rotator cuff healing concluded that PRP does not appear to have an effect on retearing rates or patient-reported outcomes when added to arthroscopic rotator cuff repair. Level of evidence: III.

27. Zhu Y, Yuan M, Meng HY, et al: Basic science and clinical application of platelet-rich plasma for cartilage defects and osteoarthritis: A review. *Osteoarthritis Cartilage* 2013;21(11):1627-1637.

   A review of the basic science behind PRP preparation as well as the biologic mechanism of action and clinical application for its use in treating cartilage defects and osteoarthritis.

28. Fortier LA, Barker JU, Strauss EJ, McCarrel TM, Cole BJ: The role of growth factors in cartilage repair. *Clin Orthop Relat Res* 2011;469(10):2706-2715.

   A systematic review of the effect of growth factors on cartilage repair found promising results, but further research is needed before routine use can be recommended.

29. Tuan RS, Chen AF, Klatt BA: Cartilage regeneration. *J Am Acad Orthop Surg* 2013;21(5):303-311.

   The basic science of cartilage regeneration and bioengineering strategies aimed at improving this process were reviewed.

30. Mei-Dan O, Carmont MR, Laver L, Mann G, Maffulli N, Nyska M: Platelet-rich plasma or hyaluronate in the management of osteochondral lesions of the talus. *Am J Sports Med* 2012;40(3):534-541.

   A randomized controlled study compared PRP and hyaluronic acid injections for the treatment of osteochondral lesions of the talus. Both injections led to improvement in pain and function, but PRP outcomes were significantly better. Level of evidence: II.

31. Siclari A, Mascaro G, Gentili C, Cancedda R, Boux E: A cell-free scaffold-based cartilage repair provides improved function hyaline-like repair at one year. *Clin Orthop Relat Res* 2012;470(3):910-919.

   A case study reported the outcomes of patients with articular cartilage defects treated with poly-gamma glutamic acid–hyaluronic acid scaffold immersed in PRP. Clinical outcomes and histologic analysis of the regenerative tissue reflected treatment benefit. Level of evidence: IV.

32. Dhollander AA, De Neve F, Almqvist KF, et al: Autologous matrix-induced chondrogenesis combined with platelet-rich plasma gel: Technical description and a five pilot patients report. *Knee Surg Sports Traumatol Arthrosc* 2011;19(4):536-542.

   A pilot study was reported with a technical description of autologous matrix-induced chondrogenesis in the treatment of chondral patellar lesions of the knee. Level of evidence: IV.

33. Filardo G, Kon E, Roffi A, Di Matteo B, Merli ML, Marcacci M: Platelet-rich plasma: Why intra-articular? A systematic review of preclinical studies and clinical evidence on PRP for joint degeneration. *Knee Surg Sports Traumatol Arthrosc* [published online November 26, 2013].

   A systematic review of intra-articular PRP injections for the treatment of arthritis suggested overall support, although the duration of the posttreatment clinical improvement was limited. Level of evidence: IV.

34. Cerza F, Carnì S, Carcangiu A, et al: Comparison between hyaluronic acid and platelet-rich plasma, intra-articular infiltration in the treatment of gonarthrosis. *Am J Sports Med* 2012;40(12):2822-2827.

   A randomized controlled study compared intra-articular PRP and hyaluronic acid injections in the treatment of gonarthrosis. Patients treated with PRP had significantly better outcomes than those treated with hyaluronic acid. Level of evidence: I.

6: Miscellaneous Topics

35. Kon E, Mandelbaum B, Buda R, et al: Platelet-rich plasma intra-articular injection versus hyaluronic acid viscosupplementation as treatments for cartilage pathology: From early degeneration to osteoarthritis. *Arthroscopy* 2011;27(11):1490-1501.

    A case control study reported on outcomes of PRP and hyaluronic acid injections for osteoarthritis. PRP injections had more and longer efficacy than hyaluronic acid injections, with reduced pain and improved function. Level of evidence: II.

36. Henning CE, Lynch MA, Yearout KM, Vequist SW, Stallbaumer RJ, Decker KA: Arthroscopic meniscal repair using an exogenous fibrin clot. *Clin Orthop Relat Res* 1990;252:64-72.

37. Zellner J, Mueller M, Berner A, et al: Role of mesenchymal stem cells in tissue engineering of meniscus. *J Biomed Mater Res A* 2010;94(4):1150-1161.

    An in vitro study of the effect of stem cells in the repair of meniscal defects found fibrocartilage-like repair tissue 14 days after application, suggesting a contribution to repair quality.

38. Ishida K, Kuroda R, Miwa M, et al: The regenerative effects of platelet-rich plasma on meniscal cells in vitro and its in vivo application with biodegradable gelatin hydrogel. *Tissue Eng* 2007;13(5):1103-1112.

39. Pujol N, Salle De Chou E, Boisrenoult P, Beaufils P: Platelet-rich plasma for open meniscal repair in young patients: Any benefit? *Knee Surg Sports Traumatol Arthrosc* 2015;23(1):51-58.

    A case control study of the efficacy of PRP in meniscal repair healing concluded that open repair of the meniscal injury improved outcomes and that PRP added to the repair site did not significantly alter the outcome. Level of evidence: III.

40. Gulotta LV, Rodeo SA: Growth factors for rotator cuff repair. *Clin Sports Med* 2009;28(1):13-23.

    The growth factors contributing to the healing process after repair of a torn rotator cuff were described.

41. Kovacevic D, Gulotta LV, Ying L, Ehteshami JR, Deng X-H, Rodeo SA: rhPDGF-BB promotes early healing in a rat rotator cuff repair model. *Clin Orthop Relat Res* [published online ahead of print October 28, 2014].

    An in vitro study of the efficacy of rhPDGF-BB in the treatment of rotator cuff tears in a rat model found improved cellular proliferation and angiogenesis but no biomechanical improvement in the healing tissue.

42. Bedi A, Maak T, Walsh C, et al: Cytokines in rotator cuff degeneration and repair. *J Shoulder Elbow Surg* 2012;21(2):218-227.

    The cytokines involved in rotator cuff degeneration and repair were described.

43. Kovacevic D, Fox AJ, Bedi A, et al: Calcium-phosphate matrix with or without TGF-β3 improves tendon-bone healing after rotator cuff repair. *Am J Sports Med* 2011;39(4):811-819.

    A controlled laboratory study investigated the effect of TGF-β3 application in a rat rotator cuff repair model. Topical application led to increased fibrocartilage formation with improved collagen organization and tendon-bone healing, with improved biomechanical strength.

44. Ide J, Kikukawa K, Hirose J, Iyama K, Sakamoto H, Mizuta H: The effects of fibroblast growth factor-2 on rotator cuff reconstruction with acellular dermal matrix grafts. *Arthroscopy* 2009;25(6):608-616.

    A controlled laboratory study investigated the effect of FGF application in a rat rotator cuff repair model. Topical application led to accelerated tendon remodeling with improved biomechanical strength.

45. Ide J, Kikukawa K, Hirose J, et al: The effect of a local application of fibroblast growth factor-2 on tendon-to-bone remodeling in rats with acute injury and repair of the supraspinatus tendon. *J Shoulder Elbow Surg* 2009;18(3):391-398.

    A controlled laboratory study of the effect of topical FGF application in a rat rotator cuff repair model found accelerated tendon remodeling and improved biomechanical strength.

46. Chan BP, Fu S, Qin L, Lee K, Rolf CG, Chan K: Effects of basic fibroblast growth factor (bFGF) on early stages of tendon healing: A rat patellar tendon model. *Acta Orthop Scand* 2000;71(5):513-518.

47. Tang JB, Cao Y, Zhu B, Xin K-Q, Wang XT, Liu PY: Adeno-associated virus-2-mediated bFGF gene transfer to digital flexor tendons significantly increases healing strength: an in vivo study. *J Bone Joint Surg Am* 2008;90(5):1078-1089.

48. Gulotta LV, Kovacevic D, Packer JD, Ehteshami JR, Rodeo SA: Adenoviral-mediated gene transfer of human bone morphogenetic protein-13 does not improve rotator cuff healing in a rat model. *Am J Sports Med* 2011;39(1):180-187.

    A controlled laboratory study of BMP-13 on rat rotator cuff repair found no effect on cartilage formation or collagen fiber organization with topical application.

49. Lamplot JD, Angeline M, Angeles J, et al: Distinct effects of platelet-rich plasma and BMP13 on rotator cuff tendon injury healing in a rat model. *Am J Sports Med* 2014;42(12):2877-2887.

    A controlled laboratory study of the effect of BMP-13 on rat rotator cuff repair found enhanced fibronectin expression with increased load-to-failure strength. Histologic improvement was found in retrieved samples.

50. Hernigou P, Poignard A, Beaujean F, Rouard H: Percutaneous autologous bone-marrow grafting for nonunions:

© 2016 American Academy of Orthopaedic Surgeons

Influence of the number and concentration of progenitor cells. *J Bone Joint Surg Am* 2005;87(7):1430-1437.

51. Hyer CF, Berlet GC, Bussewitz BW, Hankins T, Ziegler HL, Philbin TM: Quantitative assessment of the yield of osteoblastic connective tissue progenitors in bone marrow aspirate from the iliac crest, tibia, and calcaneus. *J Bone Joint Surg Am* 2013;95(14):1312-1316.

  Bone marrow aspirates from different locations were collected and centrifuged to concentrate nucleated cells, which were plated and grown in culture to identify osteoblastic progenitor cells. Progenitor cells were found to be most concentrated in iliac crest aspirates.

52. Clarke AW, Alyas F, Morris T, Robertson CJ, Bell J, Connell DA: Skin-derived tenocyte-like cells for the treatment of patellar tendinopathy. *Am J Sports Med* 2011;39(3):614-623.

  A randomized controlled study of the efficacy of autologous tenocyte-like cells in the treatment of patellar tendinopathy found that patients had significant improvement in pain and function compared with patients who received autologous plasma injection. Level of evidence: I.

53. Connell D, Datir A, Alyas F, Curtis M: Treatment of lateral epicondylitis using skin-derived tenocyte-like cells. *Br J Sports Med* 2009;43(4):293-298.

  A randomized controlled study of the efficacy of autologous tenocyte-like cells in the treatment of lateral epicondylitis found improvement in patient-reported outcome measures as well as number of tears, neovascularization, and tendon thickness.

54. Obaid H, Clarke A, Rosenfeld P, Leach C, Connell D: Skin-derived fibroblasts for the treatment of refractory Achilles tendinosis: Preliminary short-term results. *J Bone Joint Surg Am* 2012;94(3):193-200.

  A randomized controlled study of the efficacy of autologous tenocyte-like cells in the treatment of chronic Achilles tendinosis found significant improvement in pain and function. Level of evidence: I.

55. Ellera Gomes JL, da Silva RC, Silla LM, Abreu MR, Pellanda R: Conventional rotator cuff repair complemented by the aid of mononuclear autologous stem cells. *Knee Surg Sports Traumatol Arthrosc* 2012;20(2):373-377.

  A case study of arthroscopic rotator cuff repair augmented with autologous bone marrow mononuclear cells found generally positive radiographic and clinical outcomes and supported the safety of this technique. Level of evidence: IV.

56. Hernigou P, Flouzat Lachaniette CH, Delambre J, et al: Biologic augmentation of rotator cuff repair with mesenchymal stem cells during arthroscopy improves healing and prevents further tears: A case-controlled study. *Int Orthop* 2014;38(9):1811-1818.

  A cohort study comparing the results of rotator cuff repair augmented with MSCs found significant improvement in healing outcomes with bone marrow concentrate injection, as determined using follow-up MRI.

57. Steadman JR, Rodkey WG, Rodrigo JJ: Microfracture: Surgical technique and rehabilitation to treat chondral defects. *Clin Orthop Relat Res* 2001;(391, Suppl):S362-S369.

58. Wakitani S, Goto T, Pineda SJ, et al: Mesenchymal cell-based repair of large, full-thickness defects of articular cartilage. *J Bone Joint Surg Am* 1994;76(4):579-592.

59. Wakitani S, Mitsuoka T, Nakamura N, Toritsuka Y, Nakamura Y, Horibe S: Autologous bone marrow stromal cell transplantation for repair of full-thickness articular cartilage defects in human patellae: Two case reports. *Cell Transplant* 2004;13(5):595-600.

60. Wakitani S, Imoto K, Yamamoto T, Saito M, Murata N, Yoneda M: Human autologous culture expanded bone marrow mesenchymal cell transplantation for repair of cartilage defects in osteoarthritic knees. *Osteoarthritis Cartilage* 2002;10(3):199-206.

61. Nejadnik H, Hui JH, Feng Choong EP, Tai B-C, Lee EH: Autologous bone marrow-derived mesenchymal stem cells versus autologous chondrocyte implantation: An observational cohort study. *Am J Sports Med* 2010;38(6):1110-1116.

  A cohort study of chondral lesions treated with autologous chondrocyte implantation or bone marrow–derived MSCs found improvements after both treatments. Augmentation with bone marrow–derived MSCs may represent a safe alternative to autologous chondrocyte implantation. Level of evidence: III.

62. Buda R, Vannini F, Cavallo M, et al: One-step arthroscopic technique for the treatment of osteochondral lesions of the knee with bone-marrow-derived cells: Three years results. *Musculoskelet Surg* 2013;97(2):145-151.

  A case study of osteochondral lesions of the knee treated with bone marrow–derived MSCs delivered to the injury site with a scaffold found significant improvements in patient outcomes and radiographic appearance of the lesions. Level of evidence: IV.

63. Koh Y-G, Jo S-B, Kwon O-R, et al: Mesenchymal stem cell injections improve symptoms of knee osteoarthritis. *Arthroscopy* 2013;29(4):748-755.

  A case study of osteochondral lesions of the knee treated with fat pad–derived MSCs delivered through intra-articular injection found significant improvements in patient outcomes and radiographic appearance of the lesions. Level of evidence: IV.

64. Koh YG, Choi YJ, Kwon OR, Kim YS: Second-look arthroscopic evaluation of cartilage lesions after mesenchymal stem cell implantation in osteoarthritic knees. *Am J Sports Med* 2014;42(7):1628-1637.

  A case study of osteochondral lesions of the knee treated with fat-derived MSCs injected into the defect found significant improvements in patient outcomes and arthroscopic appearance of the lesions. Level of evidence: IV.

65. Kim YS, Choi YJ, Suh DS, et al: Mesenchymal stem cell implantation in osteoarthritic knees: Is fibrin glue effective as a scaffold? *Am J Sports Med* 2015;43(1):176-185.

A cohort study of the efficacy of MSCs delivered in fibrin glue for the treatment of chondral defects in arthritic knees found significant improvement in patient-reported outcome scores and arthroscopic grading of the chondral lesions. Level of evidence: III.

66. Jacobi M, Jakob RP: Meniscal repair: Enhancement of healing process, in Beaufils P, Verdonk R: *The Meniscus*. New York, NY, Springer-Verlag, 2010 , pp 129-135.

Bioengineering strategies for treatment of meniscal injuries were reviewed.

67. Nossov S, Dines JS, Murrell GA, Rodeo SA, Bedi A: Biologic augmentation of tendon-to-bone healing: Scaffolds, mechanical load, vitamin D, and diabetes. *Instr Course Lect* 2014;63:451-462.

Biologic augmentation options for tendon-bone healing were reviewed.

68. Ricchetti ET, Aurora A, Iannotti JP, Derwin KA: Scaffold devices for rotator cuff repair. *J Shoulder Elbow Surg* 2012;21(2):251-265.

Scaffold devices for rotator cuff repair augmentation and the biologic response and incorporation of these devices were reviewed.

69. Iannotti JP, Codsi MJ, Kwon YW, Derwin K, Ciccone J, Brems JJ: Porcine small intestine submucosa augmentation of surgical repair of chronic two-tendon rotator cuff tears: A randomized, controlled trial. *J Bone Joint Surg Am* 2006;88(6):1238-1244.

70. Badhe SP, Lawrence TM, Smith FD, Lunn PG: An assessment of porcine dermal xenograft as an augmentation graft in the treatment of extensive rotator cuff tears. *J Shoulder Elbow Surg* 2008;17(1, Suppl):35S-39S.

71. Barber FA, Burns JP, Deutsch A, Labbé MR, Litchfield RB: A prospective, randomized evaluation of acellular human dermal matrix augmentation for arthroscopic rotator cuff repair. *Arthroscopy* 2012;28(1):8-15.

A randomized controlled study of the safety and efficacy of an acellular human dermal matrix augmentation device for rotator cuff repairs found improved patient-reported outcomes and lower retearing rates in treated patients. Level of evidence: II.

72. Encalada-Diaz I, Cole BJ, Macgillivray JD, et al: Rotator cuff repair augmentation using a novel polycarbonate polyurethane patch: Preliminary results at 12 months' follow-up. *J Shoulder Elbow Surg* 2011;20(5):788-794.

A case study of the efficacy of a polycarbonate polyurethane patch for augmentation of a rotator cuff repair in 10 patients found significant improvements in pain and functional outcome scores. Level of evidence: IV.

73. Berruto M, Delcogliano M, de Caro F, et al: Treatment of large knee osteochondral lesions with a biomimetic scaffold: Results of a multicenter study of 49 patients at 2-year follow-up. *Am J Sports Med* 2014;42(7):1607-1617.

A case study of treatment of osteochondral lesions of the knee with a biomimetic scaffold found significant improvements in patient-reported outcome measures and high rates of lesional filling on MRI. Level of evidence: IV.

74. Crawford DC, DeBerardino TM, Williams RJ III: NeoCart, an autologous cartilage tissue implant, compared with microfracture for treatment of distal femoral cartilage lesions: An FDA phase-II prospective, randomized clinical trial after two years. *J Bone Joint Surg Am* 2012;94(11):979-989.

A randomized controlled study compared an autologous cartilage tissue implant with microfracture for the treatment of chondral lesions of the distal femur. Patients treated with the implant had superior clinical outcome scores at 2-year follow-up. Level of evidence: I.

75. Angeline ME, Gee AO, Shindle M, Warren RF, Rodeo SA: The effects of vitamin D deficiency in athletes. *Am J Sports Med* 2013;41(2):461-464.

The physiologic role of vitamin D and the potential adverse effects of vitamin D deficiency in athletes were reviewed.

76. Zhang FF, Driban JB, Lo GH, et al: Vitamin D deficiency is associated with progression of knee osteoarthritis. *J Nutr* 2014;144(12):2002-2008.

An observational study found that vitamin D deficiency was correlated with osteoarthritis.

77. Angeline ME, Ma R, Pascual-Garrido C, et al: Effect of diet-induced vitamin D deficiency on rotator cuff healing in a rat model. *Am J Sports Med* 2014;42(1):27-34.

A controlled laboratory study of the effect of vitamin D deficiency in a rat rotator cuff repair model found a decrease in biomechanical strength, with less bone formation and collagen fiber organization on histologic analysis.

78. Del Buono A, Oliva F, Osti L, Maffulli N: Metalloproteases and tendinopathy. *Muscles Ligaments Tendons J* 2013;3(1):51-57.

The role of MMPs in the pathophysiology of tendinopathy was reviewed.

79. Bedi A, Fox AJ, Kovacevic D, Deng X-H, Warren RF, Rodeo SA: Doxycycline-mediated inhibition of matrix metalloproteinases improves healing after rotator cuff repair. *Am J Sports Med* 2010;38(2):308-317.

A controlled laboratory study of the effect of locally administered doxycycline in a rat rotator cuff repair model found improved collagen formation and fiber organization on histologic analysis, with improved load-to-failure testing at 2 weeks.

80. Bedi A, Kovacevic D, Hettrich C, et al: The effect of matrix metalloproteinase inhibition on tendon-to-bone healing in a rotator cuff repair model. *J Shoulder Elbow Surg* 2010;19(3):384-391.

   A controlled laboratory study of the effect of a locally delivered MMP inhibitor in a rat rotator cuff repair model found improved collagen fiber formation and organization on histologic analysis.

81. Abate M, Schiavone C, Salini V: Sonographic evaluation of the shoulder in asymptomatic elderly subjects with diabetes. *BMC Musculoskelet Disord* 2010;11:278.

   An observational study compared rotator cuff and biceps pathology in patients with diabetes and control subjects. The patients with diabetes had higher rates of degenerative changes in the rotator cuff and biceps.

82. Clement ND, Hallett A, MacDonald D, Howie C, McBirnie J: Does diabetes affect outcome after arthroscopic repair of the rotator cuff? *J Bone Joint Surg Br* 2010;92(8):1112-1117.

   A case control study compared outcomes after rotator cuff repair in patients with or without diabetes. Those with diabetes had lower outcome scores and physical function.

83. Bedi A, Fox AJ, Harris PE, et al: Diabetes mellitus impairs tendon-bone healing after rotator cuff repair. *J Shoulder Elbow Surg* 2010;19(7):978-988.

   A controlled laboratory study of the effect of induced diabetes in a rat rotator cuff repair model found a decrease in biomechanical strength, with less bone formation and collagen fiber organization on histologic analysis.

Chapter 38

The Biology and Biomechanics of Grafts and Implants

F. Alan Barber, MD, FACS

Abstract

Biologic grafts are available for a number of applications. They are commonly used for ligament reconstruction and tendon augmentation. Allografts have a better clinical track record with better outcomes and fewer adverse events compared to xenograft and synthetic materials. For anterior cruciate ligament reconstruction allografts have proved effective, providing comparable results to autografts without the issues of donor site morbidity and more difficult rehabilitation. For patients who are not aggressive pivoting or contact athletes, and who are older than 25 years, there is no concern about allograft use. Allografts that are chemically processed or irradiated do not perform as well as deep-frozen, chemical-free, nonirradiated grafts. Acellular dermal matrix allografts can augment rotator cuff tendon healing, especially in tears greater than 3 cm in length and those with the potential for poor healing.

As suture anchor designs continue to develop, the trend is toward biodegradable and plastic anchors containing several (usually up to 3) ultra-high-molecular-weight polyethylene (UHMWPE)-containing sutures. Eyelets are commonly found at the insertion end of the anchor facilitating sliding, locking knot-tying. Screw type anchors are stronger than other designs. Glenoid anchors are smaller than rotator cuff repair anchors to more easily fit into the denser smaller glenoid bone. These smaller glenoid anchors do not provide the higher failure loads of the larger anchors but are clinically appropriate for the designed environment. Knotless anchors are primarily used for the lateral row of a double row rotator cuff repair.

Although several implants are available to assist in arthroscopic meniscal repair, the key to meniscal repair healing is a good blood supply, the absence of meniscal degeneration, and a stable knee. The current all-inside techniques use a suture-based, self-adjusting meniscal repair device with nonabsorbable UHMWPE-containing suture attached to polyether ether ketone anchors and connected by a pretied, sliding, and self-locking knot.

Keywords: biology; biomechanics; grafts; implants

Introduction

Grafts and implants are commonly used in sports medicine to repair, reconstruct, or augment ligaments, tendons, and cartilage. The options include autografts, allografts, and devices having different materials, designs,

---

Dr. Barber or an immediate family member has received royalties from DePuy-Mitek; is a member of a speakers' bureau or has made paid presentations on behalf of Conmed Linvatec and DePuy-Mitek; serves as a paid consultant to ConMed Linvatec and DePuy-Mitek; and has stock or stock options held in Johnson & Johnson.

and characteristics. The surgeon should understand the biology and biomechanics of grafts and implants as well as the strengths and weaknesses associated with their surgical applications. This information should affect preoperative discussions with the patient, the choice of surgical application, and the postoperative rehabilitation program. Several grafts and implants are available for use in the United States as related to treatment of the anterior cruciate ligament (ACL), the rotator cuff tendons, shoulder instability, and the meniscus.

Grafts in ACL Reconstruction

Reconstruction of the ACL is a common procedure that consists of replacing the torn ligament with a graft. Although different autografts have been used in the past,

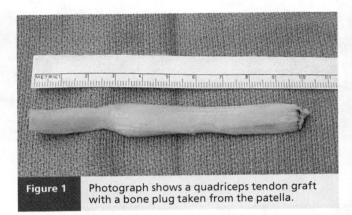

Figure 1 Photograph shows a quadriceps tendon graft with a bone plug taken from the patella.

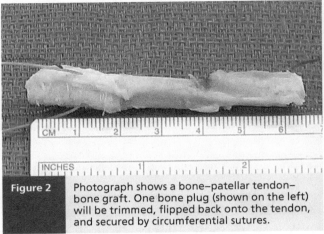

Figure 2 Photograph shows a bone–patellar tendon–bone graft. One bone plug (shown on the left) will be trimmed, flipped back onto the tendon, and secured by circumferential sutures.

bone–patellar tendon–bone (BPTB), hamstring tendon, and quadriceps tendon autografts currently are the most commonly used. Allografts from the same sources or from other tendons, such as the Achilles tendon, also are often used.

Substantially delaying or not performing an ACL reconstruction can have consequences, especially in relatively young patients. Although nonsurgical treatment of a complete ACL injury should be considered, it is associated with risks, especially in young patients. A risk of additional intra-articular damage was associated with nonsurgical treatment or delayed ACL reconstruction in 29 patients (mean age at time of injury, 15 years).[1] BPTB or hamstring tendon autograft reconstruction was performed an average 11.6 months after injury. At a mean 14.6-year follow-up (range, 10 to 20 years after surgery), the treated knees were more likely to have osteoarthritic changes than the contralateral knees. However, patients' clinical outcomes and health-related quality-of-life scores did not differ significantly from those of control subjects. The Multicenter Orthopaedic Outcomes Network study reported that ACL reconstruction is the most cost-effective treatment of an ACL tear and that it has less societal cost than nonsurgical rehabilitation, especially when the cost of work limitations and reduction in earning ability are included.[2]

Graft Biomechanics

The biomechanical properties of graft materials are influenced by graft size, graft preparation, donor age, and fixation method. To avoid damage during the healing phase, the rehabilitation program may be affected by the choice of graft. Graft strength should exceed the load-to-failure strength of the native ACL as reported in tests of relatively young cadaver specimens (average, 2,160 ± 157 N). The grafts commonly used for ACL reconstruction exceed this target. The average quadriceps tendon graft is 10 mm long (maximum length, 11 cm) and 7 mm thick, with an

ultimate load to failure of 2,352 N (Figure 1). A BPTB graft of appropriate size (10 mm long and 4 mm thick) has an ultimate load to failure of 2,977 N. In contrast, the ultimate load to failure of a strand of semitendinosus or gracilis tendon is 1,216 N or 838 N, respectively. The practice of looping the hamstring tendon creates a double-strand, triple-strand, or quadruple-strand graft with strengths of 2,422N to 4,590 N.

The manner of inserting the graft into the knee can affect how it is secured. One concern in using a BPTB graft is that excessive length of the tendon portion can lead to tunnel-graft mismatch. Rotating the graft 90° can shorten the graft and increase its strength. If the length of the tendon section of a BPTB graft exceeds 50 mm, one bone plug can be trimmed, flipped back onto the tendon, and secured by circumferential sutures (Figure 2). This technique creates a shorter graft that allows outlet fixation at both the femoral and tibial tunnels.[1] Although looping a hamstring tendon graft to create a construct with two to four strands will increase the ultimate load to failure, it is important that these separate strands be tensioned equally to maximize the graft strength and reduce stretching at nonisometric points in the joint range of motion.

Autografts

The type of graft is selected based on the patient's age and activity level as well as the preferences of the patient, family, and surgeon. The calculation of comparative costs is not straightforward. Although short-term or day-of-surgery costs may decrease if an autograft is used, a complete cost analysis must consider the entire course of treatment. If the focus is on the insurance provider within the first year, the calculation may favor the use of an autograft. If the analysis is patient focused and includes out-of-pocket costs for all physical therapy sessions, medications, and transportation as well as the cost of time lost from work, the use of an autograft may be more expensive than an allograft. If long-term costs are included in the analysis, the incidence of revision surgery must be considered. Most published discussions do not include these cost considerations, however.

Grafts harvested from the patient are the most common type of graft for ACL reconstruction in high-performance athletes. The disadvantages of using autografts include longer surgical times; donor site morbidity, such as anterior knee pain, kneeling pain, patellofemoral crepitus, anterior knee numbness, patellar fracture, tendon rupture, or muscle weakness; cosmetic concerns; and time lost from work or school.

Opinions differ as to whether a BPTB graft, multiple-strand hamstring tendon graft, or quadriceps tendon graft is superior. Several systematic reviews of randomized controlled studies have attempted to answer this question. A Cochrane Database review of 19 studies evaluated results in 1,597 young to middle-aged adults and found no statistically significant differences between BPTB and hamstring tendon grafts in functional assessments of return to activity, subjective outcome measures (Tegner activity level and Lysholm knee questionnaire scores), and the need for revision ACL reconstruction.[3] Stability tests (the KT-1000 [MEDmetric], Lachman, and pivot shift tests) consistently showed BPTB reconstruction to be more stable than hamstring tendon reconstruction. The long-term development of osteoarthritis was not analyzed, but a greater incidence of anterior knee pain was found in patients with a BPTB autograft.

Another systematic review also reported that hamstring tendon autografts were inferior to BPTB autografts for restoring knee joint stability but that patients who received a hamstring tendon autograft had less anterior knee and kneeling pain.[4] These findings were supported by a separate meta-analysis, which reported that although hamstring autografts resulted in less anterior knee pain, kneeling pain, and extension loss, the BPTB autografts resulted in lower KT-1000 arthrometer scores, and fewer positive Lachman or pivot shift tests.[5] Another meta-analysis also reported that patients who underwent BPTB reconstruction were more likely to have a stable knee (measured using the KT-1000 test) and had an almost 20% greater chance of returning to preinjury activity levels than those who underwent a semitendinosus or gracilis tendon reconstruction.[6]

Substantial knee flexion weakness and a statistically significant knee flexor deficit were reported with the use of hamstring tendon autograft.[7] Hamstring tendon autograft was reported to be more likely to lead to infection compared with BPTB autograft or allograft ($P < 0.05$), with a trend toward a greater likelihood of graft removal.[8]

In summary, the BPTB autograft provides a very secure fixation because of the presence of bone plugs at both ends of the tendon. BPTB autografts have a low failure rate and a high rate of patient satisfaction, especially in patients who want a rapid return to sports. However, the BPTB graft is associated with an increased incidence of anterior knee pain and extension loss, especially if the patient does not undergo an accelerated rehabilitation program immediately after surgery, with an emphasis on regaining full extension. Quadrupled hamstring tendon grafts also are associated with excellent outcomes, and there is less anterior knee pain and numbness than with other types of grafts. A slower return to full-pivoting sports is required, however. Quadrupled hamstring tendon grafts are more lax than BPTB grafts, especially in women. The hamstring tendon harvest leads to decreased knee flexion strength and can be a factor in graft failure. Quadriceps tendon grafting is unlikely to cause anterior knee pain or numbness, and it leads to excellent clinical outcomes. There is no more knee laxity after quadriceps tendon grafting than BPTB grafting, with no loss of knee extension.

Allografts

The use of an allograft decreases surgical time by eliminating the need for graft harvesting. Donor site morbidity and cosmetic concerns are eliminated. It is important to recognize that the rehabilitation program after allograft use must be substantially slower than the program after autograft use.

The availability of allografts sometimes is limited, and the quality can vary. The preparation of the allograft can have a significant effect on its quality and the subsequent surgical outcome. Irradiation or chemical processing significantly increases the likelihood of graft rupture.[9] ACL reconstructions using sterilized allograft had a 45% failure rate at 6-year follow-up, in sharp contrast to a 6% failure rate after autograft reconstruction.[10] Irradiated allografts were found to have greater laxity than autografts.[11] A meta-analysis comparing BPTB allografts to autografts reported no important outcome differences unless the allografts were irradiated or chemically processed.[9]

Eliminating data related to chemically processed or irradiated grafts can be difficult and requires careful reading of the research. A recent study of primary ACL reconstructions in patients no older than 18 years reported that the failure rate was 15 times greater after an allograft was used than after an autograft was used.[12] Revision surgery was required after 2 of the 59 autograft procedures and 7 of the 20 allograft procedures. Five of the allograft failures occurred approximately 6 months after surgery, and all involved irradiated or chemically processed grafts. The postsurgical motion of these allografts was not restricted, and a continuous passive motion device was used immediately after surgery. The delay in beginning an exercise program was only 1 to 2 weeks compared with the autografts. Sport-specific training began 6 months after surgery, at which point five of the seven allograft failures occurred. This study shows the need to avoid irradiated or chemically processed allografts as well as an overly aggressive rehabilitation program after allograft use. Compared with the use of autografts, successful use of allograft tissue requires the avoidance of any chemically processed grafts, avoiding grafts with any level of irradiation, and a delayed rehabilitation program.[13]

Comparison of Autografts and Allografts

Allograft reconstruction was found to allow an earlier return to sport than autograft reconstruction in patients older than 40 years.[14] A study of ACL reconstruction with BPTB allograft found no difference in subjective or objective outcomes based on whether patients were older or younger than 40 years.[15] A systematic review found that the choice of autograft or allograft did not affect ACL reconstruction outcomes but that those treated with an allograft had less laxity than those treated with an autograft (using the KT-1000 test) and that more patients with an allograft achieved a normal International Knee Documentation Committee (IKDC) Subjective Knee Evaluation Form score.[16] There was no statistical difference between allograft and autograft use in rates of ruptures or postoperative complications.

In contrast, a matched case-control study used univariate logistic regression models to find that ACL graft reconstruction was less likely to succeed in patients with a high activity level than in those with a low activity level and that ACL reconstruction was less likely to be successful if an allograft was used rather than an autograft.[17] The potential for ACL reconstruction failure in young or high-performance athletes has been a concern.[18] However, a recent prospective comparison of BPTB allograft or autograft ACL reconstruction in patients younger than 26 years found that patients who selected a graft type and followed the appropriate rehabilitation protocol had no unsuccessful procedures, no differences in functional outcome scores, and no revision procedures at an average 3-year follow-up.[13] Similar subjective and objective outcome measures were reported at an average 9 to 10 years follow-up for patients who participated in strenuous sports after undergoing autograft or fresh-frozen allograft patellar tendon ACL reconstruction.[19]

The Multicenter Orthopaedic Outcomes Network study also evaluated the effect of graft choice in ACL reconstruction.[20] Patients age 10 to 19 years were most likely to experience graft failure, irrespective of graft type, but an allograft was four times more likely to fail than an autograft. The types of allograft included anterior and posterior tibial tendon and Achilles tendon as well as BPTB, and different graft fixation techniques were used. The report did not specify whether the grafts were irradiated or chemically processed.

Considerable attention has been focused on whether the outcomes of autograft and allograft reconstructions are equivalent. A meta-analysis of 76 studies with 5,182 patients compared the use of BPTB autografts and allografts in ACL reconstruction.[21] Patients who received an autograft were found to have better outcomes (subjective IKDC, Lysholm, and Tegner scores; single-leg hop and KT-1000 tests) than those who received an allograft, but allograft use was found to lead to better rates of return to the preinjury activity level, higher overall IKDC scores, better performance on the pivot shift test, and less anterior knee pain. The allografts had a 12.7% rate of rerupture, compared with a 4.3% rate for autografts. Unfortunately, the 76 studies were not selected to eliminate irradiated or chemically processed grafts or be comparative in nature, compromising the conclusions.[21]

A systematic review found level I, II, or III evidence in nine studies that compared the use of autografts with that of nonirradiated allografts.[22] Six of the studies compared BPTB autografts and allografts, two compared hamstring tendon autografts to allografts, and one compared hamstring tendon autografts to tibialis anterior tendon allografts. No significant difference was found between the use of autografts and nonirradiated allografts in any outcome measure, including the graft failure rate.[22] Another systematic review and meta-analysis found no differences in clinical failure rates after BPTB autograft or fresh-frozen BPTB allograft was used.[23]

A systematic review and meta-analysis of five studies with a total of 504 patients compared ACL reconstructions using hamstring tendon autograft or soft-tissue allograft.[24] Some of the allografts were irradiated and chemically processed. One study reported greater laxity at follow-up in irradiated allografts than in autografts, but the meta-analysis found no significant differences between hamstring tendon autografts and soft-tissue allografts for any outcome measure, including graft laxity.[24]

Tunnel enlargement does not affect clinical outcome scores or laxity data, but it can affect graft placement and fixation in revision surgery and necessitate a two-stage procedure to allow bone grafting. The cause of tunnel enlargement after ACL reconstruction is unclear, but it usually occurs during the first few months. Tunnel enlargement can be explained by mechanical factors

© 2016 American Academy of Orthopaedic Surgeons

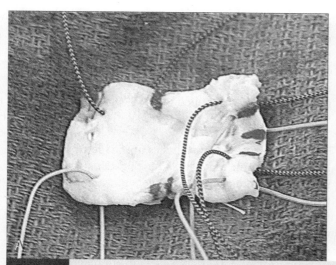
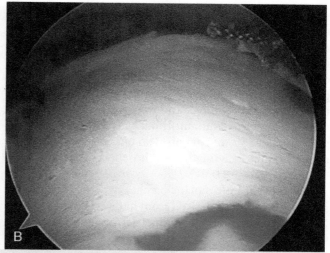

Figure 3 Images of a human dermal allograft patch for arthroscopic augmentation of rotator cuff tendon tissue that is attenuated or does not completely cover the attachment site. **A,** Photograph shows a properly sized patch is prepared by passing sutures through its periphery as well as the tendon. **B,** Arthroscopic view shows the graft passed into the joint. The sutures are tied to reinforce and augment the tendon repair. The onlay adds strength to the repair and can biologically enhance healing.

including improper graft placement, the choice of fixation method, the graft length or type, single-bundle or double-bundle reconstruction, and the effect of synovial fluid moving into the graft–tunnel wall interface. Secure fixation is important to prevent graft movement within the tunnel and allow good healing of the graft to the tunnel wall. Many types of graft fixation devices are available, and an understanding of their material properties as well as the correct technique for using them is essential.

The type of graft appears to have an effect on the development of tunnel enlargement. Hamstring tendon reconstruction can lead to substantially greater tunnel enlargement than BPTB reconstruction. A prospective comparison study found greater tunnel widening after hamstring tendon grafting than BPTB grafting as early as 4 months after reconstruction.[25] Patients with BPTB graft reconstruction had a 25% decrease in femoral tunnel size and a 2% decrease in tibial tunnel size. The graft tunnels in those with a hamstring graft were statistically larger and had increased in size; the largest increase was 73.9% in the tibial tunnel. A recent study found that at a mean 5-year follow-up after quadrupled hamstring tendon autograft reconstruction, the cross-sectional area of tunnels had more than doubled at all levels except the femoral notch level.[26] Concerns exist about the prospect of tunnel enlargement with the use of a double-bundle, double-tunnel technique, but no difference in the risk of enlargement was found based on whether a double-bundle or single-bundle technique was used.[27] The method of fixation also is important. Cortical suspension fixation allows graft motion within the tunnel and leads to

significant enlargement. A cross-pin fixation provides rigid intramedullary fixation and substantially decreases the amount of tunnel enlargement.[28]

Implants

The goal of any repair is to attach the tissue and hold it in place long enough to achieve tissue healing. A variety of implants can be used to facilitate tissue healing, including tendon patches, suture anchors, sutures, and meniscus repair devices. Rotator cuff repair is being done more frequently with the increase in the number of aging but active patients and with increasing recognition of the long-term adverse results of rotator cuff arthropathy.

The normal rotator cuff tendon has a fibrocartilage transition zone that cannot be exactly replicated by surgical repair. The best that currently can be achieved is a fibrovascular scar. Several factors affect tendon-to-bone healing, some of which are beyond the surgeon's control; these include the patient's age, smoking history, and workers' compensation status as well as the presence of fatty infiltration. The surgeon can control surgical aspects including tissue augmentation with patches, anchor and suture selection, repair technique, and postoperative rehabilitation protocol.

Rotator cuff tendon repair often involves a complete or chronic tear of degenerative, frayed, or retracted tissue. Overtensioning a tendon tear must be avoided. Augmenting the repair of a damaged tendon with an onlay graft may provide additional strength and improve the likelihood of biologic healing (Figure 3). This application is approved by the US FDA and is used for large tendon tears. The postrepair gap should be no larger than 1 cm. At 12- or 24-month follow-up, a prospective randomized controlled study found significantly decreased rates of retearing after an acellular dermal matrix allograft patch was used for augmentation of tears that involved two rotator cuff tendons and were larger than 3 cm (as documented by gadolinium-enhanced MRI).[29] The repair was intact in 85% of patients who underwent augmented repair, compared with 40% of those who did not receive augmentation ($P < 0.01$).

Several types of implant patches are available. Some allograft material is derived from human skin or tendon. Xenografts are made from animal dermis, pericardium, or small intestine submucosa. Implants made from synthetic polymers also are available. Considerations in selecting an implant patch should include tissue origin, graft source, graft processing, cross-linking, physical properties, and clinical experience.

Dermal and Tendon Allografts

GraftJacket (Wright Medical Technology) is an acellular dermal matrix allograft produced from human skin obtained from a tissue bank approved by the American Association of Tissue Banks. The skin is processed to remove epidermal and dermal cells with preservation of collagen types I, III, IV, and VII as well as elastin, chondroitin sulfate, hyaluronic acid, laminin, tenascin, proteoglycans, and fibroblast growth factor. Graftjacket allografts are available in 5 × 5 cm and 5 × 10 cm sheets with several average thicknesses. MaxForce (Wright Medical Technology) allograft is an average 1.4 mm thick (range, 1.27 to 1.78 mm), and Graftjacket MaxForce Extreme allograft is an average 2.0 mm thick (range, 1.78 to 2.25 mm). Graftjacket allografts must be hydrated for 15 to 30 minutes before implantation.

Allopatch HD (Musculoskeletal Transplant Foundation) is derived from human skin obtained from a tissue bank approved by the American Association of Tissue Banks and is an acellular human collagen matrix dermal allograft for augmentation of soft-tissue repairs. Allopatch HD is processed to preserve the biomechanical, biochemical, and matrix properties of the dermal graft. Several thicknesses are available: thin (range, 0.4 to 0.7 mm), thick (range, 0.8 to 1.7 mm), ultrathick (range, 1.8 to 3.9 mm), and extra-ultrathick (range, 4.0 to 5.0 mm). The sheets measure 2 cm × 5 cm, 5 cm × 5 cm, 4 cm × 8 cm, or 1 cm × 12 cm. Hydration is not needed, but the material must be rinsed to remove the 70% ethanol packing liquid.

RC Allograft (Arthrex) is a freeze-dried human rotator cuff tendon allograft. After donor screening, the tissue is aseptically recovered and cleaned using the AlloWash process (LifeNet Health), which includes terminal sterilization on dry ice to reduce or eliminate bacteria, marrow elements, and lipids. Some but not all forms are gamma irradiated. The thickness of the material ranges from 2 to 3 mm, and it is supplied in 2 × 3–cm sheets.

Xenografts

The available xenograft patches are made from porcine, bovine, or equine material. These products are mechanically tested under tension. In general, allograft derived from human skin is the strongest material, followed by bovine and porcine skin; porcine small intestine submucosa is the weakest patch material.[30-34] These mechanical differences can affect the durability of the patch during implantation and its effectiveness in augmenting the mechanical strength of the tendon repair.

The Restore Orthobiologic soft-tissue implant (Depuy) and CuffPatch (Arthrotek) are derived from porcine small intestine submucosa. Permacol (Covidien) and TissueMend (Stryker) are derived from porcine dermis or fetal bovine dermis, respectively. OrthAdapt (Synovis) is made from equine pericardium.

Restore, the first implant material approved by the US FDA for tendon repair, consists of more than 90% collagen with 5% to 10% lipids and a small amount of carbohydrate. The Restore implant is a circular patch 63 mm in diameter, consisting of 10 layers of porcine small intestine submucosa that are not cross-linked. It is provided dried and requires soaking for 5 to 10 minutes before use. The CuffPatch is 97% collagen and 2% elastin. Its eight layers of porcine small intestine submucosa are cross-linked using carbodiimide and sterilized using 25 kGy of gamma radiation. The material is provided as a 6.5 × 9–cm sheet that is supplied prehydrated but should be rinsed before use.

Permacol, a porcine dermal implant, is a single-layer xenograft supplied in a sterile, off-white 5 × 10 cm flat sheet of acellular cross-linked collagen and its constituent elastin fibers. The sheet is 1.0 mm thick. Cross-linking, accomplished using hexamethylene diisocyanate, increases the strength but substantially extends the degradation time of the implant. Permacol is sterilized using gamma irradiation, and it is supplied prehydrated in saline.

At 6-month follow-up, only 1 of 11 patients (5 women and 6 men, age range 52 to 78 years) who had undergone a large rotator cuff repair augmented with the Restore implant had a successful repair.[35] A study of rotator cuff repairs with or without Restore patch augmentation found a higher rate of retearing and significantly more weakness at 2-year follow-up in patients with the Restore patch.[36] The patients who received the Restore patch augmentation also had more impingement and a lower level of sports participation than those who did not receive augmentation. At a mean 13 days after surgery, 4 of 25 patients with Restore patch augmentation of a rotator cuff repair had an acute nonspecific inflammatory response requiring implant removal.[37] The Restore patch is no longer recommended for rotator cuff repair augmentation.

TissueMend is derived from fetal bovine dermis and is a single-layer graft decellularized through a series of chemical processes in which all cells, lipids, and carbohydrates are removed to reduce the risk of an inflammatory response. The result is 99% –nondenatured collagen that is not artificially cross-linked. TissueMend is manufactured as a rectangular 5 × 6 cm sheet 1.1 to 1.2 mm thick. The product is aseptically processed and sterilized in ethylene oxide, and 1 minute of hydration is required before use.

OrthAdapt, no longer on the market, was an equine pericardium xenograft cross-linked to add strength and contained 90% type I collagen and 10% type III collagen. The processed acellular pericardial tissue was not irradiated. The sheets used were 3 × 3 cm or 4 × 5 cm and approximately 0.5 mm thick.

Synthetic Grafts

The SportMesh graft (Artimplant, Biomet) is a knitted, degradable, polyurethane urea fabric constructed from Artelon scaffold fibers (Artimplant) and sterilized with 25 kGy electron beam radiation. The sheets are 4 cm × 6 cm and 0.8 mm thick (**Figure 4**). This synthetic material is soaked in saline at room temperature for 5 minutes before use. SportMesh is elastic and highly porous.

The X-Repair (Synthasome) is a woven poly-L-lactic acid (PLLA) material available in sheets measuring 12 × 40 mm with thickness of 0.8 mm. This material is elastic and was found not to contribute stiffness in an in vitro model. Human cadaver rotator cuff repairs augmented with this implant demonstrate significantly higher yield loads and ultimate failure loads.[38]

Implant Biomechanics

Biomechanical testing has been reported for several implants.[30-34] Load elongation after cyclic loading revealed that the SportMesh synthetic-material patch had significantly greater displacement during cyclic loading than any other tested graft material.[31] RC Allograft, the tested human rotator cuff tendon implant, had the least elasticity and was the most resistant to elongation. Although great elongation raises concern as to whether a graft can provide sufficient mechanical support, resistance to elongation raises concern about the potential for stress shielding during healing. Testing of ultimate load to failure found that the tested acellular human dermal allografts were

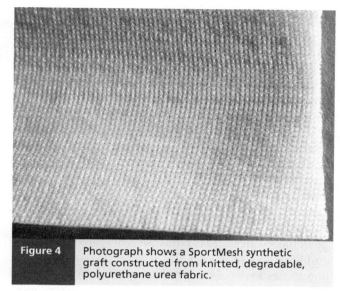

Figure 4   Photograph shows a SportMesh synthetic graft constructed from knitted, degradable, polyurethane urea fabric.

stronger than the xenograft or synthetic implants.[30-34] The acellular human dermal allografts also were stiffer than the tested equine pericardium and synthetic patches. A single vertical simple stitch was used in suture retention testing that found acellular human dermal allografts to have greater suture retention strength than xenograft and synthetic allografts.[31] The thickness of dermal grafts was related to suture retention, with a thick graft providing more strength than a thin graft.

In general, dermal allograft implants add strength to a tendon repair without stress shielding. The implants are incorporated into the repair over time, and their use was found to lead to lower rates of retearing.[29] Unlike xenograft implants, human dermal allograft implants have not been associated with inflammatory adverse events. Equally effective synthetic or tissue-engineered grafts may become available in the future, but their clinical effectiveness has not yet been established.

Suture Anchors

The primary function of a suture anchor is to securely attach suture into bone, which attaches tissue to the appropriate site and holds it in place until healing occurs, without excessive tension or loosening. The ideal suture anchor does not react to the surrounding tissue, performs its designed function for as long as needed, and disappears without a trace. Biodegradable anchors for the most part accomplish these goals and do not create difficulties related to postoperative imaging or revision procedures. Both biodegradable and nonbiodegradable (metal or plastic) anchors are subject to anchor loosening and migration, however.

© 2016 American Academy of Orthopaedic Surgeons

Suture Anchor Materials

Suture anchors were previously made from metal, but during the past 20 years biodegradable suture anchors made from other materials have become available. The initial biodegradable material was PLLA, which was followed by polymer combinations that combine lactic acid with another polymer, which usually is polyglycolic acid (PGA). The resulting copolymer, called PLLA-co-PGA, has mechanical properties comparable to those of PLLA but with more rapid degradation. A more amorphous lactide polymer can be engineered by combining different amounts of dextro (D) and levo (L) lactide monomer to create a stereoisomer. A greater percentage of the dextro component leads to a more rapid degradation and the potential for an increased inflammatory response. Several combinations of dextro and levo lactide are available. Sometimes a stereoisomer of PLLA (PDLLA) is combined with a copolymer (PLLA-co-PGA) to create an even more complex polymer with different characteristics.

Some authors have reported the development of an inflammatory synovitis associated with the use of biodegradable suture anchors resulting in the need for subsequent surgery.[39,40] An analysis of biodegradable implants without regard to the polymer type or the presence of a copolymer or stereoisomer does not consider the material characteristics of entirely different polymers. The use of the term PLLA to generically describe this group of materials ignores the substantial differences in degradation profiles, and the conclusions drawn from such analyses are inaccurate. A study of 44 shoulders requiring surgery for complications after repair of the labrum or rotator cuff stated that "gross, histologic, and MRI-visualized pathology was observed in patients in whom PLLA implants" were used.[39] In reality, the anchors in 39 shoulders were composed of levo (L)– dextro (D) lactide stereoisomers (poly–levo [70%]/dextro [30%]–lactic acid [PL70/D30LA]). The stereoisomers or copolymers of PLLA vary in biodegradable characteristics and behave differently. Only 3 of the 44 shoulders were reported to have actual PLLA anchors.

Degradation time differs among the polymers.[41-43] An inflammatory response does not develop until the long polymer chains begin to break down and release monomers. Most PLLA implants were macroscopically intact at 30-month follow-up, with no apparent inflammatory response, in contrast to the stereoisomers and copolymers of PLLA, which have markedly more rapid reabsorption patterns.[44,45] Degradation begins as these polymer chains break down and the crystalline implant becomes amorphous. Implant fragmentation releases monomers, which are phagocytosed primarily by macrophages and polymorphonuclear leukocytes. In the final degradation

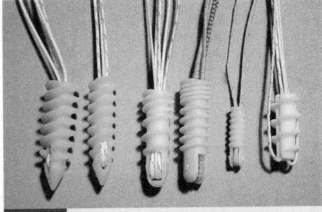

Figure 5 Photograph shows several biodegradable suture anchors constructed of biocomposite material. From left to right: the TwinFix HA 5.5 (Smith & Nephew Endoscopy), TwinFix HA 4.5 (Smith & Nephew), CrossFT BC 5.5 (ConMed-Linvatec), Healix BR 5.5 (DePuy Mitek), Gryphon BR (DePuy Mitek), and Double Play 5.0 (ArthroCare).

step, the lactic acid monomer enters the Krebs cycle and is released as carbon dioxide and water.

Inflammation is an inherent part of the degradation process. PGA is an example of a rapidly degrading polymer. The breakdown of PGA can be so rapid that acidic breakdown products incite a symptomatic local inflammatory tissue reaction within 11 weeks of implantation.[46] A sinus that discharges implant remnants sometimes develops and can persist as long as 6 months.[46] Inflammatory responses with intracapsular synovitis and granulomatous reactions in the shoulder have been reported after PGA tacks were used.[47]

Suture anchors and other implants for arthroscopic insertion are composed of different biodegradable polymers, most of which are unlikely to cause an inflammatory reaction. A recent study of 370 shoulder procedures found that an anchor-specific adverse event occurred only in 2 procedures (0.5%).[48] Only one of these adverse events was polymer related, and it occurred in a PL70/D30LA anchor that was reabsorbed too quickly, thus loosening the eyelet suture and allowing it to migrate into the joint and cause articular cartilage erosion.

The use of biocomposite materials is a recent development in biodegradable implants (Figure 5). A biocomposite combines a biodegradable polymer with a bioceramic material. Beta-tricalcium phosphate (β-TCP) is currently the most commonly used bioceramic. The other bioceramics include hydroxyapatite ($Ca_{10}(PO_4)_6(OH)_2$), calcium sulfate ($CaSO_4$), and calcium carbonate ($CaCO_3$). Combining PLLA with β-TCP blends the compressive strength and stiffness of β-TCP with the degradation

© 2016 American Academy of Orthopaedic Surgeons

profile of PLLA. The resulting biocomposite degrades more rapidly than pure PLLA, and it encourages osteoconductive ingrowth of bone into the anchor location. Osteoconductive ingrowth into the area of the implant occurs during absorption when the bioceramic releases a base that buffers the acidic monomer, thus raising the local pH toward neutral. A sclerotic bone wall is less likely to develop if the environment around the degrading implant is not acidic. The released calcium ions also encourage osteoconductive ingrowth. Biocomposite implants are replaced by a material with the radiographic appearance and density of cancellous bone.[41-43,49]

Suture-based anchors represent a new type of anchoring device. As with most shoulder anchors, one or more sutures containing No. 2 ultra-high–molecular-weight polyethylene (UHMWPE) are used. The anchor is created by adding a 1- to 3-mm-wide sleeve with a length of UHMWPE or braided polyester. The suture or sutures are woven though this sleeve. Methods of passing the suture through the sleeve create different patterns in the anchor when tension is applied.

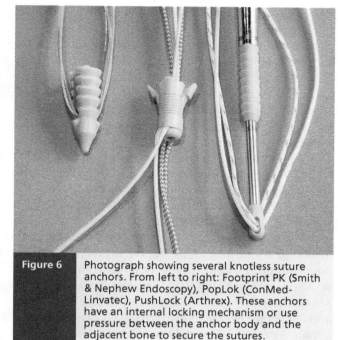

Figure 6 Photograph showing several knotless suture anchors. From left to right: Footprint PK (Smith & Nephew Endoscopy), PopLok (ConMed-Linvatec), PushLock (Arthrex). These anchors have an internal locking mechanism or use pressure between the anchor body and the adjacent bone to secure the sutures.

Biomechanical Considerations

A suture anchor in the shoulder can be a medial-row rotator cuff anchor, a lateral-row rotator cuff anchor, or a glenoid instability anchor. The design that is appropriate for a rotator cuff anchor will differ from the design appropriate for a glenoid anchor, which should be smaller, suitable for insertion into denser cortical bone, and hold fewer sutures. In contrast, a rotator cuff anchor will be larger, suitable for less dense cancellous bone, and routinely accommodate two or three sutures. Recently released suture anchors are more likely than earlier anchors to be made from a radiolucent material such as a plastic (polyether ether ketone, PEEK), a biodegradable material, or a biocomposite material. Biocomposite anchors most commonly contain β-TCP. The sutures for most anchors now contain UHMWPE, are fully threaded, and have a distal or internal eyelet.

Knotless anchors have been developed to accommodate the increasingly common use of dual-row constructs. To secure the sutures, these so-called knotless designs use an internal locking mechanism or pressure between the anchor body and the adjacent bone (Figure 6). Threaded (screw-in) and nonthreaded (push-in) knotless anchors are available. Threaded biocomposite lateral-row knotless anchors can withstand higher loads than nonthreaded knotless anchors because of the efficiency of the screw fixation design.[50]

Biomechanical studies have evaluated the effect of knots in medial-row sutures before creation of a suture bridge. Medial-row knots increase the stiffness and

stability of a dual-row repair, probably because the knotless medial-row anchor is effective in sharing the load with the lateral row. This factor is important because lateral-row anchors receive less stress than medial-row anchors. The lateral anchors of a dual-row repair take only 33% of the overall load.[51,52] This 2:1 loading ratio can cause the medial anchors to fail before the lateral-row fixation, both clinically and biomechanically, and consequently protects the lateral-row fixation.[53,54]

Medial-row anchors usually have a strong screw-in design requiring knot tying and having a higher failure load than lateral-row or glenoid anchors. These anchors also are appropriate for biceps tenodesis. Lateral-row anchors usually are a knotless design and can accommodate sutures from a medial row for a suture-bridge or transosseous technique.

Glenoid anchors for labral and shoulder instability procedures are designed to be used in relatively young patients with good-quality bone. The restricted working space and narrow glenoid contour require the use of a small anchor. Consequently, the available glenoid anchors range in diameter from less than 2 mm to 3.5 mm. Toggle anchor designs are less effective than screw-in designs in the osteoporotic bone of the greater tuberosity, but they can be used effectively in the glenoid. A relatively short anchor and shallow drilling depth are preferable in the glenoid to avoid overpenetration. If the drill is too long or the anchor penetrates into the axilla, the axillary nerve is at risk. However, a small anchor has a lower load-to-failure strength and cannot accommodate as many sutures as a larger anchor.

Few new metal anchors are being released. Instead, the current trend is toward radiolucent anchors made from PEEK, biodegradable materials including PLLA and PDL-LA, and biocomposites containing β-TCP or hydroxyapatite. Biocomposite anchors, especially those with β-TCP, are osteoconductive. Many currently available anchors were introduced several years ago or are minor variations of previous designs. The newest anchor designs typically are fully threaded, contain multiple UHMWPE sutures, and have a central or distal crossbar eyelet.

The first wholly suture-based anchor was the 1.4-mm JuggerKnot (Biomet). In the bone, the suture and sleeve are drawn up into a W shape by traction on the sutures; this W-shaped suture acts much like the toggle anchors that preceded suture-based anchors (such as RotorloC, Smith & Nephew; UltraSorb RC, Linvatec; Panalok, DePuy Mitek). As with the use of a toggle anchor, the compressed mass of suture engages the overlying cortical bone, and a space is created below the bone. Because the suture has no screw threads, ribs, fins, or expanding wings to secure itself in the cancellous bone, any slack in the suture-tissue interface can cause a piston effect against the overlying cortex, possibly leading to subcortical cavitation.

The 1.4-mm JuggerKnot had lower failure loads than other glenoid anchors; suture breaking and anchor pullout occurred with almost equal frequency.[55] The subsequently introduced 1.5- and 2.9-mm JuggerKnots have a 25-mm sleeve and significantly higher failure loads. None of the test samples failed by device pullout. In a destructive test, all of the newer JuggerKnot anchors failed by suture breaking after cyclic loading.[55]

Several other suture-based anchors are available, including the Iconix (Stryker), Y-Knot (ConMed Linvatec), SutureFix (Smith & Nephew), and Draw Tight (Parcus Medical). The three versions of the Iconix have one, two, or three No. 2 UHMWPE sutures, which are woven three times through a flat, flexible tube of braided polyester that when tensioned collapses into a cloverleaf configuration to create the anchor (Figure 7). The Y-Knot is available in 1.3- and 1.8-mm sizes for glenoid use and in a double- or triple-loaded 2.8-mm size for rotator cuff applications. The suture sleeve is compressed to form a ball configuration. In a recent laboratory test at the institution of this chapter's author, the 2.8-mm Y-Knot failed by suture breaking twice as often as by anchor pulling out of the bone; the mean resistance to failure was 500 to 600N.

Suture anchors of several sizes and designs have been mechanically evaluated. The failure mode often is related to the anchor material. For example, metal anchors are likely to be stronger than the associated suture, so

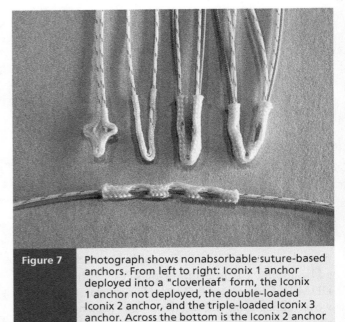

Figure 7 Photograph shows nonabsorbable suture-based anchors. From left to right: Iconix 1 anchor deployed into a "cloverleaf" form, the Iconix 1 anchor not deployed, the double-loaded Iconix 2 anchor, and the triple-loaded Iconix 3 anchor. Across the bottom is the Iconix 2 anchor without a fold.

suture breakage is common. In biodegradable anchors, the distal crossbar eyelet fails and the suture pulls out. PEEK anchors have a tendency to fail by anchor pullout. Within the suture anchor construct, the suture or the suture eyelet is more likely to fail than the anchor itself.

Anchor placement is an important consideration. Subcortical placement for the anchor is preferable to burying the anchor deeper into the bone. With cyclic loading a deeply buried anchor will shift within the cancellous bone and migrate toward the surface, thereby introducing displacement into the repair. In addition, the sutures from a deeply buried anchor will cut through the bone. In vitro testing found that this anchor motion contributed as much as one third of the total displacement of the suture anchor construct.[56] Although sutures from a deep anchor can cut a channel through the adjacent bone, the suture itself can fail as the result of abrasion by the dense cortical bone.

The design and size of the anchor have an effect on its load-to-failure strength. Several single-pull and cyclic loading load-to-failure tests found that the relatively large, fully threaded screw anchors appropriate for rotator cuff tendon repair have statistically higher failure strengths than anchors designed for glenoid placement.[57-61] However, there was no statistical difference in failure load tests of 5.5- and 6.5-mm anchors of the same design.

Clinical Considerations

Anchor Failure

Anchor failure can occur during the surgical procedure or shortly thereafter (immediate failure) or after clinical healing (late failure). Different failure issues exist for bio-degradable anchors and for metal and PEEK anchors. Immediate failure can occur at the anchor itself, as with improper insertion, breaking during insertion, pulling out from the bone, or eyelet failure; at the suture, as with breaking during suture passing or knot tying or with knot failure; or at the tissue, as with suture cutout. Late modes of failure include anchor loosening or breaking, anchor migration, and reactive changes. Inflammatory reactions related to biodegradable anchors are uncommon and tend to be polymer specific.

Improper insertion can lead to extraosseous placement of the anchor, which can cause immediate articular cartilage damage or neurovascular impingement or later damage from anchor migration. Anchor breakage during insertion can be related to the depth or angle of insertion and in some anchor designs can be related to rotation of the anchor so that the exiting sutures have an incorrect orientation.

Changing the angle of the insertion cannula while impacting an anchor can result in insertion failure. It is important to maintain an accurate alignment with the drilled hole and to avoid too much force when impacting the anchor into place. After advancing the anchor down into the cannula, it is often helpful to use finger pressure to manually seat the anchor as far as possible into the bone before using the mallet. Impacting the anchor too far down the drill hole can place it below the cortex and create difficulties related to anchor motion, suture cutting through bone, and anchor angulation with cyclic loading. In addition, removing the insertion cannula from the bone becomes more difficult.

Anchor pullout after rotator cuff repair was reported to occur in 2.4% of patients, including 0.5% of those with a tear of 3 cm or less and 11.0% of those with a tear larger than 3 cm.[62] Anchor pullout resistance is a function of the amount of contact surface at the bone-anchor interface and the friction generated. The anchor failure load increases with screw thread depth and the number of threads, which create anchor surface area. Screw-in anchors generally have a higher failure load than non–screw-in anchors. Fully threaded anchors hold better than anchors that are not fully threaded, and if deployed flush with the cortical surface, fully threaded anchors do not migrate as much.

The risk of anchor eyelet breakage has been significantly reduced by the change from prominent proximal post eyelets to distal crossbar eyelets. Although some anchors have independent suture-based eyelets, a distal crossbar eyelet at the end of a hollow central anchor core is now a common design. The distal crossbar breaks before the anchor body can be pulled from the bone, and this feature serves as a protective measure. Recent in vitro studies report anchor eyelet breakage as the principal mechanism of failure for many anchors, probably because of the use of multiple UHMWPE-containing sutures.

The causes of late failure include anchor migration and the development of inflammatory reactions. There is concern about possible anchor migration related to technical issues in arthroscopic insertion. However, open anchor insertion was associated with anchor migration as late as 7 years after insertion.[63] Both metal and biodegradable anchors have been associated with this complication. The inflammatory reactions include osteolytic changes, cyst formation, and inflammatory synovitis.[64]

Sutures

The suture has a key role in the integrity of a tissue repair. As all-arthroscopic repairs of the glenoid labrum, biceps tendon, and rotator cuff have become the standard, the importance of the suture has increased. The surgeon's challenge is to consistently approximate and hold the repaired tissue by securely tying the knot through a cannula in an aqueous environment, using knot pushers rather than the fingers. Sutures that do not hold the knot, become frayed, or are likely to break complicate this process. The sutures initially used in arthroscopic surgery were nonabsorbable braided polyester (Mersilene, Ethibond) or absorbable monofilament polydioxanone (PDS). Ethibond, a braided polyester suture, was the preferred arthroscopic suture because it was coated with polybutilate to achieve a low-friction surface with improved handling characteristics. PDS is completely reabsorbable, but the rigid monofilament imparted a memory to the suture, thus decreasing the ability to create a secure knot. PDS begins to lose breaking strength 3 weeks after implantation, retains only 40% of its original strength at 6 weeks, and has no measurable strength at 9 weeks.[65] In comparison, polyglyconate (Maxon) sutures retain no significant strength at 6 weeks, and polyglactin-910 (Vicryl) and PGA (Dexon) sutures retain only minimal breaking strength 3 weeks.[66]

These sutures were manufactured to a standard defined by the United States Pharmacopeia based on suture diameter and comparative suture-breaking strength. This system was overturned with the introduction of FiberWire (Arthrex). In this revolutionary suture, the traditional braided polyester was woven around a core of UHMWPE fibers. The combination of materials made the FiberWire suture much stronger than all others with a similar size rating. In load-to-failure testing, No. 2 FiberWire proved to be as strong as No. 5 braided polyester suture, and therefore it was much less likely to break during tying with an arthroscopic knot pusher.[57] FiberWire quickly became the suture of preference for arthroscopic applications.

To become competitive, other manufacturers introduced their own high-strength sutures, many of which were made with braided UHMWPE. The UHMWPE in all of these sutures was provided by Dyneema (DSM). Despite varied proprietary names, the braided UHMWPE suture and braided polyester suture were made of the same materials. Suture strength was further increased by elimination of the surrounding braided polyester in favor of pure braided UHMWPE. Consequently, FiberWire is substantially stronger than the earlier braided polyester sutures, but braided UHMWPE suture is substantially stronger than FiberWire.[57]

OrthoCord (Depuy Mitek), the most recently introduced suture, is a combination of braided UHMWPE with many small strands of absorbable monofilament polydioxanone; it is coated with polyglactin-910 to improve its handling characteristics. OrthoCord and FiberWire are equivalent in strength but statistically weaker than pure braided UHMWPE.[20,57,58] All of the new sutures far exceed the load-to-failure requirements for a secure tendon-to-bone repair.

The handling and feel of these new sutures differ from one another. Pure braided UHMWPE is more abrasive than FiberWire or OrthoCord, both of which have a softer feel that facilitates suture handling. Although these new sutures are strong in testing models, knots tied using them behave differently. Arthroscopic knots begin with a slip or locking knot that is followed by a series of half-hitches. Appropriately placed half-hitches should be alternated by asymmetrically applying tension to the strands with the knot pusher. The result should be a tight loop holding the tissue with a secure knot. Any clinical failure of the tied knot should be by material failure (suture breaking) rather than loop failure (knot slippage). Using a sliding locking hitch to increase internal suture resistance increases the knot complexity and can result in greater knot security. Backing up an arthroscopic knot with reverse half-hitches and post switching also is essential.

Knot slippage before material failure creates laxity in the repair. Cyclic displacement of as little as 3 to 5 mm is undesirable for healing. UHMWPE-containing sutures are more likely to slip at submaximal loads than braided polyester sutures; therefore, creating the right type of knot is especially important.[67,68] Suture surface characteristics and construction were found to affect the likelihood of knot slippage, and slippage was found to occur at very low tension levels. Two studies found that, although FiberWire was substantially stronger than braided polyester suture, more than half of the knots tied using FiberWire slipped at submaximal loads.[67,68] The Duncan loop, which does not have an internal locking loop, slipped before maximal failure 97.5% of the time. The Weston knot slipped 86%

of the time. However the SMC, Tennessee slider, Revo, and San Diego knots resisted slipping in more than 90% of the tests.[67] The conclusion was that the Duncan loop or any other knot without an internal locking loop should not be used with UHMWPE-containing suture.

Meniscus Repair

The meniscus efficiently disperses loads across the surface of the knee articular cartilage by deepening the tibial articular surface, thus increasing the weight-bearing surface area and lowering contact stresses during weight bearing. The meniscus also contributes to knee joint lubrication, stability, congruence, proprioception, and articular cartilage nutrition. An intact meniscus changes vertically oriented compression stresses into radial hoop stresses, and it serves as a secondary stabilizer for translation and rotation. The intact meniscus plays an important role in protecting an ACL-deficient knee from arthritic changes.

These important roles underscore the importance of attempting to preserve a torn meniscus. Meniscus repair is preferable if there is a good blood supply and a reasonable expectation of meniscal healing. The best candidates for meniscus repair are relatively young patients with a traumatic tear and no apparent degenerative meniscal changes, especially if they are undergoing concurrent ACL reconstruction. In general, the indications for repair are the presence of a vertical nondegenerative peripheral tear rather than a displaced bucket-handle tear, in the red-red or red-white region of the meniscus.

Four techniques have been used for meniscus repair: open, inside out, outside in, and all inside. Combinations of two of these techniques sometimes are called hybrid repairs. Inside-out and outside-in suture-based repairs are done less frequently than all-inside repairs. All-inside repairs are quicker, do not require additional incisions, and are less likely to result in neurovascular injury.

Meniscus Repair Devices

The current all-inside techniques use suture-based, self-adjusting meniscus repair devices with nonabsorbable UHMWPE-containing suture. The UHMWPE suture is much stronger than braided polyester suture and represents an important advance in the repair of meniscus tears. The suture usually is attached to nonabsorbable PEEK anchors connected by a pretied, sliding, and self-locking knot (Figure 8). These devices are inserted through an anterior arthroscopic portal, and they are passed through the meniscal fragment and into the peripheral rim. The deployed anchor is located extra-articularly on the capsule. The suture is tensioned, and

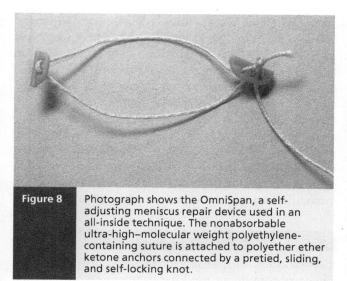

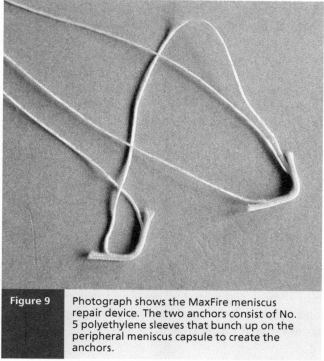

| Figure 8 | Photograph shows the OmniSpan, a self-adjusting meniscus repair device used in an all-inside technique. The nonabsorbable ultra-high–molecular weight polyethylene-containing suture is attached to polyether ether ketone anchors connected by a pretied, sliding, and self-locking knot. |

| Figure 9 | Photograph shows the MaxFire meniscus repair device. The two anchors consist of No. 5 polyethylene sleeves that bunch up on the peripheral meniscus capsule to create the anchors. |

the sliding locking knot secures the tear and maintains compression for meniscal healing.

Although older repair devices have not been removed from the market, the relatively new suture-based, self-adjusting meniscus repair devices are more often used. The available devices of this type include the Fast-Fix 360 (Smith & Nephew), OmniSpan (DePuy Mitek), Meniscal Cinch (Arthrex), the MaxFire (Biomet), Sequent (ConMed Linvatec), and CrossFix II (Cayenne Medical).

The Fast-Fix 360 has two arrow-shaped PEEK anchors connected by braided No. 2-0 UHMWPE suture containing a sliding locking knot. The rounded-handle insertion device advances the 17-gauge needle (straight, 25° curved, or 25° reverse curved) with two separate passes. The preceding version of this device (the Ultra FasT-Fix) contained a larger No. 0 UHMWPE suture. An adjustable depth limiter is on the handle as a safety feature.

The OmniSpan uses a needle (straight, 12° curved, or 27° curved) fitted onto a disposable gun. The device has a strand of No. 2-0 OrthoCord doubled between two PEEK anchors, inserted by the gun in two passes. A silicone tube on the needle provides a soft stop to limit anchor insertion at 13 mm. The sliding locking knot is located on the outside of the first PEEK anchor to be inserted, and it creates a repair with two sutures crossing on the meniscal surface between the two anchors without a knot.

The Meniscal Cinch uses a 15° curved gun loaded with two separate trocar needles. Each needle is loaded with a hollow tubular PEEK anchor connected by No. 2-0 FiberWire with a pretied sliding locking knot. After insertion of the first device, the needle associated with it is removed and handed off. The second needle is pushed

downward and clicked into position, and the second device is inserted in the same fashion as the first.

The MaxFire is a UHMWPE suture with two anchors consisting of No. 5 polyethylene sleeves that are similar to the anchors in the JuggerKnot suture anchor (Figure 9). The two anchors are inserted into the meniscus with a trigger-gun device that deploys a curved or straight needle. With traction, the deployed sleeves bunch up to create anchors on the peripheral capsule. A pretied sliding locking knot is part of the repair.

The Sequent device uses a curved needle to insert a braided No. 0 UHMWPE suture containing three, four, or seven PEEK anchors. The technique allows continuous stitching, and the anchors can be used to create a V-, W-, or box-shaped repair. The knots are created after insertion of each anchor by rotating and tensioning the insertion device to lock the suture into slots in the PEEK anchor.

The CrossFix II is an all-suture construct with no implant. The dual-pronged delivery device has two hollow, parallel 15-gauge needles (straight or 12° curved). The device has a 16-mm depth limiter. To allow the internal nitinol shuttling needle to clear the plastic sheath, 8 mm of tissue penetration is required. When exposed, the two parallel needles extend outside the plastic sheath, and a small needle shuttles a braided No. 0 UHMWPE suture with a pretied sliding Westin knot between them, creating a 3-mm mattress stitch. This system uses no suture anchor.

Biomechanical Considerations

During the postoperative rehabilitation and healing phase, meniscal repairs experience compression and shear loads but probably little if any distraction. Much higher shear loads than distraction loads can be anticipated in a suture-based repair device.[69] A comparison study of human meniscal tissue found that some suture-based, self-adjusting devices with UHMWPE-containing suture provide repair strengths comparable to those of an inside-out repair using a braided polyester or UHMWPE-containing suture.[70] The MaxFire device had substantially lower mean failure loads, completed fewer load cycles, and demonstrated greater displacement during cyclic loading. The MaxFire had a 17% failure rate related to final device tensioning during arthroscopic insertion in human cadaver menisci.[71] A meta-analysis of the biomechanical properties of meniscus repair devices and sutures found that a vertically oriented mattress suture was stronger than a horizontal mattress suture and that repairs with some meniscal devices had biomechanical properties similar to those of suture repairs.[72]

Clinical Considerations

Arthroscopic meniscus repair is a successful technique when used in appropriately selected patients. The healing rate after an isolated meniscus repair without ligament surgery is approximately 80%.[73] In early results (without revision surgery), the repair was successful in approximately 90% of patients when done in conjunction with an ACL reconstruction.[74] This rate may decline over time, but an 86% healing rate was reported at 6-year follow-up. In patients with a history of ACL reconstruction predating the meniscus injury, the success rate was lower (approximately 60%) and suggested a degenerative process.

A peripheral vertical tear is ideal for repair, but some success has been reported with other tear types. A systematic review of horizontal meniscus tear repairs found a 78% success rate when reoperation was the principal criterion.[75] Several types of tears are unlikely to heal including white-white zone tears, degenerative tears, irreducible tears, tears with rolled edges, and tears in which it is not possible to achieve a sound fixation. Chronic bucket-handle medial meniscus tears are difficult to repair, but a retrospective review of suture repairs reported encouraging results.[76] Of 24 repairs of chronic bucket-handle tears with a minimum length of 2 cm, 20 (83%) had healed at an average of 10 months after injury, based on clinical outcome scores and postoperative MRI. All of the unsuccessful repairs were isolated meniscus repairs without an associated ACL reconstruction.

Few long-term reports exist, but it appears that meniscus healing rates may deteriorate with time. The success rate of meniscus repairs using a first-generation device (Meniscus Arrow, Bionx) was found to deteriorate from approximately 91% at 2-year follow-up to 71% at 6.6-year follow-up.[77] There are few reports of second-look arthroscopy. Second-look arthroscopy was done an average 14 months after 62 all-inside meniscal repairs of red-red and red-white zone longitudinal tears using the FasT-Fix device and done at the time of ACL reconstruction.[78] The healing rate was 74%; an additional 15% were incompletely healed, and 11% had not healed. Clinical success was not equivalent to healing; only one of the unhealed repairs had mechanical symptoms at the time of the second surgery.

Summary

Biologic grafts are available for a number of applications. They are commonly used for ligament reconstruction and tendon augmentation. Allografts have a better clinical track record with better outcomes and fewer adverse events compared to xenograft and synthetic materials. ACL reconstruction allografts have proven effective, providing comparable results to autografts without the issues of donor site morbidity and more difficult rehabilitation. For patients who are not aggressive pivoting or contact athletes and who are older than 25 years, there is no concern about allograft use. Allografts that are chemically processed or irradiated do not perform as well as deep-frozen, chemical-free, nonirradiated grafts. Acellular dermal matrix allografts can augment rotator cuff tendon healing, especially in tears greater than 3 cm in length and those with the potential for poor healing.

As suture anchor designs continue to develop, the trend is toward biodegradable and plastic anchors containing several (usually up to 3) UHMWPE-containing sutures. Eyelets are commonly found at the insertion end of the anchor facilitating sliding, locking knot-tying. Screw type anchors are stronger than other designs. Glenoid anchors are smaller than rotator cuff repair anchors to more easily fit into the denser smaller glenoid bone. These smaller glenoid anchors do not offer the higher failure loads of the larger anchors but are clinically appropriate for the designed environment. Knotless anchors continue to be introduced and are principally designed for the lateral row of a double-row rotator cuff repair.

Although several implants are available to assist in arthroscopic meniscal repair, the key to meniscal repair healing is a good blood supply, the absence of meniscal degeneration, and a stable knee. The current all-inside techniques use a suture-based, self-adjusting meniscus repair device with nonabsorbable UHMWPE-containing suture attached to PEEK anchors and connected by a pretied, sliding, and self-locking knot.

Key Study Points

- BPTB allograft ACL reconstruction is an effective technique in most patients. The issue arises for the younger aggressive, noncompliant athlete who is unwilling or unable to follow a slow recovery plan.

- The use of chemically processed or irradiated allografts is associated with higher failure rates.

- Several biodegradable suture anchors made from different materials are available. More rapid polymers are more likely to develop inflammatory reactions. An appreciation that different materials behave differently is essential to the proper selection of an anchor.

Annotated References

1. Månsson O, Sernert N, Rostgard-Christensen L, Kartus J: Long-term clinical and radiographic results after delayed anterior cruciate ligament reconstruction in adolescents. *Am J Sports Med* 2015;43(1):138-145.

   ACL reconstruction in adolescents led to more osteoarthritic changes in the treated knee than in the noninvolved knee at long-term follow-up. Clinical outcomes and health-related quality of life were comparable to those of healthy control subjects. Level of evidence: IV.

2. Mather RC III, Koenig L, Kocher MS, et al; MOON Knee Group: Societal and economic impact of anterior cruciate ligament tears. *J Bone Joint Surg Am* 2013;95(19):1751-1759.

   ACL reconstruction was found to be cost-effective and to reduce societal costs relative to rehabilitation if indirect cost factors, including work status and earnings, were considered.

3. Mohtadi NG, Chan DS, Dainty KN, Whelan DB: Patellar tendon versus hamstring tendon autograft for anterior cruciate ligament rupture in adults. *Cochrane Database Syst Rev* 2011;9:CD005960.

   There was insufficient evidence to draw conclusions as to the differences in long-term functional outcome after patellar and hamstring tendon autografts were used. After patellar tendon reconstruction, knees were more likely to be stable but had more anterior issues.

4. Li S, Chen Y, Lin Z, Cui W, Zhao J, Su W: A systematic review of randomized controlled clinical trials comparing hamstring autografts versus bone-patellar tendon-bone autografts for the reconstruction of the anterior cruciate ligament. *Arch Orthop Trauma Surg* 2012;132(9):1287-1297.

   Hamstring tendon and BPTB autograft ACL reconstructions similarly restored postoperative knee joint function. Hamstring tendon autografts were inferior to BPTB

   autografts for restoring knee joint stability but were associated with fewer postoperative complications.

5. Li S, Su W, Zhao J, et al: A meta-analysis of hamstring autografts versus bone-patellar tendon-bone autografts for reconstruction of the anterior cruciate ligament. *Knee* 2011;18(5):287-293.

   BPTB autografts led to better knee stability on the KT-1000, Lachman, and pivot tests. Hamstring tendon autografts led to fewer postoperative complications, such as anterior knee pain, kneeling pain, and extension loss. No differences were found in graft failure rates.

6. Yunes M, Richmond JC, Engels EA, Pinczewski LA: Patellar versus hamstring tendons in anterior cruciate ligament reconstruction: A meta-analysis. *Arthroscopy* 2001;17(3):248-257.

7. Kim JG, Yang SJ, Lee YS, Shim JC, Ra HJ, Choi JY: The effects of hamstring harvesting on outcomes in anterior cruciate ligament-reconstructed patients: A comparative study between hamstring-harvested and -unharvested patients. *Arthroscopy* 2011;27(9):1226-1234.

   ACL reconstruction led to substantial knee flexion weakness in comparison with the unaffected knee, irrespective of hamstring tendon harvesting. The increase in knee flexor deficit in patients who underwent hamstring tendon harvest was significant in comparison with those who received an allograft. Level of evidence: III.

8. Barker JU, Drakos MC, Maak TG, Warren RF, Williams RJ III, Allen AA: Effect of graft selection on the incidence of postoperative infection in anterior cruciate ligament reconstruction. *Am J Sports Med* 2010;38(2):281-286.

   Hamstring tendon autografts have a higher incidence of infection than BPTB autografts or allografts. The use of allograft material in ACL reconstruction does not increase the risk of infection or the need for graft removal with infection. Level of evidence: III.

9. Krych AJ, Jackson JD, Hoskin TL, Dahm DL: A meta-analysis of patellar tendon autograft versus patellar tendon allograft in anterior cruciate ligament reconstruction. *Arthroscopy* 2008;24(3):292-298.

10. Gorschewsky O, Klakow A, Riechert K, Pitzl M, Becker R: Clinical comparison of the Tutoplast allograft and autologous patellar tendon (bone-patellar tendon-bone) for the reconstruction of the anterior cruciate ligament: 2- and 6-year results. *Am J Sports Med* 2005;33(8):1202-1209.

11. Sun K, Zhang J, Wang Y, et al: Arthroscopic anterior cruciate ligament reconstruction with at least 2.5 years' follow-up comparing hamstring tendon autograft and irradiated allograft. *Arthroscopy* 2011;27(9):1195-1202.

   The use of irradiated hamstring tendon allografts led to significantly more instability and joint laxity than the use of hamstring tendon autografts. However, IKDC functional and subjective scores or activity levels did not differ. Level of evidence: II.

12. Ellis HB, Matheny LM, Briggs KK, Pennock AT, Steadman JR: Outcomes and revision rate after bone-patellar tendon-bone allograft versus autograft anterior cruciate ligament reconstruction in patients aged 18 years or younger with closed physes. *Arthroscopy* 2012;28(12):1819-1825.

No significant differences in function, activity, or satisfaction were found after allograft or autograft reconstruction in patients younger than 19 years. The allografts were unsuccessful 15 times more often than the autografts. All failures occurred during the first year after reconstruction. Level of evidence: III.

13. Barber FA, Cowden CH III, Sanders EJ: Revision rates after anterior cruciate ligament reconstruction using bone-patellar tendon-bone allograft or autograft in a population 25 years old and younger. *Arthroscopy* 2014;30(4):483-491.

Reconstructions using BPTB allografts that were not irradiated or chemically processed were no more successful than those using BPTB autografts in patients no older than 25 years. Rehabilitation programs varied. Clinical outcome scores did not differ. Level of evidence: III.

14. Barrett G, Stokes D, White M: Anterior cruciate ligament reconstruction in patients older than 40 years: Allograft versus autograft patellar tendon. *Am J Sports Med* 2005;33(10):1505-1512.

15. Barber FA, Aziz-Jacobo J, Oro FB: Anterior cruciate ligament reconstruction using patellar tendon allograft: An age-dependent outcome evaluation. *Arthroscopy* 2010;26(4):488-493.

Outcomes of BPTB allograft ACL reconstruction did not subjectively or objectively differ based on whether patients were younger than 40 years or older than 40 years. Patients in both age groups had consistent results. Level of evidence: III.

16. Foster TE, Wolfe BL, Ryan S, Silvestri L, Kaye EK: Does the graft source really matter in the outcome of patients undergoing anterior cruciate ligament reconstruction? An evaluation of autograft versus allograft reconstruction results: A systematic review. *Am J Sports Med* 2010;38(1):189-199.

No specific graft source was found to be clearly superior to others. This finding led to the conclusion that the graft source has a minimal effect on the outcome of patients undergoing ACL reconstruction.

17. Borchers JR, Pedroza A, Kaeding C: Activity level and graft type as risk factors for anterior cruciate ligament graft failure: A case-control study. *Am J Sports Med* 2009;37(12):2362-2367.

Stratum-specific odds ratios revealed a multiplicative interaction between higher activity level after ACL reconstruction and allograft use, such that the odds of ACL graft failure were greatly increased. Level of evidence: III.

18. Barrett GR, Luber K, Replogle WH, Manley JL: Allograft anterior cruciate ligament reconstruction in the young, active patient: Tegner activity level and failure rate. *Arthroscopy* 2010;26(12):1593-1601.

Fresh-frozen BPTB allografts should not be used for ACL reconstruction in young patients who will return to a high activity level. The failure rate in such reconstructions was 2.6 to 4.2 times higher than if patients returned to a low activity level. Level of evidence: III.

19. Mascarenhas R, Tranovich M, Karpie JC, Irrgang JJ, Fu FH, Harner CD: Patellar tendon anterior cruciate ligament reconstruction in the high-demand patient: Evaluation of autograft versus allograft reconstruction. *Arthroscopy* 2010;26(9, Suppl):S58-S66.

In patients with high physical demands at 3- to 14-year follow-up, autograft and fresh-frozen allograft BPTB ACL reconstructions had similar patient-reported and objective outcomes. Level of evidence: III.

20. Kaeding CC, Aros B, Pedroza A, et al: Allograft Versus Autograft Anterior Cruciate Ligament Reconstruction: Predictors of Failure From a MOON Prospective Longitudinal Cohort. *Sports Health* 2011;3(1):73-81.

21. Kraeutler MJ, Bravman JT, McCarty EC: Bone-patellar tendon-bone autograft versus allograft in outcomes of anterior cruciate ligament reconstruction: A meta-analysis of 5182 patients. *Am J Sports Med* 2013;41(10):2439-2448.

ACL reconstruction with BPTB autograft led to less graft rupture or knee laxity, better results on single-leg hop tests, and greater patient satisfaction than ACL reconstruction with BPTB allografts.

22. Mariscalco MW, Magnussen RA, Mehta D, Hewett TE, Flanigan DC, Kaeding CC: Autograft versus nonirradiated allograft tissue for anterior cruciate ligament reconstruction: A systematic review. *Am J Sports Med* 2014;42(2):492-499.

A systematic review found no differences in graft failure, postoperative laxity, or outcome scores in a comparison of ACL reconstructions using autograft or nonirradiated allograft. Patients were in their late 20s and early 30s. These findings should not be extrapolated to younger, more active patients.

23. Yao LW, Wang Q, Zhang L, et al: Patellar tendon autograft versus patellar tendon allograft in anterior cruciate ligament reconstruction: A systematic review and meta-analysis. *Eur J Orthop Surg Traumatol* 2015;25(2):355-365.

A meta-analysis found no clinical differences after BPTB autograft or allograft was used in primary ACL reconstruction. Overall, more clinical failures were observed when allograft was used. Fresh-frozen allografts had results equivalent to those of autografts except in Tegner scores.

24. Cvetanovich GL, Mascarenhas R, Saccomanno MF, et al: Hamstring autograft versus soft-tissue allograft in anterior cruciate ligament reconstruction: A systematic review and meta-analysis of randomized controlled trials. *Arthroscopy* 2014;30(12):1616-1624.

© 2016 American Academy of Orthopaedic Surgeons

A review of randomized controlled studies comparing hamstring tendon autograft and soft-tissue allograft ACL reconstructions found no significant outcome differences. Level of evidence: II.

25. Clatworthy MG, Annear P, Bulow JU, Bartlett RJ: Tunnel widening in anterior cruciate ligament reconstruction: A prospective evaluation of hamstring and patella tendon grafts. *Knee Surg Sports Traumatol Arthrosc* 1999;7(3):138-145.

26. Nebelung S, Deitmer G, Gebing R, Reichwein F, Nebelung W: High incidence of tunnel widening after anterior cruciate ligament reconstruction with transtibial femoral tunnel placement. *Arch Orthop Trauma Surg* 2012;132(11):1653-1663.

    Clinical and MRI examination of 59 primary ACL reconstructions with quadrupled hamstring tendon autograft at a mean 61-month follow-up found that tunnel cross-sectional areas had more than doubled. However, knee stability or function was not affected. Level of evidence: IV.

27. Achtnich A, Stiepani H, Forkel P, Metzlaff S, Hänninen EL, Petersen W: Tunnel widening after anatomic double-bundle and mid-position single-bundle anterior cruciate ligament reconstruction. *Arthroscopy* 2013;29(9):1514-1524.

    Postoperative tunnel widening was evaluated after hamstring tendon four-tunnel double-bundle and hamstring tendon two-tunnel single-bundle ACL reconstructions. At 8-month follow-up, MRI revealed significant widening in all bone tunnels, with no difference between the types of reconstruction. Level of evidence: III.

28. Sabat D, Kundu K, Arora S, Kumar V: Tunnel widening after anterior cruciate ligament reconstruction: A prospective randomized computed tomography–based study comparing 2 different femoral fixation methods for hamstring graft. *Arthroscopy* 2011;27(6):776-783.

    After quadrupled hamstring tendon ACL reconstructions with femoral fixation using the EndoButton or Transfix, tunnel widening was measured on CT at intervals to 6 months. Tunnel widening was significantly less with the Transfix than the EndoButton. Level of evidence: II.

29. Barber FA, Burns JP, Deutsch A, Labbé MR, Litchfield RB: A prospective, randomized evaluation of acellular human dermal matrix augmentation for arthroscopic rotator cuff repair. *Arthroscopy* 2012;28(1):8-15.

    Repair of large rotator cuff tears augmented using acellular human dermal matrix led to higher outcome scores than nonaugmented repairs. On MRI, 85% of augmented repairs and 40% of nonaugmented repairs were intact (*P* < 0.01). Level of evidence: II.

30. Barber FA, Herbert MA, Coons DA: Tendon augmentation grafts: Biomechanical failure loads and failure patterns. *Arthroscopy* 2006;22(5):534-538.

31. Barber FA, Aziz-Jacobo J: Biomechanical testing of commercially available soft-tissue augmentation materials. *Arthroscopy* 2009;25(11):1233-1239.

    Acellular human collagen matrix grafts (Graftjacket or Allopatch) were stronger with cyclic loading and had greater suture retention strength than synthetic or xenograft materials (SportMesh or OrthAdapt) as well as greater stiffness.

32. Derwin KA, Baker AR, Spragg RK, Leigh DR, Iannotti JP: Commercial extracellular matrix scaffolds for rotator cuff tendon repair: Biomechanical, biochemical, and cellular properties. *J Bone Joint Surg Am* 2006;88(12):2665-2672.

33. Aurora A, McCarron J, Iannotti JP, Derwin K: Commercially available extracellular matrix materials for rotator cuff repairs: State of the art and future trends. *J Shoulder Elbow Surg* 2007;16(5, Suppl):S171-S178.

34. Derwin KA, Badylak SF, Steinmann SP, Iannotti JP: Extracellular matrix scaffold devices for rotator cuff repair. *J Shoulder Elbow Surg* 2010;19(3):467-476.

    A review of the basic science and clinical understanding of extracellular matrix scaffolds for rotator cuff repair emphasized the host immune response, scaffold remodeling, mechanical and suture retention properties, and clinical studies. Level of evidence: IV.

35. Sclamberg SG, Tibone JE, Itamura JM, Kasraeian S: Six-month magnetic resonance imaging follow-up of large and massive rotator cuff repairs reinforced with porcine small intestinal submucosa. *J Shoulder Elbow Surg* 2004;13(5):538-541.

36. Walton JR, Bowman NK, Khatib Y, Linklater J, Murrell GA: Restore orthobiologic implant: Not recommended for augmentation of rotator cuff repairs. *J Bone Joint Surg Am* 2007;89(4):786-791.

37. Malcarney HL, Bonar F, Murrell GA: Early inflammatory reaction after rotator cuff repair with a porcine small intestine submucosal implant: A report of 4 cases. *Am J Sports Med* 2005;33(6):907-911.

38. McCarron JA, Milks RA, Chen X, Iannotti JP, Derwin KA: Improved time-zero biomechanical properties using poly-L-lactic acid graft augmentation in a cadaveric rotator cuff repair model. *J Shoulder Elbow Surg* 2010;19(5):688-696.

39. McCarty LP III, Buss DD, Datta MW, Freehill MQ, Giveans MR: Complications observed following labral or rotator cuff repair with use of poly-L-lactic acid implants. *J Bone Joint Surg Am* 2013;95(6):507-511.

    Forty-four patients had macroscopic biodegradable anchor debris after shoulder débridement. Gross and histologic examination showed giant cell reactions (84%), polarizing crystalline material (100%), papillary synovitis (79%), and grade 3 or 4 chondral damage (70%). Level of evidence: IV.

40. Park MJ, Hsu JE, Harper C, Sennett BJ, Huffman GR: Poly-L/D-lactic acid anchors are associated with reoperation and failure of SLAP repairs. *Arthroscopy* 2011;27(10):1335-1340.

Bioabsorbable PL96/D4LA suture anchors were found more often than nonabsorbable anchors in unsuccessful superior labrum anterior and posterior repairs and second surgeries. The use of these suture anchors should be avoided. Level of evidence: IV.

41. Barber FA, Dockery WD, Cowden CH III: The degradation outcome of biocomposite suture anchors made from poly L-lactide-co-glycolide and β-tricalcium phosphate. *Arthroscopy* 2013;29(11):1834-1839.

A PLLA/PGA-β-TCP suture anchor (Healix BR, Depuy Synthes) was found to be completely degraded and fully reabsorbed 3 years after implantation. Osteoconductivity was observed at 71% of anchor sites and was complete or almost complete in 50%. Level of evidence: IV.

42. Barber FA, Dockery WD, Hrnack SA: Long-term degradation of a poly-lactide co-glycolide/β-tricalcium phosphate biocomposite interference screw. *Arthroscopy* 2011;27(5):637-643.

A PLLA/PGA/β-TCP interference screw (Milagro, Depuy Synthes) was found to be completely degraded and fully reabsorbed 3 years after implantation. Osteoconductivity was confirmed in 81% of patients, and the screw completely filled the prior screw site in 19%. Level of evidence: IV.

43. Barber FA, Dockery WD: Long-term absorption of beta-tricalcium phosphate poly-L-lactic acid interference screws. *Arthroscopy* 2008;24(4):441-447.

44. Martinek V, Seil R, Lattermann C, Watkins SC, Fu FH: The fate of the poly-L-lactic acid interference screw after anterior cruciate ligament reconstruction. *Arthroscopy* 2001;17(1):73-76.

45. Stähelin AC, Weiler A, Rüfenacht H, Hoffmann R, Geissmann A, Feinstein R: Clinical degradation and biocompatibility of different bioabsorbable interference screws: A report of six cases. *Arthroscopy* 1997;13(2):238-244.

46. Böstman OM, Pihlajamäki HK: Adverse tissue reactions to bioabsorbable fixation devices. *Clin Orthop Relat Res* 2000;371:216-227.

47. Edwards DJ, Hoy G, Saies AD, Hayes MG: Adverse reactions to an absorbable shoulder fixation device. *J Shoulder Elbow Surg* 1994;3(4):230-233.

48. Cobaleda Aristizabal AF, Sanders EJ, Barber FA: Adverse events associated with biodegradable lactide-containing suture anchors. *Arthroscopy* 2014;30(5):555-560.

Anchor-specific adverse events occurred in 2 of 360 procedures (0.5%). The only material-related event occurred when a PL70/D30LA anchor released the eyelet suture, which migrated into the joint and caused chondral damage. No events occurred with the use of biocomposite PLLA/β-TCP anchors. Level of evidence: IV.

49. Barber FA, Dockery WD: Long-term absorption of poly-L-lactic Acid interference screws. *Arthroscopy* 2006;22(8):820-826.

50. Barber FA, Bava ED, Spenciner DB, Piccirillo J: Cyclic biomechanical testing of biocomposite lateral row knotless anchors in a human cadaveric model. *Arthroscopy* 2013;29(6):1012-1018.

The use of threaded biocomposite knotless anchors (Healix and Bio-SwiveLock, Arthrex) led to less displacement and higher failure loads than the use of nonthreaded biocomposite anchors (PushLock). Healix knotless anchors had the lowest rate of displacement.

51. Vaishnav S, Millett PJ: Arthroscopic rotator cuff repair: Scientific rationale, surgical technique, and early clinical and functional results of a knotless self-reinforcing double-row rotator cuff repair system. *J Shoulder Elbow Surg* 2010;19(2, Suppl):83-90.

The knotless self-reinforcing dual-row repair system provided improved contact area and restored the native footprint of the rotator cuff tendon, leading to improved outcomes. Level of evidence: IV.

52. Khoury LD, Kwon YW, Kummer FJ: A novel method to determine suture anchor loading after rotator cuff repair: A study of two double-row techniques. *Bull NYU Hosp Jt Dis* 2010;68(1):25-28.

Medial anchors withstood greater loads than lateral anchors in dual-row constructs (79% versus 21%) and suture-bridge constructs (67% versus 33%). Abduction (45° to 60°) had little effect on anchor tensions. Internal and external rotation increased anterior or posterior anchor loads in both rows.

53. Yamakado K, Katsuo S, Mizuno K, Arakawa H, Hayashi S: Medial-row failure after arthroscopic double-row rotator cuff repair. *Arthroscopy* 2010;26(3):430-435.

Medial-row mattress suture pullout occurred in four patients after dual-row arthroscopic rotator cuff repair. The tendon was avulsed at the medial row, and there were exposed knots on the bony surface of the rotator cuff footprint. Level of evidence: IV.

54. Schneeberger AG, von Roll A, Kalberer F, Jacob HA, Gerber C: Mechanical strength of arthroscopic rotator cuff repair techniques: An in vitro study. *J Bone Joint Surg Am* 2002;84-A(12):2152-2160.

55. Barber FA, Herbert MA, Hapa O, et al: Biomechanical analysis of pullout strengths of rotator cuff and glenoid anchors: 2011 update. *Arthroscopy* 2011;27(7):895-905.

Load to failure was found to depend not on anchor location (cancellous or cortical bone) but on anchor type (cuff anchor or glenoid anchor). Relatively large, fully-threaded screw-in rotator cuff anchors had higher failure strengths than smaller, nonscrew glenoid anchors.

56. Mahar A, Allred DW, Wedemeyer M, Abbi G, Pedowitz R: A biomechanical and radiographic analysis of standard and intracortical suture anchors for arthroscopic rotator cuff repair. *Arthroscopy* 2006;22(2):130-135.

57. Barber FA, Herbert MA, Coons DA, Boothby MH: Sutures and suture anchors: Update 2006. *Arthroscopy* 2006;22(10):1063.e1-1063.e9.

58. Barber FA, Herbert M, Click JN: Recent suture anchor developments. *Arthroscopy* 1996;12:361-362.

59. Barber FA, Herbert MA: Suture anchors—update 1999. *Arthroscopy* 1999;15(7):719-725.

60. Barber FA, Herbert MA, Hapa O, et al: Biomechanical analysis of pullout strengths of rotator cuff and glenoid anchors: 2011 update. *Arthroscopy* 2011;27(7):895-905.

61. Barber FA, Herbert MA, Richards DP: Sutures and suture anchors: Update 2003. *Arthroscopy* 2003;19(9):985-990.

62. Benson EC, MacDermid JC, Drosdowech DS, Athwal GS: The incidence of early metallic suture anchor pullout after arthroscopic rotator cuff repair. *Arthroscopy* 2010;26(3):310-315.

   There was a minimal risk of suture anchor pullout in small- to medium-size tears, but the risk increased with tear size. Routine radiographic follow-up after the use of metallic anchors was recommended to identify anchor pullout. Level of evidence: III.

63. Goeminne S, Debeer P: Delayed migration of a metal suture anchor into the glenohumeral joint. *Acta Orthop Belg* 2010;76(6):834-837.

   Intra-articular migration of a metallic suture anchor occurred 7 years after open labral reconstruction. Surgeons should be aware of possible anchor migration in patients with sharp or persistent pain, catching sensations, or loss of mobility. Level of evidence: IV.

64. Dhawan A, Ghodadra N, Karas V, Salata MJ, Cole BJ: Complications of bioabsorbable suture anchors in the shoulder. *Am J Sports Med* 2012;40(6):1424-1430.

   Ten bioabsorbable anchor–related complications were reported to the US Food and Drug Administration in 2008, representing a small fraction of bioabsorbable anchor implantations. The use of bioabsorbable suture anchors remains safe, reproducible, and consistent. Level of evidence: IV.

65. Barber FA, Click JN: The effect of inflammatory synovial fluid on the breaking strength of new "long lasting" absorbable sutures. *Arthroscopy* 1992;8(4):437-441.

66. Barber FA, Gurwitz GS: Inflammatory synovial fluid and absorbable suture strength. *Arthroscopy* 1988;4(4):272-277.

67. Barber FA, Herbert MA, Beavis RC: Cyclic load and failure behavior of arthroscopic knots and high strength sutures. *Arthroscopy* 2009;25(2):192-199.

   Knot security and load-to-failure strength was studied in several types of sutures.

68. Abbi G, Espinoza L, Odell T, Mahar A, Pedowitz R: Evaluation of 5 knots and 2 suture materials for arthroscopic rotator cuff repair: Very strong sutures can still slip. *Arthroscopy* 2006;22(1):38-43.

69. Fisher MB, Jung HJ, McMahon PJ, Woo SL: Suture augmentation following ACL injury to restore the function of the ACL, MCL, and medial meniscus in the goat stifle joint. *J Biomech* 2011;44(8):1530-1535.

   Suture augmentation may be helpful in ACL healing in combination with functional tissue-engineering approaches by providing initial joint stability while lowering loads on the medial meniscus.

70. Barber FA, Herbert MA, Bava ED, Drew OR: Biomechanical testing of suture-based meniscal repair devices containing ultrahigh-molecular-weight polyethylene suture: Update 2011. *Arthroscopy* 2012;28(6):827-834.

   All-inside meniscal repair devices use UHMWPE suture with fixation comparable to that of vertical mattress suture repairs. The OmniSpan, Cinch, Sequent, and FasT-Fix 360 were found to be equivalent to suture repair. The MaxFire device had significantly lower loads to failure and survived less cyclic loading than other devices.

71. Likes RL, Julka A, Aros BC, et al: Meniscal repair with the MaxFire device: A cadaveric study. *Orthop Surg* 2011;3(4):259-264.

   Of 54 MaxFire devices placed in cadaver knees, 17% failed during device tensioning. Three sutures broke, one could not be reduced, and two pulled out of the meniscus.

72. M Buckland D, Sadoghi P, Wimmer MD, et al: Meta-analysis on biomechanical properties of meniscus repairs: Are devices better than sutures? *Knee Surg Sports Traumatol Arthrosc* 2015;23(1):83-89.

   A meta-analysis of 41 studies found that the loads to failure of vertically oriented meniscus repair sutures were superior to those of horizontal sutures. Some meniscal repair devices have biomechanical properties similar to those of suture repairs. Second-generation devices are significantly stronger and stiffer than first-generation devices.

73. Westermann RW, Wright RW, Spindler KP, Huston LJ, Wolf BR; MOON Knee Group: Meniscal repair with concurrent anterior cruciate ligament reconstruction: Operative success and patient outcomes at 6-year follow-up. *Am J Sports Med* 2014;42(9):2184-2192.

   Concurrent meniscal repair–ACL reconstruction was associated with an approximately 14% rate of failure at 6-year follow-up. Improvement in patient-oriented outcome scores was sustained at 6-year follow-up, and good clinical outcomes were present. Level of evidence: III.

74. Walter RP, Dhadwal AS, Schranz P, Mandalia V: The outcome of all-inside meniscal repair with relation to previous anterior cruciate ligament reconstruction. *Knee* 2014;21(6):1156-1159.

   Retrospective review of all-inside meniscal repairs with concomitant ACL reconstruction found a 9% meniscal

6: Miscellaneous Topics

reoperation rate. The rate was 37% after all-inside repair with previous ACL reconstruction. Level of evidence: IV.

75. Kurzweil PR, Lynch NM, Coleman S, Kearney B: Repair of horizontal meniscus tears: A systematic review. *Arthroscopy* 2014;30(11):1513-1519.

A systematic literature review did not support the hypothesis that surgical repair of meniscal horizontal cleave tears has an unacceptably low success rate. When reoperation was used to define failure, 77 of 98 repairs (77.8%) were successful. Level of evidence: IV.

76. Espejo-Reina A, Serrano-Fernández JM, Martín-Castilla B, Estades-Rubio FJ, Briggs KK, Espejo-Baena A: Outcomes after repair of chronic bucket-handle tears of medial meniscus. *Arthroscopy* 2014;30(4):492-496.

Repairs of chronic bucket-handle meniscal tears had good clinical outcomes and a relatively low failure rate (17%). Repairs of isolated meniscal tears were significantly less likely to succeed than repairs done in conjunction with ACL reconstruction. Level of evidence: IV.

77. Lee GP, Diduch DR: Deteriorating outcomes after meniscal repair using the Meniscus Arrow in knees undergoing concurrent anterior cruciate ligament reconstruction: Increased failure rate with long-term follow-up. *Am J Sports Med* 2005;33(8):1138-1141.

78. Tachibana Y, Sakaguchi K, Goto T, Oda H, Yamazaki K, Iida S: Repair integrity evaluated by second-look arthroscopy after arthroscopic meniscal repair with the FasT-Fix during anterior cruciate ligament reconstruction. *Am J Sports Med* 2010;38(5):965-971.

Second-look arthroscopy was used to evaluate 65 FasT-Fix meniscal repairs with concomitant ACL reconstruction; 74% were completely healed, 15% were incompletely healed, and 11% had not healed. Regardless of meniscal integrity, 83% of menisci were symptom free. Level of evidence: IV.

© 2016 American Academy of Orthopaedic Surgeons

Section 7

Medical Issues

SECTION EDITOR
Sourav K. Poddar, MD

Chapter 39

Sports Nutrition

Jacqueline R. Berning, PhD, RD, CSSD   Kelly L. Neville, MS

Abstract

Diet is a factor in human performance. No amount of training or natural ability ensures peak performance without the proper fuel for the exercising muscles. A knowledge of carbohydrate, protein, and fat consumption for athletes is imperative for sports medicine professionals who work in athletic environments. Additionally, providing science-based information and recommendations regarding hydration before, during, and after exercise can help athletes perform at their peak.

Keywords: diet and sports performance; hydration; pregame meals; recovery nutrition; competition eating

Introduction

Athletes invest a lot of time and effort in training to gain a competitive edge. Many only need to look to their diet to enhance performance; however, no amount of motivation, training, or natural ability will ensure peak performance without the proper fuel for exercising muscles. Although good eating habits cannot substitute for training and genetic aptitude, a diet focused on essential nutrients can provide energy for training, competition, recovery, and health (Figure 1). Much misinformation exists about the effects of diet and nutrients on athletic performance. A good working knowledge and understanding of sports nutrition can help team physicians and sports medicine professionals recommend diets and eating patterns that can enable their athletes to reach their athletic potential.

Ms. Neville or an immediate family member is an employee of Biogen Idec and has stock or stock options held in Amgen and Biogen. Neither Dr. Berning nor any immediate family member has received anything of value from or has stock or stock options held in a commercial company or institution related directly or indirectly to the subject of this chapter.

Energy Sources for the Muscles

Adenosine triphosphate (ATP) is the high-energy compound derived from the oxidation of macronutrients such as carbohydrates, fats, and proteins that supplies the body and the cells with energy. Muscle cells store a limited amount of ATP and depend on metabolic pathways to provide sufficient ATP for exercise and training. A resting muscle cell contains only a small amount of ATP, just enough to keep the muscles working maximally for about 2 to 4 seconds. To produce more ATP for muscle contraction over extended periods, the body uses phosphocreatine. Additionally, dietary carbohydrates and fats are used as energy sources. The breakdown of these compounds releases energy to make more ATP. The amount of ATP that is needed depends on the intensity and duration of the exercise, thus determining which energy systems become the predominant source of ATP (Table 1).

Dietary Recommendations for Athletes

Energy Availability

The number of calories needed by athletes depends on body size, body composition, and the type and length of training. Additionally, energy needs can change in season as well as out of season. To maximize health and training, athletes need to consume adequate energy to maintain or modify body weight. Many dietetic professionals now use the concept of energy availability to monitor caloric requirements. Researchers argue that this concept is more useful than that of energy balance for the athletic population.[1] Energy availability is the amount of energy left for bodily functions after the energy costs of training and competition have been calculated. Table 2 gives an example of calculations that show adequate energy availability for an athlete. It is generally agreed that athletes with an energy availability lower than 30 kcal per kg of lean body mass have a greater risk of metabolic and hormonal disruptions, including that of reproductive function. Regardless of the technique used to monitor caloric requirements, an excessive or inadequate intake of calories can result in fatigue, an increased risk of injury, a prolonged recovery period, and poor athletic performance overall.

Athletes Plates

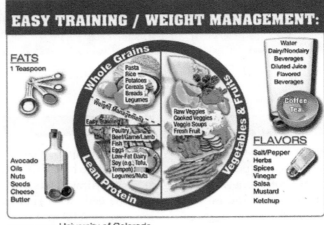

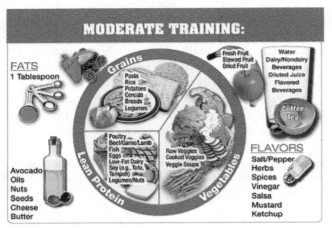

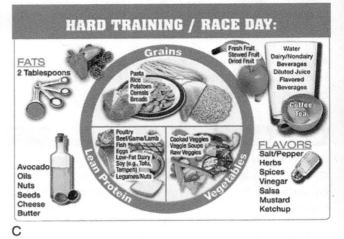

Figure 1   The athlete's plates have been designed as a food guide for athletes to follow based on the physical demands of the day. (The Athlete's Plates are a collaboration between the United States Olympic Committee Sport Dietitians and the University of Colorado [UCCS] Sport Nutrition Graduate Program, Colorado Springs, CO.)

Carbohydrates

Carbohydrates are the primary energy source for the exercising muscle. Any athlete who engages in a vigorous workout for more than 1 hour a day or works out for several hours per day may need as much as 7 to 9 g of carbohydrates per kg of body weight to maintain and replenish muscle and liver glycogen. In the past, carbohydrate recommendations often were expressed as a percentage of total calories. This percentage is poorly correlated to the amount of carbohydrate actually eaten and the fuel needed to support an athlete's training and competition; for athletes, it is important to match their carbohydrate intake to their fuel needs for training and recovery. This concept has been defined as carbohydrate availability and attempts to match increased carbohydrate intake to specific training and competition needs.[2]

Eating a variety of whole grains, fruits, and vegetables provides not only the carbohydrates that athletes need but also a range of essential vitamins, trace minerals, and fiber. Too often, athletes choose carbohydrates with high amounts of fats and sugars. Because the body has limited glycogen stores, unlimited fat stores, and typically does not use protein as an energy source during exercise, active athletes can afford to consume more calorie-dense foods from carbohydrates. Sports drinks, gels, and other foods high in sugar should be reserved for pregame and postgame refueling rather than be included in a daily meal pattern.

Table 1

Energy Systems Used in the Body to Create Adenosine Triphosphate

Energy System	Main Storage Site	When Used	Activity
Stored adenosine triphophosphate	All tissues	All the time	Sprinting 0-4 s
Phosphocreatine	All Tissues	Short bursts of activity	Shot put, high jump, bench press
Carbohydrate (anaerobic)	Muscles	High-intensity activity lasting 30 s to 2 min	200-m sprint
Carbohydrate (aerobic)	Muscles and liver	Exercise lasting 2 min to 3 h or more	Jogging, soccer, basketball, swimming
Fat (aerobic)	Muscles and fat cells	Exercise lasting more than a few minutes; greater amounts are used at lower-intensity exercise that is of long duration	Long-distance running, marathons, ultra-endurance events, cycling

Table 2

Sample Calculation of Adequate Energy Availability

Athlete's weight	53 kg
Workout expenditure	900 kcal/d
Energy intake	2500 kcal/d
Percent body fat	13%
Lean body mass	53 kg-7 kg = 46 kg
Energy availability	2500 kcal-900 kcal = 1600 kcal/46 kg lean mass = 34.8 kcal/lean mass

Protein

Protein recommendations for athletes range from 1.2 to 1.7 g of protein per kg of body weight. This amount is more than double the requirement for the sedentary adult. Protein is important for the athlete because it facilitates muscle synthesis and repair. Although most athletes exceed their protein requirement because of the added protein shakes and powders in their diets, protein requirements can be met easily through a well-planned diet. Recent research supports the consumption of approximately 25 to 30 g of protein in multiple meals throughout the day during training and off-season conditioning.[3,4] Consuming more than 40 g of protein in a single meal confers no additional benefits in boosting lean muscle mass. Protein consumption in excess of need may actually inhibit the body's ability to increase lean muscle mass.[5]

Athletes are encouraged to choose leaner sources of animal protein and to include plant sources of protein to minimize saturated fat intake. Vegetarian athletes appear to meet or exceed their protein requirements, but because plant proteins tend to be less bioavailable, vegetarians should increase their protein intake by approximately 10%.[6] An athlete following a vegetarian diet may have lower levels of muscle creatine, a nitrogenous compound found in the muscles, where it becomes phosphorylated, producing phosphocreatine. Phosphocreatine can then supply a phosphate to adenosine diphosphate to become ATP, a readily available cellular energy source. Studies have shown that elevated levels of muscle creatine increase the rate at which phosphocreatine is resynthesized and may enhance exercise performance and recovery time for short bouts of repeated maximal exercise. Several studies have shown that vegetarian athletes tend to have lower levels of muscle creatine compared with their omnivore counterparts and that vegetarians who took creatine supplements had a higher increase in resistance training and lean body mass than those in a placebo group.[7]

Vegetarian athletes gain some nutritional benefits. They consume a higher percentage of energy from carbohydrates in a diet that typically includes more fruits and vegetables compared with nonvegetarians. This may minimize the risk of free-radical damage in vegetarian athletes, offering advantages to training and health. Potential nutritional concerns for vegetarian athletes include deficits in vitamin B_{12}, iron, zinc, and calcium. Deficiencies in any of these nutrients can result in poor athletic performance. Because of the potential risk of specific dietary deficiencies of a vegetarian diet, a sports dietitian can play a key role in educating vegetarian athletes about menu planning, cooking, and food preparation to maximize their nutrient intake and athletic potential.

Fat

Fat supplies another source of energy during exercise as well as essential fatty acids and fat-soluble vitamins that are important in an athlete's diet. Most athletes fall within the range of recommended fat intake or exceed it. Athletes who consume a high-fat diet not only have adverse health effects but also may see diminished performance. Conversely, athletes who eat a very low-fat diet—less than 15% of total calories from fat—do not gain any additional performance benefits. Athletes should be encouraged to consume more heart-healthy fats, which include plant-based oils that contain monounsaturated and polyunsaturated fatty acids, and lower amounts of animal fats, which contain higher amounts of saturated fatty acids such as butter, lard, and animal fat. Trans fat intake should be kept to a minimum by limiting fried (especially deep fat–fried) foods, pastries, crackers, tortillas, croissants, biscuits, and cookies as well as stick margarine or shortening.[8]

Hydration

Sufficient fluid intake is important for everyone, but it is particularly critical for athletes, especially those training in hot and humid weather. Thirst is a late sign of dehydration. If an athlete waits to drink until thirsty, then he or she will start training in a dehydrated state. Additionally, if an athlete drinks to satisfy thirst, generally only one-half to two-thirds of fluid loss is replaced. During exercise, the goal is a loss of no more than 2% of body weight. For every pound lost during exercise, 3 cups of fluid (24 ounces) should be consumed. Athletes who are even mildly (1% to 2%) dehydrated may present with fatigue, confusion, and irritability.[9] During repeated training bouts throughout the day, weight should be monitored as a marker for hydration. In many cases, urine color charts are used as another method to determine hydration status. The rate of fluid replacement depends on the athlete's sweat rate, the duration of exercise or training, and the opportunities to consume fluids. Table 3 lists the guidelines for fluid intake before, during, and after training periods. Oral rehydration appears to be the best way to hydrate athletes, and no additional benefit appears to be conferred from intravenous fluid rehydration. Intravenous administration of fluid may be beneficial if the athlete is unable to hydrate orally.[10]

Sports Drinks

Several professional organizations, including the American College of Sports Medicine, the Academy of Nutrition and Dietetics, and the National Athletic Training Association, suggest that the consumption of a sports

Table 3
Guidelines for Recommended Fluid Intake Before, During, and After Exercise
Before Exercise
At least 2 to 4 hours before the start of exercise, drink 12 to 20 ounces of water or sports drink.
During Exercise
Consume 6 to 12 ounces of water or sports drink every 15 to 20 minutes during exercise.
After Exercise
For every pound lost, drink 16 to 24 ounces of fluid. Generally, the volume of replacement should be 1.5 times the amount of fluid lost during exercise.

drink that contains electrolytes and carbohydrates can be beneficial to athletes who train or compete for longer than 1 hour. This is especially true if the athlete has not consumed a preexercise meal, is participating in back-to-back tournament play, or has multiple workouts in 1 day. The electrolytes in these beverages aim to replace those lost in sweat, and the carbohydrates are crucial for maintaining blood glucose levels and supplying energy to the muscles as glycogen becomes depleted. Additionally, researchers have found that the consumption of sports drinks delays fatigue and maintains hydration in high-intensity activities and stop-and-go sports, such as soccer and basketball, that last less than 1 hour.[11] An ideal sports drink contains 6% to 8% carbohydrates and 110 to 165 mg of sodium and should be consumed during periods of training and competition instead of at mealtime and during other non-active times throughout the day.

Rehydrating with only water during prolonged endurance events may lead to hyponatremia. Consuming a beverage with at least 100 mg of sodium per 8 ounces will help prevent hyponatremia.

Eating During Competition and Training

The foods consumed before, during, and after competition and training can affect performance and the speed at which the body can recover. Specific guidelines are available that provide athletes with the best recommendations to ensure optimum performance.[8,10]

Before Exercise

To keep an athlete from feeling hungry before or during an athletic event, a preexercise meal should be consumed. In addition to warding off hunger, the preexercise meal maintains blood glucose levels and provides fluids for hydration. Research has shown that eating before exercise, rather than exercising in the fasted state, can improve performance.[8] Guidelines for the preexercise meal include the following strategies:

- The meal should be composed primarily of carbohydrates. This recommendation is based on digestion rates. Carbohydrates are digested in about 2 hours, with liquid emptying the fastest. Proteins take about 3 to 4 hours, and fats take 4 to 6 hours to digest and absorb. A high-fat preexercise meal may still be in the stomach of an athlete as he or she takes the field to play.

- The precompetition meal should be consumed 3 to 4 hours before play to avoid stomach distress during the event. A mixed meal of carbohydrate, protein, and fat will take longer to digest. Generally, a carbohydrate feeding of 1 g of carbohydrate per kg of body weight is appropriate 1 hour before exercise, whereas 3 to 4 g per kg of body weight can be consumed 3 to 4 hours before competition.

- Although fiber is necessary for good digestive health, it is not recommended that athletes consume high-fiber foods before competition or training because these foods may cause bloating and gastrointestinal upset.

- In the 15 to 60 minutes before competition or training, athletes may benefit from consuming a liquid carbohydrate such as a preexercise beverage or gel that contains approximately 25 g of carbohydrate. Carbohydrate sources that are high in fructose should be avoided because they slow absorption and can cause gastrointestinal upset.

- Each athlete has individual preferences, and what works for one athlete may not work for another. Personal preferences and tolerance need to be considered. If an athlete is willing to try new and unfamiliar foods, he or she should experiment with them in training sessions first.

During Exercise

Consuming carbohydrates during exercise is especially important for athletes who exercise after an overnight fast and for those who compete or train in longer events. Consuming 30 to 60 g of carbohydrates per hour can help prevent fatigue and prolong optimal endurance performance. Carbohydrates can be consumed in the form of a sports drink, energy gel, or other simple carbohydrate that is easy to digest and tolerated well by the athlete. The following guidelines for food and fluid consumption during exercise are recommended:

- Carbohydrate consumption should begin shortly after the start of exercise.

- Solid carbohydrates can be consumed during exercise;

Table 4
Determining the Hourly Sweat Rate

1. Determine body weight (in kg) before exercise
2. Determine body weight (in kg) after exercise
3. Determine fluid intake (in L) during exercise
4. Exercise duration, recorded in hours (40 min = 0.66 h)

Calculation: Sweat rate = Body weight (kg) preexercise – body weight (kg) postexercise + fluid intake/exercise time in h

Example: 125 kg – 121 kg + (2 L)/3 h = 2 L/h

however, they are digested more slowly than are liquid forms of carbohydrates. During sports such as cycling, in which less movement of the gastrointestinal tract takes place, it is easier to consume solid foods. In other sports such as running and swimming, athletes may find it easier to consume carbohydrates in liquid form.

- To maximize the absorption of carbohydrates during exercise, a combination of different sugars such as glucose, sucrose, maltodextrins, or dextrose is contained in most sports drinks. Research has shown that if an athlete needs a large amount of carbohydrates in a prolonged activity, then the combination of different sugars results in faster gastric emptying time and absorption.[12,13]

- Athletes should focus on consuming enough fluid to prevent weight loss during exercise. They should also avoid consuming too much fluid, which may result in weight gain during exercise. To consume the proper amount of fluid during exercise, an athlete should know his or her individual sweat rate. Table 4 describes how to calculate an athlete's sweat rate.

After Exercise

Proper refueling begins within 30 to 60 minutes after exercise. Refueling is more critical during a competition in which the athlete competes in multiple heats or events that occur within several hours. A postexercise recovery snack and meal promote muscle glycogen and protein synthesis. Researchers have found that glycogen synthesis is greatest immediately after exercise because the muscles tend to be insulin sensitive. Thus, consuming 1.0 to 1.5 g of carbohydrate per kg of body weight within 30 minutes after exercise and at 2-hour intervals up to 6 hours will reload the muscles with glycogen for the next day's competition or training.[14] Likewise, consuming a small amount (20 g) of protein 30 minutes after exercise stimulates protein synthesis and muscle repair.[4,11] Protein sources that have been recommended include meat, pork, chicken, turkey, egg, and dairy products. These sources appear to contain the essential amino acids, which are incorporated more readily into muscle tissue. Furthermore, research shows that leucine, an essential amino acid, is a major stimulator for the mammalian target of rapamycin pathway, which is responsible for stimulating muscle protein synthesis. Because protein and carbohydrates play a role in muscle recovery, it is important to consume both of these nutrients in a postexercise meal. In many cases, athletes consume a sports bar after exercising that is composed of only protein, but they fail to reload muscle glycogen. Similarly, an athlete who consumes a bar containing only carbohydrate fails to stimulate protein synthesis and muscle recovery. Therefore, consuming foods having a combination of carbohydrates and protein is extremely important after training. The following food combinations are examples of recovery meals and snacks recommended 30 to 60 minutes after exercise:

- A medium-size whole-grain bagel with 2 tablespoons of peanut butter and a sports drink
- An energy bar containing carbohydrates and protein and a sports drink
- A commercial recovery beverage

Within a few hours, the athlete should continue recovery by eating a meal such as:

- Two cups of whole-grain pasta with tomato sauce and 3 ounces of chicken, fish, or meat
- A turkey sandwich on wheat bread with 1 cup of fruited yogurt and a large banana

A few hours later, the athlete should eat another small snack such as:

- Two cups of whole-grain cereal with 1 cup of low-fat milk
- One piece of fruit with 2 ounces of low-fat string cheese

The recovery period is also a time to rehydrate and replace fluids and electrolytes that were lost during exercise. A simple guideline, replacing 16 to 24 ounces of fluid for every pound lost during exercise,will help start the rehydration process. In addition, consuming fluids and foods that contain electrolytes speeds the recovery rate threefold and may help prevent muscle cramps in those who are salty sweaters. It is best to consume both foods and fluids, because the combination provides nutrients that restore hydration status and the substrates for glycogen and protein synthesis.

Although recovery nutrition is highly recommended for athletes, those who will not compete or train the next day do not necessarily need to follow an optimal recovery plan. For example, a high school soccer player

in the offseason who is refining his or her soccer skills in a 2-hour practice consumes a meal a few hours after exercise along with regular eating and drinking; this is sufficient to replenish glycogen and protein synthesis before the next practice session in 3 days. Similarly, a cross-county runner who will be competing at the end of the week and goes for an easy run during the beginning of the week does not need to follow a strict recovery nutrition plan because he or she has plenty of time during the remainder of the week to restore glycogen and optimize hydration status by consuming a normal diet.

Supplements

Most athletes and consumers take supplements. Whether the benefit is real or perceived, many athletes believe that supplements will give them the winning edge. As a result, many athletes experiment with the dose and timing of supplements, hoping to gain an ergogenic benefit. Many of these dietary supplements, such as bee pollen, ginseng, artichoke hearts, and gelatin, are ineffective, whereas a few supplements, such as creatine and caffeine, may be effective only in certain scenarios. In fact, scientific support for ergogenic effectiveness exists for only a few dietary substances, including adequate fluid and electrolyte intake, carbohydrate availability, and the consumption of a variety of fruits and vegetables. From a dietary perspective, most athletes consume two to three times the amount of protein needed for optimal performance; thus protein and amino acid supplementation generally is not necessary as a means of enhancing performance. Most athletes can meet their protein requirement and all their other nutrient needs easily by consuming a healthy and varied diet. Vitamin and mineral supplementation should be used only to meet specific dietary shortcomings, such as inadequate iron or calcium intake. A risk-benefit ratio for any ergogenic aid should be calculated before the supplement is taken.

Health professionals working with athletes must approach supplement use with caution until the efficacy and safety of the supplement have been verified scientifically. The Dietary Supplement Health and Education Act of 1994 has allowed supplement manufacturers to produce a variety of supplements that do not have proven safety or efficacy without much oversight from the Food and Drug Administration. As a result, some supplements do not contain the actual substance or the amount that is listed on the label and may contain ingredients that could cause an athlete to test positive on a screen for banned drugs. Caution should be used even if the supplement has proven scientific efficacy because good manufacturing practices may not be in place, and the substance could easily be contaminated. Finally, rather than relying on a magic bullet to enhance performance, athletes should focus on optimizing their diet, training, and sleep quality. It is prudent, however, to keep open lines of communication with athletes who may be interested in taking supplements so the sports medicine practitioner can give counsel on their safety and efficacy.

Summary

A body of evidence shows that food eaten before, during, and after competition affects performance and the speed at which the athlete can recover from training or a performance. Most athletes do not have the nutrition knowledge to attain the proper balance of nutrients and energy for optimal performance. Many athletes do not eat before, during, or after exercise and then rely on supplements to meet their nutritional requirements or mistakenly use them to obtain a competitive edge.

A sports dietitian who is a registered dietitian, preferably one who is a board certified specialist in sports dietetics, can be a valuable member of the sports medicine team and can help counsel athletes on the appropriate recommendations for optimizing nutrition for performance.

Key Study Points

- Carbohydrates are the main fuel source for exercising muscle and the central nervous system. Athletes need to consume carbohydrates; however, they need only to consume enough for training and competition (carbohydrate availability) rather than consuming a certain percentage of total calories. The concept of matching carbohydrate intake to training and competition has been defined as carbohydrate availability.

- Athletes need to consume food throughout the day, rather than in one large meal. This is also true for protein consumption. Eating smaller amounts of protein (20 to 25 g) throughout the day stimulates the pathway that turns on muscle protein synthesis. Consuming large amounts of protein in one meal may comprise the amount of new muscle that can be made.

- A registered dietitian who is board certified in sports dietetics can be a valuable member of the sports medicine team because of his or her knowledge and skills to teach athletes the proper diet for performance that will allow athletes to perform at their genetic potential.

Annotated References

1. Loucks AB, Kiens B, Wright HH: Energy availability in athletes. *J Sports Sci* 2011;29(suppl 1):S7-S15.

   This article argues that the concept of energy availability is more useful for managing the diets of athletes than is the idea of energy balance and summarizes its use and the clinical consequences of low energy availability.

2. Burke LM, Hawley JA, Wong SH, Jeukendrup AE: Carbohydrates for training and competition. *J Sports Sci* 2011;29(suppl 1):S17-S27.

   This review article defines carbohydrate availability and examines the carbohydrate intake of athletes and the timing of carbohydrate consumption in relation to exercise to maintain adequate carbohydrate substrate for the muscles and central nervous system.

3. Phillips SM: A brief review of critical processes in exercise-induced muscular hypertrophy. *Sports Med* 2014;44(suppl 1):S71-S77.

   This review article examines practices of different amounts of protein ingestion and its influence on the stimulation of muscle protein synthesis (MPS). Higher protein ingestion is needed to stimulate MPS, but other factors involved are proteins that provide essential amino acids and high levels of leucine for the maximal stimulation of the mammalian target of rapamycin pathway.

4. Tipton KD, Witard OC: Protein requirements and recommendations for athletes: Relevance of ivory tower arguments for practical recommendations. *Clin Sports Med* 2007;26(1):17-36.

5. Moore DR, Robinson MJ, Fry JL, et al: Ingested protein dose response of muscle and albumin protein synthesis after resistance exercise in young men. *Am J Clin Nutr* 2009;89(1):161-168.

   This article describes a randomized study designed to yield a dose response for ingested protein in the stimulation of muscle and albumin protein synthesis. Both muscle and albumin protein syntehsis were stimulated maximally at 20 g of ingested protein.

6. Craig WJ, Mangels AR; American Dietetic Association: Position of the American Dietetic Association: Vegetarian diets. *J Am Diet Assoc* 2009;109(7):1266-1282.

   This position paper reviewed studies pertaining to vegetarianism, gave nutritional recommendations from evidence-based science, and reviewed the benefits and disadvantages of a vegetarian diet.

7. Burke DG, Chilibeck PD, Parise G, Candow DG, Mahoney D, Tarnopolsky M: Effect of creatine and weight training on muscle creatine and performance in vegetarians. *Med Sci Sports Exerc* 2003;35(11):1946-1955.

8. Rodriguez NR, DiMarco NM, Langley S; American Dietetic Association; Dietitians of Canada; American College

of Sports Medicine: Nutrition and Athletic Performance: Position of the American Dietetic Association, Dietitians of Canada, and the American College of Sports Medicine: Nutrition and athletic performance. *J Am Diet Assoc* 2009;109(3):509-527.

This position paper, composed in association with the American College of Sports Medicine and Dietitians of Canada, reviewed studies pertaining to the role of nutrition in exercise and sports. The review provides recommendations for the nutritional intake of athletes from evidence-based science.

9. D'Anci KE, Vibhakar A, Kanter JH, Mahoney CR, Taylor HA: Voluntary dehydration and cognitive performance in trained college athletes. *Percept Mot Skills* 2009;109(1):251-269.

This study investigated the cognitive and mood changes resulting from mild dehydration and glucose consumption in male and female college athletes. Dehydration was associated with higher thirst and negative moods. Subjects showed better attention with hydration.

10. American College of Sports Medicine: Selected issues for nutrition and the athlete: A team physician consensus statement. *Med Sci Sports Exerc* 2013;45(12):2378-2386.

This consensus statement provides an overview of and guide to selected issues in sports nutrition that are important to team physicians who are responsible for the care and treatment of athletes.

11. Phillips SM, Turner AP, Gray S, Sanderson MF, Sproule J: Ingesting a 6% carbohydrate-electrolyte solution improves endurance capacity, but not sprint performance, during intermittent, high-intensity shuttle running in adolescent team games players aged 12-14 years. *Eur J Appl Physiol* 2010;109(5):811-821.

This double-blind randomized study investigated the influence of consuming a 6% carbohydrate (CHO)-electrolyte drink on intermittent high-intensity performance compared with a non-CHO placebo drink. Subjects followed the Loughborough Intermittent Shuttle protocol. The time to fatigue and the volume of work performed significantly increased when CHO was ingested. No difference was seen between sprint times, however.

12. Jeukendrup AE, Moseley L: Multiple transportable carbohydrates enhance gastric emptying and fluid delivery. *Scand J Med Sci Sports* 2010;20(1):112-121.

This study compared the effects of ingesting water, a glucose solution, and a glucose plus fructose solution on gastric emptying and absorption during moderate-intensity exercise. Results showed that glucose plus fructose consumption resulted in faster emptying time and fluid delivery than glucose alone.

13. Jentjens RL, Jeukendrup AE: High rates of exogenous carbohydrate oxidation from a mixture of glucose and fructose ingested during prolonged cycling exercise. *Br J Nutr* 2005;93(4):485-492.

14. Ivy JL, Katz AL, Cutler CL, Sherman WM, Coyle EF: Muscle glycogen synthesis after exercise: Effect of time of carbohydrate ingestion. *J Appl Physiol (1985)* 1988;64(4):1480-1485.

© 2016 American Academy of Orthopaedic Surgeons

Chapter 40

Sport Psychology

Christopher M. Bader, PhD, LP, CC-AASP

Abstract

Sport psychology principles are used with a wide variety of clients or patients, from youth sport participants through the Olympic and professional ranks. Organization of the field, opportunities for collaboration, and clinical topics for further discussion with patients warrant review.

Keywords: sport psychology; athletes and mental health; injury recovery

Introduction

Sport psychology has its historical roots in the late 19th and early 20th centuries, and is a dynamic field of study concerned with endeavors that reach across clinical, educational, and research spectra. Some challenges exist within the field of sport psychology that make defining it difficult. For example, no universal definition of a "sport psychologist" exists, research typically is not widely read or understood by those outside the field, and training within the field is still debated extensively.[1-3]

Two of the major organizations focused specifically on sport psychology (as well as individuals within and outside those organizations) have attempted to address the identification of sport psychologists. The American Psychological Association (APA) includes a division (Division 47) concerned with sport and exercise psychology. This division established a proficiency for the practice of sport psychology and has stated its position that a sport psychologist should first be a licensed psychologist in his or her respective state(s) or province(s). The Association for Applied Sport Psychology (AASP) has a different audience in terms of membership, generally appealing to those with backgrounds in psychology and/or exercise science. AASP has established a distinction of Certified Consultant (indicated as "CC-AASP") within its ranks as a way to identify those in the organization who have completed specific educational requirements and mentored applied experiences.[4] As a member of APA and/or AASP, a sport psychologist is held to the ethical standards put forth in the ethical codes of the respective association. Each of those codes was created to demonstrate responsible practice by practitioners. By extension, membership in those organizations and adherence to their ethical standards should provide some protection to individuals seeking sport psychology services.

The title of sport psychologist can be somewhat confusing and misleading, depending on a person's background and use of terminology. For example, a state- or province-licensed psychologist with advanced training and supervision in the area of sports or athletics might be designated a sport psychologist. At the same time, some individuals holding the distinction of CC-AASP but not having a license to practice psychology also may use the term sport psychologist. Still others—licensed and/or certified or not—may use terms such as "sport psychology consultant," "sport psychology coach," "sport consultant," or "mental coach." Although a title may be important, the background, training, and expertise of an individual with whom a patient might choose to work is much more important.

The principles established in the practice of sport psychology can be beneficial in many fields, including surgery and medicine. Presurgical and/or postsurgical consultation with sport psychologists is being explored by physicians in many practices because of the potential to address clinical concerns before they become major clinical issues. As the understanding of preventive, as opposed to reactive, care and treatment increases, the mutually beneficial relationship between physicians and sport psychologists may prove to not only save time and money, but more importantly, also provide patients with peace of mind about their care and treatment.

Neither Dr. Bader nor any immediate family member has received anything of value from or has stock or stock options held in a commercial company or institution related directly or indirectly to the subject of this chapter.

Roles and Specialization of a Sport Psychologist

The evolving relationship between the fields of sport psychology and medicine has been well documented, as seen in the Team Physician Consensus Statement[5] that was produced by an alliance of the foremost professional medical associations and the National Collegiate Athletic Association (NCAA) Sport Science Institute (SSI)[6] publications.

In the 2014 publication, *Mind, Body and Sport*,[7] a guide to student athlete mental health from the NCAA, three prevailing models of mental health services to student athletes were discussed. Those models include the full-time employment of a sport psychologist within the athletics department, part-time use of a consultant to the athletics department, and a referral model with on-campus counseling services.[8] Each of the proposed models has advantages and disadvantages, and although these models are discussed in the context of an NCAA institution, each can be adapted for use across several settings. For example, an orthopaedic practice may have a referral-based model for its patients, in which patients are provided names and contact information for local sport psychologists before and immediately following a surgical procedure. Similarly, a hospital system may have a part-time or full-time relationship with a sport psychologist to provide services to its patients. In each of these models, the relationship between the various providers is extremely important. Trust, demonstrated knowledge, and expertise need to be present.

As the field of sport psychology continues to grow and evolve, individual providers are developing subspecialties within the field. For example, certain individuals are considered experts in the field of sport psychology and eating disorders. Additionally, emerging treatment programs specifically designed for athletes in whom eating disorders have been diagnosed and programs developed for athletes with process and chemical addiction diagnoses are now available. The areas of youth sport psychology, collegiate sport psychology, and professional or Olympic sport psychology also could be considered concentrations within the field of sport psychology, given the unique opportunities and challenges in each of those areas.

Youth Sports

Participation in youth sports has a wide range of benefits, including peer socialization, the development of self-esteem, the establishment of leadership qualities, and the promotion of health and fitness.[9] As tens of millions of young people participate in sports, meeting the needs of those athletes through sport psychology interventions (for example, workshops on various topics within the realm of sport psychology/performance enhancement) is increasingly important. It is important to encourage similar interventions to their coaches and parents or guardians as well. Approaching each group with ideas about having a positive influence on sports participation will ensure maximum benefit for youth sports participants.[10] Parents and coaches can have a great influence on their young athletes. After athletes reach a certain age, however, their parents and coaches take a backseat to their peers in terms of influential input into continued sports participation.

One way the benefits of youth sports participation can be jeopardized is by compromising the health of the young athlete through sports specialization at an early age. A direct link between early specialization and burnout is not yet clear in the research, but several risk factors are thought to be associated with that link. Through education and awareness of these potential problems, it is thought that long-term injury and burnout can be prevented.[9] Parents, coaches, physicians, and young athletes have a responsibility to participate in the prevention, treatment, and recovery from injury when it occurs. Although the clinical concerns discussed later in this chapter are seen in younger individuals, most of these problems do not fully develop until later in life. In dealing with young athletes who are injured, awareness of the possible presence of concerning symptoms is important. Additionally, resources (in the form of a handout or informational flyer, or contact information for a sport psychology professional) for the athletes and their parents are essential.

Collegiate Sports

Recently, the NCAA SSI has designated the mental health of student athletes as the main challenge to their health and safety.[7] Based on that designation, the SSI has been instrumental in publishing and disseminating information to the NCAA membership on mental health issues for student athletes.

Many schools are beginning to address the mental and physical health of collegiate student athletes before they even step onto campus. The initial transition to college encompasses several areas: academic, social, and athletic. The athletic transition can include changing roles on a team, modifying the amount of participation, or dealing with injury.[11] The academic shift can be quite an awakening as well, with some underprepared student athletes finding themselves behind before they are fully established in the academic term. Because of this potential lag, schools have begun to develop special coursework for student athletes to ease the transition.[12] The social transition can include issues surrounding relationships, social events including parties, the separation from parents or guardians, and simply fitting in on a college campus.

A student's level of athletic identity can be a major

factor during times of transition. Several recent studies relate athletic identity to career development and career maturity (one's readiness to make informed, age-appropriate career decisions and cope with career development tasks).[13] Athletic identity can be threatened when an athlete is injured. This threat to the athlete's overall identity can cause psychological issues that can impede physical recovery. When assisting a student athlete who is injured, collaboration with medical and psychological personnel can be of great benefit. It is important to involve roommates, teammates, coaches, and parents to create a positive support system throughout the process. The medical personnel (eg, physicians, athletic trainers) involved are on the front lines of monitoring potential changes in a student athlete's mental state following injury.

In addition to bodily injury, head injury, specifically concussion, has been researched and studied widely in recent years. Although deciphering the natural history of concussion remains a work in progress, there has been considerable advancement in the understanding and management of sports-related concussion. Established signs and symptoms of concussion have been developed, and guidelines are now available for coaches and athletic trainers to follow if a concussion is suspected. It is important for medical personnel to be aware of this information to minimize prolonged symptomatology. One frequently discussed psychologic symptom of concussion is depression or depressed mood, which often accompanies many of the physical symptoms of concussion.[14]

Psychologic injury, such as a severe mental health issue, often is seen for the first time during the college years. Anecdotally, an increase in the use of counseling services and in the severity of mental health issues in college students has been seen compared with years past. For example, college students, including student athletes, may experience a first bout with major depression or even a first psychotic break or episode in college. Again, medical personnel are on the front lines in detecting these issues, and fostering a positive working relationship with a clinically trained, licensed mental health provider can assist in early treatment efforts.

As mentioned previously, parents and guardians play a significant role in the lives of their student athletes. Most parents and student athletes maintain healthy boundaries during the college years; however, some situations require special considerations for the inclusion of parents or guardians. For example, when physically injured, a student athlete, who is an adult in chronological age, may still desire to have his or her parents present to help make surgical decisions and during the subsequent rehabilitation process. This provides medical and psychologic personnel another avenue of access to postsurgical student athletes, because many parents see the benefit of having a sport psychologist available, and many will encourage their student athletes to seek these services.

Underlying the transition issues and injury concerns during college are the general mental health and wellness of student athletes. Depending on the mental health status of student athletes upon entry into college, their transition and/or injury rehabilitation may be easier or more difficult.

Professional and Olympic Sports

At this developmental level of sports, the role of the sport psychologist is somewhat different. He or she may be hired by an individual player or performer or by the larger organization. Within professional sports, more organizations seem willing to hire such a provider to address the clinical and performance needs of their athletes.

For Olympic-level athletes in the United States, the US Olympic Committee (USOC) maintains a team of sport psychologists assigned to work at the various Olympic training centers and with the teams across the country. Additionally, the US National Governing Bodies may hire a sport psychologist to work specifically with their teams. The structure of the support teams within the USOC includes a sport psychologist as an integral component. Again, this arrangement is seen as useful, and when coaches help the consultant become integrated with the team, can serve to lessen the stigma associated with psychological services.[15]

Given the elite level of competition, it may be even more important to have access to a sport psychologist when considering surgery for an Olympic-level athlete. The previously mentioned intersection of injury and identity could be even more important, considering the longer and more intense involvement in the given sport.

Clinical Psychologic Concerns

Clinical concerns exist across developmental levels in sports. One of the most consistent psychologic factors associated with the risk of athletic injury is stress.[5] Psychologic support is a factor that repeatedly has been demonstrated in recent research to assist in injury rehabilitation and stress reduction.[16,17] In addition to stress, some of the most significant concerns for sport psychologists tend to be alcohol and other drugs, eating disorders, mood disorders, and anxiety disorders. These concerns can lead to higher incidences of injury and can become more pronounced in response to an injury. In addressing and/or treating clinically significant psychologic concerns, it is important to realize the benefits of having at least a consultative relationship with a psychological care provider well versed in the culture of sports.

Alcohol and Other Drugs

Although alcohol and other substance use sometimes is accepted by the general public, athletes tend to be held to different standards because of the potential for lost eligibility or participation in sports.[18] Most of the major sports leagues in the United States have begun to address substance use and abuse in their personal conduct and drug policies. When addressing student athlete use at nonprofessional levels, most of the governing organizations adopt the laws of the given country, especially for underage athletes.

Several factors—biologic, psychologic, and social—enter into an individual's potential for abuse of or dependence on a particular substance.[18] A genetic predisposition for use would represent a biologic factor influencing use. Thoughts, feelings, and behaviors surrounding use are examples of psychologic factors (for example, "One is good, two is better, and three's a party!"). People, places, and things are considered social factors influencing use.

The two most prominent substances used and abused in college are alcohol and marijuana. The current state of marijuana legalization is a complicating factor in addressing the larger issue of use or abuse, because some states have legalized marijuana for medicinal and/or recreational purposes. One of the major complicating factors is the concentration of tetrahydrocannabinol (THC) in marijuana and marijuana edibles when compared to similar products in past decades. For example, in some areas, a marijuana brownie may contain 16 servings of THC. This example illustrates the need for education about portion control when it comes to legal and illegal substances. A long history exists of athletes binging on substances, given their time in training and the biopsychosocial factors mentioned previously. Additionally, some teams have rules prohibiting use during a certain period before competition (eg, the "48- hour rule") rather than educating athletes about responsible decision making.

Asking specific questions about use, misuse, and abuse is beneficial in potentially curbing an abuse issue before it becomes a dependence issue. It also may alert a prescriber to the potential for the abuse of prescription medication following injury or surgical procedures.

Eating Disorders

The main diagnosed eating disorders are anorexia nervosa, bulimia nervosa, and binge eating disorder. Conditions also occur that do not qualify as eating disorders but are considered disordered eating; these include anorexia athletica, muscle dysmorphia/reverse anorexia, orthorexia nervosa, and obesity or being overweight.[19]

Like substance abuse, eating disorders and disordered eating have roots in genetic and sociocultural factors.

Genetics are thought to predispose to an eating disorder, but they do not tell the whole story. Sociocultural factors such as the media, the family, the peer group, and social comparison also heavily influence the development of an eating disorder. In sports, a host of additional contributing factors exist, including injury, depressive and mood disorders, weight and body-fat reduction, and performance increases. Others include the ideal of competitive thinness, wearing revealing sports attire, a contagion effect (in which an individual begins disordered eating behavior based on the perception or reality that others are doing it), subcultural expectations, and sports in which the body is seen as being judged (eg, gymnastics, diving, figure skating).[19]

Asking questions of the individual being studied seems to be key in determining the risk of or engagement in eating behaviors that could be detrimental or dangerous. A suitable time for such an evaluation is before participation in sports or before a surgical intervention. An injury that requires surgery, thus making sports participation unavailable, could trigger unhealthy or disordered eating.[19] The same scenario also could trigger a depressive or mood disorder.

Depressive and Mood Disorders

Depression is multifaceted and can affect athletic performance, academic or work performance, and social activity.[20] Major depressive disorder is in a category of mood-based disorders that also includes persistent depressive disorder (dysthymia) and premenstrual dysphoric disorder, along with other less well-known depressive disorders. Although nonathletes are affected by the symptoms of depression (eg, depressed mood, loss of interest or pleasure in activities), certain symptoms seem to be more problematic for athletes. Some indicators of depressed mood in athletes are missed rehabilitation appointments, vague or specific physical symptoms, slow or sluggish performance, and/or withdrawal from athletic participation and social opportunities.[20] Additionally, this constellation of symptoms can lead to a decline in health or performance and an increased risk of injury or suicide. At times, athletic status can be a protective factor against the development of mood disorders, insomuch as the demands on their time do not allow for extended periods of isolation. At the same time, those time demands can exacerbate an already depressed mood.[21]

When addressing depressed mood, medical and psychologic professionals should make sure to inquire about the presence of suicidal ideation. Prior to inquiry, the medical practice should ensure that it has a referral source and treatment plan in place for individuals experiencing suicidal thoughts.[22]

© 2016 American Academy of Orthopaedic Surgeons

Anxiety Disorders

Like depressive and mood disorders, anxiety disorders include a range of diagnoses, including generalized anxiety disorder, panic attacks/panic disorder, obsessive compulsive disorder, specific phobias, and posttraumatic stress disorder. Certain symptoms are common among all of these disorders, including feelings of apprehension, a sense of impending danger or doom, increased heart rate, rapid breathing, sweating, trembling, and fatigue and/or weakness. Although some of these symptoms also can result from a hard workout, in individuals with anxiety disorders, such symptoms have a negative effect on the ability to function.[23]

Athletic performance may place demands on athletes that challenge their natural reaction to an anxious presentation.[23] For example, a skier who experiences a hard fall that results in substantial injury may experience several anxiety-based symptoms when attempting to return to the mountain. If these symptoms interfere with performance, they may then meet the criteria for an anxiety disorder.

Psychiatric Issues

The presentation of these clinical concerns may call for consultation with a psychiatrist. Incorporating psychiatry into an interdisciplinary treatment plan can hasten recovery and return athletes to play with improved performance and a greater understanding of the complex nature of their presenting concerns. The early recognition of problematic symptoms is key because it shortens the time between onset and treatment, allowing a quicker resolution to the presenting concern.[24]

If clinical concerns go unaddressed, poor performance may result, thus increasing stress and potentially leading to injury. This illustrates the importance of sport psychology and the integration of service providers. One way to screen for clinical issues is to query patients about each area when they fill out the initial or preperformance physical examination paperwork. Having a qualified mental health practitioner review the answers could go a long way toward identifying and preventing additional psychiatric issues in the patient.

Summary

A brief overview of the field of sport psychology has been presented and the athlete groups that would benefit most from its principles described. It is important to consider several factors described in this chapter when treating athletes at any developmental level. Aligning the interests of those in the medical community with those of the sport psychology community can help maximize the benefit to athletes.

Key Study Points

- Several comorbid psychological factors should be considered when assessing a patient's injury or the potential for surgery.
- Consultation with a sport psychologist enhances the patient experience.

Annotated References

1. Brewer B, Van Raalte J: Introduction to sport and exercise psychology, in Brewer B, Van Raalte J, eds: *Exploring Sport & Exercise Psychology*, ed 2. Washington, DC, American Psychological Association, 2002, pp 3-9.

2. Murphy S: Preface, in Murphy S, ed: *The Sport Psych Handbook*. Champaign, IL, Human Kinetics, 2005, pp vii-viii.

3. Association for Applied Sport Psychology Abstract: *Coalition for the Advancement of Graduate Education and Training in the Practice of Sport Psychology: Voluntary Program Recognition for Sport Psychology Practice Graduate Programs*. https://www.appliedsportpsych.org/annual-conference/abstracts/20140376. Accessed June 26, 2015.

   The goal of the coalition referenced is to promote high-quality graduate training programs within the field of sport psychology.

4. Association for Applied Sport Psychology: *About Certified Consultants*. http://www.appliedsportpsych.org/certified-consultants. Accessed June 26, 2015.

   The information referenced is a site aimed at explaining the requirements and rigor involved in becoming certified through AASP.

5. American College of Sports Medicine; American Academy of Family Physicians; American Academy of Orthopaedic Surgeons; American Medical Society for Sports Medicine; American Orthopaedic Society for Sports Medicine; American Osteopathic Academy of Sports Medicine: Psychological issues related to injury in athletes and the team physician: A consensus statement. *Med Sci Sports Exerc* 2006;38(11):2030-2034.

6. National Collegiate Athletic Association: *Sport Science Institute*. http://www.ncaa.org/health-and-safety/sport-science-institute. Accessed June 26, 2015.

   NCAA SSI is a relatively new development within the NCAA. This group is devoted to activities that benefit the overall safety and wellness of the student-athletes within the NCAA.

7. Hainline B: Introduction, in Brown G, ed: *Mind, Body, and Sport: Understanding and Supporting Student-Athlete Mental Wellness*. Indianapolis, IN, National Collegiate Athletic Association, 2014.

This recent publication of the NCAA is aimed at educating professionals within NCAA member institutions.

8. Carr C, Davidson J: The psychologist perspective, in Brown G, ed: *Mind, Body, and Sport: Understanding and Supporting Student-Athlete Mental Wellness*. Indianapolis, IN, National Collegiate Athletic Association, 2014, pp 20-23.

This recent publication of the NCAA is aimed at educating professionals within NCAA member institutions. The roles of a psychologist within an athletic department and a brief history of those roles are discussed.

9. DiFiori JP, Benjamin HJ, Brenner JS, et al: Overuse injuries and burnout in youth sports: A position statement from the American Medical Society for Sports Medicine. *Br J Sports Med* 2014;48(4):287-288.

This consensus statement was offered as a systematic and evidence-based review of the literature on youth sport overuse injuries. The authors offer their summary to a wide range of possible readers including parents, athletes, coaches, and other sport scientists.

10. Smith R, Smoll F: Psychological interventions in youth sport, in Brewer B, Van Raalte J, eds: *Exploring Sport & Exercise Psychology*, ed 3. Washington, DC, American Psychological Association, 2014, pp 353-378.

The relevant literature regarding youth sport participation is reviewed. The authors also suggest interventions at various levels within the youth sport culture – interventions for parents, coaches, and athletes.

11. Petitpas A, Brewer B, Van Raalte J: Transitions of the student-athlete: Theoretical, empirical, and practical perspectives, in Etzel E, ed: *Counseling and Psychological Services for College Student-Athletes*. Morgantown, WV, Fitness Information Technology, 2009, pp 283-302.

The authors have taken the opportunity to outline the multifaceted idea of transition. They explore the various ways that student athletes can experience transition and they offer practical, research-based suggestions on how to be an effective helper to those in need.

12. Pinkney J, Tebbe C: The college student-athlete experience and academics, in Etzel E, ed: *Counseling and Psychological Services for College Student-Athletes*. Morgantown, WV, Fitness Information Technology, 2009, pp 257-282.

The impact of the 'student' part of student athlete is studied by exploring the research around academic success in student athletes. Study strategies and tips to use when working with student athletes in the area of academics are presented.

13. Savickas ML: Career maturity: The construct and its measurement. *Vocat Guid Q* 1984;32:222-231.

14. Coppell D: Post-concussion syndrome, in Brown G, ed: *Mind, Body, and Sport: Understanding and Supporting Student-Athlete Mental Wellness*. Indianapolis, IN, National Collegiate Athletic Association, 2014, pp 76-79.

This recent publication of the NCAA is aimed at educating professionals within NCAA member institutions. The nuances and difficulties associated with concussion and postconcussion including symptoms and strategies for improvement, are discussed.

15. McCann S: So you'd like a sport psychology consultant to work with your team? Three key lessons learned from Olympic teams. *Olympic Coach* 2014;25(3):26-30.

The author draws on his knowledge of working within the USOC and offers practical tools for individuals looking to hire/work with a sport psychologist. Factors that influence hiring the right person hoping to ensure success are explored.

16. Petrie T, Deiters J, Harmison R: Mental toughness, social support, and athletic identity: moderators of the life stress-injury relationship in collegiate football players. *Sport Exerc Perform Psychol* 2014;3(1):13-27.

The findings herein suggest that mental toughness moderates the relationship between positive life stress (PLS) and injury outcome. Student athletes with low levels of mental toughness and family social support miss more days to injury when experiencing high levels of PLS.

17. Ruddock-Hudson M, O'Halloran P, Murphy G: The psychological impact of long-term injury on Australian Football League. *J Appl Sport Psychol* 2014;26(4):377-394.

This study looks qualitatively and longitudinally at athletes' psychological responses to injury. The authors report the practical implications of their findings in a way that is useful for practitioners in order to benefit the athlete and their return to competition.

18. Brewer B, Petrie T: Psychopathology in sport and exercise, in Brewer B, Van Raalte J, eds: *Exploring Sport & Exercise Psychology*, ed 3. Washington, DC, American Psychological Association, 2002, pp 311-335.

19. Thompson R, Sherman R: Eating disorders: clinical and subclinical conditions, in Thompson R, Sherman R, eds: *Eating Disorders in Sport*. New York, NY, Routledge, 2010, pp 7-28.

This book provides a complete examination of eating disorders in collegiate student-athletes. Research of the disorders is reviewed and treatment suggestions and practical advice offered for individuals with disordered eating.

20. Maniar S, Sommers-Flanagan J: Clinical depression and college student-athletes, in Etzel E, ed: *Counseling and Psychological Services for College Student-Athletes*. Morgantown, WV, Fitness Information Technology, 2009, pp 323-348.

The presentation of depression in student athletes is discussed. Causes, symptoms, a litany of treatment options, and guidance for individuals who may be in a position to assist a student athlete struggling with depression are outlined.

21. Bader C: Mood disorders and depression, in Brown G, ed: *Mind, Body, and Sport: Understanding and Supporting Student-Athlete Mental Wellness.* Indianapolis, IN, National Collegiate Athletic Association, 2014, pp 38-43.

The goal of this recent publication of the NCAA is to educate professionals within NCAA member institutions. New developments, signs, symptoms, and treatment options for mood disorders, which can interfere with athletes' performance, are presented.

22. Lester D: Suicidal tendencies, in Brown G, ed: *Mind, Body, and Sport: Understanding and Supporting Student-Athlete Mental Wellness.* Indianapolis, IN, National Collegiate Athletic Association, 2014, pp 62-65.

The goal of this recent publication of the NCAA is to educate professionals within NCAA member institutions. Information, warning signs, and myths about suicide are discussed, along with possible risk factors seen in professional and student athletes.

23. Goldman S: Anxiety disorders, in Brown G, ed: *Mind, Body, and Sport: Understanding and Supporting Student-Athlete Mental Wellness.* Indianapolis, IN, National Collegiate Athletic Association, 2014, pp 34-37.

The goal of this recent publication of the NCAA is to educate professionals within NCAA member institutions. The signs/symptoms and treatment options for anxiety disorders are discussed, the disorders are described, and suggestions on how to help are offered.

24. Stull T: The psychiatrist perspective, in Brown G, ed: *Mind, Body, and Sport: Understanding and Supporting Student-Athlete Mental Wellness.* Indianapolis, IN, National Collegiate Athletic Association, 2014, pp 24-26.

The goal of this recent publication of the NCAA is aimed at educating professionals within NCAA member institutions. A psychiatric perspective is provided on some of the more commonly seen psychological disorders in student athletes.

Chapter 41

Cardiac Issues in Athletes

Kimberly G. Harmon, MD   Jonathan A. Drezner, MD

Abstract

Sudden cardiac death (SCD) is the leading cause of medical death in athletes with an estimated rate of 1 in 50,000, with higher risk in some subgroups including males, African Americans, and male basketball athletes. A thorough understanding of the epidemiology of sudden cardiac arrest and SCD in athletes is important as well as familiarity with screening methods and debate regarding detection of underlying cardiovascular disease. Recognition of the types of cardiac pathology in athletes as well as differentiation of disease from the benign changes often seen with intense training in athletes ("athlete's heart") are essential. Comprehension of issues related to return to play and restriction guidelines after diagnosis of cardiovascular disease is critical for the team physician making these decisions.

Keywords: sports cardiology; sudden cardiac death; sudden cardiac arrest; athlete

Introduction

Physical activity can have many positive physical and mental health benefits; however, in some individuals, vigorous activity can increase the risk of sudden cardiac arrest (SCA) and death. Sudden cardiac death (SCD) is the leading medical cause of death in athletes and typically is the result of undiagnosed structural or electrical

Dr. Harmon or an immediate family member has received nonincome support (such as equipment or services), commercially derived honoraria, or other non–research-related funding (such as paid travel) from SonoSite and serves as a board member, owner, officer, or committee member of the American Medical Society for Sports Medicine. Neither Dr. Drezner nor any immediate family member has received anything of value from or has stock or stock options held in a commercial company or institution related directly or indirectly to the subject of this chapter.

cardiovascular disease.[1] The ultimate objective of the preparticipation screening of athletes is the detection of "silent" cardiovascular abnormalities that can lead to SCD.[2] Distinguishing normal physiologic adaptations to exercise, collectively known as "athlete's heart," from pathology can be challenging. Electrocardiographic criteria have been developed that attempt to account for these changes and reduce the number of false-positive results while maintaining specificity.[3] A thorough understanding of the issues involved in the preparticipation examination and screening is required of sports medicine physicians. In addition, knowledge regarding the incidence of SCA in athletes, the groups at high risk for SCA, the causes of SCD in athletes, and return-to-play issues is important.

Preparticipation Examination

Twelve million competitive high school and collegiate athletes live in the United States, and most are required to have a preparticipation examination before participating in sports. The American Heart Association (AHA) recommends a 14-point screening history and physical examination[4] (Table 1), whereas the European Society of Cardiology,[5] the International Olympic Committee,[6] the Federation Internationale de Football Association, and most US professional associations recommend the addition of a 12-lead electrocardiogram (ECG), based on Italian data showing a 90% reduction in the rate of SCD with the inclusion of ECG.[7] Other studies have questioned this result, however.[8] The primary concerns cited regarding the addition of the 12-lead ECG include its cost and additional workup, high false-positive results, and the unavailability of adequate physician infrastructure for the widespread implementation of screening with ECG.

Although these concerns have been long held, a recent meta-analysis examining the history, physical examination, and electrocardiography found that the sensitivity of a 12-lead ECG was much higher than both history and physical examination, with similar specificity.[9] In addition, the false-positive rate of electrocardiography (6%) was less than that of the history (8%), or the physical examination (10%). Electrocardiography had the highest

Table 1

The 14-Element American Heart Association Recommendations for Preparticipation Cardiovascular Screening for Competitive Athletes

Medical History

Personal history

1. Chest pain/discomfort/tightness/pressure related to exertion
2. Unexplained syncope/near syncope
3. Excessive and unexplained dyspnea/fatigue or palpitations associated with exercise
4. Prior recognition of a heart murmur
5. Elevated systemic blood pressure
6. Prior restriction from participation in sports
7. Prior testing for the heart ordered by a physician

Family history

8. Premature death (sudden and unexpected or otherwise) before age 50 y attributable to heart disease in ≥ 1 relative
9. Disability from heart disease in close relative younger than 50 y
10. Hypertrophic or dilated cardiomyopathy, long QT syndrome, or other ion channelopathy, Marfan syndrome, or clinically significant arrhythmias; specific knowledge of genetic cardiac conditions in family members

Physical examination

11. Heart murmur
12. Femoral pulses to exclude aortic coarctation
13. Physical stigmata of Marfan syndrome
14. Brachial artery blood pressure (sitting position)

Data from Maron BJ, Friedman RA, Klingfield P, et al: Assessment of the 12-lead ecg as a screening test for detection of cardiovascular disease in healthy general populations of young people (12-25 years of age): A scientific statement from the American Heart Association and the American College of Cardiology. *Circulation* 2014;l30:1303-1334.

Table 2

Electrocardiographic Interpretation in Athletes: The "Seattle Criteria"

Normal ECG Findings in Athletes[a]

1) Sinus bradycardia (≥30 bpm)
2) Sinus arrhythmia
3) Ectopic atrial rhythm
4) Junctional escape rhythm
5) 1° AV block (PR interval > 200 ms)
6) Mobitz type I (Wenckebach) 2° AV block
7) Incomplete RBBB
8) Isolated QRS voltage criteria for LVH
Except: QRS voltage criteria for LVH occurring with any nonvoltage criteria for LVH such as left atrial enlargement, left axis deviation, ST segment depression, T-wave inversion, or pathologic Q waves
9) Early repolarization (ST elevation, J-point elevation, J waves, or terminal QRS slurring)
10) Convex ("domed") ST segment elevation combined with T-wave inversion in leads V1-V4 in African American or African athletes

ECG = electrocardiogram, mm = millimeter, AV = atrioventricular, ms = milliseconds, RBBB = right bundle branch block, LVH = left ventricular hypertrophy.

[a]These common training-related ECG alterations are physiologic adaptations to regular exercise, are considered normal variants in athletes, and do not require further evaluation in asymptomatic athletes.

Reproduced with permission from Drezner JA, Ackerman MJ, Anderson J, et al: Electrocardiographic interpretation in athletes: The 'Seattle criteria'. *Br J Sports Med* 2013;47[3]:122-124.

positive likelihood ratios and the lowest negative likelihood ratios for the detection of underlying cardiovascular abnormalities, suggesting that electrocardiography was the most effective strategy—and that the history and physical examination were relatively ineffective strategies—for the detection of underlying cardiovascular disease.[9] To minimize the false-positive rate, the interpretation of the ECG must take into account the physiologic adaptations of the heart to exercise. The Seattle Criteria were developed by an international group of experts in sports cardiology and have been shown to reduce the false-positive rate of ECGs in athletes to approximately 4%, while maintaining specificity[3] (Table 2).

No study has demonstrated the effectiveness of the history and physical examination alone in preventing SCD. One study examining 115 athletes with SCD revealed that only one athlete had been correctly identified at the preparticipation examination, demonstrating the relative inability of the history and physical examination to detect underlying cardiovascular disease.[10] Indeed, cost-effectiveness analysis comparing screening with ECG alone, history and physical examination alone, or electrocardiography combined with history and physical examination concluded that electrocardiography alone is the most cost-effective strategy, followed by electrocardiography combined with the history and physical examination.[11]

In many places, the infrastructure to perform and properly interpret ECGs in athletes does not exist.

Table 2 (continued)

Electrocardiographic Interpretation in Athletes: The "Seattle Criteria"

Abnormal Electrocardiogram Findings in Athletes[a]	Definition
T-wave inversion	> 1 mm in depth in two or more leads V2-V6, II and aVF, or I and aVL (excludes III, aVR, and V1)
ST segment depression	≥ 0.5 mm in depth in two or more leads
Pathologic Q waves	> 3 mm in depth or > 40 ms in duration in two or more leads (except III and aVR)
Complete left bundle branch block	QRS ≥ 120 ms, predominantly negative QRS complex in lead V1 (QS or rS), and upright monophasic R wave in leads I and V6
Intraventricular conduction delay	Any QRS duration ≥ 140 ms
Left axis deviation	-30° to -90°
Left atrial enlargement	Prolonged P wave duration of > 120 ms in leads I or II with negative portion of the P wave ≥ 1 mm in depth and ≥ 40 ms in duration in lead V1
Right ventricular hypertrophy pattern	$R-V_1 + S-V_5 > 10.5$ mm <u>AND</u> right axis deviation > 120°
Ventricular preexcitation	PR interval < 120 ms with a delta wave (slurred upstroke in the QRS complex) and wide QRS (> 120 ms)
Long QT interval[b]	QTc ≥ 470 ms (male) QTc ≥ 480 ms (female) QTc ≥ 500 ms (marked QT prolongation)
Short QT interval[b]	QTc ≤ 320 ms
Brugada-like ECG pattern	High take-off and downsloping ST segment elevation followed by a negative T wave in ≥ 2 leads in V1-V3
Mobitz type II 2° AV block	Intermittently nonconducted P waves not preceded by PR prolongation and not followed by PR shortening
3° AV block	Complete heart block
Profound sinus bradycardia	< 30 bpm or sinus pauses ≥ 3 s
Atrial tachyarrhythmias	Supraventricular tachycardia, atrial fibrillation, atrial flutter
Premature ventricular contractions	≥ 2 PVCs per 10 s tracing
Ventricular arrhythmias	Couplets, triplets, and nonsustained ventricular tachycardia

ECG = electrocardiogram, mm = millimeter, bpm = beats per minute, AV = atrioventricular, ms = milliseconds, PVC = premature ventricular contraction, RBBB = right bundle branch block, LVH = left ventricular hypertrophy.

[a] These ECG findings are unrelated to regular training or expected physiologic adaptation to exercise, may suggest the presence of pathologic cardiovascular disease, and require further diagnostic evaluation.

[b] The QT interval corrected for heart rate (QTc) ideally is measured with heart rates of 60 to 90 bpm. Consider repeating the ECG after mild aerobic activity for borderline or abnormal QTc values with a heart rate < 50 bpm.

Reproduced with permission from Drezner JA, Ackerman MJ, Anderson J, et al: Electrocardiographic interpretation in athletes: The 'Seattle criteria'. *Br J Sports Med* 2013;47[3]:122-124.

Several efforts are underway to educate providers in the interpretation of ECG in athletes, including free online training modules, available at http://learning.bmj.com/learning/course-intro/.html?courseId=10042239.

Currently, the standard of care in the United States is the AHA 14-point screening guideline, although a 12-lead ECG can be considered for patients in high-risk groups.

Table 3

Incidence of Sudden Cardiac Death

Author	Year	Country	Method	Population	Incidence	No. of years	Age Range (years)
Van Camp[53]	1996	US	Retrospective cohort	College/high school athletes	1:300,000	10	17-24
Maron[54]	1998	US	Retrospective cohort	High school athletes	1:217,000 overall	11	NA
Corrado[16]	2003	Italy	Prospective cohort study	Athletes/young people	1:47,600 athlete 1:142,900 young people	20	12-35
Eckart[20]	2004	US	Retrospective cohort	Military recruits	1:10,000	25	18-35
Drezner[55]	2005	US	Retrospective cohort	College athletes	1:67,000	3.3	NA
Gunnarson[56]	2006	Iceland	Retrospective cohort	Young people	1:68,000	30	12-35
Atkins[57]	2009	US and Canada	Prospective cohort study	Young people	1:49,000	3	12-19
Chugh[58]	2009	US	Prospective population-based	Young people	1:58,828	3	1-18
Drezner[59]	2009	US	Cross-sectional survey	High school athletes	1:23,000 SCA + SCD 1:46,000 SCD	NA	NA
Maron[14]	2009	US	Retrospective cohort	Athletes	1:163,934	27	8-39
Papadakis[23]	2009	UK	Retrospective cohort	Young people	1:55,000	4	1-35
Holst[18]	2010	Denmark	Retrospective cohort	Athletes/young people	1:82,645 athlete 1:26,595 general pop	7	12-35
Holst[18]	2010	Denmark	Retrospective cohort	Young people	1:35,000	7	1-35
Solberg[25]	2010	Norway	Retrospective cohort	Young people	1:111,111	20	15-34
Cooper[60]	2011	US	Retrospective cohort	Young people	1:32,258	NA	2-24
Eckart[21]	2011	US	Retrospective cohort	Military personnel	< 20 y - 1:29,673; 20-24 y - 1:40,983; 25-29 y - 1:30,120; 30-35 y - 1:25,000	10	18-34
Harmon[1]	2011	US	Retrospective cohort	College athletes	1:43,000	5	18-26
Margey[26]	2011	Ireland	Retrospective cohort	Young people	1:35,000	3	15-35
Marjion[61]	2011	France	Prospective	Competitive athletes	1:102,00	NA	10-35
Steinville[8]	2011	Israel	Retrospective cohort	Athletes	1st – 1:39,370 2nd– 1:37,593	24	12-44
Maron[62]	2012	US	Retrospective cohort	High school athletes	1:150,000	26	12-18
Meyer[63]	2012	US	Prospective population-based	Young people	14-24 y - 1:69.000 25-35 - 1:22,700	NA	NA
Boden[64]	2013	US	Retrospective cohort	College/ high school football	1:112,359 college 1: 312,500 high school	NA	NA
Pilmer[65]	2014	Canada	Retrospective cohort	Young people	1:128,000	5	1-19
Roberts[12]	2013	US	Retrospective cohort	High school athletes	1:416,666 last decade 1:917,000	NA	NA

© 2016 American Academy of Orthopaedic Surgeons

Table 3 (*continued*)

Incidence of Sudden Cardiac Death

Author	Year	Country	Method	Population	Incidence	Number of years	Age Range (years)
Winkel[66]	2014	Denmark	Retrospective cohort	Young people	1:90,909	7	1-18
Maron[27]	2014	US	Retrospective cohort	College athletes	1:83,000–confirmed 1:62,000–presumed	10	17-26
Toresdahl[67]	2014	US	Prospective observational	High school athletes	1:87,719 SCA+SCD	3	14-18

NA = not available, US = United States, SCA = sudden cardiac arrest, SCD = sudden cardiac death, UK = United Kingdom.

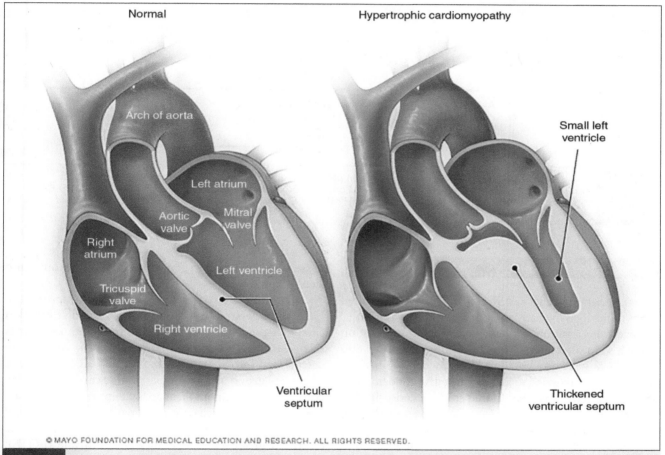

© MAYO FOUNDATION FOR MEDICAL EDUCATION AND RESEARCH. ALL RIGHTS RESERVED.

Figure 1 Drawings show a normal heart and a heart with hypertrophic cardiomyopathy. (Reproduced with permission from the Mayo Foundation for Medical Education and Research, Rochester, MN.)

Incidence of SCD in Athletes

The incidence of SCD in athletes is debated, with estimates ranging from 1:3,000 in some high-risk groups[1] to 1:917,000.[12] The cause of this discrepancy relates largely to the populations studied and the methods used for case identification.[13] Mandatory reporting of death is required in few athlete populations; thus, many studies rely on media reports, registries, and insurance claims for case identification or use unreliable population estimates. In studies using data from the mandatory reporting of death and a reliable ascertainment of the population studied, higher incidence numbers tend to be reported compared with studies relying on media reports or insurance claims for case identification[1,8,12,14-37] (Table 3). A reasonable estimate for the rate of SCD in athletes is 1:50,000, with African Americans, males, and basketball players at higher risk. The reasons for the increased risk of these subgroups are not clear.

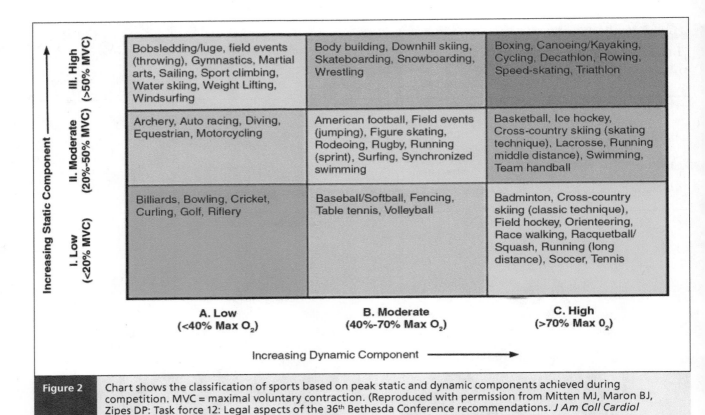

Figure 2 Chart shows the classification of sports based on peak static and dynamic components achieved during competition. MVC = maximal voluntary contraction. (Reproduced with permission from Mitten MJ, Maron BJ, Zipes DP: Task force 12: Legal aspects of the 36th Bethesda Conference recommendations. *J Am Coll Cardiol* 2005;45[8]:1373-1375.)

Causes of SCD in Athletes

The most common cause of SCD in athletes in the United States typically is hypertrophic cardiomyopathy (HCM);[14] however, this assumption has been called into question recently.[38] In a frequently quoted 2009 analysis of 690 SCDs, 36% were attributed to HCM, whereas only 3% of cases were attributed to autopsy-negative sudden unexplained death (AN-SUD).[14] In that study, 359 deaths that were considered cardiac, but for which no specific cause could be identified, were removed from this analysis with little explanation.[14] In contrast to this study, in studies of athletes from other countries[15,16,39,40] in age-matched noncompetitive athlete populations such as those in the US military[17,18] and in general populations of young people in the United States and abroad, AN-SUD represented a larger proportion of deaths and HCM a relatively smaller proportion of deaths.[19-21,41,42] A recent study of US college athletes also found AN-SUD to be most common and HCM to be more infrequent than previously predicted,[38] although a different study of the same population and examining the same autopsies, reported a higher incidence of HCM.[22] These inconsistencies highlight the need for standardized pathologic definitions, autopsies done by those with expertise in sudden cardiac death, and molecular autopsies.

Whatever the distribution of causes, it is important to have an understanding of cardiovascular diseases that can predispose athletes to SCD and the common findings related to these diseases. These conditions typically are categorized into structural and functional groups. The structural group includes hypertrophic cardiomyopathy, coronary artery anomalies, aortic rupture and/or Marfan syndrome, dilated cardiomyopathy, myocarditis and arrythmogenic right ventricular cardiomyopathy. The electrical group includes long QT syndrome (LQTS), Wolff-Parkinson-White (WPW) syndrome, Brugada syndrome, catecholaminergic polymorphic ventricular tachycardia (CPVT), and short QT syndrome. Commotio cordis is a well-described cause of SCD in athletes, occurring following impact to the chest wall during a narrow window of repolarization, leading to ventricular fibrillation.

Hypertrophic Cardiomyopathy

The prevalence of HCM is 1:500 in the general population but is found less frequently through screening in competitive athletes, approximately 1:1,000 to 1:5,000.[9,43-45]

The characteristic morphologic features of HCM include asymmetric left ventricular (LV) hypertrophy (usually involving the ventricular septum), LV wall thickness of 16 mm or more (normal is less than 12 mm; borderline is 13 to 15 mm), a ratio between the septum and free wall thickness of more than 1:3, and a nondilated left ventricle, with impaired diastolic function.[46] Histologic analysis shows a disorganized cellular architecture with cardiac myocyte disarray. An ECG will be abnormal in up to 95% of patients with HCM.[47,48] Echocardiography remains the standard to confirm the diagnosis of HCM by identifying pathologic LV wall thickness (greater than 16 mm) and a nondilated left ventricle with impaired diastolic function (Figure 1). If the diagnosis of HCM is uncertain (borderline LV wall thickness of 13 to 15 mm), MRI with gadolinium, genetic testing, or repeat echocardiography after 6 to 12 weeks of deconditioning can help distinguish HCM from athletic heart syndrome. SCD will be the presenting symptom in 80% of HCM cases, making identification through screening a priority, although some athletes may experience prodromal syncope or chest pain,[10] and some may have the characteristic murmur of HCM.[49] It is recommended that athletes with HCM compete in low-intensity sports only[50] (Figure 2).

Coronary Artery Anomalies

Athletes with coronary artery anomalies may present with symptoms of chest pain during exercise, syncope, or sudden death.[51] The most common coronary anomaly is an abnormal origin of the left coronary artery arising from the right sinus of Valsalva. Impingement of the anomalous artery with an intramural course (within the wall of the aorta) during exercise may lead to ischemia and a subsequent arrhythmia. Other features that can contribute to ischemia during exercise include an acute angled takeoff and hypoplastic ostium of the anomalous artery.

If an anomaly is suspected, transthoracic echocardiography can identify the coronary artery origins in approximately 80% to 97% of patients.[52] Advanced cardiac imaging such as CT angiography, cardiac MRI, or coronary angiography may be needed to detect coronary anomalies in some instances. Coronary artery anomalies rarely are identified through ECG. Coronary artery anomalies often can be corrected surgically, with return to play following surgical recovery.[50]

Aortic Rupture and Marfan Syndrome

Marfan syndrome is the most common inherited disorder of connective tissue that affects multiple organ systems, with a reported incidence of 2 to 3 in 10,000 individuals.[53] Marfan syndrome causes a progressive dilatation and weakness (cystic medial necrosis) of the proximal aorta that can lead to rupture and sudden death. Myxomatous degeneration of the mitral and aortic valves also can lead to valvular dysfunction. Marfan syndrome is caused by mutations in the fibrillin-1 gene, with 75% of cases inherited through autosomal dominant transmission with variable expression and 25% of cases from de novo mutations.[53] Athletes with Marfan syndrome who have nondilated aortas may participate in moderate dynamic and low static competitive sports; those with aortic root dilatation (greater than 4 cm) or prior aortic root repair should participate in low-intensity competitive sports only[50] (Figure 2).

Myocarditis

Myocarditis is another important cause of SCD. Acute inflammation of the myocardium can lead to an arrhythmogenic focus and sudden death. Coxsackie B virus is implicated in more than 50% of cases, but echovirus, adenovirus, influenza, and *Chlamydophilia pneumoniae* also have been associated with myocarditis. The acute phase of myocarditis presents with a flu-like illness, which can lead to dilated cardiomyopathy and signs and symptoms of congestive heart failure. Histologic analysis shows a lymphocytic infiltrate of the myocardium with necrosis or degeneration of adjacent myocytes. Myocardial scarring or fibrosis also can develop and can act as an arrhythmogenic focus.

Characteristic symptoms of myocarditis include a prodromal viral illness followed by progressive exercise intolerance and congestive symptoms of dyspnea, cough, and orthopnea. If myocarditis is suspected, the ECG may show diffuse low voltage, ST-T wave changes, heart block, or ventricular arrhythmias. Serologic testing may show leukocytosis, eosinophilia, an elevated erythrocyte sedimentation rate or C-reactive protein level, and increased myocardial enzymes. Echocardiography will confirm the diagnosis within the right clinical context, showing a dilated left ventricle, global hypokinesis or segmental wall abnormalities, and decreased LV ejection fraction. Cardiac MRI may demonstrate regional wall motion abnormalities and areas of late gadolinium enhancement. Athletes should be restricted from all competitive sports for 6 months following diagnosis. Return to sport may be considered after ECG, Holter monitoring, graded exercise test, enzymes, and echocardiogram have returned to normal.[50]

Arrhythmogenic Right Ventricular Cardiomyopathy

Arrhythmogenic right ventricular cardiomyopathy (ARVC) was reported as the leading cause of SCD (22%) in the Veneto region of northeastern Italy but is less commonly reported in the United States.[43] ARVC is characterized by a progressive fibrofatty replacement of the right ventricular myocardium, causing wall thinning and right ventricular dilatation. The estimated prevalence is 1 in 5,000 in the general population, and the disorder results from mutations in genes encoding for desmosomal (cell adhesion) proteins.[54]

ARVC can present with myocardial electrical instability, leading to ventricular arrhythmias, which precipitate cardiac arrest, especially during physical activity. An ECG may show right precordial T-wave inversion (beyond V1), an epsilon wave (a small terminal notch seen just beyond the QRS in V1 or V2), prolongation of QRS duration longer than 110 ms, or right bundle branch block pattern. Echocardiogram, cardiac MRI, or CT may demonstrate right ventricular dilatation and wall thinning, reduced right ventricular ejection fraction, focal right ventricular wall motion abnormalities, or right ventricular aneurysms. Fibrofatty infiltration of the right ventricle is seen best on cardiac MRI or by histologic analysis in selected cases. It is recommended that athletes with ARVC be excluded from competitive sports.[50]

Ion Channel Disorders

Ion channel disorders are primary electrical diseases of the heart predisposing to potentially lethal ventricular arrhythmias. They are characterized by mutations in ion channel proteins, leading to dysfunctional sodium, potassium, calcium, and other ion transport across cell membranes. They include disorders such as LQTS, short QT syndrome, Brugada syndrome, or familial CPVT.[55]

Long QT Syndrome

LQTS is the most common ion channelopathy and is characterized by prolongation of ventricular repolarization, as measured by the QT interval corrected for heart rate (QTc). In an asymptomatic athlete without a family history of SCD, current cutoff values for a prolonged QTc are 470 ms and 480 ms in males and females, respectively.[56] Ten gene abnormalities are recognized for LQTS involving potassium and sodium ion channels important in cardiac repolarization.[57] Most arrhythmias from LQTS are triggered by emotional or physical stress and present with syncope or near-syncope, seizures, or sudden death. Syncope is usually due to torsades de pointes, a specific form of polymorphic ventricular tachycardia. Up to 20% of patients who have LQTS and present with syncope, but in whom the diagnosis is not made and who are not treated, will experience SCD in the first year after syncope, and 50% will have SCD by 5 years.[58] Current guidelines recommend restriction from all but low-intensity competitive sports for those who have experienced an out-of-hospital cardiac arrest or syncope precipitated

by LQTS,[50] although some authors contend this guideline is too restrictive, arguing that patients should have more autonomy in decision making and that those who do return to play are unlikely to have adverse outcomes.[59]

Catecholaminergic Polyventricular Tachycardia

CPVT is a familial disorder characterized by stress-induced ventricular arrhythmias that result in SCD in children and young adults and most commonly involves a cardiac ryanodine receptor/calcium release channel mutation. CPVT can present with syncope, drowning or near drowning, seizure, or sudden death triggered by vigorous physical exertion or acute emotion. Syncope is the presenting symptom in most patients with CPVT, with the first syncopal event occurring at approximately 8 years of age.[60] A family history of syncope or sudden death is also present in 30% of cases.[60] It is recommended that athletes with CPVT be restricted from competitive sports.[50]

Wolff-Parkinson-White Syndrome

Ventricular preexcitation occurs when an accessory pathway of electrical activation bypasses the atrioventricular node. As a result, abnormal innervation of the ventricle (preexcitation) occurs, with shortening of the PR interval (less than 120 ms), slurring of the initial QRS (delta wave), and widening of the QRS (longer than 120 ms). This is evident on the ECG as the WPW syndrome pattern.[56,61]

The WPW syndrome pattern occurs in approximately 1 in 1000 athletes.[62] The presence of an accessory pathway can predispose an athlete to sudden death if the athlete also experiences atrial fibrillation. Rapid conduction of atrial fibrillation across the accessory pathway can result in ventricular fibrillation. The risk of sudden death associated with asymptomatic WPW syndrome in most population-based studies is 0.1% per year in adults.[63] Evidence suggests a higher risk of sudden death in asymptomatic children and younger adults with WPW syndrome.[64,65] Athletes with WPW should undergo further testing to stratify high-risk and low-risk pathways. High-risk pathways can be ablated with return to play after several days.[50]

Commotio Cordis

Commotio cordis is an important cause of SCD in athletes. It occurs in a structurally normal heart after the chest wall is struck with a blunt object. If the blow is sustained during a specific, narrow window of repolarization, it can lead to ventricular fibrillation.[66] In sports, commotio cordis is described most often in baseball, lacrosse, and combat sports such as karate. Biologic characteristics such as male sex, pliability of the chest wall, and genetic susceptibility play a role in commotio cordis.[66] Attempts to prevent commotio cordis include using softer "safety balls" in youth baseball. Chest protectors seem to have limited efficacy in the prevention of SCA. Early recognition and defibrillation are the keys to survival.

Athletic Heart Syndrome

Sometimes athletes are identified with larger-than-normal hearts. This finding can be secondary to pathology such as HCM or to "athlete's heart", which occurs with intensive athletic training, leading to physiologic adaptive changes including enlargement of the heart. Differentiating between the two conditions sometimes can be difficult, with serious implications and potential disqualification for those with a diagnosis of HCM. LV wall thickness is less than 13 mm in most hearts; however, between 13 and 15 mm, a physiologic "gray zone" exists, which may represent HCM or physiologic remodeling. In the past, a period of deconditioning often was recommended to assess for the regression of wall thickness. Research has demonstrated important differences between "athlete's heart" and HCM. The most reliable differentiator is the LV cavity size, which enlarges in athletes secondary to hemodynamic and neurohormonal stimuli but does not do so in HCM.[67] (Figure 1) In addition, T-wave inversion in the lateral leads is highly suggestive of HCM.

Summary

SCD is the leading cause of death in exercising athletes, occurring about 1 in every 50,000 athlete-years, although males, African Americans, and basketball players are at higher risk. Preparticipation examinations are required of most competitive athletes, and the primary objective is to screen for potentially lethal cardiovascular disorders. The AHA currently recommends a 14-point history and physical examination, although other organizations support the addition of a 12-lead ECG, particularly in high-risk groups. HCM traditionally has been thought to be the most common cause of SCD in athletes, although more recent studies have suggested AN-SUD may be a more frequent finding. Other conditions such as coronary artery abnormalities, ARVC, Marfan syndrome, and ion channel disorders are also important causes of SCD. A thorough knowledge of cardiovascular screening and pathology is important for sports physicians involved in preparticipation examinations and the care of athletes.

Key Study Points

- SCD is the leading medical cause of death in athletes with a rate of approximately 1 in 50,000 and higher risk in males, African Americans, and male basketball athletes.

- HCM is frequently cited as the most common cause of SCD; however, AN-SUD may be more common in athletes than previously thought.

- The primary objective of the PPE is the identification of previously unknown cardiovascular disorders. A standardized history and physical examination is the minimum recommended evaluation. The addition of a screening ECG significantly improves the ability to detect cardiac disorders at risk of sudden death and could be considered if proper interpretation and adequate cardiology resources are available.

- Management of many cardiovascular conditions had evolved from "identify and restrict" to identify, inform and a model of shared decision making.

Annotated References

1. Harmon KG, Asif IM, Klossner D, Drezner JA: Incidence of sudden cardiac death in National Collegiate Athletic Association athletes. *Circulation* 2011;123(15):1594-1600.

   The incidence of SCD is higher than previously reported, at 1 in 43,000 athlete years for all National Collegiate Athletic Association athletes. There are some subgroups of athletes that appear to be at higher risk including males, African Americans and male basketball athletes. Level of evidence: III.

2. Maron BJ, Douglas PS, Graham TP, Nishimura RA, Thompson PD: Task Force 1: Preparticipation screening and diagnosis of cardiovascular disease in athletes. *J Am Coll Cardiol* 2005;45(8):1322-1326.

3. Drezner JA, Ackerman MJ, Anderson J, et al: Electrocardiographic interpretation in athletes: The 'Seattle criteria'. *Br J Sports Med* 2013;47(3):122-124.

   The use of standardized criteria for interpretation of ECGs that account for the physiologic changes of training can improve sensitivity and specificity and decrease false-positive rate. Level of evidence: V.

4. Maron BJ, Friedman RA, Kligfield P, et al; American Heart Association Council on Clinical Cardiology, Advocacy Coordinating Committee, Council on Cardiovascular Disease in the Young, Council on Cardiovascular Surgery and Anesthesia, Council on Epidemiology and Prevention, Council on Functional Genomics and Translational Biology, Council on Quality of Care and Outcomes Research,

and American College of Cardiology: Assessment of the 12-lead ECG as a screening test for detection of cardiovascular disease in healthy general populations of young people (12-25 Years of Age): A scientific statement from the American Heart Association and the American College of Cardiology. *Circulation* 2014;130(15):1303-1334.

The primary purpose of cardiovascular screening is the detection of underlying disease, and this screening is recommended for athletes. A 14-point history and physical examination is recommended and where proper resources are available, ECG can be considered. Level of evidence: V.

5. Corrado D, Pelliccia A, Bjørnstad HH, et al; Study Group of Sport Cardiology of the Working Group of Cardiac Rehabilitation and Exercise Physiology and the Working Group of Myocardial and Pericardial Diseases of the European Society of Cardiology; Consensus Statement of the Study Group of Sport Cardiology of the Working Group of Cardiac Rehabilitation and Exercise Physiology and the Working Group of Myocardial and Pericardial Diseases of the European Society of Cardiology: Cardiovascular pre-participation screening of young competitive athletes for prevention of sudden death: Proposal for a common European protocol. *Eur Heart J* 2005;26(5):516-524.

6. Bille K, Figueiras D, Schamasch P, et al: Sudden cardiac death in athletes: The Lausanne Recommendations. *Eur J Cardiovasc Prev Rehabil* 2006;13(6):859-875.

7. Corrado D, Basso C, Pavei A, Michieli P, Schiavon M, Thiene G: Trends in sudden cardiovascular death in young competitive athletes after implementation of a preparticipation screening program. *JAMA* 2006;296(13):1593-1601.

8. Steinvil A, Chundadze T, Zeltser D, et al: Mandatory electrocardiographic screening of athletes to reduce their risk for sudden death proven fact or wishful thinking? *J Am Coll Cardiol* 2011;57(11):1291-1296.

In a retrospective review using two Israeli newspapers to identify athletes with sudden cardiac arrest, there was no difference noted between the time before and after the use of electrocardiography for screening. Both case identification and defining the athletic cohort by estimation temper conclusions that can be drawn from this study. Level of evidence: III.

9. Harmon KG, Zigman M, Drezner JA: The effectiveness of screening history, physical exam, and ECG to detect potentially lethal cardiac disorders in athletes: A systematic review/meta-analysis. *J Electrocardiol* 2015;48(3):329-338.

ECG is significantly more sensitive with a similar specificity to history and physical examination, with the lowest false-positive rate for the detection of cardiovascular disease in athletes. Level of evidence: III.

10. Maron BJ, Shirani J, Poliac LC, Mathenge R, Roberts WC, Mueller FO: Sudden death in young competitive athletes. Clinical, demographic, and pathological profiles. *JAMA* 1996;276(3):199-204.

11. Schoenbaum M, Denchev P, Vitiello B, Kaltman JR: Economic evaluation of strategies to reduce sudden cardiac death in young athletes. *Pediatrics* 2012;130(2):e380-e389.

The addition of ECG screening to current PPE is not cost effective. An ECG-only screening strategy is more cost effective. Level of evidence: III.

12. Roberts WO, Stovitz SD: Incidence of sudden cardiac death in Minnesota high school athletes 1993-2012 screened with a standardized pre-participation evaluation. *J Am Coll Cardiol* 2013;62(14):1298-1301.

In this retrospective review of insurance claims for SCD in Minnesota high school athletes who died while playing a school sport, it was reported found that the rate of SCD was approximately 1 in 400,000. Level of evidence: III.

13. Harmon KG, Drezner JA, Wilson MG, Sharma S: Incidence of sudden cardiac death in athletes: A state-of-the-art review. *Heart* 2014;100(16):1227-1234.

The incidence of SCD in high school athletes is between 1:50,000 and 1 in 80,000 athlete years. The incidence is college athletes is approximately 1:50,000, with high-risk groups comprising males, African Americans, and male basketball athletes. Level of evidence: V.

14. Maron BJ, Doerer JJ, Haas TS, Tierney DM, Mueller FO: Sudden deaths in young competitive athletes: Analysis of 1866 deaths in the United States, 1980-2006. *Circulation* 2009;119(8):1085-1092.

The most common cause of death in a registry was HCM (36%), followed by coronary artery anomalies (17%). Level of evidence: III.

15. Corrado D, Basso C, Rizzoli G, Schiavon M, Thiene G: Does sports activity enhance the risk of sudden death in adolescents and young adults? *J Am Coll Cardiol* 2003;42(11):1959-1963.

16. Holst AG, Winkel BG, Theilade J, et al: Incidence and etiology of sports-related sudden cardiac death in Denmark—implications for preparticipation screening. *Heart Rhythm* 2010;7(10):1365-1371.

The incidence of SCD in Danish athletes during exercise was low. The most common autopsy findings at death were arrythmogenic right ventricular cardiomyopathy, sudden unexplained death, and coronary artery disease. Level of evidence: III.

17. Eckart RE, Scoville SL, Campbell CL, et al: Sudden death in young adults: A 25-year review of autopsies in military recruits. *Ann Intern Med* 2004;141(11):829-834.

18. Eckart RE, Shry EA, Burke AP, et al; Department of Defense Cardiovascular Death Registry Group: Sudden death in young adults: An autopsy-based series of a population undergoing active surveillance. *J Am Coll Cardiol* 2011;58(12):1254-1261.

© 2016 American Academy of Orthopaedic Surgeons

The incidence of sudden unexplained death in military personnel younger than 35 years was 0.7 per 100,000. The most common cause of death in those younger than 35 years was sudden unexplained death. Level of evidence: III.

19. Papadakis M, Sharma S, Cox S, Sheppard MN, Panoulas VF, Behr ER: The magnitude of sudden cardiac death in the young: A death certificate-based review in England and Wales. *Europace* 2009;11(10):1353-1358.

    The number of cardiac and sudden deaths in the young is sufficiently high to command attention. Awareness of such deaths among primary care physicians, pathologists, and coroners should be raised. Level of evidence: III.

20. Solberg EE, Gjertsen F, Haugstad E, Kolsrud L: Sudden death in sports among young adults in Norway. *Eur J Cardiovasc Prev Rehabil* 2010;17(3):337-341.

    Myocardial infarction was the leading cause of death in Norwegian athletes age 15 to 34 years. Level of evidence: III.

21. Margey R, Roy A, Tobin S, et al: Sudden cardiac death in 14- to 35-year olds in Ireland from 2005 to 2007: A retrospective registry. *Europace* 2011;13(10):1411-1418.

    The incidence of SCD in individuals age 14 to 35 years in Ireland was 4.96 per 100,000 for males and 2.56 per 100,000 for females. Sudden arrhythmic death syndrome was the most common cause of SCD in these individuals. Level of evidence: III.

22. Maron BJ, Haas TS, Murphy CJ, Ahluwalia A, Rutten-Ramos S: Incidence and causes of sudden death in U.S. college athletes. *J Am Coll Cardiol* 2014;63(16):1636-1643.

    The incidence of SCD in college athletes, according to a review of registry and National Collegiate Athletic Association data, was 1 in 67,000. Level of evidence: III.

23. Van Camp SP, Bloor CM, Mueller FO, Cantu RC, Olson HG: Nontraumatic sports death in high school and college athletes. *Med Sci Sports Exerc* 1995;27(5):641-647.

24. Maron BJ, Gohman TE, Aeppli D: Prevalence of sudden cardiac death during competitive sports activities in Minnesota high school athletes. *J Am Coll Cardiol* 1998;32(7):1881-1884.

25. Drezner JA, Rogers KJ, Zimmer RR, Sennett BJ: Use of automated external defibrillators at NCAA Division I universities. *Med Sci Sports Exerc* 2005;37(9):1487-1492.

26. Gunnarsson G: Sudden death in the young: a 30-year nationwide study in Iceland. *Eur Soc Cardiol* 2006.

27. Atkins DL, Everson-Stewart S, Sears GK, et al; Resuscitation Outcomes Consortium Investigators: Epidemiology and outcomes from out-of-hospital cardiac arrest in children: The Resuscitation Outcomes Consortium Epistry-Cardiac Arrest. *Circulation* 2009;119(11):1484-1491.

    Age-stratified incidence and outcomes of out-of-hospital cardiac arrest in children were studied; the incidence of this condition in infants is close to that in adults but is lower in children and adolescents. Survival to discharge was reportedly more likely in children and adolescents.

28. Chugh SS, Reinier K, Balaji S, et al: Population-based analysis of sudden death in children: The Oregon Sudden Unexpected Death Study. *Heart Rhythm* 2009;6(11):1618-1622.

    Sudden cardiac arrest in children was studies over a 3-year, community-wide study. Ninety percent of deaths occurred in children younger than 1 year; most of these patients received a diagnosis of sudden infant death syndrome. Education on prevention of sudden infant death syndrome and early diagnosis of occult heart disease will play a role in prevention of sudden death in children.

29. Drezner JA, Rao AL, Heistand J, Bloomingdale MK, Harmon KG: Effectiveness of emergency response planning for sudden cardiac arrest in United States high schools with automated external defibrillators. *Circulation* 2009;120(6):518-525.

    The availability and use of automated external defibrillators is associated with high survival rates in student athletes and others who experience SCA on school grounds.

30. Cooper WO, Habel LA, Sox CM, et al: ADHD drugs and serious cardiovascular events in children and young adults. *N Engl J Med* 2011;365(20):1896-1904.

    The authors found no evidence that drugs used to treat attention deficit hyperactivity disorder contributed to an increase in serious cardiovascular events.

31. Marijon E, Tafflet M, Celermajer DS, et al: Sports-related sudden death in the general population. *Circulation* 2011;124(6):672-681.

    The authors reported that the general population experiences sports-related sudden death more often than initially suspected; prompt intervention is associated with improved survival rates.

32. Maron BJ, Haas TS, Ahluwalia A, Rutten-Ramos SC: Incidence of cardiovascular sudden deaths in Minnesota high school athletes. *Heart Rhythm* 2013;10(3):374-377.

    The risk of cardiovascular sudden death in the high school athlete population studied was small; according to autopsy data, approximately 30% of these deaths were caused by disease that could be detected during preparticipation screening.

33. Meyer L, Stubbs B, Fahrenbruch C, et al: Incidence, causes, and survival trends from cardiovascular-related sudden cardiac arrest in children and young adults 0 to 35 years of age: A 30-year review. *Circulation* 2012;126(11):1363-1372.

    Out-of-hospital cardiac arrest occurs more often in children and young adults than previously reported; future prevention programs should be guided by a thorough understanding of the causes of this occurrence.

34. Boden BP, Breit I, Beachler JA, Williams A, Mueller FO: Fatalities in high school and college football players. *Am J Sports Med* 2013;41(5):1108-1116.

   The most common causes of fatalities in high school and college football players are cardiac failure, brain injury, and heat illness, with the incidence of fatalities being higher at the college level.

35. Pilmer CM, Kirsh JA, Hildebrandt D, Krahn AD, Gow RM: Sudden cardiac death in children and adolescents between 1 and 19 years of age. *Heart Rhythm* 2014;11(2):239-245.

   Underlying causes of SCD in children and adolescents are presumed primary arrhythmia syndrome and structural heart disease. Age-specific diagnostic and prevention strategies are needed.

36. Winkel BG, Risgaard B, Sadjadieh G, Bundgaard H, Haunsø S, Tfelt-Hansen J: Sudden cardiac death in children (1-18 years): Symptoms and causes of death in a nationwide setting. *Eur Heart J* 2014;35(13):868-875.

   In a nationwide study of deaths in children over a 7-year period, more than half of those who experienced SCD had antecedent and/or prodromal symptoms. Subsequent familial screening should include diagnosis and treatment of potential inherited cardiac diseases.

37. Toresdahl BG, Rao AL, Harmon KG, Drezner JA: Incidence of sudden cardiac arrest in high school student athletes on school campus. *Heart Rhythm* 2014;11(7):1190-1194.

   Because the incidence of sudden cardiac arrest is higher than previously estimated, additional advanced cardiac screening and enhanced emergency planning in schools is required.

38. Harmon KG, Drezner JA, Maleszewski JJ, et al: Pathogeneses of sudden cardiac death in national collegiate athletic association athletes. *Circ Arrhythm Electrophysiol* 2014;7(2):198-204.

   The most common cause of death in National Collegiate Athletic Association athletes was AN-SUD (31%). HCM represented only 8% of deaths. Level of evidence: III.

39. de Noronha SV, Sharma S, Papadakis M, Desai S, Whyte G, Sheppard MN: Aetiology of sudden cardiac death in athletes in the United Kingdom: A pathological study. *Heart* 2009;95(17):1409-1414.

   Of SCDs evaluated at the National Heart and Lung Institute and Royal Brompton Hospital, most male, 81% of deaths were exertional, and the most common pathologic finding at death was a structurally normal heart. Level of evidence: III.

40. Suárez-Mier MP, Aguilera B, Mosquera RM, Sánchez-de-León MS: Pathology of sudden death during recreational sports in Spain. *Forensic Sci Int* 2013;226(1-3):188-196.

   In a study of sudden death during sports participation in the Irish population between the ages of 9 and 69 years, the most common cause of death was coronary artery disease. Death most often occurred during cycling followed by soccer. Level of evidence: III.

41. Corrado D, Basso C, Thiene G: Sudden cardiac death in young people with apparently normal heart. *Cardiovasc Res* 2001;50(2):399-408.

42. Puranik R, Chow CK, Duflou JA, Kilborn MJ, McGuire MA: Sudden death in the young. *Heart Rhythm* 2005;2(12):1277-1282.

43. Corrado D, Basso C, Schiavon M, Thiene G: Screening for hypertrophic cardiomyopathy in young athletes. *N Engl J Med* 1998;339(6):364-369.

44. Stefani L, Galanti G, Toncelli L, et al: Bicuspid aortic valve in competitive athletes. *Br J Sports Med* 2008;42(1):31-35, discussion 35.

45. Basavarajaiah S, Wilson M, Whyte G, Shah A, McKenna W, Sharma S: Prevalence of hypertrophic cardiomyopathy in highly trained athletes: Relevance to pre-participation screening. *J Am Coll Cardiol* 2008;51(10):1033-1039.

46. Maron BJ, Pelliccia A, Spirito P: Cardiac disease in young trained athletes. Insights into methods for distinguishing athlete's heart from structural heart disease, with particular emphasis on hypertrophic cardiomyopathy. *Circulation* 1995;91(5):1596-1601.

47. Maron BJ, Roberts WC, Epstein SE: Sudden death in hypertrophic cardiomyopathy: A profile of 78 patients. *Circulation* 1982;65(7):1388-1394.

48. Melacini P, Cianfrocca C, Calore C, Bovolato F, Paolo F, Quattrini F, Pelliccia F, Sharma S, McKenna W, Maron B, Pelliccia A, Corrado D: Abstract 3390: Marginal overlap between electrocardiographic abnormalities in patients with hypertrophic cardiomyopathy and trained athletes: Implications for preparticipation screening. *Circulation* 2007;116:II-765.

49. Maron BJ, Friedman RA, Kligfield P, et al; American Heart Association Council on Clinical Cardiology; Advocacy Coordinating Committee; Council on Cardiovascular Disease in the Young; Council on Cardiovascular Surgery and Anesthesia; Council on Epidemiology and Prevention; Council on Functional Genomics and Translational Biology; Council on Quality of Care and Outcomes Research, and American College of Cardiology: Assessment of the 12-lead electrocardiogram as a screening test for detection of cardiovascular disease in healthy general populations of young people (12-25 years of age): A scientific statement from the American Heart Association and the American College of Cardiology. *J Am Coll Cardiol* 2014;64(14):1479-1514.

   The primary purpose of cardiovascular screening is the detection of underlying disease and is recommended for athletes. A 14-point history and physical examination is recommended and where proper resources are available, ECG can be considered. Level of evidence: V

50. Maron BJ, Zipes DP: Introduction: Eligibility recommendations for competitive athletes with cardiovascular abnormalities-general considerations. *J Am Coll Cardiol* 2005;45(8):1318-1321.

51. Basso C, Maron BJ, Corrado D, Thiene G: Clinical profile of congenital coronary artery anomalies with origin from the wrong aortic sinus leading to sudden death in young competitive athletes. *J Am Coll Cardiol* 2000;35(6):1493-1501.

52. Pelliccia A, Spataro A, Maron BJ: Prospective echocardiographic screening for coronary artery anomalies in 1,360 elite competitive athletes. *Am J Cardiol* 1993;72(12):978-979.

53. Ammash NM, Sundt TM, Connolly HM: Marfan syndrome-diagnosis and management. *Curr Probl Cardiol* 2008;33(1):7-39.

54. Basso C, Corrado D, Thiene G: Arrhythmogenic right ventricular cardiomyopathy in athletes: Diagnosis, management, and recommendations for sport activity. *Cardiol Clin* 2007;25(3):415-422, vi.

55. Maron BJ: Sudden death in young athletes. *N Engl J Med* 2003;349(11):1064-1075.

56. Drezner JA, Ackerman MJ, Cannon BC, et al: Abnormal electrocardiographic findings in athletes: Recognising changes suggestive of primary electrical disease. *Br J Sports Med* 2013;47(3):153-167.

    This article is a review of ECG findings in athletes that are suggestive of disease. Level of evidence: V.

57. Lehnart SE, Ackerman MJ, Benson DW Jr, et al: Inherited arrhythmias: A National Heart, Lung, and Blood Institute and Office of Rare Diseases workshop consensus report about the diagnosis, phenotyping, molecular mechanisms, and therapeutic approaches for primary cardiomyopathies of gene mutations affecting ion channel function. *Circulation* 2007;116(20):2325-2345.

58. Hobbs JB, Peterson DR, Moss AJ, et al: Risk of aborted cardiac arrest or sudden cardiac death during adolescence in the long-QT syndrome. *JAMA* 2006;296(10):1249-1254.

59. Johnson JN, Ackerman MJ: Return to play? Athletes with congenital long QT syndrome. *Br J Sports Med* 2013;47(1):28-33.

    Athletes with LQTS and their families should discuss risks and benefits when faced with participation decisions. In 650 athlete years of follow-up of athletes with LQTS who chose to participate, there were no deaths. Level of evidence: III.

60. Leenhardt A, Lucet V, Denjoy I, Grau F, Ngoc DD, Coumel P: Catecholaminergic polymorphic ventricular tachycardia in children. A 7-year follow-up of 21 patients. *Circulation* 1995;91(5):1512-1519.

61. Surawicz B, Childers R, Deal BJ, et al; American Heart Association Electrocardiography and Arrhythmias Committee, Council on Clinical Cardiology; American College of Cardiology Foundation; Heart Rhythm Society: AHA/ACCF/HRS recommendations for the standardization and interpretation of the electrocardiogram: Part III: Intraventricular conduction disturbances: A scientific statement from the American Heart Association Electrocardiography and Arrhythmias Committee, Council on Clinical Cardiology; the American College of Cardiology Foundation; and the Heart Rhythm Society: Endorsed by the International Society for Computerized Electrocardiology. *Circulation* 2009;119(10):e235-e240.

62. Pelliccia A, Culasso F, Di Paolo FM, et al: Prevalence of abnormal electrocardiograms in a large, unselected population undergoing pre-participation cardiovascular screening. *Eur Heart J* 2007;28(16):2006-2010.

63. Munger TM, Packer DL, Hammill SC, et al: A population study of the natural history of Wolff-Parkinson-White syndrome in Olmsted County, Minnesota, 1953-1989. *Circulation* 1993;87(3):866-873.

64. Klein GJ, Bashore TM, Sellers TD, Pritchett EL, Smith WM, Gallagher JJ: Ventricular fibrillation in the Wolff-Parkinson-White syndrome. *N Engl J Med* 1979;301(20):1080-1085.

65. Deal BJ, Beerman L, Silka M, Walsh EP, Klitzner T, Kugler J: Cardiac arrest in young patients with Wolff-Parkinson-White syndrome. *Pacing Clin Electrophysiol* 1995;18:815.

66. Link MS: Pathophysiology, prevention, and treatment of commotio cordis. *Curr Cardiol Rep* 2014;16(6):495.

    Commotio cordis is increasing as a cause of SCD on the playing field. Prevention of commotio cordis is possible. Improved recognition and resuscitation have led to improved outcomes. Level of evidence: V.

67. Caselli S, Maron MS, Urbano-Moral JA, Pandian NG, Maron BJ, Pelliccia A: Differentiating left ventricular hypertrophy in athletes from that in patients with hypertrophic cardiomyopathy. *Am J Cardiol* 2014;114(9):1383-1389.

    Identification of HCM in young athletes is challenging when LV wall thickness is between 13 and 15 mm. In athletes with LV hypertrophy in the "gray zone" with HCM, LV cavity size appears to be the most reliable criterion to help in diagnosis, with a cutoff value of <54 mm for differentiation from athlete's heart. Other criteria, including LV diastolic dysfunction, absence of T-wave inversion on ECG, and negative family history, further aid in the differential diagnosis. Level of evidence: V.

Chapter 42

Female Athlete Triad

Marissa M. Smith, MD   Marci A. Goolsby, MD

Abstract

The female athlete triad (the Triad) is a syndrome describing the relationship between three components: energy availability, menstrual function, and bone health. The Triad can exist along a spectrum from healthy states to the severe diagnoses of eating disorder, amenorrhea, and osteoporosis. Short-term and long-term consequences of the Triad include stress fractures, infertility, and osteoporosis. These consequences can be prevented with early recognition and treatment by a multidisciplinary team. Screening for the components of the Triad is critical, and a series of questions about menstrual function, weight changes, eating behaviors, and bone injuries can help identify patients at risk. The Triad can be seen in any athlete but is more common in athletes participating in endurance, esthetic, and weight-class sports. The best treatment is prevention, but nutrition counseling and exercise modifications are the mainstays of treatment. A cumulative risk score can help guide clinicians on return to play and clearance of athletes with the Triad.

Keywords: female athlete triad; amenorrhea; oligomenorrhea; disordered eating; eating disorder; female athlete; low bone density; osteoporosis; low energy availability

Introduction

Since the enactment of Title IX of the Education Amendments of 1972, the participation of girls and women in competitive athletic endeavors has increased dramatically.

Dr. Goolsby or an immediate family member serves as a board member, owner, officer, or committee member of the American Medical Society for Sports Medicine. Neither Dr. Smith nor any immediate family member has received anything of value from or has stock or stock options held in a commercial company or institution related directly or indirectly to the subject of this chapter.

The number of high school girls involved in sports increased from less than 300,000 in 1972 to more than 3 million in 2013.[1,2]

It is well established that involvement in sports and exercise has benefits for physical and mental health, and all girls and women should be encouraged to participate in active endeavors. Participation also carries potential risk to those involved, however. One of the unique risks to the active female is the medical condition first termed the female athlete triad (the Triad) in 1992.

The Triad was originally described as the interrelationship of disordered eating, amenorrhea, and osteoporosis. Since that time, this definition has been broadened to refer to a medical condition that can involve a spectrum of disease severity (Figure 1) that includes low energy availability (EA) with or without disordered eating, a variety of menstrual irregularities, and diminished bone mineral density (BMD). It has further been established that, not only do the individual components of the Triad present along a spectrum, but only one or two of the components of the Triad may be present at any given time, an occurrence that still can have potential adverse health consequences. Understanding the range of signs and symptoms of the Triad allows early recognition and intervention for this significant medical condition.

Determining the number of women affected by the Triad is difficult because of the variability of the disease. Those with the most severe form of the Triad (eating disorder, amenorrhea, and osteoporosis) have been estimated to be between zero and 15.9%. When evaluating those with less severe components or those with only one or two components, however, the prevalence increases. Estimates are zero to 60% for menstrual disturbance, zero to 89.2% for eating disorder/disordered eating, and zero to 39.8% for low BMD.[3]

The Triad can affect women of all ages, often starting in adolescence, before or after menarche. More commonly, the Triad affects athletes involved in sports and activities that value leanness, endurance, weight class, and esthetics, such as running, gymnastics, and dancing, but it may affect any active female, making this an important topic for all health professionals to understand.

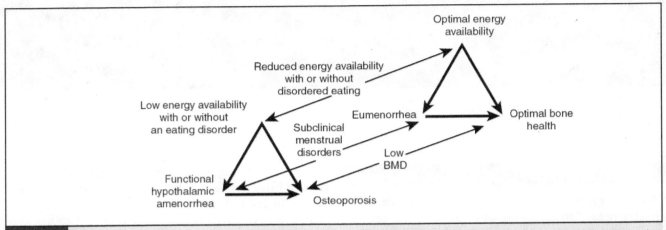

Figure 1 Diagram depicts the female athlete triad, defined as the spectrums of energy availability, menstrual function, and bone mineral density (BMD). The athlete can move along the spectrum from healthy to unhealthy states of each component. Low energy availability affects menstrual function and bone health, and menstrual dysfunction also leads to poor bone health. (Reproduced from Goolsby M, Lister J: Medical considerations and risk management: The female athlete, in Limpisvasti O, Krabak BJ, Albohm MJ, eds, et al: *The Sports Medicine Field Manual.* Rosemont, IL, American Academy of Orthopaedic Surgeons, 2015, pp 125-128. Redrawn from Nattiv A, Loucks AB, Manore NM, Sanborn CF, Sundgot-Borgen J, Warren MP; American College of Sports Medicine: American College of Sports Medicine position stand. The female athlete triad. *Med Sci Sports Exerc* 2007; 39(10):1867-1882.

Features of the Triad

Low EA

The first of the three components of the Triad is EA, defined as the difference in energy intake and exercise energy expenditure. To appropriately fuel their bodies and allow proper recovery from physical activity, athletes must have adequate EA. When EA is reduced, the risk for detrimental changes in bone health and hormonal function in girls and women is increased, leading to adverse short-term and long-term consequences such as menstrual dysfunction, infertility, an increased risk of stress fractures, early osteoporosis, and endothelial dysfunction.[4-6]

Low EA can occur for several reasons. In its most severe and pathologic form, an eating disorder, such as anorexia nervosa or bulimia nervosa, is present. Low EA also can be seen with disordered eating, such as restrictive eating and the avoidance of certain foods, without meeting the criteria for an overt eating disorder. In other cases, as a female athlete attempts to lose weight, she may reduce total caloric (energy) intake without patterns consistent with disordered eating or an eating disorder, which also can result in low EA. In addition, low EA can result from an increased caloric expenditure along with an inadvertent failure to increase intake sufficient for the energy demands of the body.

It is important to recognize that an eating disorder diagnosis is not necessary to diagnose the Triad. The most important factor is the inadequate availability of macronutrients for the body to maintain its normal function

given the increased demands of exercise. Equally important, when an athlete is suspected of having low EA, further evaluation for eating disorders is warranted, because elite athletes are at increased risk.[7]

Menstrual Dysfunction

The second component of the Triad is menstrual dysfunction. Low EA disrupts normal hormonal function, leading to menstrual irregularity.[8,9] In its most severe form, the hypoestrogenic state results in functional hypothalamic amenorrhea. The less severe spectrum of menstrual dysfunction includes oligomenorrhea, anovulatory cycles, and luteal phase dysfunction, which can develop before amenorrhea.

Estrogen and progesterone offer protection of BMD, whereas testosterone has osteoblastic properties that can increase bone growth. If the availability of these hormones becomes diminished, bone mass, bone density, and bone strength also decrease, raising the risk of low BMD and stress fractures. In addition, estrogen is protective to endothelial cells and the cardiovascular system and, although not a component of the Triad, is important to consider in the overall health of active females with menstrual dysfunction.[5]

Although seemingly easy to recognize, menstrual dysfunction often can be missed because many athletes do not realize the importance of regular menstrual cycles. It has been noted that some athletes believe that occasionally missing a menstrual cycle is normal, has no negative consequences, or is even a sign of successful training.[10] Subclinical menstrual disturbances such as luteal phase dysfunction and anovulatory cycles are frequently found in exercising women but are not readily apparent clinically.[11]

Bone Health

Low EA and hypoestrogenism negatively affect bone health, the final component of the Triad. The peak time of bone mineral deposition in girls occurs during adolescence, with bone maturity reaching its maximum genetic potential in young adulthood. After a prolonged period of low EA and menstrual dysfunction, the effect on bone may be irreversible.[9]

This change in bone health increases the risk of stress reaction, stress fractures, and early osteoporosis in women (Figure 2). This situation is cause for concern in an athlete because of the effect on her ability to perform and compete. Long-term morbidity and mortality also must be considered. It is well documented that women older than 50 years have a 50% chance of development of an osteoporosis-related fracture and that almost 30% of those experiencing a hip fracture die within 1 year of the fracture.[12-14] During adolescence and young adulthood, good nutrition and the maintenance of normal hormonal balance is thus critical for long-term health.

Screening

The active female is often unaware of the signs of the Triad and its negative consequences. Partly because of the silent nature of this disorder in its early stages, it is very important for health professionals such as athletic trainers, physical therapists, and physicians, as well as coaches, parents, and the athletes themselves to be aware of the components of the Triad and the risk factors for developing disease. Early identification of affected and at-risk athletes, along with early intervention, is important to minimize potential negative consequences.

Athletes competing in endurance sports such as long-distance running, sports that involve judging such as skating and gymnastics, and weight-class sports such as martial arts or wrestling, are traditionally at increased risk of development of the Triad. Athletes in all sports have some risk because of the possibility of low EA.[15]

Multiple organizations recommend screening female athletes during the preparticipation physical evaluation (PPE) or the yearly physical examination. The recommendation from the 2014 Female Athlete Triad Coalition (FATC) Consensus Statement is that screening of female athletes should begin during adolescence; if any part of the screening is positive for the Triad, a thorough evaluation should be undertaken.[16]

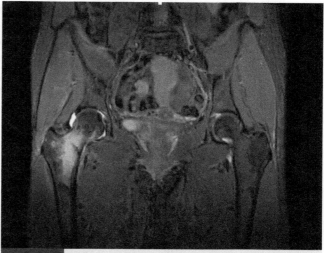

| Figure 2 | MRI shows stress fracture of the femoral neck. |

In a standard screening PPE form used by multiple American medical societies, several questions related to risk factors for the Triad are included. These questions, along with additional questions recommended by the FATC, elicit information about menstrual health, weight and nutrition, and bone health, as summarized in Table 1. Other warning signs and risk factors for the Triad, if seen, should prompt further evaluation. Some of them include involvement in sports that stress leanness and esthetics, psychosocial pressures for thinness, low self-esteem, increased training intensity especially at young ages, declining performance, mood changes, and weight loss.

Further Evaluation and Diagnosis

After it has been determined that an athlete is at risk for the Triad, a full evaluation that assesses nutrition, energy expenditure, menstrual history, and bone health is necessary. A multidisciplinary team, including a physician, a mental health professional, and a dietitian, should be involved. Many of the signs and symptoms of the Triad can be seen in other medical conditions and a complete medical evaluation for these conditions is necessary (Table 2).

Key components of the history include a nutritional history detailing eating habits, diets, and disordered eating habits such as restrictive eating, binging, or purging. Important aspects of the menstrual history include the age at menarche, the most recent menses, the frequency and pattern of the menses, any history of oligomenorrhea or amenorrhea, and the maternal menstrual history. A further history covering the incidence of stress fractures and traumatic fractures, a previous diagnosis of low BMD, and low vitamin D levels, is also important. If the patient has a history of stress fractures, details including the number of such fractures, the severity of fracture, and the site of injury are important. The involvement of the family, teammates, and coaches can provide insight into the athlete's health and behaviors such as eating small portions, doing extra workouts, not eating with others, using restrooms immediately after eating, and/or rapid changes in weight.

Table 1

Proposed Set of Screening Questions for the Female Athlete triad

Have you ever had a menstrual period?

How old were you when you had your first menstrual period?

When was your most recent menstrual period?[a]

How many periods have you had in the past 12 months?

Are you presently taking any female hormones (estrogen, progesterone, birth control pills?[a]

Do you worry about your weight?

Are you trying to gain or lose weight, or has anyone recommended that you do so?

Are you on a special diet, or do you avoid certain types of foods or food groups?

Have you ever had an eating disorder?

Have you ever had a stress fracture?

Have you ever been told you have low bone density (osteopenia or osteoporosis)?[a]

[a]. Not specifically listed on the preparticipation physical evaluation forms.

As with any thorough medical history, evaluation for the signs and symptoms of diseases that can cause similar symptoms such as thyroid disorder, polycystic ovarian disease, and hyperandrogenism should be documented. It is critical to obtain a history of the medications the patient is currently taking or has taken, especially those affecting menstruation and BMD such as oral contraceptive pills, patches, and rings, medroxyprogesterone acetate (Depo-Provera), glucocorticoids, and antiepileptic drugs. A family history of osteoporosis, fractures, menstrual dysfunction, and eating disorders can provide insight.

Physical examination findings also can help diagnose the Triad and evaluate for other causes of its components. Bradycardia, orthostatic hypotension, hypothermia, a low body mass index (BMI), and weight loss can indicate low EA. Parotid gland swelling, lanugo, enamel erosion, and calluses on the knuckles (the Russell sign) may indicate an eating disorder. Bone health can be evaluated on examination by assessing for scoliosis, kyphosis, and signs of stress fracture.

Low EA

Diagnosing low EA can be challenging because of the inherent bias in recording dietary intake, and the difficulty determining the exact caloric content of food and obtaining an accurate assessment of 24-hour energy expenditure. Multiple tools are available to help assess EA, however. A BMI less than 17.5 mg/kg^2 or a BMI less than 85% of expected body weight can indicate low EA. It is possible to have a normal body weight with low EA, however, because the body suppresses some physiologic functions to maintain the balance, leaving the patient at

Table 2

Diagnostic Testing for the Female Athlete Triad

Energy Availability	Menstrual Dysfunction	Bone Health
CBC, ESR	LH, FSH	DEXA scan for BMD
CMP	hCG (blood or urine)	Vitamin D
Albumin	Prolactin	24-hour urine calcium
T3	TSH, free T4	PTH
DEXA scan (for FFM)	Estradiol, testosterone (free and total), DHEA/S, 17-OH progesterone	
RMR	Pelvic ultrasonography	
ECG	Progesterone challenge	

CBC = complete blood count, ESR = erythrocyte sedimentation rate, CMP = complete metabolic panel, T3 = triiodothyronine, DEXA = dual-energy x-ray absorptiometry, FFM = fat-free mass, RMR = resting metabolic rate, ECG = electrocardiogram, LH = luteinizing hormone, FSH = follicle-stimulating hormone, hCG = human chorionic gonadotropin, TSH = thyroid-stimulating hormone, T4 = thyroxine, DHEA-S = dehydroepiandrosterone sulfate, OH = hydroxyprogesterone, BMD = bone mineral density, PTH = parathyroid hormone

Diagnostic studies may be indicated to evaluate for other causes and/or consequences of components of the Triad.

risk of negative physiologic consequences if not corrected. A resting metabolic rate (RMR) can be tested; if it is low or if the ratio of measured RMR to predicted RMR is less than 0.90, low EA is indicated. The more practical ways to calculate EA are based on dietary records, estimates of exercise expenditure, and measurement of fat-free mass (FFM) as described in the most recent FATC Consensus Statement.[16] Online calculators to determine EA can be found at www.femaleathletetriad.org. Studies have reported that, at less than 30 kcal/kg of FFM per day, a girl or woman is at risk of the development of menstrual dysfunction and diminished BMD; therefore, 45 kcal/kg of FFM has been recommended for physically active females to maintain normal EA.[16]

Menstrual Dysfunction

A variety of menstrual disturbances can be found in the Triad. Primary amenorrhea is diagnosed if menses has not occurred by age 15 years. Secondary amenorrhea is defined as 3 consecutive months without menses after menarche, and oligomenorrhea describes cycles longer than 35 days. Functional hypothalamic amenorrhea and other types of menstrual dysfunction are diagnoses of exclusion, and other causes to consider include outflow obstruction, pregnancy, thyroid dysfunction, hyperandrogenic syndromes, hypothalamic and pituitary disorders, primary ovarian insufficiency, and hyperprolactinemia (Table 2). Physicians in other specialties can help evaluate these patients, such as when the diagnosis of another gynecologic disorder or endocrinopathy is expected.

Bone Health

Osteoporosis is the most severe abnormality of bone health that can be found in the Triad, and evaluating for deficits in BMD and bone integrity is essential for patients at risk. The gold standard for determining BMD in children and adults is dual-energy x-ray absorptiometry (DEXA). Athletes should have a 5% to 15% higher bone density than sedentary controls.[17] In premenopausal women, the American College of Sports Medicine (ACSM) defines low BMD as a Z-score of -1.0 to -2.0, with secondary clinical risk factors for fracture such as the Triad. Osteoporosis is defined as a Z-score less than or equal to -2.0, plus secondary risk factors for fracture.[6]

The use of DEXA to evaluate bone health in the Triad is determined by risk stratification. According to the recent FATC consensus statement, having one high-risk factor for the Triad warrants DEXA evaluation[16] (Table 3). These factors include a diagnosis of an eating disorder, a BMI less than or equal to 17.5 kg/m², less than 85% of estimated weight or a weight loss greater than 10% in 1 month, menarche at age 16 years or older, any

history of fewer than 6 menstrual cycles over 12 months, 2 prior stress reactions or 1 high-risk stress reaction, or a prior Z-score less than -2.0 at least 1 year from a baseline DEXA. If moderate risk factors exist, a patient must exhibit at least two before DEXA evaluation is warranted. The location of BMD testing using DEXA varies for children and adults. In those younger than 20 years, the lumbar spine and the whole body are recommended locations. For women 20 years or older, weight-bearing sites including the spine, total hip, and femoral neck should be used. If weight-bearing sites are not available, then the radius BMD can be used in adults.[16,18,19]

Treatment

After an athlete is identified as having evidence of or risk factors for the Triad, early intervention and treatment are essential. When the condition is recognized early and treated, it is possible to prevent many of the detrimental effects of the Triad. The key to treatment is to address EA through a combination of increased energy sources and reduced energy expenditure. This protocol often requires the resources of a multidisciplinary health team, a key player being a sports dietitian to help formulate a specific diet for the individual and to help ensure compliance. A psychiatrist or sports psychologist also may be necessary if disordered eating or an eating disorder is present. As a general goal, changes should be made gradually, and often a 20% increase in caloric intake is recommended. In the recent consensus statement from the FATC, a goal of 45 kcal/kg of FFM is recommended. Furthermore, athletes need to restore lost weight or in some cases attain a higher weight than that at which amenorrhea developed.[8,20] Maximizing the intake of micronutrients such as calcium and vitamin D may be beneficial in addition to the caloric increase.

Although oral contraceptives can increase estrogen levels, they have not been shown to have a beneficial effect on BMD. Interestingly, the transdermal estrogen patch, although not an effective contraceptive, does seem to confer some benefit in improving BMD in women. At this time, estrogen or combined oral contraceptives is not the recommended solo therapy for low BMD or amenorrhea but can be used in some cases. Other bone agents, such as bisphosphonates and teriperatide, although not routinely used, could be considered in select patients, under the care of a metabolic bone specialist.

Prevention

Education is key to prevention and involves providing information about the Triad to athletes, coaches, parents,

Table 3

Female Athlete Triad Cumulative Risk Assessment

	Magnitude of Risk		
Risk Factors	Low Risk = 0 Points Each	Moderate Risk = 1 Point Each	High Risk = 2 Points Each
Low EA with or without DE/ED	☐ No dietary restriction	☐ Some dietary restriction;[a] current/past history of DE	☐ Meets DSM-V criteria for ED[b]
Low BMI	☐ BMI ≥ 18.5 **or** ≥ 90% EW[c] or weight stable	☐ BMI 17.5 < 18.5 **or** < 90% EW **or** 5 to < 10% weight loss/month	☐ BMI ≤ 17.5 **or** < 85% EW **or** ≥ 10% weight loss/month
Delayed menarche	☐ Menarche < 15 years	☐ Menarche 15 to < 16 years	☐ Menarche ≥ 16 years
Oligomenorrhea and/or amenorrhea	☐ > 9 menses in 12 months[b]	☐ 6-9 menses in 12 months[b]	☐ < 6 menses in 12 months[b]
Low BMD	☐ Z-score ≥ -1.0	☐ Z-score -1.0[d] < -2.0	☐ Z-score ≤ -2.0
Stress reaction/fracture	☐ None	☐ 1	☐ ≥ 2; ≥ 1 high risk or of trabecular bone sites[e]
Cumulative risk (total each column, then add for total score)	_____ points +	_____ points +	_____ points = _____ Total Score

BMD = bone mineral density, BMI = body mass index, DE = disordered eating, EA = energy availability, EW = expected weight, ED = eating disorder, DSM-V = Diagnostic and Statistical Manual-5.

The cumulative risk score is used to determine an athlete's clearance for sport participation.

[a] Some dietary restriction as evidenced by self-report or low/inadequate energy intake on diet logs.

[b] Current or past history.

[c] 90% EW. Absolute BMI cut-offs should not be used for adolescents.

[d] Weight-bearing sport.

[e] High-risk skeletal sites associated with low BMD and delay in return to play in athletes with one or more components of the Triad include stress reaction/fracture of trabecular sites (femoral neck, sacrum, pelvis).

Adapted with permission from the 2014 Female Athlete Triad Coalition consensus statement on treatment and return to play of the female athlete triad: 1st International Conference held in San Francisco, CA, May 2012, and 2nd International Conference held in Indianapolis, IN, May 2013. *Clin J Sport Med* 2014;24(2):96-119.

and all others involved with active girls and women. It is important to be aware of the risks, signs, and symptoms of the Triad to intervene early if symptoms do develop and to help affected athletes develop an adequate nutrition strategy and a sound exercise plan. Useful information can be found online at sites such as the FATC website (www.femaleathletetriad.org) and the International Olympic Committee Healthy Body Image website (www.olympic.org/hbi). Many other organizations also make information available to athletes, parents, coaches, and health care professionals such as ACSM, the American Medical Society for Sports Medicine, the American Academy of Pediatrics, and the American Academy of Family Physicians.

Return to Play

The first step in return to play is to appropriately treat any secondary complications such as stress fractures. For affected athletes without acute injuries, the FATC in 2014 developed a risk stratification and provided a framework for helping make return-to-play decisions[16] (Table 3 and Table 4). The cumulative risk score is used to determine an athlete's clearance for sports participation. Patients are stratified by evaluating their risk factors for the Triad and determining the number of risks in each category. The patient is designated as low, moderate, or high risk. Those deemed low risk can continue to compete and train with education to prevent increased risk of the Triad and overt disease. Those in the moderate-risk category often

Table 4

Female Athlete Triad Clearance and Return-to-Play Guidelines by Medical Risk Stratification

	Cumulative Risk Score[a]	Low Risk	Moderate Risk	High Risk
Full clearance	0–1 point	☐	N/A	N/A
Provisional/limited clearance	2–5 points	N/A	☐ Provisional clearance ☐ Limited clearance	N/A
Restricted from training and competition	≥ 6 points	N/A	N/A	☐ Restricted training/competition provisional ☐ Disqualified

[a] The Cumulative Risk Score is determined by summing the score of each risk factor (low, moderate, high risk) from the Cumulative Risk Assessment shown in Table 3.

Adapted with permission from the 2014 Female Athlete Triad Coalition consensus statement on treatment and return to play of the female athlete triad: 1st International Conference held in San Francisco, CA, May 2012, and 2nd International Conference held in Indianapolis, IN, May 2013. *Clin J Sport Med* 2014;24(2):96-119.

can have provisional clearance, which allows them to participate in physical activities, with recommendations for modifications outlined by a multidisciplinary team. These modifications can include limited or modified training, dietary plans, and psychologic therapies and can be progressed as the patient's health status improves and risks decrease. Those at high risk for the Triad or with specific significant pathology (such as stress fractures, amenorrhea, an eating disorder), are fully restricted from training and competition so the medical conditions affecting the athlete can be treated. In these circumstances, close follow-up with different members of the health care team is essential to treat and monitor the progression of the disease and its symptoms. A written treatment contract is recommended to allow the athlete to fully understand her disease, the treatment, and the expectations for follow-up and progression. If the athlete makes sufficient progress in her treatment, and her disease and risk factors for the Triad improve, she should be restratified for her risks and may eventually be cleared for participation.

Summary

The Triad can affect any female of menstruation age, causing pathologic changes to her bone health and menstrual function. The spectrum of disease can range from a healthy energy balance, normal menses, and good bone health to disordered eating, amenorrhea, and osteoporosis. Because of the detrimental health effects of this condition, it is important that all active young females be screened for the Triad, and if any component of the screening is positive, a thorough investigation should begin. After the disorder has been recognized and other causes ruled out, treatment should focus on increasing

EA to allow resumption of normal menstrual function and bone health. Further research is needed to determine the long-term consequences of the Triad, even after EA normalizes and regular menstrual function returns, and whether medications may be helpful in treatment.

Key Study Points

- The female athlete triad can affect any active girl or woman, causing short-term and long-term consequences to her health.
- Early awareness and recognition of the signs and symptoms of the Triad are important so that intervention can occur and prevent any negative health consequences.
- Low energy availability is the main target of therapy at this time. Efforts to regain adequate energy availability through increased intake and/or decreased energy utilization are essential components of treatment.

Annotated References

1. National Federation of State High School Associations: *Participation data for 1971 to 1972.* Available at: http://www.nfhs.org/ParticipationStatics/ParticipationStatics.aspx/. Accessed June 20, 2015.

   The National Federation of State High School Associations (NFHS) is the national authority for high school interscholastic athletics. Its website provides statistics for high school athletic participation in the United States from 1969 to 2014.

2. National Federation of State High School Associations: *2013-2014 High School Athletics Participation Survey.* Available at: http://www.nfhs.org/ParticipationStatics/PDF/2013-14_Participation_Survey_PDF.pdf. Updated 2014. Accessed June 20, 2015.

NFHS is the national authority for high school interscholastic athletics. Its website provides statistics for high school athletic participation in the United States from the years 1969-2014.

3. Gibbs JC, Williams NI, De Souza MJ: Prevalence of individual and combined components of the female athlete triad. *Med Sci Sports Exerc* 2013;45(5):985-996.

The authors reviewed the literature and developed a meta-analysis of the prevalence of the Female Athlete Triad and its individual components.

4. Zeni Hoch A, Dempsey RL, Carrera GF, et al: Is there an association between athletic amenorrhea and endothelial cell dysfunction? *Med Sci Sports Exerc* 2003;35(3):377-383.

5. Hoch AZ, Lal S, Jurva JW, Gutterman DD: The female athlete triad and cardiovascular dysfunction. *Phys Med Rehabil Clin N Am* 2007;18(3):385-400, vii-viii.

6. Nattiv A, Loucks AB, Manore MM, Sanborn CF, Sundgot-Borgen J, Warren MP; American College of Sports Medicine: American College of Sports Medicine position stand. The female athlete triad. *Med Sci Sports Exerc* 2007;39(10):1867-1882.

7. Sundgot-Borgen J, Torstveit MK: Prevalence of eating disorders in elite athletes is higher than in the general population. *Clin J Sport Med* 2004;14(1):25-32.

8. Gordon CM: Clinical practice. Functional hypothalamic amenorrhea. *N Engl J Med* 2010;363(4):365-371.

The author presents a review of functional hypothalamic amenorrhea including the definition, pathophysiology, diagnosis, and treatment.

9. Mallinson RJ, De Souza MJ: Current perspectives on the etiology and manifestation of the "silent" component of the Female Athlete Triad. *Int J Womens Health* 2014;6:451-467.

This study explores the current literature on the Triad, with a specific focus on bone health. The authors report on the pathophysiology of the bone changes related to the Triad, specific outcomes, and treatments of those outcomes.

10. Feldmann JM, Belsha JP, Eissa MA, Middleman AB: Female adolescent athletes' awareness of the connection between menstrual status and bone health. *J Pediatr Adolesc Gynecol* 2011;24(5):311-314.

The authors discuss the knowledge of high school athletes about menstrual dysfunction and bone health and their attitudes toward menstrual dysfunction.

11. De Souza MJ, Toombs RJ, Scheid JL, O'Donnell E, West SL, Williams NI: High prevalence of subtle and severe menstrual disturbances in exercising women: Confirmation using daily hormone measures. *Hum Reprod* 2010;25(2):491-503.

The authors present the results of a study evaluating hormonal changes that are used to detect subclinical menstrual disturbances related to exercise.

12. Johnell O, Kanis J: Epidemiology of osteoporotic fractures. *Osteoporos Int* 2005;16(Suppl 2):S3-S7.

13. Keene GS, Parker MJ, Pryor GA: Mortality and morbidity after hip fractures. *BMJ* 1993;307(6914):1248-1250.

14. Schnell S, Friedman SM, Mendelson DA, Bingham KW, Kates SL: The 1-year mortality of patients treated in a hip fracture program for elders. *Geriatr Orthop Surg Rehabil* 2010;1(1):6-14.

This study evaluated the mortality and associated mortality risk factors in a series of patients age 60 years or older with hip fracture being treated at one institution after implementing a new treatment protocol for hip fractures.

15. Torstveit MK, Sundgot-Borgen J: The female athlete triad exists in both elite athletes and controls. *Med Sci Sports Exerc* 2005;37(9):1449-1459.

16. De Souza MJ, Nattiv A, Joy E, et al; Female Athlete Triad Coalition; American College of Sports Medicine; American Medical Society for Sports Medicine; American Bone Health Alliance: 2014 Female Athlete Triad Coalition consensus statement on treatment and return to play of the female athlete triad: 1st International Conference held in San Francisco, CA, May 2012, and 2nd International Conference held in Indianapolis, IN, May 2013. *Clin J Sport Med* 2014;24(2):96-119.

The consensus statement from the FATC from the first and second international conferences gives an overview of the Triad and makes recommendations for screening, evaluation, treatment, and return to play.

17. Fehling PC, Alekel L, Clasey J, Rector A, Stillman RJ: A comparison of bone mineral densities among female athletes in impact loading and active loading sports. *Bone* 1995;17(3):205-210.

18. Crabtree NJ, Arabi A, Bachrach LK, et al; International Society for Clinical Densitometry: Dual-energy X-ray absorptiometry interpretation and reporting in children and adolescents: The revised 2013 ISCD Pediatric Official Positions. *J Clin Densitom* 2014;17(2):225-242.

The position paper from the International Society for Clinical Densitometry, as revised in 2013, describes the use of DEXA for BMD in children and adolescents and defines osteoporosis in this population.

19. International Society for Clinical Densitometry: *2013 Official Positions: Adult & Pediatric.* Available at: http://www.iscd.org/documents/2014/02/2013-iscd-official-position-brochure.pdf. Updated 2013. Accessed June 21, 2015.

© 2016 American Academy of Orthopaedic Surgeons

This position paper from the International Society for Clinical Densitometry, as revised in 2013, describes the use of DEXA for BMD density in adults and defines osteoporosis in this population.

20. Golden NH, Jacobson MS, Schebendach J, Solanto MV, Hertz SM, Shenker IR: Resumption of menses in anorexia nervosa. *Arch Pediatr Adolesc Med* 1997;151(1):16-21.

Chapter 43

Infectious Disease in the Athlete

Matthew Leiszler, MD   Kari Sears, MD   David Smith, DO

Abstract

Infectious disease in the athletic population is a common cause of morbidity and missed practice and competition in athletes. Clinicians should be familiar with common dermatologic, head and neck, pulmonary, gastrointestinal, genitourinary, and blood-borne infectious diseases to provide comprehensive care to the athlete. They also should be cognizant of the specific caveats associated with managing these illnesses in the athletic patient.

Keywords: infectious disease; athlete; sports medicine; skin infection; infectious mononucleosis; MRSA; return to play

Introduction

Athletes often are considered the healthiest segment of society, given the activity level and conditioning that many athletes maintain. However, certain aspects of athletics and team sports at times will actually increase the risk of infectious disease in athletes. An understanding of common infectious diseases in the athletic population is critical for any medical provider managing the health care of athletes.

Two main factors can play a role in infection in athletes: compromise of the immune system and exposure to potential infection. Moderate-intensity exercise appears to improve immune function, which has been shown to result in a better outcome following respiratory infection.[1] It is generally accepted that moderate-intensity exercise can improve the function of circulating cells in the innate immune system, and this seems to have a positive effect

None of the following authors or any immediate family member has received anything of value from or has stock or stock options held in a commercial company or institution related directly or indirectly to the subject of this chapter: Dr. Leiszler, Dr. Sears, and Dr. Smith.

on reducing the risk of infection. Intense exercise training, however, can have the opposite effect and increase the risk of infection, in part because of the decreased secretion of immunoglobulin A (IgA) in the saliva during intense exercise and stress, which in effect, takes down the first line of defense against infection.[2]

Managing the exposure to infection becomes particularly challenging in the team setting. Close physical contact during practices and competitions, the sharing of space, towels, and bathroom toiletries in the locker room, and team travel in congested vehicles increase the chances of transmitting contagious diseases to teammates. Prevention is therefore vital, with a focus on minimizing those risk factors that can increase transmission in the team setting. Key elements include hand hygiene, the relative isolation of infected individuals, the avoidance of shared personal items, and the adequate cleaning and disinfection of common areas. Vaccination is also an important element of prevention. Ensuring that vaccines against infectious illnesses such as influenza, meningococcal disease, and pertussis are up to date is an important element of team care. Vaccination can help to minimize the initial cases of such illnesses in a single member of a team and potential outbreaks in teammates.

As with any musculoskeletal problem, the differential diagnosis should be carefully considered, even in seemingly straightforward cases of infection. In a prospective study of elite and recreationally competitive triathletes, cyclists, and controls, nasal swabs were collected in those with symptoms of a probable upper respiratory infection. Only 30% of swabs identified an infectious cause of symptoms.[3] This underscores the importance of considering other causes, such as allergies, in athletes with upper respiratory symptoms.

In cases of infection, return-to-play guidelines include a general recommendation that fever be resolved before the athlete returns to sports participation. In many cases, however, return-to-play guidelines are not clear. The medical provider has the responsibility to ensure the safety of the athlete in question, as well as that of other athletes. This standard will help to guide return to play in areas without clear guidelines. The provider also must take into consideration the effect of illness on performance to determine if a return to sports participation is reasonable.

This chapter highlights the recent advances and the current standard of care in the prevention, diagnosis, and management of infectious diseases. In particular, the specific factors that are unique to the management of infectious disease in athletic populations are discussed. Evidence-based guidelines are presented when possible.

Bacterial Skin Infections

Although many bacterial conditions can affect athletes, commonly encountered skin infections can include methicillin-resistant *Staphylococcus aureus* (MRSA), impetigo, furunculosis, hot tub folliculitis, and pitted keratolysis.

Methicillin-Resistant *Staphylococcus aureus*

MRSA is a highly infectious strain of the bacteria *S aureus*. It was previously thought to be restricted to hospital-acquired infections following its discovery in the 1960s. During the late 1990s, MRSA became the leading cause of community-acquired bacterial infections, with approximately 30% of the general population colonized. Of all community-acquired MRSA infections, 87% to 95% are infections of the skin and soft tissue.[4] MRSA is spread via direct contact with the skin, particularly through an open, contaminated wound. The sports placing athletes most at risk for MRSA skin infections are wrestling, football, and rugby, although cases have been described among athletes from most major sports. MRSA can have a wide spectrum of presentations, ranging from streaky erythematous skin without abscess to frank necrotizing fasciitis. The most common appearance is a localized, purulent zone of tender erythema (**Figure 1**). MRSA often forms an abscess, or multiple small abscesses, over a regional but poorly defined area.

The diagnosis of MRSA often is made clinically, although a culture of purulent fluid can be obtained for confirmation. A MRSA abscess is often confused with a spider bite, because both can follow a similar clinical course. Other diagnoses to consider are infectious sebaceous cyst, septic bursitis, impetigo, and alternative bacterial etiologies. The mainstay of treatment is incision and drainage of the abscess using sterile technique. Incision and drainage alone is often sufficient for an uncomplicated clinical picture.[4] Antibiotics can be administered for concomitant large surrounding skin infection, systemic symptoms, or failure of incision and drainage alone. Treatment is based on regional resistance patterns but clindamycin or trimethoprim/sulfamethoxazole is most often effective against MRSA. Linezolid has been shown to be effective in some clinical settings, although it

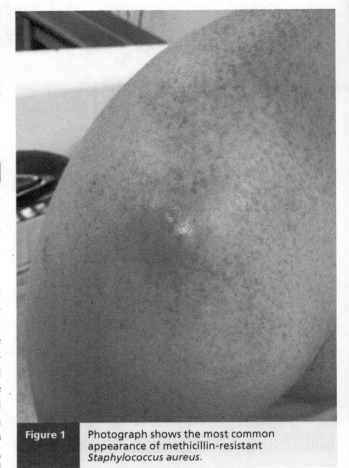

Figure 1   Photograph shows the most common appearance of methicillin-resistant *Staphylococcus aureus*.

has a larger side-effect profile. For hospitalized patients, vancomycin and daptomycin generally are adequate to treat MRSA.

An athlete with active MRSA infection of the skin can participate in most sports, assuming that the wound is adequately covered and that only minimal risk of accidental wound exposure exists during sport. Wrestling may be an exception, and return is based on state guidelines. Otherwise, return to play often is at the discretion of the athletic trainer, the coach, and the athlete. Because of the infectious nature of MRSA, substantial focus has been placed on prevention. A statewide epidemiologic study in Nebraska followed confirmed MRSA cases (of one or more individuals) in high schools and showed an increase in involvement from 4.4% of schools in 2007 to 14.4% of schools in 2008.[5] Efforts are being made to educate coaches and schools about the importance of hand hygiene and equipment cleanliness in sports.

Impetigo

Impetigo is a common superficial skin infection. Like MRSA, it is spread most often via direct contact with the skin. An athlete is most susceptible to impetigo if direct skin contact occurs during skin breakdown. Athletes in direct competition, such as wrestlers, martial artists, football players, and rugby players, are at highest risk, as are athletes with poor hygiene. Impetigo is most commonly caused by *S aureus* and less commonly by group A *Streptococcus pyogenes*.[6] Two types, bullous and nonbullous, are seen. Bullous impetigo is almost universally caused by *S aureus*. It is seen clinically as multiple thin-walled, fluid-filled vesicles that typically start as small vesicles that can coalesce to form one or more larger lesions. The blister eventually collapses, leaving behind a characteristic honey-crusted lesion. Erythematous plaques form at the base of the lesion and drain serous fluid when the crust is removed or healing. Nonbullous impetigo accounts for almost 70% of impetigo cases.[6] It begins as one or more small vesicles that do not coalesce and is more commonly associated with a classic crusting of lesions (Figure 2).

Impetigo is diagnosed clinically. Confirmatory culture of the serous fluid can be performed if the diagnosis is unclear. It can appear similar to tinea, especially in nonbullous cases. Tinea almost never appears on the lips, as impetigo can, however. The differential diagnosis also should include erysipelas, inflammatory or viral dermatoses, and (much less commonly) pemphigus vulgaris. The treatment of impetigo has two components: the removal of the crusting and antibiotic therapy. In all cases, the lesions must be kept clean and should be washed directly with soap and warm water to remove the crusting and serous fluid. Antibacterial soap is not necessary, although it is not discouraged. The first-line therapy for impetigo should be a topical antibiotic that supplies coverage for both *Staphylococcus* and *Streptococcus* bacteria. Mupirocin and fusidic acid are both effective first-line treatment options. Mupirocin is highly effective against all *Staphylococcus* and *Streptococcus* strains, except group D streptococcus. Bacterial resistance is low, at near 0.3%.[6] Fusidic acid is slightly less effective against *Streptococcus* and is not marketed in the United States. Over-the-counter compound antibiotic ointments are not recommended because of multidrug resistance, desensitization from overuse, and side effects of contact dermatitis in 6% to 8% of cases.[6] Although topical preparations are more effective and carry fewer side effects, oral antibiotic therapy is sometimes used. Oral options may include dicloxacillin and cephalexin; erythromycin is used if the patient is allergic to penicillin.

The National Athletic Trainers Association (NATA) recommends that any suspicious lesions should be tested and cultured for antimicrobial sensitivity. Return-to-play criteria require the appearance of no new lesions for at least 48 hours, completion of 72 hours of antibiotic

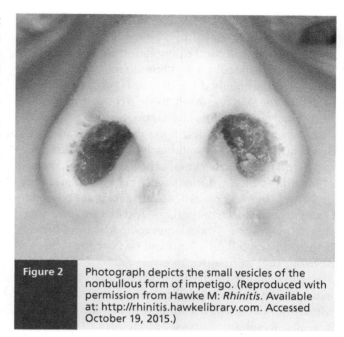

Figure 2 Photograph depicts the small vesicles of the nonbullous form of impetigo. (Reproduced with permission from Hawke M: *Rhinitis*. Available at: http://rhinitis.hawkelibrary.com. Accessed October 19, 2015.)

therapy, and no further drainage or exudate from the wound site. Simply covering active lesions is not sufficient to allow return to competition.

Folliculitis and Furunculosis

Folliculitis and furunculosis are closely related disease processes. Folliculitis is a superficial infection of the hair follicle, whereas furunculosis relates to the deep follicular base. Folliculitis and furunculosis typically are caused by *S aureus*, except in special cases.

Hot tub folliculitis is contracted, as the name implies, after exposure to wet environments. *Pseudomonas aeruginosa* commonly can colonize hot tubs, swimming pools, and wet heating pads in athletic training rooms. Athletes can be exposed when submerged in the water and are at particular risk with open or broken skin. *Pseudomonas* is known to thrive on moist surfaces and carries a high antibiotic resistance profile. A study conducted at a Division I university indicated that 96% of *Pseudomonas* isolates from athletic hot tubs and swimming pools displayed multidrug resistance.[7] Hot tub folliculitis presents as multiple pruritic pustules with a follicular appearance. In some cases, pustules can have a subtle green appearance. Symptoms typically develop 6 hours to 2 days after exposure and are confined to the skin that was exposed.[7,8] In severe cases, the athlete may experience systemic symptoms such as malaise, fever, and chills.

Furunculosis is frequently described as an abscess or boil. Furuncles are most common in areas of increased friction and heat such as the groin, axillae, or gluteal folds. Presentation may be similar to that of MRSA-related abscesses, although MRSA is implicated in only approximately 20% of cases.[8]

A history and physical examination are often adequate to diagnose furunculosis and hot tub folliculitis. Culture may be accurate only if the wound is pyogenic, because swabbing the skin is unlikely to yield the pathogenic bacteria. Hot tub folliculitis often is observed in a "dunked" distribution with a discrete horizontal demarcation. The differential diagnosis should include acne vulgaris, contact dermatitis, impetigo, and urticaria. The management of folliculitis and furuncles should begin with placement of a warm compress over the area to encourage consolidation. Large furuncles may require incision and drainage if they do not resolve. Topical mupirocin may be of benefit.[8] If surrounding cellulitis is present or systemic symptoms develop, oral antibiotics to cover *Staphylococcus* and *Streptococcus* can be given, usually for 10 to 14 days. The management of hot tub folliculitis is largely supportive. Most mild cases are self-limited and resolve over 1 to 2 weeks. Resultant abscesses rarely form. If symptoms are severe or lesions are widespread, antibiotic therapy can be prescribed and directed to combat *Pseudomonas*. Antibiotics usually are reserved for severe cases because of the multidrug resistance displayed.[7]

The return-to-play criteria are identical to those for impetigo. The athlete should have no new lesions for 48 hours, take 72 hours of directed antibiotics (if indicated), and have no drainage from active lesions. The lesions should not be covered to allow play.

Pitted Keratolysis

Pitted keratolysis is a noncontagious superficial infection of the feet and, rarely, the hands. This condition is characterized by well-defined, 1 to 3 mm, discrete pits along the soles of the feet. Lesions become pronounced when the feet are moist or are submerged in water. Gram-positive bacteria, chiefly *Corynebacterium* and *Actinomyces* species, commonly are implicated. Although athletes with hyperhidrosis are most at risk, tight-fitting or infrequently changed socks or gloves are also predisposing factors. Figure skaters and ice hockey players may be at increased risk because of the prolonged time spent in skates in wet environments.

The diagnosis is based on clinical examination. In addition to skin pitting, athletes may often present with excessive sweating and odor. Coral red fluorescence under the Wood lamp may be seen but is limited to cases in which *Corynebacterium* causes surrounding erythrasma. Treatment with several topical modalities has been investigated, although evidence is lacking. Topical clindamycin or erythromycin has been the mainstay of therapy since the 1980s. Topical bactroban also has been effective. A

small case study has shown some efficacy with topical clindamycin 1% and benzoyl peroxide 5%, when used with a drying agent.[9] The management includes avoiding tight-fitting socks and shoes. Cotton or moisture-wicking socks should be used when possible. Good hygiene is imperative, and footwear, especially skates, should be kept clean and dry. The application of roll-on antiperspirant containing 20% aluminum chloride to the feet may be helpful. A 2012 study performed on the Dutch army demonstrated that a combination of preventive measures, topical antibiotics, and the treatment of hyperhidrosis should be the mainstay of treatment.[10] Pitted keratolysis is not communicable and should not warrant disqualification from sports participation.

Viral Skin Infections

Although athletes are susceptible to many viral infections, verruca (the common wart), molluscum contagiosum, and herpes gladiatorum and zoster are among the most common. These infections can be difficult to treat, which emphasizes the importance of prevention to minimize disruption in sports participation.

Verruca

Verruca is an extremely common infection caused by the human papilloma virus (HPV). Studies show the prevalence is estimated at 5% to 20% in children and young adults, although data vary widely among the general population. More than 100 types of HPV have been identified, and the virus can cause warts on various parts of the body. The virus lies dormant on surfaces and often is spread by barefoot contact with pool decks, in locker rooms, and by direct unintentional scraping.

Verruca often is diagnosed clinically. A lesion is described as a discrete, hyperkeratotic papule that often is raised. Multiple black dots representing thrombosed capillaries are often noted. The differential diagnosis includes corns and calluses, which are often difficult to distinguish. Dermoscopy has been used to successfully differentiate and gauge treatment efficacy. Although warts often are left untreated intentionally, they can cause substantial morbidity if located in a painful area, such as on the plantar surface of the foot. Multiple treatments have been studied, all with varyied degrees of efficacy. Lesions often are pared to expose the capillary beds, allowing the penetrance of medication. Topical salicylic acid and cryotherapy are the most viable treatment options.[11] A Cochrane clinical review shows that salicylic acid treatment has the most consistent evidence in terms of efficacy and low side-effect profile and is more effective on plantar warts. Although cryotherapy is widely used, it is often painful and less effective on plantar warts.[11] Both treatments have been shown to be largely more effective than placebo, whereas duct tape occlusion has not.[12] Lesions can ultimately be difficult to eradicate; thus, prevention is extremely important. Injection of *Candida albicans* antigen at the base of the wart may be a consideration for resistant warts.

The athlete may resume sports participation if the lesions are covered. Topical salicylic acid can be used with an occlusive dressing on top. Pain tolerance should be a consideration if cryotherapy is used before participation.

Molluscum Contagiosum

Molluscum contagiosum is caused by the molluscum contagiosum virus (MCV), a virus in the poxvirus family. It infects only the skin, growing in the epidermis. Although the incidence and prevalence are highly variable, molluscum contagiosum is more common among young children and adolescents living in close quarters. The virus is transmitted by direct contact with skin or infected water. A higher transmission risk is demonstrated in those who use swimming pools and who live in warmer climates. MCV also can be transmitted sexually or while shaving.[13]

Molluscum is a clinical diagnosis. Infection appears as a collection of discrete, umbilicated papules, ranging from 1 to 5 mm in diameter. The lesions are flesh colored, raised, and round (**Figure 3**). In immunocompetent individuals, fewer than 20 lesions usually are present in a cluster, although larger clusters have been observed. Infection is rarely present on the palms, the soles, or the mucosal areas but can be seen on the genitals when sexually transmitted. When lesions are broken, a thick, white material may be expressed. The differential diagnosis includes verruca, cystic lesions, and granulomatous conditions and can be aided by examination with a dermatoscope if necessary. Although MCV infection often resolves spontaneously, full clearance can take 6 to 9 months. In athletes, the treatment is often destructive, using cryotherapy or curettage, or topical, using imiquimod, cantharadin, or potassium hydroxide (KOH) 5% solution. The athlete can return to play immediately if lesions are curetted and covered during competition.[14]

Herpes Simplex Virus

Herpes simplex infection can particularly problematic in athletes. The herpes simplex virus (HSV) is the parent virus responsible for herpes gladiatorum and herpes zoster in addition to many other conditions. HSV is transmitted via direct contact and can rapidly infect a large number of teammates if not recognized quickly. A 2003 University of Minnesota study found a 33% likelihood of transmission from an infected wrestler to the wrestling partner.[15]

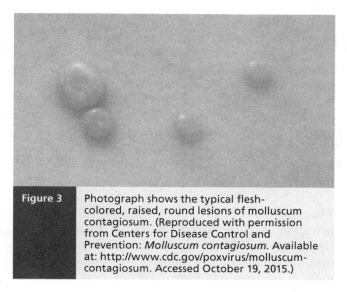

Figure 3 Photograph shows the typical flesh-colored, raised, round lesions of molluscum contagiosum. (Reproduced with permission from Centers for Disease Control and Prevention: *Molluscum contagiosum.* Available at: http://www.cdc.gov/poxvirus/molluscum-contagiosum. Accessed October 19, 2015.)

Prevalence varies widely and is population dependent, age dependent, and sport dependent.

Herpes gladiatorum, caused by HSV-1, can carry an incubation period of 3 to 10 days, which varies depending on the host's immune response. An infected athlete often experiences a prodromal phase, which can range from subtle malaise to a flu-like illness.[14] An HSV outbreak of the skin occurs after this prodromal phase, presenting as widespread 2- to 5-mm vesicles, which often are clustered on an erythematous base. Areas affected are the trunk, arms, legs, and head. Vesicles can erupt and are virulent. In late stages of infection, vesicles can become crusted.

In the early stage of infection, the diagnosis is not always obvious. The differential diagnosis includes folliculitis, acne, dermatitis, and impetigo. Clinical diagnosis often is made and is easier with a clear prodromal history. Viral culture is helpful but can take days to obtain; thus a Tzanck preparation of vesicular fluid can be helpful in the short term.[14] Oral acyclovir and valacyclovir are the most effective treatments of HSV, although acyclovir is more cost effective. Acyclovir is dosed five times daily, however, which could create a compliance issue compared with valacyclovir, which has a twice-daily dosing. Oral antivirals are ineffective when lesions are fully formed and crusting.[14] The prevention of herpes gladiatorum infection is largely based on hygiene, education, and the recognition of at-risk athletes. Antiviral prophylaxis has been found to be helpful to prevent eruptions in those with recurrent herpes labialis or in those who have had a documented mass exposure.[15] National Collegiate Athletic Association and NATA guidelines state that athletes with HSV-1 infection may not return to competition until lesions have a dried adherent crust, and the athlete has been receiving oral antiviral treatment for at least 5 days.[14]

Herpes Zoster

Herpes zoster is less common among athletes but can carry substantial morbidity if not recognized. Herpes zoster, commonly known as shingles, can present with or without a significant viral prodrome. After exposure, the herpes zoster virus lies dormant in a dorsal spinal root ganglion. Herpes zoster carries the highest incidence of all neurologic diseases, with a lifetime incidence of 30% among all persons.[16] The skin eruption associated with a zoster outbreak can occur weeks to many years after initial exposure. When skin eruption does occur it often is preceded by exposure to a significant stressor or illness. The rash seen in herpes zoster is characteristic of a herpetic rash, in that vesicles erupt on an erythematous base (Figure 4). The pattern of eruption is different, however, in that it follows a specific unilateral dermatome specific to the dormant infection site in the spinal root ganglion. The rash is usually painful, often exquisitely so.

The diagnosis is similar to that of herpes gladiatorum and other HSV types. Clinical diagnosis is usually sufficient and can be aided by a Tzanck preparation and culture if the diagnosis is uncertain. The differential diagnosis includes folliculitis, impetigo, acne, and dermatitis. Treatment with oral antivirals is considered first line and should be initiated within 72 hours of rash eruption to increase the healing response and reduce pain. Acyclovir, famciclovir, and valacyclovir all are approved and well-tolerated treatment options. Postherpetic neuralgia is a complication that may arise after an episode of shingles. Prevention with early antiviral treatment is essential because the pain can be significant. Postherpetic neuralgia has been successfully treated with gabapentin or controlled-release oxycodone, both of which show some benefit during the initial 8 days of treatment.

Although shingles cannot be passed from one person to another, the varicella zoster virus can be spread from a person with active shingles to someone not previously infected or vaccinated against varicella zoster or chickenpox. In this case, chickenpox, but not shingles, may develop in the new contact. NATA does not have a consensus statement regarding return to play for athletes with herpes zoster. Shingles is less contagious than chickenpox, and risk of transmission is low even in the active blister phase if the lesions are covered.

Fungal Skin Infections

Fungal skin infections are common among athletes. Most fungal skin infections in athletes are caused by tinea (mycoses of the skin), and the dermatophytes *Tricophyton rubrum* and *Tricophyton tonsurans* are the most common agents. Fungal infections are often opportunistic, placing

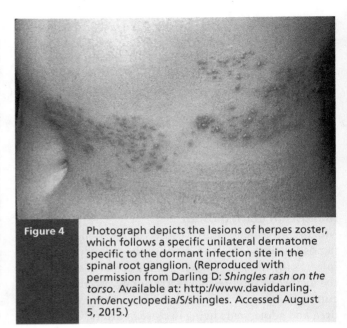

Figure 4 Photograph depicts the lesions of herpes zoster, which follows a specific unilateral dermatome specific to the dormant infection site in the spinal root ganglion. (Reproduced with permission from Darling D: *Shingles rash on the torso.* Available at: http://www.daviddarling.info/encyclopedia/S/shingles. Accessed August 5, 2015.)

those with compromised immune systems and poor hygiene at higher risk.

Tinea Pedis

Tinea pedis, or athlete's foot, is common in athletes and in the general population, affecting approximately 15% of the population worldwide and is more common in adolescents and men. Tinea pedis is transmitted easily in warm, moist communal areas such as showers and locker rooms; the fungus incubates in the moist, warm environment of a shoe. *T rubrum* is implicated in most cases, although *Trichophyton mentagrophytes* is most common in athletes. Infection causes macerated skin, itching, flaking, and scaling of the feet and commonly spreads to the interdigital areas. Severe tinea pedis can cause cracking of the skin and can result in concomitant cellulitis and onychomycosis. Rarely, a hypersensitivity response to the dermatophyte can develop in athletes, resulting in an inflammatory or vesicular eruption.

Clinical examination alone is sufficient for diagnosis. To confirm the diagnosis, a KOH preparation of skin scrapings can be performed. Fungal culture can be helpful in recalcitrant cases. The differential diagnosis includes *Candida* infection, dyshidrotic eczema, psoriasis, and contact dermatitis. Both topical and oral agents have shown to be effective. Topical agents are prescribed for 1 to 6 weeks, depending on the agent used. Ketoconazole 2% and clotrimazole 1% are good initial topical choices. Topical sertaconazole has demonstrated efficacy against interdigital tinea pedis when used once daily for 4 weeks.[17] Oral agents, although effective, can cause an increase in transaminase levels depending on the agent used. Recurrence of tinea pedis is common, and athletes should be educated about prevention. Keeping the feet clean and dry, using moisture-wicking socks, and wearing sandals in communal areas are important for prevention. Aluminum chloride foot powder can be used as a drying agent. NATA return-to-competition guidelines recommend that clearance be given when lesions have adequately responded to treatment or can be covered securely.[14]

Tinea Cruris

Tinea cruris is a fungal infection of the groin region. Commonly known as jock itch, tinea cruris is an opportunistic fungal infection that infects athletes for reasons similar to those of tinea pedis. *T rubrum*, *T metagrophytes*, and *C albicans* are the most common infectious agents. Athletes wearing jock straps or tight-fitting clothing are most at risk, because the fungus incubates and proliferates in the warm, moist regions of the groin folds. Males are affected most often. Like tinea pedis, tinea cruris causes pruritic, macerated skin that is often erythematous, flaky, and peeling. A well-defined, hyperpigmented area of skin can indicate infection.

Often, the diagnosis is clinical. A KOH preparation also can be used when the diagnosis is in question or if no strictly demarcated area of skin is present. A Wood lamp can be used if erythrasma is suspected, under which the rash would glow a pathognomonic red. The differential diagnosis should include contact dermatitis, intertrigo, acanthosis nigricans, erythrasma, and (rarely) Hailey-Hailey disease (familial benign pemphigus). Topical therapy is usually sufficient. A 2014 meta-analysis reviewed over 18,000 cases of tinea cruris and corporis. Data from this analysis showed that many topical agents have acceptable cure rates.[18] Terbinafine and 1% naftifine are effective. Many combination antifungal/steroid preparations are used but supporting data are limited. Prevention strategies are aimed at decreasing moisture and heat in the groin. Clean, dry athletic supporters and support shorts should be worn, and athletes should shower immediately after engaging in activity. In those with tinea pedis, care should be taken when using towels, because fungi can spread to other regions. Clearance may be given if the lesions are responding to treatment or can be securely covered.[14]

Tinea Corporis

Tinea corporis is a fungal infection of the trunk, arms, legs, or neck, commonly known as ringworm. Tinea corporis is also an opportunistic dermatophyte infection. The infection is transmitted by skin-to-skin contact, placing wrestlers at higher risk. It is caused most commonly by *T. rubrum* and *T. tonsurans*; the latter is most commonly

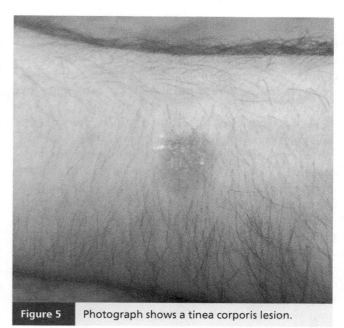

Figure 5 Photograph shows a tinea corporis lesion.

seen among wrestlers. Like other forms of tinea, tinea corporis fungi prefer warm, moist environments in which they incubate and replicate. Tight-fitting clothing, wet and humid conditions, and excessive sweating are risk factors. The lesions appear in a superficial, loose, circular pattern and often have an erythematous, scaly component peripherally (**Figure 5**). Tinea corporis eruption is often pruritic.

Clinical examination is also sufficient to diagnose tinea corporis in most cases. A KOH preparation and fungal culture of skin scrapings also can be used to confirm the diagnosis. As with tinea cruris, treatment with a topical or oral agent is effective. Evidence supports using topical terbinafine and naftifine, although many azole agents are also effective. Treatment is usually effective at 2 weeks; higher cure rates occur at 4 weeks.[18] Tinea corporis is contagious and can be passed easily among teammates, particularly on wrestling teams. Tinea corporis also can be passed from an infected household pet. Prevention includes using clean, dry clothing and towels, wearing loose-fitting clothing, and avoiding direct contact with an affected person or pet. Athletes with tinea infection should be allowed to play if lesions are securely covered or are responding to treatment with a topical or oral agent, although wrestling rules usually require a minimum of 72 hours of topical therapy before return to play.[14]

Eye, Ear, Nose, and Throat Infections

Conjunctivitis

Conjunctivitis is a frequent problem among athletes and has many causes, both infectious and noninfectious.

Allergic conjunctivitis is the most common cause, followed closely by the infectious causes. Although conjunctivitis is the most common cause of a red eye, the clinician also must consider the less common but more serious causes, including keratitis, uveitis, iritis, and acute glaucoma.[19]

Viral conjunctivitis is the most common cause of infectious conjunctivitis in adults, and up to 90% of cases are caused by adenoviruses. It is usually bilateral and presents with conjunctival irritation and sometimes watery discharge (Figure 6). Treatment is usually symptomatic, using cold compresses, antihistamines, and artificial tears. Antibiotics are not helpful for viral conjunctivitis and may promote antibiotic resistance. Potential complications can include epidemic keratoconjunctivitis and pharyngoconjunctival fever. Because viral conjunctivitis is highly contagious, athletes participating in contact sports such as rugby and football should be withheld from participation until symptoms resolve. Good handwashing technique and cleaning of equipment is important in preventing the spread of infection to other athletes, especially for athletes who use shared equipment, such as gymnasts, weightlifters, and basketball players. Multiple reports exist of adenovirus outbreaks in swimming pools, so swimmers and divers should be kept out of the water until their symptoms resolve.[20] Symptoms usually resolve within 7 days; athletes with persistent symptoms should be referred for a more comprehensive eye examination. One recent study showed that using combination dexamethasone/iodine drops might reduce the duration of symptoms by 2 days compared with placebo.[21] Using topical steroids in the setting of a corneal ulcer can result in corneal melt and loss of vision, and is not currently recommended.[19]

Bacterial conjunctivitis occurs most frequently in the winter months. The combination of bilateral discharge, an absence of itching, and no prior history of conjunctivitis is highly suggestive of a bacterial etiology. *Streptococcus* and *Staphylococcus* are the most commonly isolated bacteria in culture-proven disease, and MRSA is becoming increasingly common. Treatment with topical antibiotics is recommended, and no significant difference in treatment success exists with broad-spectrum antibiotic options. Appropriate choices include tobramycin, fluoroquinolones, and combination drops. Athletes participating in contact sports should be held from competition until treatment is complete.

Otitis Media

Acute otitis media (AOM) is most frequently a complication of viral upper respiratory infection (URI) and resultant eustachian tube dysfunction. The diagnostic criteria for AOM include otalgia with a mildly bulging

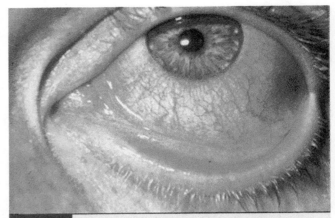

Figure 6 Photograph depicts the typical presentation of viral conjunctivitis. (Reproduced with permission from Jacobs DS: Conjunctivitis, in Trobe J, ed: *UpToDate*. Waltham, MA, Wolters Kluwer, 2014. Available at http://www.uptodate.com/contents/conjunctivitis. Accessed October 19, 2015.)

tympanic membrane or a moderate to severe bulging tympanic membrane (Figure 7). AOM is much more common in children than in adults, and few data exist to guide treatment in adults. Athletes often present with otalgia, aural fullness, possibly fever, and a recent URI. Antibiotic treatment in children is reserved for those younger than 2 years or those with symptoms that persist over 48 to 72 hours. It is reasonable to extend those recommendations to athletes and reserve antibiotic treatment for those with persistent or severe symptoms or those with frank tympanic membrane perforation. The most common causative organisms remain *Streptococcus pneumoniae*, *Haemophilus influenzae*, and *Moraxella catarrhalis*; amoxicillin is the first-line choice for antibiotic treatment.[22]

With a few exceptions, most athletes with otitis media will be able to continue competition. Adequate pain control can be achieved with NSAIDs and acetaminophen. Potential symptoms that can affect performance include balance problems and temporary hearing loss. Decongestants and nasal steroids have not been shown to relieve effusion related to AOM, and can have deleterious side effects.[23] Special attention should be paid to divers, who may experience significant changes in middle ear pressure if submerged beyond a few feet. Athletes with persistent symptoms of middle ear effusion should be evaluated for other potential causes.

Otitis Externa

Otitis externa is an acute inflammatory condition of the external ear canal that is almost exclusively caused by a bacterial infection (Figure 8). It occurs more frequently in a moist environment, so athletes who participate in water

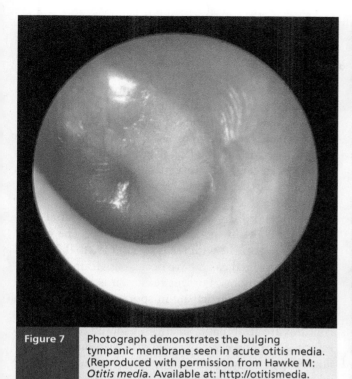

Figure 7 Photograph demonstrates the bulging tympanic membrane seen in acute otitis media. (Reproduced with permission from Hawke M: *Otitis media*. Available at: http://otitismedia. hawkelibrary.com. Accessed October 19, 2015.)

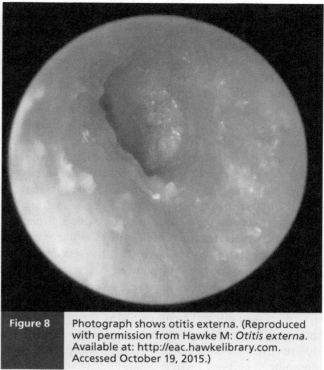

Figure 8 Photograph shows otitis externa. (Reproduced with permission from Hawke M: *Otitis externa*. Available at: http://eac.hawkelibrary.com. Accessed October 19, 2015.)

sports and those competing in warm, humid climates are more susceptible. Although infections are often polymicrobial, the most frequent causative organisms are *P aeruginosa* and *S aureus*. Antibiotic therapy must include coverage for these common pathogens. Therapy for otitis externa should be topical rather than systemic, because much higher local drug concentrations can be achieved with drops placed in the ear. Although it is clear that topical therapy is superior to systemic therapy, no convincing evidence shows that antimicrobial drops are more effective than other topical therapies such as antiseptic or steroid drops. The choice of topical therapy largely is determined by the provider's comfort and familiarity with available treatments. Adequate pain control is important, because acute otitis externa can be an extremely painful condition. NSAIDs are often effective for pain control, but stronger pain medications may be needed for the first 48 to 72 hours.

Athletes with otitis externa should receive at least 7 days of treatment. Those participating in water sports should complete treatment before returning to competition. If tightly fitting earplugs can be used, participation may be allowed when symptoms resolve. Acidifying eardrops used before and/or after swimming may help to prevent otitis externa in athletes with recurrent episodes. The addition of a systemic antibiotic with pseudomonal coverage should be considered in athletes with an extension of infection outside the external ear canal or in those who do not respond to topical treatment alone.[24]

Pharyngitis

Acute pharyngitis, like most URIs, is caused most frequently by viral pathogens. It is important to consider bacterial causes, however, most commonly group A β-hemolytic streptococcus (GABHS). GABHS and viral pharyngitis often can be distinguished from each other by their accompanying symptoms. Viral pharyngitis often occurs with a sore throat, cough, coryza, conjunctivitis, ulcerative stomatitis, or rash. In addition to a sore throat, GABHS pharyngitis may be associated with abdominal pain, fever, headache, and tender anterior cervical chain lymphadenopathy. The well-established Centor criteria can help clinicians determine who should be evaluated for GABHS with a rapid antigen test. GABHS most often occurs in children aged 5 to 15 years, so it is more likely to affect younger athletes than those in college or older. Athletes presenting with 0 or 1 of the Centor criteria—which include exudative tonsillitis, fever, tender anterior cervical adenopathy, and absence of cough—are unlikely to have GABHS and should not be tested. Athletes with two or more criteria should be tested for GABHS and treated if appropriate.

The mainstay of treatment of GABHS pharyngitis continues to be penicillin. Cephalexin and clindamycin are appropriate second-line choices for those who are allergic to penicillin. Treatment may reduce the duration of symptoms by 1 to 2 days. Athletes may participate in sports if symptoms are well controlled and hydration and nutrition status are adequate to perform rigorous physical activity.

Mononucleosis

Infectious mononucleosis (IM) is a clinical syndrome resulting from acute infection with the Epstein-Barr virus. Up to 90% of adults have serologic evidence of previous exposure to Epstein-Barr virus, although many of those infections never manifest or demonstrate the severe symptoms that can be associated with IM. The incidence of IM is highest in those age 15 to 25 years, making this problem particularly evident in college populations and collegiate athletic teams. Although no evidence exists that athletes are more susceptible to IM, the risks related to splenic rupture and the almost universal recommendation for a period of limited exercise make it a particularly frustrating diagnosis for college athletes.

The classic clinical findings of IM include a prodromal syndrome of headache, malaise, fatigue, and fever, followed by pharyngitis and lymphadenopathy. Other common symptoms include palatal petechiae (25%) and rash (10% to 40%). Pharyngitis is often exudative and frequently is accompanied by significant tonsillar hypertrophy. Physical examination also should include a careful abdominal examination to evaluate for splenomegaly. Palpation and percussion for splenomegaly should be a routine part of the physical examination in an athlete with possible IM despite a poor sensitivity of 20% to 70%.

Several laboratory tests can be used to aid in the diagnosis of IM. The presence of more than 10% atypical lymphocytes—in the setting of a relative lymphocytosis—suggests IM. A complete blood count also may reveal other nonspecific signs of a viral infection such as mild thrombocytopenia and leukocytosis. The heterophile antibody test has a reported sensitivity of 79% to 95% and a specificity of 82% to 99%, but results may be falsely negative if the test is performed early in the course of the illness. Repeat testing may be useful if clinical suspicion is high but initial tests are inconclusive. Epstein-Barr virus antibody tests are also available to confirm acute, subacute, or prior infection. Viral capsid antigens IgM and IgG are present early in the infection, and positive results are highly suggestive of an acute infection. The presence of nuclear antigen suggests prior infection.

As for most viral illnesses, the treatment of IM is primarily supportive. NSAIDs and acetaminophen are usually effective in controlling fever and pain. Athletes with severe symptoms or dehydration may benefit temporarily from corticosteroids, although no evidence exists to show that they provide any lasting benefit in the overall disease course. Patients who have profound tonsillar hypertrophy with resultant or impending airway compromise should receive corticosteroids and be monitored in a setting where advanced airway management is readily available. No indication for using antiviral medications exists in patients with a competent immune system. A high incidence of coinfection with group A streptococcus is present, and it is appropriate to treat patients who test positive with antibiotics. Amoxicillin use in patients with IM can cause a diffuse maculopapular rash, so it is prudent to consider an antibiotic from a different class, if possible.[25]

Splenic rupture is the most concerning potential complication of IM in the athletic population. The overall incidence in patients with IM is about 0.1% to 0.2%, and most documented cases have occurred within the first 3 weeks of symptoms. For this reason, it is recommended that athletes not participate in sports for 3 weeks from the onset of symptoms. Approximately 50% of splenic ruptures are atraumatic, so athletes should be advised to refrain from any exertional activity. Although ultrasonography of the spleen can determine its size, it is unclear whether that information should change clinical decision making. One study evaluated the average spleen size of tall, healthy athletes and revealed that the normal spleen size in a tall, healthy athlete is much larger than that in the average-size population, making the benefit of ultrasonography even less clear in taller athletes.[26] Although documentation of an enlarged spleen may provide some objective support when informing an athlete he or she may not compete, no data yet support a return to sports participation earlier than 3 weeks based on spleen size. Athletes may return to activity 3 weeks after the onset of symptoms if they are asymptomatic and afebrile. Although some authors report starting light activity before the 3-week mark, no literature is currently available that supports return to contact sports within 3 weeks of symptom onset, irrespective of spleen size or laboratory values.[27]

Pulmonary Infections

Bronchitis

Bronchitis is an inflammatory condition of the tracheobronchial tree resulting in a cough, which is often productive. It is caused most often by a virus but can occasionally be caused by atypical bacterial organisms. The most common causative organisms are similar to those that cause URIs. Rhinovirus, adenovirus, parainfluenza, and influenza A and B are the most common viral etiologies. Of those, only influenza may benefit from antiviral therapy. Potential bacterial causes include *Bordetella pertussis*, *Mycoplasma pneumoniae*, and *Chlamydophila pneumoniae*.

The clinical signs and symptoms of bronchitis overlap with other respiratory diseases. Athletes usually report a productive cough. They also may have wheezing related to airway inflammation, fever, and dyspnea on exertion. The color or quantity of the sputum cannot reliably differentiate bronchitis from pneumonia. The symptoms resolve with no specific therapy in most patients. Although no clear evidence shows that any therapy consistently improves symptoms, some patients may benefit from a short course of bronchodilators or antitussives.

Antibiotic therapy should be reserved for patients who are not improving or those who have underlying medical problems such as asthma, chronic obstructive pulmonary disease, or immunosuppression. Most athletes improve without antibiotic therapy, and few have true risk factors for a bacterial etiology. The early identification of athletes at risk for influenza is important. Treatment with antiviral medications including oseltamivir and zanamivir can be initiated within 48 hours of symptom onset and may reduce the length of symptomatology. The team physician also should consider whether prophylaxis with antiviral medications is appropriate for teammates or close contacts of a student athlete with influenza.[28]

If antibiotics are used for the treatment of bronchitis, amoxicillin, doxycycline, and azithromycin are reasonable choices. It is important to discuss potential antibiotic side effects with an athlete before medication is provided, particularly before administering a drug that is unlikely to substantially alter the disease course.

Pneumonia

Pneumonia is an infection of the lung parenchyma that results in several clinical findings. Athletes with pneumonia may report any combination of cough, chest pain, fever, general malaise, dyspnea at rest or on exertion, or reduced exercise tolerance. Physical examination can reveal tachycardia, tachypnea, crackles, rales, or tactile fremitus. No combination of clinical findings can reliably distinguish pneumonia from other respiratory illnesses; therefore, evidence of pneumonia on chest radiograph or other imaging is required for the diagnosis of pneumonia.

The appropriate treatment of pneumonia requires knowledge of the likely causative organisms. In the population of generally healthy athletes with community-acquired pneumonia, the most likely organisms are *S pneumoniae*, *H influenzae*, and *M pneumoniae*. First-line choices for antibiotic coverage include azithromycin, clarithromycin, or doxycycline. Athletes with risk factors for hospital-acquired pneumonia or significant comorbidities and those who recently have traveled internationally may require more broad antibiotic coverage.[29] The return to activity for athletes should be undertaken slowly and gradually. Athletes may increase activity as tolerated when antibiotic therapy is completed but should be advised that the recovery after pneumonia may be much longer than that after a routine URI.

Gastrointestinal and Genitourinary Infections

Gastrointestinal Infection

Acute gastrointestinal (GI) infection, or gastroenteritis, is the second most common condition in athletes after respiratory infection. Although acute GI illness generally is self-limited, the primary concern in athletes is dehydration. For traveling athletes, diarrhea is a common concern and a challenge when away from their home resources. Acute GI illness is related most often to a viral, bacterial, or protozoal etiology, with viral illness being the most common cause.

Viruses cause most cases of gastroenteritis, which occur most often in the winter months. The most common viruses identified include norovirus and rotavirus, and each virus causes millions of GI illnesses in the United States each year. The incubation period tends to be relatively short (24 to 60 hours), as does the duration (12 to 60 hours). The diagnosis is usually clinical, and the condition is characterized by diarrhea of short duration. Nausea, vomiting, and fever with abdominal discomfort also may be present. The treatment is generally symptomatic, although in athletes, intravenous fluids may be beneficial for acute dehydration secondary to diarrhea, vomiting, and intolerance of oral fluids. In addition, loperamide can be considered to prevent further diarrhea if the episode is clearly of viral etiology without blood in the stool, and it may help to minimize dehydration. If vomiting is occurring often, an antiemetic may be warranted.

For athletic teams, a major concern is the high rate of transmission with minimal contact. This has been demonstrated in a documented outbreak among 13 National Basketball Association teams, as well as in 9 members of a teenage girls' soccer team, who contracted the same norovirus strain from touching a reusable grocery bag or consuming its contents.[30,31] Transmission may be fecal-oral or secondary to exposure to vomit and, potentially, fomites, so members of the team who are ill should consider using a single restroom separate from that of healthy teammates. Encouraging the use of hand soap rather than hand sanitizer, especially during the winter months, is vital to minimizing outbreaks among teams. Team physicians also may consider holding ill athletes from competition for 24 to 72 hours to minimize transmission.

Most GI illnesses do not need studies for diagnosis. Only about 1.5% to 6.0% of all GI illnesses are bacterial in nature.[32] Patients with blood or pus in the stool with persistent fever, severe pain, pregnancy, or recent antibiotic use should be evaluated for bacterial causes of gastroenteritis, however. Patients with at least four loose stools per day for more than 3 days are considerably more likely to have an important pathogen.[33] Tests should include stool studies for fecal leukocytes and culture, and practitioners also should consider testing for ova and parasites if risk factors are present. *Clostridium difficile* testing is indicated if antibiotics have been used recently. Obtaining an adequate history is important; the history should include queries about recent meals, travel, camping and outdoor activity, natural water exposure, the frequency of stools, pets, and contact with others having similar symptoms.

Bacteria can cause GI illness in one of three ways: by the production of toxins, by direct invasion of the bowel with secondary inflammation, or by a combination of both. Inflammatory gastroenteritis includes infection with *Campylobacter*, *Shigella*, *Salmonella*, enterohemorrhagic *Escherichia coli*, and *C difficile* (Table 1). Rapid-onset diarrhea related to food intake also can help narrow the diagnosis. Diarrhea from *S aureus* or *Bacillus cereus* typically occurs within 6 hours of ingestion, because of a preformed toxin. Infection with *Clostridium perfringens* occurs at 8 to 16 hours after ingestion. Patients with signs of bacterial infection after recent antibiotic use should undergo stool testing for *C difficile* and treatment if the test is positive. Probiotics may play a role in reducing the risk of antibiotic-associated diarrhea.[34]

Protozoal infections are less common, but can include *Cryptosporidium parvum*, *Giardia lamblia*, and *Entameoba histolytica* (Table 1).

Genitourinary or Sexually Transmitted Infection

Sexually transmitted infections (STIs) have been described as a hidden epidemic, partially because of the reluctance of society to openly address sexual health. This is even more critical in some athletic populations that may demonstrate an increased likelihood of risky sexual behavior. Older male high school athletes as well as male and female collegiate athletes are more likely to demonstrate risk-taking behavior than are their peers, including having multiple sexual partners and not practicing safe sex.[35,36] Therefore, understanding how to identify, treat, and prevent common STIs is essential to the sports medicine provider.

HPV is the most common STI in the United States. Most men and women in the United States will be infected with HPV at some point in their lives. HPV usually resolves with time and causes no morbidity, although some subtypes can progress to genital warts, and other subtypes have been linked to several cancers, including cervical, anal, and some oropharyngeal cancers.

Genital warts typically are caused by HPV 6 and HPV 11 and may present as cauliflower-like, flat, papular, or keratotic lesions on the penis, vulva, perineum, or mucosal surfaces. In general, cryotherapy or trichloracetic acid is used to destroy the lesions, although biopsy should be considered in lesions that are atypical or if the diagnosis is not confirmed. Approximately 70% of all cervical cancers are caused by HPV types 16 and 18. HPV vaccines are directed at high-risk subtypes, and have been shown to be effective.[37,38] Vaccination is recommended for both males and females at age 11 or 12 years, and for those not vaccinated previously, the vaccine is approved through age 21 years for males and age 26 years for females.

Chlamydia trachomatis is the second most common STI in the United States, although more than half of cases are undiagnosed. Chlamydia infections are asymptomatic in 90% of women and 60% of men, and it primarily affects those between the ages of 15 and 25 years.[39] Of those who are not treated, the infection resolves spontaneously in about 30%, but the rest remain persistently infected or pelvic inflammatory disease eventually develops. Infection with chlamydia increases an individual's risk of HIV contraction. It is therefore recommended that women younger than 25 years be screened annually for chlamydia. Screening has been shown to reduce the incidence of pelvic inflammatory disease by 50%.[40] Symptomatic women often present with cervical inflammation or yellow, cloudy discharge from the cervical os, and symptomatic men may present with discharge from the penis. Urine testing is effective and has largely replaced the more invasive swab test. Treatment is simple and effective, with azithromycin single-dose oral therapy as the primary option. Those with a positive test should abstain from intercourse for at least 7 days after treatment, and partners of infected individuals having sexual contact within the past 60 days should be tested or treated presumptively.

Neisseria gonorrhoeae infection is less common than is chlamydia, but it can be difficult to distinguish from chlamydia initially on presentation. Both men and women may have discharge, although women may be more likely to be asymptomatic. If a high clinical suspicion for *N gonorrhoeae* or chlamydia is present, providers may consider treating for both. The treatment of *N gonorrhoeae* is generally effective with a single dose of ceftriaxone, although resistance to ceftriaxone is possible. Frequently, coinfection with chlamydia is present, and the US Centers for Disease Control and Prevention (CDC) therefore recommends treatment with both ceftriaxone

Table 1

Overview of the Etiologies of Nonviral Gastroenteritis

Causative Agent	Important Characteristics	Treatment Options (in Addition to Supportive Therapy)
Campylobacter	Results from ingestion of meat, poultry, dairy products Usually self-limited, resolves in 5–7 days	Only small subset of patients benefit from antibiotics Azithromycin and erythromycin are most likely to be beneficial
Shigella	More common in children younger than 5 years More common in developing countries Bloody diarrhea	Antibiotics may shorten course Ciprofloxacin (caution: may cause tendinitis) Ceftriaxone Azithromycin
Salmonella	Results from ingestion of poultry, dairy products, reptile exposure Outbreaks with peanut products and raw produce	Ciprofloxacin (caution: may cause tendinitis) Ceftriaxone Azithromycin
Enterohemorrhagic E. coli	More common than enterotoxigenic E coli in United States Releases toxins; can cause systemic complications Most common serotype is O157:H7 10% of patients with O157:H7 develop hemolytic uremic syndrome	Azithromycin
Enterotoxigenic E coli	Most common cause of traveler's diarrhea	Likely needs antibiotics Ciprofloxacin (caution: may cause tendinitis) Ceftriaxone Azithromycin
Clostridium difficile	Associated with antibiotic use Laboratory: stool enzyme immunoassay for toxins A and B Admission recommended unless no systemic symptoms and no organ dysfunction	Discontinue current antibiotic agent Treat with oral metronidazole Vancomycin (resistant or recurrent cases)
Cryptosporidium parvum (protozoan parasite)	Can transmit via bird or cattle feces leeching through soil into water supply; can transmit human to human Causes "rice water diarrhea" (similar to cholera) Laboratory: stool microscopy detection of oocysts or stool test for Cryptosporidium antigen	Self-limited, usually resolves with symptomatic care Nitazoxanide for persistent cases
Giardia lamblia (flagellated protozoan parasite)	Fecal-oral transmission Campers drinking from streams, especially in the mountains Pools can be a source Laboratory: stool microscopy detection of cysts or trophozoites	Metronidazole Pregnancy, first trimester: Paromomycin
Entamoeba histolytica	Diarrhea over 1 week Weight loss and abdominal tenderness Can develop liver abscess, rarely, brain abscess Laboratory: stool test for Entamoeba histolytica antigen	Treat with metronidazole initially. Follow with luminal agent paromomycin to eradicate colon infection.

E coli = Escherichia coli

and azithromycin in cases of a positive *N gonorrhoeae* test. Genital tract infection with *N. gonorrhea* can disseminate to other areas of the body and cause skin and synovial infections, underscoring the importance of prompt, adequate treatment.

Blood-Borne Infectious Illness

With the rapid escalation in the prevalence and knowledge of illnesses such as HIV infection and hepatitis over the past 30 years, blood-borne illnesses and their potential for transmission have been a major concern for athletes and medical care providers. Fortunately, the risk of transmission during sports activity is relatively low. Of the three blood-borne illnesses discussed in this section, hepatitis B is 10 times more likely to be transmitted than hepatitis C, and 100 times more likely to be transmitted than HIV.[41]

Hepatitis B has a higher risk of transmission because of the higher levels of infectious virus in the blood. Documented cases have been reported of transmission in sumo wrestlers and Olympic wrestlers, although these cases were noted in areas with a high prevalence of hepatitis B in the general population.[42,43] Hepatitis B is most likely to be transmitted via perinatal mother-to-child exposure, parenteral exposure, or sexual intercourse; infection via mucosal contact with infected blood or blood products is less likely. Most of those infected with hepatitis B are asymptomatic, or the infection clears spontaneously, but complications such as liver failure, cirrhosis, and hepatocellular carcinoma are possible. The diagnosis is made primarily on serologic markers, and treatment is based on chronicity, age, the severity of disease, the likelihood of response, and potential adverse events. The hepatitis B vaccine is a routine part of the childhood vaccination series and should be considered for adults with risk factors based on lifestyle or potential occupational exposure.

Hepatitis C is much more likely to be contracted by athletes from parenteral exposure than during sports activity or sexual intercourse. Therefore, athletes who are involved in blood doping, steroid use, or other illicit drug use are at the highest risk of hepatitis C infection.[44] Of patients exposed to hepatitis C, chronic infection develops in 55% to 85% ; of those with chronic infection, most are asymptomatic. The workup initially includes testing for antibodies to determine infection, followed by viral genotyping and viral load testing to determine treatment options.

HIV continues to be an important illness worldwide, but with adequate medical treatment including antiretroviral therapy, it is not the rapidly terminal illness it once was. Although many well-known athletes have received an HIV diagnosis, only one case is thought to have been transmitted during sports activity.[45] Athletes are much more likely to contract HIV during non–sport-related activity, such as blood doping and intravenous drug use, than by participating in sports.[41]

Meningitis

In the athletic team setting, meningitis is one of the more concerning diagnoses, given the potential for transmission and the severity of illness. Most commonly, the cause of meningitis is viral or cannot be determined (aseptic meningitis). Bacterial illness is infrequent, but can produce substantial mortality, with complications including neurologic sequelae. Because of the early difficulty in differentiating between the two etiologies, the clinician must suspect a bacterial cause initially.[46]

Outbreaks among sports teams, most commonly American football teams, have been reported. Echovirus and coxsackie virus, both in the *Enterovirus* genus, have been isolated in most of these cases.[47,48] These viruses are spread primarily via fecal-oral transmission, but also can be spread via respiratory secretions, leading to possible transmission during the sharing of water bottles among teammates.

Symptoms of meningitis include nausea, vomiting, photophobia, malaise, and drowsiness. These symptoms may be present in viral and bacterial meningitis but are usually more severe in bacterial meningitis. The classic triad of signs of bacterial meningitis is fever, neck stiffness, and altered mental status, but all three signs are present in only 44% of cases.[49] It is important to evaluate for nuchal rigidity and to determine the presence of meningeal signs, including the Kernig and the Brudzinski signs. A thorough skin examination should be performed to evaluate for hemorrhagic lesions associated with meningococcal meningitis. Lumbar puncture is the most important diagnostic test in those suspected to have meningitis, although in some cases, CT of the head should be performed before lumbar puncture.[50] In addition, blood should be drawn for culture as early as possible.

Treatment initially includes antimicrobial therapy until bacterial meningitis can be ruled out. The Infectious Diseases Society of America guidelines suggest that antimicrobial therapy should be instituted as soon as the diagnosis of bacterial meningitis is suspected or proven and not delayed to await the results of lumbar puncture or imaging studies.[50] After a diagnosis is determined, treatment depends on the specific etiology of meningitis.

In the team setting, preventive measures are vital if meningitis has been diagnosed in a single athlete. These measures should include consistent handwashing, disinfecting shared areas, using single-use cups instead of communally served drinks, and isolating the athlete with meningitis.[46] The CDC recommends vaccination for meningococcal disease at ages 11 to 12 years, with a booster at age 16 years.

Summary

Infectious diseases in athletes can be common causes of time lost from training or competition. Certain factors relating to immune function and potential exposures can alter an athlete's risk for infectious diseases. The medical team must therefore be proficient in the diagnosis and management of these conditions to safely guide return-to-play decisions for athletes. Preventive measures should be taken when possible to reduce the risks of initial infections and outbreaks among members of athletic teams.

Key Study Points

- Infectious disease illnesses constitute a substantial level of morbidity in athletes, and a familiarity with these illnesses will aid sports medicine physicians in caring for their athletes.

- Maximizing preventative efforts in both hygiene and environmental exposures is effective to decrease risks of several infectious disease illnesses, including gastroenteritis and MRSA.

- Early identification and relative isolation of athletes with communicable diseases including influenza and gastroenteritis will help prevent rapid spread within the team setting.

Annotated References

1. Martin SA, Pence BD, Woods JA: Exercise and respiratory tract viral infections. *Exerc Sport Sci Rev* 2009;37(4):157-164.

   The authors proposed a model detailing modulation of immune function due to moderate exercise and the corresponding effect on respiratory viral infections.

2. Walsh NP, Gleeson M, Shephard RJ, et al: Position statement. Part one: Immune function and exercise. *Exerc Immunol Rev* 2011;17:6-63.

   A position statement from experts in the field is presented regarding the current understanding of the effect of exercise on immune function.

3. Spence L, Brown WJ, Pyne DB, et al: Incidence, etiology, and symptomatology of upper respiratory illness in elite athletes. *Med Sci Sports Exerc* 2007;39(4):577-586.

4. Malachowa N, Kobayashi SD, DeLeo FR: Community-associated methicillin-resistant Staphylococcus aureus and athletes. *Phys Sportsmed* 2012;40(2):13-21.

   This review article outlined MRSA among athletes with regard to epidemiology and virulence, with special attention given to outpatient management and prevention strategies.

5. Buss BF, Connolly S: Surveillance of physician-diagnosed skin and soft tissue infections consistent with methicillin-resistant Staphylococcus aureus (MRSA) among Nebraska high school athletes, 2008-2012. *J Sch Nurs* 2014;30(1):42-48.

   Data compiled from this survey-based 2014 study showed MRSA rates among Nebraska high school students over a 4-year span across different sports.

6. Pereira LB: Impetigo - review. *An Bras Dermatol* 2014;89(2):293-299.

   This review article detailed the etiologies, types, and clinical presentation of impetigo and provided a broad outline of available treatment options.

7. Lutz JK, Lee J: Prevalence and antimicrobial-resistance of Pseudomonas aeruginosa in swimming pools and hot tubs. *Int J Environ Res Public Health* 2011;8(2):554-564.

   This surveillance study collected *Pseudomonas* samples from hot tubs and pools to measure antibiotic susceptibility and resistance patterns. Level of evidence: III.

8. Levy JA: Common bacterial dermatoses: Protecting competitive athletes. *Phys Sportsmed* 2004;32(6):33-39.

9. Vlahovic TC, Dunn SP, Kemp K: The use of a clindamycin 1%-benzoyl peroxide 5% topical gel in the treatment of pitted keratolysis: A novel therapy. *Adv Skin Wound Care* 2009;22(12):564-566.

10. van der Snoek EM, Ekkelenkamp MB, Suykerbuyk JC: Pitted keratolysis; physicians' treatment and their perceptions in Dutch army personnel. *J Eur Acad Dermatol Venereol* 2013;27(9):1120-1126.

    This cross-sectional questionnaire conducted among physicians assessed deployability and the perceived efficacy of treatment of Dutch soldiers.

11. Kwok CS, Gibbs S, Bennett C, Holland R, Abbott R: Topical treatments for cutaneous warts. *Cochrane Database Syst Rev* 2012;9:CD001781.

    This article is the updated comprehensive Cochrane review detailing all available data regarding the treatment of cutaneous warts, including comprehensive comparative data and practice suggestions. Level of evidence: II.

12. Wenner R, Askari SK, Cham PM, Kedrowski DA, Liu A, Warshaw EM: Duct tape for the treatment of common warts in adults: A double-blind randomized controlled trial. *Arch Dermatol* 2007;143(3):309-313.

13. Chen X, Anstey AV, Bugert JJ: Molluscum contagiosum virus infection. *Lancet Infect Dis* 2013;13(10):877-888.

    This review article outlined the condition's clinical features, management, and epidemiology, and provided a detailed review of molluscum contagiosum virus virology, immunology, and genetic patterns.

14. Zinder SM, Basler RS, Foley J, Scarlata C, Vasily DB: National athletic trainers' association position statement: Skin diseases. *J Athl Train* 2010;45(4):411-428.

    This National Athletic Trainers' Association 2010 comprehensive position statement on skin diseases in athletes included overviews of individual disease processes, potential treatments, and return-to-play guidelines.

15. Anderson BJ: The epidemiology and clinical analysis of several outbreaks of herpes gladiatorum. *Med Sci Sports Exerc* 2003;35(11):1809-1814.

16. Dworkin RH, Barbano RL, Tyring SK, et al: A randomized, placebo-controlled trial of oxycodone and of gabapentin for acute pain in herpes zoster. *Pain* 2009;142(3):209-217.

    This randomized controlled trial studied postherpetic neuralgia and the effect of oxycodone against gabapentin and placebo over 28 days of treatment. Level of evidence: II.

17. Weinberg JM, Koestenblatt EK: Treatment of interdigital tinea pedis: Once-daily therapy with sertaconazole nitrate. *J Drugs Dermatol* 2011;10(10):1135-1140.

    This small trial showed that sertaconazole is an effective once daily topical treatment of interdigital tinea pedis, which may promote adherence to therapy. Level of evidence: II.

18. El-Gohary M, van Zuuren EJ, Fedorowicz Z, et al: Topical antifungal treatments for tinea cruris and tinea corporis. *Cochrane Database Syst Rev* 2014;8:CD009992.

    This systematic review of the existing literature from 1946 to 2013 outlined and compared available topical treatments of tinea cruris and tinea corporis. Level of evidence: I.

19. Azari AA, Barney NP: Conjunctivitis: A systematic review of diagnosis and treatment. *JAMA* 2013;310(16):1721-1729.

    This review article summarized the most recent information regarding all types of conjunctivitis. Level of evidence: II.

20. Artieda J, Pineiro L, Gonzalez M, et al: A swimming pool-related outbreak of pharyngoconjunctival fever in children due to adenovirus type 4, Gipuzkoa, Spain, 2008. *Euro Surveill* 2009;14(8).

    This article presented a case series of 59 children in whom pharyngoconjunctival fever caused by adenovirus developed as a result of poorly disinfected swimming pools in Spain. Level of evidence: IV.

21. Pinto RD, Lira RP, Abe RY, et al: Dexamethasone/povidone eye drops versus artificial tears for treatment of presumed viral conjunctivitis: A randomized clinical trial. *Curr Eye Res* 2014;13:1-8.

    This randomized controlled trial investigated the effect of a dexamethasone/povidone-iodine eye drop on the symptoms and duration of viral conjunctivitis. It showed that, compared with artificial tears, dexamethasone/povidone-iodine drops reduced the duration of conjunctivitis by about 2 days but caused more stinging. Level of evidence: II.

22. Harmes KM, Blackwood RA, Burrows HL, Cooke JM, Harrison RV, Passamani PP: Otitis media: Diagnosis and treatment. *Am Fam Physician* 2013;88(7):435-440.

    This review article reported the current recommendations for the diagnosis and treatment of acute otitis media and otitis media with effusion.

23. Bonney AG, Goldman RD: Antihistamines for children with otitis media. *Can Fam Physician* 2014;60(1):43-46.

    This review article discussed the use of decongestants, antihistamines, or both, for otitis media in children. The authors concluded that no consistent evidence shows that decongestants or antihistamines are beneficial in the symptomatic treatment or faster resolution of otitis media.

24. Rosenfeld RM, Schwartz SR, Cannon CR, et al: Clinical practice guideline: Acute otitis externa. *Otolaryngol Head Neck Surg* 2014;150(1, Suppl)S1-S24.

    This review article presented comprehensive guidelines for the diagnosis and treatment of acute otitis externa, with a complete review of the current literature. Level of evidence: V.

25. Putukian M, O'Connor FG, Stricker P, et al: Mononucleosis and athletic participation: An evidence-based subject review. *Clin J Sport Med* 2008;18(4):309-315.

    This review article provided all the current information regarding guidelines for the safe return to play after infectious mononucleosis. The authors concluded that athletes should be held from sports participation until asymptomatic. There are some studies that suggest return to contact activity before 3 weeks is safe.

26. McCorkle R, Thomas B, Suffaletto H, Jehle D: Normative spleen size in tall healthy athletes: Implications for safe return to contact sports after infectious mononucleosis. *Clin J Sport Med* 2010;20(6):413-415.

    This cohort study investigated the average spleen size of tall healthy athletes compared with those having the accepted average adult spleen sizes. The findings concluded that tall athletes had much larger spleens than those with the published average sizes and that spleen size may not reflect pathology in tall athletes. Level of evidence: IV.

27. Becker JA, Smith JA: Return to play after infectious mononucleosis. *Sports Health* 2014;6(3):232-238.

    In this clinical review on the evidence for return to play after infectious mononucleosis, the key conclusions include the unreliability of spleen size in guiding return to play, individualization in determining the return to play, and the recommendation that athletes be asymptomatic before returning to sports.

28. Worrall G: Acute bronchitis. *Can Fam Physician* 2008;54(2):238-239.

29. Smoot MK, Hosey RG: Pulmonary infections in the athlete. *Curr Sports Med Rep* 2009;8(2):71-75.

    This review article summarizes recent information and recommendations on community-acquired pneumonia and bronchitis in athletes.

30. Desai R, Yen C, Wikswo M, et al: Transmission of norovirus among NBA players and staff, winter 2010-2011. *Clin Infect Dis* 2011;53(11):1115-1117.

    This case series documented an outbreak of norovirus among teammates and between teams in the National Basketball Association. Level of evidence: IV.

31. Repp KK, Keene WE: A point-source norovirus outbreak caused by exposure to fomites. *J Infect Dis* 2012;205(11):1639-1641.

    This case review documents an outbreak of norovirus affecting several members of a soccer team, in which a contaminated grocery bag and its contents were implicated as the source of infection, suggesting that fomites can become airborne and lead to infection. Level of evidence: V.

32. Guerrant RL, Van Gilder T, Steiner TS, et al; Infectious Diseases Society of America: Practice guidelines for the management of infectious diarrhea. *Clin Infect Dis* 2001;32(3):331-351.

33. Dryden MS, Gabb RJ, Wright SK: Empirical treatment of severe acute community-acquired gastroenteritis with ciprofloxacin. *Clin Infect Dis* 1996;22(6):1019-1025.

34. Kale-Pradhan PB, Jassal HK, Wilhelm SM: Role of Lactobacillus in the prevention of antibiotic-associated diarrhea: A meta-analysis. *Pharmacotherapy* 2010;30(2):119-126.

    This article is a meta-analysis examining the use of the probiotic *Lactobacillus* to reduce the risk of diarrhea secondary to antibiotic use. Level of evidence: I.

35. Nattiv A, Puffer JC, Green GA: Lifestyles and health risks of collegiate athletes: A multi-center study. *Clin J Sport Med* 1997;7(4):262-272.

36. Wetherill RR, Fromme K: Alcohol use, sexual activity, and perceived risk in high school athletes and non-athletes. *J Adolesc Health* 2007;41(3):294-301.

37. FUTURE II Study Group: Quadrivalent vaccine against human papillomavirus to prevent high-grade cervical lesions. *N Engl J Med* 2007;356(19):1915-1927.

38. Paavonen J, Naud P, Salmerón J, et al; HPV PATRICIA Study Group: Efficacy of human papillomavirus (HPV)-16/18 AS04-adjuvanted vaccine against cervical infection and precancer caused by oncogenic HPV types (PATRICIA): Final analysis of a double-blind, randomised study in young women. *Lancet* 2009;374(9686):301-314.

    An analysis of a randomized, double-blind trial assessing the efficacy of HPV-16/18 ASO4-adjuvanted vaccine against HPV infections is presented. Primary outcome showed high efficacy against CIN2+ associated with HPV 16/18. Level of evidence: I.

39. Hennrikus E, Oberto D, Linder JM, Rempel JM, Hennrikus N: Sports preparticipation examination to screen college athletes for Chlamydia trachomatis. *Med Sci Sports Exerc* 2010;42(4):683-688.

    This article is a prospective prevalence study reporting the rate of chlamydia based on random urine testing in college athletes. Level of evidence: II.

40. Scholes D, Stergachis A, Heidrich FE, Andrilla H, Holmes KK, Stamm WE: Prevention of pelvic inflammatory disease by screening for cervical chlamydial infection. *N Engl J Med* 1996;334(21):1362-1366.

41. Gutierrez RL, Decker CF: Blood-borne infections and the athlete. *Dis Mon* 2010;56(7):436-442.

    This review article focused on hepatitis B, hepatitis C, the risks of transmission in athletic activity, and recommendations for prevention in athletic settings.

42. Bae SK, Yatsuhashi H, Takahara I, et al: Sequential occurrence of acute hepatitis B among members of a high school Sumo wrestling club. *Hepatol Res* 2014;44(10):E267-E272.

    This case report discussed a hepatitis B infection most likely transmitted between two members of a Sumo wrestling team and a coach. Level of evidence: V.

43. Bereket-Yücel S: Risk of hepatitis B infections in Olympic wrestling. *Br J Sports Med* 2007;41(5):306-310, discussion 310.

44. Aitken C, Delalande C, Stanton K: Pumping iron, risking infection? Exposure to hepatitis C, hepatitis B and HIV among anabolic-androgenic steroid injectors in Victoria, Australia. *Drug Alcohol Depend* 2002;65(3):303-308.

45. Torre D, Sampietro C, Ferraro G, Zeroli C, Speranza F: Transmission of HIV-1 infection via sports injury. *Lancet* 1990;335(8697):1105.

46. Ewald AJ, McKeag DB: Meningitis in the athlete. *Curr Sports Med Rep* 2008;7(1):22-27.

47. Moore M, Baron RC, Filstein MR, et al: Aseptic meningitis and high school football players. 1978 and 1980. *JAMA* 1983;249(15):2039-2042.

48. Baron RC, Hatch MH, Kleeman K, MacCormack JN: Aseptic meningitis among members of a high school football team. An outbreak associated with echovirus 16 infection. *JAMA* 1982;248(14):1724-1727.

49. van de Beek D, de Gans J, Spanjaard L, Weisfelt M, Reitsma JB, Vermeulen M: Clinical features and prognostic factors in adults with bacterial meningitis. *N Engl J Med* 2004;351(18):1849-1859.

50. Tunkel AR, Hartman BJ, Kaplan SL, et al: Practice guidelines for the management of bacterial meningitis. *Clin Infect Dis* 2004;39(9):1267-1284.

© 2016 American Academy of Orthopaedic Surgeons

Chapter 44

Facial Injuries

Jeffrey A. Housner, MD, MBA   Laurie D. Donaldson, MD

Abstract

Because of the nature of current sports activities, the clinician who cares for the athlete must be prepared to recognize and assess a variety of injuries that can occur to the face. A comprehensive framework is necessary to guide the evaluation, treatment, and triage of injuries to the skin, eyes, ears, teeth, and bones sustained as a result of facial trauma. Life-threatening injuries are given priority and must be ruled out initially. Injuries that require emergency department evaluation and/or specialty consultation warrant immediate attention. The objectives for management include parallel goals: the restoration of normal function and the attainment of acceptable cosmetics. The prevention of facial injuries, particularly dental trauma, remains a critical component of the preservation of facial structures. Return-to-play considerations also should be discussed.

Keywords: facial trauma; facial injuries; sports

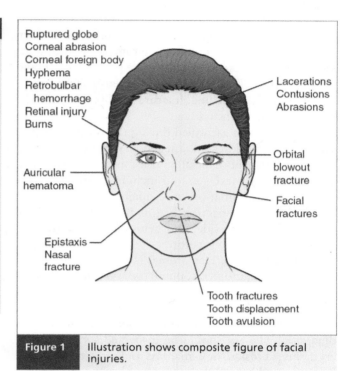

Figure 1 Illustration shows composite figure of facial injuries.

Introduction

Facial trauma is common in sports activities, yet the true incidence of all facial injuries sustained during sports participation is unknown. Sports injuries to the face occur in a variety of settings and can be treated with minimal intervention that is not reported or recorded by traditional surveillance methods.[1] A 2014 comprehensive review determined that sports accidents were the causative factor in approximately 10% of all maxillofacial fractures worldwide.[2] Participation in many types of sports can result in facial injuries, with a higher occurrence noted during rugby, soccer, cycling, basketball, skiing, and ice hockey.[3-6] Most injuries occur in boys and men between the ages of 10 and 29 years.[7] The mechanism of injury is usually self-evident and results from contact with the ground (for example, the field, floor, or mat); with the head, elbow, fist, or foot of an opponent; or with equipment such as a ball, puck, stick, or post. Facial injuries can result in significant physical disfigurement and can have devastating psychologic effects. Therefore, expedient and effective treatment is needed to promote optimal healing and minimize psychologic trauma. An organized and sequential evaluation, undertaken while considering a broad differential diagnosis (Figure 1), is necessary for the prompt recognition of facial injuries and the appropriate triage and treatment.

Initial Assessment

Disfiguring facial injuries can be distracting to the patient and the clinician. Nevertheless, clinicians must focus on

Neither of the following authors nor any immediate family member has received anything of value from or has stock or stock options held in a commercial company or institution related directly or indirectly to the subject of this chapter: Dr. Housner and Dr. Donaldson.

the basics of trauma care (the primary survey) and address all life-threatening injuries before performing a complete facial examination. As part of the primary survey, and while maintaining cervical spine immobilization, an evaluation for airway compromise, impaired breathing, hemorrhagic shock, and an altered level of consciousness should be performed immediately. The unconscious athlete should be assumed to have a cervical spine injury. If the athlete is conscious, query to ensure no neck pain or cervical tenderness is present. Any injury above the clavicle is assumed to involve the cervical spine until proven otherwise. When ongoing reports of neurologic symptoms or cervical spine tenderness are present, cervical spine precautions should be undertaken. The initial assessment also should focus on the control of bleeding, fracture stabilization, and the recognition of a concussion.

After problems identified during the primary survey are adequately addressed, a secondary survey, including careful assessment of facial injuries, must be performed. The secondary survey should include a systematic approach and examination of all major facial structures and functions. Inspection begins by viewing the face from the front, the side, and below. It is important to assess for asymmetry before swelling begins and distorts facial features. Hematoma, lacerations, erythema, a sunken globe, proptosis, pupillary asymmetry, redness or bleeding within the eye, a widening of the midface, depression of the zygomatic arch, septal deviation, and septal hematoma should be noted to guide the differential diagnosis. The ear should be inspected for laceration, erythema, abrasion, or hematoma and assessment should be performed behind the ear for any bruising (the Battle sign), which indicates basilar skull fracture. An intraoral examination should be performed to look for lacerations or missing teeth. The facial bones, temporomandibular joints, muscles, and areas of suspected injury should be palpated for tenderness, crepitus, swelling, instability, dislocation, fracture, and foreign bodies. The lips, the cheeks, and the floor of the mouth should be bimanually palpated. A bimanual examination of the maxilla and mandible is performed to assess for fracture or instability.

Ocular movements are assessed for range of motion. If range of motion is limited, this sign could suggest an extraocular muscle entrapment that can occur with an orbital fracture. Diplopia or visual disturbance with extraocular movements could suggest muscle entrapment or injury to cranial nerve III, IV, or VI. Sensation should be checked at the forehead, cheek, and jaw to test cranial nerve V. Motor function can be tested by having the athlete raise his or her eyebrows, shut the eyelids tight, smile widely, and pucker the lips. If the athlete is able to perform these functions, cranial nerve VII is likely intact. Finally,

whispering or rubbing the fingertips near the ear can test hearing. An oto-ophthalmoscope also should be used to assess for blood or fluid in the external canal that could indicate basilar skull fracture. The tympanic membrane also can be viewed for rupture, which can occur during trauma. In addition, the oto-ophthalmoscope can be used to look into the nose for septal hematoma.

Soft-Tissue Injuries

Contusions

Facial contusions are common injuries in the athlete, ranging from mild to severe. Treatment is primarily supportive, directed at treating pain and swelling. Cryotherapy typically is used—with caution to avoid cold burning the skin—to help reduce swelling and discomfort. Most contusions resolve within a few weeks without any further intervention.

Abrasions

Abrasions, defined as wounds to the superficial layers of the skin, are also common soft-tissue injuries. Because of the mechanism of injury, abrasions involve more surface area than they do depth. As a consequence, they are not amenable to suture closure. Healing occurs via the reepithelialization of the skin layers. Abrasions are managed by removing any foreign debris and by thorough cleansing and irrigation with soap and water. A nonadherent dressing can be applied to help prevent contamination and to promote healing.

Lacerations

Careful exploration of every laceration should be performed to determine its severity, to remove debris, and to assess for damage to underlying muscles, tendons, nerves, blood vessels, or bone. The goals of laceration repair are to achieve hemostasis, avoid infection, restore function, and achieve optimal cosmetic results. Definitive laceration management depends on the time elapsed since injury, the extent and location of the wound, the available laceration repair materials, and the skill of the physician. The decision to allow the wound to heal by secondary intention or to close it is based on clinical judgment.[8] The decision to perform primary closure or refer to subspecialty care ultimately is based on the physician's level of expertise, experience, and comfort with managing the laceration.[9] Laceration wounds should be irrigated with normal saline or tap water.[10] Povidone iodine solution, hydrogen peroxide, and detergents should not be used because their toxicity to fibroblasts impedes healing in wounds that penetrate the dermis.[8] The wound can be irrigated with any method that delivers sufficient volume and pressure.

The necessary volume of fluid will vary, based on the size of the wound and the degree of contamination. A common delivery method consists of discharging the fluid from a syringe through a needle or angiocatheter. A useful on-field tip is to repeatedly puncture a quarter-sized area of a bottle of normal saline with a needle. The wound can then be showered by squeezing the bottle.

Primary repair is usually the preferred treatment of facial lacerations. In general, facial lacerations without risk factors for infection can be closed within 24 hours if appropriately cleansed.[8] Laceration repair follows common wound-closure principles of aseptic technique and universal body fluid precautions. Optimal cosmetic results can be achieved by using the finest suture possible, depending on skin thickness and wound tension. Suture material larger than No. 6-0 is rarely used on the face. Most facial lacerations can be closed with acceptable cosmetic result using a single interrupted or running closure technique and nylon suture. Lacerations involving the lacrimal apparatus, parotid gland, facial nerve, or vermillion border of the lip should be repaired only by an experienced practitioner. If the laceration is too complex, the athlete should be referred to a surgical subspecialist. Sutures placed on the face should be removed in 5 to 7 days. Skin staples should not be used on the face but can be considered for use on the scalp.

Eyelid lacerations are an important subtype of facial lacerations. Superficial, simple lacerations that are horizontal and follow the skin lines usually heal well without suturing. More complicated eyelid lacerations should be referred to subspecialty care for evaluation and management.

Local anesthesia with lidocaine 1% or bupivacaine 0.25% is appropriate for small wounds. Anesthetics that contain epinephrine should not be used on the nose or ears. The sting of anesthetic injections can be reduced by injecting slowly, warming the anesthetic, or buffering it with sodium bicarbonate (1 mL of sodium bicarbonate per 10 mL of anesthetic).[11] Although local anesthetic injected directly around the wound border usually provides adequate anesthesia, a selected facial nerve block can provide more effective anesthesia without distorting the wound edges. In a nerve block, anesthesia is injected directly adjacent to the nerve supplying the surgical field. Three useful nerve blocks invaluable for facial laceration repair are the supraorbital, infraorbital, and mental. All three nerves lie on an imaginary straight vertical line that passes through the pupil and the corner of the mouth (**Figure 2**). The supraorbital nerve, which provides sensation to the lateral forehead, emerges from the supraorbital foramen along the orbital rim. The supraorbital notch can be palpated along the superior orbital rim.

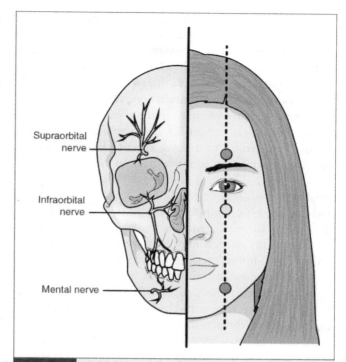

Figure 2 Illustration shows the alignment of the supraorbital notch, the infraorbital foramen, and the mental foramen in a vertical line passing through the pupil and the corner of the mouth.

The infraorbital nerve, which provides sensation to the upper lip, cheek, and lateral nose, emerges from the infraorbital foramen just below the inferior border of the orbit. The mental nerve, which provides sensation to the lower lip and chin, exits from the mental foramen of the mandible. All of these nerve blocks can be approached transdermally using a 25-gauge or 27-gauge needle gently advanced through the skin. The infraorbital and mental nerves also can be approached intraorally with less discomfort to the patient.[12] The upper lip (for infraorbital nerve block) or lower lip (for mental nerve block) is retracted and the small-gauge needle is pierced into the fold where the gingiva and buccal mucosa meet. The needle is advanced slowly less than 1 cm along the periosteum until met by external pressure from a guide finger directly palpating the nerve. Conceptually, this approach may sound unpleasant, but in practice, less pain occurs than with a transdermal approach, and the procedure is more technically straightforward. Generally, only 1 to 2 mL of anesthetic agent is needed to anesthetize the nerve for the three previously described nerve blocks.

Tissue adhesives, such as 2-octylcyanoacrylate, present another option for laceration repair. They are comparable with sutures in cosmetic results, dehiscence rates, and infection risk.[13,14] Tissue adhesives can be applied more quickly, however, without anesthesia, and they need little or no follow-up.[9] Tissue adhesives can be used for the closure of simple lacerations less than 4 cm in length that do not involve areas of high skin tension. To close the wound, the edges are approximated and the adhesive is applied in a thin layer. Three to four layers are applied, waiting 30 seconds between applications. Extreme caution should be exercised when using adhesive close to the eye.

Epistaxis

Because the blood supply to the nose is extensive, the athlete who sustains trauma to the nose usually presents with epistaxis, which may or may not be associated with a nasal bone fracture. Epistaxis generally occurs because of microdisruption to the Kiesselbach plexus in the anteroinferior septum. Bleeding can be controlled by applying pressure with the fingers to the nasal alae tightly against the septum for 10 to 15 minutes or by using nasal packing with cotton or gauze. In cases that do not respond to direct pressure, many otolaryngologists recommend initial treatment with two sprays of oxymetazoline to hasten hemostasis, although few published data exist to support the practice.[15] In severe cases, when the source of the bleeding can be identified, chemical cautery with silver nitrate can be considered after determining that topical anesthesia is adequate. Bleeding from posterior nasal sources usually originates from a branch of the sphenopalatine artery and may require posterior packing. If bleeding is not controlled, the athlete must be seen by a subspecialist for definitive treatment.

Facial Fractures

The diagnosis of a facial fracture can be determined via the clinical history, along with physical examination, and confirmed with imaging. The initial treatment includes elevation of the head, ice application, and analgesic pain medication. Facial fractures should be referred to subspecialty care as soon as possible. Nondisplaced nasal fractures can be treated symptomatically.

Nasal Fractures

The nose is the most prominent projection on the face; therefore, it is the site of one of the most common facial bone fractures.[16] The best time to examine the nose is within the first few hours after the injury, before significant swelling occurs and when the injury can be visualized more clearly. Nasal fractures generally present with an obvious nasal deformity, tenderness to palpation,

epistaxis, and/or periorbital ecchymosis. Closed reduction with adequate pain control and/or sedation can be attempted for displaced but otherwise uncomplicated nasal fractures evaluated within 6 hours.[17] Some otolaryngologists prefer to wait 3 to 7 days to allow the swelling to resolve, however. At the time of injury, the athlete may be unable to determine whether his or her appearance will be acceptable because of the degree of swelling over the nasal bridge.[16] The athlete with a suspected nasal fracture should be evaluated carefully for concomitant injuries to the midface or skull. Clear rhinorrhea from the nose should raise suspicion for cerebrospinal fluid leakage, which indicates fracture to the cribriform plate. The septum should be examined for deviation and/or septal hematoma. If present, a septal hematoma must be drained to prevent abscess formation and/or the development of a collapsed nasal bridge, also called a saddle-nose deformity.

Maxillary Fractures

The Le Fort classification commonly is used to describe the fracture pattern of maxillary fractures (Figure 3). Although these fractures rarely present exactly in the classically described form, they typically demonstrate significant components of one or more of the fracture patterns. A Le Fort I fracture is a transverse fracture through the maxilla only. The fracture line runs horizontally above the teeth and just below the nose. This pattern results in the separation of the palate and tooth-bearing portion of the maxilla from the rest of the face. On visual inspection, facial distortion may be present in the form of an elongated face, swelling, and ecchymosis. On examination, a step-off deformity of the palate and/or mobility of the maxilla when the upper teeth are grasped and moved in an anterior-posterior direction may be evident. A Le Fort II fracture is a pyramid-shaped fracture involving more of the midface traversing the nose, infraorbital rim, and orbital floor, and proceeding laterally through the lateral buttress and posteriorly through the pterygomaxillary buttress. These fractured bones may be impacted backward and upward, or the fragment may be floating free. The maxilla and nasal complex will move as a unit when the upper teeth are grasped and shifted from front to back. In a Le Fort III fracture, the facial skeleton is separated from the cranium, which can result in complete craniofacial dissociation if bilateral. The fracture line runs through the bridge of the nose and extends along the medial wall of the orbit, across the floor of the orbit, through the lateral orbital wall, and then out across the zygomatic arch. Manipulation of the palate results in movement of the zygomatic bones.

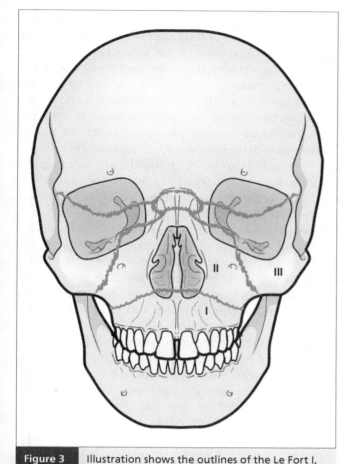

Figure 3 Illustration shows the outlines of the Le Fort I, II, and III fractures of the maxilla.

Orbital Blowout Fractures

Orbital blowout fractures occur when blunt trauma to the globe results in collapse of the inferior orbital wall. The force of the trauma creates increased pressure to all walls of the orbit, but the orbital floor is most susceptible to fracture because of its thin, eggshell-like construct. In addition, the orbital floor receives minimal support from the air-filled, mucosa-lined maxillary sinus sitting beneath it. Orbital blowout fractures frequently present with periorbital swelling and ecchymosis. The injured athlete should be asked about diplopia and examined for limited upward gaze; both findings usually are due to entrapment of the inferior rectus muscle. Infraorbital hypoesthesia can result if damage has occurred to the infraorbital nerve that runs through the inferior wall of the orbit. Enophthalmos can develop secondary to herniation (acute) or necrosis (subacute) of periorbital fat. If extraocular movements are limited with a suspected orbital blowout fracture, immediate CT scan is indicated to evaluate for strangulation of the extraocular muscles, which results in muscle necrosis.[18]

Zygomatic Fractures

In addition to forming the cheekbones of the face, the zygoma, or zygomatic arch, forms a portion of the lateral and inferior orbital rim and provides an attachment point for the superior portion of the masseter muscle. Thus, zygomatic fractures can affect vision, jaw function, and facial cosmetics.[19] Zygomatic fractures generally occur from blunt trauma to the face and cheek. Signs and symptoms may include subconjunctival hemorrhage, swelling or ecchymosis over the zygoma, periorbital ecchymosis, a depressed malar eminence and orbital rim, paresthesia in the distribution of the infraorbital nerve, emphysema in the orbit or overlying soft tissue of the cheek, trismus, malposition of the globe, or diplopia.

Mandibular Fractures and Dislocations

Mandibular fractures are relatively common sports injuries, comprising up to 40% to 50% of all sports-related maxillofacial fractures.[3,6,20] Two common symptoms described by patients are pain and the feeling that the teeth no longer correctly meet. The teeth are very proprioceptive secondary to nerve fibers around the periodontal ligament, so even a small shift generates an abnormal feeling of malocclusion. Other signs and symptoms can include swelling, bleeding, tenderness, numbness (because the inferior alveolar nerve runs along the jaw and can be compressed by a fracture), trismus, and a step-off deformity at the fracture site. An intraoral sublingual hematoma is pathognomonic for a mandibular fracture.[21] Stabilization for transport can be facilitated by using a Barton bandage (Figure 4).

Mandibular dislocations frequently result from a lateral blow to the jaw while the mouth is open. The injury is observed most often in sports such as basketball and hockey, in which a high incidence of elbow trauma occurs to the face. Generally, the mandible is displaced anterior to the eminence of the mandibular fossa. The athlete presents with an obvious deformity in the temporomandibular region and is unable to close the mouth. On the field, anterior mandibular dislocations can be reduced using a variety of methods without procedural sedation or local anesthesia. The classic reduction technique is performed with the athlete seated on the floor, the ground, or a chair, facing the clinician with the head stabilized. The athlete is asked to open his or her mouth widely against resistance; this motion reduces the muscle tone of the elevator muscles through reciprocal inhibition and allows concurrent manual reduction. In a simultaneous maneuver, the clinician exerts maximal downward reduction force using gloved thumbs on the patient's lower molars or mandibular ridge while exerting steady and constant downward pressure by moving

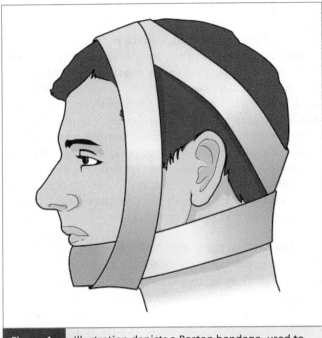

Figure 4 Illustration depicts a Barton bandage, used to stabilize the mandible during patient transport. (Reproduced from Lanzi GL: Facial and dental injuries, in Limpisvasti O, Krabak BJ, Albohm MJ, Wadsworth LT, Herring SA, Provencher MT: *The Sports Medicine Field Manual.* Rosemont, IL, American Academy of Orthopaedic Surgeons, 2015, pp 187-196.)

Athletes with an auricular hematoma report substantial pain or pressure at the external ear, perhaps out of proportion to the visible trauma. Later, swelling, loss of the external ear landmarks, or fluctuance palpated at the external ear consistent with hematoma may be present. If an athlete sustains an auricular hematoma and is able to tolerate pain, he or she may be allowed to continue sports participation, with advisement about the risk of further injury to the ear. Acutely, an untreated hematoma can enlarge and rupture. Chronically, an untreated auricular hematoma can result in a disfiguring cauliflower ear, resulting from pressure necrosis and the formation of new cartilage and fibrous tissue.

If an auricular hematoma is suspected, early recognition and treatment are important. An otolaryngologist can be consulted for definitive treatment. Before the blood within the hematoma coagulates, it should be decompressed as soon as possible through aspiration or incision and drainage. This step should be followed by the placement of a protective molding, worn for 3 to 7 days. If adequate coverage/protection is not possible, the athlete should be restricted from play until evidence of healing is present. Otherwise, repeated injury can lead to recurrent bleeding and hematoma. Antibiotics often are prescribed to prevent infection, especially if incision and drainage are performed. In high-risk sports such as wrestling, a protective ear covering should be worn to prevent reinjury. All wrestlers should be encouraged to wear protective gear at all times during practice and competition.

Eye Injuries

Of the 100,000 eye injuries resulting from sports each year, an estimated 42,000 are treated in the emergency department, and 13,500 athletes end up legally blind.[23,24] Of sports-related eye injuries, 90% can be prevented by wearing protective equipment.[25] Sports commonly responsible for injury to the eye include baseball, basketball, softball, racquetball, football, and soccer.[25]

The evaluation of eye injuries can be approached systematically. First, visual acuity should be assessed with a handheld Snellen chart, followed by visual field testing. At the same time, extraocular movements can be confirmed. Pupil size should be assessed for reactivity to light and accommodation. The relative afferent pupillary defect can be assessed with the swinging flashlight test. If the pupil paradoxically dilates when exposed to light, injury to the optic nerve or retina is suggested. Conjunctival erythema, hyphema, and laceration should be visualized. Finally, the facial bones should be inspected and palpated to assess for associated bony injury.

the mandible down, then posteriorly, and then up, with the rest of the fingers and the hand around the jaw and chin, levering upward. The downward pressure clears the condyle of the articular eminence, whereas the posterior pressure repositions the condyle within the mandibular fossa.[22] If the maneuver is unsuccessful, the athlete may need procedural sedation and should be transported to an emergency department.

Ear Injuries/Auricular Hematoma

Blunt trauma to the ear is common in sports such as wrestling, boxing, rugby, and mixed martial arts. Shearing forces occur at the external ear as it sustains direct contact with surfaces such as the floor or a mat. These forces cause blood to accumulate in the subperichondrial space, creating an auricular hematoma. The perichondrium supplies nutrients to the underlying cartilage, and if the hematoma separates the underlying cartilage from the perichondrium, necrosis occurs. This disrupted vascular supply to the external ear cartilage also increases the risk of infection.

Corneal Abrasion

Corneal abrasions are one of the most common eye injuries encountered in sport. They occur from blunt trauma, such as injury from a fingernail or a stick. The symptoms of corneal abrasion are sharp pain, a foreign body sensation, tearing, redness, and possibly reduced vision. The diagnosis can be confirmed with fluorescein dye instilled into the eye by touching the strip to the inner lower lid and using a Wood lamp or a blue light from an ophthalmoscope. A corneal scratch will be highlighted by the fluorescein dye.

If the abrasion is small (for example, from a finger poke), supportive care only may be needed. Corneal abrasion is treated with topical antibiotics and cycloplegics.[26] Eye patches no longer are recommended for more than 1 day because they can lead to loss of vision and have not been proven to help with pain.[26,27] Contact lens wearers should discontinue using contacts until the antibiotics are discontinued and should be considered for referral to an ophthalmologist for close follow-up because of a higher risk of infection. Most corneal abrasions resolve within 24 to 48 hours; if the abrasion is still symptomatic after this time, the athlete should be referred to an ophthalmologist.

Corneal Foreign Body

Foreign bodies acquired from environmental debris and particles can present with symptoms similar to a corneal abrasion. If a foreign body is suspected, the upper lid should be everted and the lower lid pulled out to assess for foreign body. The eye can be irrigated with saline, or a moistened cotton swab can be used to remove the foreign body if visible. If the particle cannot be extracted, an evaluation in the emergency department or by an ophthalmologist should be obtained. Topical antibiotics typically are not used for corneal foreign bodies but can be considered in unhygienic or wilderness settings.[28] Athletes with a corneal abrasion or corneal foreign body can return to play if the pain is tolerated and no loss of vision has occurred.[29]

Ruptured Globe

A ruptured globe occurs during high-velocity trauma from a missile object such as a hockey puck or stick, bat, racquet ball, or baseball. A ruptured globe can result from a blunt blow or penetrating injury. The cornea, sclera, or both can be disrupted partially or fully (open globe rupture). Athletes will present with a history of a direct blow or trauma, severe pain, visual disturbance, and decreased extraocular movements. Subconjunctival hemorrhage that is present 360° around the cornea is highly suspicious for a ruptured globe.[30] A hyphema is present in many cases. A sunken and distorted eye, pupil irregularity, and leakage of vitreous material may be present. Alternatively, in a closed globe rupture without a full-thickness tear through the cornea and sclera, the globe may look normal.

A ruptured globe requires emergent evaluation in the emergency department and should be treated as an ocular emergency. On transport, a rigid eye shield, or the lower half of a Styrofoam cup if a shield is not available, should be placed, and manipulation or pressure on the eye should be avoided. These injuries have a high rate of vision loss. Ruptured globes are not always obvious on physical examination; therefore, a high index of suspicion should be maintained, and referral to an ophthalmologist should be considered for any athlete with significant high-velocity trauma to the eye.[29]

Hyphema

Blunt trauma such as a projectile object or a fist punch also can result in a hyphema. The shearing forces on the blood vessels of the iris cause rupture, with leakage of blood into the anterior chamber. Layering of blood at the inferior iris can be seen, and the pupil may be irregular or sluggish. Vision may be blurred if the hyphema is large, and pain and photophobia may be present. Most hyphemas layer over less than one-third of the anterior chamber. If severe, however, blood can fill the entire anterior chamber, creating an 8-ball hyphema. All hyphemas require urgent ophthalmology evaluation because of possible complications and their association with other intraocular injury. Occasionally, hospitalization is required. Typical treatment includes an eye patch and shield, rest, and elevation of the head of the bed. Most hyphemas resolve within a few days, but rebleeding occurs in approximately 25% of cases within the first 3 to 5 days. Rebleeding is associated with corneal staining, possible increased intraocular pressures, and a poorer prognosis. For this reason, aspirin and NSAIDs should be avoided. In athletes with sickle cell disease, caution should be exercised because sickling can occur where blood accumulates in the anterior chamber. In athletes with sickle cell trait, an association with secondary bleeding, increased intraocular pressures, and permanent visual impairment is present.[31] All players with hyphema need clearance by an ophthalmologist before returning to play because of the risk of rebleeding, which can permanently affect vision.

Retrobulbar Hemorrhage

Blunt trauma to the eye, which often occurs in sports, can lead to bleeding in the closed orbital space. The resulting increased pressure leads to decreased perfusion and ischemia as well as a compartment syndrome of the eye. The optic nerve and retina will be damaged from ischemia. Elevated intraocular pressure lasting longer than 90 minutes can lead to blindness.[32] Physical examination may reveal periorbital bruising, reduced vision, proptosis, pain, and a relative afferent pupillary defect. A high index of suspicion should be maintained because this injury needs to be treated emergently to avoid irreversible ischemia and subsequent blindness. The treatment consists of surgical decompression.

Retinal Injury

Retinal injury also can occur as a result of blunt trauma. The athlete may report severe pain or reduced vision. Flashing lights and floaters are symptoms specific to retinal injury and should prompt urgent ophthalmologic evaluation.[30]

Burns and Radiation Exposure

In athletic events held at high altitude, on water, or on snow, ultraviolet burns to the conjunctiva and cornea can occur. Athletes present with severe eye pain, tearing, photophobia, and eyelid spasms. With fluorescein dye, a fine punctate staining pattern will be seen. Treatment consists of systemic analgesics and topical antibiotics. These injuries can be prevented by using ultraviolet ray-blocking, shatter-resistant eyewear.

Dental Injuries

The incidence of sports-related dental trauma varies from 14% to 57%, depending on the type and competitive level of the sport.[33] These injuries can result from contact or noncontact forces transmitted to the teeth. Studies have shown that sports such as basketball, biking, ice hockey, rugby, baseball, and wrestling are common culprits of dental trauma in males.[33-35] In females, the highest risk for dental trauma occurs during basketball and field hockey.[35]

The tooth consists of a crown that is visible above the gum line and the root, which is imbedded in the alveolar socket of the jaw bone and secured in place by the periodontal ligament. The tooth is made up of multiple layers: the enamel, which is the hard white outer covering; dentin, a softer layer of yellowish connective tissue; and pulp, which contains the neurovascular bundle.

Tooth Fractures

Crown fractures commonly occur to the permanent anterior teeth. A class I fracture, or simple chipped tooth, involves the outer enamel only. The athlete may notice a rough edge of the tooth, which should not be painful or

sensitive. These injuries do not require urgent evaluation and can be seen by a dentist nonemergently to smooth out the enamel. Class II fractures expose the yellow dentin and are suitable for outpatient care by a dentist. If a fracture of the crown has occurred, with dentin or pulp visible, the athlete will report pain when exposed to cold, air, or palpation. Class III fractures expose the dental pulp, seen as a red line or dot, and are exquisitely painful. If the broken fragment is located, it should be placed in a solution such as milk, saline, or commercial balanced salt solution. These more severe injuries require urgent evaluation by a dentist or endodontist.

Root fractures occur much less frequently than crown fractures. The diagnosis of a root fracture typically is made solely by radiographic appearance. A root fracture should be suspected if mobility of the root segment is present without movement of the apical segment on palpation, however. Root fractures should be treated emergently to preserve pulp vitality.

Tooth Displacement

A tooth can become displaced from a direct or indirect blow that results in stretching or rupture of the periodontal ligament. The tooth may be luxated out of the socket (extruded), compressed into the socket (intruded or impacted, appearing shorter than adjacent teeth), or there may be buccal or lingual lateral displacement. An extruded or laterally displaced tooth should be repositioned as quickly as possible. If the tooth is intruded, however, it should not be manipulated in the field.

Tooth Avulsion

A tooth avulsion is a dental emergency, and every attempt should be made to replace the tooth as quickly as possible. The eventual vitality of the tooth depends directly on the time lapsed before reimplantation.[36] If treatment is delayed more than 2 hours, only a 5% chance of tooth survival exists.[37] Every effort should be made to attempt reimplantation of the tooth within 20 minutes for the greatest chance of survival.[38] The tooth should be located, with attempts made to preserve its vitality. Only the crown should be handled to avoid damage to the fragile periodontal ligament. If debris is present on the tooth, it should be rinsed gently with saline, water, or milk. If the athlete is conscious, the tooth should be repositioned into the alveolar socket. The athlete can then gently bite on sterile gauze in preparation for transport to the emergency department and/or dentist. If the tooth cannot be repositioned, it can be placed in a commercial tooth saving kit such as milk or commercial balanced salt solution. Tooth avulsions involving primary teeth in youth should not be replaced in the alveolar socket.

Prevention

Facial Protection

Protective facial devices can lower the risk of facial injuries significantly. Prior to 1959, before facemasks were mandatory in American football, 50% of injuries were defined as facial or dental trauma. In 1988, the incidence declined to 1.4%.[39] The rules governing protective equipment vary by sport as well as by participant level of play. In the National Collegiate Athletic Association, athletes currently are required to wear facemasks for facial protection in men's lacrosse, football, men's and women's ice hockey, and fencing. Goalkeepers in women's lacrosse and catchers in softball and baseball also are required to wear facemasks.[40] Although debate continues in the world of hockey regarding the appropriate level of facial protection, a substantial reduction in facial injuries has been demonstrated when a full facemask is worn versus a half shield.[41,42]

Mouth Guards

Mouth guards protect the teeth and dissipate energy from a direct blow, which significantly reduces the risk of dental injury. The Academy for Sports Dentistry recommends using a properly fitted mouth guard professionally fabricated for fit and function for all contact and collision sports.[43] Over-the-counter mouth guards can provide a small degree of protection and remain an appropriate choice for many youth sports because of their easy availability and low cost.

Eye Protection

Athletes need to be counseled on the importance of eye protection, because most eye injuries in sports can be prevented with proper eye protection.[25] When categorizing sports based on the risk to the eye in the unprotected player, only two sports were considered eye safe: track and field (with the exception of javelin and discus, unless good field supervision is present) and gymnastics.[44] All athletes involved in organized sports should be advised to wear appropriate eye protection. The American Society for Testing and Materials has standardized specifications for eye protection in racket sports, women's lacrosse, field hockey, basketball, baseball, soccer, skiing, and snowboarding. These standards can be reviewed at: http://www.astm.org/Standards/F803.htm.

The American Academy of Pediatrics and the American Academy of Ophthalmology recommend that all functionally one-eyed athletes (having less than 20/40 vision in the affected eye with corrected vision) wear appropriate eye protection for all sports. It is also recommended that they not participate in boxing or full-contact martial arts. For sports that require a facemask or helmet, it is recommended that sport goggles also be worn if the facemask becomes displaced and while sitting on the bench.

Summary

Facial injuries are common in many sports activities. Every injury should be approached methodically, including an initial evaluation for life-threatening injuries, followed by an assessment tailored to the nature, severity, and location of the injury. A broad differential diagnosis should be entertained to recognize injury patterns and determine the urgency of treatment. A low threshold for subspecialty consultation should be upheld for significant injuries to the face, eyes, and mouth. Facial and oral protection is vital in preventing disfiguring and/or vision-altering injuries.

Key Study Points

- A thorough evaluation of all facial injuries should be performed, including a broad differential diagnosis to consider injury to the skin, eyes, ears, bones, and soft tissue.
- Depending on the severity of facial injuries, emergency services and subspecialty consultation should be implemented when indicated.

Annotated References

1. Hendrickson CD, Hill K, Carpenter JE: Injuries to the head and face in women's collegiate field hockey. *Clin J Sport Med* 2008;18(5):399-402.

2. Boffano P, Kommers SC, Karagozoglu KH, Forouzanfar T: Aetiology of maxillofacial fractures: A review of published studies during the last 30 years. *Br J Oral Maxillofac Surg* 2014;52(10):901-906.

   This systematic review of 69 articles published worldwide over the past 30 years evaluated the incidence of maxillofacial injuries from all causes, including sports activities. Level of evidence: V.

3. Antoun JS, Lee KH: Sports-related maxillofacial fractures over an 11-year period. *J Oral Maxillofac Surg* 2008;66(3):504-508.

4. Exadaktylos AK, Eggensperger NM, Eggli S, Smolka KM, Zimmermann H, Iizuka T: Sports related maxillofacial injuries: The first maxillofacial trauma database in Switzerland. *Br J Sports Med* 2004;38(6):750-753.

5. Maladière E, Bado F, Meningaud JP, Guilbert F, Bertrand JC: Aetiology and incidence of facial fractures sustained during sports: A prospective study of 140 patients. *Int J Oral Maxillofac Surg* 2001;30(4):291-295.

6. Mourouzis C, Koumoura F: Sports-related maxillofacial fractures: A retrospective study of 125 patients. *Int J Oral Maxillofac Surg* 2005;34(6):635-638.

7. Romeo SJ, Hawley CJ, Romeo MW, Romeo JP, Honsik KA: Sideline management of facial injuries. *Curr Sports Med Rep* 2007;6(3):155-161.

8. Hollander JE, Singer AJ: Laceration management. *Ann Emerg Med* 1999;34(3):356-367.

9. Forsch RT: Essentials of skin laceration repair. *Am Fam Physician* 2008;78(8):945-951.

10. Fernandez R, Griffiths R: Water for wound cleansing. *Cochrane Database Syst Rev* 2012;2:CD003861.

    This systematic review assessed the infection and healing rates of water and various other solutions used for wound cleansing.

11. Scarfone RJ, Jasani M, Gracely EJ: Pain of local anesthetics: Rate of administration and buffering. *Ann Emerg Med* 1998;31(1):36-40.

12. Ferrera PC, Chandler R: Anesthesia in the emergency setting: Part II. Head and neck, eye and rib injuries. *Am Fam Physician* 1994;50(4):797-800.

13. Quinn J, Wells G, Sutcliffe T, et al: A randomized trial comparing octylcyanoacrylate tissue adhesive and sutures in the management of lacerations. *JAMA* 1997;277(19):1527-1530.

14. Singer AJ, Hollander JE, Valentine SM, Turque TW, McCuskey CF, Quinn JV; Stony Brook Octylcyanoacrylate Study Group: Prospective, randomized, controlled trial of tissue adhesive (2-octylcyanoacrylate) vs standard wound closure techniques for laceration repair. *Acad Emerg Med* 1998;5(2):94-99.

15. Krempl GA, Noorily AD: Use of oxymetazoline in the management of epistaxis. *Ann Otol Rhinol Laryngol* 1995;104(9 Pt 1):704-706.

16. Higuera S, Lee EI, Cole P, Hollier LH Jr, Stal S: Nasal trauma and the deviated nose. *Plast Reconstr Surg* 2007;120(7, Suppl 2)64S-75S.

17. Mondin V, Rinaldo A, Ferlito A: Management of nasal bone fractures. *Am J Otolaryngol* 2005;26(3):181-185.

18. Reehal P: Facial injury in sport. *Curr Sports Med Rep* 2010;9(1):27-34.

    This review article described the evaluation, treatment, and prevention of the facial injuries that can occur as a result of sports participation.

19. Kelley P, Hopper R, Gruss J: Evaluation and treatment of zygomatic fractures. *Plast Reconstr Surg* 2007;120(7, Suppl 2)5S-15S.

20. James RB, Fredrickson C, Kent JN: Prospective study of mandibular fractures. *J Oral Surg* 1981;39(4):275-281.

21. Springer I, Haerle F: Sublingual hematoma: Pathognomonic of fracture of the mandible, in Haerle F, Champy M, Terry B, eds: *Atlas of Craniofacial Osteosynthesis: Microplates, Miniplates, and Screws*, ed 2. Stuttgart, Germany, Thieme Medical Publishers, 2009, pp 10-11.

    A specific chapter in this atlas of craniofacial disorders focused n the clinical finding of a sublingual hematoma and how it is believed to be pathognomonic for a mandibular fracture.

22. Chan TC, Harrigan RA, Ufberg J, Vilke GM: Mandibular reduction. *J Emerg Med* 2008;34(4):435-440.

23. Napier SM, Baker RS, Sanford DG, Easterbrook M: Eye injuries in athletics and recreation. *Surv Ophthalmol* 1996;41(3):229-244.

24. United States Consumer Product Safety Commission: *Sports and Recreational Eye Injuries*. Washington, DC, U.S. Consumer Product Safety Commission, 2000.

25. Goldstein MH, Wee D: Sports injuries: An ounce of prevention and a pound of cure. *Eye Contact Lens* 2011;37(3):160-163.

    This review of the available literature covered sports-related ocular trauma and its prevention.

26. Fraser S: Corneal abrasion. *Clin Ophthalmol* 2010;4:387-390.

    This article discussed up-to-date treatment options for corneal abrasions.

27. Turner A, Rabiu M: Patching for corneal abrasion. *Cochrane Database Syst Rev* 2006;2(2):CD004764.

28. Ellerton JA, Zuljan I, Agazzi G, Boyd JJ: Eye problems in mountain and remote areas: Prevention and onsite treatment—official recommendations of the International Commission for Mountain Emergency Medicine ICAR MEDCOM. *Wilderness Environ Med* 2009;20(2):169-175.

    This article is a consensus opinion from the International Commission for Mountain Emergency Medicine. Practical advice is given regarding the management of eye problems in remote, high altitude, or wilderness settings. Prevention of eye problems in these settings is discussed.

29. Trobe JD: Ophthalmic trauma, in *The Physicians' Guide to Eye Care*, ed 3. San Francisco, CA, American Academy of Ophthalmology, 2006, pp 75-92.

30. Pokhrel PK, Loftus SA: Ocular emergencies. *Am Fam Physician* 2007;76(6):829-836.

© 2016 American Academy of Orthopaedic Surgeons

31. Nasrullah A, Kerr NC: Sickle cell trait as a risk factor for secondary hemorrhage in children with traumatic hyphema. *Am J Ophthalmol* 1997;123(6):783-790.

32. Hayreh SS, Kolder HE, Weingeist TA: Central retinal artery occlusion and retinal tolerance time. *Ophthalmology* 1980;87(1):75-78.

33. Ashley P, Di Iorio A, Cole E, Tanday A, Needleman I: Oral health of elite athletes and association with performance: A systematic review. *Br J Sports Med* 2015;49(1):14-19.

    This systematic review article of the available literature examined the overall oral health of athletes, including a subsection on oral/dental trauma. Level of evidence: V.

34. Soporowski NJ, Tesini DA, Weiss AI: Survey of orofacial sports-related injuries. *J Mass Dent Soc* 1994;43(4):16-20.

35. Lee-Knight CT, Harrison EL, Price CJ: Dental injuries at the 1989 Canada games: An epidemiological study. *J Can Dent Assoc* 1992;58(10):810-815.

36. Andreasen JO, Andreasen FM, Skeie A, Hjørting-Hansen E, Schwartz O: Effect of treatment delay upon pulp and periodontal healing of traumatic dental injuries — a review article. *Dent Traumatol* 2002;18(3):116-128.

37. Howe AS: Craniomaxillofacial injuries, in Seidenberg PH, Beutler AI, eds: *The Sports Medicine Resource Manual.* Philadelphia, PA, Saunders Elsevier, 2008, pp 253-271.

38. Barrett EJ, Kenny DJ: Avulsed permanent teeth: A review of the literature and treatment guidelines. *Endod Dent Traumatol* 1997;13(4):153-163.

39. Welbury RR, Murray JJ: Prevention of trauma to teeth. *Dent Update* 1990;17(3):117-121.

40. 2014-15 NCAA Sports Medicine Handbook, Protective Equipment, August 2014, pp. 104-108.

    This official handbook of the National Collegiate Athletic Association and sports medicine contains a section on protective equipment discussing the specific safety equipment required in individual sports.

41. Benson BW, Mohtadi NG, Rose MS, Meeuwisse WH: Head and neck injuries among ice hockey players wearing full face shields vs half face shields. *JAMA* 1999;282(24):2328-2332.

42. Stuart MJ, Smith AM, Malo-Ortiguera SA, Fischer TL, Larson DR: A comparison of facial protection and the incidence of head, neck, and facial injuries in Junior A hockey players. A function of individual playing time. *Am J Sports Med* 2002;30(1):39-44.

43. Academy for Sports Dentistry Position Statement: *A properly fitted mouthguard.* Available at: http://www.academyforsportsdentistry.org/position-statement. Accessed: July 20, 2015.

    This official position statement from the Academy for Sports Dentistry covers the qualifications of a Team Dentist, mouth guard recommendations, sports dentistry in the dental school curriculum, and a smokeless tobacco position statement.

44. Vinger PF: A practical guide for sports eye protection. *Phys Sportsmed* 2000;28(6):49-69.

Chapter 45

Abdominal Injuries

Stephen R. Paul, MD   Sagir Girish Bera, DO, MPH, MS   Brenden J. Balcik, MD

Abstract

Abdominal injuries make up a small percentage of sports-related injuries, with a recent 10-year review demonstrating an incidence of 0.56% of pediatric sports-related injuries due to abdominal or testicular trauma. Despite the relatively low incidence, the outcome of abdominal injuries can be poor, even including death, making the diagnosis, management, and treatment of such injuries of the utmost importance. The most commonly injured organs from blunt abdominal trauma are the spleen, kidney, intestines, and liver. These injuries can result from direct or indirect trauma, often presenting without overt signs of trauma. Frequently, symptoms can present with a delayed onset or not at all and therefore, knowledge of the mechanism of injury is important. Athletes with suspected abdominal injuries should be directed to a facility appropriately equipped to manage such injuries, with access to CT, angiography, on-demand surgical capabilities, and ability for continuous monitoring. Management decisions are determined by the hemodynamic status of the athlete. CT in most cases is the diagnostic modality of choice, with Focused Assessment with Sonography for Trauma examination used in the initial workup. In the hemodynamically stable athlete, the treatment of choice is nonsurgical. Many organ systems have grading systems based on CT scans. There is no consensus for return-to-play decisions and often the degree of injury is a factor. In all cases, attention to the readiness of the athlete to return to play should be based on normalization of their physical findings—laboratory examination, hemodynamic status with evidence of continued injury—and psychologic preparedness.

None of the following authors or any immediate family member has received anything of value from or has stock or stock options held in a commercial company or institution related directly or indirectly to the subject of this chapter: Dr. Paul, Dr. Bera, and Dr. Balcik.

Keywords: abdominal injuries; blunt abdominal trauma

Introduction

Blunt abdominal trauma (BAT) in sports is not very common. Furthermore, high-quality research performed in randomized controlled trials (RCTs) and clear undisputed guidelines for return to play after injury are few. Most statistical analysis of sports injuries fails to identify abdominal injuries as a reportable category.[1] Many review articles in the literature cite the incidence of sports-related abdominal trauma as being as high as 10%.[2] The incidence actually may be quite a bit lower, however. In a 10-year review of the National Pediatric Trauma Registry, of 81,923 cases of trauma, 6.64% were related to sports injuries, with only 0.56% due to abdominal or testicular trauma.[3]

According to recently published studies on abdominal injuries (those that involve the spleen, kidney, intestines, and liver, as well as abdominal contusions and abdominal muscle tears), no organ system reaches even 1% of all injuries reported. Discrepancies exist about which organ is injured most commonly in BAT and about the differences in adult and pediatric populations. Generally, however, the abdominal organs most commonly injured are the spleen, liver, and kidney. The pancreas, bladder, gastrointestinal tract and diaphragm were injured less often.

Although abdominal injuries are not the most common injuries in sports, the outcome of an abdominal injury can be catastrophic.[4] Therefore, every sports medicine practitioner should be familiar with the presentation, evaluation, identification, and treatment of traumatic abdominal injuries.

The mechanism of abdominal injuries is related to force mechanics: high-velocity forces, along with well-placed direct contact with lower velocity forces, cause injury. Abdominal injuries can result from collisions in sports such as football, soccer, or skiing; from well-placed local contact with a lacrosse ball, hockey stick, or bicycle handlebars; or from rapid deceleration such as during falls while snowboarding, surfing, or playing extreme

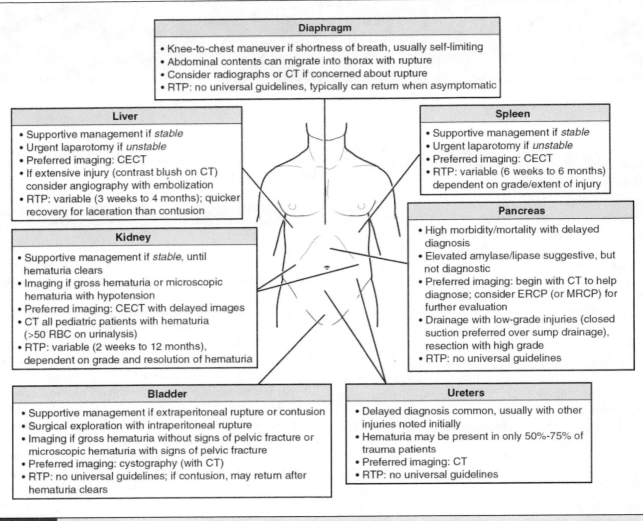

Diaphragm
- Knee-to-chest maneuver if shortness of breath, usually self-limiting
- Abdominal contents can migrate into thorax with rupture
- Consider radiographs or CT if concerned about rupture
- RTP: no universal guidelines, typically can return when asymptomatic

Liver
- Supportive management if *stable*
- Urgent laparotomy if *unstable*
- Preferred imaging: CECT
- If extensive injury (contrast blush on CT) consider angiography with embolization
- RTP: variable (3 weeks to 4 months); quicker recovery for laceration than contusion

Spleen
- Supportive management if *stable*
- Urgent laparotomy if *unstable*
- Preferred imaging: CECT
- RTP: variable (6 weeks to 6 months) dependent on grade/extent of injury

Kidney
- Supportive management if *stable*, until hematuria clears
- Imaging if gross hematuria or microscopic hematuria with hypotension
- Preferred imaging: CECT with delayed images
- CT all pediatric patients with hematuria (>50 RBC on urinalysis)
- RTP: variable (2 weeks to 12 months), dependent on grade and resolution of hematuria

Pancreas
- High morbidity/mortality with delayed diagnosis
- Elevated amylase/lipase suggestive, but not diagnostic
- Preferred imaging: begin with CT to help diagnose; consider ERCP (or MRCP) for further evaluation
- Drainage with low-grade injuries (closed suction preferred over sump drainage), resection with high grade
- RTP: no universal guidelines

Bladder
- Supportive management if extraperitoneal rupture or contusion
- Surgical exploration with intraperitoneal rupture
- Imaging if gross hematuria without signs of pelvic fracture or microscopic hematuria with signs of pelvic fracture
- Preferred imaging: cystography (with CT)
- RTP: no universal guidelines; if contusion, may return after hematuria clears

Ureters
- Delayed diagnosis common, usually with other injuries noted initially
- Hematuria may be present in only 50%-75% of trauma patients
- Preferred imaging: CT
- RTP: no universal guidelines

Figure 1 Illustration shows abdominal injuries from blunt trauma. RTP = return to play, CECT = contrast-enhanced CT, ERCP = endoscopic retrograde cholagniopancreatography, MRCP = magnetic resonance cholangiopancreatography.

sports.[5-7] Differences exist between pediatric and adult BAT. In children, the diaphragm is more horizontal, so the abdominal organs are more anterior and inferior compared with those of adults and are therefore more exposed to injury. Additionally, in children, the rib cage is more pliable and there is less protective musculature and fat present to protect the internal organs.

Early suspicion for and recognition of blunt trauma to the abdominal contents, along with appropriate management, can be life saving. Awareness of the mechanism of injury and performing repeated assessments are essential. After the athlete is stabilized, quick transport to an emergency facility equipped for in-depth assessment and appropriate management is important if intra-abdominal injury is suspected.

In this chapter, discussion will be limited to the hemodynamically stable athlete without signs of peritonitis. Additionally, unless noted otherwise, the nonsurgical treatment or observation will be the preferred treatment of choice in a facility equipped for ongoing clinical monitoring with the availability of angiography, imaging, and on-demand urgent surgical capabilities. Key issues related to blunt abdominal trauma in a sports setting are presented in Figure 1.

General Sideline Approach

Awareness of the mechanism of injury and a high index of suspicion are paramount when identifying abdominal injuries. Direct contact will often result in abdominal wall trauma with outwards signs such as contusions, abrasions, and hematomas, and also may involve underlying organs. Indirect trauma from rapid deceleration often show no visible outward signs of trauma and may involve the internal organs such as the spleen, liver, kidney, and hollow viscera.

Any athlete with a suspected abdominal injury should be removed from play for a comprehensive evaluation. Repeat examinations are essential and should include inspection for signs of trauma, peritonitis (guarding, rebound tenderness, rigidity, and pain with jostling of the abdomen), and shock, along with any progression of pain in terms of quality, radiation, localization, provocation timing, and severity. Vital signs should be taken, along with a general survey performed according to Advanced Trauma Life Support guidelines to include the spine, thorax, and pelvis. Often, abdominal injuries present innocuously, with delayed symptoms or worsening pain occurring later. Symptoms presenting hours to days later may be due to hollow viscous perforation and abscess formation.

Specific signs can be seen in abdominal trauma. The Kehr sign, presenting as pain referred to the left shoulder, can signal splenic injury. Signs of hemoperitoneum include the Saegesser sign (phrenic nerve pressure, producing neck pain), the Ballance sign (fixed left flank dullness), the Cullen sign (a periumbilical bluish discoloration), and the Grey Turner sign (a bluish discoloration of the left flank).

Further Evaluation

In the emergency department, most patients with sports abdominal injury are evaluated based on whether they are hemodynamically stable or unstable. If the patient is stable, CT with contrast is the gold standard, the goal being to reduce unnecessary laparotomies.[4,8-11] If the patient is hemodynamically unstable, Focused Assessment with Sonography for Trauma (FAST) examinations often are done initially to determine whether exploratory laparotomy is needed. Diagnostic peritoneal lavage (DPL), because of its invasive nature, lack of specific information about organ injury, inability to determine retroperitoneal injuries, and substantial false-positive rate (leading to unnecessary laparotomies) has been replaced by FAST. FAST examinations are cost effective, quick, and especially useful in hemodynamically unstable patients because they involve no radiation exposure and rely on identification of intraperitoneal fluid and injuries.[8] The sensitivity of the FAST examination is user-dependent and not very high when the examination is performed by less experienced clinicians. Sensitivities reported in the literature are 46% for the liver, 50% for the spleen and renal injury 44%.[10]

Additionally, 5% to 37% of intra-abdominal organs injured are without free peritoneal fluid.[9]

No RCTs exist that screen for high-energy blunt abdominal trauma to determine whether CT should be done selectively or routinely.[11] A Cochrane review found no RCT-based evidence to support the use of ultrasonography in algorithms for blunt abdominal trauma. There was no evidence that the use of ultrasonography in algorithms improved mortality, reduced diagnostic time with better precision, or reduced unnecessary interventional procedures.[9] In clinical practice, the FAST examination remains an integral tool in the initial workup for blunt abdominal trauma to help assess the need for laparotomy, especially in a hemodynamically unstable patient. FAST also is used in the patient with clinical suspicion of high-energy blunt trauma in whom CT should be avoided.[8-10]

The sports medicine physician should be able to infer which organs have been injured from observation and the mechanism of injury involved. This knowledge can assist in the diagnostic evaluation and workup. Most of the literature on BAT concerns multiorgan injury, but not necessarily that resulting from sport-related injury. In clinical presentations with a high index of suspicion for injury, a focused examination will alert the clinician to possible intra-abdominal injury, leading to an appropriate diagnosis and treatment.

Types of Abdominal Injuries

Diaphragmatic Spasm

Diaphragmatic spasm was first reported in 1947 and is usually the result of a blow to the epigastrium, causing a spasm of the diaphragm muscle, and resulting in difficulty breathing accompanied by chest or abdominal pain.[12] The athlete experiences "getting the wind knocked out." This injury is self-limiting, and the initial treatment is enabling relaxation of the diaphragm by flexing the hips, stretching the torso, and loosening any tight-fitting outerwear. The athlete may return to play after resolution of symptoms.

Abdominal Wall Injuries

The incidence of abdominal wall injuries has been reported to be between 0.7% and 7%, including injuries to the torso.[13] These injuries may involve a contusion or strain to the abdominal wall and musculature, which includes the rectus abdominis, internal and external oblique, and transverse abdominis muscles. These muscles protect the abdominal contents and aid in trunk flexion and compression of the abdominal space, pulling the chest down to aid respiration. The lower abdominal muscles are important for pelvic stabilization and for supporting the core as an aid in upper extremity function.

Contusion of the abdominal wall can occur by a direct blow or while straining the muscles with indirect force, such as in a forceful contraction of the muscles. The athlete often will report anterior abdominal pain, which is worsened with trunk extension, contraction of the abdominal muscles in flexion or rotation, or during a supine leg raise. The pain may present as an "acute abdomen," rigid and with guarding. The abdominal wall should be palpated to localize the pain. The pain is reproduced with tensing of the abdominal muscles (the Carnett sign),[14] trunk flexion and rotation, and raising of the leg when supine—all of which involve use of the abdominal muscles, which can discriminate between injury of the abdominal musculature and the parietal peritoneum and underlying visceral structures. The pain may be relieved with passive trunk flexion.[13] The workup is limited to examination only if no other worrisome signs are present. Treatment consists of relative rest (allowing the trunk to remain partially flexed and limiting trunk extension and rotation), ice, and analgesics. Progression to abdominal wall stretching and return to play when the athlete regains full range of motion without pain usually occur within 1 to 2 weeks.

Rectal Sheath Hematoma

Rectal sheath hematoma (RSH) is an injury of the abdominal wall that often is self-limiting and benign, but may require additional workup and invasive treatment. The mechanism of injury is similar to that of the previously described abdominal wall injuries but usually involves more force. The inferior epigastric artery loosely courses between the rectus abdominis muscle and posterior rectus sheath. It must move with muscle contraction and therefore is susceptible to tearing with enough force. RSH has a presentation similar to that of other abdominal wall injuries, with abdominal pain worsened by contraction of the abdominal muscles. If the pain is severe, it may be accompanied by nausea and vomiting. Often, a mass may be palpable at or below the level of injury. A delayed presentation may be periumbilical ecchymosis (the Cullen sign).

In a large or enlarging hematoma, evaluation and ligation of the epigastric artery may be necessary. Initially, ultrasonography can be useful, but it is not reliable for determining the accurate location of the source of bleeding; therefore, CT is recommended.[4,13] Treatment of RSH is supportive, including relaxed trunk flexion, ice, and analgesics. As permitted, gentle stretching of the abdominal wall may be performed.

Injuries to the Spleen

The spleen is reported to be the most frequently injured organ from BAT in sports.[5,15-17] The incidence is low, however, and improved diagnostic evaluation and nonsurgical treatment methods have led to fewer intra-abdominal complications and improved mortality.[15,17,18] Because undiagnosed splenic trauma still carries high morbidity and mortality,[16,19] the sports medicine practitioner should be able to recognize the condition and its characteristics.

The spleen resides in the left upper quadrant below the diaphragm and, in adults, is protected by the costal margins of ribs 9 through 12. When enlarged, or as a normal variant in children, the spleen can extend beyond the costal margins. The spleen is encapsulated and can contain a large amount of blood, which can delay signs of trauma. Injuries to the spleen during sports activity occur from a direct blow to the left upper quadrant or from deceleration injuries during high-speed activities or falls. Certain preexisting conditions, including infections (eg, infectious mononucleosis), hematologic disorders, and fever can cause splenic enlargement and facilitate splenic injury.[17]

Clinical symptoms of splenic injury can include sharp abdominal pain in the left upper quadrant and generalized abdominal pain or distension with or without signs of peritonitis. Pain may be referred to the left shoulder (the Kehr sign) because of peritoneal irritation of the diaphragm. Rib pain on the left side and signs of trauma or fracture may be present. If blood extravasates into the peritoneal cavity, signs of peritonitis and shock may ensue. A potential difficulty in diagnosis may stem from bleeding being contained by the splenic capsule. After sharp pain from the initial injury, symptoms may ease until they present in a delayed fashion, a situation that can be catastrophic. A high level of suspicion for splenic injury should be maintained by the sideline physician, resulting in prompt transport to an appropriate trauma center for workup.

In the hemodynamically unstable patient, the FAST examination (or DPL if FAST is unavailable) plays a role before laparotomy. Contrast CT is the diagnostic study of choice for splenic trauma in the hemodynamically stable patient.[18,20] The grading of splenic injuries follows the American Association for the Surgery of Trauma (AAST) organ grading system, the Spleen Injury Scale. Capsular containment, the depth of parenchymal involvement, and the location and degree of laceration are important components.[21] Grade I (small) hematomas have less than 10% of surface area or capsular laceration and less than 1 cm of parenchymal depth. Grade II (moderate) hematomas involve 10% to 50% of surface area or an intraparenchymal depth of less than 5 cm and have capsular laceration measuring 1 to 3 cm not involving a trabecular vessel. Grade III (large) hematomas have more than 50% of surface area or are expanding, have greater than or equal to 5 cm of intraparenchymal depth or are expanding, and involve a laceration more than 3 cm of parenchymal depth or involve trabecular vessels. Grade IV (large with partial devascularization) lacerations involve segmental or hilar vessels with more than 25% devascularization of the spleen. Grade V (total devascularization) represents a completely shattered spleen or laceration of the hilar vasculature with major devascularization. Although not used to a substantial degree or reported in the literature, the Baltimore CT grading system is an alternative classification methodology that incorporates vascular injuries to aid the assessment for use of angiography and embolization.[22]

The presence of a vascular contrast blush, the pooling of contrast within or around the injured organ noted on CT, can represent active bleeding. Debate exists about the optimal management of this condition. The Eastern Association for the Surgery of Trauma (EAST) Practice Management Guidelines[18] state (level III evidence) that contrast blush noted on CT is not by itself an absolute indication for laparotomy or angiographic intervention. The authors concur that other factors need to be accounted for, such as patient age, the grade of injury, and hemodynamic status.

Nonsurgical management includes initial monitoring and activity restriction with serial hematocrit measurements. The timing and frequency of these interventions have not been standardized by research to date. The grade of injury plays a role. In grade I injuries, monitoring should be performed in a supervised environment, with discharge as early as day 1 or 2 if the hematocrit levels and the patient remain stable. Patients with grade II injuries should be rested in an inpatient, monitored bed. Those with grade III or higher injuries should be kept in an intensive care unit for variable lengths, with a minimum total stay of at least 3 days.[18,23]

Repeat CT in the management of splenic injuries is also controversial.[24] Most authors recommend against repeating CT for lower grade (grade I or II) injuries. In those with higher grades of injury or with evidence of continued bleeding or symptoms, repeat CT can be indicated. Also, in elite, high-level athletes, repeat CT can be done for higher grade injuries to help with return to activities, but it is not recommended. Also, ultrasonography may be used to serially document healing and to help satisfy return-to-play recommendations if the findings on ultrasound correlate with CT findings.[25] The mean time to healing was studied using ultrasonography in splenic injuries graded by CT in children.[26] The ultrasonographic organ grading system differs from that of AAST in that the ultrasonographic system contains four grades, with grade III equivalent to the AAST grades II and IV, and

the ultrasound grade IV equivalent to the AAST grade V[26] (Table 1).

The time for return to play is not consistent in the literature. Factors to consider are healing time for the spleen and the potential for rebleeding. The incidence of delayed splenic rupture has been reported to be 1% to 8% in adults and only zero to 7.5% in pediatric patients.[17] The risk of splenectomy in the 180 days following discharge home was 1.4%.[18,27] Consultation with the surgeon is recommended. The following ranges are suggested for the return to full activity, but not necessarily to contact sports. In grade I and II injuries, the time to return ranged from less than 6 weeks to 6 months. For grade III injuries, the time to return ranged from 6 weeks to 6 months. Grade IV and V injuries resulted in a return of from 2 or 3 to 6 months, with 5% of those surveyed restricted longer than 6 months.[18] A case series describes hockey players with grade III injuries who were allowed to return to play at 2 months without complications.[25]

It is interesting to note that, after splenectomy, athletes often return to activity sooner than those treated nonsurgically.[17,25] An important consideration for patients who have undergone splenectomy is having the appropriate pneumococcal, *Haemophilus influenzae* type B, and *Neisseria meningitides* vaccines. Patients who have undergone splenectomy are also at increased risk for protozoan infections such as babesisosis and malaria and for *Capnocytophaga canimorsus* after dog bites.[17]

The recommendations for the management of splenic injury are listed in Table 2.

Table 1

CT Grade and Healing Time Noted With Ultrasonography for Splenic Injury in Children

Grade of Injury (Buntain System)	Equivalent AAST Grade	Healing by US (mean time, weeks)[a]
I	I	3.1 +/– 3.06
II	I	8.21 +/– 3.86
III	III, IV	12.11 +/– 54.32
IV	V	20.71 +/– 7.72

AAST = American Association for the Surgery of Trauma, US = ultrasonography.

[a]Healing time noted by Lynch et al at time of discharge ultrasound comparing grade of injury by two systems of splenic injury.

Data from Lynch JM, Meza MP, Newman B, Gardner MJ, Albanese CT: Computed tomography grade of splenic injury is predictive of the time required for radiographic healing. *J Pediatr Surg* 1997;32(7):1093-1095, discussion 1095-1096.

Table 2

Recommendations for Managing Splenic Injury

Recommendations	Level of Evidence
Patients hemodynamically unstable or with diffuse peritonitis should have urgent laparotomy.	1
In the hemodynamically stable patient without peritonitis, routine laparotomy is NOT indicated.	2
Nonsurgical management trial is not contraindicated in hemodynamically stable patients regardless of severity of injury grade, neurologic status, presence of associated injuries, or age > 55.	2
In hemodynamically stable patient without peritonitis, CECT should be performed.	2
Nonsurgical management for splenic injuries should take place only in a setting equipped to monitor the patient and perform serial examinations and with an operating room on standby for urgent laparotomy.	2

CECT = contrast-enhanced CT.

Data from Stassen NA, Bhullar I, Cheng JD, et al; Eastern Association for the Surgery of Trauma: Selective nonoperative management of blunt splenic injury: An Eastern Association for the Surgery of Trauma practice management guideline. *J Trauma Acute Care Surg* 2012;73(5, Suppl 4) S294-S300.

Injuries to the Liver

The liver is reportedly the most commonly injured intra-abdominal organ from all trauma.[5,28] Common injuries include hematoma or laceration of the subcapsular or intraparenchymal tissue. Evaluation may demonstrate right upper quadrant abdominal pain, referred pain, and possible injury to the ribs.

In a review article of EAST Practice Management Guidelines, level II evidence recommendations for liver trauma were summarized.[29] Evaluation with contrast-enhanced CT remains the gold standard for the diagnosis of liver injuries in the stable patient without signs of peritonitis. Angiography with embolization should be considered when evidence of active bleeding (a contrast blush noted in the parenchyma) is present on CT. The success rate for nonsurgical management has been reported to be between 82% and 100%.[28] The use of liver function tests to determine diagnostic and treatment paradigms has been studied.[30-32] Most of these studies have been small and/or retrospective. Therefore, no consensus exists on the use of elevated liver enzymes to aid in the diagnosis of liver injury, given varied results and thresholds.[28]

The organ injury grading system according to the AAST criteria has been used to aid in the diagnosis and management of liver injury.[21] The system grades injury based on the location and the extent of lesions noted on CT. Grades III or higher include subscapular hematoma greater than 50%, intraparenchymal hematoma greater than 10%, or a laceration deeper than 3 cm. In general, the higher the grade, the more anatomic disruption is noted. For example, grade I has minimal disruption,

whereas grade V has massive disruption.

The duration of hospital observation has been proposed to be at least 24 hours for grades I and II and at least 36 hours for grades III and higher.[33] The overall success rate for nonsurgical management was 94%; failures were related to the development of peritonitis from concomitant bowel injuries or hemorrhage attributed to a source other than the liver.

Complications, reportedly low at 0% to 11%, often present later in the clinical course as abdominal pain, jaundice, nausea, vomiting, or biliary peritonitis.[33] These complications include bile leaks, bile peritonitis, hepatic abscess, bilious ascites, and hemobilia.[29] Intervention with endoscopic retrograde cholangiopancreatography (ERCP), angiography, percutaneous drains, or laparoscopy may be needed for the management of these complications.

Current evidence does not support the need for routine, follow-up CT before or after discharge.[24,34] Follow-up CT would be recommended if clinically indicated for hemodynamic deterioration or signs of peritonitis.

Return to play also has been linked to the degree of injury. For isolated liver injury involving a simple laceration or subscapular hematoma, healing has been reported to take 2 to 4 months. A higher grade injury may take up to 6 months to heal.[25] The healing times of liver injury were evaluated by ultrasonographic follow-up[35] (Table 3). It was noted that healing time was faster for lacerations than for hematomas. The authors of a 2011 study noted that the average length of inpatient stay after isolated liver injury was 2.2 days.[33] The protocol used in that study allowed light activity after the second day. Patients were restricted from contact sports for 3 months.

Only limited, high-quality literature is available regarding activity restrictions and return to play after liver injury.[5,24,25,29] The American Pediatric Surgical Association recommends 'normal' age-appropriate activity restriction correlated with CT staging ranging from 3 to 6 weeks for stages I to IV, respectively.[34] Importantly, this recommendation of age-appropriate activity restriction was not an endorsement for the time required to safely return to contact sports. Most studies and review articles that do address return to play in contact sports recommend tailoring the return-to-play decisions based on the athlete's degree of injury recovery, the normalization of liver enzymes, and readiness in terms of physiologic conditioning and mental fitness, with an informed consent approach.

Table 4 outlines the recommendations for the management of liver injury.[29]

Injuries to the Kidney

In BAT, the kidney is the third most common organ injured in adults and the most common organ injured in children, according to the pediatric literature.[3] Overall, the kidney is the most commonly injured organ in the genitourinary tract and comprises 1.5% of all trauma.[36] Of all renal injuries, 90% to 95% are from BAT. Most injuries to the kidneys (95% to 98%) are mild, however, and can be treated nonsurgically.[37]

The kidney is a retroperitoneal organ, protected by the lower ribs, the abdominal muscles, and the latissimus dorsi and paravertebral muscles of the back. Mechanisms of injury to the kidneys include direct blows, punctures from a fractured rib, or deceleration from a high velocity, because the kidney is partially mobile. Sports and other activities in which these types of injury are seen include bicycling, all-terrain vehicle riding, playground falls, motor vehicle racing, skateboarding, in-line skating, horseback riding, gymnastics, and contact sports such as football, soccer, and rugby.

Pediatric patients reportedly are more susceptible than adults to kidney injury in BAT because of the physical differences between the kidneys of children and those of

Table 3

Liver Healing Time Noted With Ultrasonography Per CT Stage of Injury

CT Stage	Hematoma (days)	Laceration (days)
I	6	—
II	45	29
III	108	34
IV	—	78

Data from Tiberio GA, Portolani N, Coniglio A, et al: Evaluation of the healing time of non-operatively managed liver injuries. *Hepatogastroenterology* 2008;55(84):1010-1012.

Table 4

Recommendations for Managing Liver Injury

Recommendations	Level of Evidence
BAT patients who are hemodynamically unstable or who have diffuse peritonitis should undergo urgent laparotomy.	1
BAT patients who are hemodynamically stable without peritonitis should undergo CECT.	2
The severity of liver injury by grade, neurologic status, age greater than 55 years, and/or the presence of other associated injuries are NOT absolute contraindications for nonsurgical management that is hemodynamically stable.	2
Angiography with embolization should be considered in hemodynamically stable patients with evidence of active extravasation (contrast blush on CT).	2
Nonsurgical management should be considered in liver injuries only in a facility that offers monitoring, serial clinical examinations, and urgent operating room availability on standby.	2

BAT = blunt abdominal trauma, CECT = contrast-enhanced computed tomography.

Data from Stassen NA, Bhullar I, Cheng JD, et al; Eastern Association for the Surgery of Trauma: Nonoperative management of blunt hepatic injury: An Eastern Association for the Surgery of Trauma practice management guideline. *J Trauma Acute Care Surg* 2012;73(5, Suppl 4) S288-S293.

adults. The kidney is proportionately larger in dimension to body size in childhood. In children, the kidney is also more exposed because it is situated lower in the abdomen and is less protected by the ribcage; also, children have a lower amount of perirenal fat and weaker abdominal musculature.[38] It has been noted in one study that older children had a higher number of blunt trauma injuries during sports than did younger athletes.[3] This finding stands in contrast to the expected greater number of injuries in younger patients, according to another study.[38] The discrepancy may be explained by the distinction between trauma caused by incidents occurring outside of sports (eg, motor vehicle accidents, falls, penetrating trauma) and those occurring from BAT in sports. It has been theorized that the older athletes played with more speed and mass and had greater force in collisions than did their younger counterparts.[3]

Renal injury in adults is manifested by gross or microscopic hematuria, hypotension, and signs of trauma such as abdominal or flank pain, rib fractures and contusions to the abdomen, flank, or ribs.[39] CT is ordered if an adult presents with gross hematuria, microscopic hematuria with hypotension, and penetrating injury, with a suspected mechanism for renal injury. If microscopic hematuria without hypotension is present, observation with frequent examinations and laboratory studies are required. Pediatric patients may not be hypotensive with renal injuries; therefore, the threshold for ordering imaging studies is lower than in adults. CT is ordered for all pediatric patients if hematuria, defined as having more than 50 red blood cells per high-power field present on urinalysis, a mechanism for renal injury, and abdominal/flank symptoms are present.[41] Using these criteria, no injuries were missed on CT.[39,40]

Contrast three-phase CT renal protocol is helpful in establishing the diagnosis, directing treatment, identifying other injuries, and defining the anatomy of lacerations and devascularized renal parenchyma, as well as urinary extravasation or retroperitoneal bleeding.[40] The AAST organ grading system[21] correlates CT findings (the extent and grade of kidney injury) with the treatment recommendations.[41]

Grade I injuries include contusions or subcapsular hematoma that are nonexpanding, with no parenchymal laceration. Grade II injuries are classified as a nonexpanding perirenal hematoma confined to the retroperitoneum or a laceration less than 1.0 cm of the depth of the renal cortex, without urinary extravasation. A grade III injury is a laceration less than 1.0 cm of the parenchymal depth of the renal cortex not involving the collecting system and without urinary extravasation. A grade IV injury is a parenchymal laceration extending through the renal cortex, the medulla, and the collecting system or the main renal artery, or a vein injury with contained hemorrhage. A grade V injury is a completely shattered kidney or an avulsion of the renal hilum, with associated devascularization of the kidney.[21]

Nonsurgical management initially consists of bed rest with close observation and frequent serial examinations, urinalysis, and hematocrits. As gross hematuria clears, light activity is permitted. Most kidney injuries are grades I and II and respond to nonsurgical management. Many grade III injuries also are treated with nonsurgical management.[18,36] Debate exists regarding the optimal treatment of grade IV injury but treatment often starts with nonsurgical management, with consideration for diagnostic angiography for renal embolization. Indications for laparotomy include hemodynamic instability, other associated abdominal injuries, an expanding or pulsatile perirenal hematoma or mass, renal pelvis injury, and grade V injuries.[42,43]

Return to play depends on the grade of injury and the resolution of microscopic hematuria, with minor injuries taking 2 to 6 weeks and major injury taking 6 to 12 months.[42] Renal injuries in the National Football League over 14 years were reviewed and it was noted that contusions were the most common injuries and that injuries occurred 10 times more often in games than in practice.[44] No reported loss of kidney function and no reinjury of the kidneys occurred after resumption of play. Return to play was reported as occurring 2 to 6 weeks from the date of most contusions, with lacerations taking 8 weeks. More severe injuries were reimaged.

Table 5 outlines the recommendations for the management of kidney injury.[43]

Athletes With a Solitary Kidney

Recommendations exist for allowing athletes with a solitary kidney to participate in sports. The PPE Preparticipation Physical Evaluation Monograph, 4th edition, gives a qualified "yes" for allowing participation in contact sports.[45] "If the athlete chooses to play in a sport that may place a solitary kidney at increased risk for damage, a full explanation should be given to the athlete, his or her parent(s) or guardian(s), and the coaches. The explanation should include the controversial use of available protection (flak or shock-absorbing jacket), which has not been proved to reduce the risk of injury, potential serious long-term consequences of potential injury, and treatment of injuries if they occur."[45] Studies have shown that most kidney injuries resulting in loss occurred as a result of motor vehicle accidents, pedestrian and motor vehicle accidents, and falls. No kidneys were lost from injury during participation in contact sports. The only

Table 5

Recommendations for Managing Kidney Injury

Recommendations[a]

1. Hemodynamic stability should be assessed on admission.

2. Findings on physical examination such as hematuria; pain, abrasions, and bruising of the flank; fractured ribs; abdominal tenderness; and abdominal mass or distension could indicate renal injury.

3. Urine from a patient suspected of renal trauma should be evaluated for hematuria by visual examination and dipstick.

4. Patients with hematuria (gross or microscopic) and hypotension should undergo CT.

5. CECT with delayed images is the gold standard for diagnosis and grading of renal injuries in hemodynamically stable patients.

6. Hemodynamically stable patients with blunt renal trauma should be treated nonsurgically until gross hematuria clears.

CECT = contrast-enhanced CT.

[a] Grade of all recommendations is A.

Data from Summerton DJ, Djakovic N, Kitrey ND, et al: Guidelines on urological trauma. 2014 European Association of Urology. Available at: http://uroweb.org/guideline/urological-trauma/. Accessed July 25, 2015.

kidneys lost to injury during sports participation occurred in high-speed sports such as skiing, sledding, and in-line skating.[40,46]

Injury to the Bladder

Bladder trauma is also uncommon in sports and has an overall incidence of 1.6% of all BAT, with 44% having at least one other associated intra-abdominal injury.[46,47] This factor may explain the high mortality rate of 10% to 22% associated with traumatic bladder injuries.[48] An estimated 2% to 11% of patients with pelvic fractures sustain bladder injuries,[47] and fracture of the pelvis increased the risk of bladder rupture from 1.6% to 5.7%.[48] Serious bladder injury in sports is infrequent, however. In adults older than 20 years, the emptied bladder is protected anteriorly by the pelvic ring and posteriorly by the peritoneum and lower abdominal contents. As the bladder fills, it rises out of the protective pelvic ring. Importantly, in children, the bladder is located in the abdomen because the bony pelvis is not developed, leaving children more susceptible to injury.

The bladder can sustain three types of injuries: contusion, extraperitoneal rupture, or intraperitoneal rupture.

The mechanism of injury can assist in making the diagnosis. Typical mechanisms include rapid deceleration, high-velocity impact, and collision, as well as penetration.[49] Examples of sports reported to cause bladder injury are motor vehicle racing, horseback riding, bull riding, high-speed alpine sports, gymnastics, martial arts, rugby, and football.

The most common type of bladder rupture is extraperitoneal, with an incidence of 70% to 90%, resulting from pelvic ring rupture that causes bony fragments to penetrate and rupture the bladder near the anterolateral aspect of the base of the bladder.[49] Urine then leaks into the perivesicular space and can even track into the thigh, scrotum, or perineum. The next most common type of bladder rupture is intraperitoneal, with an incidence of 15% to 25%, in which the bladder ruptures near the dome (the weakest part of the bladder) when distended and exposed out of its pelvic protection.[49] This type of injury often is caused by blunt force. Here, the urine can leak into paracolic gutters and in between loops of bowel. A combined intraperitoneal and extraperitoneal type of rupture of the bladder, having an incidence of 5% to 12%, also is seen.[49]

Cardinal symptoms of bladder rupture include gross hematuria, abdominal pain, and difficult or absent voiding. Gross hematuria is present 95% of the time, particularly if an associated pelvic fracture is present. Only microscopic hematuria is noted, however, 5% to 15% of the time.[43] The clinician also may note bruises to the abdomen, signs of trauma, and distension, as well as swelling of the thigh, scrotum, or perineum.

The workup for bladder rupture starts with suspicion, based on the mechanism of injury and presenting symptoms. According to the European Association of Urology position statement, when signs of trauma are present, cystography should be obtained if the following factors are seen: (1) gross hematuria without pelvic fracture, (2) microscopic hematuria with pelvic fracture, or (3) isolated microscopic hematuria. The presence of gross hematuria and signs of pelvic fracture are absolute indications for cystography.[43] Cystography with CT is preferred in the setting of other suspected trauma, for example, to visualize the kidneys and ureters.

Treatment is based on the location and type of injury as well as concomitant injuries. Most uncomplicated extraperitoneal ruptures may be treated nonsurgically with a catheter and antibiotics. Often, when open reduction and internal fixation is done for the pelvic ring, surgical repair of the bladder is performed to prevent further contamination of the surgical site. Also, if the neck of the bladder is ruptured, surgical repair often is indicated. Intraperitoneal ruptures are treated with surgical exploration and repair.

Although often unreported, bladder contusions are probably more common if no sustained hematuria is present. Most bladder contusions are self-limiting, and require a diagnosis of exclusion. The injury represents a partial tear of the bladder mucosa. The mechanism of injury is a flaccid bladder reverberating on itself. A presentation of atraumatic hematuria warrants evaluation for other causes of hematuria such as infection, medication, nephrolithiasis, malignancy, sickle cell disease, and rhabdomyolysis. The presence of microtraumatic bladder contusions should be noted. In this setting, the trauma is repetitive and reportedly mild. An example would be distance running, in which the empty bladder reverberates against itself. The result can be asymptomatic hematuria, and after exclusion of other causes, the treatment is rest and hydration until the resolution of the hematuria.[49,50] A partially filled bladder can help mitigate this potential sequela of repetitive microtrauma causing asymptomatic hematuria.

No published guidelines exist for return to play after bladder rupture. Therefore, as for other BAT to intra-abdominal organs, the clinician should wait until the athlete is asymptomatic and physically and mentally ready to resume graded return-to-play activities. Ideally, this progression would be managed with the consultation of an appropriate urologic specialist. The EAST recommendations for the treatment of bladder injuries state that nonsurgical treatment of blunt extraperitoneal rupture of the bladder has outcomes similar to those of primary suturing, with level III evidence.[51]

Injury to the Ureters

Ureter injury is rare, accounting for only 1.0% to 2.5% of urinary tract injuries. Of the injuries to the ureters, only approximately one-third result from blunt trauma; most are related to motor-vehicle accidents due to deceleration forces.[43] When the ureters are injured, other accompanying abdominal-pelvic injuries usually are present.

The mechanism of injury in BAT is deceleration, in which the renal pelvis can be sheared from the ureter. The diagnosis often is delayed. Hematuria may be present only in 50% to 75% of patients presenting with trauma.[52] A high index of suspicion is needed to diagnose ureter injuries. When they are suspected, CT is useful in demonstrating the extravasation of contrast, ascites, hydronephrosis, urinoma, or dilation of the ureter.[43] Treatment varies, based on the degree of injury and the associated injuries. Stenting is useful when indicated.

No literature on return-to-play standards exist. Therefore, the clinician should wait until the athlete is asymptomatic and physically and mentally ready to resume graded return-to-play activities, after consultation with an appropriate specialist.

Table 6

Eastern Association for the Surgery of Trauma Guidelines for Managing Pancreatic Trauma

Recommendations for Treatment[a]

Delay in Dx or main pancreatic duct injury causes increased morbidity.

CT is suggestive but not diagnostic of pancreatic injury.

Amylase/lipase levels are suggestive but not diagnostic of pancreatic injury.

Grade 1 and 2 injuries can be managed by drainage alone.

Grade 3 injuries should be managed with resection and drainage.

Closed suction is preferred to sump suction.

Dx = diagnosis.

[a] Level of evidence for all treatment recommendations is III.

Data from Bokhari F, Phelan H, Holevar M, et al: EAST, Eastern Association for the Surgery of Trauma: Pancreatic trauma, diagnosis and management of. 2009. Available at: https://www.east.org/resources/treatment-guidelines/pancreatic-trauma-diagnosis-and-management-of

Injury to the Pancreas

The pancreas is the fourth most commonly injured organ in BAT, but its treatment presents a dilemma for the sports medicine practitioner. High morbidity and mortality are associated with a delay in diagnosis and management. Also, the diagnostic workup is less proven and clear than that for other organs. Furthermore, the pancreas is retroperitoneal, so most signs and symptoms of abdominal organ injury may not apply to the pancreas. Scant good literature exists to help the clinician diagnose and manage pancreatic injuries related to BAT. The EAST review found no RCTs, and most studies reviewed were small, retrospective, and without controls.[53] The best recommendations supported were of level III evidence at best[53] (Table 6).

The incidence of pancreatic injury in BAT has been reported in similar ranges for the pediatric and adult populations, 2% to 10% and 3% to 12%, respectively.[54,55] Most traumatic pancreatic injury results from penetrating trauma (such as gunshot or knife wounds) or blunt mechanisms. As described previously, the pancreas is retroperitoneal, and in sports, the usual mechanism of injury is compression against the spine, commonly at the junction between the head and the body of the pancreas. These injuries have been reported in soccer, football, rugby, and karate and from bicycle handlebars directly compressing the pancreas. In children and lean adults, the pancreas may be more exposed.[55] The complications of pancreatic injury are associated with the organ's proximity to other structures (such as the aorta, superior mesenteric artery, vena cava, duodenum, and bowel). Complications have been reported in 19% to 55% of all pancreatic injuries and include pancreatic pseudocyst, fistula, and pancreatitis.[54]

The sports medicine practitioner needs to have a high level of suspicion and be aware of the mechanism of injury, because abdominal pain and peritoneal signs—if initially present—often will diminish over a short time, usually within 6 to 8 hours.[55] CT, which is helpful but not diagnostic, is not the best modality for accurate staging. Furthermore, common pancreatic duct injuries can be missed on CT.[53] Additional studies can help diagnose pancreatic injuries. ERCP can identify duct injuries and be therapeutic, allowing stent placement. It is invasive, however, and has a potential for further complications, including iatrogenic pancreatitis, gastrointestinal tract perforation, and hemorrhage. Magnetic resonance cholangiopancreatography has gained favor as a noninvasive alternative to ERCP, with equally good results in identifying pancreatic duct anatomy and without the potential complications of ERCP.[55]

Pancreatic enzymes have been investigated as a diagnostic aid. Studies performed before the EAST summary was published were lacking in the use of controls, were not randomized, and had low numbers of subjects.[53] Conclusions from these limited studies showed that elevation of serum amylase and lipase were suggestive of pancreatic injury but did not possess adequate sensitivity or specificity to diagnose pancreatic injury.[53] Additionally, when concomitant craniofacial trauma was present, the likelihood of falsely elevated salivary amylase levels existed.[57] A more recent prospective cohort study with some controls demonstrated combined serum amylase and lipase predicted pancreatic injury with a sensitivity of 100% and a specificity of 85%.[56] It was noted that significant elevation in amylase was observed in pancreas and bowel injuries, whereas elevation of lipase showed specificity of pancreatic injury with or without injury to the bowel. These findings were time dependent, only being valid if measured longer than 6 hours postinjury. Higher grade injuries were associated with higher levels of amylase and lipase. The cutoffs were greater than 100 IU for serum amylase and greater than 250 IU for serum lipase.

The classification of pancreatic injuries follows the AAST grading system and is based on pancreatic duct involvement.[21] Grade I and II injuries have minor to major contusion and minor to major laceration, respectively, without duct involvement or tissue loss. Grade III injury includes distal transection or parenchymal injury with duct involvement. Grade IV involves proximal transection or parenchymal injury involving the ampulla, and grade V represents massive disruption of the head of the pancreas.

Management largely is based on the suspected involvement of the ducts, but again, few good-quality studies exist, and consensus is lacking, especially for grade IV to V injury. The informal consensus is to treat grade I and II injuries with nonsurgical management, using closed drainage if necessary. In grade III injuries with duct involvement, management ranges from suturing the duct or placing stents to resection. Outcomes vary, and the rate of complications, including fistula formation and abscesses, varies, with higher rates noted for drainage alone than for resection. The management of grade IV and higher injuries remains controversial, with poor clarity in the literature. Resection with drainage is used often, as are more complicated surgical procedures such as pancreaticoduodenectomy (the Whipple procedure) and Roux-en-Y pancreaticojejunostomy.[54] The surgical management of higher grade pancreatic injuries is beyond the scope of this chapter. The consensus is that earlier intervention for higher grade injuries reduces morbidity, however.

Return-to-play guidelines are not discussed in the literature. Thus, return-to-play decisions should be based on tissue healing, the normalization of symptoms and laboratory assessment, the resolution of complications if present, and in general, the athlete's physical and mental readiness to resume a stepwise increase in levels of activity.

Gastrointestinal Tract Injury

Traumatic injury to the gastrointestinal tract is not common, and the literature on the subject is limited to case reports and concomitant treatment of other organ injuries in BAT. Gastrointestinal tract injury is noted in 5% to 7% of laparotomies performed for BAT. In penetrating trauma, gastrointestinal tract injury is fairly common and is seen in 80% of presenting cases.[56]

The causes of injury include contusion, which can lead to rupture or tears of the bowel or viscera and mesenteric vessels. Several mechanisms for injury have been proposed, including crushing of the gastrointestinal tract between the blunt object and the spine, as well as rapid deceleration that causes shear forces between the fixed and mobile gastrointestinal tract segments, which often is where mesenteric tears occur, causing bleeding. Also described is a burst injury pattern, resulting from the pressure gradient between closed loops of bowel on impact. Sports in which gastrointestinal tract injuries reportedly occur include soccer, football, horseback riding, high-speed alpine sports or motor vehicle racing, and cycling, from handlebar penetration.[16]

Presenting symptoms can be unreliable and may include signs of peritonitis, abdominal pain, and emesis. Often, symptoms are absent or delayed until leakage occurs, causing peritoneal irritation or hemodynamic compromise. Maintaining clinical suspicion for gastrointestinal tract injury is important, based on the mechanisms described.[16] Laparotomies performed solely on clinical symptoms were reported to have false-negative rates of 40%.[57] Close observation, serial examinations, and the monitoring of hemodynamic status are essential.[56]

In the hemodynamically stable patient, FAST examinations may show hemoperitoneum or pneumoperitoneum, leading to laparotomy. CT with contrast is recommended if clinical suspicion exists, along with an applicable mechanism of injury and serial examination findings. Definitive treatment involves surgical management.[56]

No recommendations for return to play exist in the literature. So again, in consultation with the surgeon, return to play is achieved in a graded fashion when the athlete is physically and mentally prepared.

Diaphragmatic Rupture

Diaphragmatic rupture occurs mainly from BAT or penetrating trauma, although most studies demonstrate a higher occurrence from penetrating trauma.[58-60] The incidence of diaphragmatic rupture ranges from 4% to 8%, with mortality, usually from associated injuries, as high as 1% to 28%.[59,61,62] A dearth of sports medicine literature related to diaphragmatic rupture exists; most articles are case reports. The mechanism of injury is rapid deceleration, often with a caudally directed force. Sports in which diaphragmatic rupture has been reported include skiing, snowboarding, luge, skeleton, swimming, and diving. One case report of a spontaneous, atraumatic rupture during Pilates was presumed to result from deep-breathing exercises.[63]

The pressure gradient between the thoracic and abdominal cavities allows the contents of the abdomen to invade the thorax after a tear. The organs most likely to herniate are the stomach and the bowel, and most organs do so on the left hemidiaphragm, in a 3:1 ratio.[59,62] The liver acts as a barrier to the bowel contents on the right because of tears and herniation. Associated injuries include fractured ribs, lung contusion and tears, and laceration of the liver and bowel.

Diagnosis is difficult in the absence of associated injuries, because a diaphragmatic tear often fails to cause blood loss or signs of peritonitis; therefore, isolated tears may present initially as being hemodynamically stable. Possible associated symptoms can include tachypnea, dyspnea, chest pain, and signs of intestinal obstruction. Bowel sounds may be heard in the left thorax more than

in the right thorax, with decreased breath sounds in the affected hemithorax.[61]

Radiographs may be helpful in the diagnosis, although the sensitivity is approximately 50% on initial examination and may increase up to 62% on delayed chest radiographs.[58] Useful signs on radiographs include loss of normal hemidiaphragm contours, observation of viscus in the hemidiaphragm, and mediastinal shift. FAST examination may identify abnormal diaphragm motility but is not relied on for diagnosis.[61] CT is helpful to identify diaphragmatic tear and often is used to better delineate other potential injuries to organs.[64] In clinically stable patients, MRI can aid in the subtleties of diagnosis. Management most often includes surgical exploration and repair with nonabsorbable sutures.

No literature exists addressing the return to play after diaphragmatic rupture. The sports medicine practitioner should apply the same approach as that used for other organs for return to play when no guidelines are available.

Summary

Abdominal trauma, although rare, is still associated with a substantial risk of morbidity and mortality. The sports medicine practitioner should be aware of the mechanism of injury and, when a high level of suspicion for abdominal trauma exists, should refer the patient to an appropriate facility for observation, workup, and management, as indicated. Although ultrasonography should still be part of the diagnostic workup, in a hemodynamically stable patient contrast-enhanced CT is the preferred study. Nonsurgical management is successful in most mild to moderate grade injuries. In these cases, little need for follow-up CT exists, especially for the determination of readiness for return to activity. Poor evidence exists from randomized controlled studies regarding the time of observation, return to activity, and return to play, and additional studies are needed. Finally, return-to-play decisions should be made when the athlete is asymptomatic, with informed consent regarding the risk of reinjury. Assessment of the physical and mental readiness of the athlete is of paramount importance.

© 2016 American Academy of Orthopaedic Surgeons

Key Study Points

- Athletes suspected of having abdominal injuries often based on knowledge of the mechanism of injury should be immediately removed from play and evaluated for blunt abdominal trauma. Signs and symptoms, if present, often have a delayed onset.

- In children, the kidney and bladder often are injured more commonly than in adults.

- The imaging study of choice for the hemodynamically stable athlete is a CT scan with contrast. FAST examinations are helpful in the hemodynamically stable athlete in many cases to avoid laparotomies.

- Nonsurgical management is typically the treatment of choice for most blunt abdominal injuries in a hemodynamically stable patient. Evaluation and treatment for blunt abdominal trauma should be in a facility with capabilities for CT scanning, angiography, surgery and continuous monitoring on demand.

- Blunt abdominal trauma involving the pancreas poses a dilemma: high morbidity and mortality with no good means of evaluation (CT scan, laboratory results, and physical examination findings are not diagnostic).

- Return-to-play decisions, although there is no consensus, are based on the location and extent of injury, and repeat CT scans are not recommended for most blunt abdominal trauma.

Annotated References

1. Comstock RD, Collins CL, Currie DW: National high school sports-related injury surveillance study 2012-2013. University of Colorado, Denver, CO. Available at: http://www.ucdenver.edu/academics/colleges/PublicHealth/research/ResearchProjects/piper/projects/RIO/Documents/2012-13.pdf. Accessed on July 25, 2015.

   This surveillance report by high school athletic trainers is the most recent published data collection of the high school sports-related injury surveillance system, with an online reporting system. Level of evidence: III.

2. Bergqvist D, Hedelin H, Karlsson G, Lindblad B, Mätzsch T: Abdominal trauma during thirty years: Analysis of a large case series. *Injury* 1981;13(2):93-99.

3. Wan J, Corvino TF, Greenfield SP, DiScala C: Kidney and testicle injuries in team and individual sports: Data from the national pediatric trauma registry. *J Urol* 2003;170(4 Pt 2):1528-1532, discussion 1531-1532.

4. Walter KD: Radiographic evaluation of the patient with sport-related abdominal trauma. *Curr Sports Med Rep* 2007;6(2):115-119.

5. Rifat SF, Gilvydis RP: Blunt abdominal trauma in sports. *Curr Sports Med Rep* 2003;2(2):93-97.

6. Machida T, Hanazaki K, Ishizaka K, et al: Snowboarding injuries of the abdomen: Comparison with skiing injuries. *Injury* 1999;30(1):47-49.

7. Geddes R, Irish K: Boarder belly: Splenic injuries resulting from ski and snowboarding accidents. *Emerg Med Australas* 2005;17(2):157-162.

8. Ballantyne B, Ling A, Pazionis A, Roebotham RW: The current role of focused assessment with Sonography for trauma (FAST) in the ever-evolving approach to abdominal trauma. *UWOMJ* 2012;81(1):20-22.

   This review article summarizes the diagnostic approach to the blunt abdominal trauma patient. Level of evidence: V.

9. Stengel D, Bauwens K, Rademacher G, Ekkernkamp A, Güthoff C: Emergency ultrasound-based algorithms for diagnosing blunt abdominal trauma. *Cochrane Database Syst Rev* 2013;7(No. CD004446):CD004446.

   This Cochrane review of trauma algorithms includes ultrasound for blunt abdominal trauma. The authors found insufficient evidence of quality studies randomized controlled trials to justify using ultrasound-based clinical decision making. Level of evidence: II.

10. Sato M, Yoshii H: Reevaluation of ultrasonography for solid-organ injury in blunt abdominal trauma. *J Ultrasound Med* 2004;23(12):1583-1596.

11. Van Vugt R, Keus F, Kool D, Deunk J, Edwards M: Selective computed tomography (CT) versus routine thoracoabdominal CT for high-energy blunt-trauma patients. *Cochrane Database Syst Rev* 2013;12(No. CD009743):CD009743.

   This Cochrane review assesses the difference between routine CT and selective CT in the management of blunt high-energy trauma. The authors found no RCTs to support either method. Level of evidence: I.

12. Wolf S: Sustained contraction of the diaphragm, the mechanism of a common type of dyspnea and precordial pain. *J Clin Invest* 1947;26(6):1201.

13. Johnson R: Abdominal wall injuries: Rectus abdominis strains, oblique strains, rectus sheath hematoma. *Curr Sports Med Rep* 2006;5(2):99-103.

14. Suleiman S, Johnston DE: The abdominal wall: An overlooked source of pain. *Am Fam Physician* 2001;64(3):431-438.

15. Olthof DC, van der Vlies CH, Scheerder MJ, et al: Reliability of injury grading systems for patients with blunt splenic trauma. *Injury* 2014;45(1):146-150.

This retrospective study looks at intra-rater and inter-rater reliability, comparing the AAST grading system and the Baltimore grading system using CT for splenic trauma. The Baltimore CT grading system was developed in 2007 and predicts the need for angiography, embolization, or surgery. Both grading systems appear to be equally reliable, but because the Baltimore system incorporates vascular injury, it may be superior in the clinical management of blunt splenic injuries. Level of evidence: III.

16. Wegner S, Colletti JE, Van Wie D: Pediatric blunt abdominal trauma. *Pediatr Clin North Am* 2006;53(2):243-256.

17. Gannon EH, Howard T: Splenic injuries in athletes: A review. *Curr Sports Med Rep* 2010;9(2):111-114.

   This review article summarizes the current approach to splenic injuries in athletes and addresses the return-to-play conundrum. Level of evidence: V.

18. Stassen NA, Bhullar I, Cheng JD, et al; Eastern Association for the Surgery of Trauma: Selective nonoperative management of blunt splenic injury: An Eastern Association for the Surgery of Trauma practice management guideline. *J Trauma Acute Care Surg* 2012;73(5, Suppl 4)S294-S300.

   The practice management guidelines committee of the Eastern Association for the Surgery of Trauma made recommendations for the nonsurgical treatment of splenic injuries based on the level of evidence. They summarized the areas of poor consensus and the need for future research. Level of evidence: III.

19. Bhangu A, Nepogodiev D, Lal N, Bowley DM: Meta-analysis of predictive factors and outcomes for failure of non-operative management of blunt splenic trauma. *Injury* 2012;43(9):1337-1346.

   This systematic review with meta-analysis analyzes the predictive factors and outcomes of the failure of nonsurgical management in splenic trauma. Level of evidence: III.

20. Gomez D, Haas B, Al-Ali K, Monneuse O, Nathens AB, Ahmed N: Controversies in the management of splenic trauma. *Injury* 2012;43(1):55-61.

   The authors surveyed 70 experts in trauma care from 10 countries to explore the controversies in the nonsurgical management of splenic trauma including, imaging, angioembolization, and nonsurgical management in special populations. Level of evidence: IV.

21. Moore EE, Cogbill TH, Jurkovich GJ, Malangoni MA, Jukovich GJ, Champion HR: Scaling system for organ specific injuries. *Curr Opin Crit Care* 1996;2:450-462.

22. Olthof DC, van der Vlies CH, Joosse P, van Delden OM, Jurkovich GJ, Goslings JC; PYTHIA Collaboration Group: Consensus strategies for the nonoperative management of patients with blunt splenic injury: A Delphi study. *J Trauma Acute Care Surg* 2013;74(6):1567-1574.

   This is a study using the Delphi method of polling experts in their field, in this case, blunt splenic trauma. This study notes the consensus of approach and does not summarize

randomized controlled studies. The authors did note that, among practitioners, a lack of consensus remains regarding the time to return to play, with recommendations ranging from 4 weeks to 3 months, depending on the grade of injury and activity status. Level of evidence: IV.

23. Izu BS, Ryan M, Markert RJ, Ekeh AP, McCarthy MC: Impact of splenic injury guidelines on hospital stay and charges in patients with isolated splenic injury. *Surgery* 2009;146(4):787-791, discussion 791-793.

   This retrospective study compares the cost and hospitalization stay before and after implementation of treatment guidelines for nonsurgical management in splenic injury. The authors found no cost difference but did find a substantial difference in the length of hospital stay, which was shorter after implementing the guidelines. Level of evidence: III.

24. Sharma OP, Oswanski MF, Singer D: Role of repeat computerized tomography in nonoperative management of solid organ trauma. *Am Surg* 2005;71(3):244-249.

25. Juyia RF, Kerr HA: Return to play after liver and spleen trauma. *Sports Health* 2014;6(3):239-245.

   This article reviews the literature on return to play after liver and spleen injuries (grade C recommendations). Level of evidence: III.

26. Lynch JM, Meza MP, Newman B, Gardner MJ, Albanese CT: Computed tomography grade of splenic injury is predictive of the time required for radiographic healing. *J Pediatr Surg* 1997;32(7):1093-1095, discussion 1095-1096.

27. Zarzaur BL, Vashi S, Magnotti LJ, Croce MA, Fabian TC: The real risk of splenectomy after discharge home following nonoperative management of blunt splenic injury. *J Trauma* 2009;66(6):1531-1536, discussion 1536-1538.

   This prospective cohort study looks at the number of blunt splenic trauma patients who were readmitted after being treated nonsurgically and discharged home. The authors found that 8.5% of those readmitted within 180 days (1.4% of the total discharged home) had undergone splenectomy. Of interest, 64% were readmitted within 1 week of discharge. Level of evidence: III.

28. Holmes JF, Sokolove PE, Brant WE, et al: Identification of children with intra-abdominal injuries after blunt trauma. *Ann Emerg Med* 2002;39(5):500-509.

29. Stassen NA, Bhullar I, Cheng JD, et al; Eastern Association for the Surgery of Trauma: Nonoperative management of blunt hepatic injury: An Eastern Association for the Surgery of Trauma practice management guideline. *J Trauma Acute Care Surg* 2012;73(5, Suppl 4)S288-S293.

   The practice management guidelines committee for the Eastern Association for the Surgery of Trauma made recommendations for the nonsurgical treatment of liver injuries based on the level of evidence. The areas of poor consensus were summarized and the need for future research was discussed. Level of evidence: II.

30. Karam O, La Scala G, Le Coultre C, Chardot C: Liver function tests in children with blunt abdominal traumas. *Eur J Pediatr Surg* 2007;17(5):313-316.

31. Puranik SR, Hayes JS, Long J, Mata M: Liver enzymes as predictors of liver damage due to blunt abdominal trauma in children. *South Med J* 2002;95(2):203-206.

32. Tian Z, Liu H, Su X, et al: Role of elevated liver transaminase levels in the diagnosis of liver injury after blunt abdominal trauma. *Exp Ther Med* 2012;4(2):255-260.

    This retrospective study evaluates using liver enzymes to predict the presence and severity of liver injury. Level of evidence: III.

33. Parks NA, Davis JW, Forman D, Lemaster D: Observation for nonoperative management of blunt liver injuries: How long is long enough? *J Trauma* 2011;70(3):626-629.

    This retrospective review of trauma patients with blunt liver injuries looks at the length of observation. Level of evidence: III.

34. Stylianos S; The APSA Trauma Committee: Evidence-based guidelines for resource utilization in children with isolated spleen or liver injury. *J Pediatr Surg* 2000;35(2):164-167, discussion 167-169.

35. Tiberio GA, Portolani N, Coniglio A, et al: Evaluation of the healing time of non-operatively managed liver injuries. *Hepatogastroenterology* 2008;55(84):1010-1012.

36. van der Vlies CH, Olthof DC, van Delden OM, et al: Management of blunt renal injury in a level 1 trauma centre in view of the European guidelines. *Injury* 2012;43(11):1816-1820.

    This is a retrospective review of the management of renal trauma patients over 4 years. Level of evidence: III.

37. Viola TA: Closed kidney injury. *Clin Sports Med* 2013;32(2):219-227.

    This is a review article of kidney trauma. Level of evidence: V.

38. Brown CK, Dunn KA, Wilson K: Diagnostic evaluation of patients with blunt abdominal trauma: A decision analysis. *Acad Emerg Med* 2000;7(4):385-396.

39. Bernard JJ: Renal trauma: Evaluation, management, and return to play. *Curr Sports Med Rep* 2009;8(2):98-103.

    This review article assessed at renal injuries and conditions, from microscopic hematuria to blunt trauma. Level of evidence: V.

40. Holmes FC, Hunt JJ, Sevier TL: Renal injury in sport. *Curr Sports Med Rep* 2003;2(2):103-109.

41. Santucci RA, McAninch JW, Safir M, Mario LA, Service S, Segal MR: Validation of the American Association for the Surgery of Trauma organ injury severity scale for the kidney. *J Trauma* 2001;50(2):195-200.

42. Nicola R, Menias CO, Mellnick V, Bhalla S, Raptis C, Siegel C: Sports-related genitourinary trauma in the male athlete. *Emerg Radiol* 2015;22(2):157-168.

    This review article discusses male genitourinary trauma. Level of evidence: V.

43. Summerton DJ, Djakovic N, Kitrey ND, et al: Guidelines on urological trauma. 2014 (update on 2013 published guidelines). European Association of Urology. Available at: http://uroweb.org/guideline/urological-trauma/. Accessed July 25, 2015.

    These updated guidelines, published online, summarize the literature and recommend an evidence-based approach to managing urologic trauma. Level of evidence: III.

44. Brophy RH, Gamradt SC, Barnes RP, et al: Kidney injuries in professional American football: Implications for management of an athlete with 1 functioning kidney. *Am J Sports Med* 2008;36(1):85-90.

45. Bernhardt D, Roberts WO, eds: *PPE Preparticipation Physical Evaluation*, ed 4. Elk Grove Village, IL, American Academy of Pediatrics, May 2010. https://www.aap.org/en-us/about-the-aap/Committees-Councils-Sections/Council-on-sports-medicine-and-fitness/Documents/PPE-4-forms.pdf

46. Johnson B, Christensen C, Dirusso S, Choudhury M, Franco I: A need for reevaluation of sports participation recommendations for children with a solitary kidney. *J Urol* 2005;174(2):686-689, discussion 689.

47. Gomez RG, Ceballos L, Coburn M, et al: Consensus statement on bladder injuries. *BJU Int* 2004;94(1):27-32.

48. McGeady JB, Breyer BN: Current epidemiology of genitourinary trauma. *Urol Clin North Am* 2013;40(3):323-334.

    This review article summarizes the major injuries to the genitourinary system. Level of evidence: V.

49. Guttmann I, Kerr HA: Blunt bladder injury. *Clin Sports Med* 2013;32(2):239-246.

    This article reviews the literature and summarizes the pathophysiology, diagnosis, and management of common bladder injuries. Level of evidence: V.

50. Bryan ST, Coleman NJ, Blueitt D, Kilmer NI: Bladder problems in athletes. *Curr Sports Med Rep* 2008;7(2):108-112.

51. Holevar M, Ebert J, Luchette F, et al: Genitourinary trauma, management of. Management guidelines for the management of genitourinary trauma, the EAST Practice Management Guidelines Work Group. Published 2004; east.org. Available at: https://www.east.org/education/practice-management-guidelines/genitourinary-trauma-management-of

52. Brandes S, Coburn M, Armenakas N, McAninch J: Diagnosis and management of ureteric injury: An evidence-based analysis. *BJU Int* 2004;94(3):277-289.

53. Bokhari F, Phelan H, Holevar M, et al: EAST, Eastern Association for the Surgery of Trauma: Pancreatic trauma, diagnosis and management of. Published 2009 Available at: https://www.east.org/resources/treatment-guidelines/pancreatic-trauma-diagnosis-and-management-of Accessed on July 25, 2015.

These management guidelines accompany a review and summary of the literature, providing evidenced-based recommendations for the recognition and management of pancreatic injury from trauma. Level of evidence: III.

54. Haugaard MV, Wettergren A, Hillingsø JG, Gluud C, Penninga L: Non-operative versus operative treatment for blunt pancreatic trauma in children. *Cochrane Database Syst Rev* 2014;2(No CD009746):CD009746.

This Cochrane review compares nonsurgical management with the surgical treatment of pancreatic injuries from trauma. Summaries in the literature are not based on RCTs. Level of evidence: II.

55. Echlin PS, Klein WB: Pancreatic injury in the athlete. *Curr Sports Med Rep* 2005;4(2):96-101.

56. Mahajan A, Kadavigere R, Sripathi S, Rodrigues GS, Rao VR, Koteshwar P: Utility of serum pancreatic enzyme levels in diagnosing blunt trauma to the pancreas: A prospective study with systematic review. *Injury* 2014;45(9):1384-1393.

This prospective cohort study looks at the AAST CT grading of injury, ultrasonography, and pancreatic enzymes. The authors also systematically reviewed the literature for comparisons to their findings. Level of evidence: III.

57. Hughes TM, Elton C: The pathophysiology and management of bowel and mesenteric injuries due to blunt trauma. *Injury* 2002;33(4):295-302. Medline http://dx.doi.org/10.1016/S0020-1383(02)00067-0

58. Gelman R, Mirvis SE, Gens D: Diaphragmatic rupture due to blunt trauma: Sensitivity of plain chest radiographs. *AJR Am J Roentgenol* 1991;156(1):51-57.

59. Hanna WC, Ferri LE, Fata P, Razek T, Mulder DS: The current status of traumatic diaphragmatic injury: Lessons learned from 105 patients over 13 years. *Ann Thorac Surg* 2008;85(3):1044-1048.

60. Okada M, Adachi H, Kamesaki M, et al: Traumatic diaphragmatic injury: Experience from a tertiary emergency medical center. *Gen Thorac Cardiovasc Surg* 2012;60(10):649-654.

This retrospective look at traumatic diaphragm injuries over 12 years identifies the factors affecting mortality and morbidity. Level of evidence: III.

61. Shehata SM, Shabaan BS: Diaphragmatic injuries in children after blunt abdominal trauma. *J Pediatr Surg* 2006;41(10):1727-1731.

62. Simpson J, Lobo DN, Shah AB, Rowlands BJ: Traumatic diaphragmatic rupture: Associated injuries and outcome. *Ann R Coll Surg Engl* 2000;82(2):97-100.

63. Yang YM, Yang HB, Park JS, Kim H, Lee SW, Kim JH: Spontaneous diaphragmatic rupture complicated with perforation of the stomach during Pilates. *Am J Emerg Med* 2010;28(2):259.e1-259.e3.

This article presents a case report of a unique presentation of diaphragmatic rupture without trauma. Level of evidence: V.

64. Nchimi A, Szapiro D, Ghaye B, et al: Helical CT of blunt diaphragmatic rupture. *AJR Am J Roentgenol* 2005;184(1):24-30.

Chapter 46

Heat Illness and Hydration

Alexander E. Ebinger, MD

Abstract

Heat illness is a frequently encountered disease state in athletes. The sports clinician should understand the diagnosis, recognition, and treatment of the spectrum of pathologies related to this condition.

Keywords: heat illness; heatstroke; hydration; hyponatremia

Introduction

Exertional heat-related illness (EHRI) is a frequently encountered but preventable issue. It remains, however, one of the leading causes of death in athletes every year.[1,2] EHRI refers to a spectrum of disease states. Most commonly encountered in American football, the risk of heat illness is present for athletes across a variety of sports, especially for those exercising in warm, humid climates and in events with a prolonged length of participation. This risk also extends to nonathletes, notably those with jobs requiring strenuous exertion, including military personnel, firefighters, and outdoor laborers. It is important for the clinician to comprehend how the body's thermoregulatory system responds to the effects of exercise. This understanding will enable the physician to provide recommendations about ways to recognize, treat, and prevent heat-related illness. This chapter discusses the clinical presentation and pathophysiology of the continuum of heat illness, the implications for performance, and the recommendations for treatment and prevention.

Neither Dr. Ebinger nor any immediate family member has received anything of value from or has stock or stock options held in a commercial company or institution related directly or indirectly to the subject of this chapter.

Background and Epidemiology

The incidence of heat illness is likely underreported. Estimating from data collected between 2005 and 2009, high school athletes had exertional heat illness at a rate of 1.2 to 1.6 occurrences per 100,000 athlete-exposures.[3] This report likely underreported the true incidence of heat illness, because only participants losing at least 1 day of activity were included. Heatstroke is among the leading causes of death among high school athletes.[2] American football maintains the highest rate of heat illness and injury with a rate 10 to 11 times more frequent than that of other sports.[3,4] August is the peak time of year for exertional heat injury because of the initiation of practices in hot, humid conditions in unacclimatized individuals.[5] Among high school football players, the highest rates occurred in offensive linemen, defensive linemen, and linebackers.[4] Since 1995, 52 football players have died from exertional heatstroke.[2] In 2011 alone, five cases of heatstroke death occurred in high school athletes. In 2012 and 2013 combined, only one death attributed to heatstroke was reported.[2] Despite the association with hot weather conditions, heat illness also can occur in cool climates and even has been reported in swimmers.[6,7]

Pathophysiology

Exercising muscles generate increased metabolic energy. This increased energy production creates excess heat, which must be transferred to the environment to maintain normothermia, defined as a body temperature of 37°C. The preoptic nucleus of the hypothalamus regulates body temperature, with a range of 37°C plus or minus 1°C. When body temperature exceeds the preferred threshold, the body works to dissipate heat by one of four mechanisms: evaporation, conduction, convection, or radiation. Evaporation is the primary mechanism by which exercising athletes dissipate heat. Water vaporizes from either the respiratory tract or the skin via sweat. Evaporation is limited by environmental humidity, and a water vapor pressure gradient must exist for heat to be transferred via this method. When relative humidity exceeds 75%, evaporation becomes an ineffective method for heat loss.

Conduction is the direct transfer of heat from the body by direct contact of a colder entity. Conduction is therefore dependent on relative temperature. If the temperature of a given object exceeds body temperature, no heat loss via conduction may occur. Convection is the transfer of heat to a gas or liquid moving over a body; it also depends on relative temperature. If the temperature of the air or liquid is greater than body temperature, no heat loss via convection may occur. Radiation is heat loss by electromagnetic waves; no direct contact is required.

Heat loss requires a functioning cardiovascular system. As body temperature rises, cardiac output rises, the vasodilation of peripheral blood vessels occurs, and blood flow to the skin increases. These processes allow core heat to be transferred to the periphery, where the heat can be transferred to the external environment. Many elements play a role in this process. One of the main factors is hydration status. Circulating plasma volume is directly affected by hydration status, and individuals who are dehydrated have a reduced circulating plasma volume. Sweat generation and respiratory losses further complicate volume depletion during exercise. Volume depletion reduces stroke volume and cardiac output, inhibiting peripheral blood flow and, thus, heat dissipation. It is estimated that for every 1% of body mass lost from dehydration, core body temperature rises 0.12°C to 0.25°C.[8] This elevation can lead to cardiorespiratory compromise and neurologic injury and is further described in the next paragraphs.

Trained and acclimatized athletes experience several physiologic changes that help prevent heat illness. Increased plasma volume, an increased rate of sweat production, increased cutaneous vasodilation, decreased urinary and sweat sodium concentrations, reduced heart rate for a set workload, and a decreased sweat-production threshold are all adaptations that reduce the occurrence of heat illness.[9] Additionally, maximum sweat rates can vary by age, level of physical fitness, and conditioning. Elite adult athletes can sweat up to 3 L/h (Figure 1).

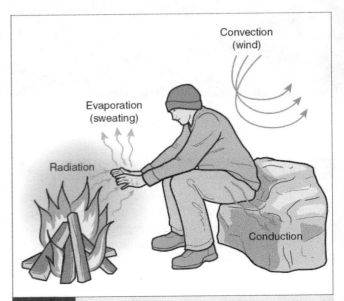

Figure 1 Illustration shows the four mechanisms of heat dissipation: radiation, evaporation, convection, and conduction.

Table 1

Medications and Other Substances Associated With Exercise-Related Heat Illness

Stimulants (amphetamines, ephedra, levothyroxine, methylphenidate)

Anticholinergics

Antihistamines

Cardiovascular drugs (β-blockers, calcium channel blockers, diuretics)

Illegal drugs (cocaine, heroin, lysergic acid diethylamide [LSD], phencyclidine [PCP], methamphetamine)

Laxatives

Alcohol

Caffeine

Risk Factors

Significant variability for heat tolerance exists among individuals because of a combination of genetic, adaptive, and neuroendocrine factors. Environmental stress, poor baseline physical fitness, a lack of heat acclimatization, inappropriate clothing, previous episodes of heat illness, and a lack of understanding of heat-related illness are all risk factors for EHRI. Another possible risk factor for heat illness is a lack of sleep.[10] Chronic medical problems including obesity, cardiovascular disease, peripheral vascular disease, poorly controlled diabetes, and hypertension are risk factors for EHRI. Acute medical issues such as diarrhea, recent febrile illness, and sunburn also may predispose to EHRI. Additionally, certain medications may predispose to heat illness (Table 1). Protective equipment such as helmets and shoulder pads as well as restrictive clothing can reduce the heat dissipation capacity, leading to an increase in EHRI. Furthermore, football players may exhibit up to double the sweat rates of cross-country runners, leading to dehydration.[11] At one time, children were thought to be at greater risk for heat illness, given their larger ratio of body surface to mass, but recent literature has shown this assumption to be incorrect.[12]

Consideration must be given to the environmental heat stress placed on exercising athletes. The wet bulb globe temperature (WBGT) is a measure of environmental heat stress, which takes into account ambient air temperature, radiant heat, and percent humidity. The equation for determining WBGT is:

WBGT = (0.1) dry bulb temperature + (0.2) globe temperature + (0.7) wet bulb temperature

Dry bulb temperature measures the ambient air temperature, globe temperature measures the radiant heat, and wet bulb temperature measures the relative humidity. The greatest weight is placed on wet bulb temperature, a reflection of evaporation being the most critical method of heat dissipation.

WBGT is used to guide exercise participation. The greatest risk for heat-related illness occurs when the WBGT exceeds 28°C.[13] Individual variation exists despite these guidelines, and nonacclimatized individuals may experience heat-related illness at a WBGT lower than 28°C (Table 2). Conversely, cardiovascularly fit and heat-acclimatized individuals may be able to continue to exercise with minimal difficulty even when the WBGT exceeds 28°C, with caution.

Heat Illness/Heat Injury/Heatstroke

Heat illness is a spectrum of disease, ranging from mild symptoms such as muscle cramping to more severe symptoms such as neurologic dysfunction, end-organ failure, and death. Some controversy exists about the exact classification of heat illness and the effects directly attributable to heat.[9,14]

Among the milder forms of exercise-related heat illness are heat edema, heat rash, and exercise-related muscle cramps. Heat edema is simply edema presenting in dependent body parts during exercise. Heat rash is a papulovesicular pruritic rash that presents with exercise. Heat cramps are common in athletes exercising in hot, humid weather. Despite their association with heat, muscle cramps occur independent of ambient temperature and are poorly understood. They are thought to be related to sweat loss and dehydration, sodium depletion, electrolyte imbalance, and muscle fatigue.[15-17] Predisposing factors include heavy sweating (worse in those with high sweat-sodium concentrations), preexercise dehydration, insufficient sodium intake before and during exercise, and a lack of acclimatization. Heat cramps may be preceded by muscle fasciculations and may be a precursor to heat exhaustion. For the diagnosis of heat cramps, the core temperature must remain normal, and no other, more severe, signs may be present.

Heat syncope is a more serious condition. Again, controversy exists as to whether heat syncope, more appropriately termed exercise-associated collapse (EAC), is truly a heat-related illness. Heat does not directly cause the syncopal event, because core body temperature is not elevated, although heat indirectly contributes through peripheral vasodilatory effects. Athletes undergoing EAC experience syncope directly after finishing an event. The pathologic cause for EAC is blood pooling in the periphery via blood vessel vasodilation requisite for heat dissipation. Skeletal muscle contractions augment venous return during exercise. When a sudden decline of skeletal muscle contraction occurs, such as at the end of a race, an abrupt reduction in venous return and a concomitant decrease in cardiac output occur, leading to a syncopal event. Heat syncope is not associated with an increase in core temperature and does not produce persistent neurologic deficits after measures are taken to improve venous return (ie, laying the athlete flat and elevating the legs). Physicians must be careful to distinguish EAC from other causes of neurologic dysfunction such as heatstroke or hyponatremia. This distinction requires a careful evaluation of the circumstances surrounding the collapse, an adequate physical examination, and potentially, an evaluation of core body temperature and a measurement of serum sodium. Additionally, consideration must be given to other etiologies of syncope such as arrhythmia or underlying heart disease, particularly in older individuals. Any syncopal event that is not associated with a sudden reduction in exercise intensity needs to be carefully examined for alternative causes of collapse.

Heat exhaustion is the presence of extreme weakness without neurologic dysfunction. Should any confusion be present, it is very transient. Athletes often demonstrate tachycardia and profuse sweating. Additional symptoms may include headache, cramps, nausea, vomiting, and diarrhea. An elevation in core temperature may occur, but it is less than 40°C (104°F), which is the key differentiation point between heat exhaustion and heatstroke. The skin may be cool and clammy, and occasionally, hypotension may be present.

Exertional heatstroke (EHS) manifests as a multisystem dysfunction, including the presence of central nervous system dysfunction such as confusion, headache, an altered level of consciousness, seizure, or unresponsiveness. This dysfunction is the result of central nervous system damage at the cellular level. In addition to neurologic dysfunction, a core temperature greater than 40°C must be present to establish the diagnosis. Athletes are often tachycardic and hypotensive and have many other overlapping features such as nausea, vomiting, weakness, dizziness, and dehydration. Historically, the absence of sweating was pathognomonic for heatstroke; however,

Table 2

Wet Bulb Globe Temperature Levels for the Modification or Cancellation of Athletic Workouts or Competition in Healthy Adults

WBGT (°F)	WBGT (°C)	Continuous Activity and Competition	Training and Noncontinuous Activity for Nonacclimatized, Unfit, High-Risk Individuals[a]	Training and Noncontinuous Activity for Acclimatized, Fit, Low-Risk Individuals[a,b]
≤50.0	≤10.0	Generally safe; exertional heatstroke can occur associated with individual factors	Normal activity	Normal activity
50.1-65.0	10.1-18.3	Generally safe; exertional heatstroke can occur	Normal activity	Normal activity
65.1-72.0	18.4-22.2	Risk of exertional heatstroke and other heat illness begins to rise; high-risk individuals should be monitored or not compete	Increase rest/work ratio; monitor fluid intake	Normal activity
72.1-78.0	22.3-25.6	Risk for all competitors is increased	Increase rest/work ratio and decrease total duration of activity	Normal activity; monitor fluid intake
78.1-82.0	25.7-27.8	Risk for unfit, nonacclimatized individuals is high	Increase rest/work ratio; decrease intensity and total duration of activity	Normal activity; monitor fluid intake
82.1-86.0	27.9-30.2	Cancel level for exertional heatstroke risk	Increase rest/work ratio to 1:1, decrease intensity and total duration of activity; limit intense exercise; watch at-risk individuals carefully	Plan intense or prolonged exercise with discretion[c]; watch at-risk individuals carefully
86.1-90.0	30.1-32.2	NA	Cancel or stop practice and competition	Limit intense exercise[c] and total daily exposure to heat and humidity; watch for early signs and symptoms
≥90.1	>32.3	NA	Cancel exercise	Cancel exercise, uncompensable heat stress[d] exists for all athletes[c]

WBGT = wet bulb globe temperature; NA = not applicable.

[a] While wearing shorts, a T-shirt, socks, and sneakers.

[b] Acclimatized to training in the heat for at least 3 weeks.

[c] Differences in local climate and individual heat acclimatization status may allow activity at higher levels than outlined in the table, but athletes and coaches should consult with sports medicine staff and should be cautious when exceeding these limits.

[d] Internal heat production exceeds heat loss, and core body temperature rises continuously, without a plateau. Adapted from Joy SM: Heat and Hydration, in Kibler WB, ed: *Orthopaedic Knowledge Update Sports Medicine,* ed 4. Rosemont, IL, American Academy of Orthopaedic Surgeons, 2009, p 383.

Data from Casa DJ, Armstrong LE: Exertional heatstroke: A medical emergency, in Armstrong LE, ed: *Exertional Heat Illness.* Champaign, IL, Human Kinetics, 2005, pp 26-56.

Spectrum of Heat Illness

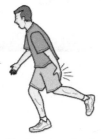

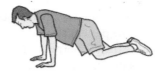

Heat cramps/rash

Symptoms:
Painful cramping/pruritic rash.

Physical examination:
Tense muscle/ papulovesicular rash.

Treatment:
Depends on clinical situation. Consider hydration, temporary removal from sport until symptoms improve.

Heat syncope/exercise-associated collapse

Symptoms:
Presyncopal vs syncopal event.

Physical examination:
Varies depending on cause. No persistent neurological deficits should be present with improved venous return. If confusion persists, consider other more serious causes of syncope.

Treatment:
Removal from play, rehydration depending on cause: 3% saline, Advanced Cardiovacular Life Support.

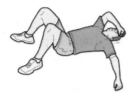

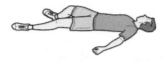

Heat exhaustion

Symptoms:
Extreme weakness without neurologic dysfunction, headache, nausea, cramps, vomiting. If any confusion, must be transient.

Physical examination:
No persistent altered mental status. May be tachycardic Temp < 40°C.

Treatment:
Remove from play. Hydrate. Continued reevaluation.

Heatstroke

Symptoms:
Confusion, altered mental status, seizure, unresponsive.

Physical examination:
Tachycardic, hypotensive.
Temp > 40°C, ± sweating.

Treatment:
Aggressive cooling, emergency medical service; transport to emergency department. Intravenous fluids.

Figure 2 Illustration shows the spectrum of heat illness.

sweating may be present and does not exclude heatstroke. Unrecognized or untreated EHS may progress to multisystem organ failure, cardiac arrhythmia, acute respiratory distress syndrome, disseminated intravascular coagulation, and ultimately, death (Figure 2).

Management of Heat-Related Illnesses

Recognition of EHS is of paramount importance. Evaluation begins following BLS/ACLS (Basic Life Support/ Advanced Cardiac Life Support) protocol, with airway, breathing, and circulation assessment followed by an assessment of neurologic function. Measurement of the core temperature and serum sodium are also key in diagnosis and illness severity stratification. If the temperature is elevated, especially if it is greater than 40°C, immediate and aggressive cooling must be instituted. Emergency medical services (EMS) should be activated. If symptoms are attributable to a certain diagnosis of heatstroke, immediate cooling should be performed before transport. If the diagnosis is uncertain, the temperature is not elevated, or severe hyponatremia is not present, the patient should be transported immediately to the nearest emergency department. Removal from the heat is important, along with immediate clearance of all items preventing heat dissipation (shoulder pads, running tights, shoes). Cooling measures such as ice-cold towels on the axilla, groin, and neck, fanning, cooling blankets, and cold-water immersion (36°F to 50°F) all are appropriate therapies for reducing core body temperature. Cold-water immersion is the mainstay of treatment for heatstroke because it provides the quickest method for lowering core body temperature. The exact temperature at which cooling should take place is a matter of current debate.[18] Cooling should be discontinued when core body temperature reaches 101°F to 102°F, and continuous careful monitoring of the patient's mental status and vital signs should occur during cooling and after the cooling process stops. An estimate of core temperature reduction is 1°C for every 5 minutes (1°F for every 3 minutes) of cold-water immersion. Rectal and gastrointestinal probe temperature provide the only satisfactory measurement of core body temperature; other measurements (oral, aural, temporal, axillary) should not be used to guide treatment. If cooling is initiated before transport, transfer to the closest emergency department can occur when the rectal temperature reaches 102°F. Antipyretic agents play no current role in exercise-related heat illness. If available, intravenous fluids may be given. Oral volume repletion may take place if the patient's mental status is sufficient. Return-to-activity guidelines suggest that athletes refrain from exercise for at least 7 days after the event and follow up with a physician 1 week after the event for further evaluation and testing.[19]

Management of the milder forms of heat illness depends on the clinical situation. Heat exhaustion requires removal of the athlete from competition. If the temperature is elevated, core temperature reduction methods may be instituted, although as previously stated, body temperature by definition does not exceed 40°C. Volume repletion may be achieved via enteral fluid administration or, if the patient is unable to tolerate liquids by mouth, administration of intravenous fluids. Individuals experiencing heat exhaustion should be held out of competition for at least 24 hours, longer if symptoms have not completely resolved. Muscle cramps may be treated with rest,

fluid resuscitation, massage, and ice baths. Prevention of muscle cramping generally focuses on maintaining hydration status throughout participation.

Exercise-Associated Hyponatremia

Exercise-associated hyponatremia (EAH) is a potentially severe electrolyte disturbance related to prolonged exercise. EAH is defined as a serum or plasma sodium level below the normal reference range, which typically is less than 135 mg/dL, occurring during or up to 24 hours after prolonged physical activity.[20] Clinical manifestations of EAH range from nonspecific symptoms such as weakness, dizziness, nausea, and headache to more severe symptoms including seizures, confusion, coma, and death. The incidence of hyponatremia is estimated to be between 0% and 18% in marathons and triathlons.[21] Two of the main risk factors for EAH are excessive fluid intake during a race and failure to suppress antidiuretic hormone (ADH) release during exercise.[22] Most cases of EAH occur due to ingestion of large amounts of hypotonic fluid, including free water, over a prolonged period of exertion. Increased ingestion of hypotonic fluids leads to dilutional hyponatremia. Normally, a compensatory mechanism for hyponatremia is suppression of ADH release. Failure to suppress ADH diminishes the body's capacity to get rid of free water.[23] Persistent hyponatremia may lead to seizures, cerebral edema, and coma in addition to respiratory arrest and death.

Event staff should be equipped to measure point-of-care serum sodium levels. Mild symptoms with documented hyponatremia may be managed by removal from participation and fluid restriction. Severe symptoms require intravenous hypertonic saline (100 mL of 3% saline) and transport to the nearest emergency department. Strategies to prevent the overingestion of hypotonic fluids include participant education about fluid type and drinking rates and increasing the distances between marathon hydration stations.

Prevention of Heat Illness

Numerous strategies can help to prevent exercise-related heat illness. The first steps are recognition of the climate conditions that predispose to heat illness and allowing athletes to acclimatize to hot and humid conditions. This is achieved by gradual increases in practice intensity and duration and the gradual introduction of items that limit heat dissipation such as helmets and shoulder pads. Prevention of dehydration is key to the prevention of heat illness.

As previously discussed, WBGT can be used by

physicians, coaches, and event coordinators to gauge the risk of heat illness. Participants—and even spectators—should be made aware of the implications of elevated WBGTs. When WBGT exceeds 28°C, event organizers should seriously consider canceling events or modifying them so they start earlier in the morning or later at night. A worldwide precedent was set when the 2014 Fédération Internationale de Football Association (FIFA) World Cup mandated water breaks for players and officials because of elevated WBGT. Heat acclimatization is a crucial component of the prevention of EHRI. The NCAA (National Collegiate Athletic Association) has implemented guidelines for heat acclimatization.

Individual risk factors should be acknowledged. Athletes who have previously experienced EHRI should be identified and closely monitored. Medical conditions that predispose to EHRI should be noted. Medications that may contribute to EHRI should be identified and, depending on the underlying medical condition, could be changed to a different medication, or the athlete could be monitored for signs of heat illness. Educating medical personnel about the prevention of dehydration is important. The medical training staff should understand how to recognize heat-related illness and have measures set up to treat EHRI, including shady areas, ample cool fluids, bags of ice, and if available, intravenous fluids. Rapid body cooling with cold-water immersion should be readily available. Most importantly, early activation of the EMS system should be emphasized. A written action plan can be an important component of treating EHRI.

Individual efforts to combat heat illness include maintenance of the preexercise hydration status. One easily available estimate of dehydration is day-to-day weight measurement. For every 1 kg of body mass loss, 1 L of fluid replacement should be initiated within 2 hours of exercise. Preparticipation maintenance of hydration is essential to performance. A balance must be struck between the ingestion of free water, sodium, and carbohydrate-containing beverages. Research suggests cool or cold beverages are preferred over those at room temperature, and carbohydrate-containing beverages are more palatable, which may induce fluid consumption. Dietary sodium is required to maintain extracellular fluid osmolality. This typically can be achieved through consuming a normal diet. Free water ingestion without adequate sodium will lead to a decrease in the plasma sodium concentration. Preexercise hyperhydration is not currently known to be of measurable benefit, although it possibly could serve to restore euvolemia in dehydrated athletes.

Summary

EHRI is a potentially deadly but preventable condition. The recognition and modification of external and internal risk factors is important in reducing the danger of EHRI. This process includes maintaining hydration status before and during exercise and being cognizant of the environmental conditions. For athletes, coaches, organizers, and physicians, recognizing and understanding the spectrum of EHRI is important.

Key Study Points

- Early therapy is key to the management of EHRI.
- EHS is a medical emergency, and cold-water immersion is the gold standard of care.
- EMS activation should not be delayed, particularly if the diagnosis is uncertain.
- Core temperature (rectal temperature) is requisite for the diagnosis of heat injury.

Annotated References

1. Maron BJ, Doerer JJ, Haas TS, Tierney DM, Mueller FO: Sudden deaths in young competitive athletes: Analysis of 1866 deaths in the United States, 1980-2006. *Circulation* 2009;119(8):1085-1092.

   This is a report of sudden deaths in high school athletes from a national registry. Data were collected from 1980 to 2006.

2. Kucera K, Klossner D, Colgate B, Cantu R: *Annual Survey of Football Injury Research 1931-2013. American Football Coaches Association; National Collegiate Athletic Association; National Federation of State High School Associations.* National Athletic Trainers' Association, Carrolton, TX, 2014.

   This study examined the incidence and characteristics of heat-related illness among high school athletes from 2005 to 2009.

3. Yard EE, Gilchrist J, Haileyesus T, et al: Heat illness among high school athletes—United States, 2005-2009. *J Safety Res* 2010;41(6):471-474.

   This is a report of high school football deaths from 1931 to 2013, including their direct and indirect relationship to football as well as the type of injury.

4. Kerr ZY, Casa DJ, Marshall SW, Comstock RD: Epidemiology of exertional heat illness among U.S. high school athletes. *Am J Prev Med* 2013;44(1):8-14.

   This retrospective analysis of National High School Sports-Related Injury Surveillance Study data reported the incidence, geography, and timing of exertional heat-related illnesses.

5. Boden BP, Breit I, Beachler JA, Williams A, Mueller FO: Fatalities in high school and college football players. *Am J Sports Med* 2013;41(5):1108-1116.

   This epidemiological analysis reported the causes of high school and college football deaths from 1990 to 2010.

6. Mountjoy M, Junge A, Alonso JM, et al: Sports injuries and illnesses in the 2009 FINA World Championships (Aquatics). *Br J Sports Med* 2010;44(7):522-527.

   A prospective recording and analysis reported the frequency and characteristics of injuries and illnesses sustained during the 2009 *Fédération Internationale de Football Association* (FINA) World Championships.

7. Macaluso F, Barone R, Isaacs AW, Farina F, Morici G, Di Felice V: Heat stroke risk for open-water swimmers during long-distance events. *Wilderness Environ Med* 2013;24(4):362-365.

   This article presented a review of the risks of heat illness in open-water swimmers.

8. Casa DJ, Stearns RL, Lopez RM, et al: Influence of hydration on physiological function and performance during trail running in the heat. *J Athl Train* 2010;45(2):147-156.

   This semirandomized crossover analysis reported the effects of hydration status on physiologic function and performance in athletes during trail running.

9. Nichols AW: Heat-related illness in sports and exercise. *Curr Rev Musculoskelet Med* 2014;7(4):355-365.

   This review of the current concepts surrounding heat illness in sports and exercise included pathophysiology, clinical syndromes, effects of hydration status, and risk-reduction strategies.

10. Rav-Acha M, Hadad E, Epstein Y, Heled Y, Moran DS: Fatal exertional heat stroke: A case series. *Am J Med Sci* 2004;328(2):84-87.

11. Sawka MN, Burke LM, Eichner ER, Maughan RJ, Montain SJ, Stachenfeld NS; American College of Sports Medicine: American College of Sports Medicine position stand. Exercise and fluid replacement. *Med Sci Sports Exerc* 2007;39(2):377-390.

12. Bergeron MF, Devore C, Rice SG; Council on Sports Medicine and Fitness and Council on School Health; American Academy of Pediatrics: Policy statement—Climatic heat stress and exercising children and adolescents. *Pediatrics* 2011;128(3):e741-e747.

   This is a policy statement from an expert panel on heat stress in children.

13. Armstrong LE, Casa DJ, Millard-Stafford M, Moran DS, Pyne SW, Roberts WO; American College of Sports Medicine: American College of Sports Medicine position stand.

Exertional heat illness during training and competition. *Med Sci Sports Exerc* 2007;39(3):556-572.

14. Noakes TD: A modern classification of the exercise-related heat illnesses. *J Sci Med Sport* 2008;11(1):33-39.

15. Casa DJ, Clarkson PM, Roberts WO: American College of Sports Medicine roundtable on hydration and physical activity: Consensus statements. *Curr Sports Med Rep* 2005;4(3):115-127.

16. Eichner ER: The role of sodium in 'heat cramping'. *Sports Med* 2007;37(4-5):368-370.

17. Bergeron MF: Exertional heat cramps: Recovery and return to play. *J Sport Rehabil* 2007;16(3):190-196.

18. Casa DJ, Armstrong LE, Kenny GP, O'Connor FG, Huggins RA: Exertional heat stroke: New concepts regarding cause and care. *Curr Sports Med Rep* 2012;11(3):115-123.

   Novel concepts regarding treatment of EHS were presented in this article.

19. O'Connor FG, Casa DJ, Bergeron MF, et al: American College of Sports Medicine Roundtable on exertional heat stroke—return to duty/return to play: Conference proceedings. *Curr Sports Med Rep* 2010;9(5):314-321.

   This is a report on an expert conference convened to discuss relevant exertional heat illness issues such as potential long-term consequences, the concept of thermotolerance, and the role of thermal tolerance testing in return-to-play decisions.

20. Hew-Butler T, Ayus JC, Kipps C, et al: Statement of the Second International Exercise-Associated Hyponatremia Consensus Development Conference, New Zealand, 2007. *Clin J Sport Med* 2008;18(2):111-121.

21. Hoffman MD, Hew-Butler T, Stuempfle KJ: Exercise-associated hyponatremia and hydration status in 161-km ultramarathoners. *Med Sci Sports Exerc* 2013;45(4):784-791.

   This study represents a 5-year analysis that attempted to define the relationship between postrace blood sodium ([Na]) concentration and change in body weight; to examine the interactions among EAH incidence, ambient temperature, and hydration state; and to explore the effect of hydration status on performance.

22. Hew-Butler T: Arginine vasopressin, fluid balance and exercise: Is exercise-associated hyponatraemia a disorder of arginine vasopressin secretion? *Sports Med* 2010;40(6):459-479.

   This article is a review of the role of arginine vasopressin and the effects of exercise.

23. Hew-Butler T, Jordaan E, Stuempfle KJ, et al: Osmotic and nonosmotic regulation of arginine vasopressin during prolonged endurance exercise. *J Clin Endocrinol Metab* 2008;93(6):2072-2078.

© 2016 American Academy of Orthopaedic Surgeons

Section 8

The Young Athlete

SECTION EDITOR
Matthew D. Milewski, MD

Chapter 47

Osteochondritis Dissecans

Kevin G. Shea, MD   Ted J. Ganley, MD

Abstract

Osteochondritis dissecans most commonly affects the knee, ankle, and elbow, and is typically seen in young, active populations. It is important to review the epidemiology, presenting clinical complaints, and nonsurgical and surgical treatment options for osteochondritis dissecans for optimal patient outcomes.

Keywords: osteochondritis dissecans; cartilage reconstruction; cartilage repair

Introduction

Osteochondritis dissecans (OCD), first described in the 19th century, affects a substantial number of young athletes and can result in pain, mechanical symptoms, and development of intra-articular loose bodies of osteocartilagenous tissue. A contemporary definition of OCD is a "focal, idiopathic alteration of subchondral bone with risk for instability and disruption of adjacent articular cartilage that may result in premature osteoarthritis."[1] Contemporary research refers to the OCD lesion as progeny bone and the surrounding normal tissue as parent bone.

The etiology of OCD remains unknown, although many causes have been proposed, including acute trauma, overuse, and genetic and vascular causes. Ischemia is

Dr. Shea or an immediate family member serves as an unpaid consultant to Clinical Data Solutions; and serves as a board member, owner, officer, or committee member of the American Academy of Orthopaedic Surgeons, the American Orthopaedic Society for Sports Medicine, the North Pacific Orthopedic Society, and the Pediatric Orthopaedic Society of North America. Neither Dr. Ganley nor any immediate family member has received anything of value from or has stock or stock options held in a commercial company or institution related directly or indirectly to the subject of this chapter.

thought to be present in some cases, although this has not been confirmed in all cases, based on histologic studies.[2] OCD is called osteochondrosis in animals and is quite common in horses and pigs. Veterinary animal model research, including detailed anatomic evaluation of the condyle vascularity of the knee, suggests a vascular etiology in most cases.[3]

Location of OCD

Although numerous studies confirm that the most common location for OCD is the knee joint, the ankle and elbow joints are also commonly affected. OCD is relatively rare in other joints, but has also been reported in the hip and shoulder. Epidemiologic studies evaluating OCD in large populations have demonstrated that the knee is the most common location. Within the knee, OCD is located in the medial femoral condyle (64% of cases), the lateral femoral condyle (32% of cases), and the patella, trochlear groove, and tibial plateau (less than 4% of cases).[4] Approximately 50% of lesions appeared on the right side, 43% appeared on the left side, and only 7% were bilateral; however, other studies have suggested that bilateral cases may be as prevalent as 30%. OCD was not identified in patients age 2 to 5 years, but was seen in patients age 6 to 11 years, and was most common in patients age 12 to 19 years. Patients age 12 to 19 years were almost four times more likely to have a diagnosis of OCD of the knee compared with those age 6 to 11 years. Males had a 3.8-fold higher risk of the development of OCD of the knee than females. This condition was also more common in African American populations than in Caucasian, Hispanic, or Asian populations.

Another large population-based study reviewed OCD of the ankle. As with knee OCD, ankle OCD was not reported in those younger than 5 years, and was increasingly common in those between age 12 and 19 years.[5] Females had a higher risk of OCD of the talus than males. On the basis of race and ethnicity, non-Hispanic whites had the highest relative risk for disease, and African Americans had the lowest risk.

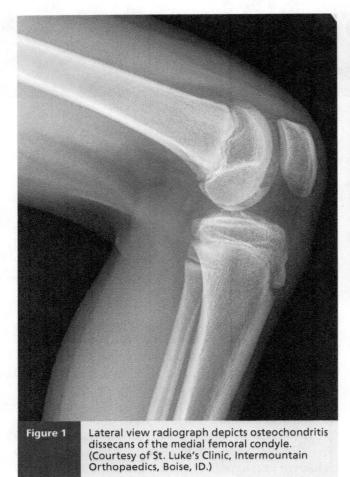

Figure 1   Lateral view radiograph depicts osteochondritis dissecans of the medial femoral condyle. (Courtesy of St. Luke's Clinic, Intermountain Orthopaedics, Boise, ID.)

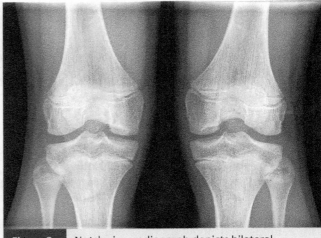

Figure 2   Notch view radiograph depicts bilateral osteochondritis dissecans of the medial femoral condyles. (Courtesy of St. Luke's Clinic, Intermountain Orthopaedics, Boise, ID.)

OCD of the Knee

In 2011, the American Academy of Orthopaedic Surgeons published a clinical practice guideline on OCD of the Knee, which reviewed important clinical questions for evaluation and treatment. Few higher level prospective studies are available on this topic, and few long-term follow-up studies are available.[6] Multicenter prospective cohorts and randomized trials will be critical to develop a better understanding of the outcomes and best treatment options for this condition.

Clinical Presentation

Many patients with OCD of the knee present with fairly benign symptoms. Lesions that are stable and remain in situ may lack swelling or mechanical symptoms. Some patients may only report activity-related pain. The symptoms may overlap with growing pains and patellofemoral pain, for example. With more advanced lesions, symptoms can be much more substantial, including swelling, mechanical complaints, and reports of occasional limping. The examination can reveal swelling and some

mechanical complaints similar to those of a meniscus injury, especially in more advanced cases, but many patients will have minimal to no findings on examination. In most patients, the pain is localized to the anterior knee region around the femoral condyle. Many will have an entirely normal gait pattern with walking and/or running. Multifocal lesions of the knee are less common, but can occur in some cases.[7]

Imaging Evaluation

Standard AP and lateral knee radiographs (Figure 1) alone may not identify OCD lesions. The use of notch and Merchant view radiographs can help identify more lesions. Up to 30% of OCD cases may be bilateral, so imaging evaluation of both knees may be advantageous (Figure 2). For those with more advanced lesions or in cases in which surgical treatment is considered, MRI sequences can assist with surgical planning. Historically, alignment has not been evaluated in patients with OCD, but research suggests lower extremity alignment may be a consideration for some patients.[8] Specifically, varus and valgus mechanical axis alignment of the knee may be associated with OCD of the medial and lateral condyle, respectively.

Classification

Numerous classification systems for OCD of the knee exist, although validation of these systems remains a concern. Classification systems using MRI have been proposed to help assess lesion stability and the potential for healing. MRI criteria for OCD instability have been proposed (high T2-weighted signal intensity rim, surrounding cysts, high T2-weighted signal intensity cartilage fracture line, and fluid-filled osteochondral defects), although the capability of MRI to accurately predict lesion stability in skeletally immature patients has been questioned[9] (Figure 3). Arthroscopic classification systems exist, although future studies on reliable, validated systems are necessary.[10] A multicenter OCD study group has developed and validated arthroscopic[11] and radiologic[12] classification systems for OCD. Ultimately, the validated classifications system may be important for prospective trials and registry-based outcomes for the treatment of OCD. Arthroscopic classification systems are the gold standard for evaluating lesion size, cartilage condition, and fragment stability, and therefore may be more definitive for treatment decisions.

Treatment

Nonsurgical treatment in skeletally immature patients, especially for those with substantial growth remaining, may have a better prognosis for healing. In cases in which the patient does not have substantial mechanical symptoms, and the MRI sequences do not show signs of substantial instability, a nonsurgical program can be used. Predicting stability on MRI can be challenging, especially in younger patients.[13] Healing rates greater than 50% to 60% have been reported for appropriately selected patients.[14] An ideal nonsurgical treatment option has not yet been demonstrated, but activity restrictions that include a period of casting or the use of an unloading brace can improve healing rates. Activity changes for 4 to 6 months or longer may be necessary to obtain adequate healing in these patients.[14,15] Research on healing predictors could help determine the best treatment options and help with patient-centered decision making.[15] These predictors can include age, presence of cyst-like lesions, mechanical symptoms, and lesion size.

For patients in whom nonsurgical treatment has failed, different treatment options exist.[16] Most literature published on knee OCD relates to condyle location, but several recent series were published on patellar and trochlear OCD, which are relatively rare.[17,18] For stable lesions, treatment options include both transarticular and retroarticular drilling[19,20]; studies have demonstrated excellent healing with both techniques.[21,22] Retroarticular drilling can be more technically challenging in some locations, and increased radiation use during the procedure can also be a limitation, but the clinical outcomes are excellent. Ultrasonographic guidance for percutaneous drilling has been described, although this approach does not allow for direct evaluation of cartilage/lesion stability; therefore, its use may be limited to cases in which cartilage lesion instability is a potential concern.[23]

Retroarticular drilling and bone grafting with minimally invasive techniques have been described[24,25] for

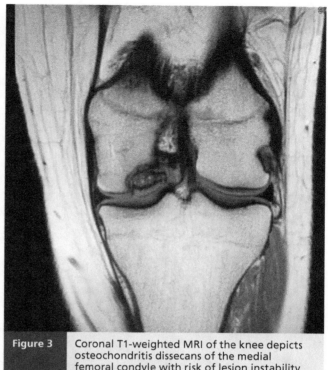

Figure 3 Coronal T1-weighted MRI of the knee depicts osteochondritis dissecans of the medial femoral condyle with risk of lesion instability. (Courtesy of St. Luke's Clinic, Intermountain Orthopaedics, Boise, ID.)

more advanced, stable lesions, and allow placement of bone grafting behind the lesion using minimally invasive techniques with arthroscopic and C-arm fluoroscopic guidance. Longer term follow-up and larger study sizes will be necessary to confirm treatment outcomes.

For patients with unstable lesions, or those close to or beyond skeletal maturity, more advanced treatment options may be necessary (Figure 4). Fragment excision may not have ideal outcomes,[26] and attempts to salvage the native cartilage and bone can provide a better prognosis.[26-28] These options include drilling, which may be combined with different approaches to bone grafting, and internal fixation with an attempt to salvage the native cartilage tissue.[19,29,30] Numerous studies have shown successful outcomes in patients who undergo lesion stabilization, especially in younger patients.[27,31] Prospective cohorts and randomized clinical trials will be necessary to fully evaluate these techniques because most are retrospective case series.

Hardware selection is debated in the literature, with proponents of both metallic and bioabsorbable fixation devices.[18,32-34] (Table 1) Numerous reconstruction and salvage techniques with their inherent limitations and biases have been studied in smaller case series. Osteochondral autograft transplantation (OAT) has been evaluated in retrospective cases series.[35,36] Biologic fixation was advocated based on the use of small osteochondral autografts. A prospective study on OCD compared microfracture with osteochondral autograft implantation.[37] Both groups improved functionally after surgery, but patients in the osteochondral implantation group had better results at an average follow-up of 4.2 years. Osteochondral autograft combined with screw fixation has also been described.[38] One study suggested that donor site morbidity for osteochondral autografts may not be significant in young patients,[39] but some adult studies have shown symptoms at OAT harvest sites.

The treatment of defects using autologous cartilage implantation (ACI) has also been evaluated. Several studies reported good outcomes using ACI techniques.[40,41] The use of cell-free, biomimetic osteochondral scaffold has been studied, with promising results reported at short-term follow-up. Bulk osteochondral allografts have been described, showing good results at short-term and longer term follow-up.[42-44]

OCD of the Elbow

Clinical Presentation and Imaging Evaluation

OCD of the elbow and Panner disease may represent different stages of a related condition. Historically, Panner disease has been described in younger patients (younger than 10 years), and in many cases, it will resolve with time. OCD of the elbow is thought to develop in older patients, and in many cases, these lesions do not heal. In many athletes, the cause of these conditions is thought to be related to overload of the lateral elbow compartment, and perhaps to the limitations of elbow vascularity. The contribution of vascular etiology to OCD has been proposed for both the knee and elbow, and secondary overload can also enhance the risk of development and/or progression of the condition.

Many young patients with OCD of the elbow present with relatively minor symptoms, including occasional mechanical symptoms, minimal loss of motion, and occasional effusion. Baseball, gymnastics, and other overhead sports pose a relatively high risk for this condition.[45] In some cases, the only notable physical examination finding may be a loss of 5° to 10° of extension compared with the contralateral elbow. Most OCD lesions are identified using plain radiography. Some cases can be better seen using MRI, which is also good at identifying substantial bone edema, loose bodies, or more subtle lesions not

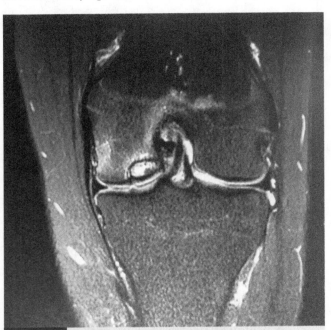

Figure 4 Coronal T2-weighted MRI of the knee depicts osteochondritis dissecans of the medial femoral condyle with risk of lesion instability. (Courtesy of St. Luke's Clinic, Intermountain Orthopaedics, Boise, ID.)

Table 1

Bioabsorbable Versus Metal Implants for OCD Fixation

Implant	Advantages	Disadvantages
Bioabsorbable	Removal may not be necessary Do not produce substantial artifact with MRI	Concerns about strength and implant failure Incomplete absorption Backing out from bone May result in substantial cyst formation around implants
Metal	Do not leave cystic lesions during screw absorption Titanium screws may induce less MRI artifact	May produce substantial artifact on MRI studies Removal may be necessary if close to cartilage surface and not recessed within stable bone Backing out from bone

OCD = osteochondritis dissecans.

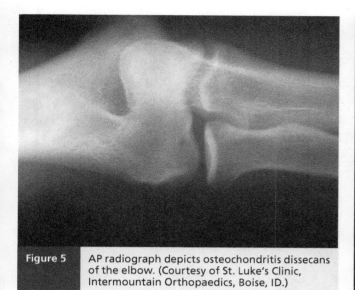

Figure 5 AP radiograph depicts osteochondritis dissecans of the elbow. (Courtesy of St. Luke's Clinic, Intermountain Orthopaedics, Boise, ID.)

fully appreciated on radiography (**Figures 5, 6, and 7**). Newer techniques may be valuable for cartilage evaluation, including those using ultrasonography, and may be complementary to other forms of advanced imaging in the future.[46]

Treatment Options

Younger patients with substantial growth remaining may respond well to activity modifications, and in some cases, both rest and shorter periods of immobilization can be beneficial. For throwing athletes, switching to another position with less throwing demands can be helpful, such as having a pitcher or catcher switch to first base. For those who do not respond to activity modifications and/or restrictions, surgical treatment is an option. Larger lesions, including those that expand to involve the lateral wall of the capitellum, as well as those with intra-articular loose bodies, can progress to surgical treatment more frequently than small lesions (**Figure 8**). The staging system developed in 2011 can help with the evaluation and management of this condition.[47] Most published series on elbow OCD are based on level IV evidence or case series, so treatment recommendations are not based on higher levels of evidence.[48,49] Arthroscopic débridement with and without drilling has shown reasonable outcomes in shorter term follow-up, although longer term follow-up for throwing sports, gymnastics, and other high-demand, upper extremity sports are limited.[50,51]

Uncontained lesions can have a worse prognosis than contained lesions.[52] OAT harvest from the knee and mosaicplasty procedures have been examined for the treatment of larger, uncontained lesions.[53,54] Larger lesions may have a worse prognosis,[55] and access to the joint for certain lesion sizes and locations can be technically challenging.

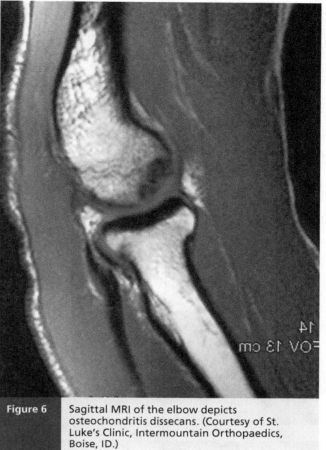

Figure 6 Sagittal MRI of the elbow depicts osteochondritis dissecans. (Courtesy of St. Luke's Clinic, Intermountain Orthopaedics, Boise, ID.)

New techniques, including the use of oblique grafts, have been developed to address challenges to joint access.[56] A 2011 study provided an excellent review of surgical treatment options.[47]

OCD of the Talus

The etiology of OCD of the talus remains unknown, although many talar lesions are associated with a history of trauma. A history of trauma may be less likely with posteromedial lesions.[57]

Clinical Presentation and Imaging Evaluation

Many patients with talar OCD present with symptoms of ankle pain alone, without substantial swelling or mechanical symptoms in early stages of the condition. In patients with a history of ankle sprain and anterolateral lesions, patients may have tenderness over the lateral aspect of the talus. The Berndt and Hardy classification system for radiographic staging of talar OCD is currently in use. In addition to plain radiography (**Figures 9 and 10**), MRI can be a useful tool to evaluate the extent of the lesion, as well

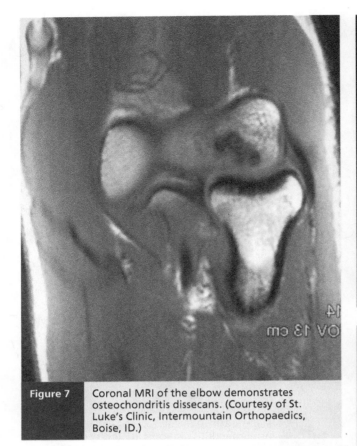

Figure 7 Coronal MRI of the elbow demonstrates osteochondritis dissecans. (Courtesy of St. Luke's Clinic, Intermountain Orthopaedics, Boise, ID.)

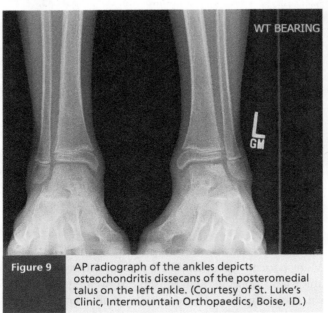

Figure 9 AP radiograph of the ankles depicts osteochondritis dissecans of the posteromedial talus on the left ankle. (Courtesy of St. Luke's Clinic, Intermountain Orthopaedics, Boise, ID.)

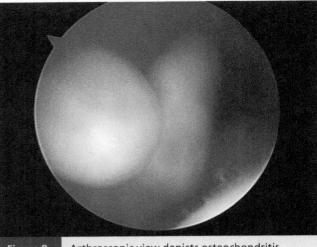

Figure 8 Arthroscopic view depicts osteochondritis dissecans of the elbow with intra-articular free bodies. (Courtesy of St. Luke's Clinic, Intermountain Orthopaedics, Boise, ID.)

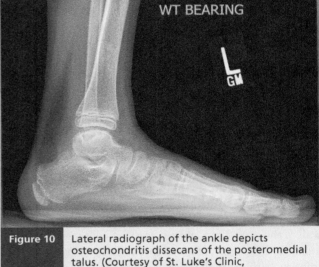

Figure 10 Lateral radiograph of the ankle depicts osteochondritis dissecans of the posteromedial talus. (Courtesy of St. Luke's Clinic, Intermountain Orthopaedics, Boise, ID.)

Treatment Options

A systematic review for the treatment of talar OCD revealed almost exclusively level IV case series evidence, and no strong recommendations could be made for specific treatment options given the limitations of the evidence.[59] Many of the case series had limited follow-up (≤3 years), which further limits the understanding of the surgical outcomes and the effect on patient function.

In patients with stable lesions and in those without mechanical symptoms and effusions, nonsurgical treatment (activity modifications, immobilization) is an option, and healing has been reported in some series using this approach. Published series of nonsurgical treatment

as the condition of the cartilage. MRI for postoperative evaluation may be limited, and several series have shown improvement in clinical function despite persistent MRI abnormalities after surgery.[58]

are limited. A case series in children showed relatively low rates of healing with nonsurgical treatment, and surgical intervention was recommended if healing did not occur within 6 months.[60]

Drilling of the talus has been described using several techniques including direct arthroscopic visualization. Access to the posteromedial region of the talus is limited, even with the ankle in full plantar flexion. Access to this region can be gained by using several approaches, including retrograde drilling techniques (including the use of three-dimensional imaging guidance) and transmalleolar drilling.

Treatment using osteochondral autograft transfer from the knee has been described in several studies, including one with a mean short-term follow-up of 2.5 years.[61] In this series, older patients were more likely to have substantial symptoms at the knee joint after graft harvest, and caution was recommended for use of this procedure in older patients. Malleolar osteotomy has been described as a technique to gain access for OAT graft placement, and relatively low rates of wound healing complications and delayed union of the osteotomy site have been described.[58] In 2014, an excellent review of treatment options for OCD of the talus was published.[62]

Summary

Treatment of knee, elbow, and talar OCD will continue to evolve, and determining the optimal treatment will continue to challenge researchers. Multicenter study designs, including prospective cohorts and randomized clinical trials, may provide adequate power to determine optimal outcomes.

Key Study Points

- Treatment of OCD continues to evolve, and multicenter studies will be essential to develop higher levels of evidence for optimal treatment protocols.
- For patients with lesions that do not heal with nonsurgical measures that include activity modification, surgery can improve joint function in the short term.

Annotated References

1. Edmonds EW, Shea KG: Osteochondritis dissecans: Editorial comment. *Clin Orthop Relat Res* 2013;471(4):1105-1106.

   The purpose of this symposium was to highlight what is and what is not understood regarding the histology,

   natural history, outcomes, and treatment of OCD. OCD is a focal, idiopathic alteration of subchondral bone with risk for instability and disruption of adjacent articular cartilage that may result in premature osteoarthritis.

2. Shea KG, Jacobs JC Jr, Carey JL, Anderson AF, Oxford JT: Osteochondritis dissecans knee histology studies have variable findings and theories of etiology. *Clin Orthop Relat Res* 2013;471(4):1127-1136.

   Future studies with consistent methodology are necessary to draw major conclusions about the histology and progression of OCD lesions. Inconsistent histologic findings have resulted in a lack of consensus regarding the presence of osteonecrosis, whether the necrosis is primary or secondary, the association of cartilage degeneration, and the etiology of OCD. Level of evidence: III.

3. Olstad K, Hendrickson EH, Carlson CS, Ekman S, Dolvik NI: Transection of vessels in epiphyseal cartilage canals leads to osteochondrosis and osteochondrosis dissecans in the femoro-patellar joint of foals; a potential model of juvenile osteochondritis dissecans. *Osteoarthritis Cartilage* 2013;21(5):730-738.

   Transection of blood vessels within epiphyseal cartilage canals resulted in necrosis of vessels and chondrocytes (ischemic chondronecrosis) in foals. The ischemic hypothesis for the pathogenesis of OCD has been reproduced experimentally in foals.

4. Kessler JI, Nikizad H, Shea KG, Jacobs JC Jr, Bebchuk JD, Weiss JM: The demographics and epidemiology of osteochondritis dissecans of the knee in children and adolescents. *Am J Sports Med* 2014;42(2):320-326.

   In this population-based cohort study of pediatric OCD of the knee, male patients had a much greater incidence of OCD and almost four times the risk of OCD compared with female patients. Also, patients age 12 to 19 years had 3 times the risk of OCD of the knee as compared with 6- to 11-year-old children. Level of evidence: IV.

5. Kessler JI, Weiss JM, Nikizad H, et al: Osteochondritis dissecans of the ankle in children and adolescents: Demographics and epidemiology. *Am J Sports Med* 2014;42(9):2165-2171.

   In this population-based cohort study of pediatric ankle OCD, female patients had a greater incidence of OCD and a 1.5 times greater risk for ankle OCD compared with male patients. Teenagers had nearly seven times the risk for ankle OCD compared with children 6 to 11 years of age. Level of evidence: IV.

6. Chambers HG, Shea KG, Carey JL: AAOS Clinical Practice Guideline: Diagnosis and treatment of osteochondritis dissecans. *J Am Acad Orthop Surg* 2011;19(5):307-309.

   Clinical questions regarding evaluation and treatment of OCD of the knee are presented.

7. Backes JR, Durbin TC, Bentley JC, Klingele KE: Multifocal juvenile osteochondritis dissecans of the knee: A case series. *J Pediatr Orthop* 2014;34(4):453-458.

Lesions located on the medial femoral condyle healed at a statistically significant greater rate than other locations within the knee. Sex, age, and associated discoid menisci had no effect on healing prognosis. Level of evidence: IV.

8. Jacobi M, Wahl P, Bouaicha S, Jakob RP, Gautier E: Association between mechanical axis of the leg and osteochondritis dissecans of the knee: Radiographic study on 103 knees. *Am J Sports Med* 2010;38(7):1425-1428.

An association was found between medial condyle OCD and varus axis, and between lateral condyle OCD and valgus axis. This evokes higher loading of the affected knee compartment than of the unaffected knee compartment; therefore, axial alignment may be a cofactor in OCD of the femoral condyles. Level of evidence: IV.

9. Kijowski R, Blankenbaker DG, Shinki K, Fine JP, Graf BK, De Smet AA: Juvenile versus adult osteochondritis dissecans of the knee: Appropriate MR imaging criteria for instability. *Radiology* 2008;248(2):571-578.

When used together, the criteria were 100% sensitive and 11% specific for instability in juvenile OCD lesions and 100% sensitive and 100% specific for instability in adult OCD lesions. Previously described MRI criteria for OCD instability have high specificity for adult but not juvenile lesions of the knee. Level of evidence: IV.

10. Jacobs JC Jr, Archibald-Seiffer N, Grimm NL, Carey JL, Shea KG: A review of arthroscopic classification systems for osteochondritis dissecans of the knee. *Clin Sports Med* 2014;33(2):189-197.

Currently, no arthroscopic classification system has been universally accepted. A future classification system should be developed that reconciles the discrepancies among the current systems and provides a clear, consistent, and reliable method for classifying OCD lesions of the knee during arthroscopy. Level of evidence: IV.

11. Carey JL, Grimm NL: Treatment algorithm for osteochondritis dissecans of the knee. *Orthop Clin North Am* 2015;46(1):141-146.

For unstable yet salvageable OCD lesions, the senior author's preferred treatment is fixation with bone grafting. For unstable and unsalvageable OCD lesions, the senior author's preferred treatment is autologous chondrocyte implantation with bone grafting. Level of evidence: V.

12. Wall EJ, Polousky JD, Shea KG, et al; Research on Osteo-Chondritis Dissecans of the Knee (ROCK) Study Group: Novel radiographic feature classification of knee osteochondritis dissecans: A multicenter reliability study. *Am J Sports Med* 2015;43(2):303-309.

Many diagnostic features of femoral condyle OCD lesions can be reliably classified on plain radiographs, supporting their future testing in multifactorial classification systems and multicenter research to develop prognostic algorithms. Other radiographic features should be excluded, however, because of poor reliability. Level of evidence: III.

13. Samora WP, Chevillet J, Adler B, Young GS, Klingele KE: Juvenile osteochondritis dissecans of the knee: Predictors of lesion stability. *J Pediatr Orthop* 2012;32(1):1-4.

MRI continues to be reliably sensitive to juvenile OCD lesions and a good predictor of low-grade, stable lesions. However, MRI predictability of high-grade, unstable juvenile OCD lesions is less reliable. Level of evidence: IV.

14. Wall EJ, Vourazeris J, Myer GD, et al: The healing potential of stable juvenile osteochondritis dissecans knee lesions. *J Bone Joint Surg Am* 2008;90(12):2655-2664.

In two-thirds of skeletally immature patients, 6 months of nonsurgical treatment that includes activity modification and immobilization results in progressive healing of stable OCD lesions. Lesions with an increased size and associated swelling and/or mechanical symptoms at presentation are less likely to heal. Level of evidence: III.

15. Krause M, Hapfelmeier A, Möller M, Amling M, Bohndorf K, Meenen NM: Healing predictors of stable juvenile osteochondritis dissecans knee lesions after 6 and 12 months of nonoperative treatment. *Am J Sports Med* 2013;41(10):2384-2391.

A 6-month period of surgical treatment with or without casting might be appropriate if the healing potential is greater than 48%. A 12-month period of nonsurgical treatment may be successful if the cyst-like lesion is less than 1.3 mm in length as assessed on MRI. Level of evidence: II.

16. Yang JS, Bogunovic L, Wright RW: Nonoperative treatment of osteochondritis dissecans of the knee. *Clin Sports Med* 2014;33(2):295-304.

Prognosis and treatment depend on the stability of the lesion and the age of the patient. Skeletally immature patients with stable lesions are amenable for nonsurgical treatment. Nonsurgical treatment is less predictable in skeletally mature patients and patients with unstable lesions. Level of evidence: IV.

17. Kramer DE, Yen YM, Simoni MK, et al: Surgical management of osteochondritis dissecans lesions of the patella and trochlea in the pediatric and adolescent population. *Am J Sports Med* 2015;43(3):654-662.

Surgical treatment of patellofemoral OCD in children and adolescents produces a high rate of satisfaction and return to sports. Female sex, prolonged duration of symptoms, and internal fixation may be associated with worse outcomes. Level of evidence: IV.

18. Wall EJ, Heyworth BE, Shea KG, et al: Trochlear groove osteochondritis dissecans of the knee patellofemoral joint. *J Pediatr Orthop* 2014;34(6):625-630.

MRI aids in the diagnosis and staging of trochlear groove OCD lesions, as almost half of these lesions may not be identifiable on radiographs, and one-quarter are associated with OCD lesions in other locations of the same knee. Multiple surgical treatments can be used to achieve healing or resolution of symptoms in stable and unstable lesions; however, a larger comparative study is needed to make specific recommendations. Level of evidence: IV.

19. Abouassaly M, Peterson D, Salci L, et al: Surgical management of osteochondritis dissecans of the knee in the paediatric population: A systematic review addressing surgical techniques. *Knee Surg Sports Traumatol Arthrosc* 2014;22(6):1216-1224.

The most common techniques to treat OCD were transarticular drilling for stable lesions and bioabsorbable pin fixation for unstable lesions. The key findings were that most lesions healed postoperatively, irrespective of technique, and that good-quality trials are required to more appropriately compare the effectiveness of techniques. Level of evidence: IV.

20. Edmonds EW, Albright J, Bastrom T, Chambers HG: Outcomes of extra-articular, intra-epiphyseal drilling for osteochondritis dissecans of the knee. *J Pediatr Orthop* 2010;30(8):870-878.

Extra-articular, intraepiphyseal drilling of OCD lesions produced excellent results over the historical controls using intra-articular drilling for those patients in whom initial conservative management failed. This technique avoids intraoperative damage to the overlying intact articular cartilage and promotes osseous healing by fenestration of the sclerotic rim surrounding the OCD lesion. Level of evidence: IV.

21. Adachi N, Deie M, Nakamae A, Ishikawa M, Motoyama M, Ochi M: Functional and radiographic outcome of stable juvenile osteochondritis dissecans of the knee treated with retroarticular drilling without bone grafting. *Arthroscopy* 2009;25(2):145-152.

This study shows that retroarticular drilling without bone grafting leads to improved clinical outcomes and high healing rates. Retroarticular drilling is recommended for patients with stable juvenile OCD of the knee in whom initial nonsurgical treatment has failed. Level of evidence: IV.

22. Boughanem J, Riaz R, Patel RM, Sarwark JF: Functional and radiographic outcomes of juvenile osteochondritis dissecans of the knee treated with extra-articular retrograde drilling. *Am J Sports Med* 2011;39(10):2212-2217.

Retrograde extra-articular drilling provided clinical and radiographic improvement in most juveniles with OCD lesions in whom nonsurgical treatment has failed. This method serves to decompress the lesion and allow revascularization without disrupting the articular cartilage surface in stable OCD lesions. Level of evidence: IV.

23. Berná-Serna JD, Martinez F, Reus M, Berná-Mestre JD: Osteochondritis dissecans of the knee: Sonographically guided percutaneous drilling. *J Ultrasound Med* 2008;27(2):255-259.

A 14-year-old boy had OCD of the external femoral condyle. Conventional radiography, MRI, and sonography revealed the osteochondral lesion. On the basis of the good results obtained in the case, it is thought that sonographically guided percutaneous drilling may be a good alternative to arthroscopic drilling in cases of early OCD lesions without displacement of the fragment. Level of evidence: IV.

24. Lebolt JR, Wall EJ: Retroarticular drilling and bone grafting of juvenile osteochondritis dissecans of the knee. *Arthroscopy* 2007;23(7):794.e1-794.e4.

The authors presented an effective technique for retroarticular drilling and bone grafting of juvenile OCD. Major advantages of this technique include the ease of harvest/transfer of autograft, readily available instrumentation to perform the procedure, and the ability to avoid violation of stable articular cartilage. Level of evidence: IV.

25. Lykissas MG, Wall EJ, Nathan S: Retro-articular drilling and bone grafting of juvenile knee osteochondritis dissecans: A technical description. *Knee Surg Sports Traumatol Arthrosc* 2014;22(2):274-278.

The goal of surgery in stable juvenile OCD is to promote revascularization and reossification of the osteochondral fragment by creating channels, linking the subchondral bone to the OCD lesion. The proposed technique represents a promising adjunct for the management of stable juvenile OCD lesions that fail to heal after 3 to 6 months of nonsurgical treatment and for nondisplaced, unstable OCD lesions that undergo internal fixation. Level of evidence: IV.

26. Murray JR, Chitnavis J, Dixon P, et al: Osteochondritis dissecans of the knee; long-term clinical outcome following arthroscopic debridement. *Knee* 2007;14(2):94-98.

The authors reviewed 32 knees in 26 patients who had previously undergone arthroscopic debridement for symptomatic OCD of the knee. Patients undergoing excision of OCD fragments did worse than those in whom the fragment was preserved; however, the risk of further surgery was raised if a fragment was left in situ during initial surgery. Level of evidence: IV.

27. Magnussen RA, Carey JL, Spindler KP: Does operative fixation of an osteochondritis dissecans loose body result in healing and long-term maintenance of knee function? *Am J Sports Med* 2009;37(4):754-759.

Surgical fixation of grade IV OCD loose bodies results in stable fixation. At an average of 9 years after surgery, patients had no symptoms of osteoarthritis pain and had normal function in activities of daily living. However, patients reported substantially reduced knee-related quality of life. Surgical fixation of OCD loose bodies is a better alternative to lesion excision. Level of evidence: IV.

28. Trinh TQ, Harris JD, Flanigan DC: Surgical management of juvenile osteochondritis dissecans of the knee. *Knee Surg Sports Traumatol Arthrosc* 2012;20(12):2419-2429.

Surgical treatment of juvenile OCD has substantially improved clinical and radiographic outcomes at short-, mid-, and long-term follow-up. No difference in clinical or radiographic outcome was demonstrated in comparing different surgical techniques, with the exception of poorer results with isolated fragment excision. Level of evidence: IV.

29. Adachi N, Deie M, Nakamae A, Okuhara A, Kamei G, Ochi M: Functional and radiographic outcomes of unstable juvenile osteochondritis dissecans of the knee treated with lesion fixation using bioabsorbable pins. *J Pediatr Orthop* 2015;35(1):82-88.

The fixation of the unstable juvenile OCD lesions with bioabsorbable pins demonstrated improved clinical outcomes and radiographic high healing rates at a mean of 3.3 years of follow-up. This procedure is advocated for patients with unstable juvenile OCD lesions of sufficient quality to enable fixation, which will preserve the normal contour of the distal femur. Level of evidence: IV.

30. Carey JL, Grimm NL: Treatment algorithm for osteochondritis dissecans of the knee. *Clin Sports Med* 2014;33(2):375-382.

For unstable yet salvageable OCD lesions, the senior author's preferred treatment is fixation with bone grafting. For unstable and unsalvageable OCD lesions, the senior author's preferred treatment is autologous chondrocyte implantation with bone grafting. Level of evidence: IV.

31. Kocher MS, Czarnecki JJ, Andersen JS, Micheli LJ: Internal fixation of juvenile osteochondritis dissecans lesions of the knee. *Am J Sports Med* 2007;35(5):712-718.

Given the relatively high healing rate, good functional outcome, and low complication rate, the authors advocate internal fixation of unstable juvenile OCD lesions of the knee, even for detached lesions and in patients with a history of surgery for the OCD lesion. Level of evidence: IV.

32. Camathias C, Festring JD, Gaston MS: Bioabsorbable lag screw fixation of knee osteochondritis dissecans in the skeletally immature. *J Pediatr Orthop B* 2011;20(2):74-80.

There was substantial improvement in knee function scores, with all patients reporting improvement or much improvement in function. Simple arthroscopic fixation of OCD with SmartScrews is proposed as an effective treatment in the pediatric population leading to a rapid recovery of premorbid function. Level of evidence: IV.

33. Grimm NL, Ewing CK, Ganley TJ: The knee: Internal fixation techniques for osteochondritis dissecans. *Clin Sports Med* 2014;33(2):313-319.

For the athlete with a newly diagnosed OCD of the knee, the first step in formulating a treatment plan is determining the stability of the lesion. Determining the most appropriate method for fixation depends on several variables and should include the athlete's level of play, sport, and overall goals. Level of evidence: IV.

34. Camathias C, Gögüs U, Hirschmann MT, et al: Implant failure after biodegradable screw fixation in osteochondritis dissecans of the knee in skeletally immature patients. *Arthroscopy* 2015;31(3):410-415.

This series reported a 23% rate of failure/fracture of bioabsorbable screws associated with OCD lesion fixation. Level of evidence: IV.

35. Miniaci A, Tytherleigh-Strong G: Fixation of unstable osteochondritis dissecans lesions of the knee using arthroscopic autogenous osteochondral grafting (mosaicplasty). *Arthroscopy* 2007;23(8):845-851.

Autogenous osteochondral grafting of unstable OCD lesions in the knee is a reliable and minimally invasive technique that provides a stable biologic fixation using autogenous bone graft and has few complications. Level of evidence: IV.

36. Miura K, Ishibashi Y, Tsuda E, Sato H, Toh S: Results of arthroscopic fixation of osteochondritis dissecans lesion of the knee with cylindrical autogenous osteochondral plugs. *Am J Sports Med* 2007;35(2):216-222.

Biologic fixation of OCD lesions with cylindrical osteochondral autograft provided healing of the osteochondral fragments. Level of evidence: IV.

37. Gudas R, Simonaityte R, Cekanauskas E, Tamosiūnas R: A prospective, randomized clinical study of osteochondral autologous transplantation versus microfracture for the treatment of osteochondritis dissecans in the knee joint in children. *J Pediatr Orthop* 2009;29(7):741-748.

At an average of 4.2 years follow-up, a prospective, randomized, clinical study in children younger than 18 years showed significant superiority of the mosaic-type OAT over microfracture for the treatment of OCD defects in the knee. However, the study has shown that both microfracture and OAT provide encouraging clinical results for children younger than 18 years. Level of evidence: I.

38. Lintz F, Pujol N, Pandeirada C, Boisrenoult P, Beaufils P: Hybrid fixation: Evaluation of a novel technique in adult osteochondritis dissecans of the knee. *Knee Surg Sports Traumatol Arthrosc* 2011;19(4):568-571.

This promising technique combines biologic fixation using an autograft osteochondral plug with metallic screw fixation. Level of evidence: IV.

39. Nishimura A, Morita A, Fukuda A, Kato K, Sudo A: Functional recovery of the donor knee after autologous osteochondral transplantation for capitellar osteochondritis dissecans. *Am J Sports Med* 2011;39(4):838-842.

A time lag in recovery was reported between postoperative symptoms and muscle power at 3 months. However, harvesting osteochondral grafts did not have adverse effects on donor knee function in young athletes at 2 years following osteochondral autograft transplantation for capitellar OCD. Level of evidence: IV.

40. Filardo G, Kon E, Berruto M, et al: Arthroscopic second generation autologous chondrocytes implantation associated with bone grafting for the treatment of knee osteochondritis dissecans: Results at 6 years. *Knee* 2012;19(5):658-663.

Second-generation ACI associated with bone grafting is a valid treatment option for knee OCD and may offer a good, stable clinical outcome at a mean follow-up of 6 years. Additional studies are needed to confirm the results over time, and to determine if the improvement is only symptomatic, or if this procedure may also prevent or delay further knee degeneration. Level of evidence: IV.

41. Krishnan SP, Skinner JA, Carrington RW, Flanagan AM, Briggs TW, Bentley G: Collagen-covered autologous chondrocyte implantation for osteochondritis dissecans of the knee: Two- to seven-year results. *J Bone Joint Surg Br* 2006;88B(2):203-205.

The study included 37 patients who were evaluated at a mean follow-up of 4.08 years. The age at the time of collagen-covered ACI determined the clinical outcome for juvenile-onset disease ($P = 0.05$), whereas the size of the defect was the major determinant of outcome in adult-onset disease ($P = 0.01$). Level of evidence: III.

42. Lyon R, Nissen C, Liu XC, Curtin B: Can fresh osteochondral allografts restore function in juveniles with osteochondritis dissecans of the knee? *Clin Orthop Relat Res* 2013;471(4):1166-1173.

The authors suggested that fresh osteochondral allografts restored short-term function in patients whose juvenile OCD did not respond to standard treatments. Level of evidence: IV.

43. Murphy R, Pennock AT, Bugbee WD: Osteochondral allograft transplantation of the knee in pediatric and adolescent population. *Am J Sports Med* 2014;42(3):635-640.

With 88% good/excellent results and 80% salvage rate of clinical failures with an additional allograft, osteochondral allograft transplantation is a useful treatment option in pediatric and adolescent patients. Level of evidence: IV.

44. Murphy RT, Pennock AT, Bugbee WD: Osteochondral allograft transplantation of the knee in the pediatric and adolescent population. *Am J Sports Med* 2014;42(3):635-640.

Osteochondral allograft transplantation was shown to be a useful treatment option in pediatric and adolescent patients, with 88% good/excellent results and 80% salvage rate of clinical failures with an additional allograft. Level of evidence: IV.

45. Nissen CW: Osteochondritis dissecans of the elbow. *Clin Sports Med* 2014;33(2):251-265.

OCD affects the elbow of many young, skeletally immature athletes. There is a predilection for those involved in overhead-dominant sports and sports that require the arm to be a weight-bearing limb. Level of evidence: IV.

46. Nishitani K, Nakagawa Y, Gotoh T, Kobayashi M, Nakamura T: Intraoperative acoustic evaluation of living human cartilage of the elbow and knee during mosaicplasty for osteochondritis dissecans of the elbow: An in vivo study. *Am J Sports Med* 2008;36(12):2345-2353.

The OCD lesion had lower signal intensity than did the intact part of the capitellum. Although the macroscopic view looked intact, the radial head cartilage was degenerated as measured acoustically. Level of evidence: IV.

47. Ahmad CS, Vitale MA, ElAttrache NS: Elbow arthroscopy: Capitellar osteochondritis dissecans and radiocapitellar plica. *Instr Course Lect* 2011;60:181-190.

Radiocapitellar plica can cause chondromalacic changes on the radial head and capitellum, with symptoms including painful clicking and effusions. Arthroscopic plica resection is indicated when nonsurgical treatment fails. Level of evidence: IV

48. Chen NC: Osteochondritis dissecans of the elbow. *J Hand Surg Am* 2010;35(7):1188-1189.

Both reconstruction and arthroscopic débridement yield notable improvement after surgery. There is some evidence that reconstruction yields better results than débridement for larger defects at mid-term follow-up. Level of evidence: IV.

49. de Graaff F, Krijnen MR, Poolman RW, Willems WJ: Arthroscopic surgery in athletes with osteochondritis dissecans of the elbow. *Arthroscopy* 2011;27(7):986-993.

This review suggests that surgical treatment must be considered for athletes with OCD after a period of unsuccessful nonsurgical therapy. Nevertheless, larger studies with enhanced methodologic quality and longer follow-up should be performed to support this conclusion. Level of evidence: III.

50. Arai Y, Hara K, Fujiwara H, Minami G, Nakagawa S, Kubo T: A new arthroscopic-assisted drilling method through the radius in a distal-to-proximal direction for osteochondritis dissecans of the elbow. *Arthroscopy* 2008;24(2):237.e1-237.e4.

With this technique, the entire OCD lesion can be vertically drilled under arthroscopic guidance. This method is minimally invasive, and an early return to sports could be possible. Level of evidence: IV.

51. Rahusen FT, Brinkman JM, Eygendaal D: Results of arthroscopic debridement for osteochondritis dissecans of the elbow. *Br J Sports Med* 2006;40(12):966-969.

The clinical outcome after arthroscopic debridement for OCD of the elbow shows good results, with pain relief during activities of daily living and sport. The function of the elbow, as reflected by the modified Andrews elbow scoring system score, improved from poor to excellent. Level of evidence: IV.

52. Shi LL, Bae DS, Kocher MS, Micheli LJ, Waters PM: Contained versus uncontained lesions in juvenile elbow osteochondritis dissecans. *J Pediatr Orthop* 2012;32(3):221-225.

At short-term follow-up, uncontained elbow OCD lesions have greater flexion contracture when compared with contained lesions. Elbow OCD lesions also have higher rates of joint effusion and are broader and shallower. Level of evidence: IV.

53. Yamamoto Y, Ishibashi Y, Tsuda E, Sato H, Toh S: Osteochondral autograft transplantation for

osteochondritis dissecans of the elbow in juvenile baseball players: Minimum 2-year follow-up. *Am J Sports Med* 2006;34(5):714-720.

Osteochondral autograft transplantation is a useful treatment for reattachment of the lesion as well as osteochondral resurfacing of elbow OCD. Level of evidence: IV.

54. Iwasaki N, Kato H, Ishikawa J, Masuko T, Funakoshi T, Minami A: Autologous osteochondral mosaicplasty for osteochondritis dissecans of the elbow in teenage athletes. *J Bone Joint Surg Am* 2009;91(10):2359-2366.

The mean clinical score described by Timmerman and Andrews (with a maximum of 200 points) improved significantly from 131 +/- 23 points preoperatively to 191 +/- 15 points postoperatively (*P* < 0.0001). The current midterm results indicate that mosaicplasty can provide satisfactory clinical outcomes for teenage athletes with advanced capitellar OCD lesions. Level of evidence: IV.

55. Nobuta S, Ogawa K, Sato K, Nakagawa T, Hatori M, Itoi E: Clinical outcome of fragment fixation for osteochondritis dissecans of the elbow. *Ups J Med Sci* 2008;113(2):201-208.

Fragment fixation for OCD of the humeral capitellum was effective in patients whose lesion thickness was less than 9 mm. Fixation by flexible wire or thread and revascularization by drilling for the fragment were considered to be insufficient for large lesions with a thickness of 9 mm or more. Level of evidence: IV.

56. Miyamoto W, Yamamoto S, Kii R, Uchio Y: Oblique osteochondral plugs transplantation technique for osteochondritis dissecans of the elbow joint. *Knee Surg Sports Traumatol Arthrosc* 2009;17(2):204-208.

This procedure addresses some of the challenges associated with the placement of osteochondral autografts in the elbow joint, due to the smaller size of and limited access to the capitellum. Level of evidence: IV.

57. Canale ST, Belding RH: Osteochondral lesions of the talus. *J Bone Joint Surg Am* 1980;62(1):97-102.

Long-term results indicated that few lesions unite when treated nonsurgically. Degenerative changes in the ankle joint, whether symptomatic or not, were common (50% of the ankles) regardless of the type of treatment. Level of evidence: IV.

58. Woelfle JV, Reichel H, Javaheripour-Otto K, Nelitz M: Clinical outcome and magnetic resonance imaging after osteochondral autologous transplantation in osteochondritis dissecans of the talus. *Foot Ankle Int* 2013;34(2):173-179.

OAT was reported as a safe procedure with good clinical results for talar OCD. Because an abnormal MRI finding was not necessarily diagnostically conclusive, MRI might be of limited value in postoperative follow-up. Level of evidence: IV.

59. Zwingmann J, Südkamp NP, Schmal H, Niemeyer P: Surgical treatment of osteochondritis dissecans of the talus: A systematic review. *Arch Orthop Trauma Surg* 2012;132(9):1241-1250.

Although OCD of the talus represents a frequently observed orthopaedic pathology, evidence concerning surgical treatment of talar OCD is still lacking. From this study of more than 1,100 patients, no strong recommendations can be given based on scientific evidence. Level of evidence: IV.

60. Perumal V, Wall E, Babekir N: Juvenile osteochondritis dissecans of the talus. *J Pediatr Orthop* 2007;27(7):821-825.

In skeletally immature patients, few juvenile OCD of the talus lesions respond to 6 months of nonsurgical treatment. Surgery should be adopted if pain persists and if the patient is not willing to modify activities. Level of evidence: IV.

61. Woelfle JV, Reichel H, Nelitz M: Indications and limitations of osteochondral autologous transplantation in osteochondritis dissecans of the talus. *Knee Surg Sports Traumatol Arthrosc* 2013;21(8):1925-1930.

OAT is a safe procedure with good clinical results in talar OCD. Because advanced age is associated with increased donor site morbidity, indications for OAT in older patients should be carefully considered. Because no other variables affected the clinical outcome of OAT adversely, no contraindications exist for OAT (for example, in osteochondral lesions requiring more than one graft, lateral lesions, patients with body mass index greater than 25 kg/m², preexisting osteoarthritis, or unsuccessful previous surgery). Level of evidence: IV.

62. Talusan PG, Milewski MD, Toy JO, Wall EJ: Osteochondritis dissecans of the talus: Diagnosis and treatment in athletes. *Clin Sports Med* 2014;33(2):267-284.

OCD of the talus is a subset of osteochondral lesions of the talus that also includes osteochondral fractures, osteonecrosis, and degenerative arthritis. Osteochondral lesions of the talus can be associated with ankle injury. This article discusses the anatomy, pathoanatomy, history, physical examination, imaging, management algorithm, and outcomes of surgical treatment of osteochondral lesions in these patients. Level of evidence: IV.

© 2016 American Academy of Orthopaedic Surgeons

Chapter 48

Anterior Cruciate Ligament Tears in Skeletally Immature Athletes

Benton E. Heyworth, MD   Melissa A. Christino, MD

Abstract

Anterior cruciate ligament (ACL) tears are becoming increasingly common injuries in young athletes, with surgical treatment in the skeletally immature knee posing unique challenges. Surgical intervention using physeal-sparing or physeal-respecting techniques are the preferred treatment strategies and have been shown to be successful at restoring knee stability and functionality while avoiding iatrogenic growth disturbance or deformity. Because of the uniquely high activity level of children and adolescents, establishing reliable strategies to prevent ACL tear and retear, still in their nascent stages for this age group, requires special attention and advancement.

Keywords: anterior cruciate ligament; ACL; pediatric sports; sports injuries; pediatric ACL

Introduction

Anterior cruciate ligament (ACL) tears in children and adolescents, previously perceived as a rare clinical entity, are now increasingly common injuries being treated by orthopaedic surgeons throughout the United States and internationally. Sports-related injuries in children have increased as a result of higher participation rates, higher levels of competition, and earlier focus on individual sports.[1,2] Whereas tibial spine avulsion fractures were

---

Dr. Heyworth or an immediate family member serves as a board member, owner, officer, or committee member of the American Orthopaedic Society for Sports Medicine and the Pediatric Orthopaedic Society of North America. Neither Dr. Christino nor any immediate family member has received anything of value from or has stock or stock options held in a commercial company or institution related directly or indirectly to the subject of this chapter.

historically considered the pediatric equivalent of an adult ACL tear, intrasubstance ACL ruptures are occurring more commonly in skeletally immature patients of varied age.[3] Because children have important anatomic and physiologic differences from adults, treatment algorithms for young athletes with ACL tears have evolved to respect these differences.

The Growing Athlete

The physes, or growth plates, generate the longitudinal growth of the human skeleton. In children, the cartilaginous physes are open, or biologically active, and are therefore vulnerable to metabolic or mechanical injury that can cause angular deformity of the extremity or growth arrest. The two growth plates around the knee are the fastest growing physes in the lower extremity and are vulnerable to growth disturbance resulting from surgical intervention for ACL reconstruction. The distal femoral physis accounts for approximately 10 mm of growth per year, and the proximal tibial physis accounts for approximately 6 mm of growth per year. Skeletal maturity is attained after the growth plates of the long bones have closed, or ossified, and this generally occurs after puberty (in girls, at approximately age 14.5 years; in boys, at approximately age 16.5 years).[4-7] Females grow for approximately 2 years after menarche, and their peak height velocity occurs at approximately 11.5 years; the peak height velocity for males occurs later, at approximately 13.5 years. Based on the presence or absence of secondary sex characteristics at the onset of puberty, physiologic maturity can be estimated using the Tanner staging system.[8] However, because of challenges in assessing Tanner stage in adolescents and preadolescents in the office setting, as well as recent literature demonstrating large interobserver variability among sports medicine surgeons using this system,[9] the standard of care for the assessment of skeletal maturity has evolved to include radiographs of the left hand to determine bone age, with estimates of skeletal age using

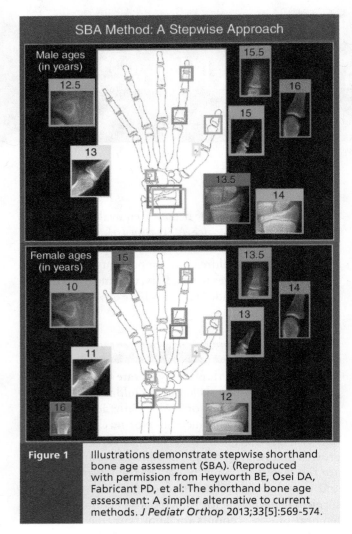

Figure 1 Illustrations demonstrate stepwise shorthand bone age assessment (SBA). (Reproduced with permission from Heyworth BE, Osei DA, Fabricant PD, et al: The shorthand bone age assessment: A simpler alternative to current methods. *J Pediatr Orthop* 2013;33[5]:569-574.

the Greulich and Pyle Atlas[10] or more efficient shorthand methods derived from the atlas[11] (**Figure 1**).

Despite the rapid growth changes occurring around the time of puberty, the position of the ACL footprint on the lateral femoral condyle within the intercondylar notch is unchanged and remains close to the distal femoral physis. A cadaver study showed the distance from the femoral ACL footprint to the distal femoral physis remained constant (slightly less than 3 mm) from fetal stages through adolescence.[12] Although this relationship does not change with age and growth, anatomic variations about the knee exist during development. An MRI study of adolescent patients with open physes showed that intercondylar notch volume was substantially smaller in a population of patients with ACL tears than in those without; notch volume was also found to be substantially smaller in girls than in boys.[13] The anatomic variations

in notch volume can therefore increase predisposition to ACL injury.

When considering surgical intervention in growing children and adolescents, it is paramount to avoid iatrogenic injury to the growth plate that can cause growth disturbance. One rabbit model demonstrated that although disruption of 3% of the cross-sectional surface area of the distal femoral growth plate did not cause growth disturbance, disruption of 7% or more caused substantial growth disturbance.[14] A subsequent rabbit study showed that although 3% physeal disruption in the distal femur did not cause growth disturbance, both valgus angulation and growth arrest were observed with 4% cross-sectional disruption in the proximal tibial physis.[15] Because physeal volume increases with age, the percentage of physeal disruption from a given reamer size was less in the older children studied.[16] Moreover, tunnel diameter and graft size had the largest effect on determining the volume of growth plate disruption in children age 10 to 15 years because of nonlinear variable relationships. Similarly, a computer simulation model showed that because the volume of physeal damage influenced growth arrest, the effects of double-bundle drilling on the distal femoral physis should be avoided in skeletally immature patients.[17] A recent clinical MRI study in skeletally immature patients suggested that some degree of physeal disruption occurs with partial transphyseal and all-epiphyseal reconstruction techniques, which are described in greater detail later in this chapter.[18] However, at short-term follow-up, this disruption had not translated into clinically significant sequelae of altered alignment or limb-length discrepancy. Overgrowth has also been a reported concern in prepubescent children undergoing ACL reconstruction.[19-21] Minimizing iatrogenic damage to the distal femoral and proximal tibia physes, if not avoiding them altogether, remains a central objective in the management of ACL injuries in children with substantial growth remaining.

Diagnosis

Patient History/Mechanism of Injury

The mechanism of injury for ACL tears in skeletally immature patients is similar to that of adults, in whom either contact or noncontact knee twisting injuries occur. Patients often report hearing a "pop," followed by substantial effusion and pain. ACL tears were identified in 22% of patients age 10 to 14 years and in 40% of patients age 15 to 18 years who presented with an acute hemarthrosis.[22] Young patients can also have a delayed presentation, with reports of continued pain, instability, and effusions after a remote injury. Patients with a delayed presentation may have been evaluated previously for their injury but the diagnosis of an ACL tear may not have been considered because of their age.

Risk Factors

Recent evidence suggests that pediatric and adolescent patients who engage in high activity levels and year-round sport specialization may be at increased risk for the development of ACL injuries.[1,2,23] Females younger than 18 years have been noted to sustain more overuse and soft-tissue sports injuries compared with males,[24,25] and females are significantly more likely to sustain ACL tears than males.[26,27] Because of age-based differences in the ratio of collagen types in the ligaments, skeletally immature children generally have more ligamentous laxity than adults, and laxity has also been proposed as a risk factor for ACL tears.[28]

Physical Examination

In the first 3 to 4 weeks following an ACL injury in a child, the physical examination usually reveals an effusion, decreased range of motion, and varied ability to comfortably bear weight. In skeletally immature patients with open physes, Salter-Harris physeal fractures should always be included in the differential diagnosis, and bony palpation of the growth plates and varus/valgus stability testing should be performed. The presence of hypermobility or generalized ligamentous laxity should be assessed, and the stability of the contralateral knee tested because greater variability exists in ligamentous examination results in children than in adults. Standing leg alignment should also be assessed and documented; however, in the acute postinjury setting, this may have to be performed with the patient supine. Anterior drawer, Lachman, and pivot shift test results will be asymmetric from the contralateral knee in a patient with a complete ACL tear. Some evidence exists that in the rare partial ACL tear, which can primarily involve one bundle of the ligament, a positive pivot shift test result correlates highly with disruption of the posterolateral bundle.[29] The patient also may demonstrate other findings on physical examination consistent with concomitant knee injuries such as meniscal tears, chondral injuries, or other ligamentous injuries. Depending on the age and comfort level of the child, level of cooperation with the examination can vary, and the most reliable examination will be under general anesthesia, making it a critical confirmatory step before all knee procedures.

Imaging

Knee radiographs should be obtained to rule out bony abnormalities such as fractures, tibial spine avulsions, osteochondral injuries, or physeal injuries. However, MRI is the imaging test of choice to confirm a suspected ACL tear. Because the diagnostic efficacy of MRI in evaluating children's knees has previously been questioned,[30] 3T MRI has more recently been shown to have a high level of accuracy in diagnosing ACL tears in children and teenagers, and therefore can be valuable if there are questionable or equivocal findings with lower resolution studies.[31] A PA radiograph of the left hand should be obtained, and the bone age determined with the Greulich and Pyle Atlas[10] or a shorthand method.[11] This information is used for ACL preoperative planning purposes to determine whether a physeal-sparing, physeal-respecting, partial transphyseal, or traditional transphyseal reconstruction technique should be used.

Associated Injuries

Additional knee injuries are common in children and adolescents with ACL tears, including meniscal tears, chondral injuries, and ligamentous injuries.[32] In a review of 124 skeletally immature patients with acute ACL tears, the prevalence of meniscal tears was 69.3%, and lateral meniscal tears were more common than medial meniscus tears, as with adults.[33] Another study demonstrated that children with ACL tears and open physes had similar rates of meniscal tears and chondral injuries compared with children with closed physes.[34] Medial meniscus tears have been associated with greater patient weight and age older than 15 years, and patients with both an ACL tear and a meniscal tear are at higher risk for chondral injury in the affected meniscal compartment.[35] Delay in ACL surgery in children has also been associated with higher rates and severity of medial meniscus tears and chondral injuries,[35,36] and the number of instability episodes has been found to be an independent predictor of subsequent intra-articular injury.[37,38]

Nonsurgical Management

Historically, children with ACL tears were treated by delaying ACL reconstruction until skeletal maturity to avoid the potential risk of physeal damage during reconstruction that could result in longitudinal growth disturbance or deformity. However, multiple recent studies have continued to substantiate more historic evidence, which suggested that nonsurgical management of pediatric ACL injuries, even with bracing and attempted activity modification, has poor results because of undue risk of meniscal and chondral injuries, even in the first 1 to 2 years after injury.[32,33,35,36,39-43] A recent meta-analysis suggested that early surgical treatment of pediatric ACL injuries has more favorable outcomes than nonsurgical or delayed surgical management.[44] Nonsurgical management of ACL injuries in the skeletally immature should be reserved for patients with low-grade partial ACL tears in knees without instability, particularly without rotational instability,[45] and for patients who have substantial medical or psychologic barriers to surgery or compliance with postoperative rehabilitation.

Surgical Management

Surgical management of ACL tears in active, skeletally immature patients has become the preferred treatment strategy to stabilize the knee, thereby protecting the knee from cartilage and meniscal injuries, and more safely allowing functional participation in activities with cutting and/or pivoting exposures.[46,47] In adolescents approaching skeletal maturity who have minimal growth remaining (skeletal age: older than 13 years for girls, older than 14 years for boys), traditional transphyseal ACL reconstruction can be considered because the potential for clinically significant growth arrest is minimal at this stage of maturity.[48] For younger patients, traditional techniques, particularly those involving the placement of graft bone plugs (for example, patellar tendon) or implants across the physis, can adversely affect the growing athlete's physis.[15-17] Multiple techniques have been described to avoid growth complications in prepubescent patients, which involve minimal to no growth plate violation and fixation away from the physes (Figure 2).

Recent high-level evidence suggests that allograft has a higher failure rate in young patients than autograft, and should therefore ideally be avoided in children undergoing ACL reconstruction.[49,50] Patellar tendon grafts, which involve use of bone plugs on the graft, are generally also a suboptimal graft choice in young children because of the greater potential of forming a tethering bony bridge across the growth plate if bone plugs are placed or fixed in the area of the physis. Thus, hamstring or iliotibial band (ITB) autograft are the most common graft choices. Physeal-sparing techniques have demonstrated successful clinical results, with few reported instances of growth disturbance.

Extraphyseal

The outcomes of a combined intra-articular/extra-articular reconstruction using ITB autograft were described in 44 skeletally immature patients with a follow-up period longer than 5 years[51,52] (Figure 2, A). In this technique, the ITB remains attached to the Gerdy tubercle distally and a free limb of graft tissue is harvested proximally, tubularized, wrapped around the posterior lateral femoral condyle, and passed through the intercondylar notch in the over-the-top position and under the intermeniscal

ligament in a small trough in the proximal tibial epiphysis. For femoral fixation, the graft is sutured to the posterolateral periosteum of the lateral femoral condyle and capsular tissue, and tibial fixation is achieved by suturing the free graft end to the metaphyseal tibial periosteum distal to the proximal tibial growth plate. With tendon-to-bone healing of the graft in the epiphyseal tibial trough over time, tibial fixation eventually approximates the native ACL footprint. Excellent results have been reported with this technique, with no reported instances of growth disturbance, a low graft failure rate, and a revision rate of 4.5%.

Although the extra-articular ITB technique can place the ACL graft in a relatively less anatomic position than other described techniques, biomechanical studies have suggested that ITB reconstruction restores anterior-posterior and rotational stability to a greater degree than all-epiphyseal and over-the-top transtibial techniques, possibly to the point of overconstraint, although the implant-based fixation approach in these adult cadaver models does not mirror the periosteal suture fixation inherent in the described technique.[53] Importantly, the ITB technique precludes the need for implants, protects physeal function according to medium-term follow-up studies, and optimizes future options for revision in case of retear, which appears to be rare. Figure 3 is an algorithmic approach to pediatric ACL injuries that is currently used.[52] Longer term and higher volume studies are needed to further elucidate the outcomes for this technique.

All-Epiphyseal

Several techniques for all-epiphyseal reconstruction have been described in small series. Although the drilling of femoral and tibial epiphyseal tunnels can facilitate more anatomic positioning of the ACL graft relative to its native footprint, imaging guidance and technical precision are required to position tunnels within the epiphyseal bone while avoiding injury to the physis or articular cartilage. A technique has been described in which femoral and tibial epiphyseal tunnels are established using fluoroscopic guidance, and a quadruple hamstring autograft is secured with suspensory fixation on the femur and a screw-and-post construct on the tibial metaphysis[54] (Figure 2, B). A In a series of 12 patients, excellent postoperative stability and functional outcomes were reported. Femoral and tibial interference screws were used for epiphyseal fixation and demonstrated that the use of intraoperative CT scan with three-dimensional reconstruction can help avoid physeal injury[55] (Figure 2, C). An all-inside, all-epiphyseal, triple-looped semitendinosus technique has been described that used retrograde drilling with fluoroscopic guidance and adjustable-loop, suspensory

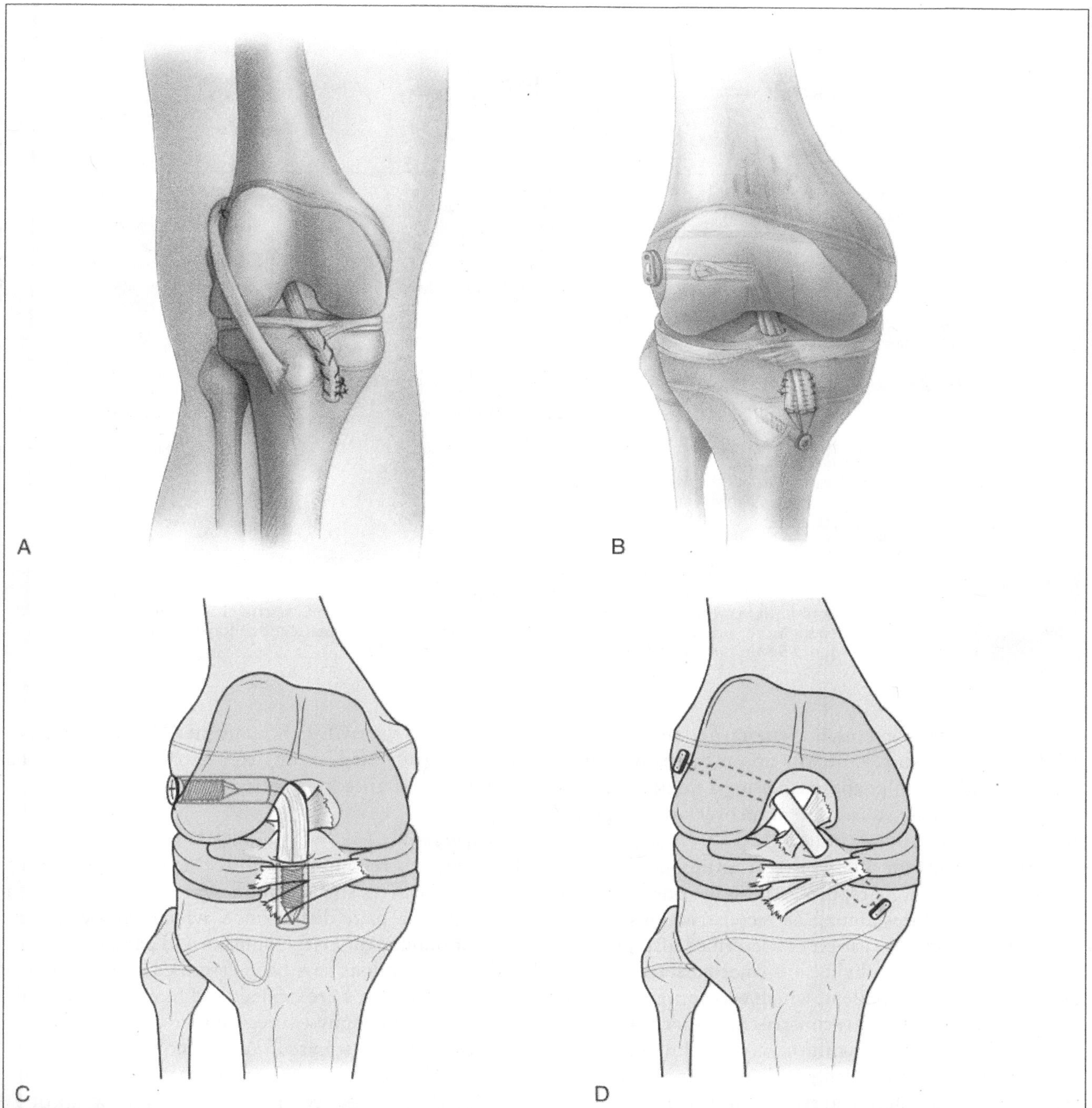

Figure 2 Illustrations depict anterior cruciate ligament reconstruction techniques to avoid growth complications in prepubescent patients. **A,** The Micheli technique of intra-articular/extra-articular extraphyseal reconstruction using iliotibial band autograft. (Reproduced with permission from Kocher MS, Garg S, Micheli LJ: Physeal sparing reconstruction of the anterior cruciate ligament in skeletally immature prepubescent children and adolescents: Surgical technique. *J Bone Joint Surg Am* 2006;88[Suppl 1 Pt 2]:283-293.) **B,** The all-epiphyseal technique with tibial metaphyseal screw-post fixation. (Reproduced with permission from Anderson AF: Transepiphyseal replacement of the anterior cruciate ligament using quadruple hamstring grafts in skeletally immature patients. *J Bone Joint Surg Am* 2004;86[suppl 1 pt 2,]:201-209.) **C,** The all-epiphyseal technique with femoral and tibial epiphyseal interference screw fixation. **D,** The all-epiphyseal technique with femoral and tibial blind epiphyseal sockets and suspensory fixation.

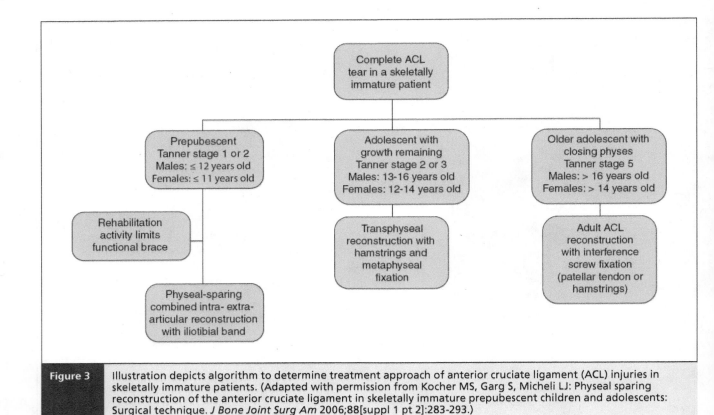

Figure 3 Illustration depicts algorithm to determine treatment approach of anterior cruciate ligament (ACL) injuries in skeletally immature patients. (Adapted with permission from Kocher MS, Garg S, Micheli LJ: Physeal sparing reconstruction of the anterior cruciate ligament in skeletally immature prepubescent children and adolescents: Surgical technique. *J Bone Joint Surg Am* 2006;88[suppl 1 pt 2]:283-293.)

fixation constructs on both the femoral and tibial sides[56,57] (**Figure 2, D**). Two-year follow-up outcomes have been reported with a similar approach using a single hamstring graft with interference screw fixation over suture tape and relatively shorter, blind tunnels.[58,59]

Revision rates for all-epiphyseal techniques have not been comprehensively reported, although one study noted two graft failures among 28 reconstructions (7%) at 2-year follow-up.[58] A case report described distal femoral valgus deformity and slight limb-length discrepancy in a skeletally immature patient, which was appreciated after revision all-epiphyseal reconstruction that followed a graft failure associated with the same technique.[60] MRI was performed in 15 patients at 6 and 12 months following all-inside all-epiphyseal reconstruction and it was reported that although no physeal disruption was noted on the femoral side with this technique, 10 patients demonstrated a small amount of tibial physeal compromise (mean, 2.1%), which was not associated with clinically appreciable growth disturbance.[18] Substantial limb-length discrepancy resulting from overgrowth has been reported in two cases, with more mild limb-length discrepancies seen in four additional patients.[20]

Biomechanical studies suggest that the all-epiphyseal technique enhances anterior stability of the knee compared to the ACL-deficient state.[53,57,61] However, results have suggested incomplete restoration of rotational stability[53] and knee kinematics.[57]

Transphyseal

Transphyseal reconstruction in prepubescent patients typically involves smaller, more vertical tunnels to minimize growth plate disturbance, which can occur with large or oblique tunnels. Complete and partial transphyseal reconstructions have been described, in which one or both growth plates are drilled, and fixation is generally placed in the metaphyseal region to avoid the physis.

Seventeen transphyseal ACL reconstructions were performed in prepubescent patients, with no evidence of growth disturbance at an average follow-up of 70 months.[62] Several reports have described good clinical results at final follow-up and no cases of growth disturbance following transphyseal reconstruction;[63-67] other reports have described cases of limb-length discrepancy, angular deformity, or overgrowth within series of transphyseal reconstructions.[21,68,69] One case report described two cases of limb-length discrepancy secondary to overgrowth in children who underwent partial transphyseal ACL reconstruction using autogenous ITB, with over-the-top suture fixation on the femoral side and tibial placement through a transphyseal tunnel with metaphyseal metal staple fixation.[19] An MRI study of 43 pubescent patients with open physes at the time of transphyseal reconstruction demonstrated that bone tunnels comprised less than 3% of the growth plate, but areas of focal physeal disruption and bony bridging were seen in 12% of patients. No clinical evidence of growth disturbance was observed in these patients, which was likely related to the limited growth remaining of the study population.[70] Another MRI study showed that partial transphyseal reconstruction caused tibial physeal disturbances in an average of 5.4% of the physis, without clinical evidence of growth compromise.[18] Given the continued practice by some surgeons of transphyseal reaming in the skeletally immature, comparative evidence assessing outcomes of these techniques relative to newer physeal-sparing techniques will be particularly beneficial.

Surgical Outcomes and Rehabilitation

Young children with high activity levels are at risk for primary ACL tears as well as subsequent injuries and ACL graft re-tears. Although multiple studies have suggested that age younger than 20 years is a risk factor for revision in general,[50,71,72] one study demonstrated that skeletally immature patients have rates of early revision and early reoperation similar to those of older adolescents with closed physes.[34] Younger patients have also been shown to have a higher risk of undergoing contralateral ACL reconstruction.[71] In a recent large-scale cohort study, adolescence and playing soccer were risk factors independently associated with higher revision rates, and the two risk factors combined demonstrated a threefold increase in the likelihood of revision surgery.[73] Adolescents with an ACL reconstruction have a sixfold higher incidence of subsequent ACL injury on either the surgical or contralateral knee compared with healthy control patients, and 29.5% of the 78 adolescent patients studied sustained a second ACL injury within 24 months of return to sport.[74]

Meniscal repairs in adolescents undergoing ACL reconstruction have been shown to be substantially more successful than isolated meniscal repairs.[26] A study of meniscal repairs in patients younger than 18 years showed a 74% overall healing rate of meniscal repairs associated with ACL reconstruction. Simple tears had a healing rate of 84%, and complex tears, bucket-handle tears, medial meniscus tears, and skeletal immaturity were found to be risk factors for failed repair.

Return to sport among skeletally immature athletes is reported to be between 6 and 9 months in most series. However, substantial strength and functional deficits were found in skeletally immature patients more than

1 year following ACL reconstruction, suggesting these patients may require longer rehabilitation efforts.[75] Recent literature also suggested that perioperative femoral nerve blocks in pediatric patients may be associated with postoperative functional strength deficits, and a decreased likelihood of meeting return-to-sport criteria 6 months postsurgery.[76] Proper rehabilitation is critical to preventing further injury or graft re-tear with return to activity. Pediatric athletes may be the age group most likely to prefer returning to a high activity level following ACL reconstruction. This not only places them at risk for reinjury, but it also can predispose a high risk for mood disturbance, depression, threatened athletic identity, and fear of reinjury following ACL injury.[77] A pediatric patient's emotional response to injury and rehabilitation can be important prognostically and should be closely observed.

Injury prevention can play an important role in the pediatric population. Universal neuromuscular injury prevention training programs have been advocated as cost-effective interventions that could potentially decrease the incidence of ACL tears in this age group by 63%.[78] Programs focusing on strengthening, proximal muscle control, and varied exercise modalities have been successful in reducing ACL injuries in young females.[79]

Although physeal-sparing or transphyseal techniques provide young athletes with safe surgical options for ACL reconstruction with good surgical outcomes, preventing the initial ACL injury and minimizing the likelihood of reinjury in this young, extremely active population remains a priority for optimizing the long-term health of pediatric athletes.

Summary

ACL tears in skeletally immature patients are increasingly common injuries in a challenging patient population. Various surgical techniques have successfully restored knee stability and allowed continued participation in sports and activities, while minimizing injury to growing physes. Longer term outcomes for these techniques have yet to be described, but prevention strategies to minimize initial injuries as well as recurrent injuries following ACL reconstruction may be valuable in such a young, active population. Further studies are needed to better elucidate the natural history of ACL tears in young athletes.

Key Study Points

- ACL tears in skeletally immature patients are becoming increasingly common injuries.

- In the setting of a large effusion or suspected hemarthrosis in a young patient who has sustained a knee contact injury or twisting mechanism, because of the high frequency of ACL tears, physical examination and MRI should be directed toward assessing for intra-articular injury.

- Nonsurgical management, which was historically pursued for pediatric ACL injuries, has been associated with high rates of meniscal or chondral injury in young athletic or physically active patients.

- Multiple physeal-sparing or physeal-respecting surgical techniques have been described and shown to be successful in restoring knee stability in skeletally immature patients, including extraphyseal reconstruction using ITB autograft, all-epiphyseal reconstruction techniques with hamstring autograft and various fixation options, and transphyseal reconstruction that minimizes growth plate disturbance.

- Young athletes are at higher risk for rerupture and revision surgery than their adult counterparts, including contralateral limb ACL tears.

- Injury prevention programs may play a valuable role in preventing ACL injuries in young patients.

Annotated References

1. Dodwell ER, Lamont LE, Green DW, Pan TJ, Marx RG, Lyman S: 20 years of pediatric anterior cruciate ligament reconstruction in New York State. *Am J Sports Med* 2014;42(3):675-680.

   This population-based study quantitatively examined the increasing rates of ACL injuries diagnosed in young patients in the state of New York between 1990 and 2009.

2. Mall NA, Paletta GA: Pediatric ACL injuries: Evaluation and management. *Curr Rev Musculoskelet Med* 2013;6(2):132-140.

   This review highlights current concepts related to the diagnosis, management, and treatment of ACL injuries in pediatric patients.

3. Ganley TJ. Knee injuries in kids: Why the increase? Available at: http://www.medscape.com/viewarticle/755155. Accessed August 5, 2015.

   Over a 12-year period (1999 to 2011), the incidence of meniscal tears, tibial spine fractures, and ACL ruptures all increased at Children's Hospital of Philadelphia; however,

   a more than 400% increase in ACL ruptures occurred compared with tibial spine fractures during this time.

4. Anderson M, Green WT, Messner MB: Growth and predictions of growth in the lower extremities. *J Bone Joint Surg Am* 1963;45:1-14.

5. Anderson M, Messner MB, Green WT: Distribution of lengths of the normal femur and tibia in children from one to eighteen years of age. *J Bone Joint Surg Am* 1964;46:1197-1202.

6. Pritchett JW: Longitudinal growth and growth-plate activity in the lower extremity. *Clin Orthop Relat Res* 1992;275:274-279.

7. Paley D, Bhave A, Herzenberg JE, Bowen JR: Multiplier method for predicting limb-length discrepancy. *J Bone Joint Surg Am* 2000;82(10):1432-1446.

8. Tanner JM, Whitehouse RH: Clinical longitudinal standards for height, weight, height velocity, weight velocity, and stages of puberty. *Arch Dis Child* 1976;51(3):170-179.

9. Slough JM, Hennrikus W, Chang Y: Reliability of Tanner staging performed by orthopedic sports medicine surgeons. *Med Sci Sports Exerc* 2013;45(7):1229-1234.

   High intraobserver and interobserver variability were observed when Tanner staging was performed by orthopaedic surgeons based on clinical photographs, suggesting that this may not be a reliable method to guide surgical decision making.

10. Greulich WW, Pyle SI: *Radiographic Atlas of Skeletal Development of the Hand and Wrist*, ed 2. Stanford, CA, Stanford University Press, 1959.

11. Heyworth BE, Osei DA, Fabricant PD, et al: The shorthand bone age assessment: A simpler alternative to current methods. *J Pediatr Orthop* 2013;33(5):569-574.

    A shorthand bone age method was developed based on certain radiographic parameters. This method of quantifying skeletal maturity was found to be simple, reliable, and efficient. Level of evidence: III.

12. Behr CT, Potter HG, Paletta GA Jr: The relationship of the femoral origin of the anterior cruciate ligament and the distal femoral physeal plate in the skeletally immature knee. An anatomic study. *Am J Sports Med* 2001;29(6):781-787.

13. Swami VG, Mabee M, Hui C, Jaremko JL: Three-dimensional intercondylar notch volumes in a skeletally immature pediatric population: A magnetic resonance imaging-based anatomic comparison of knees with torn and intact anterior cruciate ligaments. *Arthroscopy* 2013;29(12):1954-1962.

    This MRI study in adolescent patients with sports injuries showed that three-dimensional notch volume was smaller in girls than in boys, and was also smaller in knees with ACL tears compared with ACL-intact knees. Level of evidence: III.

14. Mäkelä EA, Vainionpää S, Vihtonen K, Mero M, Rokkanen P: The effect of trauma to the lower femoral epiphyseal plate. An experimental study in rabbits. *J Bone Joint Surg Br* 1988;70(2):187-191.

15. Guzzanti V, Falciglia F, Gigante A, Fabbriciani C: The effect of intra-articular ACL reconstruction on the growth plates of rabbits. *J Bone Joint Surg Br* 1994;76(6):960-963.

16. Kercher J, Xerogeanes J, Tannenbaum A, Al-Hakim R, Black JC, Zhao J: Anterior cruciate ligament reconstruction in the skeletally immature: An anatomical study utilizing 3-dimensional magnetic resonance imaging reconstructions. *J Pediatr Orthop* 2009;29(2):124-129.

    This study used a custom software model to assess the volume of physeal disruption with simulated transphyseal drilling. Graft radius was found to be the most critical factor affecting the volume of physeal injury. Level of evidence: IV.

17. Shea KG, Grimm NL, Belzer JS: Volumetric injury of the distal femoral physis during double-bundle ACL reconstruction in children: A three-dimensional study with use of magnetic resonance imaging. *J Bone Joint Surg Am* 2011;93(11):1033-1038.

    Three-dimensional MRI models of children's knees demonstrated that double-bundle surgical techniques substantially increased the volume of physeal injury with tunnel drilling, and could increase the risk of growth disturbance.

18. Nawabi DH, Jones KJ, Lurie B, Potter HG, Green DW, Cordasco FA: All-inside, physeal-sparing anterior cruciate ligament reconstruction does not significantly compromise the physis in skeletally immature athletes: A postoperative physeal magnetic resonance imaging analysis. *Am J Sports Med* 2014;42(12):2933-2940.

    Physeal-specific MRI in 23 skeletally immature patients was used to evaluate the volume of physeal disturbance with all-epiphyseal and partial transphyseal ACL reconstructions. Tibial physeal disturbance occurred with both techniques but was noted to be minor and did not result in any clinical growth disturbances. Level of evidence: IV.

19. Chotel F, Henry J, Seil R, Chouteau J, Moyen B, Bérard J: Growth disturbances without growth arrest after ACL reconstruction in children. *Knee Surg Sports Traumatol Arthrosc* 2010;18(11):1496-1500.

    This case report describes two cases of overgrowth in pediatric patients following ACL reconstruction using an over-the-top ITB autograft with a transtibial tunnel. Level of evidence: V.

20. Koch PP, Fucentese SF, Blatter SC: Complications after epiphyseal reconstruction of the anterior cruciate ligament in prepubescent children. *Knee Surg Sports Traumatol Arthrosc* 2014 [Epub ahead of print].

    This retrospective review discusses outcomes and complications following all-epiphyseal reconstructions in 12 prepubescent patients. Substantial overgrowth was seen in two patients and minor limb-length discrepancies were seen in four additional patients. Level of evidence: IV.

21. McIntosh AL, Dahm DL, Stuart MJ: Anterior cruciate ligament reconstruction in the skeletally immature patient. *Arthroscopy* 2006;22(12):1325-1330.

22. Abbasi D, May MM, Wall EJ, Chan G, Parikh SN: MRI findings in adolescent patients with acute traumatic knee hemarthrosis. *J Pediatr Orthop* 2012;32(8):760-764.

    This study reviewed the knee MRIs of 131 young patients who presented with a history of acute knee trauma and effusion seen on MRI. ACL tears were present in 22% of younger patients (age range, 10 to 14 years) compared with 40% of older patients (age range, 15 to 18 years). Level of evidence: III.

23. Stracciolini A, Casciano R, Levey Friedman H, Meehan WP III, Micheli LJ: Pediatric sports injuries: An age comparison of children versus adolescents. *Am J Sports Med* 2013;41(8):1922-1929.

    This study examined sports injuries in children and adolescents presenting to a large academic medical center from 2000 to 2009. A substantial percentage of injuries required surgical intervention, and older children tend to sustain higher amounts of overuse injuries. Level of evidence: III.

24. Stracciolini A, Casciano R, Levey Friedman H, Stein CJ, Meehan WP III, Micheli LJ: Pediatric sports injuries: A comparison of males versus females. *Am J Sports Med* 2014;42(4):965-972.

    This study examined sex differences in sports injuries in children and adolescents. Females were found to sustain a higher percentage of overuse injuries and more injuries to the lower extremity. Level of evidence: III.

25. Stracciolini A, Casciano R, Friedman HL, Meehan WP III, Micheli LJ: A closer look at overuse injuries in the pediatric athlete. *Clin J Sport Med* 2015;25(1):30-35.

    This cross-sectional study examined sex differences in overuse sports injuries. Females sustained more overuse injuries than males, but a large proportion of this sex discrepancy was attributable to differences in the types of sports played.

26. Agel J, Arendt EA, Bershadsky B: Anterior cruciate ligament injury in national collegiate athletic association basketball and soccer: A 13-year review. *Am J Sports Med* 2005;33(4):524-530.

27. Prodromos CC, Han Y, Rogowski J, Joyce B, Shi K: A meta-analysis of the incidence of anterior cruciate ligament tears as a function of gender, sport, and a knee injury-reduction regimen. *Arthroscopy* 2007;23(12):1320-1325.e6.

28. Kim SJ, Kumar P, Kim SH: Anterior cruciate ligament reconstruction in patients with generalized joint laxity. *Clin Orthop Surg* 2010;2(3):130-139.

Generalized ligamentous laxity is a risk factor for ACL tears as well as inferior outcomes following reconstruction. This paper discusses the issues related to surgical decision making in the setting of laxity.

29. Yoon KH, Lee SH, Park SY, Kang DG, Chung KY: Can physical examination predict the intraarticular tear pattern of the anterior cruciate ligament? *Arch Orthop Trauma Surg* 2014;134(10):1451-1457.

This study examined the correlation between physical examination findings and arthroscopic tear patterns. Pivot shift test results were found to be a reliable predictor of posterolateral bundle tear or complete ACL tear.

30. Kocher MS, DiCanzio J, Zurakowski D, Micheli LJ: Diagnostic performance of clinical examination and selective magnetic resonance imaging in the evaluation of intraarticular knee disorders in children and adolescents. *Am J Sports Med* 2001;29(3):292-296.

31. Schub DL, Altahawi F, F Meisel A, Winalski C, Parker RD, M Saluan P: Accuracy of 3-Tesla magnetic resonance imaging for the diagnosis of intra-articular knee injuries in children and teenagers. *J Pediatr Orthop* 2012;32(8):765-769.

In patients younger than 20 years, 3T MRIs were found to have high sensitivity and specificity for diagnosing ACL injuries. Level of evidence: II.

32. Moksnes H, Engebretsen L, Risberg MA: Prevalence and incidence of new meniscus and cartilage injuries after a nonoperative treatment algorithm for ACL tears in skeletally immature children: A prospective MRI study. *Am J Sports Med* 2013;41(8):1771-1779.

This prospective study examined 40 skeletally immature patients with ACL tears who followed a nonsurgical treatment course. The incidence of new meniscal injuries after initial diagnostic MRI was 19.5%, and 32% of nonsurgically treated patients required subsequent surgical ACL reconstruction.

33. Samora WP III, Palmer R, Klingele KE: Meniscal pathology associated with acute anterior cruciate ligament tears in patients with open physes. *J Pediatr Orthop* 2011;31(3):272-276.

In this retrospective review of 124 skeletally immature patients, meniscal injury accompanied ACL rupture in 69.3% of patients, with lateral meniscus tears being more common in children with open physes. Level of evidence: IV.

34. Csintalan RP, Inacio MC, Desmond JL, Funahashi TT: Anterior cruciate ligament reconstruction in patients with open physes: Early outcomes. *J Knee Surg* 2013;26(4):225-232.

This large retrospective study compared patients with closed physes with patients with open physes and ACL tears and reported no significant differences in the prevalence of chondral or meniscal injuries, early revision surgery, or reoperation rates following ACL reconstruction.

35. Dumont GD, Hogue GD, Padalecki JR, Okoro N, Wilson PL: Meniscal and chondral injuries associated with pediatric anterior cruciate ligament tears: Relationship of treatment time and patient-specific factors. *Am J Sports Med* 2012;40(9):2128-2133.

Pediatric patients who underwent ACL reconstruction more than 150 days after injury had higher rates of medial meniscal tears compared with those treated before 150 days postinjury. Level of evidence: III.

36. Lawrence JT, Argawal N, Ganley TJ: Degeneration of the knee joint in skeletally immature patients with a diagnosis of an anterior cruciate ligament tear: Is there harm in delay of treatment? *Am J Sports Med* 2011;39(12):2582-2587.

In a series of 70 patients younger than 14 years, a delay in surgical treatment greater than 12 weeks was associated with higher rates of irreparable medial meniscal tears and lateral compartment chondral injuries. Level of evidence: III.

37. Funahashi KM, Moksnes H, Maletis GB, Csintalan RP, Inacio MC, Funahashi TT: Anterior cruciate ligament injuries in adolescents with open physis: Effect of recurrent injury and surgical delay on meniscal and cartilage injuries. *Am J Sports Med* 2014;42(5):1068-1073.

This review of young patients with ACL tears showed no significant association between time to surgery and meniscal/chondral injury; however, an increased number of substantial encounters was associated with combined meniscal and cartilage injury. Level of evidence: III.

38. Kluczynski MA, Marzo JM, Bisson LJ: Factors associated with meniscal tears and chondral lesions in patients undergoing anterior cruciate ligament reconstruction: A prospective study. *Am J Sports Med* 2013;41(12):2759-2765.

This case-control study showed that male sex predicted meniscal tears, age and obesity predicted chondral injuries, and number of instability episodes was an independent predictor of intra-articular injury. Level of evidence: III.

39. Guenther ZD, Swami V, Dhillon SS, Jaremko JL: Meniscal injury after adolescent anterior cruciate ligament injury: How long are patients at risk? *Clin Orthop Relat Res* 2014;472(3):990-997.

In adolescent patients, medial meniscal tears were found to increase steadily in frequency more than 1 year after ACL injury. Level of evidence: IV.

40. Kocher MS, Saxon HS, Hovis WD, Hawkins RJ: Management and complications of anterior cruciate ligament injuries in skeletally immature patients: Survey of the Herodicus Society and The ACL Study Group. *J Pediatr Orthop* 2002;22(4):452-457.

41. Frosch KH, Stengel D, Brodhun T, et al: Outcomes and risks of operative treatment of rupture of the anterior cruciate ligament in children and adolescents. *Arthroscopy* 2010;26(11):1539-1550.

This meta-analysis of case series examined clinical outcomes and risks of ACL surgery in pediatric patients, and

8. The Young Athlete

showed low rates of graft failure after ACL reconstruction in young patients. Level of evidence: IV.

42. Cipolla M, Scala A, Gianni E, Puddu G: Different patterns of meniscal tears in acute anterior cruciate ligament (ACL) ruptures and in chronic ACL-deficient knees. Classification, staging and timing of treatment. *Knee Surg Sports Traumatol Arthrosc* 1995;3(3):130-134.

43. Henry J, Chotel F, Chouteau J, Fessy MH, Bérard J, Moyen B: Rupture of the anterior cruciate ligament in children: Early reconstruction with open physes or delayed reconstruction to skeletal maturity? *Knee Surg Sports Traumatol Arthrosc* 2009;17(7):748-755.

    Skeletally immature patients who delayed ACL reconstruction until skeletal maturity were found to have higher rates of medial meniscal tears and subsequent meniscectomies when compared with patients who underwent reconstruction while skeletally immature.

44. Ramski DE, Kanj WW, Franklin CC, Baldwin KD, Ganley TJ: Anterior cruciate ligament tears in children and adolescents: A meta-analysis of nonoperative versus operative treatment. *Am J Sports Med* 2014;42(11):2769-2776.

    This meta-analysis of pediatric patients with ACL tears showed that nonsurgical or delayed management resulted in more knee instability and inability to return to previous activity levels, thus favoring early surgical stabilization of ACL tears in the pediatric population.

45. Kocher MS, Micheli LJ, Zurakowski D, Luke A: Partial tears of the anterior cruciate ligament in children and adolescents. *Am J Sports Med* 2002;30(5):697-703.

46. Fabricant PD, Jones KJ, Delos D, et al: Reconstruction of the anterior cruciate ligament in the skeletally immature athlete: a review of current concepts: AAOS exhibit selection. *J Bone Joint Surg Am* 2013;95(5):e28.

    This paper comprehensively reviews current literature regarding ACL tears in skeletally immature athletes. Surgical reconstruction in young patients has yielded successful surgical outcomes.

47. Frank JS, Gambacorta PL: Anterior cruciate ligament injuries in the skeletally immature athlete: Diagnosis and management. *J Am Acad Orthop Surg* 2013;21(2):78-87.

    This review article discusses the unique characteristics of managing the pediatric ACL tear. Natural history, growth-related considerations, current literature, and surgical options are described.

48. Vavken P, Murray MM: Treating anterior cruciate ligament tears in skeletally immature patients. *Arthroscopy* 2011;27(5):704-716.

    This systematic literature review suggests that surgical management of ACL tears in skeletally immature patients is the treatment of choice, and nonsurgical management can result in further meniscal and/or chondral intra-articular damage. Level of evidence: IV.

49. Engelman GH, Carry PM, Hitt KG, Polousky JD, Vidal AF: Comparison of allograft versus autograft anterior cruciate ligament reconstruction graft survival in an active adolescent cohort. *Am J Sports Med* 2014;42(10):2311-2318.

    In adolescent patients, graft type and postoperative knee laxity were predictors of graft survival, and autograft was recommended in young patients undergoing primary ACL reconstruction. Level of evidence: III.

50. Kaeding CC, Aros B, Pedroza A, et al: Allograft versus autograft anterior cruciate ligament reconstruction: Predictors of failure from a MOON prospective longitudinal cohort. *Sports Health* 2011;3(1):73-81.

    Young patients (age range, 10 to 19 years) were found to have an increased risk of ACL graft failure following reconstruction, and allograft was associated with a substantially higher risk of failure when compared with autograft.

51. Kocher MS, Garg S, Micheli LJ: Physeal sparing reconstruction of the anterior cruciate ligament in skeletally immature prepubescent children and adolescents. *J Bone Joint Surg Am* 2005;87(11):2371-2379.

52. Kocher MS, Garg S, Micheli LJ: Physeal sparing reconstruction of the anterior cruciate ligament in skeletally immature prepubescent children and adolescents. Surgical technique. *J Bone Joint Surg Am* 2006;88(Suppl 1 Pt 2):283-293.

53. Kennedy A, Coughlin DG, Metzger MF, et al: Biomechanical evaluation of pediatric anterior cruciate ligament reconstruction techniques. *Am J Sports Med* 2011;39(5):964-971.

    Biomechanical test results comparing all-epiphyseal, transtibial over-the-top, and extra-articular ITB techniques showed that ITB reconstruction best restored anteroposterior stability of the knee and rotational control.

54. Anderson AF: Transepiphyseal replacement of the anterior cruciate ligament using quadruple hamstring grafts in skeletally immature patients. *J Bone Joint Surg Am* 2004;86(Pt 2, Suppl 1):201-209.

55. Lawrence JT, Bowers AL, Belding J, Cody SR, Ganley TJ: All-epiphyseal anterior cruciate ligament reconstruction in skeletally immature patients. *Clin Orthop Relat Res* 2010;468(7):1971-1977.

    This report described a physeal-sparing, all-epiphyseal ACL reconstruction technique, which uses all-epiphyseal tunnels with interference screw fixation, as well as the use of three-dimensional intraoperative CT to minimize the risk of growth disturbance. Level of evidence: IV.

56. McCarthy MM, Graziano J, Green DW, Cordasco FA: All-epiphyseal, all-inside anterior cruciate ligament reconstruction technique for skeletally immature patients. *Arthrosc Tech* 2012;1(2):e231-e239.

    This paper describes a physeal-sparing, all-inside, all-epiphyseal ACL reconstruction, with retrograde epiphyseal tunnel drilling and suspensory fixation of autogenous hamstring graft.

57. McCarthy MM, Tucker S, Nguyen JT, Green DW, Imhauser CW, Cordasco FA: Contact stress and kinematic analysis of all-epiphyseal and over-the-top pediatric reconstruction techniques for the anterior cruciate ligament. *Am J Sports Med* 2013;41(6):1330-1339.

In this biomechanical cadaver study, all-epiphyseal and over-the-top reconstruction techniques were found to restore anterior and rotational stability to the ACL-deficient knee, but they did not restore normal knee kinematics to the ACL-intact knee.

58. Cassard X, Cavaignac E, Maubisson L, Bowen M: Anterior cruciate ligament reconstruction in children with a quadrupled semitendinosus graft: Preliminary results with minimum 2 years of follow-up. *J Pediatr Orthop* 2014;34(1):70-77.

This paper described the outcomes following an all-epiphyseal technique using retroreamed sockets and short, quadruple semitendinosus grafts with terephthalate tape. Good outcomes were reported using this technique in skeletally immature patients with no instances of growth disturbance.

59. Collette M, Cassard X: The Tape Locking Screw technique (TLS): A new ACL reconstruction method using a short hamstring graft. *Orthop Traumatol Surg Res* 2011;97(5):555-559.

This technique paper describes the Tape Locking Screw ACL reconstruction, using short retrograde tunnel sockets, short single hamstring graft, and interference screw fixation over terephthalate tape strips.

60. Lawrence JT, West RL, Garrett WE: Growth disturbance following ACL reconstruction with use of an epiphyseal femoral tunnel: A case report. *J Bone Joint Surg Am* 2011;93(8):e39.

This case report documents a case of valgus deformity and slight leg-length discrepancy in a skeletally immature patient who underwent revision all-epiphyseal ACL reconstruction after failure of the same technique. No surgical intervention was required for treatment.

61. Sena M, Chen J, Dellamaggioria R, Coughlin DG, Lotz JC, Feeley BT: Dynamic evaluation of pivot-shift kinematics in physeal-sparing pediatric anterior cruciate ligament reconstruction techniques. *Am J Sports Med* 2013;41(4):826-834.

This cadaver study simulated pivot shift test results to assess stability following physeal-sparing ACL reconstruction techniques. All-epiphyseal, extra-articular ITB, and transtibial over-the-top techniques all resulted in improved knee stability compared with the ACL-deficient state.

62. Streich NA, Barié A, Gotterbarm T, Keil M, Schmitt H: Transphyseal reconstruction of the anterior cruciate ligament in prepubescent athletes. *Knee Surg Sports Traumatol Arthrosc* 2010;18(11):1481-1486.

This study compared surgical and nonsurgical treatment of ACL tears in immature patients who were Tanner stage 1 or 2: 58% of nonsurgically treated patients required later surgery because of instability, and those treated surgically with transphyseal reconstruction demonstrated better clinical results and functional outcomes.

63. Kocher MS, Smith JT, Zoric BJ, Lee B, Micheli LJ: Transphyseal anterior cruciate ligament reconstruction in skeletally immature pubescent adolescents. *J Bone Joint Surg Am* 2007;89(12):2632-2639.

64. Cohen M, Ferretti M, Quarteiro M, et al: Transphyseal anterior cruciate ligament reconstruction in patients with open physes. *Arthroscopy* 2009;25(8):831-838.

Twenty-six skeletally immature patients underwent transphyseal ACL reconstruction with autogenous hamstring graft, and were found to have good clinical outcomes with no instances of substantial growth disturbance.

65. Kim SJ, Shim DW, Park KW: Functional outcome of transphyseal reconstruction of the anterior cruciate ligament in skeletally immature patients. *Knee Surg Relat Res* 2012;24(3):173-179.

This retrospective review assessed outcomes of transphyseal ACL reconstruction in 25 skeletally immature patients who had reached skeletal maturity by final follow-up. Average follow-up was 6 years, and patients reported good functional outcomes and no substantial leg length or limb alignment abnormalities.

66. Redler LH, Brafman RT, Trentacosta N, Ahmad CS: Anterior cruciate ligament reconstruction in skeletally immature patients with transphyseal tunnels. *Arthroscopy* 2012;28(11):1710-1717.

Eighteen skeletally immature pubescent patients underwent transphyseal ACL reconstruction. At a mean follow-up of 43.4 months, patients demonstrated excellent clinical functional outcomes with no instances of graft re-tear or growth disturbance. Level of evidence: IV.

67. Kumar S, Ahearne D, Hunt DM: Transphyseal anterior cruciate ligament reconstruction in the skeletally immature: Follow-up to a minimum of sixteen years of age. *J Bone Joint Surg Am* 2013;95(1):e1.

Thirty-two skeletally immature patients who underwent transphyseal ACL reconstruction were retrospectively studied with a minimum follow-up of 4 years. Patients had satisfactory clinical and functional outcomes, and one case of mild valgus deformity was reported, but this was not functionally important.

68. Lipscomb AB, Anderson AF: Tears of the anterior cruciate ligament in adolescents. *J Bone Joint Surg Am* 1986;68(1):19-28.

69. Liddle AD, Imbuldeniya AM, Hunt DM: Transphyseal reconstruction of the anterior cruciate ligament in prepubescent children. *J Bone Joint Surg Br* 2008;90(10):1317-1322.

70. Yoo WJ, Kocher MS, Micheli LJ: Growth plate disturbance after transphyseal reconstruction of the anterior cruciate

ligament in skeletally immature adolescent patients: An MR imaging study. *J Pediatr Orthop* 2011;31(6):691-696.

This MRI study and retrospective review of 43 adolescent patients who underwent transphyseal ACL reconstruction showed that focal physeal disruption was present in 11.6% of patients after reconstruction, most commonly at the tibial physis. No patient demonstrated evidence of clinical growth disturbance.

71. Wasserstein D, Khoshbin A, Dwyer T, et al: Risk factors for recurrent anterior cruciate ligament reconstruction: A population study in Ontario, Canada, with 5-year follow-up. *Am J Sports Med* 2013;41(9):2099-2107.

This cohort study of patients age 15 to 60 years showed that young age (range, 15 to 19 years) and use of allograft were associated with increased risk of revision ACL reconstruction. Young age was also associated with a higher risk for contralateral ACL injury and reconstruction. Level of evidence: III.

72. Magnussen RA, Lawrence JT, West RL, Toth AP, Taylor DC, Garrett WE: Graft size and patient age are predictors of early revision after anterior cruciate ligament reconstruction with hamstring autograft. *Arthroscopy* 2012;28(4):526-531.

Among 338 patients undergoing primary ACL reconstruction, hamstring autograft size less than 8 mm and age younger than than 20 years were associated with high revision rates. Level of evidence: III.

73. Andernord D, Desai N, Björnsson H, Ylander M, Karlsson J, Samuelsson K: Patient predictors of early revision surgery after anterior cruciate ligament reconstruction: A cohort study of 16,930 patients with 2-year follow-up. *Am J Sports Med* 2015;43(1):121-127.

This prospective cohort study reported that adolescents and soccer players had an increased risk of revision surgery after ACL reconstruction, and the combination of these two predictors had an almost threefold higher risk for revision surgery. Level of evidence: II.

74. Paterno MV, Rauh MJ, Schmitt LC, Ford KR, Hewett TE: Incidence of Second ACL Injuries 2 Years After Primary ACL Reconstruction and Return to Sport. *Am J Sports Med* 2014;42(7):1567-1573.

In young athletes (mean age, 17.3 years) with primary ACL reconstructions, 29.5% of patients sustained a second ACL injury within 24 months of return to sport, and patients who have undergone ACL reconstruction had a higher risk of another ACL tear compared with control patients. Level of evidence: II.

75. Greenberg EM, Greenberg ET, Ganley TJ, Lawrence JT: Strength and functional performance recovery after anterior cruciate ligament reconstruction in preadolescent athletes. *Sports Health* 2014;6(4):309-312.

Young patients with all-epiphyseal ACL reconstructions were reviewed for their strength and functional performance measures following rehabilitation. Substantial strength and functional deficits were found in some patients at 7 months as well as more than 1 year postoperatively. Level of evidence: IV.

76. Luo TD, Ashraf A, Dahm DL, Stuart MJ, McIntosh AL: Femoral nerve block is associated with persistent strength deficits at 6 months after anterior cruciate ligament reconstruction in pediatric and adolescent patients. *Am J Sports Med* 2015;43(2):331-336.

In patients 18 years or younger who underwent ACL reconstruction, femoral nerve blocks were associated with strength deficits at 6 months compared with control patients, and patients without a block were four times more likely to meet return-to-sport criteria at 6 months. Level of evidence: III.

77. Christino MA, Fantry AJ, Vopat BG: Psychological aspects of recovery following anterior cruciate ligament reconstruction. *J Am Acad Orthop Surg* 2015;23(8):501-509.

This review summarizes the current literature regarding psychologic sequelae of ACL tears. Psychologic factors can have important effects on athletes' injury experiences and rehabilitation.

78. Swart E, Redler L, Fabricant PD, Mandelbaum BR, Ahmad CS, Wang YC: Prevention and screening programs for anterior cruciate ligament injuries in young athletes: A cost-effectiveness analysis. *J Bone Joint Surg Am* 2014;96(9):705-711.

Using a decision-analysis model, neuromuscular training programs for young athletes were proposed to be a cost-effective strategy for preventing ACL injuries and reducing costs associated with ACL injury.

79. Sugimoto D, Myer GD, Barber Foss KD, Hewett TE: Specific exercise effects of preventive neuromuscular training intervention on anterior cruciate ligament injury risk reduction in young females: Meta-analysis and subgroup analysis. *Br J Sports Med* 2015;49(5):282-289.

This systematic review found that preventive neuromuscular training efficacy in young female athletes was increased with strengthening exercises, proximal control exercises, and multiple exercise techniques.

Patellofemoral Instability and Other Common Knee Issues in the Skeletally Immature Athlete

Aristides I. Cruz Jr, MD   Matthew D. Milewski, MD

Abstract

The skeletally immature athlete often presents with sports- and activity-related conditions that are unique to this patient population. The immature skeleton presents unique sites of injury and pathology in children principally because of the presence of open cartilaginous growth centers. These growth centers represent areas of weakness that predispose these athletes to injury. The orthopaedic surgeon must take special care in treating certain injuries in those with open physes and apophyses in this patient population.

Keywords: pediatric knee; patellar dislocation; anterior knee pain; knee; immature athlete; patellofemoral instability; tibial spine avulsion; discoid meniscus; osteochondrosis

Introduction

Knee injuries in the skeletally immature athlete are among the most commonly encountered problems in the clinician's office and are the result of both overuse and acute trauma. There are four common knee pathologies in this population: patellofemoral instability, tibial spine (eminence) avulsion fracture, discoid lateral meniscus, and knee osteochondroses (Osgood-Schlatter disease and Sinding-Larsen-Johansson [SLJ] disease).

Dr. Cruz or an immediate family member serves as a board member, owner, officer, or committee member of the Pediatric Orthopaedic Society of North America. Dr. Milewski or an immediate family member serves as a board member, owner, officer, or committee member of the Pediatric Orthopaedic Society of North America.

Patellofemoral Instability

Patellofemoral instability with lateral patellar dislocation or subluxation is a common disorder of the knee in skeletally immature athletes. In the child or adolescent athlete, properly treating the cause of instability is important for return to play and to prevent recurrence. Skeletally immature patients should receive special consideration because the presence of open physes influences evaluation and treatment.

Epidemiology

The incidence of patellofemoral instability in the United States is estimated to be 2.29 per 100,000 person-years,[1] with the peak incidence occurring between 15 and 19 years of age. The rates of instability are equal between males and females, and 51.9% of instability events occur during athletic activity. Nonsurgical treatment of first-time dislocators is successful 62% of the time.[2] Ligamentous laxity or joint hypermobility can also influence outcome after patellar dislocation, with better functional results in those without hypermobility.[3]

Diagnosis, Anatomy, and Biomechanics

The primary restraint to lateral patellar dislocation is the medial patellofemoral ligament (MPFL), which resists lateral translation of the patella. Injury to this ligament predisposes patients to recurrent dislocation. The MPFL zone of injury after acute patellar dislocation varies.[4] One study showed that MPFL injury most commonly involves the patellar attachment (61%), followed by femoral attachment injury (12%), injury to both attachments (12%), and midsubstance injury (9%). Six percent of patients had no identifiable injury. The MPFL zone of injury following acute patellar dislocation differs when comparing skeletally mature and immature patients.[5] Patellar-side MPFL injury is more common in skeletally immature patients (79%) than in skeletally mature patients (54%).

In skeletally immature patients, the location of the MPFL femoral attachment is important because it is near the distal femoral physis. One study showed that the femoral insertion of the MPFL is distal to the physis.[6] Additionally, because of the flare of the medial aspect of the distal femoral physis, the femoral insertion of the MPFL can appear to be closer to the physis than it actually is on a lateral radiograph (Figure 1). An MRI study found that the MPFL femoral insertion was distal to the physis in 86% of patients, 7% were located at the same level as the physis, and 7% were located proximal to the physis.[4] On average, the femoral insertion of the MPFL was 5 mm distal to the physis, and 36% of patients had a femoral insertion within 5 mm of the physis. In skeletally immature cadavers,[7] the center of the MPFL origin was found to be distal to the distal femoral physis in all specimens. The proximal extent of the MPFL origin footprint was found to extend above the physis in older specimens.

The distal attachment of the extensor mechanism also should be considered when evaluating patients with patellofemoral instability. A commonly used parameter for assessing the distal attachment of the extensor mechanism is the tibial tubercle–trochlear groove (TT-TG) distance. An increased TT-TG distance is associated with patellar instability in pediatric and adolescent patients.[8] The type of imaging modality is also an important consideration when measuring TT-TG distance: MRI can potentially underestimate the TT-TG distance compared with CT.[9]

Patellar height should also be assessed because patella alta can be associated with patellofemoral instability. Whether this relationship is causative is unclear, and several studies have shown that patellar height decreases following MPFL reconstruction.[10,11] Accurate measurement of patellar height in skeletally immature patients can be challenging because of incomplete ossification centers. A 2010 study[12] showed that the Insall-Salvati ratio is most reliable in patients with near-complete ossification, and that the Koshino Index[13] may be more applicable but less valid in younger children. The Caton-Deschamps index may be a simpler, more reliable method for determining patellar height in skeletally immature patients[14] (Figure 2).

Trochlear dysplasia is associated with recurrent instability even after MPFL reconstruction. In a 2014 study, only 43% of patients returned to sports participation after MPFL reconstruction if they also had severe trochlear dysplasia.[15] In this series, all patients with severe dysplasia had recurrent instability compared with 9.3% of those with mild dysplasia.

Treatment

No clear evidence supports surgical over nonsurgical treatment of acute patellar dislocation.[16] The primary

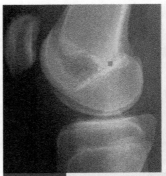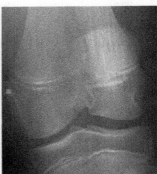

Figure 1 Medial patellofemoral ligament insertion site in a skeletally immature patient. (Reproduced with permission from Nelitz M1, Dreyhaupt J, Reichel H, Woelfle J, Lippacher S: Anatomic reconstruction of the medial patellofemoral ligament in children and adolescents with open growth plates: Surgical technique and clinical outcome. *Am J Sports Med* 2013;41[1]:58-63.)

absolute indication for surgical treatment of acute patellar dislocation is the presence of an osteochondral loose body.[17]

For chronic patellar instability in the child or adolescent athlete, it is important to keep multiple factors in mind when deciding on treatment. One algorithm uses physeal status, Q-angle, trochlear morphology, and TT-TG distance to determine the optimal procedure for treating patients with chronic instability.[18] Medial imbrication is recommended for skeletally immature patients, with or without soft-tissue distal realignment (Roux-Goldthwait procedure), depending on TT-TG distance. MPFL reconstruction is recommended for skeletally mature patients, with or without distal realignment (tibial tubercle osteotomy). Additionally, trochleoplasty is recommended in those with severe trochlear dysplasia. A slightly different treatment algorithm has been proposed that accounts for rotational alignment and patellofemoral chondral lesions.[19] Surgical treatment options for chronic patellofemoral instability in the child or adolescent athlete are also listed in Figure 3.

MPFL Reconstruction

Several surgical techniques for MPFL reconstruction have been described for skeletally immature patients. A 2013 study describes an MPFL reconstruction technique with bioabsorbable screw fixation distal to the distal femoral physis and a looped graft through the patella[20] (Figure 4). A 2014 study describes an MPFL reconstruction technique using a pedicled quadriceps tendon autograft.[21] Double-bundle, anatomic MPFL reconstruction is also described with two tunnels drilled into the patella.[20] A 2011 study described MPFL reconstruction in skeletally

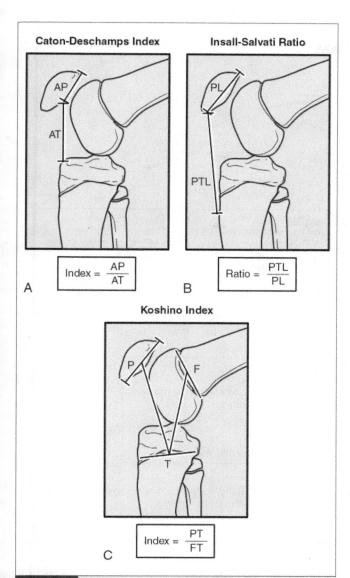

Figure 2 Illustrations depict methods of assessing patellar height in skeletally immature patients. **A,** The Caton-Deschamps index: calculated by dividing the articular facet length of the patella (AP) by the distance between the inferior aspect of the patellar articular facet and the anterior corner of superior aspect of the tibial epiphysis (AT). **B,** The Insall-Salvati ratio: calculated by dividing the patellar tendon length (PTL) by the patellar length (PL). **C,** The Koshino index: calculated by dividing the distance from the center of the patella to the center of the tibial physis (PT) by the distance from the center of the femoral physis to the center of the tibial physis (FT).

immature patients using patellar tunnels, with graft tenodesis to the adductor magnus to avoid drilling a tunnel near the distal femoral physis.[22] To date, no study has directly compared MPFL reconstruction techniques in skeletally immature patients. During MPFL reconstruction in

skeletally immature patients, careful attention should be given to femoral fixation to minimize the risk of physeal damage, and the amount of patellar drilling should be minimized.

Video 49.1: A Surgical Technique for Medial Patellofemoral Ligament Reconstruction in the Skeletally Immature. Henry B. Ellis, MD, Philip L. Wilson, MD (14 min)

Distal Realignment

In the setting of an abnormal TT-TG distance, distal realignment in addition to MPFL reconstruction/proximal realignment should be considered. Skeletally immature patients present a challenge when considering distal realignment because tibial tubercle osteotomy (such as the Fulkerson procedure) is contraindicated. A technique of distal realignment with transfer of the tibial tubercle periosteum has been described to avoid injury to the tibial tubercle apophysis.[23] The Galeazzi procedure involves tenodesis of the semitendinosus tendon to the patella while preserving its distal attachment. This procedure is designed to provide a checkrein for lateral patellar tracking; however, it is "nonanatomic." An 82% rate of recurrent subluxation/dislocation at an average follow-up of 70 months has been reported in patients who underwent a Galeazzi procedure.[24] Additionally, 35% of patients underwent additional procedures to treat persistent symptoms. The so-called 3-in-1 procedure involves lateral retinacular release, vastus medialis advancement, and transfer of the medial third of the patellar ligament to the medial collateral ligament. Although this procedure has been shown to be safe and reliable, isokinetic strength testing of the surgical limb has shown persistent weakness compared with the contralateral limb.[25] The Roux-Goldthwait procedure involves lateral retinacular release and transfer of the lateral half of the patellar ligament medially. This procedure has shown good results in small series.[26,27]

Trochleoplasty

The femoral trochlea provides a lateral buttress to resist patellar dislocation, and trochlear dysplasia can predispose patients to instability. A 2013 study reported success treating recurrent instability in patients whose surgery for patellofemoral instability had failed, by treating the underlying trochlear dysplasia with trochleoplasty.[28] A 2013 study described successful outcomes following combined MPFL reconstruction and trochleoplasty in patients with patellofemoral instability in the setting of trochlear dysplasia.[29] A 2011 study reported on trochleoplasty to

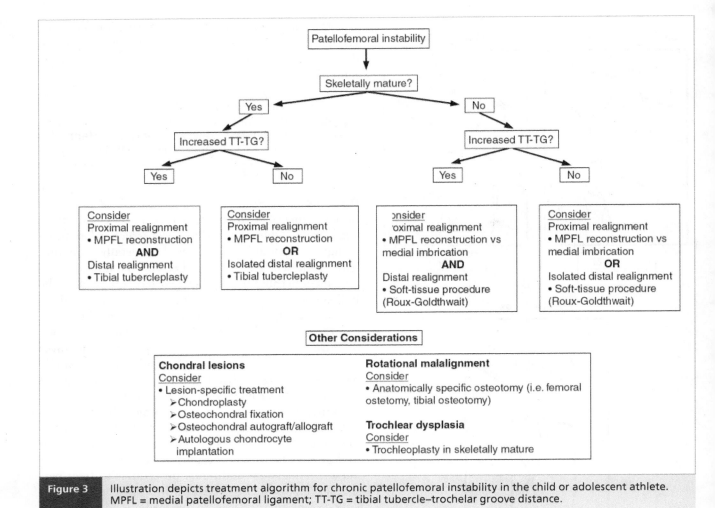

Figure 3   Illustration depicts treatment algorithm for chronic patellofemoral instability in the child or adolescent athlete. MPFL = medial patellofemoral ligament; TT-TG = tibial tubercle–trochelar groove distance.

treat trochlear dysplasia in patients with patellofemoral instability and concluded that trochleoplasty is useful and reliable; however, improved postoperative knee pain is less predictable.[30]

Complications

Complications following surgery for patellofemoral instability include recurrent instability, stiffness, patellar fracture, patellofemoral arthrosis, and persistent pain. A 2013 study reported a 16.2% complication for MPFL reconstruction in patients younger than 21 years.[31] Forty-seven percent of complications were secondary to technical factors and considered preventable. Female sex and bilateral MPFL reconstruction were risk factors associated with postoperative complications. Another 2013 study reported that subjective outcomes and recurrence rates were worse in patients with trochlear dysplasia or an increased TT-TG distance in which isolated MPFL reconstruction was performed, further emphasizing the importance of treating associated pathology.[32] A systematic review in 2014 showed that recurrence rates can be higher in MPFL repair (26.9%) or medial retinacular repair/plication (16.5%) compared with MPFL reconstruction (6.6%).[33]

Tibial Spine Avulsion Fractures

Tibial spine (eminence) avulsion fractures occur when the anterior cruciate ligament (ACL) avulses from its insertion on the proximal tibia epiphysis. Generally, tibial spine avulsion fractures are seen in younger patients between age 8 and 14 years.[34] Associated intra-articular injuries are common, and the rate of meniscal or collateral ligament damage associated with these injuries is estimated to be between 3.8% and 40.0%.[35-37]

Diagnosis, Anatomy, and Biomechanics

The ACL insertion on the tibia involves the anterior recess between the medial and lateral intercondylar eminences. In skeletally immature patients, avulsion fracture occurs

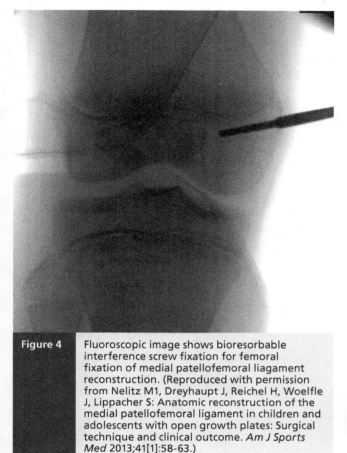

Figure 4 Fluoroscopic image shows bioresorbable interference screw fixation for femoral fixation of medial patellofemoral liagament reconstruction. (Reproduced with permission from Nelitz M1, Dreyhaupt J, Reichel H, Woelfle J, Lippacher S: Anatomic reconstruction of the medial patellofemoral ligament in children and adolescents with open growth plates: Surgical technique and clinical outcome. *Am J Sports Med* 2013;41[1]:58-63.)

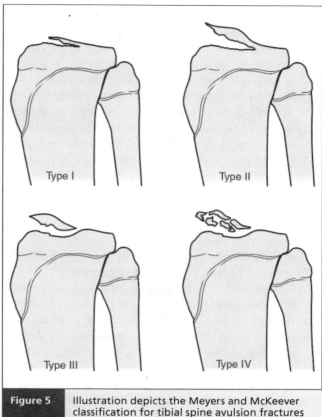

Figure 5 Illustration depicts the Meyers and McKeever classification for tibial spine avulsion fractures with the Zaricznyj modification.

because of tension failure of the incompletely ossified tibial eminence. Appropriate treatment of these injuries is important because nonanatomic healing can result in loss of appropriate ACL tension and cause functional instability. Additionally, a displaced bone fragment can block range of motion (particularly in extension) and result in pain and limitation in activity or difficulty with sports participation.

The most common classification system for tibial spine avulsion fractures uses lateral radiographs of the injured knee (Figure 5). Type I fractures have minimal displacement, type II fractures have displacement of the anterior third to half of the tibial spine but have an intact posterior hinge, and type III fractures are completely displaced.[38] The classification was later modified and a type IV fracture was added to describe comminuted and rotated fractures.[39]

CT can help evaluate residual displacement after closed reduction of tibial spine avulsion fractures as well as assess fragment size and comminution. MRI in the setting of tibial spine avulsion fracture is controversial. The advantages of MRI include the ability to evaluate concomitant injuries or soft-tissue interposition (such as

intermeniscal ligament or meniscal entrapment) beneath the tibial spine fracture. In a 2011 study, 90% of tibial spine fractures had subchondral bone bruises and 40% had meniscal tears seen on MRI.[36] A 2015 study found associated soft-tissue or other injury (including meniscal entrapment, meniscal tear and chondral injury) in 59% of patients with tibial spine avulsion fractures.[37] Cartilaginous tibial eminence fractures have recently been described and are defined by a double-PCL sign on MRI in patients 5 to 8 years old.[40] One disadvantage of MRI in pediatric patients is the possible need for sedation to obtain high-quality images. Additionally, if surgery is indicated for a displaced tibial spine fracture, evaluation under anesthesia and diagnostic arthroscopy can directly evaluate intra-articular injury, obviating the need for MRI.

Treatment

The treatment of tibial spine avulsion fractures depends on the amount of displacement, comminution, and associated injuries. Nonsurgical treatment consisting of closed reduction and immobilization in extension is recommended for type I fractures and type II fractures in which adequate closed reduction is obtained. Close follow-up after closed reduction is needed to ensure maintenance of reduction. Immobilization is recommended for 6 weeks, followed by gradual and progressive range of motion.

Recently, two systematic reviews compared nonsurgical and surgical treatment of tibial spine avulsion fractures. A 2014 study reported that nonsurgical treatment of completely displaced tibial spine fractures resulted in a higher rate of nonunion as well as increased knee laxity and greater loss of motion.[41] A 2015 study echoed these findings and reported clinical instability in 70% of patients treated nonsurgically versus 14% clinical instability in surgically treated patients.[42] A higher rate of subsequent ACL reconstruction was also reported in patients who were treated nonsurgically.

Surgical treatment consists of either open or arthroscopic reduction and internal fixation. Arthroscopically assisted tibial spine fracture treatment allows for full evaluation of intra-articular contents and concomitant procedures for other diagnosed pathology. Various fixation options are available, including solid screws, cannulated screws, bioabsorbable screws, suture fixation, suture anchors, or any combination. Suture anchors have become widely used in shoulder arthroscopy, and these techniques and skills have been translated to the treatment of tibial spine avulsion fractures.[43,44] An advantage of suture anchor fixation is the ability to spare the physis in skeletally immature patients. Another possible advantage includes the ability to provide suture bridge compression across the tibial spine fragment analogous to rotator cuff double-row repairs.[43]

Suture fixation of tibial spine avulsion fractures has been described since the mid 1990s, and the development of arthroscopic techniques using suture fixation are continually refined.[45,46] Using this technique, sutures are passed through the base of the ACL along with a chondral fragment. These sutures are brought down through drill holes in the proximal tibial metaphysis and tied over a bone bridge or to a screw and post (Figure 6). Different devices have been used for suture passage such as labral repair hooks or suture passers along with meniscal repair devices.[45] Drill holes can be placed using a standard tibial ACL guide.[46]

Biomechanical studies have studied various screw, suture, and suture anchor fixation techniques. One study found antegrade screw fixation was better than suture fixation in a cadaver model;[47] however, other studies have reported contemporary suture fixation techniques as superior to screw fixation.[48,49] In one study, fixation was stronger with braided, nonabsorbable suture than with 4.0-mm cannulated screw fixation with a washer.[48] A 2013 study compared physeal-sparing suture fixation techniques and found that ultra-high–molecular-weight

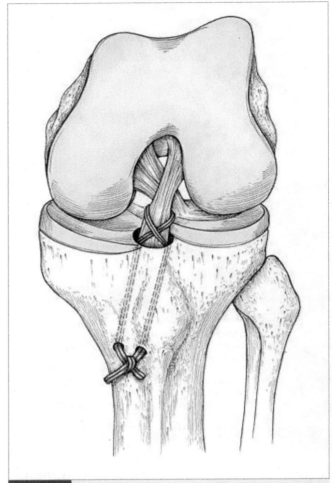

Figure 6 Illustration demonstrating suture fixation to repair a tibial eminence fracture. (Reproduced from LaFrance RM, Giordano B, Goldblatt J, et al: Pediatric tibial eminence fractures: Evaluation and management. *J Am Acad Orthop Surg* 2010;18[7]:395-405.)

polyethylene (UHMWPE) suture fixation was stronger than polydioxanone suture (PDS) or single-screw fixation and more consistent than suture anchor fixation.[49] Most recent studies support UHMWPE suture fixation as having the strongest initial fixation strength combined with cyclic loading strength to resist the rigors of early mobilization.

Complications

Common complications after treatment of tibial spine avulsion fractures include loss of motion, residual laxity, growth arrest, and angular deformity. Nonunion has also been reported.[50] Residual laxity has been reported in 10% of knees managed surgically and 22% of knees managed nonsurgically.[51] Loss of motion or arthrofibrosis after

© 2016 American Academy of Orthopaedic Surgeons

tibial spine avulsion fracture is one of the most common and difficult complications to treat. A 2012 study found that early range of motion (within 4 weeks of surgery) resulted in quicker return to activity and a 12-fold decrease in the rate of arthrofibrosis.[52] A 2010 study reported on complications related to reoperation for arthrofibrosis after treatment of tibial spine fractures.[53] Distal femoral physeal fracture and subsequent growth arrest were described in 12.5% of patients who underwent manipulation under anesthesia for arthrofibrosis following treatment of tibial spine avulsion fracture. This highlights two important principles regarding arthrofibrosis after tibial spine avulsion fracture: that prevention of stiffness after surgical treatment is essential and requires stable fixation with immediate rehabilitation, and arthroscopic lysis of adhesions before manipulation is essential to help prevent physeal fracture.

Discoid Lateral Meniscus

Discoid lateral meniscus is a common cause of knee symptoms in children. Young children with discoid lateral meniscus can present with snapping knee syndrome, in which an unstable discoid lateral meniscus causes intermittent snapping or popping of the knee. This condition is often unaccompanied by a history of traumatic injury. In young children, the snapping can be asymptomatic; in older children, the snapping is more likely to cause pain with activity.

Etiology

Compared with the normal meniscus, the discoid meniscus has an abnormal shape, is inherently different at a molecular level, and may have abnormal peripheral attachments resulting in microinstability or macroinstability. The discoid meniscus encompasses more surface area on top of the tibial articular surface compared with a normal meniscus with a semilunar shape. The discoid meniscus is also thicker than normal, especially within its central aspect (away from the periphery) and is altered at the molecular level with more haphazardly arranged circumferential collagen fibers compared with normal menisci.[54] The abnormal shape and morphology of the discoid meniscus as well as the disorganization within the collagen network can contribute to meniscal tears and degeneration.

Classification

The Watanabe classification, the most commonly used system to classify discoid lateral menisci (**Figure 7**), is based on arthroscopic appearance and stability. Type I (complete) discoid lateral meniscus is stable to arthroscopic

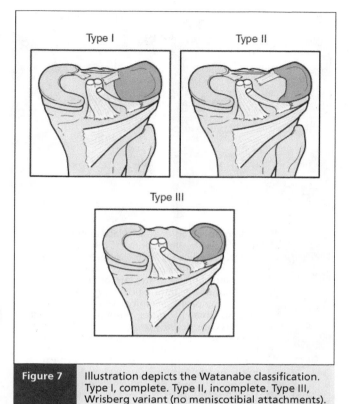

Figure 7 Illustration depicts the Watanabe classification. Type I, complete. Type II, incomplete. Type III, Wrisberg variant (no meniscotibial attachments).

probing, block-shaped, and covers the entire tibial plateau. Type II (incomplete) is stable to arthroscopic probing and covers up to 80% of the tibial plateau. Type III (Wrisberg variant) is characterized by instability on probing. Type III is devoid of posterior meniscotibial attachments and is attached posteriorly only to the meniscofemoral ligament of Wrisberg, resulting in posterior horn instability.

Instability of the discoid lateral meniscus is increasingly recognized as an important aspect of arthroscopic evaluation. A 2004 study reviewed 112 patients (128 knees) with a mean age of 10 years who underwent arthroscopic evaluation and treatment of discoid lateral meniscus.[55] Peripheral rim instability was present in 28% of discoid lateral menisci; instability was more common in complete than in incomplete discoid lateral menisci (38.9% versus 18.2%) and in younger patients (age, 8.2 years versus 10.7 years). Additionally, the most common location for peripheral rim instability was the anterior third (47.2%), followed by the posterior third (38.9%) and the middle third (11.1%). In a 2007 study, 28 consecutive patients underwent arthroscopic treatment of discoid lateral meniscus.[56] Meniscal instability was found in 77% of knees, with anterior horn instability in 53%, posterior instability in 16%, and combined anterior and posterior instability in 6%. Of 23 unstable menisci, 22 were treated with arthroscopic saucerization and suture

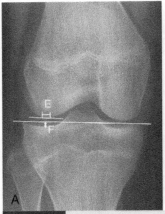
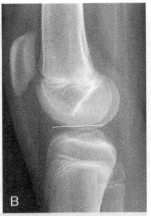

Figure 8 Radiographs depict discoid lateral meniscus **A,** AP view shows squaring of the lateral femoral condyle (E), which is the amount of straight articular surface of condyle (short line), and cupping of the lateral tibial plateau (F), measured from the tibial joint line (long line) to the proximal limit of the lateral tibial plateau (arrow). A measurement greater than 1 mm is considered a positive result. **B,** Lateral view shows the lateral femoral condylar notch, from the tangential line (line), which meets the smooth contour of the articular surface to the notch. A value greater than 1 mm is deemed positive. (Reproduced with permission from Choi SH, Ahn JH, Kim KI, et al: Do the radiographic findings of symptomatic discoid lateral meniscus in children differ from normal control subjects? *Knee Surg Sports Traumatol Arthrosc* 2015;23[4]:1128-1134.)

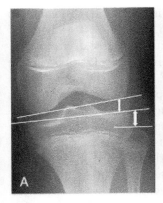
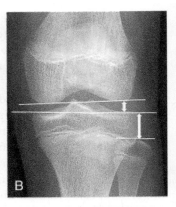
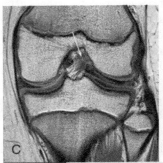
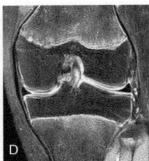

Figure 9 **A,** AP radiograph demonstrates widened lateral joint space (thin arrow) and elevated fibular head (thick arrow). **B,** AP radiograph shows normal lateral joint space (short arrow) and fibular head height (long arrow). **C,** Coronal MRI shows complete type I discoid lateral meniscus (arrow). **D,** Coronal MRI shows normal lateral meniscus shape. (Reproduced with permission from Choi SH, Ahn JH, Kim KI, et al: Do the radiographic findings of symptomatic discoid lateral meniscus in children differ from normal control subjects? *Knee Surg Sports Traumatol Arthrosc* 2015;23[4]:1128-1134.)

stabilization. Careful intraoperative examination of discoid lateral menisci is advocated, and meniscal stabilization (in addition to saucerization and treating meniscal tears) is recommended when instability is present.

Imaging

Standard radiographs are usually normal in children with discoid lateral meniscus, although there may be subtle radiographic findings. When compared with patients without deformity, children with discoid lateral menisci may have differences in the height of the lateral tibial spine, lateral joint space distance, height of the fibular head, and obliquity of the lateral tibial plateau[57] (Figures 8 and 9).

A 2009 study retrospectively examined knee MRIs of patients with discoid lateral meniscus who were treated with arthroscopy, and a new MRI classification scheme to facilitate the diagnosis of meniscal pathology was proposed.[58] The patients' MRI findings were described based on the relationship of the lateral meniscus to the lateral tibial plateau (no shift, anterocentral shift, posterocentral shift, central shift). Those with a shift on preoperative MRI were substantially more likely to have undergone

meniscal repair during arthroscopic treatment, and the direction of the shift correlated with the repair location.

A retrospective review of 69 patients who had undergone arthroscopic treatment of discoid lateral menisci was conducted to determine whether meniscal displacement or deformation on MRI was correlated with meniscus tear.[59] The aforementioned proposed classification[58] was modified and described the concept of "morphologic change" when diagnosing a tear in discoid lateral menisci. A morphologic change was diagnosed if a difference greater than 70% was noted in meniscal thickness between the anterior/posterior and medial/lateral portions of the meniscus. A morphologic change was also diagnosed if the meniscus crossed the lateral tibial spine on coronal MRI sequences or went beyond the tibial plateau margin on sagittal sequences. All types of tears (except radial tears) found on arthroscopy were associated with some sort of morphologic change on preoperative MRI.

When compared with signal intensity change on MRI, morphologic change was better at predicting the presence of a discoid lateral meniscus tear in children.

Treatment

Support is increasing for meniscal reshaping and/or partial meniscectomy for the treatment of symptomatic discoid lateral meniscus rather than total or subtotal excision. Stabilization of the meniscus is increasingly recognized as important if it is determined to be unstable during arthroscopy.[55,56] A retrospective case-control study of 51 patients compared patients who were treated with arthroscopic meniscal saucerization alone versus those who underwent saucerization plus stabilization.[60] The average patient age was 11.7 years and the average follow-up was 15 months. No significant differences were noted between treatment groups regarding postoperative knee range of motion, complications, or self-reported functional scores. Short-term clinical outcomes for patients with symptomatic discoid menisci requiring surgical intervention were good, and most patients had complete relief of symptoms and reliable restoration of both knee motion and function with a relatively low complication rate. The addition of meniscal stabilization did not affect the clinical outcomes in those who demonstrated meniscal instability.

The timing of treatment can influence cartilage health and meniscal reparability in patients with a discoid lateral meniscus tear. A 2014 study investigated the relationship between isolated discoid lateral meniscus tears and the presence of articular cartilage lesions in 252 consecutive patients.[61] Articular cartilage lesions were present in 26.6% of patients. Multivariable logistic regression analysis revealed that in addition to sex and body mass index, preoperative symptoms lasting longer than 6 months increased the likelihood of finding articular cartilage lesions at arthroscopy. Osteochondritis dissecans (OCD) lesions within the lateral femoral condyle can also be associated with the presence of a discoid lateral meniscus.[62] A 2013 study reviewed meniscal tear patterns in children and adolescents and found that those treated within 3 months of symptom onset were more likely to have reparable tears compared with those who were treated more than 6 months after onset.[63]

Knee Osteochondroses

Osteochondrosis is characterized by a disturbance in endochondral ossification in a previously normal endochondral growth center. Osteochondroses have been reported in almost every growth center of the body. Two common osteochondroses affecting the skeletally immature knee are Osgood-Schlatter disease and SLJ disease

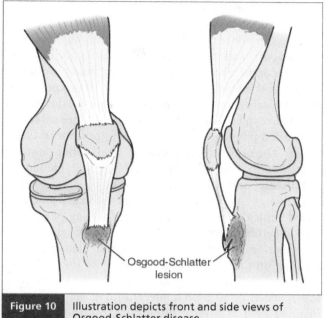

Osgood-Schlatter lesion

Figure 10 Illustration depicts front and side views of Osgood-Schlatter disease.

(although not a true osteochondrosis), which affect the tibial tubercle apophysis and the inferior pole of the patella, respectively. Both disorders have relatively predictable clinical presentations and are commonly self-limited conditions. Managing patient and parent expectations are as important as properly managing the condition itself.

Osgood-Schlatter Disease

Osgood-Schlatter disease is a traction apophysitis of the tibial tubercle apophysis that commonly affects children who are undergoing rapid growth (Figure 10). The exact cause of Osgood-Schlatter disease is unknown but it is likely an overuse syndrome in the developing skeleton. The condition occurs when stress is placed on the developing tibial tubercle apophysis by the extensor mechanism and commonly occurs in the running or jumping athlete. A cross-sectional study of 956 adolescent students between 12 and 15 years old found a 9.8% prevalence of Osgood-Schlatter disease (11.0% in boys and 8.3% in girls).[64] Using multivariable logistic regression analysis, a significant association was found between Osgood-Schlatter disease and participation in sports activity and rectus femoris tightness. This provides further support for the proposed etiology of Osgood-Schlatter disease as an overuse syndrome as well as a rationale for treatment with physical therapy–guided stretching exercises.

Clinical Presentation

Patients with Osgood-Schlatter disease present with pain and swelling over the tibial tubercle and may report increased pain with running, jumping, and kneeling activities. Tenderness to palpation, swelling, and prominence of the tibial tubercle as well as tightness of the quadriceps and hamstrings can be appreciated on physical examination. Pain can be reproduced with resisted knee extension. A detailed physical examination is important to differentiate Osgood-Schlatter disease from other common conditions that cause knee pain such as patellar tendinitis, SLJ disease, and pes anserine bursitis.

Although Osgood-Schlatter disease can often be diagnosed clinically, plain radiographic imaging of the knee should be obtained to rule out other potential causes of knee pain, especially if the presentation is atypical. Depending on the severity and chronicity of the condition, elevation, radiolucency, and fragmentation of the tibial tubercle can be seen on a lateral radiograph. Advanced imaging such as MRI is often unnecessary to establish the diagnosis.

Treatment

Osgood-Schlatter disease is generally a self-limited condition and initial treatment should focus on symptomatic care (NSAIDs, analgesics), activity modification (rest, avoiding aggravating activities), and physical therapy (focusing on quadriceps, hamstring, and iliotibial band stretching and strengthening). The symptoms of Osgood-Schlatter disease can persist until closure of the tibial tubercle apophysis, and although many patients will be asymptomatic after they reach adulthood, up to 60% can still have some residual pain over the tibial tubercle with kneeling.[65]

More invasive treatment can be considered for recalcitrant Osgood-Schlatter disease. A large series of male military recruits reviewed the long-term outcomes after surgical treatment for unresolved Osgood-Schlatter disease.[66] The patients underwent isolated residual ossicle removal, isolated tibial tubercle resection, or combined ossicle removal and tibial tubercle resection. After a median-duration follow-up of 10 years, 87% of patients reported no restrictions in everyday activities or at work and 75% had returned to their preoperative level of sports activity. Thirty-eight percent reported a complete absence of pain with kneeling. More recently, hyperosmolar dextrose injection was examined for the treatment of recalcitrant cases of Osgood-Schlatter disease.[67] In this study, 54 patients with refractory Osgood-Schlatter disease were randomly assigned to either usual care (physical therapy) or double-blind injection of 1% lidocaine solution with or without 12% dextrose. Injections were administered monthly for 3 months. At 1-year follow-up, those who received injections that contained 12% dextrose were more likely to be able to participate in sports asymptomatically compared with those who were treated with 1% lidocaine injection alone or usual care.

SLJ Disease

SLJ disease is analogous to Osgood-Schlatter disease. Osgood-Schlatter disease is an osteochondrosis of the tibial tubercle apophysis; SLJ disease involves the inferior pole of the patella. Because there is no apophysis of the inferior pole of the patella, SLJ disease can be more accurately described as an enthesitis rather than a true osteochondrosis. SLJ disease traditionally presents in slightly younger patients than Osgood-Schlatter disease.

Clinical Presentation

Patients with SLJ disease typically have pain with activities that require running and jumping, similar to those with Osgood-Schlatter disease. Symptoms are only present during the offending activity and often resolve with rest. Physical examination reveals maximum tenderness with or without swelling over the inferior pole of the patella located over the insertion of the patellar ligament. Careful history should assess the acuity of symptoms and physical examination should examine for any palpable defect at this location or the inability to perform a straight leg raise. An acute or traumatic onset of pain associated with a palpable defect and inability to perform a straight leg raise should increase suspicion for a patellar sleeve fracture rather than SLJ disease.

Plain radiographic imaging of the knee can reveal calcification or ossification at the inferior pole of the patella (**Figure 11**). Radiographs can also help rule out other causes of knee pain such as fractures, Osgood-Schlatter disease, and bipartite patella. As with Osgood-Schlatter disease, SLJ disease can usually be diagnosed clinically and advanced imaging such as MRI is usually not necessary.

Treatment

SLJ disease often has a self-limited course with resolution of symptoms after maturation of the inferior pole of the patella. As with Osgood-Schlatter disease, treatment should focus on symptom control with NSAIDs or analgesic medication, activity modification, physical therapy, and rest. A brief period of immobilization in a cylinder cast or knee extension brace can be considered for select patients. Late sequelae of SLJ are rare and one case report exists of a fracture through a previously united ossicle.[68] Surgical excision of symptomatic, nonunited ossicles of the inferior pole of the patella can be considered

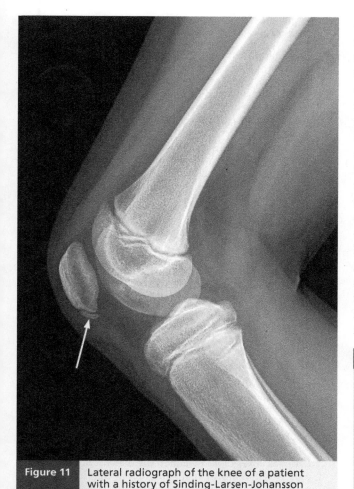

Figure 11 Lateral radiograph of the knee of a patient with a history of Sinding-Larsen-Johansson disease (arrow).

of motion and rehabilitation to prevent loss of motion and arthrofibrosis. Discoid lateral meniscus is a potential cause of knee pathology in the pediatric patient. History and physical examination remain the cornerstones of diagnosis; however, recent advances in imaging techniques and interpretation, specifically MRI, can aid in evaluation and treatment. Good treatment results have been obtained with arthroscopic reshaping (saucerization) of the discoid lateral meniscus to a more normal contour. Additionally, the importance of evaluating for and treating meniscal instability is increasingly recognized and associated articular cartilage lesions are relatively common. Osgood-Schlatter disease and SLJ disease are common conditions of the knee in the juvenile athlete. Both conditions typically have a self-limited course and respond to a period of rest, anti-inflammatory and/or analgesic medication, activity modification, and physical therapy. Symptoms usually resolve by the time patients reach skeletal maturity but surgery can be considered for recalcitrant cases.

Key Study Points

- Respect of physeal anatomy is important when evaluating and treating patellofemoral instability in skeletally immature athletes.
- Assessing and addressing meniscal instability is an important aspect of treating symptomatic discoid lateral meniscus.
- Knee overuse syndromes in children and adolescents are common, and most respond to nonsurgical treatment.

for recalcitrant cases in adults. To date, no study has investigated the use of injection therapy for the treatment of SLJ disease.

Summary

Patellofemoral instability in the child and adolescent athlete is a common cause of knee dysfunction. Properly assessing and treating the many factors that can contribute to instability is essential to a successful outcome. Tibial spine avulsion fracture is a unique injury to the ACL attachment. Prompt diagnosis and treatment are essential to restore normal knee mechanics. Nonsurgical treatment is recommended for nondisplaced fractures or for those that reduce anatomically with closed reduction. Surgical intervention is recommended for displaced fractures using various open and arthroscopic techniques. Biomechanical studies support the use of all suture fixation. Stable fixation is needed to ensure the ability to begin early range

Annotated References

1. Waterman BR, Belmont PJ Jr, Owens BD: Patellar dislocation in the United States: Role of sex, age, race, and athletic participation. *J Knee Surg* 2012;25(1):51-57.

    The authors of this study queried The National Electronic Injury Surveillance System for all patellar dislocations presenting to emergency departments from 2003 to 2008. The incidence of patellar dislocation was 2.29 per 100,000 person-years in the US; equal rates were found between males and females with peak incidence between 15 and 19 years of age and 51.9% occurred during athletic activity. Level of evidence: II.

2. Lewallen LW, McIntosh AL, Dahm DL: Predictors of recurrent instability after acute patellofemoral dislocation in pediatric and adolescent patients. *Am J Sports Med* 2013;41(3):575-581.

This case-control study compared nonsurgical treatment with surgical treatment of first-time patellar dislocation in pediatric and adolescent patients and reported a 62% success rate for nonsurgical treatment and a 31% success rate in skeletally immature patients with trochlear dysplasia. Fifty percent of patients with recurrent instability required surgical intervention to gain stability. Level of evidence: III.

3. Howells NR, Eldridge JD: Medial patellofemoral ligament reconstruction for patellar instability in patients with hypermobility: A case control study. *J Bone Joint Surg Br* 2012;94(12):1655-1659.

   This case-control study examined the influence of hypermobility on clinical outcome following MPFL reconstruction. Functional results were better in nonhypermobile patients and although hypermobility is not a contraindication to MPFL reconstruction, patients with hypermobility should be counseled on postoperative expectations. Level of evidence: III.

4. Kepler CK, Bogner EA, Hammoud S, Malcolmson G, Potter HG, Green DW: Zone of injury of the medial patellofemoral ligament after acute patellar dislocation in children and adolescents. *Am J Sports Med* 2011;39(7):1444-1449.

   This cohort study examined MPFL zone of injury after acute patellar dislocation. The zone in the pediatric population was found to be the patellar attachment in 61%, the femoral attachment in 12%, and both attachments in 12%. The remaining 15% had injury at multiple locations or no identifiable injury. Level of evidence: II.

5. Felus J, Kowalczyk B: Age-related differences in medial patellofemoral ligament injury patterns in traumatic patellar dislocation: Case series of 50 surgically treated children and adolescents. *Am J Sports Med* 2012;40(10):2357-2364.

   The study examined 50 consecutive patients (age range, 10.5 to 17.5 years) who underwent surgery for first-time patellar dislocation. MPFL injury was present in 94%, most commonly at the patellar attachment (66%), followed by the midsubstance fiber area (50%) and the femoral attachment (32%); 46% had injury in more than one location. Patellar-side injury was more common in skeletally immature versus mature patients (79% versus 54%). Level of evidence: IV.

6. Nelitz M, Dornacher D, Dreyhaupt J, Reichel H, Lippacher S: The relation of the distal femoral physis and the medial patellofemoral ligament. *Knee Surg Sports Traumatol Arthrosc* 2011;19(12):2067-2071.

   This retrospective radiographic review of 27 patients who had a history of patellofemoral instability (mean age, 14.3 years) examined the relationship of the femoral origin of the MPFL to the medial aspect of the distal femoral physis. The femoral origin of the MPFL was a median of 6.4 mm distal to the physis. Level of evidence: IV.

7. Shea KG, Polousky JD, Jacobs JC Jr, et al: The relationship of the femoral physis and the medial patellofemoral ligament in children: A cadaveric study. *J Pediatr Orthop* 2014;34(8):808-813.

   This anatomic study examined the relationship of the distal femoral physis to the MPFL in six skeletally immature cadaver knee specimens. All subjects had a center of MPFL origin footprint at or below the distal femoral physis. The proximal extent of the MPFL origin footprint was found to extend above the physis in two older specimens.

8. Pennock AT, Alam M, Bastrom T: Variation in tibial tubercle-trochlear groove measurement as a function of age, sex, size, and patellar instability. *Am J Sports Med* 2014;42(2):389-393.

   This study examined TT-TG variations as a function of patient age and size in a population with patellar instability compared with those without instability. An elevated TT-TG was found in both pediatric and adolescent patients with patellar instability, with measurement varying as a function of patient age and height (TT-TG increased by 0.12 cm for each 1-cm increase in height). Level of evidence: III.

9. Camp CL, Stuart MJ, Krych AJ, et al: CT and MRI measurements of tibial tubercle-trochlear groove distances are not equivalent in patients with patellar instability. *Am J Sports Med* 2013;41(8):1835-1840.

   This study examined the reliability of TT-TG distance measurements on MRI and CT. Although TT-TG distance can be measured with excellent interrater reliability on both MRI and CT, MRI tended to underestimate TT-TG distance compared with CT. Level of evidence: II.

10. Lykissas MG, Li T, Eismann EA, Parikh SN: Does medial patellofemoral ligament reconstruction decrease patellar height? A preliminary report. *J Pediatr Orthop* 2014;34(1):78-85.

    The authors examined preoperative and postoperative lateral knee radiographs of 38 adolescents who underwent MPFL reconstruction between 2005 and 2011. Patients who underwent MPFL reconstruction showed a significantly greater decrease in patellar height measurements compared with control patients. Level of evidence: III.

11. Fabricant PD, Ladenhauf HN, Salvati EA, Green DW: Medial patellofemoral ligament (MPFL) reconstruction improves radiographic measures of patella alta in children. *Knee* 2014;21(6):1180-1184.

    The authors examined patellar height measurements (using the Insall-Salvati ratio, modified Insall-Salvati ratio, and Caton-Deschamps index) in 27 children (mean age, 14.9 years) who underwent isolated MPFL reconstruction. Preoperative and postoperative patellar height indices were measured. Isolated MPFL reconstruction was associated with consistently improved patellar height measurements to within normal childhood ranges. Level of evidence: IV.

12. Park MS, Chung CY, Lee KM, Lee SH, Choi IH: Which is the best method to determine the patellar height in children and adolescents? *Clin Orthop Relat Res* 2010;468(5):1344-1351.

© 2016 American Academy of Orthopaedic Surgeons

In this study, 108 children and adolescents were evaluated using MRI and lateral knee radiographs. Insall-Salvati, Blackburne-Peel, and Koshino-Sugimoto methods were used to determine patellar height. The Insall-Salvati ratio appeared most reliable in patients older than 13 years with almost complete ossification. For younger patients, the Kushino-Sugimoto method was the only applicable and most reliable (but less valid) method. Level of evidence: I.

13. Koshino T, Sugimoto K: New measurement of patellar height in the knees of children using the epiphyseal line midpoint. *J Pediatr Orthop* 1989;9(2):216-218.

14. Thévenin-Lemoine C, Ferrand M, Courvoisier A, Damsin JP, Ducou le Pointe H, Vialle R: Is the Caton-Deschamps index a valuable ratio to investigate patellar height in children? *J Bone Joint Surg Am* 2011;93(8):e35.

The authors of this study examined lateral knee radiographs of 300 healthy patients divided into 10 groups based on age. The mean Caton-Deschamps index was 1.06 ± 0.21 with excellent intra- and interobserver reliability. The Caton-Deschamps index is a simple, reliable index for evaluating patellar height in children and is an alternative to the Insall-Salvati ratio and Koshino-Sugimoto method. Level of evidence: I.

15. Hopper GP, Leach WJ, Rooney BP, Walker CR, Blyth MJ: Does degree of trochlear dysplasia and position of femoral tunnel influence outcome after medial patellofemoral ligament reconstruction? *Am J Sports Med* 2014;42(3):716-722.

The authors of this study examined the relationship between the degree of trochlear dysplasia and femoral tunnel position on outcome after MPFL reconstruction in a 68 patients (72 knees). Mean follow-up was 31.3 months. Multivariable regression analysis demonstrated that the distance of the femoral tunnel to the anatomic position predicted clinical outcome. Additionally, all patients with severe trochlear dysplsia (N = 7) had recurrent dislocation compared with only 9.3% (N = 5) of patients with mild dysplasia. Level of evidence: IV.

16. Petri M, Liodakis E, Hofmeister M, et al: Operative vs conservative treatment of traumatic patellar dislocation: Results of a prospective randomized controlled clinical trial. *Arch Orthop Trauma Surg* 2013;133(2):209-213.

This multicenter, randomized controlled trial compared outcomes after nonsurgical and surgical treatment in 20 patients (mean age 24.6 years) after first-time patellar dislocation. No significant difference was reported between groups; however, a tendency toward better Kujala score and lower dislocation rates existed for patients treated surgically. Post hoc power analysis revealed that the study was likely underpowered. Level of evidence: I.

17. Hennrikus W, Pylawka T: Patellofemoral instability in skeletally immature athletes. *Instr Course Lect* 2013;62:445-453.

This report reviewed the evaluation and treatment of patellofemoral instability in skeletally immature athletes.

18. Cootjans K, Dujardin J, Vandenneucker H, Bellemans J: A surgical algorithm for the treatment of recurrent patellar dislocation. Results at 5 year follow-up. *Acta Orthop Belg* 2013;79(3):318-325.

This report retrospectively reviewed 110 patients who underwent several procedures for recurrent patellofemoral instability. Based on the results, an algorithm was described using physeal status, Q angle, and TT-TG distance when determining optimal surgical treatment. Level of evidence: IV.

19. Luhmann SJ, O'Donnell JC, Fuhrhop S: Outcomes after patellar realignment surgery for recurrent patellar instability dislocations: A minimum 3-year follow-up study of children and adolescents. *J Pediatr Orthop* 2011;31(1):65-71.

This study examined 23 pediatric and adolescent patients (27 knees) who underwent patellar realignment surgery for patellar instability. At a mean follow-up of 5 years, 93% of patients reported persistent improvement in knee function, and pain and recurrent instability was infrequent (7%). Despite the low rate of recurrent instability, patient-reported outcome measures were lower than expected (mean International Knee Documentation Committee (IKDC) score, 65.5). Level of evidence: III.

20. Nelitz M, Dreyhaupt J, Reichel H, Woelfle J, Lippacher S: Anatomic reconstruction of the medial patellofemoral ligament in children and adolescents with open growth plates: Surgical technique and clinical outcome. *Am J Sports Med* 2013;41(1):58-63.

In this case series, 21 consecutive skeletally immature patients with recurrent patellar instability underwent physeal-respecting, double-bundle MPFL reconstruction. The average age at surgery was 12.2 years, the average follow-up was 2.8 years. Significantly improved Kujala scores were reported postoperatively compared with preoperative scores. Level of evidence: IV.

21. Nelitz M, Williams SR: Anatomic reconstruction of the medial patellofemoral ligament in children and adolescents using a pedicled quadriceps tendon graft. *Arthrosc Tech* 2014;3(2):e303-e308.

The authors described an MPFL reconstruction technique using a pedicled quadriceps tendon autograft. The advantages of this technique include the avoidance of drilling patellar tunnels, a single incision, and sparing of the hamstring tendons for reconstruction of any future ligamentous injuries. Level of evidence: IV.

22. Yercan HS, Erkan S, Okcu G, Ozalp RT: A novel technique for reconstruction of the medial patellofemoral ligament in skeletally immature patients. *Arch Orthop Trauma Surg* 2011;131(8):1059-1065.

The authors present a technique for MPFL reconstruction in skeletally immature patients using semitendinosis autograft passed through patellar bone tunnels and tenodesed to the adductor magnus tendon to avoid drilling tunnels near the distal femoral physis. Level of evidence: IV.

23. Savarese E, Bisicchia S, Carotenuto F, Ippolito E: A technique for treating patello-femoral instability in immature patients: The tibial tubercle periosteum transfer. *Musculoskelet Surg* 2011;95(2):89-94.

   The authors describe a distal realignment procedure for treating patellofemoral instability in skeletally immature patients using transfer of the tibial tubercle periosteum instead of performing tibial tubercle osteotomy. Level of evidence: IV.

24. Grannatt K, Heyworth BE, Ogunwole O, Micheli LJ, Kocher MS: Galeazzi semitendinosus tenodesis for patellofemoral instability in skeletally immature patients. *J Pediatr Orthop* 2012;32(6):621-625.

   In this retrospective review, 28 skeletally immature patients (34 knees) underwent the Galeazzi procedure for patellofemoral instability between 1990 and 2006. Approximately 82% of patients experienced recurrent subluxation or dislocation and 35% had secondary intervention. Despite the high recurrence rate, the Galeazzi procedure can still be a reasonable temporizing procedure before patients reach skeletal maturity. Level of evidence: IV.

25. Oliva F, Ronga M, Longo UG, Testa V, Capasso G, Maffulli N: The 3-in-1 procedure for recurrent dislocation of the patella in skeletally immature children and adolescents. *Am J Sports Med* 2009;37(9):1814-1820.

   In this review, 25 skeletally immature patients (mean age at operation, 13.5 years) underwent surgical intervention with the 3-in-1 procedure (lateral release, vastus medialis advancement, and medial transfer of lateral third of the patellar ligament) for recurrent patellar dislocation. At mean follow-up of 3.8 years, patients had significant increases in postoperative Kujala scores and modified Cincinnati scores. Level of evidence: IV.

26. Marsh JS, Daigneault JP, Sethi P, Polzhofer GK: Treatment of recurrent patellar instability with a modification of the Roux-Goldthwait technique. *J Pediatr Orthop* 2006;26(4):461-465.

   In this retrospective cohort, 20 patients (30 knees) with recurrent patellar instability underwent the modified Roux-Goldthwait procedure and lateral release. Mean follow-up was 6.2 years. Using Insall criteria, 26 knees had excellent results, 3 were good, and 1 was fair. Level of evidence: IV.

27. Biglieni L, Fiore M, Coviello M, Felli L: Patellar instability: Combined treatment with Goldthwait technique and arthroscopic lateral release. *Musculoskelet Surg* 2011;95(2):95-99.

   In this retrospective cohort, 19 adolescent patients (20 knees) underwent the Roux-Goldthwait procedure and arthroscopic lateral release for treatment of recurrent patellofemoral instability. At a mean follow-up of 6.8 years, there were 11 excellent results, 6 good, 2 fair, and 1 poor based on the Cox grading system and the Bray score. Level of evidence: IV.

28. Dejour D, Byn P, Ntagiopoulos PG: The Lyon's sulcus-deepening trochleoplasty in previous unsuccessful patellofemoral surgery. *Int Orthop* 2013;37(3):433-439.

   In this retrospective cohort, 22 patients (24 knees) underwent trochleoplasty for recurrent patellar dislocation associated with trochlear dysplasia. At a mean follow-up of 66 months, pain decreased in 72% of patients and the apprehension sign was negative in 75%. Significant decreases were reported in sulcus angle, TT-TG distance, and lateral patellar tilt compared with preoperative measurements. A significant increase in mean postoperative Kujala score was also reported. Level of evidence: IV.

29. Nelitz M, Dreyhaupt J, Lippacher S: Combined trochleoplasty and medial patellofemoral ligament reconstruction for recurrent patellar dislocations in severe trochlear dysplasia: A minimum 2-year follow-up study. *Am J Sports Med* 2013;41(5):1005-1012.

   This study examined 23 patients (26 knees; mean age, 19.2 years) who had patellofemoral instability and severe trochlear dysplasia treated with combined trochleoplasty and MPFL reconstruction. At a mean follow-up of 2.5 years, no recurrent dislocations were reported, and Kujala, IKDC, and visual analog scale scores all had significant improvements compared with preoperative values. Level of evidence: III.

30. Fucentese SF, Zingg PO, Schmitt J, Pfirrmann CW, Meyer DC, Koch PP: Classification of trochlear dysplasia as predictor of clinical outcome after trochleoplasty. *Knee Surg Sports Traumatol Arthrosc* 2011;19(10):1655-1661.

   In this retrospective review, 38 patients (44 knees) underwent trochleoplasty for patellar instability. Patient outcomes were compared based on the type of trochlear dysplasia and trochleoplasty was found to be a useful, reliable surgical technique to improve patellofemoral instability in patients with trochlear dysplasia. The overall results depended directly on the type of dysplasia, with a substantially better clinical outcome in types B and D. Level of evidence: III.

31. Parikh SN, Nathan ST, Wall EJ, Eismann EA: Complications of medial patellofemoral ligament reconstruction in young patients. *Am J Sports Med* 2013;41(5):1030-1038.

   In this retrospective case series, all patients who underwent MPFL reconstruction between 2005 and 2011 were examined for postoperative complications. A total of 179 knees were identified; 38 complications were described in 29 knees (16.2%). Major complications (34 of 38) included recurrent instability in 8 patients, stiffness in 8, patellar fracture in 6, and patellofemoral arthrosis and/or pain in 5. Eighteen (47%) complications were determined to be secondary to technical factors and considered preventable. Level of evidence: IV.

32. Wagner D, Pfalzer F, Hingelbaum S, Huth J, Mauch F, Bauer G: The influence of risk factors on clinical outcomes following anatomical medial patellofemoral ligament (MPFL) reconstruction using the gracilis tendon. *Knee Surg Sports Traumatol Arthrosc* 2013;21(2):318-324.

In this prospective case series, 50 patients with chronic patellofemoral instability underwent MPFL reconstruction. Clinical data, radiographs, and MRIs were prospectively evaluated pre-operatively and postoperatively to detect risk factors for patellofemoral instability. A low rate of recurrent dislocation (2%) was reported. MRI showed good integration of the reconstructed MPFL and a positive effect on patellar tilt (decreased tilt). A negative relationship was found between the degree of trochlear dysplasia and outcomes. Level of evidence: IV.

33. Matic GT, Magnussen RA, Kolovich GP, Flanigan DC: Return to activity after medial patellofemoral ligament repair or reconstruction. *Arthroscopy* 2014;30(8):1018-1025.

This systematic review examined return to activity after MPFL repair or reconstruction in 10 articles and identified 402 patients who met inclusion criteria. Recurrent dislocation was higher in patients who underwent MPFL repair rather than reconstruction; however, repair and reconstruction had similar postsurgical Tegner scores. Level of evidence: IV.

34. Zionts L: Fractures and Dislocations about the Knee, in Green NE, Swionkowski MR, eds: *Skeletal Trauma in Children* .Philadelphia, WB Saunders, 2009, pp 452-455.

35. Johnson AC, Wyatt JD, Treme G, Veitch AJ: Incidence of associated knee injury in pediatric tibial eminence fractures. *J Knee Surg* 2014;27(3):215-219.

This retrospective case series reviewed pediatric tibial eminence fractures to examine the incidence of associated knee pathology. Twenty pediatric patients treated surgically for tibial eminence fracture over a 10-year period at a single institution were identified. Six patients (30%) had associated meniscal tears with meniscal tear occurring more commonly in type III versus type II fractures. Two patients sustained associated ligamentous injury and none had associated chondral defects. Level of evidence: IV.

36. Shea KG, Grimm NL, Laor T, Wall E: Bone bruises and meniscal tears on MRI in skeletally immature children with tibial eminence fractures. *J Pediatr Orthop* 2011;31(2):150-152.

In this retrospective case series, 20 skeletally immature children with tibial eminence fractures underwent MRI examination of the knee. Subchondral bone contusions were seen in 18 (90%). Lesion location included the lateral femoral condyle (80%), lateral tibial plateau (75%), medial femoral condyle (60%), and medial tibial plateau (30%). Meniscal tears were present in eight (40%) patients, four each in the medial and lateral menisci. Level of evidence: IV.

37. Mitchell JJ, Sjostrom R, Mansour AA, et al: Incidence of meniscal injury and chondral pathology in anterior tibial spine fractures of children. *J Pediatr Orthop J Pediatr Orthop* 2015;35(2):130-135.

In this retrospective review, of 58 children who sustained a tibial spine fracture between 1996 and 2011, 59% children had an associated soft-tissue or other bony injury diagnosed using MRI or arthroscopy. The most commonly associated injuries were meniscal entrapment, meniscal tears, and chondral injury. No associated injuries with type I fractures were reported. Of type II fractures, 29% had meniscal entrapment, 33% had meniscal tears, and 7% demonstrated chondral injury. Of type III fractures, 48% had meniscal entrapment, 12% had meniscal tears, and 8% had chondral injury. Level of evidence: IV.

38. Meyers MH, McKeever FM: Fracture of the intercondylar eminence of the tibia. *J Bone Joint Surg Am* 1959;41-A(2):209-220, discussion 220-222.

39. Zaricznyj B: Avulsion fracture of the tibial eminence: Treatment by open reduction and pinning. *J Bone Joint Surg Am* 1977;59(8):1111-1114.

40. Chotel F, Seil R, Greiner P, Chaker MM, Berard J, Raux S: The difficult diagnosis of cartilaginous tibial eminence fractures in young children. *Knee Surg Sports Traumatol Arthrosc* 2014;22(7):1511-1516.

This retrospective case series described cartilaginous tibial eminence fracture in six patients. Radiographs were normal in four and showed thin ossification in two. MRI was negative for ACL rupture; however, four had a double-PCL sign. Patients were referred for treatment at a median of 6 months (range, 2.5 to 48.0 months) after injury with symptoms related to nonunion, ossification, and secondary enlargement of the avulsed fragment. The authors emphasized a high index of suspicion when evaluating these patients to avoid missed or delayed diagnosis of this rare entity. Level of evidence: IV.

41. Gans I, Baldwin KD, Ganley TJ: Treatment and management outcomes of tibial eminence fractures in pediatric patients: A systematic review. *Am J Sports Med* 2014;42(7):1743-1750.

In this systematic review of studies examining tibial eminence fractures in children and adolescents, 26 articles were identified that met inclusion criteria, including 1 level III article and 25 level IV articles. The level of evidence supporting various treatments for tibial eminence fractures in children and adolescents is low, with insufficient evidence to conclude the superiority of open versus arthroscopic treatment or screw versus suture fixation techniques. Type III and IV fractures heal with greater laxity and greater loss of range of motion after treatment. Level of evidence: IV.

42. Bogunovic L, Tarabichi M, Harris D, Wright R: Treatment of tibial eminence fractures: A systematic review. *J Knee Surg* 2015;28(3):255-262.

This systematic review examined outcomes of nonsurgically and surgically treated tibial eminence fractures. Sixteen studies met inclusion criteria. The pooled mean age of patients was 23 years; mean follow-up was 35 months. Clinical instability was seen in 70% of patients treated nonsurgically and 14% of patients treated surgically. The rate of ACL reconstruction was higher in nonsurgically treated patients. Suture fixation was associated with improvements in clinical measures of stability and decreased need for hardware removal compared with screw fixation; however, no difference was reported in patient perceived stability and need for ACL reconstruction between the two treatment methods. Level of evidence: IV.

43. Kim JI, Kwon JH, Seo DH, Soni SM, Muñoz M, Nha KW: Arthroscopic hybrid fixation of a tibial eminence fracture in children. *Arthrosc Tech* 2013;2(2):e117-e120.

   The authors describe an arthroscopic technique for treating tibial eminence fractures in children by using a bioabsorbable suture anchor in addition to all-inside arthroscopic suture fixation to the intermeniscal ligament and tibial periosteum.

44. Sawyer GA, Hulstyn MJ, Anderson BC, Schiller J: Arthroscopic suture bridge fixation of tibial intercondylar eminence fractures. *Arthrosc Tech* 2013;2(4):e315-e318.

   The authors describe an arthroscopic technique for treating tibial eminence fractures in children with an all-inside, all-epiphyseal suture bridge technique using anchors.

45. Ochiai S, Hagino T, Watanabe Y, Senga S, Haro H: One strategy for arthroscopic suture fixation of tibial intercondylar eminence fractures using the Meniscal Viper Repair System. *Sports Med Arthrosc Rehabil Ther Technol* 2011;3:17.

   In this retrospective case series, five patients (mean age 28.8 years) underwent arthroscopic suture fixation of tibial eminence fractures using an all-inside meniscal repair system. Surgical results were assessed using plain radiographs, postoperative range of motion, and Lysholm scores. At latest follow-up, all fractures maintained reduction obtained at surgery and postoperative Lysholm scores showed good results. Level of evidence: IV.

46. Kluemper CT, Snyder GM, Coats AC, Johnson DL, Mair SD: Arthroscopic suture fixation of tibial eminence fractures. *Orthopedics* 2013;36(11):e1401-e1406.

   This retrospective case series evaluated the clinical outcomes of an arthroscopic suture fixation technique in 17 tibial eminence fractures treated between 1998 and 2010. Average patient age was 16.8 years (range, 13 to 37 years) and average follow-up was 25 months (range, 2 months to 13 years). Postoperatively, all fractures were radiographically healed, and all patients had stable Lachman and negative pivot shift test results. Two patients had 3° of extension loss and one patient lost more than 10° of knee flexion. Level of evidence: IV.

47. Tsukada H, Ishibashi Y, Tsuda E, Hiraga Y, Toh S: A biomechanical comparison of repair techniques for anterior cruciate ligament tibial avulsion fracture under cyclic loading. *Arthroscopy* 2005;21(10):1197-1201.

48. Bong MR, Romero A, Kubiak E, et al: Suture versus screw fixation of displaced tibial eminence fractures: A biomechanical comparison. *Arthroscopy* 2005;21(10):1172-1176.

49. Anderson CN, Nyman JS, McCullough KA, et al: Biomechanical evaluation of physeal-sparing fixation methods in tibial eminence fractures. *Am J Sports Med* 2013;41(7):1586-1594.

   This biomechanical laboratory study of skeletally immature porcine knees examined the strength and resistance to displacement of physeal-sparing techniques used to fix tibial eminence fractures. Four treatment groups: UHMWPE suture–suture button, suture anchor, PDS–suture button, and screw fixation. Physeal-sparing fixation of tibial eminence fractures with UHMWPE suture button is biomechanically superior to both PDS–suture button and single-screw fixation at the time of surgery and provides more consistent fixation than suture anchors.

50. Abdelkafy A, Said HG: Neglected ununited tibial eminence fractures in the skeletally immature: Arthroscopic management. *Int Orthop* 2014;38(12):2525-2532.

   In this prospective case series, 13 patients (average age [± SD] at surgery, 10 ± 2.6 years) with neglected, nonunited tibial eminence fractures were treated with arthroscopic reduction and suture fixation. At an average follow-up of 10.8 months, 12 patients had grade A objective IKDC score and 1 had grade B. All patients showed radiographic union and anatomic reduction at 12.4 weeks postoperatively. Eleven patients had clinical stability based on Lachman, anterior drawer, and pivot shift test results and no patient reported subjective instability. Level of evidence: IV.

51. Aderinto J, Walmsley P, Keating JF: Fractures of the tibial spine: Epidemiology and outcome. *Knee* 2008;15(3):164-167.

52. Patel NM, Park MJ, Sampson NR, Ganley TJ: Tibial eminence fractures in children: Earlier posttreatment mobilization results in improved outcomes. *J Pediatr Orthop* 2012;32(2):139-144.

   In this retrospective case-control study, 40 patients (40 knees; mean age, 12 years; range, 5 to 17 years) underwent treatment of tibial eminence fractures. When compared with patients who initiated postoperative range of motion within 4 weeks of treatment, those who started range of motion later than 4 weeks required more days to return to full activity and were 12 times more likely to develop arthrofibrosis ($P = 0.029$). Even when accounting for other factors in multivariable regression analysis, earlier initiation of range of motion was associated with earlier return to full activity. After definitive treatment of tibial eminence fractures, early range of motion results in a more rapid return to full activity. Level of evidence: III.

53. Vander Have KL, Ganley TJ, Kocher MS, Price CT, Herrera-Soto JA: Arthrofibrosis after surgical fixation of tibial eminence fractures in children and adolescents. *Am J Sports Med* 2010;38(2):298-301.

   In this retrospective case series, 32 patients underwent surgical treatment of tibial eminence fractures: 24 patients required reoperation for loss of flexion ($N = 9$), loss of extension ($N = 4$), or both ($N = 11$). Manipulation under anesthesia resulted in distal femoral fractures and subsequent growth arrest in 3 patients; 29 patients achieved near-full knee motion at final follow-up. Manipulation under anesthesia for arthrofibrosis should only be performed following treatment of tibial eminence fractures in conjunction with lysis of adhesions. Level of evidence: IV.

54. Papadopoulos A, Kirkos JM, Kapetanos GA: Histomorphologic study of discoid meniscus. *Arthroscopy* 2009;25(3):262-268.

Intact, complete lateral discoid meniscus samples were examined from 10 patients who had undergone arthroscopic saucerization and compared with control samples of intact lateral menisci excised during knee arthroplasty procedures. Histomorphologic scoring showed substantial disorganization of the circular collagen network in discoid menisci compared with control patients, especially along the posterior third of the specimens. Additionally, a heterogeneous course of the circumferentially arranged collagen fibers was shown in the discoid meniscus group. Level of evidence: I.

55. Klingele KE, Kocher MS, Hresko MT, Gerbino P, Micheli LJ: Discoid lateral meniscus: Prevalence of peripheral rim instability. *J Pediatr Orthop* 2004;24(1):79-82.

56. Good CR, Green DW, Griffith MH, Valen AW, Widmann RF, Rodeo SA: Arthroscopic treatment of symptomatic discoid meniscus in children: Classification, technique, and results. *Arthroscopy* 2007;23(2):157-163.

57. Choi SH, Ahn JH, Kim KI, et al: Do the radiographic findings of symptomatic discoid lateral meniscus in children differ from normal control subjects? *Knee Surg Sports Traumatol Arthrosc* 2015;23(4):1128-1134.

Radiographic findings were examined in 78 consecutive children (91 knees) who underwent arthroscopic surgery for discoid lateral meniscus. Substantial differences in the mean height of the lateral tibial spine, lateral joint space distance, height of the fibular head, and obliquity of the lateral tibial plateau were found between those with a discoid lateral meniscus and age- and sex-matched control patients. Several plain radiographic findings in children with symptomatic discoid lateral meniscus were different than in matched control patients. Level of evidence: II.

58. Ahn JH, Lee YS, Ha HC, Shim JS, Lim KS: A novel magnetic resonance imaging classification of discoid lateral meniscus based on peripheral attachment. *Am J Sports Med* 2009;37(8):1564-1569.

This retrospective cohort study of 67 patients (82 knees) examined preoperative MRIs of patients who had undergone surgery for discoid lateral meniscus. A new MRI classification of discoid lateral meniscus was proposed based on the peripheral attachment. An association was noted between discoid lateral menisci classification and rate of meniscus repair. Additionally, meniscus repair location was associated with the type of classification on MRI. Level of evidence: II.

59. Yoo WJ, Lee K, Moon HJ, et al: Meniscal morphologic changes on magnetic resonance imaging are associated with symptomatic discoid lateral meniscal tear in children. *Arthroscopy* 2012;28(3):330-336.

This retrospective cohort study of 69 patients (79 knees) examined whether meniscal displacement or deformation on MRI was associated with meniscus tear in discoid lateral meniscus. All tear types (except radial tears) found on arthroscopy were associated with some morphologic change in the discoid lateral meniscus as evaluated using preoperative MRI. Morphologic change as opposed to signal intensity change on MRI had greater sensitivity for detecting tears in discoid lateral menisci. Level of evidence: IV.

60. Carter CW, Hoellwarth J, Weiss JM: Clinical outcomes as a function of meniscal stability in the discoid meniscus: A preliminary report. *J Pediatr Orthop* 2012;32(1):9-14.

This retrospective case-control study of 51 patients (57 knees; mean age, 11.7 years) compared patients who underwent discoid lateral meniscus saucerization alone versus saucerization + stabilization. At a mean follow-up of 15 months, no substantial difference was reported between the groups when evaluating postoperative outcome measures of range of motion, complications, and IKDC, Tegner, and Lysholm scores. Short-term results for patients with symptomatic discoid menisci requiring surgery are favorable and the addition of meniscal stabilization for those with meniscal instability does not negatively affect outcome. Level of evidence: III.

61. Fu D, Guo L, Yang L, Chen G, Duan X: Discoid lateral meniscus tears and concomitant articular cartilage lesions in the knee. *Arthroscopy* 2014;30(3):311-318.

This prospective case series of 252 patients evaluated from 2010 to 2012 who had undergone surgery for discoid lateral meniscus characterized articular cartilage lesions found during arthroscopy. The most common location of cartilage lesions was the lateral tibial plateau (11.6%) and multivariable logistic regression analysis showed that body mass index (> 23 kg/m²), sex (female), and course of symptoms (> 6 months) were associated with cartilage lesions. Level of evidence: IV.

62. Kamei G, Adachi N, Deie M, et al: Characteristic shape of the lateral femoral condyle in patients with osteochondritis dissecans accompanied by a discoid lateral meniscus. *J Orthop Sci* 2012;17(2):124-128.

This retrospective case-control study examining 58 patients (63 knees; mean age, 17.7 years) compared knees that had OCD of the lateral femoral condyle and those without OCD. The OCD group had a significantly larger intercondylar prominence ratio. Level of evidence: III.

63. Shieh A, Bastrom T, Roocroft J, Edmonds EW, Pennock AT: Meniscus tear patterns in relation to skeletal immaturity: Children versus adolescents. *Am J Sports Med* 2013;41(12):2779-2783.

This retrospective cross-sectional study of 293 patients (age range, 10 to 19 years) compared meniscal tear patterns between children (open growth plates) and adolescents. Overall, 14% of tears were of the discoid meniscus (*N* = 46). Discoid tears comprised 25% of tears in children but only 7% of tears in adolescents. Children accounted for 70% of all discoid meniscus tears and 41% required peripheral rim repair in addition to saucerization. Concomitant ligament injury was more common in adolescents (51% versus 28%). Level of evidence: III.

64. de Lucena GL, dos Santos Gomes C, Guerra RO: Prevalence and associated factors of Osgood-Schlatter syndrome

in a population-based sample of Brazilian adolescents. *Am J Sports Med* 2011;39(2):415-420.

This cross-sectional study examined 956 adolescent students (mean age (± SD), 13.7 ± 1.04 years) from 2008 to 2009 in the school system of Natal, Brazil. The prevalence of Osgood-Schlatter disease was 9.8%. Multivariable logistic regression analysis showed that factors significantly associated with Osgood-Schlatter disease were regular participation in sports and shortening of the rectus femoris muscle. Level of evidence: III.

65. Krause BL, Williams JP, Catterall A: Natural history of Osgood-Schlatter disease. *J Pediatr Orthop* 1990;10(1):65-68.

66. Pihlajamäki HK, Mattila VM, Parviainen M, Kiuru MJ, Visuri TI: Long-term outcome after surgical treatment of unresolved Osgood-Schlatter disease in young men. *J Bone Joint Surg Am* 2009;91(10):2350-2358.

This retrospective cohort study examined 107 consecutive military recruits (117 knees) who had undergone surgery for unresolved Osgood-Schlatter disease. The rate of surgically treated, unresolved Osgood-Schlatter disease was 42 per 100,000 military recruits. After a median follow-up of 10 years, 87% reported no restrictions in everyday activity or at work and 75% returned to their preoperative level of sports. Six patients experienced minor postoperative complications and two had undergone reoperation for treatment of Osgood-Schlatter disease. Level of evidence: IV.

67. Topol GA, Podesta LA, Reeves KD, Raya MF, Fullerton BD, Yeh HW: Hyperosmolar dextrose injection for recalcitrant Osgood-Schlatter disease. *Pediatrics* 2011;128(5):e1121-e1128.

This randomized, controlled trial of 54 patients (65 knees; age range, 9 to 17 years) with recalcitrant Osgood-Schlatter disease compared treatment with hyperosmolar dextrose injection with placebo. Both experimental and control groups returned to unaltered sport activity at 3 months. At 1 year, asymptomatic sport was more common in the experimental group than the placebo group and usual care. Hyperosmolar dextrose injection over the apophysis and patellar tendon origin was safe and well tolerated in this population and resulted in more rapid and frequent achievement of unaltered sport and asymptomatic sport compared with usual care. Level of evidence: I.

68. Freedman DM, Kono M, Johnson EE: Pathologic patellar fracture at the site of an old Sinding-Larsen-Johansson lesion: A case report of a 33-year-old male. *J Orthop Trauma* 2005;19(8):582-585.

Video Reference

49.1: Ellis HB, Wilson PL: Video. *A Surgical Technique for Medial Patellofemoral Ligament Reconstruction in the Skeletally Immature.* Texas Scottish Rite Hospital, Dallas, TX, 2013.

© 2016 American Academy of Orthopaedic Surgeons

Chapter 50

Special Considerations in Head Injuries in Adolescent Athletes

Regina Kostyun, MSEd, ATC   Carl W. Nissen, MD   Imran Hafeez, MD

Abstract

The perception of athletic head injuries is drastically changing in youth sports. Although the majority of head injuries are not life threatening, milder head injuries can lead to long-lasting impairment if misdiagnosed or left untreated. Clinicians are taking the lead in responding to these head injuries with a conservative approach, ensuring all symptoms and dysfunction have fully resolved before discussing return to sport. Coaches and parents are being called on to increase their education and awareness of these injuries, therefore helping to increase quick identification of head injuries and decrease the likelihood of further harm in young athletes.

Keywords: adolescent; head injury; concussion; clinical management; return to school; return to sport; concussion education

Introduction

Injuries sustained to the head during sports participation fall along a spectrum of severity. Although most closed head injuries are considered mild in nature with subsequent dysfunctions demonstrating transient characteristics, life-threatening and catastrophic injuries do occur. Physicians involved in the care of young athletes, especially those engaged in on-field care and return-to-play decisions,

Dr. Nissen or an immediate family member serves as a board member, owner, officer, or committee member of the American Orthopaedic Society for Sports Medicine. Neither of the following authors nor any immediate family member has received anything of value from or has stock or stock options held in a commercial company or institution related directly or indirectly to the subject of this chapter: Ms. Kostyun and Dr. Hafeez.

must be vigilant and mindful of the head injury continuum and implement a conservative management approach for these adolescents. Although sports-related concussions are the predominant head injury in a young athletic population, physicians must remain attentive to the potential for catastrophic head injuries and be able to execute seamless provision of care during a life-threatening event.

Epidemiology

Participation in organized sports is increasing among young individuals. The National Federation of State High School Associations estimates that approximately 7.6 million high school student athletes participate annually in organized sports. When middle school, youth, and recreational athletes are included, the number increases to 27 million participants.[1] However, the increased participation in organized sports has also contributed to an increase in sport-related injuries. Injuries to the head have long been recognized as a concern in contact sports and account for approximately 7% of all sport-related injuries in young athletes.[2,3] Dating back to the turn of the century when American football, due to a series of catastrophic injuries, was proposed to be banned by President Roosevelt, these injuries, their recognition, and appropriate treatment have been a topic of much concern. With current increased knowledge and understanding of these head injuries, along with the widespread availability of modern radiologic techniques, the diagnosis and management of these conditions has improved. Although protective gear has improved drastically over the past 50 years, intracranial bleeds appear to be on the rise in the young athletic population for unexplained reasons.[4] One-third of adolescents who present to the emergency department with intracranial hemorrhages and cervical spine fractures sustain their injury while participating in a sport.[5] Although the concern over intracranial bleeds remains high, even more concerning over the past decade is the recognition of concussions in this age group. Increased involvement in sports combined with improved identification of concussion injuries has resulted in a 4.2-fold increase in the number of diagnosed concussions sustained at the high school level over the past decade.[6] During a similar time frame, emergency departments have seen a 200% increase in the number of adolescent patients treated for concussions[7] with the most common cause of injury related to sports participation.[8]

The sharp increase of diagnosed sports-related concussions paired with the concern surrounding the possible long-term consequences of head injuries in the adolescent population has become a source of public concern. The amplified focus from clinicians, researchers, and sports organizations on this injury has resulted in an acute awareness of concussions not only from the medical community but also from the media and government sectors. This new era of improved understanding regarding head injuries has resulted in a new level of scrutiny and concern. This heightened awareness has established a platform of education and awareness with the goal of reducing the severity of head injuries.

Definition and Mechanism of Injury

Head injuries can be defined as diffuse or focal, with each classification of injury having its own unique clinical sequelae.[9] Diffuse injuries, such as shearing injuries, result in microtrauma to the connective system of the brain; focal injuries result in macrotrauma to vessels and other tissues within the brain.

Concussions, diffuse head injuries, are defined as a "trauma-induced transient alteration in mental status that may or may not involve loss of consciousness."[10] Concussions are caused by trauma, either direct or indirect. Direct trauma occurs to the head. Indirect trauma is absorbed by the body and transferred to the head.[11] The resultant linear and rotational forces sustained to the brain are thought to generate transient disturbances in brain function.[12] This temporary intrusion in brain function generally occurs in the absence of a structural injury. Diffuse changes in metabolic function and subsequent energy imbalance results in the signs and symptoms that make up the clinical presentation of a concussion.

Recent concern has been raised about the possible sequela following subconcussive impacts an individual sustains, not only during a single sports season but cumulatively over his or her athletic career.[13] These potential subconcussive forces, as well as the cumulative number of impacts sustained over a given season, have been measured in adolescent football and ice hockey players.[14,15] However, a pathologic impact magnitude or number of cumulative blows has not yet been identified and the exact mechanism of concussion remains unclear. Impact location has also been shown to have poor prognostic and clinical value in an adolescent population.[16]

Focal head injuries include intracranial hematomas, such as subdural, epidural, intracerebral, or subarachnoid hemorrhages (Figure 1). These injuries should be considered in all instances of head trauma, especially in high-energy impacts to the head. Subdural hemorrhage, bleeding between the dura mater and the brain, is most commonly seen in athletes who participate in contact sports. Bleeding into the space between the dura mater and the inner surface of the skull, or epidural hemorrhage, can occur when an unhelmeted athlete is struck in the head. Intracerebral hemorrhages or contusions commonly seen in the orbitofrontal lobes as a result of a coup-contrecoup injury are rare in sports-related trauma. Subarachnoid hemorrhage, or bleeding in the subarachnoid space, is commonly caused by shearing stress between the arachnoid membrane and pia mater. Subarachnoid hemorrhages are often associated with indirect trauma to the head as the resultant rotational forces are transmitted from the body to the head.

Intracranial hemorrhages can evolve quickly and without rapid identification and treatment, substantial morbidity can occur. Although these injuries are rare in young athletes, certain contact and high-risk sports are more prone to these potentially catastrophic injuries.[17] Of the sports commonly played by young athletes, football, ice hockey, lacrosse, soccer, gymnastics, diving, track and field, and wrestling carry the highest risk of life-threatening injury to the head.[18]

On-Field Management and Initial Care

Sideline assessments of injuries no longer focus on severity grading; instead, initial evaluations are used to identify the presence of a concussion and as a screening tool to detect cervical spine instability, intracranial hemorrhaging, or other critical pathologies.[19,20] Differentiating between emergent and nonthreatening conditions can be challenging immediately following the injury. A 2013 systematic review of clinical tests used during the assessment of a head injury, either on-field or within 24 hours of the injury, supports a comprehensive, systematic, multifaceted approach for the on-field evaluation of an adolescent athlete to improve the chances of a positive outcome.[21] Because the progression of injuries, especially intracranial bleeds, can lead to devastating outcomes, subsequent assessments should be completed to help identify worsening symptoms or a neurologic decline that would indicate a severe injury.

Initial evaluation of the athlete should begin with an assessment of airway, breathing, and circulation. The

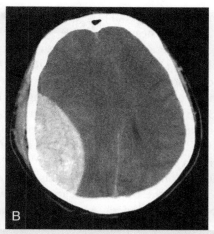
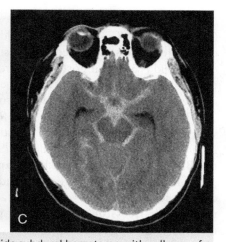

Figure 1 Magnetic resonance images of intracranial hemorrhages. (**A**) A large left-side subdural hematoma with collapse of the ventricle and midline shift. (**B**) A right-side acute epidural hematoma with midline shift. Note the soft-tissue reaction at the site of the direct blow to the head. (**C**) A right-side subarachnoid hematoma.

need for an artificial airway should be determined, especially in an unconscious athlete. Loss of consciousness can place an athlete at increased risk of aspiration as well as impair breathing, which may lead to hypoventilation and subsequent injury to the central nervous system.[9] Evaluation of the cervical spine should occur after the athlete's airway, breathing, and circulation have been assessed. Cervical instability or spinal cord injury should be assumed in an unconscious athlete, and proper stabilization should occur before the athlete is transported to a higher level of care. In the case of either a cervical spine or head injury, when the athlete is participating in a helmeted sport, the facemask should be removed and the helmet should remain on when the athlete is boarded and transported to the nearest medical facility. This procedure also should be followed if the initial evaluation determines that focal neurologic impairments exist.

Athletes with prolonged loss of consciousness, decreased mental status, severe headache, or persistent vomiting following head trauma are suspected of having a focal injury, such as an intracranial hemorrhage, and should undergo further evaluation. The presence of unilateral signs or symptoms or a Glasgow Coma Scale (GCS) score of 13 or lower also requires immediate acceleration to a higher level of care.

Conscious athletes without findings of focal neurologic injuries should be evaluated for a concussion following head trauma. Understanding the mechanism of injury, recognizing the presenting signs and symptoms, and assessing cognitive impairments make the clinical diagnosis of a concussion. The most commonly used sideline assessments include an inventory of current signs and symptoms, an assessment of postural stability, and a brief assessment of cognitive function in conjunction with a

Table 1	
Commonly Used Sideline and Follow-up Concussion Assessment Tools	
On-Field Assessments	**Postdiagnosis Assessments**
Sports Concussion Assessment Tool (SCAT3)	Post-Concussion Symptom Scale
Sports Concussion Assessment Tool for children (childSCAT3)	Balance Error Scoring System
Standardized Assessment of Concussion	**Neurocognitive testing**
Post-Concussion Symptom Scale	Immediate Post-Concussion and Cognitive Testing (ImPACT)
Balance Error Scoring System	Axon Sports Computerized Cognitive Assessment Tool (CCAT)
King-Devick test	HeadMinder

thorough history. No single 'best' tool is available for the diagnosis of a concussion; therefore, sports medicine professionals should use a combination of assessment tools, both on-field and during follow-up evaluations (Table 1).

The symptoms of a concussion can be classified into four domains: somatic, cognitive, emotional, and sleep. Symptom checklists can be used during the on-field evaluation as a systematic approach of asking definitive yes-or-no questions for individual concussion symptoms despite the concern of underreporting by adolescent athletes.[21] Two of the most commonly used symptom checklists include the Post-Concussion Symptom Scale and the symptom evaluation list in the Sports Concussion Assessment Tool (SCAT3) and SCAT3 for children (childSCAT3). The most commonly discussed and recognized sign of a concussion on the field is a loss of postural control during the acute phase of a concussion, with several medical societies recommending the use of postural assessments acutely.[11,12,21] The Balance Error Scoring System (BESS) is the most widely used sideline assessment of static balance[22,23] and is included in the SCAT3 and childSCAT3. However, the BESS has been examined primarily in a collegiate population, with little research conducted on athletes of high school age and younger. In addition, the BESS may be unsuccessful in identifying persistent balance dysfunctions. A brief assessment of cognitive function, although more challenging, is appropriate and included in most sideline assessment tools. The use of computerized neurocognitive testing for sideline assessment has not been well investigated. Therefore, the application of these tools during an on-field evaluation is not commonplace and cannot be recommended at this time.[21] The use of the King-Devick test to assess oculomotor function in collegiate and professional athletes is supported in the literature,[24,25] although its use has not been investigated in high school and younger athletes. Immediate removal from all physical activity should occur if signs or symptoms consistent with a concussion are present during the on-field evaluation following a traumatic event.[11,26]

Many youth sports and town leagues do not have access to medical care on the sideline during practices or games. In these situations, the clinicians in pediatric emergency departments often provide the first medical evaluation of a young athlete with a suspected concussion. During the past decade, emergency department providers have substantially increased their awareness of concussions and most physicians follow published guidelines when managing concussion patients. These guidelines recommend that serial follow-up assessments with a medical provider should occur for continued care until the concussion has resolved. Pediatric emergency department clinicians[27] and athletic trainers[22] have recently demonstrated similar referral patterns for adolescent patients to follow up with their primary care providers for further management of concussion symptoms. In many instances in the past, the young athlete was simply watched by the athletic trainer or told by emergency department personnel to rest for a week and then return to play. This change in concussion management is important because clinicians completing the initial assessment are now recommending follow-up care to ensure resolution of symptoms and recovery from the injury instead of initially predicting recovery at the moment of injury and recommending arbitrary dates for return to school and return to play.

Concussion Management Team

Although concussions are considered mild in relation to other head injuries, this does not diminish their complexity.[10-12,26,28] As research continues to improve the understanding of this multifaceted injury, sports medicine practitioners are being called on to collaborate with other professionals to create a multidisciplinary concussion management team to provide better care for adolescent athletes.[11,22,26,29] This team, composed of medical professionals with experience in concussions, oversees the education and awareness of concussions at the youth level, provides a cohesive network to increase identification of this injury, provides prompt implementation of rest, and oversees a safe, successful return to academics as well as athletics. This team supports the adolescent with the emotional challenges of sustaining a concussion as well as the social and mental difficulties associated with persistent concussion symptoms.[30] Since 2010, multiple professional societies, including the American Medical Society for Sports Medicine[12] and the American Academy of Orthopaedic Surgeons,[31] have released position statements describing their role within this team.

The members of the concussion management team can vary with an individual's recovery time. If an adolescent recovers rapidly from his or her concussion, the team may consist of only a few members. However, if an adolescent experiences persistent symptoms with a protracted recovery, the concussion management team will need to include other medical professionals such as neurologists, neuropsychologists, sports medicine physicians, psychologists, physical therapists, athletic trainers, school nurses, school guidance counselors, and school faculty members. Irrespective of the formal titles of the individuals comprising the team, all members must remain current on the literature given the rapid increase in understanding of concussion and the noteworthy changes to the current best practice management models for adolescents.[22,32]

In the secondary school setting, athletic trainers are the best prepared and trained medical providers to evaluate a head injury with a suspected concussion.[33] The main focus for athletic trainers should be to ensure the adolescent athlete is properly assessed and receives guidance and education regarding acute concussion management. The establishment of a concussion management team and written concussion policy within the school establishes lines of communication between all involved team members to ensure the health and safety of the student athlete with a concussion.[11,26] The concussion management team is essential for facilitating the smooth transition of the student athlete with concussion back into the academic environment.[22] The possibility for a smooth return of the student athlete to the classroom is greatly enhanced with a well-functioning and interactive management team, reducing the far-reaching, negative consequences possible in young athletes.[34]

Clinical Management

Imaging

Neuroimaging is a key factor in determining the severity of injury and the expediency with which medical care must be delivered for focal head injuries. When assessing head injury, the main indicators for neuroimaging are focal neurologic deficit, altered mental status, vomiting, and parental anxiety.[27] The concern over radiation exposure in adolescents over the past decade has led to more specific guidelines as to when radiologic evaluation is appropriate in instances of head trauma. Clinical decision rules, such as the Canadian CT Head Rule and the New Orleans Criteria, should be used to help determine the need for neuroimaging following blunt head trauma (Table 2). When neuroimaging is required in a young athlete, MRI may be a safer alternative to CT; MRI has been shown to be as sensitive as CT in detecting intracranial hemorrhage and reducing radiation exposure in pediatric patients.[35]

Standard neuroimaging provides essentially no clinical information regarding isolated concussion injuries. Alterations in brain function as a result of a concussion have been thought to occur in the absence of structural injury due to a substantial number of normal CT and MRI scans obtained from these patients.[11,36] Advancements in neuroimaging may soon dispute this commonly accepted statement.[37] Currently, work is being completed to investigate the role of diffusion tensor imaging, functional MRI, and magnetic resonance spectroscopy regarding concussion management, specifically in the area of quantifying the severity of injury.[36]

Clinical Management Plan for Concussions

Current recommendations for management after the initial diagnosis include a series of follow-up assessments until resolution of concussion symptoms and impairments, followed by a closely monitored progression back to full academic activity and unrestricted play to ensure a smooth and safe recovery.[11,26] Cognitive and physical activity modification is often determined from the information gained from these assessments as well as discussion with the adolescent athlete and his or her parents. Given the complexity of concussions, an individualized management plan should be created for each adolescent athlete.

A short-term period of rest from cognitive and physical exertion followed by a gradual and systematic increase in

Table 2	
Clinical Prediction Rules for Patients With Blunt Head Trauma	
Canadian CT Head Rule	**New Orleans CT Head Criteria**
Head CT is required for minor head injury patients with any one of these findings	Head CT is required for blunt trauma patients with LOC, GCS score 15, normal neurologic examination, and any of the following criteria:
GCS score < 15 at 2 hours after injury	Headaches
Suspected open or depressed skull fracture	Vomiting
Any sign of basal skull fracture (hemotympanum, "raccoon eyes", Battle sign, CSF otorrhea/rhinorrhea)	Age older than 60 years
Vomiting ≥ 2 episodes	Drug or alcohol intoxication
Age 65 years or older	Deficits in short-term memory
Amnesia before impact ≥ 30 minutes	Physical evidence of trauma above the clavicles
Dangerous mechanism of injury (fall from elevation, struck by vehicle)	Seizure
100% sensitive, 60% specific[76]	82% sensitive, 26% specific[76]

CSF = cerebrospinal fluid, GCS = Glasgow Coma Scale, LOC = loss of consciousness.

these activities continues to be the foundation of appropriate concussion management.[11] Student athletes who do not rest and continue to engage in activities that provoke their concussion symptoms have demonstrated longer recovery times.[38-40] Conversely, complete abstinence from cognitive and light aerobic activities, especially for an extended period, has not been shown to be beneficial.[39]

Return to Learn

Adolescents with concussions benefit from a gradual reentry plan to help facilitate a smooth return to the academic environment.[34] When a student athlete has been cleared to return to the classroom, the individual may still be affected by the concussion, yet appears well to teachers, school administrators, and peers.[41] A reentry plan should address classroom accommodations as well as environmental adjustments, depending on the student athlete's symptoms and cognitive difficulties. The main focus for the concussion management team during the return-to-learn phase is to balance the need for the individual to be in the classroom with the appropriate accommodations and adjustments to decrease the potential for recurrent or persistent symptoms.

Return to Play

Current return-to-play guidelines are based largely on the resolution of concussion symptoms and progression through increasingly demanding exertional exercise without provocation of symptoms. The potential exists for adverse outcomes if an adolescent athlete is allowed to return to contact or collision activities too soon. This may be evident in the percentage of recurrent injuries that occur within a short time from the original injury.[6,16] Recent investigations have found lingering motor performance measurement deficits in adolescent concussion patients who have appeared to fully recover clinically from their injury.[42,43] This highlights the possibility that motor control may have a different recovery trajectory compared with symptom resolution or return of normal neurocognitive function.

Recovery Patterns

Adolescents may demonstrate longer recovery patterns following a concussion than adults. It has been shown that 68% to 98% of adolescent athletes will recover within 1 month from their concussion.[44-47] However, a subset of patients will continue to experience concussion symptoms longer than 4 weeks.[40,47] Females as well as adolescents with a previous history of concussion, previous diagnosis of migraine headaches, learning disability, or attention deficit hyperactivity disorder may be predisposed to a longer recovery course.[16,47,48] The substantial variation in recovery length supports the implementation of an individualized management plan. Concussions cannot be generalized and each injury will be different.

Additional Management Strategies

For most adolescents who recover from a concussion within a few weeks, the treatment plan may only need to include a short period of rest and activity modification until resolution of symptoms. In the situation in which persistent symptoms or impairments continue to plague the individual, additional treatment options including medication, dietary changes, physical therapy, sub-threshold exercise, and emotional support should be considered and implemented into the management plan.

Medications have a limited but specific role in concussion management if the individual continues to note unrelenting symptoms that have persisted past the accepted recovery length for an adolescent athlete, and if the individual's symptoms negatively affect his or her quality of life.[11,49] Given the lack of well-controlled studies on the use of certain medications for symptom management, care should be taken when prescribing these agents to a young population.[49] Sleep disturbances may be the most common postconcussion symptom often treated with medications, followed by persistent headaches, cognitive difficulties, and emotional changes. The most recent International Consensus Statement on Concussion in 2012[11] notes the unique situations in which pharmacologic therapies are warranted during concussion management but strongly warns against returning an athlete to contact or collision activities if medications are still being used because of the potential to cover or hide lingering symptoms.

Increasing evidence supports using subsymptom threshold aerobic exercise as rehabilitation for a possible physiologic dysfunction following a concussion.[50-52] In addition, subsymptom threshold aerobic exercise can also help ease feelings of depression or anxiety in adolescent athletes who have been completely removed from their team and have lost their sense of identity as an athlete.

Preseason Preparation

An Emergency Action Plan is a document that outlines how to triage a life-threatening or catastrophic event. An Emergency Action Plan should be in place for every venue that supports athletic play and reviewed by all members of the medical and coaching staff on a yearly basis to ensure a rapid and seamless execution of care if an adolescent athlete is injured.[53]

In many cases, use of a structured preparticipation examination can enhance the management of an adolescent athlete who suffers a concussion during a sporting season. The preparticipation examination typically includes a screening neurologic examination along with baseline neurocognitive assessments. Baseline assessments are becoming increasingly prevalent in the secondary school setting.[22] In situations in which neurocognitive baseline assessments are implemented in a group testing environment, a standardized approach toward test administration, proper supervision of the testing environment, and appropriate education of the student athlete on the purpose of this type of testing is necessary to ensure valid scores.[54,55] Even when these steps are taken to improve the validity of the baseline examinations, the tests should be reviewed by an experienced user of the neurocognitive examinations to confirm their validity. Neurocognitive baseline assessments completed in a group setting may be inappropriate for certain adolescents, especially those with a diagnosis of attention deficit hyperactivity disorder or learning disabilities.[55,56]

Specific Concerns in a Youth Population

Individuals with persistent symptoms following a concussion tend to be classified as having postconcussion syndrome. However, postconcussion syndrome is inadequately defined, the etiology is poorly understood, and the term is commonly interchanged with "postconcussion symptoms." The argument has been made that the transition from concussion to postconcussion syndrome should occur at the point when typical concussion symptoms should have resolved in the targeted population.[57] Given the fact that adolescent athletes have substantial variation in recovery lengths, defining the point where concussion symptoms should typically resolve is challenging.

Concerns exist for adolescent athletes returning to sports while still symptomatic from their concussions. The National Center for Catastrophic Injury Research has data that suggest a possible risk factor for a catastrophic injury is the presence of a recent head injury.[3,58] Although incredibly rare, second-impact syndrome should be considered by sports medicine physicians given its relevance to a youth population. Second-impact syndrome is typically a repeat injury that occurs when an athlete has not fully recovered from a previous injury, resulting in diffuse cerebral swelling with delayed catastrophic deterioration, and on occasion brainstem herniation.[59] Second-impact syndrome is a poorly understood injury because the only literature that exists on this topic consists of case reports. Second-impact syndrome has been documented in 14- to 18-year-olds in whom death occurs from diffuse cerebral edema and possible herniation as the brain loses its ability to autoregulate intracranial and cerebral perfusion pressure. It has been assumed that several of these athletes continued to participate in sports while symptomatic from a recent concussion when the structural injury was sustained.[60] To help prevent second-impact syndrome from occurring, strict guidelines forbid athletes from participating in collision or contact activities while symptomatic from a concussion. Although some experts refute the presence of second-impact syndrome, sports medicine clinicians acknowledge concern about adverse long-term neurologic sequelae following repeat impacts to the head in a symptomatic individual. This finding highlights the need for proper education, especially for the athlete, to disclose symptoms to those involved in his or her care.

Another concerning factor with prematurely returning an adolescent athlete to contact and collision activities is the risk of chronic traumatic encephalopathy (CTE).

CTE, a neurodegenerative disease postulated to occur from repetitive trauma, was originally identified in the 1960s. Until recently, CTE has been diagnosed postmortem in retired professional athletes and military personnel. Current theory links CTE with chronic repetitive head trauma, although causation has not yet been confirmed. Research on CTE is in its infancy and current reports represent a basic appearance of this injury within contact sports.[13] Additional work in this area must identify risk factors for the development of CTE.

Injury Prevention

Reducing the frequency of adolescent concussions continues to be a prevailing mission for sports medicine providers, researchers, and sports organizations. Although improvements in helmet design have helped decreased the risk of skull fractures,[61] helmets as well as other types of protective equipment (headbands, mouth guards) have not been shown to result in decreased concussion occurrence rates.[62] Recent changes to contact and collision activities in youth hockey[63] and similar proposed changes to youth football and youth soccer may yield promising results, although empirical data have not yet confirmed a reduction in the overall number of sustained concussions. These organizations are following the precedents of collegiate football programs that have decreased the amount of contact that occurs during practices.

Concussion awareness paired with state legislation has recently become the main focus of protecting adolescent athletes.[64] A national focus has been placed on appropriate and conservative management of young student athletes.[65] This emphasis has pushed for legislative guidelines to protect young athletes from the mismanagement of concussion injuries.[32] As of November 2014, all states have passed legislation on concussion management in adolescent athletes. The laws in each state and the discussion surrounding them have emphasized the importance of creating protocols and concussion treatment plans. Each law indicates that the athletes, coaches, parents, and medical staff at the youth level are responsible for being aware of the issues surrounding concussions and their management.[65] However, only 41 states require adolescent athletes to complete formal concussion education, and 39 require parents to complete formal concussion education. Educational programs exist and several states have developed their own concussion education curriculum. These programs as well as private programs often include resources such as the US Centers for Disease Control and Prevention's Heads Up Toolkit, Sports Legacy Institute Community Educators courses, ThinkFirst, and Brain 101 and have been shown to increase awareness and early appropriate management in youth sports.[66,67] These programs often have a specific population as their target audience. The Heads Up Toolkit targets parents and coaches, and the Sport Legacy Institute program specifically targets athletes and provides real-life concussion experiences.

Adolescent athletes, particularly those who participate in town or recreational leagues, are usually not the target population of legislation and often are not exposed to the same level of education. Parents of football athletes 5 to 15 years of age may struggle to correctly identify concussion symptoms, with most parents failing to recognize sleep disturbances and emotional distress as resulting from a concussion.[68]

The extensive educational programs in most states are directed in large part toward high school students. The purpose of these programs is to raise awareness and improve the initial recognition and treatment of concussions because these student athletes are still reluctant to report possible injury.[69,70] Approximately 50% of student athletes do not report their injuries to coaches or medical staff.[71] Although high school student athletes can correctly identify certain concussion symptoms such as dizziness, headaches, and confusion,[70,72] other symptoms such as nausea, amnesia, sleep disturbances, emotional or personality changes, and the delayed onset of symptoms are less well known to this population.[69,70,72] Student athletes commonly cite self-misdiagnosing a bell-ringer or concussion injury as an injury not serious enough to warrant medical attention,[70] as well as internal pressure to avoid letting down teammates[73,74] or parents[75] as reasons for not reporting their injury. Although these educational initiatives cannot prevent all concussions, the hope is that early, proper diagnosis of concussions will decrease the possibility and hopefully the actual incidence of second-impact, multiimpact, and recurrent injuries, or overlapping concussion syndrome. Therefore, continuation and improvement of concussion awareness and educational programs is important.

Recent studies have investigated the relationship between a student athlete's socioeconomic framework and disclosure of concussion injuries.[69,70] The socioeconomic framework of adolescent athletes is complex and includes the individual behaviors and traits of the athletes, the strength of their peer networks, their social environment, and even the policies of their sport's organization.[69] Coaches who are properly educated on the current management of adolescent athletes with a concussion have the ability to not only increase identification of these injuries but also ensure a sports environment of compliance of the athlete with appropriate and safe return to play.[69]

Summary

Participation in athletic activities will always pose a threat of head injury to adolescent athletes. Clinicians must be prepared to rapidly and effectively triage care for an adolescent athlete who suffers a life-threatening head injury. In the case of a sports-related concussion, clinicians must take a conservative stance on appropriately resting and slowly progressing an adolescent athlete back to cognitive and physical activities once the concussion has fully resolved. Given the difficulty of eliminating the risk of head injuries during sport, clinicians can help educate coaches, parents, and athletes on the proper steps to take in the event of a head injury in a young athlete to mitigate the chance of further injury.

Key Study Points

- Head injuries are common in the adolescent population. Prompt recognition of catastrophic versus nonemergent injuries and subsequent triage of care is paramount to avoiding long-term problems.

- A concise and structured approached to an on-field assessment of a head injury paired with the development and rehearsal of an Emergency Action Plan will help ensure smooth and seamless delivery of care in the event of a life-threatening event.

- Concussions are complex injuries that require a multidisciplinary group of health care professionals to oversee care and management until full resolution of symptoms. The establishment of a concussion management team at school helps ensure the safe and full return of the student athlete with a concussion to the classroom and the athletic field.

- Education of all involved in adolescent sports, including the athletes themselves, is perhaps the most important area where improvements can be made toward prevention of head injury.

Annotated References

1. DiFiori JP, Benjamin HJ, Brenner J, et al: Overuse injuries and burnout in youth sports: A position statement from the American Medical Society for Sports Medicine. *Clin J Sport Med* 2014;24(1):3-20.

2. Kelly KD, Lissel HL, Rowe BH, Vincenten JA, Voaklander DC: Sport and recreation-related head injuries treated in the emergency department. *Clin J Sport Med* 2001;11(2):77-81.

This descriptive epidemiologic study outlines the occurrence of sport-related injuries in adolescents from data collected from a nationwide sample of emergency departments. During a single year, emergency department visits for concussion care totaled $154.8 million.

3. Nalliah RP, Anderson IM, Lee MK, Rampa S, Allareddy V, Allareddy V: Epidemiology of hospital-based emergency department visits due to sports injuries. *Pediatr Emerg Care* 2014;30(8):511-515.

4. Forbes JA, Zuckerman SL, He L, et al: Subdural hemorrhage in two high-school football players: Post-injury helmet testing. *Pediatr Neurosurg* 2013;49(1):43-49.

   In this case report, the biomechanical testing results on the football helmets worn by two athletes who suffered subdural hemorrhages during play revealed both helmets were deemed compliant per National Operating Committee on Standards for Athletic Equipment standards. The authors raise concern that even with protective equipment passing helmet safety specifications, catastrophic head injuries still occur in high school football.

5. Meehan WP III, Mannix R: A substantial proportion of life-threatening injuries are sport-related. *Pediatr Emerg Care* 2013;29(5):624-627.

   This large retrospective study of emergency department visits over a 10-year span revealed that 40% of catastrophic injuries sustained by pediatric and adolescent patients are related to sports participation. The authors discuss the possibility of preventing life-threatening injuries in this population by advocating for rule changes, better coaching education, and properly fitted protective equipment.

6. Lincoln AE, Caswell SV, Almquist JL, Dunn RE, Norris JB, Hinton RY: Trends in concussion incidence in high school sports: A prospective 11-year study. *Am J Sports Med* 2011;39(5):958-963.

   This descriptive epidemiological study prospectively gathered concussion injury rates for 25 high schools over a 10-year period. Their results revealed a 4.2-fold increase in diagnosed concussions in 12 varsity sports, with football and girls soccer having the highest incidence rates.

7. Bakhos LL, Lockhart GR, Myers R, Linakis JG: Emergency department visits for concussion in young child athletes. *Pediatrics* 2010;126(3):e550-e556.

   This retrospective review reports on data collected by the National Electronic Injury Surveillance System on 100 US based hospitals. Over a 4-year collection period, children 8 to 19 years of age accounted for 502,000 emergency department visits with a diagnosis of concussion. Nearly half of all diagnosed concussions were sports related.

8. Simon TD, Bublitz C, Hambidge SJ: External causes of pediatric injury-related emergency department visits in the United States. *Acad Emerg Med* 2004;11(10):1042-1048.

9. Morris SA, Jones WH, Proctor MR, Day AL: Emergent treatment of athletes with brain injury. *Neurosurgery* 2014;75(suppl 4):S96-S105.

A comprehensive review of life-threatening head injuries in athletes is presented. This article reviews current sideline emergency management, transportation, and management of protective equipment when caring for an athlete with a head injury.

10. Broglio SP, Cantu RC, Gioia GA, et al; National Athletic Trainer's Association: National Athletic Trainers' Association position statement: Management of sport concussion. *J Athl Train* 2014;49(2):245-265.

11. McCrory P, Meeuwisse WH, Aubry M, et al: Consensus statement on concussion in sport: The 4th International Conference on Concussion in Sport, Zurich, November 2012. *J Athl Train* 2013;48(4):554-575.

12. Harmon KG, Drezner JA, Gammons M, et al: American Medical Society for Sports Medicine position statement: Concussion in sport. *Br J Sports Med* 2013;47(1):15-26.

13. Stern RA, Riley DO, Daneshvar DH, Nowinski CJ, Cantu RC, McKee AC: Long-term consequences of repetitive brain trauma: Chronic traumatic encephalopathy. *PM R* 2011;3(10, suppl 2)S460-S467.

    This review article discusses the emerging evidence on chronic traumatic encephalopathy and highlights the need for additional research to help identify the population at risk as well as the clinical presentation and evolution of the disease.

14. Reed N, Taha T, Keightley M, et al: Measurement of head impacts in youth ice hockey players. *Int J Sports Med* 2010;31(11):826-833.

    The purpose of this pilot study was to describe the biomechanical measures of head impacts, as measured by the Head Impact Telemetry System, to young male ice hockey athletes. A secondary purpose was to investigate how athlete and game characteristics may influence the frequency and magnitude of head impacts. The authors followed 13 13- to 14-year-old ice hockey athletes for a single season. Their findings showed that the wing position demonstrated a significantly higher number of impacts to their heads (10.9 hits) than a defense (5.95 hits) and centers (6.45) position per game. The wing position also experienced a significantly greater rotational acceleration during hits than center positions. Low magnitude hits with a linear acceleration less than 30 g comprised the majority of hits (83.1%) sustained at all positions.

15. Broglio SP, Martini D, Kasper L, Eckner JT, Kutcher JS: Estimation of head impact exposure in high school football: Implications for regulating contact practices. *Am J Sports Med* 2013;41(12):2877-2884.

    Several football organizations have debated a rule change that would reduce the weekly number of contact practices in hopes of mitigating the number of subconcussive blows sustained by athletes, yet limited data exist to support this movement. The authors of this cross-sectional study examined magnitude and frequency data collected on 42 high school football athletes wearing the Head Impact Telemetry System in their helmets over a single season. Although athletes continue to sustain the greatest number and highest magnitude of blows to their head during games, the findings of this study suggest an 18% reduction in the number of sustained head blows when limiting contact practice to once per week.

16. Kerr ZY, Collins CL, Mihalik JP, Marshall SW, Guskiewicz KM, Comstock RD: Impact locations and concussion outcomes in high school football player-to-player collisions. *Pediatrics* 2014;134(3):489-496.

   The purpose of this study was to describe concussion outcomes in terms of impact location during player-to-player contact in high school football athletes. Data retrieved from the RIO system for the 2008–2013 high school football seasons revealed 2,526 concussions that were sustained from player-to-player contact. Impact location had no association with injury recurrence, number of reported symptoms, symptom resolution, or length of time until return to play. Loss of consciousness was found to occur more often with top-of-the-head blows, which emphasizes the importance of proper tackling mechanics.

17. Zemper ED: Catastrophic injuries among young athletes. *Br J Sports Med* 2010;44(1):13-20.

   This comprehensive review of catastrophic injuries sustained by young athletes identified football, cheerleading, ice hockey, gymnastics, wrestling, and lacrosse as the sports that carry the highest risk of injury. On average, 24 football athletes sustain a catastrophic injury every year. Previous head injury, lack of appropriate protective gear, and inexperienced coaching have all been identified as risk factors.

18. Proctor MR, Cantu RC: Head and neck injuries in young athletes. *Clin Sports Med* 2000;19(4):693-715.

19. Ellis MJ, Leddy JJ, Willer B: Physiological, vestibulo-ocular and cervicogenic post-concussion disorders: An evidence-based classification system with directions for treatment. *Brain Inj* 2015;29(2):238-248.

   This systematic review discusses an evidence-based approach toward treating physiologic, vestibulo-ocular, and cervicogenic impairments and dysfunctions following a concussion.

20. Eckner JT, Kutcher JS: Concussion symptom scales and sideline assessment tools: A critical literature update. *Curr Sports Med Rep* 2010;9(1):8-15.

   Because of the complexity of concussion injuries, a single assessment tool cannot accurately diagnose a concussion. Rather, a multifaceted assessment approach is advocated.

21. McCrea M, Iverson GL, Echemendia RJ, Makdissi M, Raftery M: Day of injury assessment of sport-related concussion. *Br J Sports Med* 2013;47(5):272-284.

   This comprehensive review of assessment tools used during the acute phase of a concussion suggests the diagnosis of a concussion be made from the information obtained from a cluster of tools instead of reliance on a single tool.

22. Williams RM, Welch CE, Weber ML, Parsons JT, Valovich McLeod TC: Athletic trainers' management practices and referral patterns for adolescent athletes after sport-related concussion. *Sports Health* 2014;6(5):434-439.

   An online survey of 851 athletic trainers in the secondary school setting, with a response rate of 25.9%, revealed 77.8% refer adolescent athletes with a concussion to a physician for care. The authors note collaboration of care within the secondary school setting can be improved because only 37.1% of athletic trainers shared concussion management with the school nurse, and 12.5% were the sole health care provider.

23. Guskiewicz KM: Balance assessment in the management of sport-related concussion. *Clin Sports Med* 2011;30(1):89-102, ix.

   Loss of postural control indicates neurologic impairment. Therefore, an assessment of an athlete's balance should be incorporated into the clinical examination for a concussion. Balance impairments, seen acutely following a concussion, may resolve within a few days.

24. Galetta KM, Brandes LE, Maki K, et al: The King-Devick test and sports-related concussion: Study of a rapid visual screening tool in a collegiate cohort. *J Neurol Sci* 2011;309(1-2):34-39.

   This study compared preseason to postseason King-Devick test scores in 219 collegiate athletes. Although a mild learning effect was observed, as postseason scores were better than preseason scores, in healthy collegiate athletes, in 10 athletes who suffered a concussion during the playing season their sideline King-Devick scores were significantly worse than their preseason scores.

25. Galetta MS, Galetta KM, McCrossin J, et al: Saccades and memory: Baseline associations of the King-Devick and SCAT2 SAC tests in professional ice hockey players. *J Neurol Sci* 2013;328(1-2):28-31.

   This prospective study describes the relationship between the Standard Assessment of Concussion (SAC) and King-Devick tests during preseason baseline testing in 27 professional ice hockey players. The authors suggest a relationship between immediate memory and saccadic eye motion because lower SAC memory scores were found with slower King-Devick time scores.

26. Giza CC, Kutcher JS, Ashwal S, et al: Summary of evidence-based guideline update: evaluation and management of concussion in sports: report of the Guideline Development Subcommittee of the American Academy of Neurology. *Neurology* 2013;80(24):2250-2257.

   The authors present a systematic review of risk factors for sustaining a concussion, the predictive abilities of diagnostic tools and clinical presentations in identifying severe or prolonged impairments, and interventions that reduce recovery times.

27. Kinnaman KA, Mannix RC, Comstock RD, Meehan WP III: Management of pediatric patients with concussion

by emergency medicine physicians. *Pediatr Emerg Care* 2014;30(7):458-461.

The purpose of this study was to identify strategies implemented by emergency medicine physicians when caring for young individuals with concussions. The majority of physicians (81%) reported using published guidelines from the American Academy of Neurology and the International Conference on Concussion in Sport when managing concussion patients, and 86% recommended follow-up care to ensure complete resolution of symptoms.

28. Guskiewicz KM, Register-Mihalik J, McCrory P, et al: Evidence-based approach to revising the SCAT2: Introducing the SCAT3. *Br J Sports Med* 2013;47(5):289-293.

The SCAT3 is a collection of the most sensitive and reliable concussion assessments currently available. A systematic and streamlined way of assessing impairments following a concussion is provided.

29. Halstead ME, Walter KD; Council on Sports Medicine and Fitness: American Academy of Pediatrics. Clinical report—sport-related concussion in children and adolescents. *Pediatrics* 2010;126(3):597-615.

30. Echemendia RJ, Iverson GL, McCrea M, et al: Role of neuropsychologists in the evaluation and management of sport-related concussion: An inter-organization position statement. *Arch Clin Neuropsychol* 2012;27(1):119-122.

31. Herring SA, Cantu RC, Guskiewicz KM, et al; American College of Sports Medicine: Concussion (mild traumatic brain injury) and the team physician: A consensus statement—2011 update. *Med Sci Sports Exerc* 2011;43(12):2412-2422.

32. Moreau WJ, Nabhan DC: Development of the 2012 American Chiropractic Board of Sports Physicians position statement on concussion in athletics. *J Chiropr Med* 2013;12(4):269-273.

33. Meehan WP III, Taylor AM, Proctor M: The pediatric athlete: Younger athletes with sport-related concussion. *Clin Sports Med* 2011;30(1):133-144, x.

This review article highlights the lack of data on youth athletes and sport-related concussions. Given the differences and variations of concussions between adults and adolescents, youth athletes need to be included as their own subgroup and require their own set of management strategies.

34. Diaz AL, Wyckoff LJ: NASN position statement: Concussions—the role of the school nurse. *NASN Sch Nurse* 2013;28(2):110-111.

35. Roguski M, Morel B, Sweeney M, et al: Magnetic resonance imaging as an alternative to computed tomography in select patients with traumatic brain injury: A retrospective comparison. *J Neurosurg Pediatr* 2015;15(5):529-534.

In this retrospective review of 574 pediatric patients admitted to an emergency department for head trauma and who subsequently underwent both MRI and CT examinations, only 30 patients had postivie findings. In the subset of patients with positive findings, the authors showed that there was no significant difference between MRI and CT in detecting intracranial injury.

36. Difiori JP, Giza CC: New techniques in concussion imaging. *Curr Sports Med Rep* 2010;9(1):35-39.

Visualizing and quantifying concussion injuries continues to be challenging given the lack of information provided by standard neuroimaging. This review discusses the recent advancements that have been made to help provide clinicians with objective data obtained from innovative neuroimaging techniques.

37. Cubon VA, Putukian M, Boyer C, Dettwiler A: A diffusion tensor imaging study on the white matter skeleton in individuals with sports-related concussion. *J Neurotrauma* 2011;28(2):189-201.

Structural injuries following a concussion are not commonly visualized on MRI and CT but may be detected using diffusion tensor imaging (DTI). The authors report the findings of using DTI on patients with concussions, moderate to severe traumatic brain injury, and severe traumatic brain injury compared with age-matched controls. They suggest DTI may be sensitive enough to detect mild and severe injury to white matter fiber tracks.

38. Moser RS, Glatts C, Schatz P: Efficacy of immediate and delayed cognitive and physical rest for treatment of sports-related concussion. *J Pediatr* 2012;161(5):922-926.

This small retrospective study of 49 high school and collegiate athletes who suffered a concussion demonstrated a week of cognitive and physical rest was beneficial in reducing symptoms regardless of when the rest period was implemented.

39. Majerske CW, Mihalik JP, Ren D, et al: Concussion in sports: Postconcussive activity levels, symptoms, and neurocognitive performance. *J Athl Train* 2008;43(3):265-274.

40. Brown NJ, Mannix RC, O'Brien MJ, Gostine D, Collins MW, Meehan WP III: Effect of cognitive activity level on duration of post-concussion symptoms. *Pediatrics* 2014;133(2):e299-e304.

The results of a prospective study on 335 adolescent and young athletes being treated for a sport-related concussion demonstrated those individuals who did not restrict their cognitive activities during the recovery phase of their concussion had a longer time until symptom resolution and clearance back to sport than individuals who limited their cognitive involvements. The authors note the results of this study support the recommendation of cognitive rest and highlight their results that complete abstinence from cognitive activities was not associated with quicker recovery times.

41. Halstead ME, McAvoy K, Devore CD, Carl R, Lee M, Logan K; Council on Sports Medicine and Fitness; Council on School Health: Returning to learning following a concussion. *Pediatrics* 2013;132(5):948-957.

42. Powers KC, Kalmar JM, Cinelli ME: Recovery of static stability following a concussion. *Gait Posture* 2014;39(1):611-614.

   The authors set out to investigate center of pressure characteristics during static stance in nine collegiate football players cleared to return to play following concussion and nine age- and position-matched healthy control teammates. The football players who had clinically recovered from their concussion demonstrated persistent anterior-posterior balance control deficits and may reflect lingering vestibular impairments that are difficult to detect with current clinical assessments.

43. Howell DR, Osternig LR, Chou LS: Return to activity after concussion affects dual-task gait balance control recovery. *Med Sci Sports Exerc* 2015;47(4):673-680.

   The authors set out to investigate the center of mass characteristics during a dual-task gait analysis in 19 adolescent athletes with concussions and 19 uninjured matched controls. At the time of clinical recovery and return to sport, the adolescents with concussion continued to demonstrate increased displacement and velocity during a dual-task gait compared with the healthy controls. The authors suggest recovery of gait balance control may not coincide with symptom resolution and return of normal neurocognition.

44. Lau BC, Collins MW, Lovell MR: Cutoff scores in neurocognitive testing and symptom clusters that predict protracted recovery from concussions in high school athletes. *Neurosurgery* 2012;70(2):371-379, discussion 379.

   ImPACT scores of 108 male high school football athletes were analyzed to determine if certain symptom clusters could identify athletes who demonstrated a protracted recovery following their concussion. The results of this study reveal certain symptom clusters may have prognostic value in identifying resolution of symptoms and return of working neurocognitive function following a concussion.

45. Meehan WP III, d'Hemecourt P, Comstock RD: High school concussions in the 2008-2009 academic year: Mechanism, symptoms, and management. *Am J Sports Med* 2010;38(12):2405-2409.

   This descriptive epidemiologic study of 544 concussions collected during a single academic year demonstrated high school athletes were less likely to return to sport within 1 week of their injury when computerized neuropsychological testing was implemented into the clinical management.

46. Zuckerman SL, Lee YM, Odom MJ, Solomon GS, Forbes JA, Sills AK: Recovery from sports-related concussion: Days to return to neurocognitive baseline in adolescents versus young adults. *Surg Neurol Int* 2012;3:130.

   In this retrospective, observational study of 100 high school and 100 collegiate athletes, neurocognitive recovery was delayed in younger athletes compared with older athletes. Postinjury ImPACT scores for verbal memory, visual memory, reaction time, and symptoms for younger athletes took longer to return back to baseline ImPACT scores than older athletes following a concussion injury.

47. Eisenberg MA, Andrea J, Meehan W, Mannix R: Time interval between concussions and symptom duration. *Pediatrics* 2013;132(1):8-17.

   In this prospective cohort study of 280 adolescents recovering from a recent concussion, individuals with a previous concussion were symptomatic for a longer period of time than individuals experiencing their first concussion. The authors of this study suggest proceeding with caution when discussing return-to-play decisions given the risk of prolonged symptoms during repeat injuries.

48. Castile L, Collins CL, McIlvain NM, Comstock RD: The epidemiology of new versus recurrent sports concussions among high school athletes, 2005-2010. *Br J Sports Med* 2012;46(8):603-610.

   This study compared the epidemiology of first-time versus recurrent concussions in athletes at 100 high schools nationally over a 5-year period. Data were collected on 2,417 concussions, of which 292 were repeat injuries. The results suggest high school athletes who suffer multiple concussions demonstrated a longer time until symptom resolution and were withheld from sport participation for a longer duration. A significant number of athletes suffered a repeat concussion when returned to sport within 3 weeks of their original injury.

49. Meehan WP III: Medical therapies for concussion. *Clin Sports Med* 2011;30(1):115-124, ix.

   This study reviewed the efficacy of pharmacological treatment of a sport-related concussion. To date, medications have not been shown to increase healing from a concussion injury. Rather, certain medications may have usefulness in aiding patients with chronic headaches, sleep disturbances, and emotional changes as they recover from concussion.

50. Baker JG, Freitas MS, Leddy JJ, Kozlowski KF, Willer BS: Return to full functioning after graded exercise assessment and progressive exercise treatment of postconcussion syndrome. *Rehabil Res Pract* 2012;2012:705309.

   The results of this small pilot study suggest individuals with postconcussion syndrome may be experiencing chronic symptoms that are not the result of ongoing physiologic dysfunctions that occur during the initial onset of a concussion. The authors suggest that postconcussion syndrome should be considered as a constellation of disorders.

51. Leddy JJ, Cox JL, Baker JG, et al: Exercise treatment for postconcussion syndrome: A pilot study of changes in functional magnetic resonance imaging activation, physiology, and symptoms. *J Head Trauma Rehabil* 2013;28(4):241-249.

   Clinicians have found postconcussion syndrome challenging to treat, given the complexity and lack of a specific etiology around the chronicity of symptoms. The authors of this pilot study sought to understand how an aerobic exercise treatment may influence brain activation patterns, measured by functional MRI, in patients with post-concussion syndrome. Five females with postconcussion syndrome demonstrated functional MRI activation patterns similar to age- and sex-matched controls during a math task after completing two sessions of the Balke treadmill protocol. The results suggest a controlled progression of aerobic exercise may be beneficial at improving brain activation in patients with postconcussion syndrome.

52. Leddy JJ, Sandhu H, Sodhi V, Baker JG, Willer B: Rehabilitation of Concussion and Post-concussion Syndrome. *Sports Health* 2012;4(2):147-154.

   This comprehensive review on rehabilitation techniques for concussion symptoms and dysfunctions identified therapeutic benefits from certain types of therapies, such as cognitive behavioral and aerobic exercise therapies, when administered appropriately.

53. Andersen J, Courson RW, Kleiner DM, McLoda TA: National Athletic Trainers' Association Position Statement: Emergency Planning in Athletics. *J Athl Train* 2002;37(1):99-104.

54. Moser RS, Schatz P, Neidzwski K, Ott SD: Group versus individual administration affects baseline neurocognitive test performance. *Am J Sports Med* 2011;39(11):2325-2330.

   This study evaluated the differences in baseline neurocognitive testing in high school athletes tested in a group compared with an individual setting. Of the 331 athletes who completed baseline ImPACT testing, the 165 athletes who tested in a group setting demonstrated significantly lower scores in all four composites. The authors stressed the importance of ensuring athletes complete baseline testing in properly supervised and quiet testing environments.

55. Vaughan CG, Gerst EH, Sady MD, Newman JB, Gioia GA: The relation between testing environment and baseline performance in child and adolescent concussion assessment. *Am J Sports Med* 2014;42(7):1716-1723.

   When properly trained test administrators follow a standardized protocol and adequately supervise the testing environment, high school athletes can effectively complete baseline neurocognitive testing in a group setting. The results of this study demonstrated no significant differences between ImPACT scores for 313 athletes tested individually and 626 athletes tested in groups of 15.

56. Elbin RJ, Kontos AP, Kegel N, Johnson E, Burkhart S, Schatz P: Individual and combined effects of LD and ADHD on computerized neurocognitive concussion test performance: Evidence for separate norms. *Arch Clin Neuropsychol* 2013;28(5):476-484.

   Given the unknown potential influence learning disabilities and attention deficit disorders may have on baseline computerized neurocognitive testing, the authors of this study compared baseline scores between athletes with and without self-reported learning disabilities and attention deficit disorders. Athletes who self-reported either diagnosis or a combination of each demonstrated lower composite scores and reported a higher number of symptoms.

57. Jotwani V, Harmon KG: Postconcussion syndrome in athletes. *Curr Sports Med Rep* 2010;9(1):21-26.

58. Boden BP, Tacchetti RL, Cantu RC, Knowles SB, Mueller FO: Catastrophic head injuries in high school and college football players. *Am J Sports Med* 2007;35(7):1075-1081.

59. McCrory P, Berkovic S: Second impact syndrome. *Neurology* 1998;50(3):677-683.

60. Thomas M, Haas TS, Doerer JJ, et al: Epidemiology of sudden death in young, competitive athletes due to blunt trauma. *Pediatrics* 2011;128(1):e1-e8.

   The authors analyzed retrospectively collected data over a 30-year period with the aim of determining the epidemiology and frequency of sudden death in athletes age 21 years and younger. Blunt trauma resulted in an average of nine deaths per year, which the authors noted was significantly less than cardiovascular-related deaths. The head and neck were the most commonly involved areas, with football contributing the largest number of deaths.

61. McIntosh AS, Andersen TE, Bahr R, et al: Sports helmets now and in the future. *Br J Sports Med* 2011;45(16):1258-1265.

   The authors present a systematic review of the current literature on helmet design, helmet standards, and the constraints around creating a helmet to prevent concussions, and identified knowledge deficits in several areas and thus stressed the need for further research.

62. Benson BW, McIntosh AS, Maddocks D, Herring SA, Raftery M, Dvorák J: What are the most effective risk-reduction strategies in sport concussion? *Br J Sports Med* 2013;47(5):321-326.

   This comprehensive review presents evidence that demonstrates protective equipment and neck strengthening have not been proven to reduce the chance of concussion. The authors stress the need for well-designed, sport-specific, prospective studies on this topic.

63. Brooks A, Loud KJ, Brenner JS, et al; Council on Sports Medicine and Fitness: Reducing injury risk from body checking in boys' youth ice hockey. *Pediatrics* 2014;133(6):1151-1157.

64. Adler RH, Herring SA: Changing the culture of concussion: Education meets legislation. *PM R* 2011;3(10, Suppl 2)S468-S470.

65. Tomei KL, Doe C, Prestigiacomo CJ, Gandhi CD: Comparative analysis of state-level concussion legislation and review of current practices in concussion. *Neurosurg Focus* 2012;33(6):E11, 1-9.

   This study was a comparative analysis of 43 states with existing concussion legislation. Legislation was directed specifically toward youth and school-aged athletes, excluding athletes participating at the collegiate level. The targeted population, education and training of individuals, and criteria for removal and return to play vary significantly from state to state. Interestingly, no state required the athlete to complete formal education. Rather, responsibilities for athlete safety were placed on coaches, parents, and appropriate health care providers.

66. Covassin T, Elbin RJ, Sarmiento K: Educating coaches about concussion in sports: evaluation of the CDC's "Heads Up: concussion in youth sports" initiative. *J Sch Health* 2012;82(5):233-238.

As increasingly more states are enacting legislation to protect youth athletes from the consequences of concussion management, an increasing amount of responsibility is being placed on youth sport coaches, many of whom are volunteers. The results of this survey of 336 youth sport coaches support access to the Centers for Disease Control and Prevention's "Heads Up" tool kit for improved concussion awareness and education as well as response to concussions when they occur on the field.

67. Bagley AF, Daneshvar DH, Schanker BD, et al: Effectiveness of the SLICE Program for Youth Concussion Education. *Clin J Sport Med* 2012;22(5):385-389.

The SLICE program curriculum was shown to successfully improve concussion recognition and athletes' response in the event of a concussion injury during play when administered to elementary middle and high school students. Females and athletes older than 13 years demonstrated the greatest improvements between prepresentation and postpresentation assessments.

68. Mannings C, Kalynych C, Joseph MM, Smotherman C, Kraemer DF: Knowledge assessment of sports-related concussion among parents of children aged 5 years to 15 years enrolled in recreational tackle football. *J Trauma Acute Care Surg* 2014;77(3, suppl 1)S18-S22.

This study evaluated the results of a survey on concussion knowledge completed by parents with children playing youth tackle football. There were no parents who were able to correctly identify all signs and symptoms associated with a concussion, despite half of the parents reporting they had received some form of formal education on concussions.

69. Kerr ZY, Register-Mihalik JK, Marshall SW, Evenson KR, Mihalik JP, Guskiewicz KM: Disclosure and non-disclosure of concussion and concussion symptoms in athletes: Review and application of the socio-ecological framework. *Brain Inj* 2014;28(8):1009-1021.

The results of this literature review focused on the socio-ecological framework for disclosing concussion. Although the majority of research has been on the intrapersonal and interpersonal factors, gaps in the literature exist on the influence of policy levels on disclosure of concussion symptoms.

70. Register-Mihalik JK, Guskiewicz KM, McLeod TC, Linnan LA, Mueller FO, Marshall SW: Knowledge, attitude, and concussion-reporting behaviors among high school athletes: A preliminary study. *J Athl Train* 2013;48(5):645-653.

A survey of 167 high school athletes demonstrated that increased concussion knowledge was associated with increased reporting of symptoms to the school's medical staff or parents. However, the authors reported that 40% of concussions and 13% of bell-ringers are still unreported as a result of the athlete undervaluing the severity of the injury.

71. Register-Mihalik JK, Linnan LA, Marshall SW, Valovich McLeod TC, Mueller FO, Guskiewicz KM: Using theory to understand high school aged athletes' intentions to report sport-related concussion: Implications for concussion education initiatives. *Brain Inj* 2013;27(7-8):878-886.

The authors of this study sought to understand the challenges facing athletes when deciding whether or not to disclose concussion symptoms. In a sample of 167 high school athletes, athletes with a promoting attitude toward concussion reporting as well as the positive influences from coaches and teammates were identified as key factors for concussion reporting. This highlights the need to not only educate athletes about concussions, but suggests the need for a sporting environment that promotes and rewards reporters.

72. Cournoyer J, Tripp BL: Concussion knowledge in high school football players. *J Athl Train* 2014;49(5):654-658.

The authors of this cross-sectional study administered a survey to 334 varsity football athletes to determine the level of understanding high schoolers in Florida had on concussions following newly enacted concussion-education legislation. The results of this study suggest that concussion education on symptom identification and ultimately consequences of mismanagement should not be placed on the parents alone because 25% of athletes reported never discussing concussions with their parents and 60% correctly identified brain hemorrhage and death as possible consequences.

73. Bloodgood B, Inokuchi D, Shawver W, et al: Exploration of awareness, knowledge, and perceptions of traumatic brain injury among American youth athletes and their parents. *J Adolesc Health* 2013;53(1):34-39.

Educational endeavors aimed at increasing concussion knowledge and highlighting the importance of early identification of symptoms in high school and youth athletes as well as their parents are on the rise. The authors of this study surveyed 252 young athletes and 300 parents to identify current views and knowledge regarding concussion injuries. Certain subgroups, specifically parents of children age 10 to 13 years, athletes age 13 to 15 years, and mothers and parents who use the Internet several times a day, seem to have more awareness and concern regarding concussion injuries.

74. Chrisman SP, Quitiquit C, Rivara FP: Qualitative study of barriers to concussive symptom reporting in high school athletics. *J Adolesc Health* 2013;52(3):330-335.e3.

Educational endeavors aimed at increasing concussion knowledge and highlighting the importance of early identification of symptoms in high school athletes are on the rise. The authors of this qualitative focused group study of 50 high school athletes determined that although these athletes had appropriate knowledge regarding concussion injuries, withdrawal from play or lack of coach approachability seemed to be barriers toward reporting symptoms.

75. Sarmiento K, Mitchko J, Klein C, Wong S: Evaluation of the Centers for Disease Control and Prevention's concussion initiative for high school coaches: "Heads Up: Concussion in High School Sports". *J Sch Health* 2010;80(3):112-118.

High school coaches who completed the US Centers for Disease Control and Prevention's Heads Up toolkit between 2005 and 2006 were surveyed on their knowledge, attitudes, and behaviors toward concussion injuries. High school coaches found the toolkit to be comprehensive and useful, but noted their most difficult barrier in dealing with a concussion injury was overly competitive athletes and their parents who viewed a concussion as a weakness and disputed the potential risks associated with continued play.

76. Bouida W, Marghli S, Souissi S, et al: Prediction value of the Canadian CT head rule and the New Orleans criteria for positive head CT scan and acute neurosurgical procedures in minor head trauma: A multicenter external validation study. *Ann Emerg Med* 2013;61(5):521-527.

At the conclusion of this 3-year prospective study, the results demonstrated that the Canadian CT Head Rule had higher sensitivity and specificity of predicting neurosurgical intervention than the New Orleans Criteria in patients with mild head injuries. The authors suggest the use of such clinical decision rules may help reduce the frequency of unnecessary CT.

Chapter 51

Shoulder and Elbow Injuries in the Skeletally Immature Athlete

Eric W. Edmonds, MD

Abstract

The skeletally immature athlete is susceptible to a unique set of injuries in the shoulder and elbow compared with skeletally mature athletes; however, a few injuries are shared that bridge the developmental distance, irrespective of physeal patency. The injuries that occur in the skeletally immature shoulder and elbow can be defined as overuse, fracture, or instability (with the clear acknowledgment that these pathologies can overlap in this young population, especially regarding etiology, treatment, and outcomes). Recent developments in surgeons' understanding of the assessment of these injuries, treatment of these injuries, and even potential outcomes of injuries have been reported.

Keywords: childhood shoulder labrum and tendon tears; capitellar OCD; youth elbow ulnar collateral ligament injury; imaging of child elbow; labral tears; rotator cuff tears; osteochondritis dissecans

Introduction

Defining skeletal immaturity is an important place to begin the discussion of injuries in skeletally immature athletes. The proximal humeral physis closes between age 14 and 17 years in girls and between age 16 and 18 years in boys;[1] the distal humeral physes and proximal forearm physes have a wide range of variability that culminates in

Dr. Edmonds or an immediate family member is a member of a speakers' bureau or has made paid presentations on behalf of Arthrex and Orthopediatrics; has received research or institutional support from Inion; and serves as a board member, owner, officer, or committee member of the American Academy of Orthopaedic Surgeons, the American Orthopaedic Society for Sports Medicine; and the Pediatric Orthopaedic Society of North America.

overall closure at approximately age 16 years.[2] Therefore, most of this chapter discusses children younger than 16 years.

When young athletes sustain an injury that is considered to be a result of overuse, they are most often engaged in an activity involving overhead activity, including, but not limited to, baseball, softball, volleyball, tennis, gymnastics, and water polo.[3] However, the more traumatic injuries that involve fractures and dislocations appear to be associated with higher impact sports such as football, wrestling, and batting in baseball. An additional concern regarding the shoulder is a current trend that younger children (mean age, 9 years) sustain proximal humerus fractures, and teenagers (mean age, 15.5 years) sustain dislocations and separations.[3]

However, the spectrum of injury that can be seen within this young cohort goes beyond simple fracture and dislocation. In the shoulder, proximal humeral epiphysiolysis (Little Leaguer's shoulder), partial rotator cuff tears, internal impingement pathology with labral tears, and complications associated with multidirectional instability can all be seen.[1] Similarly, the elbow is susceptible to medial epicondylitis (Little Leaguer's elbow spectrum) and valgus overload syndrome, ruptures of the anterior bundle of the medial ulnar collateral ligament, capitellar osteochondritis dissecans (OCD), and Panner disease.[1] With many of these periphyseal upper extremity injuries, the skeletally immature athlete is at risk for growth disruption and deformity if the pathology is not appropriately identified and treated.[3]

Shoulder

Treatment of the shoulder requires an ability to assess pathology within the joint itself. A study that evaluated the intra-articular pathology seen arthroscopically in the skeletally immature athlete found that 94% of children treated using this approach had labral pathology present.[4] Moreover, almost one-fourth (23%) of the labral pathology involved the posterior labrum separately or in conjunction with superior extension. In this same cohort, 28% had a partial rotator cuff tendon tear that predominantly involved the supraspinatus tendon. Although complete rotator cuff tendon tears can occur in this age group, none were seen within the study population.

Imaging of the shoulder in the skeletally immature has not changed much in the past decade.[5] Plain radiographic films with contralateral images are recommended for the assessment of proximal humerus epiphysiolysis (also known as Little Leaguer's shoulder), and MRI is warranted to assess for injuries to the anterior and posterior labrum. Additionally, the use of magnetic resonance arthrography can help identify anterior labrum periosteal sleeve avulsions and humeral avulsions of the glenohumeral ligaments. Humeral avulsions of the glenohumeral ligaments can be missed during surgical assessment; therefore, preoperative identification is important. The evaluation of the shoulder via magnetic resonance arthrography still has limitations. A study assessing the ability to identify partial rotator cuff tendon tears in the adolescent cohort demonstrated that the diagnostic accuracy of magnetic resonance arthrography in this group was 72%.[6] A high false-negative rate suggested that the study could be specific, but not sensitive, for diagnosis.

Overuse Injuries

Most overuse injuries to the shoulder involve throwing or overhead activities, and most recent studies on this subject involve baseball.[7,8] A 2010 review highlighted some of the changes seen in overuse of the throwing arm in the skeletally immature.[7] With substantial time throwing, even in children as young as 8 years, an increase in external rotation and a decrease in internal rotation at the shoulder can be clinically identified. Humeral remodeling can occur throughout development until the physis closes. This remodeling can result in up to 15° of humeral retroversion at maturity compared with the contralateral side, either by forcing rotation or reducing the amount of normal rotational development. This change is considered by some studies to be beneficial to the mechanics of throwing, but for this chapter, it highlights the torsional force being applied to the proximal physis of the humerus. This force could, at least in part, result in epiphysiolysis.

Epiphysiolysis tends to peak between age 13 and 16 years in boys,[7] and the treatment is always nonsurgical. Although described in boys, there is no reason the condition might not develop in girls, especially now that girls are joining youth baseball leagues. These patients are prevented from throwing for a period of 6 weeks to 3 months, at which point a gradual throwing program is begun so long as they remain symptom free. Most throwing programs start by increasing the distance thrown (long-toss program), followed by a short-toss program that increases velocity. These programs are 90% successful in eliminating symptoms indefinitely as long as rotator cuff and periscapular muscle strengthening, capsular stretching exercises, and good throwing mechanics are emphasized.[7]

Although it is important to recognize epiphysiolysis and treat it appropriately to reduce the risk of physeal closure, it is even more important to educate families on how to avoid overusing the arm, thus preventing the injury. A 10-year prospective study was performed to help identify the risk factors associated with this injury.[8] Pitchers between 9 and 14 years old were evaluated, and the study found that pitching more than 100 innings within 1 calendar year was associated with a 3.5-fold higher risk of injuring the arm. Although a trend toward increased rates of injury in those who played both pitcher and catcher positions was noted, this was not significant, nor was the risk factor of throwing curveballs for those younger than 13 years. The best educational approach was to limit the number of innings pitched in 1 year and to encourage play at positions other than pitcher and catcher to reduce the risk of injury.

Fractures

Injuries to the osseous structures of the shoulder consist predominantly of proximal humerus fractures, clavicle fractures, and injuries associated with a Bankart lesion. Treatment of clavicle fractures in the skeletally immature patient is quite controversial and only one comparative study published in 2010 reported better radiographic results in the surgical cohort than in the nonsurgical cohort.[9] Two studies attempted to evaluate the potentially detrimental effects of leaving a displaced clavicle fracture unreduced. One study identified teenagers with a malunited clavicle fracture and tested them on a work simulator machine, using the uninjured shoulder as an internal control.[10] At a mean follow-up of 2 years, no differences were found in shoulder range of motion, but slight decreases were noted in maximal shoulder external rotation strength (8%; $P = 0.04$) and abduction endurance strength (11%; $P = 0.04$). However, all children returned to at least their preinjury level of sports participation. In a similar study performed on a slightly younger cohort using a different work simulator, no substantial difference was detected in abduction or adduction torque or in the power between affected and unaffected shoulders.[11] In addition, minimal effects were seen via the outcome questionnaire and only one child required corrective osteotomy. Further investigation will be required to determine whether or not the skeletally immature athlete with a displaced clavicle fracture will have any complications with or without surgical management.

© 2016 American Academy of Orthopaedic Surgeons

In contrast to the clavicle, substantially more information exists regarding the treatment of proximal humerus fractures and their ability to remodel over time. A recent study compared the outcomes of displaced proximal humerus fractures (Neer grade III or IV) treated with and without surgery.[12] This study found no difference in the occurrence of complications, rate of return to activity, or cosmetic satisfaction in a matched cohort of skeletally immature patients (Figure 1). However, a trend was noted for seeing less than desirable outcomes in the nonsurgical patients older than 12 years: for every 1-year increase in age at the time of fracture, the likelihood increased by a factor of 3.8 to have a less than desirable outcome.

The treatment has been updated for the adolescent apophysis avulsion injury of the lesser tuberosity, which is uncommon. Patients treated with either suture anchors or transosseous sutures can achieve pain relief and expect full return of internal rotation strength, with a return to sports activity at a mean of 4.4 months postoperatively, although return of external rotation strength can be delayed until 6 months postoperatively.[13]

Instability

Many adolescent athletes at the cusp of skeletal maturity will preferentially dislocate their shoulder rather than sustain a fracture. A clear trend is noted in the North American literature to treat patients of all ages with arthroscopic stabilization rather than with open surgical intervention.[14] A recent multicenter study evaluated the potential complications associated with shoulder arthroscopy in children.[15] Minor complications reported in this population were consistent with readmission for pain control, broken pain pump catheter, injury to the cephalic vein, allergic reactions to skin prep, transient dysesthesias, headaches, bronchitis, syncope, transient hypotension, and uvula swelling. An additional procedure, outside of the planned protocol, was performed in 2.5% of patients for these minor complications.

Regarding the actual treatment of adolescent traumatic anterior instability of the shoulder, a recent level III study compared open and arthroscopic treatment in this age group.[16] In 99 subjects (approximately two thirds were treated arthroscopically), no substantial difference was found between the two cohorts, and a 21% redislocation rate was noted in this population. Irrespective of surgical technique, a survival curve demonstrated that the repairs have a 2-year survival rate of 86% and a 5-year survival rate of only 49%. This young population, in contrast to the historic results seen in the adult population, does not seem to have successful outcomes regarding shoulder instability. The reasons for this increased recurrent instability rate have not been proved, but it is possible that the

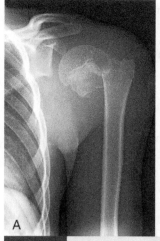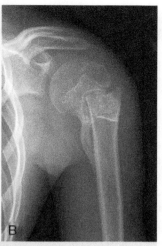

Figure 1 AP radiographs of a displaced proximal humerus fracture sustained after a fall in an 11-year-old boy. **A,** View obtained after fall. **B,** View obtained after 6 weeks of nonsurgical treatment demonstrates abundant callous and remodeling. (Copyright San Diego Pediatric Orthopedics, San Diego, CA.)

young age of the cohort has a tendency toward augmented levels of physical activity (both a greater rate of activity and an increased level of risk behavior).

Even the presence of benign hypermobility can be the source of pathology and injury in the young shoulder.[1,17] In addition to labral tears, adolescent shoulders appear to be susceptible to partial rotator cuff tendon tears, in a mechanism consistent with internal impingement. A 2013 study demonstrated evidence of 53 teenagers (15 girls, 38 boys) with partial rotator cuff tears sustained from overhead sports, including a large cohort of female water polo players. Nonsurgical management failed in almost 60% of tears; but, during surgery, 70% of those tears in which initial physical therapy treatment failed were found to have associated pathology, including labral tears.[17]

Elbow

As with the shoulder, the evaluation of injury in the skeletally immature elbow has been updated several times during the past 5 years. The best approach to analyzing the immature elbow in these athletes is to perform a segmental analysis of the lateral, medial, and posterior structures.[18] This allows assessment of the variety of potentially injured structures (bone, ligaments, cartilage, physes, and apophyses) in a systematic manner with less risk of missing a potential site of pathology. The injuries most pertinent to the orthopaedic surgeon includes OCD, Little Leaguer's elbow (medial epicondylitis), medial epicondyle fractures, and ulnar collateral ligament injuries.[19] Many of these injuries can be included under the umbrella of valgus overload: tension is placed on the medial (and potentially, posterior) structures and compression is placed on the lateral (and potentially, posterior) structures.

A 2010 study on assessing changes in the elbows of children with a known throwing history and who were experiencing medial-side pain demonstrated a difference in the ability of plain radiography and MRI to help identify the source of pain.[20] Although a few children demonstrated slight hypertrophy (widening) of the medial epicondyle apophysis and fragmentation, most MRIs demonstrated those same changes as well as edema within the flexor-prontator muscle mass tendon, strain to the ulnar collateral ligament, and edema within the apophysis without widening. However, even with these additional findings noted on MRI, the clinical management was not altered.

Overuse Injuries

Although the medial structures get the most attention regarding overuse, recent publications have focused on the lateral side of the elbow and the treatment of capitellar OCD.[21-24] Currently, a wide array of techniques seem to be available for the treatment of symptomatic elbow OCD.

In 2010, two studies were published regarding the best treatment of the skeletally immature patient. One study indicated that arthroscopic débridement alone had good midterm outcomes (mean, 3.6 years) regarding symptoms of pain and function.[21] This assessment was based on the ability to return to sport and the mean Disabilities of the Arm, Shoulder and Hand score (8.6 of 100), irrespective of the lesion grade. However, the other study suggested that the removal of loose bodies alone was insufficient and that establishing a good lateral shoulder to the capitellum was more important.[22] An osteochondral autograft from the rib was used to reconstruct this aspect of the capitellum when required. Substantially improved outcomes were reported using a modified elbow rating system, but some children did not return to sport and the overall cohort had a reduced arc of motion.

Other articles have been published examining different surgical treatments in this skeletally immature cohort. In 2012, an algorithmic treatment for OCD lesions was implemented that included retroarticular (transhumeral) drilling, fragment fixation, and débridement with good, but not excellent, results.[23] In this small series, 20% of elbows required a second surgery to manage symptomatic OCD. In contrast to the 2010 study on rib autograft utilization,[22] the 2012 series[23] reported an improvement in the postoperative elbow arc of motion, predominately with extension. In 2013, the results of a slightly larger series[24] agreed with earlier publications that lateral-edge OCD had worse outcomes, but also agreed with the more recent 2012 publication that not every child does well after OCD treatment. This latest study used drilling to stimulate healing in patients in the stable OCD group and incorporated an osteochondral autograft (essentially, a mosaicplasty) to secure the unstable lesions. The arc of motion was improved postoperatively, but only 80% of children returned to sports at 1 year and 50% of the lateral-edge OCD cases required reoperation. The definite treatment of capitellar OCD in the skeletally immature is still undetermined, but these recent publications indicate a need to identify the appropriate treatment of the specific OCD (location and stability occupy divergent paths in an algorithm).

Fractures

The treatment of fractures of the humeral medial epicondyle has been debated since the 1970s, but some important developments have occurred within the past 5 years. In 2010, two papers highlighted a problem in performing accurate radiographic assessment of this fracture. The first study reported poor interobserver and intraobserver reliability in assessing fracture displacement.[25] With disagreement defined as a measurement difference of 2 mm or more, the study disagreed with 26% of its own measurements, with 54% of its AP radiographic measurements, with 87% of its lateral radiographic measurements, and with 64% of its oblique radiographic measurements. Some recommendations were provided regarding the best methodology to keep measurements consistent, but the amount of perceived displacement should not be a criterion for choosing treatment of these fractures. The other study suggested that although all literature on medial epicondyle fractures uses AP radiographs, new evidence using three-dimensional CT displaces this modality as the primary methodology for measuring displacement.[26] When measuring displacement on plain radiography and CT, significantly different findings were reported (Table 1), and AP and lateral radiographs were not sufficient or accurate enough to measure medial epicondyle fracture displacement. Therefore, these two papers potentially negate any results or conclusions from outcome papers published before 2010.

In response, a study published in 2013 evaluated the capability of the internal oblique radiographs to accurately help define the displacement of humeral medial epicondyle fractures. Observers were 60% accurate in predicting the true displacement on internal oblique films (when position was controlled at 45° and trigonometry was applied to the measured displacement).[27] This methodology is time-consuming and still not accurate, implying that better methods for defining displacement are still needed

© 2016 American Academy of Orthopaedic Surgeons

for this fracture type. A recent cadaver study suggests that the use of a new axial image can provide improved understanding of the true displacement[28] (Figure 2).

Despite not having a validated, accurate, and low-radiation methodology for determining fracture displacement, some data are available regarding the outcomes of treatment. Keeping in mind that the results of past studies using AP radiographs to define criteria for treatment should be questioned, the outcomes from the treatment of children with minimally displaced fractures, but not associated with a dislocation event, can potentially be used. In a 2013 study comparing surgical and nonsurgical treatment with a minimum 2-year follow-up, no differences were demonstrated in Disabilities of the Arm, Shoulder and Hand scores between the treatment cohorts.[29] This study identified that one half of each cohort required physical therapy and that one half of surgical cases reported some transient numbness. To date, this is the only comparative study with outcomes between treatment groups in the skeletally immature patient with a medial epicondyle fracture.

Instability

Potentially related to overuse injuries, elbow instability in the skeletally immature group is more commonly

Table 1			
Measurements of Minimally Displaced Medial Epicondyle Fractures			
Plane of Displacement	**Radiograph**	**3D CT**	**_P_ Value**
Coronal (AP)	3.5 mm	0.3 mm	< 0.001
Sagittal (lateral)	0.9 mm	8.8 mm	< 0.001
Internal oblique	6.6 mm	8.8 mm	0.037

Substantial differences can be seen in measurements between perceived displacement on AP radiographs and actual measurements on three-dimensional (3D) CT scans of minimally displaced medial epicondyle fractures.

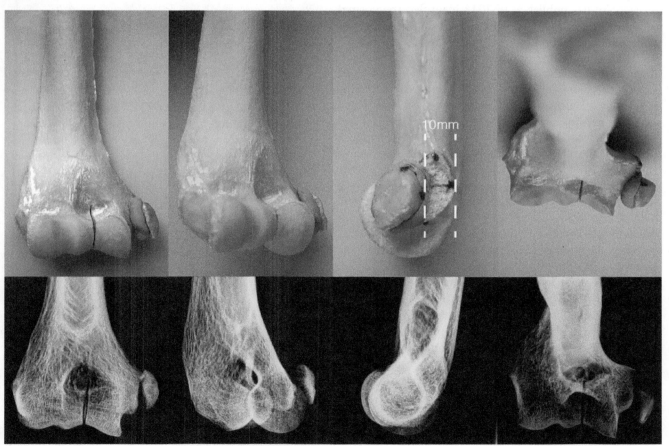

AP   Internal Oblique   Lateral   Distal Humerus Axial

Figure 2 Radiographs and photographs obtained from cadavers demonstrate the elbow views more commonly obtained for medial epicondyle fracture assessment. Note the inability to accurately assess displacement that follows the muscle vector pull. (Copyright San Diego Pediatric Orthopedics, San Diego, CA.)

associated with a traumatic event. Injuries can occur either medially[30] or laterally.[31] A large study on the reconstruction of medial ulnar collateral ligament tears (with subcutaneous ulnar nerve transposition) reported that valgus stability could be restored and 83% of overhead athletes returned to competition.[30] Perhaps more importantly, at a minimum 2-year follow-up, complications were found in 20% of the cohort, 4% of which were major (ulnar nerve injuries, medial epicondyle fractures, and reoperation for osteophyte formation). Posterolateral rotatory instability is much less common. A series of nine children reported that posterolateral rotatory instability was often diagnosed in a delayed manner, and that any child with a contracture of unclear etiology should be considered for this pathology.[31] Surgical correction is technically difficult (especially considering that often the surgery was initially being performed for a contracture release), and ligament reconstruction can risk injury to the lateral physes and apophyses. Therefore, preoperative identification of the injury is paramount for safe treatment.

Two studies published in 2013 identified the normal attachment of the anterior bundle of the medial ulnar collateral ligament relative to the apophysis of the medial epicondyle.[32,33] Both publications report that the ligament inserts on the apophysis or epicondyle itself, and not on the condyle (Figure 3). The importance of this is not yet fully defined, but it could play a role in the decision-making process for treating displaced medial epicondyle fractures (especially if the epicondyle fracture occurred secondary to an elbow dislocation event).

Summary

The skeletally immature athlete is at risk for injury in the shoulder or elbow through overuse, fracture, or instability. Most recent publications have highlighted the understanding of radiographic assessment or lack thereof, and have emphasized advancements in understanding treatment of this young, extremely active group. Surgeons can translate adult pathology to the skeletally immature, but they need to be cognizant of the physes and apophyses around the shoulder and elbow and how they play a role in injury. MRI appears to be a good modality to help discover underlying injuries in this age group when contralateral plain radiography is otherwise negative.

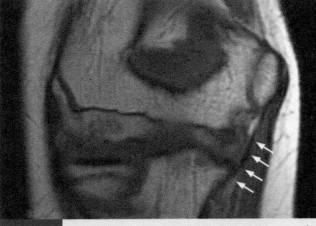

Figure 3 Coronal T1-weighted MRI demonstrates normal attachment of the anterior bundle of the medial ulnar collateral ligament (arrows) on the medial epicondyle ossification. (Copyright San Diego Pediatric Orthopedics, San Diego, CA.)

Key Study Points

- Using contralateral plain radiographs can help identify injuries to the physis or apophyses of either the shoulder or elbow in the skeletally immature. MRI can safely assess the injury if plain radiographs are not helpful.

- The treatment of capitellar OCD is evolving, but the lateral shoulder (buttress) of the capitellum appears to be important to overall success in treatment.

- The treatment of clavicle fractures and medial epicondyle fractures is still being evaluated and the definitive care in the skeletally immature is still being debated.

- Shoulder instability surgery in the adolescent cohort may not result in the long-term success seen in the young adult population, perhaps because of the increased activity level in this age group.

- Ulnar collateral ligament reconstruction has good outcomes for a large proportion of the young athlete population, but families should be aware that approximately 20% may experience complications, require additional surgery, or not be able to return to a higher level of play.

Annotated References

1. Chen FS, Diaz VA, Loebenberg M, Rosen JE: Shoulder and elbow injuries in the skeletally immature athlete. *J Am Acad Orthop Surg* 2005;13(3):172-185.

2. Maylahn DJ, Fahey JJ: Fractures of the elbow in children; review of three hundred consecutive cases. *J Am Med Assoc* 1958;166(3):220-228.

3. Dashe J, Roocroft JH, Bastrom TP, Edmonds EW: Spectrum of shoulder injuries in skeletally immature patients. *Orthop Clin North Am* 2013;44(4):541-551.

   This epidemiologic study of all children presenting to a single institution describes the spectrum of shoulder pathology seen, ranging from fractures to tumors. Level of evidence: IV.

4. Edmonds EW, Roocroft JH, Parikh SN: Spectrum of operative childhood intra-articular shoulder pathology. *J Child Orthop* 2014;8(4):337-340.

   This multicenter study evaluated the pathology spectrum seen in skeletally immature patients treated with shoulder arthroscopy. Level of evidence: IV.

5. May MM, Bishop JY: Shoulder injuries in young athletes. *Pediatr Radiol* 2013;43(Suppl 1):S135-S140.

   Increased levels of competition in younger athletes has resulted in more shoulder injuries, and advances in cross-sectional imaging is important in guiding treatment. Level of evidence: IV.

6. Edmonds EW, Eisner EA, Kruk PG, Roocroft JH, Dwek JD: Diagnostic shortcomings of magnetic resonance arthrography to evaluate partial rotator cuff tears in adolescents. *J Pediatr Orthop* 2015;35(4):407-411.

   In this study, diagnostic accuracy of magnetic resonance arthrography in adolescent partial rotator cuff injuries was 72%; therefore, clinical suspicion is an important factor in determining management. Level of evidence: III.

7. Leonard J, Hutchinson MR: Shoulder injuries in skeletally immature throwers: Review and current thoughts. *Br J Sports Med* 2010;44(5):306-310.

   This review reported that although pediatric athletes sustain soft-tissue injuries, growth plate injuries are much more common. Therefore, injury prevention should target proper throwing mechanics and reduced exposure. Level of evidence: IV.

8. Fleisig GS, Andrews JR, Cutter GR, et al: Risk of serious injury for young baseball pitchers: A 10-year prospective study. *Am J Sports Med* 2011;39(2):253-257.

   In this study, risk of injury to young pitchers over 10 years of activity was 5%. Reduction of innings pitched per year can be beneficial. Throwing curveballs does not appear to directly affect risk of injury. Level of evidence: III.

9. Vander Have KL, Perdue AM, Caird MS, Farley FA: Operative versus nonoperative treatment of midshaft clavicle fractures in adolescents. *J Pediatr Orthop* 2010;30(4):307-312.

   This retrospective review of adolescents treated surgically (versus nonsurgically) reported that surgically treated clavicle fractures experienced significantly faster radiographic union and that alignment and length were restored better, placing patients in the nonsurgical cohort at risk for malunion. Level of evidence: III.

10. Schulz J, Moor M, Roocroft J, Bastrom TP, Pennock AT: Functional and radiographic outcomes of nonoperative treatment of displaced adolescent clavicle fractures. *J Bone Joint Surg Am* 2013;95(13):1159-1165.

    In this study, no substantial deficiencies were found in adolescent malunited clavicle fractures with intermediate follow-up, as measured using functional test results and patient-derived outcome questionnaire. Level of evidence: IV.

11. Bae DS, Shah AS, Kalish LA, Kwon JY, Waters PM: Shoulder motion, strength, and functional outcomes in children with established malunion of the clavicle. *J Pediatr Orthop* 2013;33(5):544-550.

    Skeletally immature patients with malunited clavicle fractures in this study did not have clinically meaningful loss of shoulder motion or abduction/adduction strength, and indications for surgery need to be developed for this age group. Level of evidence: IV.

12. Chaus GW, Carry PM, Pishkenari AK, Hadley-Miller N: versus nonoperative treatment of displaced proximal humeral physeal fractures: A matched cohort. *J Pediatr Orthop* 2015;35(3):234-239.

    This matched cohort study demonstrated no differences in function, complications, return to full activity, or cosmesis of children treated either with or without surgery for proximal humerus physeal fractures. However, a trend for less-than-desirable outcomes was noted in children older than 12 years treated nonsurgically. Level of evidence: III.

13. Vezeridis PS, Bae DS, Kocher MS, Kramer DE, Yen YM, Waters PM: Surgical treatment for avulsion injuries of the humeral lesser tuberosity apophysis in adolescents. *J Bone Joint Surg Am* 2011;93(20):1882-1888.

    High-energy injuries sustained during sports can cause avulsion fractures of the humeral lesser tuberosity, and a degree of clinical suspicion is necessary for diagnosis so that surgical intervention can be performed in a timely manner. Level of evidence: IV.

14. Zhang AL, Montgomery SR, Ngo SS, Hame SL, Wang JC, Gamradt SC: Arthroscopic versus open shoulder stabilization: Current practice patterns in the United States. *Arthroscopy* 2014;30(4):436-443.

    Since 2009, the incidence of shoulder stabilization surgery in the United States has doubled and almost 90% are performed via arthroscopy. Level of evidence: IV.

15. Edmonds EW, Lewallen LW, Murphy M, Dahm D, McIntosh AL: Peri-operative complications in pediatric and adolescent shoulder arthroscopy. *J Child Orthop* 2014;8(4):341-344.

    Using very strict criteria, this study reported a 2.5% rate of major complications associated with shoulder arthroscopy, most of which involved pain and complications with anesthesia compared with direct surgical complications. Level of evidence: IV.

16. Shymon SJ, Roocroft J, Edmonds EW: Traumatic anterior instability of the pediatric shoulder: A comparison of arthroscopic and open bankart repairs. *J Pediatr Orthop* 2015;35(1):1-6.

    In this comparison of arthroscopic and open treatment of anterior traumatic shoulder instability, no substantial differences in outcomes were seen. However, the rate of redislocation was 21% in this adolescent cohort with a 5-year survival of only 49%, irrespective of technique. Level of evidence: III.

17. Eisner EA, Roocroft JH, Moor MA, Edmonds EW: Partial rotator cuff tears in adolescents: Factors affecting outcomes. *J Pediatr Orthop* 2013;33(1):2-7.

    This study reported that isolated partial articular-side rotator cuff tendon injuries can be treated successfully with physical therapy; however, in the presence of associated pathology, surgical intervention is often needed. Level of evidence: III.

18. Dwek JR, Chung CB: A systematic method for evaluation of pediatric sports injuries of the elbow. *Pediatr Radiol* 2013;43(Suppl 1):S120-S128.

    This study determined that the pediatric elbow is best assessed by compartmentalizing the radiographic evaluation to the lateral, medial, and posterior compartments, thereby separately considering all injuries associated with the common forces experienced at each location during sports participation. Level of evidence: V.

19. Zellner B, May MM: Elbow injuries in the young athlete—an orthopedic perspective. *Pediatr Radiol* 2013;43(Suppl 1):S129-S134.

    In this report, valgus overload caused most elbow injuries in the child athlete, with capitellar OCD, medial epicondyle injuries and ulnar collateral ligament injuries become more frequent. Level of evidence: IV.

20. Wei AS, Khana S, Limpisvasti O, Crues J, Podesta L, Yocum LA: Clinical and magnetic resonance imaging findings associated with Little League elbow. *J Pediatr Orthop* 2010;30(7):715-719.

    This study reported that MRI demonstrates more pathology than plain radiography in childhood baseball players, but the findings do not appear to change clinical management. Level of evidence: III.

21. Schoch B, Wolf BR: Osteochondritis dissecans of the capitellum: Minimum 1-year follow-up after arthroscopic debridement. *Arthroscopy* 2010;26(11):1469-1473.

    In this study, the treatment of capitellar OCD in children with isolated arthroscopic débridement resulted in improved outcome scores, but also a clear risk of reduced activity level secondary to the elbow. Level of evidence: IV.

22. Mihara K, Suzuki K, Makiuchi D, Nishinaka N, Yamaguchi K, Tsutsui H: Surgical treatment for osteochondritis dissecans of the humeral capitellum. *J Shoulder Elbow Surg* 2010;19(1):31-37.

    The treatment of capitellar OCD in children with cartilage restoration, especially reconstruction of the lateral margin, results in improved functional scores, but also results in overall reduction in the postoperative total arc of the elbow. Level of evidence: IV.

23. Tis JE, Edmonds EW, Bastrom T, Chambers HG: Short-term results of arthroscopic treatment of osteochondritis dissecans in skeletally immature patients. *J Pediatr Orthop* 2012;32(3):226-231.

    The treatment of capitellar OCD in children with arthroscopically assisted débridement and transhumeral drilling of the lesion had good short-term outcomes for resolution if the lesion was stable, but fixation and persistent issues existed if the overlying cartilage was unstable. Level of evidence: IV.

24. Kosaka M, Nakase J, Takahashi R, et al: Outcomes and failure factors in surgical treatment for osteochondritis dissecans of the capitellum. *J Pediatr Orthop* 2013;33(7):719-724.

    The treatment of capitellar OCD in children with osteochondral peg fixation and osteochondral autograft transplantation can improve outcome scores, but success is inversely related to lesion size. Level of evidence: IV.

25. Pappas N, Lawrence JT, Donegan D, Ganley T, Flynn JM: Intraobserver and interobserver agreement in the measurement of displaced humeral medial epicondyle fractures in children. *J Bone Joint Surg Am* 2010;92(2):322-327.

    Intra- and interobserver agreement is poor in measuring humeral medial epicondyle fracture displacement on conventional radiographs. Level of evidence: IV.

26. Edmonds EW: How displaced are "nondisplaced" fractures of the medial humeral epicondyle in children? Results of a three-dimensional computed tomography analysis. *J Bone Joint Surg Am* 2010;92(17):2785-2791.

    Standard radiographs are not sufficient or accurate enough to measure the medial displacement of medial humeral epicondylar fractures because displacement occurs in the anterior direction. Level of evidence: I.

27. Gottschalk HP, Bastrom TP, Edmonds EW: Reliability of internal oblique elbow radiographs for measuring displacement of medial epicondyle humerus fractures: A cadaveric study. *J Pediatr Orthop* 2013;33(1):26-31.

    Using a standard 45° internal oblique radiograph of the elbow can help determine the displacement of medial humerus epicondyle fractures when the measurement is

© 2016 American Academy of Orthopaedic Surgeons

multiplied by 1.4, with good observer reliability. Level of evidence: II.

28. Souder CD, Farnsworth CL, McNeil NP, Bomar JD, Edmonds EW: The Distal Humerus Axial View: Assessment of Displacement in Medial Epicondyle Fractures. *J Pediatr Orthop* 2015;35(5):449-454.

    This cadaver study demonstrated improved accuracy of measuring the displacement of medial epicondyle humerus fractures using a newly described axial image compared with the standard views of the elbow. Level of evidence: II.

29. Lawrence JT, Patel NM, Macknin J, et al: Return to competitive sports after medial epicondyle fractures in adolescent athletes: Results of operative and nonoperative treatment. *Am J Sports Med* 2013;41(5):1152-1157.

    This retrospective comparison reported no difference in outcomes between surgical or nonsurgical management for medial epicondyle humerus fractures. However, evidence exists that fractures associated with a dislocation can be best treated surgically. Level of evidence: IV.

30. Cain EL Jr, Andrews JR, Dugas JR, et al: Outcome of ulnar collateral ligament reconstruction of the elbow in 1281 athletes: Results in 743 athletes with minimum 2-year follow-up. *Am J Sports Med* 2010;38(12):2426-2434.

    Four-fifths of adolescents treated with ulnar collateral ligament reconstruction and subcutaneous ulnar nerve

transposition returned to their previous level of competition or higher in less than 1 year with stability. Level of evidence: IV.

31. Lattanza LL, Goldfarb CA, Smucny M, Hutchinson DT: Clinical presentation of posterolateral rotatory instability of the elbow in children. *J Bone Joint Surg Am* 2013;95(15):e105.

    This study reported that posterolateral rotatory instability can occur in children, and the most common clinical finding is elbow contracture. Level of evidence: IV.

32. Larsen N, Moisan A, Witte D, et al: Medial ulnar collateral ligament origin in children and adolescents: An MRI anatomic study. *J Pediatr Orthop* 2013;33(6):664-666.

    This MRI study demonstrated the insertion of the anterior bundle of the medial ulnar collateral ligament to be on the medial epicondyle (mean, 3.1 mm medial to the physis). Level of evidence: IV.

33. Zell M, Dwek JR, Edmonds EW: Origin of the medial ulnar collateral ligament on the pediatric elbow. *J Child Orthop* 2013;7(4):323-328.

    This MRI study on the anterior bundle of the medial ulnar collateral ligament found it to insert at a mean of 3.0 mm medial to the physis and that boys had a wider ulnar collateral ligament than girls (4.05 mm versus 3.72 mm). Level of evidence: IV.

Chapter 52

Strength Training and Conditioning in Young Athletes

Tracy L. Zaslow, MD, FAAP, CAQSM

Abstract

Strength training programs may be implemented as part of a comprehensive physical activity program and can provide many benefits to the entire range of youth when implemented properly. It is important for sports medicine physicians to have an understanding of strength training and its common misconceptions, and the health benefits of and current evidence-based recommendations regarding strength training during childhood and adolescence.

Keywords: youth; adolescents; young athlete; strength training; weight training; resistance training

Introduction

The current trends for children's physical activity include a wide spectrum from the high-level athlete at risk for overuse injury and overtraining to the inactive child at risk for obesity and long-term health problems. Strength training programs can provide many benefits to the entire spectrum of youth when implemented properly. This chapter defines strength training, discusses common misconceptions, highlights the health benefits of and reviews current evidence-based recommendations regarding strength training during childhood and adolescence.

Physical Activity and Strength Training

Physical activity is essential for normal growth and development in children and a physically active lifestyle

Neither Dr. Zaslow nor any immediate family member has received anything of value from or has stock or stock options held in a commercial company or institution related directly or indirectly to the subject of this chapter.

sets the foundation for lifelong activity and disease prevention.[1] The World Health Organization recognizes physical inactivity as the fourth-leading risk factor for global mortality for noncommunicable diseases.[2] Currently it is recommended that children and adolescents (age range, 6 to 17 years) participate in 60 minutes or more of physical activity per day.[3] Physical activity guidelines recommend that age-appropriate physical activity include: aerobic activity of 60 minutes or more of moderate- to vigorous-intensity physical activity (this can include either moderate-intensity aerobic activity such as brisk walking, or vigorous-intensity activity such as running; and strength training that should incorporate vigorous-intensity activities, including those that strengthen muscle and bone, at least three times per week (for this age group, bone-loading activities can be performed as part of playing games, running, turning or jumping).[2]

Strength (or resistance) training refers to a specialized method of conditioning whereby an individual is working against a wide range of resistance loads to enhance health, fitness, and performance.[4] Resistance training includes exercises using body weight, weight machines, free weights (barbells and dumbbells), elastic bands, and medicine balls. Resistance training should not be confused with weight lifting, which involves explosive but highly controlled movements that require technical skill.[5] Guidelines for youth strength training have been provided by multiple organizations including the American Academy of Pediatrics Council on Sports Medicine and Fitness, the National Strength and Conditioning Association, the American College of Sports Medicine, the American Medical Society for Sports Medicine, the American Orthopaedic Society for Sports Medicine, and the National Athletic Trainers Association. Recommendations are summarized throughout this chapter.

Is strength training safe and effective for children and adolescents? Previously, strength training was discouraged in young athletes because of currently unsupported concerns regarding growth plate injury, flexibility impairment, and presumed ineffectiveness. Adverse effects of strength training programs on growth have not been demonstrated in children as young as 6 years.[6] Decreased flexibility has only been confirmed in one study that incorporated soccer agility training with strength training;[7] other studies have demonstrated improved[8,9] or unchanged flexibility outcomes.[10] Additionally, prior concerns were based on limited injury rate data with weight lifting or weight equipment that did not account for proper supervision, proper use of weight equipment, and type of training. Previous studies examining acute resistance training injuries[11] have highlighted the fact that such injuries occur primarily with the implementation of inappropriate training load, supervision by unqualified instructors, or without adequate supervision.[12] Strength training was not previously recommended because the development of muscle strength was believed to be impossible without circulating androgen levels before puberty; however, more recent strength training studies using programs of adequate intensity and duration have demonstrated strength gains substantially greater than those expected from normal growth and maturation.[13,14]

Ultimately, substantial scientific evidence has established that strength training provides health, performance, and injury prevention benefits for children and adolescents[4,15,16] Because muscular strength is an essential component of motor skill performance,[17] developing competence and confidence to perform resistance exercise during growth years can have important long-term implications for health fitness and performance.

Health Benefits of Strength Training

Physical activity is essential for normal growth and development through childhood and adolescence. Participation in age-appropriate fitness programs can improve cardiovascular health, aid weight management, strengthen bone, improve psychosocial well-being, enhance motors skills, and prevent sports-related injury. Developing confidence, appropriate strength, and competence to perform fundamental motor skills through activities that consolidate skill and health-related fitness can also provide the foundation to maximize the efficacy of neuromuscular conditioning during preadolescence with long-term implications for health, fitness, and sports performance.[18] Additionally, the inclusion of an appropriately supervised strength training program during physical education classes does not have any adverse effects on after-school performance in adolescent athletes.[19]

Cardiovascular Health

With increasing rates of youth obesity, resistance training is an important tool to potentially improve healthy body composition. Traditionally, youth with obesity have been encouraged to participate in aerobic activities; however, excess weight limits their ability to perform high-impact physical activity (such as running) and increases the risk for musculoskeletal overuse injuries. Additionally, youth with obesity often lack the motor skills and confidence to pursue rigorous physical activity. Therefore, resistance training can be an excellent entry point for this population to enable them to build the strength, skills, and fitness to enable further pursuit of more intense exercise.[20]

Several studies demonstrated that children and adolescents with obesity or at risk for obesity and who participated in resistance or circuit (combined resistance and aerobic training) programs improved their body composition.[4] Resistance training programs have been shown to not only decrease body fat but substantially increase insulin sensitivity in adolescent males at risk for obesity.[21] Increased insulin sensitivity remained substantial after adjustment for changes in total body fat and total lean mass, indicating resistance training may have resulted in qualitative skeletal muscle changes, enhancing insulin activity.

Although no direct correlation exists between regular physical activity and reducing blood pressure in normotensive youth, limited data suggest that resistance training using submaximal loads can be an effective intervention for hypertensive adolescents.[22]

The effects of resistance training on blood lipoproteins in children and adolescents are not well documented. Resistance training has been shown to have a positive effect on blood lipid profile in children and adolescents when compared with an inactive group.[4,23] However, recommendations to improve blood lipid profiles in youth with dyslipidemia emphasizes the importance of a comprehensive health program that includes regular physical activity, nutrition education, and behavioral counseling.[24]

Bone Health

Previously, important and likely inappropriate concerns existed regarding potential damage to growth plates from resistance training and high-impact exercise; however, resistance training has not been shown to have a detrimental effect on linear growth in children and adolescents.[25] Not only are these concerns not supported by the medical literature, but these traditional fears have actually been replaced by evidence indicating that the ideal time to build bone mass is childhood and is achieved by participating in weight-bearing activities.[26,27] Further evidence indicates that mechanical stress applied to developing growth plates from appropriate resistance training with moderate- to high-intensity resistance exercise promotes bone growth and formation to optimize bone mineral accrual during

© 2016 American Academy of Orthopaedic Surgeons

childhood and adolescence.[28-30] Ultimately, although bone mass is influenced by genetics, engaging in regular resistance training in conjunction with adequate nutritional intake (calcium, vitamin D, and calories) promotes normal bone formation and growth and can maximize bone mineral density during childhood and adolescence.[27,31] Developing healthy regular physical activity habits promotes continuation of these habits into adulthood and ultimately could reduce the risk of developing adult diseases later in life.

Psychosocial Health

The medical literature examining the psychological benefits of strength training is sparse and findings are equivocal. Initial studies did not demonstrate resistance training–induced psychologic benefits for healthy youth[11]; however, other studies have demonstrated improvements in psychologic well-being,[32] mood, and self-appraisal[13] in youth who engaged in physical activity programs that included resistance training. Further research indicates that self-concept and self-perception are related to an individual's physical activity level.[33-35] Specific studies evaluating self-concept and self-perception with specific resistance training programs also demonstrated improvements.[36,37] Overall, age-appropriate resistance training focused on enjoyment and self-improvement positively affects the psychologic well-being of youth.

However, intense training with excessive pressure to perform at levels beyond their ability and/or without appropriate rest intervals, can negatively affect youth. Furthermore, inappropriate coaching, unethical training practices, or emphasis on lean physique can result in abuse of performance-enhancing drugs,[38] restrictive eating behaviors,[39] or burnout (overtraining syndrome).[4,40]

Injury Risk

Resistance training programs that are developmentally appropriate and well supervised can be an excellent tool to decrease injury. Children actually have a lower risk of resistance training–related injuries such as strains and sprains than adults;[41] however, appropriate supervision with attention to postural alignment and technical competency is essential. Physical inactivity is a known risk factor for activity-related injury;[41] thus, youth who regularly participate in age-appropriate fitness programs that include resistance exercise may be less likely to sustain injury. Building this essential foundation of physical fitness is even more important in sedentary youth whose musculoskeletal fitness may be ill-prepared for the demands of recreational games and sports practice.[12,42]

Additionally, for the highly competitive athlete, incorporating appropriate resistance training programs into regular conditioning has been shown to decrease injury risk in multiple sports including soccer, football, and rugby.[43,44] Strength training programs have been implemented to prevent specific overuse injuries such as rotator cuff and scapular stabilization for overhead throwing athletes and quadriceps/hamstring exercises for running/sprinting athletes. Well-supervised comprehensive resistance training programs designed to treat abnormal biomechanics that develop during adolescence, especially in female athletes, have demonstrated efficacy for diminishing injury rates (specifically, anterior cruciate ligament injury in female athletes).[45,46] Resistance training programs implemented early in preadolescent girls can induce an increase in muscle power, strength, and coordination that mirrors the natural neuromuscular spurt that occurs in boys.[42,47,48]

Special Populations

Females have a natural propensity for the development of poor neuromuscular adaptations with muscular growth during puberty that predispose female athletes to increased injury risk.[48-50] Participation in resistance training by female athletes has been shown to demonstrate safer movement mechanics and decreased injury rates.[45,46] Certain medical conditions can be exacerbated by strength training and must be considered before recommending a strength training program[51-53] (Table 1). Consultation with the appropriate specialist can help determine participation risks, which can be minimal and lower than those associated with a sedentary lifestyle.

Guidelines for Strength Training

Prior to beginning a formal strength training program, a medical evaluation (such as the Preparticipation Physical Evaluation) is recommended to evaluate injury risk factors and medical history and to discuss training goals and expectations.

Appropriate Exercises

Exercises incorporated into youth strength training programs must be specifically selected to be appropriate for the developmental age and current fitness level for the individual. Emphasis on technique fundamentals and close supervision during training are essential. In addition to selecting the appropriate exercises, equipment of the correct size must be selected for the athlete to safely execute correct technique; most strength training and gym equipment are adult size and do not have weight increments appropriate for children. Therefore, although free

Table 1

Medical Conditions to Consider Before Strength Training

Complex congenital heart disease: Those with mild congenital heart disease may be safe for all activities; however, those with moderate to severe forms or who have undergone surgery may be more limited. Cardiologic consultation is indicated before clearance to participate in strength training and physical activity programs.

Coronary artery anomalies

Hypertrophic cardiomyopathy: Disease manifestation can change during adolescence and repeated evaluations are recommended.

Carditis: Inflammation of the heart can predispose to sudden death with exertion.

Systemic pulmonary hypertension

Uncontrolled hypertension: Those with hypertension (>5 mm Hg higher than the 99th percentile for age, sex, and height) should avoid heavy weight lifting, power lifting, body building, and sports with a high static component. Workup is indicated for those with >95th percentile for age, sex, and height.

Acquired heart disease including acute rheumatic fever with carditis

Underlying disease

Ehlers-Danlos syndrome: The vascular form can predispose to cardiovascular risks; all forms are at increased risk for joint injury because of associated ligamentous laxity.

Marfan syndrome: Aortic aneurysm can cause sudden death.

Kawasaki disease (coronary artery vasculitis)

Systemic or HLA-B27–associated arthritis requires cardiovascular assessment for possible cardiac complications during exercise.

Juvenile dermatomyositis or systemic lupus erythematosus with cardiac involvement requires cardiac assessment before clearance.

Fever: Rarely, fever can accompany myocarditis or other conditions that make typical exercise dangerous.

Splenomegaly: Increased spleen size, especially when associated with mononucleosis, predisposes to increased risk of splenic rupture.

Anthracycline use: The cardiotoxic effects of anthracycline increase risk of cardiac problems and resistance training must be considered with caution; strength training that avoids isometric contractions may be permitted.[52,53]

Obesity: Because of increased risk of cardiovascular strain and injury, appropriate acclimatization and gradual activity implementation are important.

weights require better balance, control, and technique, they can provide appropriate weight increments and are preferred for young children in a supervised strength training program.

When determining which exercises to incorporate into a program, many factors must be considered, including baseline fitness level, technical expertise, coaching proficiency, equipment availability, and training goals. For children and adolescents with a low training age (that is, minimal training experience and/or poor technical competency), exercise programs should be designed to promote the development of muscular strength and enhance overall fundamental skill competency.[5] Neuromuscular coordination is most susceptible to change during childhood, resulting in the development of motor competency.[54] "Starter" programs can include basic body weight exercises such as squatting, lunging, pressing, and pulling movements. After these technical skills are mastered and appropriate strength is developed, free weight exercises including weight lifting and plyometrics are incorporated. For technically competent youth, free weight resistance training with close supervision is recommended over machine-based resistance training because adult equipment is often not sized appropriately and weight increments are too large for youth. Additionally, studies in the adult population demonstrate less muscle activation in machine-based resistance training than in free weight resistance training,[55,56] further supporting the recommendation to use free weight resistance exercises.

Volume and Intensity

Determining the appropriate volume and intensity of a strength training program is essential. Volume refers to the number of times an exercise is performed within a training session multiplied by the resistance used (kilograms).[5] Intensity refers to the resistance to be overcome during a repetition.[5] Although these variables are inversely related, both must be considered to develop an appropriate program that promotes technical skill acquisition and strength while minimizing injury risk. If intensity is too high, the participant is unlikely to perform the exercise with correct technique, increasing the risk of injury; if the volume is excessive, overtraining can occur.

An individual's one repetition maximum (1RM) is defined as the maximum amount of weight an individual can displace at one time. 1RMs are used in research settings to assess baseline strength levels, and one study demonstrated no injury with properly supervised 1RM testing in healthy children.[57] Currently, 1RM strength testing is not endorsed as an appropriate measure before skeletal maturity by the American Academy of Pediatrics Council of Sports Medicine.[52] Additionally, 1RM test results are not a practical means of assessment for physical education classes with a large number of participants and minimal time where supervision is limited. Simple field-based measures such as the vertical jump, long jump, and hand grip strength have been correlated to 1RM strength values and are a more practical means of assessing muscular strength in school and recreational settings.[58] Irrespective of 1RM load or strength assessment evaluation measure chosen, ultimately, an individual's technical competency (the ability to perform the exercise with appropriate technique) is the most important factor to consider when designing an appropriate program.

Strength Training Program Progression

Training programs for youth without experience in resistance training are recommended to include a range of exercises and movement patterns and to begin at low volume (one to two sets) and low to moderate training intensities (up to 60% 1RM).[59] To ensure safe, correct technique, it is recommended that youth initially perform a low number of repetitions (one to three), with concurrent cueing during each repetition. However, not all exercises need to be performed for the same number of sets and repetitions; the specific program design depends on individual goals and the level of technical competency and strength. As skills are mastered with correct technique, the program can be advanced to increase the sets, the repetitions per set, and the intensity; these program changes must be made gradually to minimize injury risk and to maximize learning and strength gains. Participants

must be supervised as the program progresses to monitor for fatigue and continued technical competency during training sessions that can result in poor technique and increased injury risk.

Rest Intervals During Training Sessions

Rest intervals are an important component of any training program. Rest is essential to prevent fatigue-related, poor implementation of technique and increased risk for injury. In a research setting, children recover more quickly from fatigue-inducing resistance training and are less likely to sustain muscle damage than adults.[60,61] Current recommendations are for rest periods of approximately 1 minute; however, longer rest periods (range, 2 to 5 minutes) may be appropriate with increases in intensity and exercises that require advanced technical skill, force, or power production (such as weightlifting or plyometric exercises).[5] Additionally, despite the faster recovery rate in children, youth must always be closely supervised to evaluate for continued attention and execution of proper technique throughout a training session. Last, 8 hours or more of sleep per night has been correlated to a lower injury occurrence rate, and thus, adequate sleep must be encouraged to minimize injury risk.[62]

Training Frequency

Because youth are actively growing and developing, allowing appropriate rest and recovery time is essential. When developing a resistance training program, the timing frequency (number of sessions performed per week) must be selected carefully. Studies indicate that two to three sessions per week enable muscular strength development in children and adolescents.[4,14] Training frequency can increase as children progress to adulthood and increase competitive intensity; however, resistance training programs should be incorporated to complement the training program, and not as an additional training session, to minimize overtraining and overuse injury.

Repetition Velocity

Repetition velocity refers to how fast a specific movement is performed. Initially, when training experience is limited and/or a child is learning a new technique, the movement is best performed at a moderate rate to ensure correct technique (posture, position, alignment) and maximize control. However, after a technique is mastered, greater movement velocities should be used to promote the development of motor recruitment patterns and firing intensities.[63] Additionally, repetition velocities can vary within a session depending on the goal and experience for each individual exercise. Ultimately, incorporating high-velocity movements is especially important during the growing years when neural plasticity and motor coordination are most sensitive to change.

Summary

The health, fitness, and performance benefits of strength training for children and adolescents are extensive. To maximize the safety and efficacy of strength training programs for youth, attention must focus on the following: Programs must include appropriate supervision from qualified professionals; programs must address the needs, goals, and abilities of younger populations; and programs are ideally developed for the individual according to biologic age, training age, motor skill competency, psychosocial maturity, technical proficiency, and existing strength levels.

The health and fitness benefits of strength training provide essential muscle strength and motor skills to decrease the risk for poor health outcomes later in life. Additionally, programs have been shown to reduce sports-related injuries and are a key component of preparatory training programs for aspiring young athletes. Ultimately, youth strength training programs are an opportunity to enjoy physical fitness while developing technical skill and competency at an appropriate intensity and volume to build a healthy fitness foundation for life.

Key Study Points

- The myth that strength training is harmful has been dispelled.
- Strength training can be an important part of training for young athletes, can promote lifelong fitness, and reduce sports-related injuries.
- Strength training programs must include appropriate supervision, address the needs of younger populations, and be tailored to the biologic and training age of the athlete.

Annotated References

1. Rowland TW: Promoting physical activity for children's health: Rationale and strategies. *Sports Med* 2007;37(11):929-936.

2. World Health Organization: *Global Recommendations on Physical Activity for Health.* Geneva, WHO Press, 2010.

   Activity recommendations for three age groups (ranges: 5 to 17 years, 18 to 64 years, and 65 years and older) are presented.

3. U.S. Department of Health and Human Services: *Physical Activity Guidelines for Americans.* Washington, DC, US Department of Health and Human Services, 2008.

4. Faigenbaum AD, Kraemer WJ, Blimkie CJ, et al: Youth resistance training: Updated position statement paper from the national strength and conditioning association. *J Strength Cond Res* 2009;23(5, Suppl):S60-S79.

   An updated report is presented on recommendations on youth resistance training regarding: potential risks and concerns, potential health and fitness benefits, types and amount of resistance training needed, and program design considerations for optimizing long-term training adaptations.

5. Lloyd RS, Faigenbaum AD, Stone MH, et al: Position statement on youth resistance training: The 2014 International Consensus. *Br J Sports Med* 2014;48(7):498-505.

   Scientific evidence supports participation in appropriately designed youth resistance training programs that are supervised and instructed by qualified professionals. Health, fitness, and performance benefits associated with training for children and adolescents are outlined.

6. Ramsay JA, Blimkie CJ, Smith K, Garner S, MacDougall JD, Sale DG: Strength training effects in prepubescent boys. *Med Sci Sports Exerc* 1990;22(5):605-614.

7. Christou M, Smilios I, Sotiropoulos K, Volaklis K, Pilianidis T, Tokmakidis SP: Effects of resistance training on the physical capacities of adolescent soccer players. *J Strength Cond Res* 2006;20(4):783-791.

8. Lillegard WA, Brown EW, Wilson DJ, Henderson R, Lewis E: Efficacy of strength training in prepubescent to early postpubescent males and females: Effects of gender and maturity. *Pediatr Rehabil* 1997;1(3):147-157.

9. Weltman A, Janney C, Rians CB, Strand K, Katch FI: The effects of hydraulic-resistance strength training on serum lipid levels in prepubertal boys. *Am J Dis Child* 1987;141(7):777-780.

10. Faigenbaum AD, Milliken LA, Loud RL, Burak BT, Doherty CL, Westcott WL: Comparison of 1 and 2 days per week of strength training in children. *Res Q Exerc Sport* 2002;73(4):416-424.

11. Padres E, Eliakim A, Costantini N, et al: The effect of long-term resistance training on anthropometric measures, muscle strength, and self-concept in pre-pubertal boys. *Pediatr Exerc Sci* 2001;13:357-372.

12. Faigenbaum AD, Myer GD: Resistance training among young athletes: Safety, efficacy and injury prevention effects. *Br J Sports Med* 2010;44(1):56-63.

   Resistance training can be a safe, effective, and worthwhile activity for children and adolescents provided that qualified professionals supervise all training sessions and provide age-appropriate instruction on proper lifting procedures and safe training guidelines.

13. Annesi JJ, Westcott WL, Faigenbaum AD, Unruh JL: Effects of a 12-week physical activity protocol delivered by YMCA after-school counselors (Youth Fit for Life) on fitness and self-efficacy changes in 5-12-year-old boys and girls. *Res Q Exerc Sport* 2005;76(4):468-476.

14. Behringer M, Vom Heede A, Yue Z, Mester J: Effects of resistance training in children and adolescents: A meta-analysis. *Pediatrics* 2010;126(5):e1199-e1210.

   A greater number of training sessions per week is associated with greater strength gains after resistance training, and long-term interventions are more beneficial than short ones. The ability to gain muscular strength correlates to increase with age and maturation status. Level of evidence: I.

15. American College of Sports Medicine: *ACSMs Guidelines for Exercise Testing and Prescription,* ed 8. Philadelphia, PA, Lippincott Williams and Wilkins, 2010.

   This manual summarizes recommended procedures for exercise testing and exercise prescription in healthy and sick patients.

16. Behringer M, Vom Heede A, Matthews M, Mester J: Effects of strength training on motor performance skills in children and adolescents: A meta-analysis. *Pediatr Exerc Sci* 2011;23(2):186-206.

   After resistance training, younger patients and nonathletes showed greater gains in motor performance. Thus, resistance training can provide an effective way for enhancing motor performance in children and adolescents. Level of evidence: I.

17. Malina RM, Bouchard C, Bar-Or O: *Growth, Maturation and Physical Activity.* Champaign, IL, Human Kinetics, 2004, pp 3-20.

18. Myer GD, Faigenbaum AD, Stracciolini A, Hewett TE, Micheli LJ, Best TM: Exercise deficit disorder in youth: A paradigm shift toward disease prevention and comprehensive care. *Curr Sports Med Rep* 2013;12(4):248-255.

   Exercise-deficient children need to be identified early in life and treated with appropriate exercise programs to target movement and physical problems. If the opportunity is missed, later interventions to promote healthy lifestyles choices will be more difficult to achieve.

19. Faigenbaum AD, McFarland JE, Buchanan E, Ratamess NA, Kang J, Hoffman JR: After-school fitness performance is not altered after physical education lessons in adolescent athletes. *J Strength Cond Res* 2010;24(3):765-770.

   The after-school fitness performance of 20 adolescent athletes was assessed following three different physical education lessons (aerobic training, resistance training, and basketball skill training). The study concluded that an exercise lesson does not have an adverse effect on after-school fitness performance.

20. Sothern MS, Loftin JM, Udall JN, et al: Safety, feasibility, and efficacy of a resistance training program in preadolescent obese children. *Am J Med Sci* 2000;319(6):370-375.

21. Shaibi GQ, Cruz ML, Ball GD, et al: Effects of resistance training on insulin sensitivity in overweight Latino adolescent males. *Med Sci Sports Exerc* 2006;38(7):1208-1215.

22. Hagberg JM, Ehsani AA, Goldring D, Hernandez A, Sinacore DR, Holloszy JO: Effect of weight training on blood pressure and hemodynamics in hypertensive adolescents. *J Pediatr* 1984;104(1):147-151.

23. Sung RY, Yu CW, Chang SK, Mo SW, Woo KS, Lam CW: Effects of dietary intervention and strength training on blood lipid level in obese children. *Arch Dis Child* 2002;86(6):407-410.

24. Hoelscher DM, Kirk S, Ritchie L, Cunningham-Sabo L; Academy Positions Committee: Position of the Academy of Nutrition and Dietetics: Interventions for the prevention and treatment of pediatric overweight and obesity. *J Acad Nutr Diet* 2013;113(10):1375-1394.

   Guidance and recommendations are presented for levels of intervention targeting obesity prevention and treatment from preschool children to adolescents.

25. Malina RM: Weight training in youth-growth, maturation, and safety: An evidence-based review. *Clin J Sport Med* 2006;16(6):478-487.

26. Gunter KB, Almstedt HC, Janz KF: Physical activity in childhood may be the key to optimizing lifespan skeletal health. *Exerc Sport Sci Rev* 2012;40(1):13-21.

   Physical activity during childhood conveys optimal benefits to bone mass, size, and structure. These benefits persist beyond activity cessation. Currently, the most effective interventions to enhance skeletal development have been school based.

27. Vicente-Rodríguez G: How does exercise affect bone development during growth? *Sports Med* 2006;36(7):561-569.

28. Álvarez-San Emeterio C, Antuñano NP, López-Sobaler AM, González-Badillo JJ: Effect of strength training and the practice of Alpine skiing on bone mass density, growth, body composition, and the strength and power of the legs of adolescent skiers. *J Strength Cond Res* 2011;25(10):2879-2890.

   In this study, Alpine skiing combined with strength training proved to have a positive effect on the power and percentage of muscle mass in legs, as well as on the bone density in the lumbar spine compared with sedentary individuals.

29. Hind K, Burrows M: Weight-bearing exercise and bone mineral accrual in children and adolescents: A review of controlled trials. *Bone* 2007;40(1):14-27.

30. Yu CC, Sung RY, So RC, et al: Effects of strength training on body composition and bone mineral content in children who are obese. *J Strength Cond Res* 2005;19(3):667-672.

31. Turner CH, Robling AG: Designing exercise regimens to increase bone strength. *Exerc Sport Sci Rev* 2003;31(1):45-50.

32. Yu CC, Sung RY, Hau KT, Lam PK, Nelson EA, So RC: The effect of diet and strength training on obese children's physical self-concept. *J Sports Med Phys Fitness* 2008;48(1):76-82.

33. Altintaş A, Aşçi FH: Physical self-esteem of adolescents with regard to physical activity and pubertal status. *Pediatr Exerc Sci* 2008;20(2):142-156.

34. Dunton GF, Schneider M, Graham DJ, et al: Physical activity, fitness, and physical self-concept in adolescent females. *Pediatr Exerc Sci* 2006;18:240-251.

35. Knowles AM, Niven AG, Fawkner SG, Henretty JM: A longitudinal examination of the influence of maturation on physical self-perceptions and the relationship with physical activity in early adolescent girls. *J Adolesc* 2009;32(3):555-566.

In this study, 150 early adolescent girls were observed. A decrease in overall physical activity over 12 months was not influenced by age maturation, but variance in physical activity was partially accounted for by physical self-perception.

36. Lubans DR, Aguiar EJ, Callister R: The effects of free weights and elastic tubing resistance training on physical self-perception in adolescents. *Psychol Sport Exerc* 2010;11:497-504.

In this study, 108 adolescents were divided into two resistance training groups (free weights and elastic tubing) and a control group. Those in the resistance training groups improved their body composition. Resistance training is feasible and effective for improving aspects of health-related fitness.

37. Velez A, Golem DL, Arent SM: The impact of a 12-week resistance training program on strength, body composition, and self-concept of Hispanic adolescents. *J Strength Cond Res* 2010;24(4):1065-1073.

The health and fitness of 28 Hispanic adolescents (divided randomly into control and resistance training groups) was assessed before and after intervention. Resistance training resulted in important psychologic and physiologic improvement.

38. Hoffman JR, Faigenbaum AD, Ratamess NA, Ross R, Kang J, Tenenbaum G: Nutritional supplementation and anabolic steroid use in adolescents. *Med Sci Sports Exerc* 2008;40(1):15-24.

39. Nattiv A, Loucks AB, Manore MM, Sanborn CF, Sundgot-Borgen J, Warren MP; American College of Sports Medicine: American College of Sports Medicine position stand. The female athlete triad. *Med Sci Sports Exerc* 2007;39(10):1867-1882.

40. Brenner JS; American Academy of Pediatrics Council on Sports Medicine and Fitness: Overuse injuries, overtraining, and burnout in child and adolescent athletes. *Pediatrics* 2007;119(6):1242-1245.

41. Bloemers F, Collard D, Paw MC, Van Mechelen W, Twisk J, Verhagen E: Physical inactivity is a risk factor for physical activity-related injuries in children. *Br J Sports Med* 2012;46(9):669-674.

Sex, age, and level of physical activity are independent risk factors for physical activity–related injuries in children. Injury risk substantially declined with an increase in weekly exposure, the most active kids had the lowest injury risk.

42. Myer GD, Faigenbaum AD, Ford KR, Best TM, Bergeron MF, Hewett TE: When to initiate integrative neuromuscular training to reduce sports-related injuries and enhance health in youth? *Curr Sports Med Rep* 2011;10(3):155-166.

Integrative neuromuscular training (INT) may be most beneficial if initiated during preadolescence. If maintained throughout childhood and adolescence, INT will likely improve movement biomechanics, minimize risk of sports-related injury, and promote positive health outcomes during adulthood.

43. Soligard T, Myklebust G, Steffen K, et al: Comprehensive warm-up programme to prevent injuries in young female footballers: Cluster randomised controlled trial. *BMJ* 2008;337:a2469.

44. Emery CA, Meeuwisse WH: The effectiveness of a neuromuscular prevention strategy to reduce injuries in youth soccer: A cluster-randomised controlled trial. *Br J Sports Med* 2010;44(8):555-562.

In this study, 744 youth soccer players were randomized into soccer-specific neuromuscular program and control groups. The overall injury rate was lower in the neuromuscular program group.

45. Myer GD, Ford KR, McLean SG, Hewett TE: The effects of plyometric versus dynamic stabilization and balance training on lower extremity biomechanics. *Am J Sports Med* 2006;34(3):445-455.

46. Myer GD, Sugimoto D, Thomas S, Hewett TE: The influence of age on the effectiveness of neuromuscular training to reduce anterior cruciate ligament injury in female athletes: A meta-analysis. *Am J Sports Med* 2013;41(1):203-215.

An association was found between neuromuscular training and reduction of anterior cruciate ligament injury incidence. It may be optimal to start with neuromuscular programs during early adolescence.

47. Myer GD, Ford KR, Palumbo JP, Hewett TE: Neuromuscular training improves performance and lower-extremity biomechanics in female athletes. *J Strength Cond Res* 2005;19(1):51-60.

48. Hewett TE, Myer GD, Ford KR, et al: Biomechanical measures of neuromuscular control and valgus loading of the knee predict anterior cruciate ligament injury risk in female athletes: A prospective study. *Am J Sports Med* 2005;33(4):492-501.

49. Ford KR, Shapiro R, Myer GD, Van Den Bogert AJ, Hewett TE: Longitudinal sex differences during landing in knee abduction in young athletes. *Med Sci Sports Exerc* 2010;42(10):1923-1931.

For this study, 315 subjects were tested in two sessions, 1 year apart. The knee abduction angle of females was substantially increased during rapid adolescent growth, as well as their knee abduction motion and moments during the subsequent year after rapid adolescent growth, compared with males.

50. Hewett TE, Myer GD, Ford KR: Decrease in neuromuscular control about the knee with maturation in female athletes. *J Bone Joint Surg Am* 2004;86-A(8):1601-1608.

51. Rice SG; American Academy of Pediatrics Council on Sports Medicine and Fitness: Medical conditions affecting sports participation. *Pediatrics* 2008;121(4):841-848.

52. American Academy of Pediatrics Council on Sports Medicine and Fitness, McCambridge TM, Stricker PR: Strength training by children and adolescents. *Pediatrics* 2008;121(4):835-840.

53. Steinherz LJ, Steinherz PG, Tan CT, Heller G, Murphy ML: Cardiac toxicity 4 to 20 years after completing anthracycline therapy. *JAMA* 1991;266(12):1672-1677.

54. Borms J: The child and exercise: An overview. *J Sports Sci* 1986;4(1):3-20.

55. Schwanbeck S, Chilibeck PD, Binsted G: A comparison of free weight squat to Smith machine squat using electromyography. *J Strength Cond Res* 2009;23(9):2588-2591.

Electromyographic activity was increased in the gastrocnemius, biceps femoris, and vastus medialis during the free-weight squat versus machine squat. No substantial difference was reported for any other muscles.

56. Schick EE, Coburn JW, Brown LE, et al: A comparison of muscle activation between a Smith machine and free weight bench press. *J Strength Cond Res* 2010;24(3):779-784.

Subjects were tested in two training sessions. The free-weight bench press demonstrated greater muscle activation than the Smith machine for muscle groups tested.

57. Faigenbaum AD, Milliken LA, Westcott WL: Maximal strength testing in healthy children. *J Strength Cond Res* 2003;17(1):162-166.

58. Castro-Piñero J, Ortega FB, Artero EG, et al: Assessing muscular strength in youth: Usefulness of standing long jump as a general index of muscular fitness. *J Strength Cond Res* 2010;24(7):1810-1817.

In this study, 94 children underwent upper and/or lower extremity strength tests. The standing long jump (SLJ) was strongly associated with lower and upper body muscular strength tests. Thus, SLJ could be considered a general index of muscular fitness in youth.

59. Ratamess NA, Alvar BA, Evetoch TK, et al; American College of Sports Medicine: American College of Sports Medicine position stand. Progression models in resistance training for healthy adults. *Med Sci Sports Exerc* 2009;41(3):687-708.

The optimal characteristics of strength-specific programs include the use of concentric, eccentric, and isometric muscle actions and the performance of bilateral and unilateral single- and multiple-joint exercises. In addition, it is recommended that strength programs sequence exercises to optimize the preservation of exercise intensity.

60. Faigenbaum AD, Ratamess NA, McFarland J, et al: Effect of rest interval length on bench press performance in boys, teens, and men. *Pediatr Exerc Sci* 2008;20(4):457-469.

61. Zafeiridis A, Dalamitros A, Dipla K, Manou V, Galanis N, Kellis S: Recovery during high-intensity intermittent anaerobic exercise in boys, teens, and men. *Med Sci Sports Exerc* 2005;37(3):505-512.

62. Milewski MD, Skaggs DL, Bishop GA, et al: Chronic lack of sleep is associated with increased sports injuries in adolescent athletes. *J Pediatr Orthop* 2014;34(2):129-133.

Hours of sleep per night and grade in school were the best independent predictors of injury in this study. Sleep deprivation was associated with injuries. Thus, promoting adequate amount of sleeping hours may help in the protection against sports-related injuries. Level of evidence: III.

63. Young WB: Transfer of strength and power training to sports performance. *Int J Sports Physiol Perform* 2006;1(2):74-83.

Section 9

Imaging

SECTION EDITOR
Cree M. Gaskin, MD

Chapter 53

MRI of the Glenohumeral Joint

James Derek Stensby, MD

Abstract

MRI and magnetic resonance arthrography of the shoulder are valuable tools in the assessment of the rotator cuff, labroligamentous complex, and rotator interval. Knowledge of the added benefits of MRI in comparison to other imaging modalities, the common pitfalls and normal variants, and added benefit of intra-articular contrast and abduction-external rotation positioning strengthen the preoperative assessment in patients presenting with shoulder pain and instability.

Keywords: glenohumeral joint; labrum; MRI; rotator cuff

Introduction

MRI of the glenohumeral joint is done without contrast, with intravenous contrast as an indirect arthrogram, or with intra-articular contrast. The choice of technique varies by institution and clinical indication. In the typical MRI protocol, images are acquired in the axial, oblique sagittal, and oblique coronal planes. Some institutions use the oblique or angled axial plane to target the antero-inferior glenoid labrum. The benefits of intra-articular administration of contrast in direct magnetic resonance arthrography (MRA) include capsular distension, which improves visualization of the labrum, capsule, ligaments, biceps tendon, articular cartilage, and articular side of the rotator cuff.[1] MRA also allows simultaneous administration of intra-articular anesthetic and steroids to provide diagnostic information and therapeutic benefit, without decreasing the image contrast.[2]

The absolute contraindications to MRA include the presence of cellulitis or joint infection or a history of

Neither Dr. Stensby nor any immediate family member has received anything of value from or has stock or stock options held in a commercial company or institution related directly or indirectly to the subject of this chapter.

ipsilateral reflex sympathetic dystrophy. Anticoagulation therapy and a history of contrast allergy are relative contraindications.[1] The most severe complication is joint infection, which occurs in approximately 1 of every 40,000 patients.[3] The most common complication is pain, on average beginning 16 hours after the injection and resolving over 2 days.[4] A survey of 202 patients who underwent shoulder MRA found that 1% of patients described the pain as worse than expected and 40% described MRA as more tolerable than MRI.[5]

The Rotator Cuff

MRI and MRA are excellent tools for evaluating the rotator cuff because they offer better soft-tissue contrast than other imaging studies. A meta-analysis of the accuracy of preoperative imaging in detecting full-thickness rotator cuff tears found sensitivity of 95.4% and specificity of 98.9% for MRA, compared with sensitivity of 92.1% and specificity of 92.9% for conventional MRI.[6] Preoperative identification of partial-thickness rotator cuff tears was less robust; with MRA, sensitivity was 85.9% and specificity was 96%, and with conventional MRI sensitivity was 63.6% and specificity was 91.7%.[6] Each of the imaging planes allows specific aspects of the rotator cuff anatomy and pathology to be assessed. Oblique sagittal images are best for assessing the anterior fibers of the supraspinatus tendon, the anterior-posterior dimension of any rotator cuff tear, the coracoacromial arch, and the rotator cuff musculature. The oblique coronal plane is best for the supraspinatus and infraspinatus tendons, the transverse dimension of any tear, retraction of the myotendinous junction, and the medial extent of a delaminating tear. The axial plane is best for assessing the subscapularis tendon.

A full-thickness rotator cuff tear is identified if fiber discontinuity spans the entire thickness of the tendon, with the defect isointense to fluid on T2-weighted sequences or matching gadolinium signal intensity on MRA.[7] A partial tear is diagnosed if the fluid- or gadolinium-filled area of fiber discontinuity spans only a portion of the tendon thickness.[8] Articular-side thickening of the supraspinatus and infraspinatus (presumably the rotator cable) on images obtained in the neutral position was found to suggest the presence of a partial-thickness articular-side rotator cuff tear[9] (Figure 1). Conversely, the rotator cable was reliably identified in the absence of a rotator cuff tear on images obtained in the abduction-external rotation (ABER) position. The description of a full-thickness tear should include its location, the tendons involved, its anterior-posterior size, and the extent of retraction. The description of a partial-thickness tear should include not only location and size but also the percentage of tendon thickness that is affected and whether the tear involves the articular or bursal surface.[10]

Preoperative identification of rotator cuff pathology can be improved by understanding the features that distinguish rotator cuff tendinopathy from tendon tears, the most common location of rotator cuff tears, and the pitfalls of MRI of the rotator cuff. On MRI, rotator cuff tendinopathy appears as increased thickness and increased signal intensity. T2-weighted fat-suppressed sequences are useful for distinguishing tendinopathy from a tendon tear, which is isointense to fluid. An evaluation of degenerative tears in 360 shoulders found the rotator cuff segment 15 to 16 mm posterior to the rotator cuff interval to be the most common location of tears.[11] This segment's location in the center of the rotator crescent may make it more prone to tearing and initiation of a degenerative tear.

Recent studies identified several MRI pitfalls. Increased signal intensity in the substance of the tendon cannot be used in isolation to diagnose rotator cuff pathology because increased signal may result from variations in histology or the magic angle artifact, which usually is seen in the distal tendon.[12] MRI evaluation of the subscapularis tendon was found to be less robust than MRI evaluation of other rotator cuff tendons.[13] Specificity and positive predictive value for subscapularis tears both were 100% compared with arthroscopy, but sensitivity was only 39% and accuracy was only 69%.[13] These data support the premise that MRA, fat suppression, and image interpretation by a fellowship-trained musculoskeletal radiologist are useful in the preoperative diagnosis of subscapularis tears. Identification of a cyst in or adjacent to the lesser tuberosity should prompt a careful assessment of the subscapularis.[14] The difficulties in evaluating the subscapularis tendon include volume averaging of the superior margin of the tendon and the adjacent rotator cuff interval mimicking a tear, difficulty in differentiating an intrasubstance or concealed tear from an articular-side tear, and an irregular contour of the tendon surface caused by tendinopathy and leading to a false-positive diagnosis of a tear.[15]

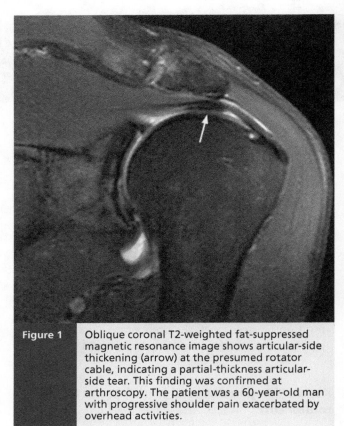

Figure 1 Oblique coronal T2-weighted fat-suppressed magnetic resonance image shows articular-side thickening (arrow) at the presumed rotator cable, indicating a partial-thickness articular-side tear. This finding was confirmed at arthroscopy. The patient was a 60-year-old man with progressive shoulder pain exacerbated by overhead activities.

The Labrum and Labral Instability

The fibrocartilaginous labrum assists in stabilizing the glenohumeral joint by increasing the surface area of the articulation, deepening the articular cavity, and serving as a site of attachment for the capsuloligamentous complex and biceps tendon. The normal labrum has uniform low signal intensity with a roughly triangular configuration on all MRI sequences. The labrum may have a sharp or rounded free edge. Increased signal within the labrum may be an artifact caused by volume averaging or magic angle (on short echo time sequences). The labrum is best assessed with MRA, which increases the conspicuity of tears with a combination of joint distension, separation of the soft-tissue support structures, and extension of contrast into any defect. The superior and inferior aspects of the labrum are best assessed on oblique coronal images, and axial images offer the best views of the anterior and posterior labrum. Angled or oblique axial images may yield the best views of the anteroinferior and posterosuperior aspects of the labrum. The glenohumeral ligaments are best evaluated using a combination of axial and sagittal images. Any anteroinferior bone loss is best detected on oblique sagittal images. MRI is slightly

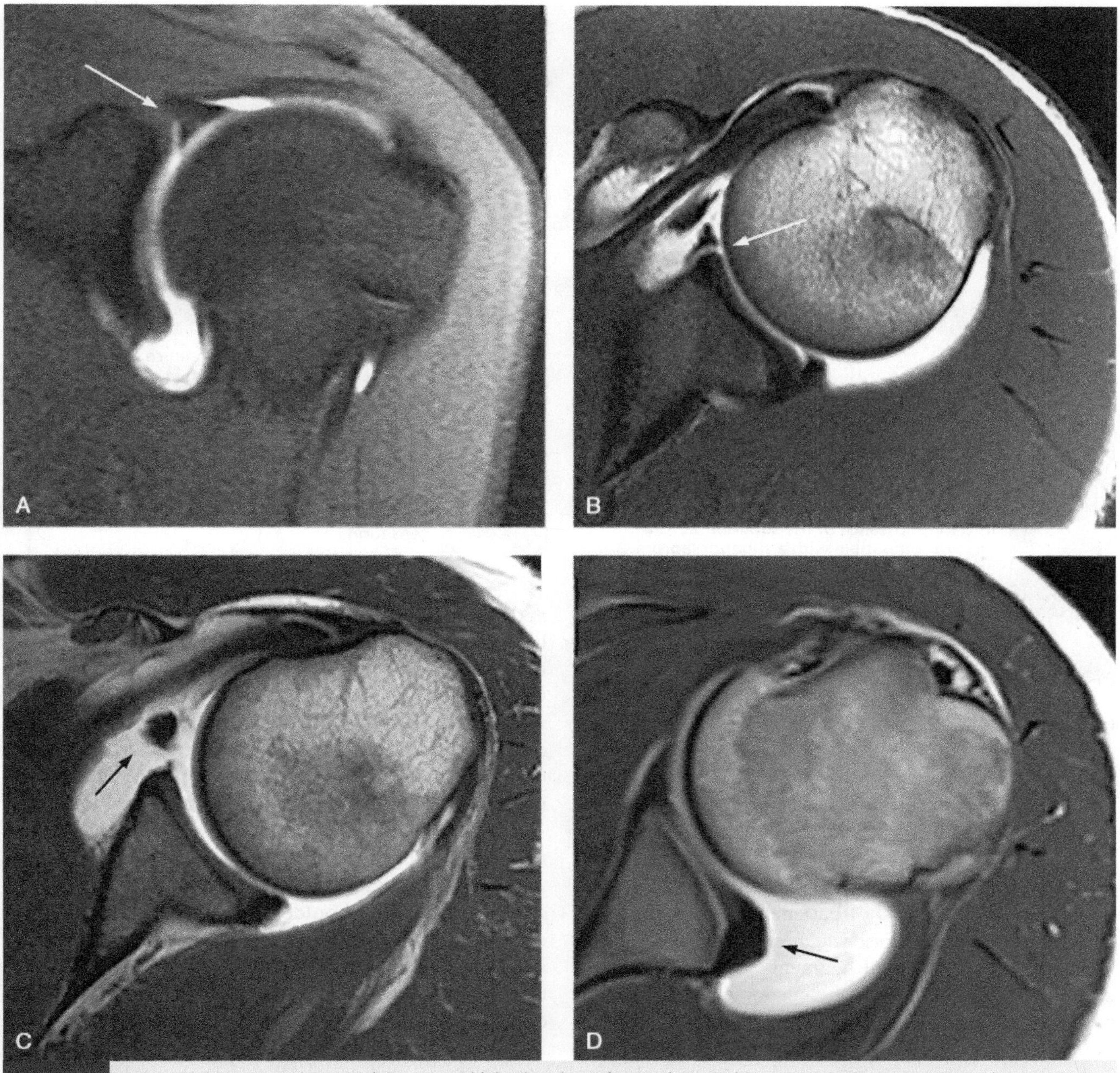

Illustration

Figure 2 Magnetic resonance images show normal labral variants (arrows). **A,** A thin curvilinear contrast extension between the glenoid and superior labrum, anterior to the biceps anchor, which is consistent with a sublabral sulcus. **B,** A sublabral foramen with contrast extension between the glenoid and anterosuperior labrum, above the midglenoid. **C,** A Buford complex with an absent anterosuperior labrum and a thick middle glenohumeral ligament. **D,** A hypertrophic posteroinferior labrum secondary to mild glenoid hypoplasia.

inferior to CT for assessing glenoid bone loss when compared to arthroscopically proven defects.[16]

An understanding of the many normal variants of the labrum can prevent a false-positive diagnosis of a labral tear. Most labral variants are found in the superior and anterosuperior labrum. The sublabral sulcus or recess is a common variant that can be mistaken for a superior labrum anterior and posterior tear. The sulcus, which is seen in as many as 73% of patients, has a smooth, well-defined margin, parallels the glenoid and does not extend posterior to the biceps-labral anchor[17] (Figure 2, A). If the contrast or abnormal signal extends into the substance of the superior labrum, it can be preoperatively distinguished from a tear (Figure 3). In the anterosuperior

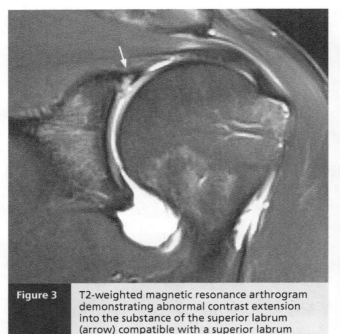

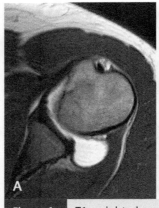

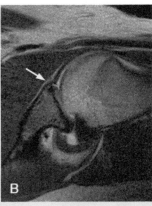

Figure 3 T2-weighted magnetic resonance arthrogram demonstrating abnormal contrast extension into the substance of the superior labrum (arrow) compatible with a superior labrum anterior to posterior tear. The patient was a 50-year-old man who presented with a 3-month history of right shoulder pain that worsened with abduction. The patient underwent arthroscopic repair after conservative management failed.

Figure 4 T1-weighted magnetic resonance arthrogram of the anteroinferior labrum in the standard (**A**) and abduction-external rotation (**B**) positions. Linear T1 hyperintense contrast (arrow) interposed between the glenoid and the nondisplaced labrum in (**B**) is compatible only with a Perthes lesion. The patient was an 18-year-old woman who played volleyball and had shoulder pain, swelling, and a popping sensation.

quadrant, the labrum may not be firmly adherent to the glenoid, and contrast or fluid can be interposed into this sublabral foramen (Figure 2, *B*). The sublabral foramen may extend and become contiguous with the sublabral recess, but it should not extend into the biceps-labral anchor or anteriorly below the midglenoid. The Buford complex, another anterosuperior labral variant, is found on arthroscopy in 1.5% of patients as a focally absent labrum in the anterosuperior quadrant with a thick, cord-like middle glenohumeral ligament[18] (Figure 2, *C*). An additional variant that may be encountered in the evaluation of the labrum is labral hypertrophy in the setting of posterior glenoid hypoplasia (Figure 2, *D)*.

Several imaging techniques can be used in evaluating the anteroinferior labrum. The most complete evaluation is obtained with MRA in both the standard and ABER positions. The Perthes lesion, a nondisplaced avulsion of the labrum with stripping of the medial periosteum, is best seen on sequences obtained in the ABER position[19,20] (Figure 4). The anterior labral periosteal sleeve avulsion lesion, which is a medially displaced avulsion of the labrum and attached glenohumeral ligament with intact scapular periosteum, is best identified on MRI in the standard position.[19] Although MRA has been the standard for evaluation of the labrum, a recent comparison study found that multidetector computed tomographic

arthrography (CTA) offered better evaluation of the labroligamentous complex, cartilage, and osseous injuries than MRA.[21] The authors concluded that although CTA is less expensive, has fewer contraindications, and requires less time than MRA, it does not offer a complete evaluation of the extra-articular structures, is less reliable than MRA for evaluating the middle glenohumeral ligament, and exposes the patient to radiation.

There has been recent emphasis on preoperative identification of a humeral avulsion of the glenohumeral ligament (HAGL) because this lesion may be a cause of failed surgery to correct shoulder instability (Figure 5). The difficulty of identifying a HAGL lesion arthroscopically increases the importance of preoperative imaging detection.[22] Unfortunately, HAGL lesions often are not detected on MRI. A recent study reported that 26% of HAGL lesions could not be identified on MRI despite knowledge of the surgical findings.[23] All of the patients had a history of anterior dislocation or instability. Additional injuries, the most common of which were Hill-Sachs fracture and subscapularis tendon tear, were identified in 95% of patients. In a patient with relevant history or after noncontributory conventional MRI, MRA can aid in the preoperative diagnosis of a HAGL lesion.[22,23]

The Biceps Tendon and Rotator Cuff Interval

Lesions of the biceps tendon and rotator cuff interval can be a source of pain. These lesions usually occur in conjunction with rotator cuff pathology, but they also

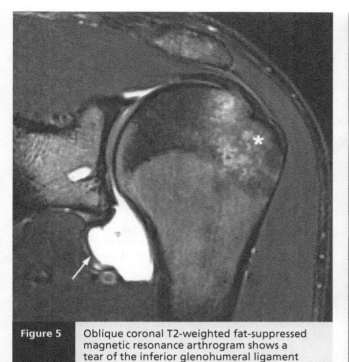

Figure 5 Oblique coronal T2-weighted fat-suppressed magnetic resonance arthrogram shows a tear of the inferior glenohumeral ligament at its humeral attachment, which has led to an abnormal double contour (arrow). Edema in the humeral head (asterisk) resulted from dislocation and anterior impaction. The patient was a 21-year-old man who played hockey, had a history of labral repair, and had a recurrent dislocation.

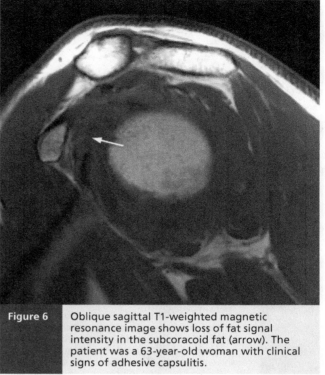

Figure 6 Oblique sagittal T1-weighted magnetic resonance image shows loss of fat signal intensity in the subcoracoid fat (arrow). The patient was a 63-year-old woman with clinical signs of adhesive capsulitis.

can occur in isolation. Proton density–weighted sequences with fat suppression have the greatest sensitivity for detecting tendon degeneration, although tendon caliber change is more specific.[24] Diagnosing partial tears of the biceps tendon at the entrance to the bicipital groove can be challenging on MRI or MRA without directed effort. Biceps tendon partial tears at the groove entrance show abnormal signal intensity, but half have an associated caliber change, and evaluation in all imaging planes aids in identification of a biceps groove entrance lesion.[25] The biceps pulley, which is composed of the superior glenohumeral ligament and coracohumeral ligament in combination with the subscapularis, holds the biceps tendon in place. MRA was found to have sensitivity of 82% to 89% and specificity of 87% to 98% in the evaluation of the biceps pulley.[26] Diagnostic criteria included nonvisualization or discontinuity of the superior glenohumeral ligament, medial subluxation of the biceps tendon on axial images, biceps tendinopathy, and inferior displacement on oblique sagittal images.

The rotator cuff interval is a triangular region bounded medially by the coracoid process, superiorly by the anterior margin of the supraspinatus, and inferiorly by the superior margin of the subscapularis. In the rotator cuff interval the anterior capsule is supported by both the superior glenohumeral ligament and the coracohumeral ligament. The biceps tendon traverses the rotator cuff interval, where it is held in place by the biceps pulley, before exiting the joint via the bicipital groove. The complex anatomy of the rotator cuff interval is best assessed with MRA because joint distension can separate the components of the rotator cuff interval. Abnormalities of the rotator cuff interval can lead to a restricted range of motion or instability. Adhesive capsulitis is a common condition characterized by painful and restricted range of motion that is exacerbated at night. The MRI findings in adhesive capsulitis include thickening of at least 4 mm in the coracohumeral ligament, thickening of the joint capsule in the rotator cuff interval, and obliteration of the subcoracoid fat[27] (Figure 6). Conversely, a capacious rotator cuff interval capsule may be seen in the setting of instability. With MRA all five patients with a surgically identified rotator cuff interval lesion had contrast extension to the undersurface of the coracoid process[28] (Figure 7). The rotator cuff interval was found to be significantly larger in patients with chronic anterior instability.[29]

Summary

MRI and MRA offer an excellent means of assessing internal derangement of the glenohumeral joint and the

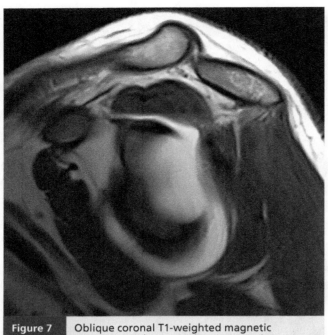

Figure 7 Oblique coronal T1-weighted magnetic resonance arthrogram shows a capacious capsule in the rotator cuff interval with contrast extension to the undersurface of the coracoid anteriorly. The patient was a 14-year-old girl who had been injured in a cheerleading accident. Preoperative examination under anesthesia confirmed both anterior and posterior instability.

rotator cuff, and they can be bolstered by tailoring the technique to the specific clinical concern. Knowledge of MRI techniques, artifacts, normal variants, and pitfalls adds power to this clinical tool.

Key Study Points

- MRA improves sensitivity and specificity for both full (95.4% / 89.9% versus 92.1% / 92.9%) and partial (85.9% / 96% versus 63.6% / 91.7%) in comparison with arthroscopy.
- MRA in the ABER position improves evaluation of the inferior labrum and identification of Perthes lesions.
- Preoperative assessment of the subscapularis, the humeral attachment of the glenohumeral ligament, and the biceps tendon at its entrance to the bicipital groove is challenging.
- Knowledge of the normal labral variants improves the preoperative MRI evaluation.
- MRI findings of adhesive capsulitis include thickening of the coracohumeral ligament, thickening of the joint capsule in the rotator interval, and obliteration of subcoracoid fat.

Annotated References

1. Rhee RB, Chan KK, Lieu JG, Kim BS, Steinbach LS: MR and CT arthrography of the shoulder. *Semin Musculoskelet Radiol* 2012;16(1):3-14.

   MRA technique, indications, contraindications, and imaging protocols were reviewed, with relevant anatomy and pathology.

2. Ugas MA, Huynh BH, Fox MG, Patrie JT, Gaskin CM: MR arthrography: Impact of steroids, local anesthetics, and iodinated contrast material on gadolinium signal intensity in phantoms at 1.5 and 3.0 T. *Radiology* 2014;272(2):475-483.

   The signal intensity of MRA phantoms containing varying concentrations of gadolinium, iodinated contrast, local anesthetic, and corticosteroids were studied.

3. Newberg AH, Munn CS, Robbins AH: Complications of arthrography. *Radiology* 1985;155(3):605-606.

4. Giaconi JC, Link TM, Vail TP, et al: Morbidity of direct MR arthrography. *AJR Am J Roentgenol* 2011;196(4):868-874.

   A survey of 155 consecutive patients determined the frequency, intensity, and time course of pain after direct MRA.

5. Binkert CA, Zanetti M, Hodler J: Patient's assessment of discomfort during MR arthrography of the shoulder. *Radiology* 2001;221(3):775-778.

6. de Jesus JO, Parker L, Frangos AJ, Nazarian LN: Accuracy of MRI, MR arthrography, and ultrasound in the diagnosis of rotator cuff tears: A meta-analysis. *AJR Am J Roentgenol* 2009;192(6):1701-1707.

   A meta-analysis of 65 studies evaluated the sensitivity and specificity of direct MRA, standard MRI, and ultrasound in the evaluation of full- and partial-thickness rotator cuff tears.

7. Farley TE, Neumann CH, Steinbach LS, Jahnke AJ, Petersen SS: Full-thickness tears of the rotator cuff of the shoulder: Diagnosis with MR imaging. *AJR Am J Roentgenol* 1992;158(2):347-351.

8. Kassarjian A, Bencardino JT, Palmer WE: MR imaging of the rotator cuff. *Radiol Clin North Am* 2006;44(4):503-523, vii-viii.

9. Sheah K, Bredella MA, Warner JJ, Halpern EF, Palmer WE: Transverse thickening along the articular surface of the rotator cuff consistent with the rotator cable: Identification with MR arthrography and relevance in rotator cuff evaluation. *AJR Am J Roentgenol* 2009;193(3):679-686.

   A retrospective review of 54 patients compared arthroscopy with MRA in standard and ABER positions for identification of the rotator cable as an indicator of rotator cuff tears.

© 2016 American Academy of Orthopaedic Surgeons

10. Ellman H: Diagnosis and treatment of incomplete rotator cuff tears. *Clin Orthop Relat Res* 1990;254:64-74.

11. Kim HM, Dahiya N, Teefey SA, et al: Location and initiation of degenerative rotator cuff tears: An analysis of three hundred and sixty shoulders. *J Bone Joint Surg Am* 2010;92(5):1088-1096.

   A retrospective review of 360 shoulder ultrasound examinations determined the most common location of partial- and full-thickness rotator cuff tears.

12. Tuite MJ: Magnetic resonance imaging of rotator cuff disease and external impingement. *Magn Reson Imaging Clin N Am* 2012;20(2):187-200, ix.

   External impingement and its MRI characteristics were reviewed.

13. Adams CR, Schoolfield JD, Burkhart SS: Accuracy of preoperative magnetic resonance imaging in predicting a subscapularis tendon tear based on arthroscopy. *Arthroscopy* 2010;26(11):1427-1433.

   A retrospective review compared the sensitivity and specificity of MRI and arthroscopy for the diagnosis of subscapularis tears in 90 consecutive patients. Level of evidence: III.

14. Wissman RD, Kapur S, Akers J, Crimmins J, Ying J, Laor T: Cysts within and adjacent to the lesser tuberosity and their association with rotator cuff abnormalities. *AJR Am J Roentgenol* 2009;193(6):1603-1606.

   A retrospective review of 1,000 shoulder MRI examinations correlated the presence of MRI-visualized humeral head cysts in various locations with the presence of rotator cuff tears.

15. Gyftopoulos S, O'Donnell J, Shah NP, Goss J, Babb J, Recht MP: Correlation of MRI with arthroscopy for the evaluation of the subscapularis tendon: A musculoskeletal division's experience. *Skeletal Radiol* 2013;42(9):1269-1275.

   A retrospective review of 286 patients compared the sensitivity and specificity of MRI and arthroscopy in the evaluation of the subscapularis. Discordant findings were reviewed to identify pitfalls in the MRI evaluation.

16. Lee RK, Griffith JF, Tong MM, Sharma N, Yung P: Glenoid bone loss: Assessment with MR imaging. *Radiology* 2013;267(2):496-502.

   A retrospective study compared MRI of glenoid bone loss with CT and arthroscopy in 166 patients.

17. Smith DK, Chopp TM, Aufdemorte TB, Witkowski EG, Jones RC: Sublabral recess of the superior glenoid labrum: Study of cadavers with conventional nonenhanced MR imaging, MR arthrography, anatomic dissection, and limited histologic examination. *Radiology* 1996;201(1):251-256.

18. Williams MM, Snyder SJ, Buford D Jr: The Buford complex: The "cord-like" middle glenohumeral ligament and absent anterosuperior labrum complex. A normal anatomic capsulolabral variant. *Arthroscopy* 1994;10(3):241-247.

19. Tian CY, Cui GQ, Zheng ZZ, Ren AH: The added value of ABER position for the detection and classification of anteroinferior labroligamentous lesions in MR arthrography of the shoulder. *Eur J Radiol* 2013;82(4):651-657.

   A retrospective study compared gold-standard arthroscopy with MRI in the standard and ABER positions for evaluation of the anteroinferior labrum.

20. Wischer TK, Bredella MA, Genant HK, Stoller DW, Bost FW, Tirman PF: Perthes lesion (a variant of the Bankart lesion): MR imaging and MR arthrographic findings with surgical correlation. *AJR Am J Roentgenol* 2002;178(1):233-237.

21. Acid S, Le Corroller T, Aswad R, Pauly V, Champsaur P: Preoperative imaging of anterior shoulder instability: Diagnostic effectiveness of MDCT arthrography and comparison with MR arthrography and arthroscopy. *AJR Am J Roentgenol* 2012;198(3):661-667.

   A retrospective study compared direct MRI and CTA in the evaluation of anterior instability. Arthroscopy was considered the gold standard.

22. George MS, Khazzam M, Kuhn JE: Humeral avulsion of glenohumeral ligaments. *J Am Acad Orthop Surg* 2011;19(3):127-133.

   Clinical findings, imaging findings, and treatment of HAGL lesions were reviewed.

23. Magee T: Prevalence of HAGL lesions and associated abnormalities on shoulder MR examination. *Skeletal Radiol* 2014;43(3):307-313.

   Imaging findings and associated injuries in 23 consecutive patients with surgically confirmed HAGL lesions were retrospectively reviewed.

24. Buck FM, Grehn H, Hilbe M, Pfirrmann CW, Manzanell S, Hodler J: Degeneration of the long biceps tendon: Comparison of MRI with gross anatomy and histology. *AJR Am J Roentgenol* 2009;193(5):1367-1375.

   MRI and histologic findings of biceps tendinopathy in 15 cadaver specimens were compared.

25. Gaskin CM, Anderson MW, Choudhri A, Diduch DR: Focal partial tears of the long head of the biceps brachii tendon at the entrance to the bicipital groove: MR imaging findings, surgical correlation, and clinical significance. *Skeletal Radiol* 2009;38(10):959-965.

   A retrospective study compared arthroscopy and MRI of partial tears of the biceps tendon at the biceps groove entrance in 16 patients.

26. Schaeffeler C, Waldt S, Holzapfel K, et al: Lesions of the biceps pulley: Diagnostic accuracy of MR arthrography of the shoulder and evaluation of previously described and new diagnostic signs. *Radiology* 2012;264(2):504-513.

   A retrospective study evaluated the accuracy of MRA in the diagnosis of lesions of the biceps pulley in 80 consecutive patients, in comparison with arthroscopy.

27. Mengiardi B, Pfirrmann CW, Gerber C, Hodler J, Zanetti M: Frozen shoulder: MR arthrographic findings. *Radiology* 2004;233(2):486-492.

28. Vinson EN, Major NM, Higgins LD: Magnetic resonance imaging findings associated with surgically proven rotator interval lesions. *Skeletal Radiol* 2007;36(5):405-410.

29. Kim KC, Rhee KJ, Shin HD, Kim YM: Estimating the dimensions of the rotator interval with use of magnetic resonance arthrography. *J Bone Joint Surg Am* 2007;89(11):2450-2455.

© 2016 American Academy of Orthopaedic Surgeons

Chapter 54

MRI of the Elbow

Nicholas C. Nacey, MD

Abstract

Radiography, CT, ultrasound, and MRI all are used in elbow imaging to assess patients with pain. However, MRI is the best imaging modality for evaluating soft-tissue structures in the elbow. The common flexor/extensor tendons, biceps tendon, collateral ligaments, and nerves all are commonly injured structures that are easily evaluated with MRI.

Keywords: elbow; MRI

Introduction

Radiography, CT, ultrasound, and MRI each have a role in elbow imaging. Radiographs of the elbow should be obtained if the patient has acute traumatic injury or chronic pain. CT can be helpful in identifying mineralized intra-articular loose bodies or delineating the anatomy of a complex intra-articular fracture. Ultrasound soft-tissue evaluation in the elbow is most useful in evaluating the distal biceps and the common flexor and extensor tendons.[1] Ultrasound allows dynamic imaging, which may be useful in evaluating for ulnar nerve subluxation or a snapping triceps.

In general, MRI is the imaging modality best suited for evaluating soft-tissue structures in the elbow including ligaments, tendons, cartilage, and nerves. Conventional MRI sequences should be obtained in all three planes using T1-weighted and fluid-sensitive sequences (short tau inversion recovery or T2-weighted sequences with fat suppression). Magnetic resonance arthrography (MRA) is particularly beneficial in the evaluation of osteochondral

Neither Dr. Nacey nor any immediate family member has received anything of value from or has stock or stock options held in a commercial company or institution related directly or indirectly to the subject of this chapter.

lesions, loose bodies, and ulnar collateral ligament (UCL) injury in a throwing athlete.[2] Coronal studies should be obtained along a line connecting the medial and lateral epicondyles, and sagittal studies should be perpendicular to the coronal studies.[3] MRI units with a 3-Tesla magnetic field strength can generate high signal-to-noise ratios and are able to demonstrate a more detailed depiction of normal anatomy compared to a 1.5-Tesla unit. Caution is necessary, however, because 3-Tesla imaging can show mild signal alterations of tendons, ligaments, and nerves of the elbow that may not be symptomatic.[4]

Tendons

The common extensor and flexor tendons are best seen on fluid-sensitive coronal and axial studies. Normal tendon should be hypointense on all sequences, except that so-called magic angle artifact occasionally occurs on short echo time sequences, such as T1-weighted and proton density sequences, when normal tendon fibers are oriented 55° from the main magnetic field. Mildly hyperintense or intermediate signal on fluid-sensitive studies within one of these tendons is consistent with tendinosis. A diagnosis of tendinosis on the basis of short echo time sequences requires caution because of the potential for false diagnosis related to magic angle artifact. The presence of magic angle artifact can be confirmed by identifying the normal hypointense appearance of the tendon on T2-weighted or short tau inversion recovery sequences. Hyperintense signal that matches the signal intensity of joint fluid is consistent with tendon tearing[5] (Figure 1). Muscle edema from an associated strain may be seen adjacent to an area of common extensor-flexor tendinosis or tearing. High signal intensity from reactive edema in the adjacent bone sometimes can be seen but need not be present. The extensor carpi radialis brevis is the most commonly injured component of the common extensor tendon, and the pronator teres and flexor carpi radialis are the most commonly injured components of the common flexor tendon. Evaluating the underlying collateral ligament is

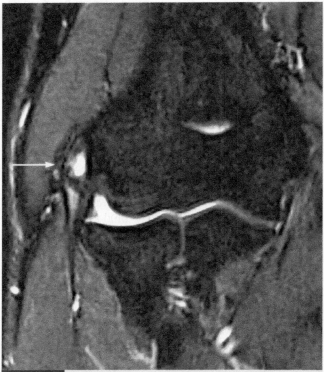

Figure 1 A coronal fluid-sensitive MRI study showing an internal cleft of fluid in the common extensor tendon (arrow), consistent with a high-grade partial tear. The untorn portions of the tendon are thickened and show internal intermediate signal that is not as bright as the fluid signal of the tear, consistent with underlying tendinosis.

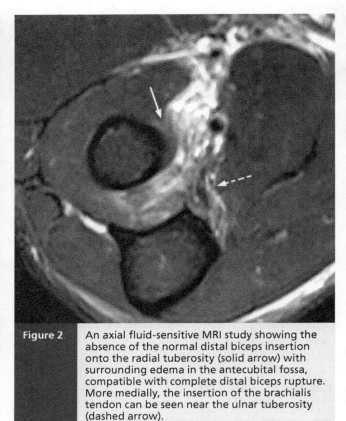

Figure 2 An axial fluid-sensitive MRI study showing the absence of the normal distal biceps insertion onto the radial tuberosity (solid arrow) with surrounding edema in the antecubital fossa, compatible with complete distal biceps rupture. More medially, the insertion of the brachialis tendon can be seen near the ulnar tuberosity (dashed arrow).

critical because tendon débridement in the presence of an undetected ligament injury can lead to elbow instability.[6]

The distal biceps tendon lies anterior to the brachialis tendon and has a much longer tendon segment.[7] Axial studies should extend just distal to the radial tuberosity to ensure that the entire tendon insertion is included. Absence of the biceps tendon at its insertion is consistent with a complete rupture (Figure 2). The distal biceps tendon may have a bifurcated appearance near its insertion on the radial tuberosity because of separation of the short and long heads.[8] Distal biceps tendon tears may proximally retract if there is injury to the lacertus fibrosus. For presurgical planning, sagittal MRI studies can easily measure the extent of tendon stump retraction.[9] Tendinosis and a partial tear of the distal biceps tendon can occur. The distal biceps tendon has no tendon sheath but instead a bicipitoradial bursa is interposed between the tendon and underlying bone. The bursa may become enlarged and inflamed if there is associated biceps pathology.[6] The curving distal biceps tendon sometimes has intermediate signal on T1- or proton density–weighted studies as a result of magic angle artifact; this artifact

is not seen on T2-weighted studies.[10] Positioning the patient in elbow flexion, shoulder abduction, and forearm supination (the FABS position) can improve visualization of the biceps tendon.[7] The triceps tendon normally has a striated appearance because three muscular components contribute to its fibers.[10] Triceps tears usually are best seen on sagittal studies near the insertion of the triceps on the olecranon. Small avulsion fractures or fractured enthesophytes often are present but are best seen on radiographs.[11,12]

Ligaments

The anterior bundle of the UCL, which is the primary stabilizer of the medial side of the elbow, often is injured in throwing athletes. The anterior bundle is best seen on coronal studies. The humeral attachment typically is broader than the distal attachment on the sublime tubercle of the ulna. The posterior bundle of the UCL is less often injured than the anterior bundle and is best seen on axial studies as the floor of the cubital tunnel just deep to the ulnar nerve. With MRA, a tear of the UCL appears as ligament thinning or thickening with associated T2-weighted hyperintense fluid signal or T1-weighted hyperintense signal from gadolinium contrast. In a full-thickness tear, fluid or

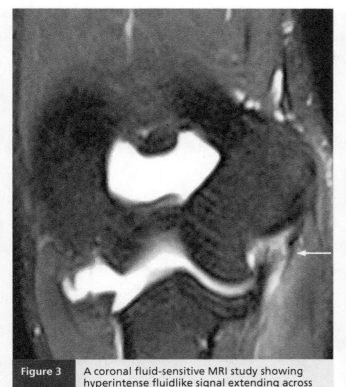

Figure 3 A coronal fluid-sensitive MRI study showing hyperintense fluidlike signal extending across the entire thickness of the ulnar collateral ligament anterior bundle near its humeral attachment (arrow), consistent with a full-thickness tear. The distal insertion of the ligament on the sublime tubercle of the ulna appears intact.

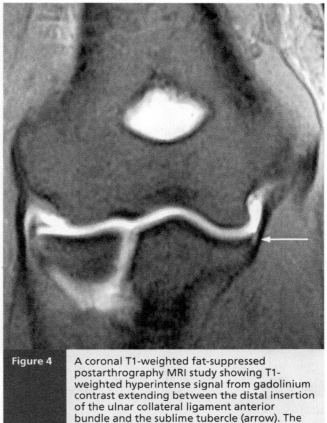

Figure 4 A coronal T1-weighted fat-suppressed postarthrography MRI study showing T1-weighted hyperintense signal from gadolinium contrast extending between the distal insertion of the ulnar collateral ligament anterior bundle and the sublime tubercle (arrow). The presence of the T sign suggests partial-thickness undersurface tearing.

contrast extends across the entire thickness of the ligament and possibly into the adjacent soft tissues[13] (**Figure 3**). Contrast extending between the distal attachment of the UCL anterior bundle and the sublime tubercle (called a T sign) is compatible with a partial-thickness undersurface tear in throwing athletes with medial instability[14] (**Figure 4**). However, anatomic correlation studies found that the T sign can be a normal variant if the gap is less than 3 mm, especially if the patient is older than 75 years.[15,16] In a reconstructed UCL, an enlarged appearance may be normal, with internal intermediate signal of the graft relative to the native UCL. Graft interruption and laxity with a T2-weighted hyperintense fluid signal or gadolinium contrast extending across the graft is compatible with recurrent tearing, however.[17,18]

The lateral ligament complex consists of the radial collateral ligament (RCL), lateral ulnar collateral ligament (LUCL), and annular ligament. The proximal attachment of the RCL and LUCL to the humerus lies just deep to the common extensor tendon, with the RCL just anterior to the LUCL origin. The RCL extends distally to attach to the annular ligament. The LUCL passes along the posterior aspect of the radial head and neck and the annular ligament to eventually insert on the supinator crest of the ulna.[3] The distal aspect of the LUCL can be difficult to see on MRI because of its oblique course; most LUCL tears occur at the humeral attachment, however[16] (**Figure 5**). RCL and LUCL tears appear as fluid signal or gadolinium contrast extending across a portion of the ligament in a partial-thickness tear or the entire thickness of the ligament in a full-thickness tear. LUCL injury often is associated with posterolateral rotatory instability or a prior elbow dislocation.[19,20]

A synovial fringe (a symptomatic plica) sometimes can be found in the radiocapitellar compartment. The diagnostic use of MRI can be problematic because the synovial fringe sometimes has a similar appearance in people with and without symptoms.[21] A synovial fringe thickness of more than 3 mm and coverage of more than one third of the radial head are believed to be the most specific signs of synovial fringe syndrome. Possible associated findings include increased signal within the plica, signal changes in the surrounding bone marrow, and radiocapitellar chondral loss.[22]

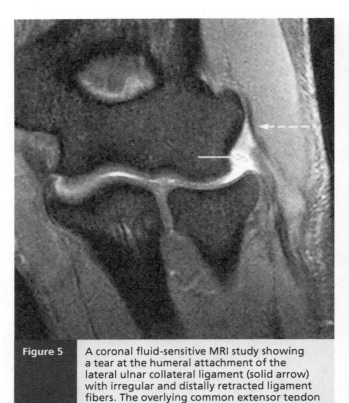

Figure 5 A coronal fluid-sensitive MRI study showing a tear at the humeral attachment of the lateral ulnar collateral ligament (solid arrow) with irregular and distally retracted ligament fibers. The overlying common extensor tendon is thinned, compatible with partial tearing (dashed arrow).

Bones and Cartilage

Two normal, common osseous elbow variants of the elbow are important to note. Cortical irregularity sometimes is seen along the posterior aspect of the capitellum at the bare area without overlying cartilage. This variant, sometimes called a capitellar pseudodefect, can mimic an osteochondral lesion on far-posterior coronal MRI.[23,24] In addition, a central trochlear ridge that is devoid of overlying cartilage can be seen on sagittal MRI and should not be mistaken for a chondral defect.[23,24]

An osteochondral lesion often occurs in the capitellum more anteriorly than the capitellar pseudodefect, typically in older children with fused physes.[25] A capitellar osteochondral lesion is seen on MRI as abnormal signal intensity in the subchondral bone with potential overlying chondral abnormality. Stability of the osteochondral lesion is determined by the presence of focal cartilage interruption and fluid signal or cystic change along the deep aspect of the lesion in the subchondral bone[26] (Figure 6). MRA can be used to determine fragment instability; extension of T1-weighted hyperintense signal from gadolinium contrast along the deep aspect of the lesion is indicative of instability. In children with unfused physes, Panner disease is an osteochondrosis caused by necrosis

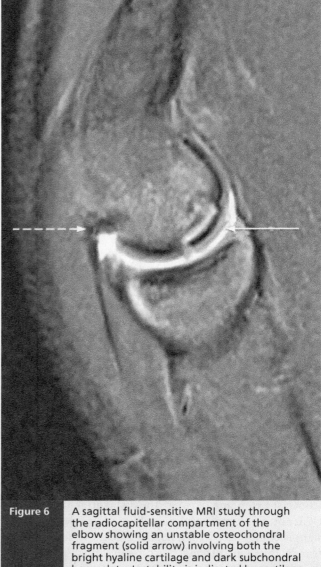

Figure 6 A sagittal fluid-sensitive MRI study through the radiocapitellar compartment of the elbow showing an unstable osteochondral fragment (solid arrow) involving both the bright hyaline cartilage and dark subchondral bone plate. Instability is indicated by cartilage fissures at the margins of the osteochondral fragment with T2-weighted hyperintense fluid signal tracking along the deep aspect of the lesion. The osteochondral fragment is on the anterior aspect of the capitellum. A normal pseudodefect of the capitellum is seen as an irregular area of bone more posteriorly on the capitellum where there is no overlying cartilage (dashed arrow).

and regeneration of the unfused capitellar ossification center. Heterogeneous T1- and T2-weighted signals with associated fragmentation of the capitellar ossification center are characteristic MRI findings in Panner disease.[27]

MRI may be clinically indicated to evaluate for radiographically occult or subtle fractures, most commonly in the radial head or neck in adults and the supracondylar

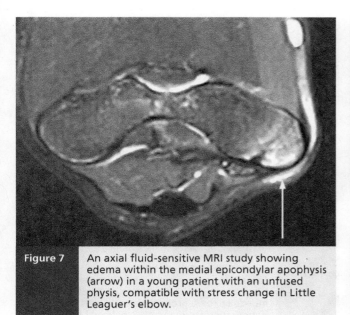

Figure 7   An axial fluid-sensitive MRI study showing edema within the medial epicondylar apophysis (arrow) in a young patient with an unfused physis, compatible with stress change in Little Leaguer's elbow.

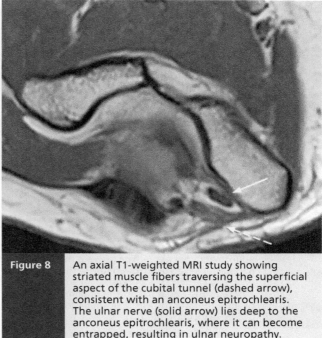

Figure 8   An axial T1-weighted MRI study showing striated muscle fibers traversing the superficial aspect of the cubital tunnel (dashed arrow), consistent with an anconeus epitrochlearis. The ulnar nerve (solid arrow) lies deep to the anconeus epitrochlearis, where it can become entrapped, resulting in ulnar neuropathy.

region in children.[12] Bone contusions often are present after dislocation and can be seen on MRI.[2] An avulsive stress injury to the medial epicondyle, sometimes called Little Leaguer's elbow, can occur before physeal fusion in a young throwing athlete.[14] Edemalike signal from recurrent avulsive stress can be seen on fluid-sensitive MRI within the medial epicondylar apophysis as well as its associated physis (Figure 7). The physis may appear to be abnormally widened.

Cartilage abnormalities can be seen on MRI, although they may be difficult to diagnose because of the intrinsically thin nature of elbow cartilage. In throwing athletes, cartilage defects and/or osteophyte formation can be seen along the medial aspect of the olecranon with posteromedial olecranon impingement as a component of valgus overload syndrome.[14] Intra-articular loose bodies are easily seen on conventional MRI sequences or MRA.

Nerves

The ulnar nerve is the nerve most commonly entrapped at the elbow. The ulnar nerve courses through the cubital tunnel formed anteriorly by the medial epicondyle and UCL posterior bundle, laterally by the olecranon, and posteriorly by the arcuate ligament. The ulnar nerve travels between the humeral and ulnar heads of the flexor carpi ulnaris muscles along the distal aspect of the cubital tunnel; in the more proximal portion there should only be thin, low-signal (ie, dark) arcuate ligament along the superficial aspect of the tunnel without any overlying muscle fibers. Any muscle fibers in this area are from an accessory muscle known as the anconeus epitrochlearis,

which can be associated with ulnar neuropathy[28] (Figure 8). Any mass lesion within the cubital tunnel, such as a ganglion cyst or osteophytes, creates a predisposition to neuropathy. The ulnar nerve also is subject to neuropathy from a mechanical etiology because of valgus overload in throwing athletes.[14] The ulnar nerve normally shows mild hyperintensity on T2-weighted studies in individuals without symptoms. Any nerve enlargement, distortion of the normal nerve fascicles, or extreme hyperintensity on T2-weighted studies suggests neuropathy.[29] Ulnar nerve abnormalities are best seen on axial studies. If scanning is continued distally into the forearm, denervation changes consisting of muscle edemalike signal or fatty atrophy can be seen in the flexor carpi ulnaris and the ulnar half of the flexor digitorum profundus.[30]

The radial nerve courses just deep to the brachioradialis muscle until it approaches the proximal aspect of the supinator muscle (the arcade of Frohse). At this level, the nerve splits into an anterior superficial sensory branch and a posterior deep motor branch (also called the posterior interosseous nerve). MRI can be helpful in identifying an underlying mass causing neuropathy, such as a lipoma or ganglion cyst. Other common causes of radial neuropathy are difficult to distinguish on MRI and include a thickened arcade of Frohse and prominent radial recurrent arteries (the leash of Henry).[29] A normal radial nerve can be difficult to see on conventional MRI sequences, but because of underlying neuropathy may be more visible if it becomes pathologically enlarged or

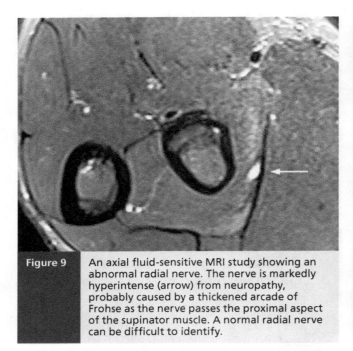

Figure 9 An axial fluid-sensitive MRI study showing an abnormal radial nerve. The nerve is markedly hyperintense (arrow) from neuropathy, probably caused by a thickened arcade of Frohse as the nerve passes the proximal aspect of the supinator muscle. A normal radial nerve can be difficult to identify.

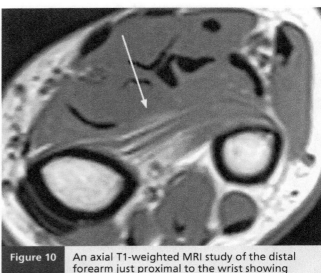

Figure 10 An axial T1-weighted MRI study of the distal forearm just proximal to the wrist showing fatty atrophy of the pronator quadratus muscle (arrow), probably caused by chronic denervation from an abnormality of the anterior interosseous nerve.

hyperintense with T2 weighting (**Figure 9**). Denervation changes may be seen in the innervated territory of the supinator and extensor musculature.[30]

The median nerve courses through the anteromedial elbow along with the brachial artery and vein. Common causes of median neuropathy include entrapment between the two heads of the pronator teres muscle, a thickened bicipital aponeurosis, and a fibrous arch of the flexor digitorum superficialis muscle, all of which are difficult to see on MRI.[28] One abnormality that can be detected by imaging is a normal-variant supracondylar spur with an associated Struthers ligament. The supracondylar spur can be well seen on radiographs, and the relationship between the spur and the Struthers ligament with the median nerve can be deciphered using MRI.[23] The median nerve gives off a motor branch called the anterior interosseous nerve, which innervates the flexor pollicis longus, pronator quadratus, and radial half of the flexor digitorum profundus.[29,30] Pathology within the anterior interosseous nerve itself can be difficult to directly observe on MRI, but denervation changes consisting of edema and/or fatty atrophy within the innervated muscles can suggest the diagnosis (Figure 10).

Summary

MRI is the imaging modality best suited for evaluating soft-tissue structures in the elbow. Common indications include common flexor or extensor tendinopathy, distal biceps tear, UCL or lateral ligamentous complex injuries, osteochondral lesion evaluation, and nerve pathology.

MRA is particularly beneficial in the evaluation of osteochondral lesions, loose bodies, and UCL injury in a throwing athlete.

Key Study Points

- The origins of the common flexor and extensor tendons should be homogenously hypointense on all sequences; intermediately hyperintense signal within the tendon origin on a fluid-sensitive sequence is seen in tendinosis, whereas signal hyperintensity approaching that of joint fluid is consistent with tearing.

- Partial-thickness UCL anterior bundle tears demonstrate ligament thinning or thickening with associated T2-weighted hyperintense fluid signal or T1-weighted hyperintense signal from gadolinium contrast if MRA is performed. Gadolinium tracking deep to the anterior bundle insertion on the sublime tubercle can be seen as a subtle finding of partial-thickness undersurface tears seen only with MRA. In a full-thickness tear, fluid or contrast extends across the entire thickness of the ligament and possibly into the adjacent soft tissues.

- MRI can accurately demonstrate denervation findings in the musculature of the elbow and proximal forearm. However, MRI is often unable to detect the precise pathology within the affected nerve, particularly in the radial and median nerves.

Annotated References

1. Radunovic G, Vlad V, Micu MC, et al: Ultrasound assessment of the elbow. *Med Ultrason* 2012;14(2):141-146.

   The use of ultrasound in elbow imaging was reviewed, with an emphasis on normal tendon and ligament appearance and pathology as well as dynamic maneuvers used in elbow imaging.

2. Dewan AK, Chhabra AB, Khanna AJ, Anderson MW, Brunton LM: MRI of the elbow: Techniques and spectrum of disease. *J Bone Joint Surg Am* 2013;95(14):e99, 1-13.

   Common MRI findings in the elbow were outlined, with an emphasis on recent articles and clinical experience.

3. Terada N, Yamada H, Toyama Y: The appearance of the lateral ulnar collateral ligament on magnetic resonance imaging. *J Shoulder Elbow Surg* 2004;13(2):214-216.

4. Del Grande F, Aro M, Farahani SJ, Wilckens J, Cosgarea A, Carrino JA: Three-Tesla MR imaging of the elbow in non-symptomatic professional baseball pitchers. *Skeletal Radiol* 2015;44(1):115-123.

   A retrospective analysis described common findings on 3-Tesla elbow MRI in asymptomatic professional baseball pitchers, including collateral ligament thickening and ulnar nerve abnormalities.

5. Walz DM, Newman JS, Konin GP, Ross G: Epicondylitis: Pathogenesis, imaging, and treatment. *Radiographics* 2010;30(1):167-184.

   The normal anatomy of the common flexor and extensor tendons was described, with pathologic findings as seen on MRI and ultrasound as well as treatment options.

6. Hayter CL, Adler RS: Injuries of the elbow and the current treatment of tendon disease. *AJR Am J Roentgenol* 2012;199(3):546-557.

   Common elbow pathologic findings on MRI were described, with percutaneous treatment options including corticosteroid injection, percutaneous tenotomy, and platelet-rich plasma injection.

7. Chew ML, Giuffrè BM: Disorders of the distal biceps brachii tendon. *Radiographics* 2005;25(5):1227-1237.

8. Dirim B, Brouha SS, Pretterklieber ML, et al: Terminal bifurcation of the biceps brachii muscle and tendon: Anatomic considerations and clinical implications. *AJR Am J Roentgenol* 2008;191(6):W248-W255.

9. Blease S, Stoller D, Safran M, Li A, Fritz R: The elbow, in Stoller D, ed: *Magnetic Resonance Imaging in Orthopaedics and Sports Medicine,* ed 3. Baltimore, MD, Wolters Kluwer, 2007, pp 1463-1625.

10. Mallisee TA, Boynton MD, Erickson SJ, Daniels DL: Normal MR imaging anatomy of the elbow. *Magn Reson Imaging Clin N Am* 1997;5(3):451-479.

11. Koplas MC, Schneider E, Sundaram M: Prevalence of triceps tendon tears on MRI of the elbow and clinical correlation. *Skeletal Radiol* 2011;40(5):587-594.

    A retrospective study found a higher than expected 3.8% rate of triceps tendon injury in patients referred for elbow MRI. Most injuries consisted of a partial tear.

12. Sheehan SE, Dyer GS, Sodickson AD, Patel KI, Khurana B: Traumatic elbow injuries: What the orthopedic surgeon wants to know. *Radiographics* 2013;33(3):869-888.

    Radiographic findings in common elbow fractures were described, with appropriate use of cross-sectional imaging. It is critical for the radiologist to convey certain elbow trauma findings to the orthopaedic surgeon.

13. Beltran LS, Bencardino JT, Beltran J: Imaging of sports ligamentous injuries of the elbow. *Semin Musculoskelet Radiol* 2013;17(5):455-465.

    The imaging manifestations of sports-related injuries to the medial and lateral collateral ligament complex were reviewed, with normal anatomy, injury biomechanics, and appropriate treatment.

14. Ouellette H, Bredella M, Labis J, Palmer WE, Torriani M: MR imaging of the elbow in baseball pitchers. *Skeletal Radiol* 2008;37(2):115-121.

15. Munshi M, Pretterklieber ML, Chung CB, et al: Anterior bundle of ulnar collateral ligament: Evaluation of anatomic relationships by using MR imaging, MR arthrography, and gross anatomic and histologic analysis. *Radiology* 2004;231(3):797-803.

16. Hughes T, Chung C: Elbow ligaments and instability, in Chung C, Steinbach L, eds: *MRI of the Upper Extremity: Shoulder, Elbow, Wrist, and Hand.* Philadelphia, PA, Wolters Kluwer, 2010, pp 402-430.

    This thorough textbook focuses on upper extremity MRI.

17. Wear SA, Thornton DD, Schwartz ML, Weissmann RC III, Cain EL, Andrews JR: MRI of the reconstructed ulnar collateral ligament. *AJR Am J Roentgenol* 2011;197(5):1198-1204.

    Despite the complex appearance of the reconstructed UCL, MRI can show ligament discontinuity compatible with postsurgical tear. MRA generally should be used to increase joint distention and show any insinuation of intra-articular gadolinium contrast through the ligament defect.

18. MacMahon PJ, Murphy DT, Zoga AC, Kavanagh EC: Postoperative imaging of the elbow, wrist, and hand. *Semin Musculoskelet Radiol* 2011;15(4):340-356.

    Surgery of the elbow, wrist, and hand were reviewed for radiologists, with the postsurgical appearance. There is particular focus on ulnar collateral ligament reconstruction.

19. Schaeffeler C, Waldt S, Woertler K: Traumatic instability of the elbow: Anatomy, pathomechanisms and presentation on imaging. *Eur Radiol* 2013;23(9):2582-2593.

The types of elbow instability and their imaging manifestations were discussed, including posterolateral rotatory instability, valgus instability, complex instability, and dislocation injuries.

20. Schreiber JJ, Potter HG, Warren RF, Hotchkiss RN, Daluiski A: Magnetic resonance imaging findings in acute elbow dislocation: Insight into mechanism. *J Hand Surg Am* 2014;39(2):199-205.

   A retrospective study of patients with elbow dislocation found that complete ligamentous tears were more common on the medial than the lateral side. On the lateral side, tears were more common in the LUCL than in the RCL.

21. Ruiz de Luzuriaga BC, Helms CA, Kosinski AS, Vinson EN: Elbow MR imaging findings in patients with synovial fringe syndrome. *Skeletal Radiol* 2013;42(5):675-680.

   This small retrospective study compared MRI findings in patients with diagnosed synovial fringe syndrome with those in normal control subjects. No findings were statistically significantly different between the groups, although there was a notable difference in plica thickness; thickness greater than 2.6 mm was associated with synovial fringe syndrome.

22. Cerezal L, Rodriguez-Sammartino M, Canga A, et al: Elbow synovial fold syndrome. *AJR Am J Roentgenol* 2013;201(1):W88-W96.

   The clinical presentation, imaging findings, and treatment of synovial fold syndrome were reviewed. Synovial fold syndrome can be clinically confused with other causes of lateral elbow pain, such as lateral epicondylitis, and it also can be misdiagnosed on imaging because of its variable appearance, which often is not related to symptoms.

23. Stein JM, Cook TS, Simonson S, Kim W: Normal and variant anatomy of the elbow on magnetic resonance imaging. *Magn Reson Imaging Clin N Am* 2011;19(3):609-619.

   The normal anatomy of the elbow on MRI was reviewed, with an emphasis on osseous and nonosseous variants that can mimic pathology.

24. Sampaio ML, Schweitzer ME: Elbow magnetic resonance imaging variants and pitfalls. *Magn Reson Imaging Clin N Am* 2010;18(4):633-642.

   Common findings on MRI of the elbow can be misinterpreted as pathologic by an inexperienced interpreter.

25. Bancroft LW, Pettis C, Wasyliw C, Varich L: Osteochondral lesions of the elbow. *Semin Musculoskelet Radiol* 2013;17(5):446-454.

   A pictorial review shows radiographic and MRI findings of osteochondral lesions of the elbow, particularly in the capitellum, with an emphasis on relevant classification systems.

26. Kijowski R, De Smet AA: MRI findings of osteochondritis dissecans of the capitellum with surgical correlation. *AJR Am J Roentgenol* 2005;185(6):1453-1459.

27. Helms C, Major N, Anderson M, Kaplan P, Dussault R: Elbow, in *Musculoskeletal MRI,* ed 2. Philadelphia, PA, Elsevier, 2009, pp 224-243.

28. Linda DD, Harish S, Stewart BG, Finlay K, Parasu N, Rebello RP: Multimodality imaging of peripheral neuropathies of the upper limb and brachial plexus. *Radiographics* 2010;30(5):1373-1400.

   Anatomy, clinical findings, and imaging findings associated with common neuropathies of the upper extremity were reviewed, with the use of ultrasound or MRI in conjunction with electrophysiologic testing.

29. Andreisek G, Crook DW, Burg D, Marincek B, Weishaupt D: Peripheral neuropathies of the median, radial, and ulnar nerves: MR imaging features. *Radiographics* 2006;26(5):1267-1287.

30. Kim SJ, Hong SH, Jun WS, et al: MR imaging mapping of skeletal muscle denervation in entrapment and compressive neuropathies. *Radiographics* 2011;31(2):319-332.

   Distinguishing intrinsic abnormalities within small nerves may be difficult on MRI, but denervation changes consisting of edema and/or fatty atrophy can be seen within the innervated distribution. Nerve distribution maps were reviewed for commonly affected nerves throughout the body, including the elbow.

Chapter 55

Imaging of the Hip

Jennifer L. Pierce, MD

Abstract

Understanding the imaging of the hip joint can provide further detail and information needed to accurately diagnose the complexity of hip pain. MRI is an important modality for the evaluation of both intra-articular etiologies of hip pain such as labrochondral abnormalities and extra-articular etiologies such as ischiofemoral and iliopsoas impingements.

Keywords: acetabular labrum; femoroacetabular impingement; hip cartilage; hip imaging; MRI

Introduction

Imaging of the hip has evolved substantially as a result of new concepts in hip morphology and biomechanics as well as the increasing number of arthroscopic hip procedures being performed.[1] Radiography, CT, ultrasound, and MRI are valuable diagnostic tools. Specific considerations are pertinent in evaluating a painful hip joint in patients who may have ischiofemoral impingement, iliopsoas impingement, or an abnormality of the hip labrum or cartilage in femoroacetabular impingement (FAI).

Ischiofemoral Impingement

Pain and other symptoms of ischiofemoral impingement syndrome are caused by entrapment of the quadratus femoris muscle between the ischial tuberosity and the lesser trochanter.[2] Narrowing of the ischiofemoral space can result from variable positioning of the lower extremity or a congenital or acquired deformity as with fracture, bursitis, or enthesopathy at the lesser trochanter

Neither Dr. Pierce nor any immediate family member has received anything of value from or has stock or stock options held in a commercial company or institution related directly or indirectly to the subject of this chapter.

or ischial tuberosity.[2,3] Because competitive sports often require repetitive, complex movements and great hip exertion, ischiofemoral impingement commonly occurs in athletes.[2,4] Multiple studies found substantial narrowing of the ischiofemoral space in patients with abnormal impingement of the quadratus femoris.[2,4,5] The normal lesser trochanter–ischial tuberosity interval has been reported to be approximately 2 cm; this distance allows rotation of the femur without improper friction or contact with the ischial tuberosity, hamstrings, and quadratus femoris.[2] However, data are limited and vary on normal values for the ischiofemoral space or abnormal values that warrant a diagnosis of ischiofemoral impingement. With internal rotation of the hip, ischiofemoral space was measured at 13 mm (± 5 mm) in patients with ischiofemoral impingement, compared with 23 mm (± 8 mm) in control subjects.[2] When the interval was measured with the hip in neutral position, the ischiofemoral space was 12.9 mm (±3.7 mm) in patients with symptoms and 29.3 mm (± 5.9 mm) in control subjects.[4]

Radiographs in patients with ischiofemoral impingement typically are normal. Bone production, sclerosis, or cystic change occasionally can be seen along the ischial tuberosity or lesser trochanter. MRI is the preferred modality for revealing ischiofemoral space narrowing and edema of the quadratus femoris muscle. Axial fluid-sensitive images, such as T2-weighted fat-suppressed and short tau inversion recovery studies, are especially useful for this purpose.[6] Other MRI findings associated with ischiofemoral impingement include bursae formation along the quadratus femoris or obturator externus, ischial tuberosity or lesser trochanter bone changes, and abnormality of the hamstring tendons[2,4] (Figure 1). Muscle strain and tearing of the quadratus femoris can appear similar to that of ischiofemoral impingement and should be considered if there is no narrowing of the ischiofemoral space.[5]

Iliopsoas Impingement

Iliopsoas impingement is a source of hip pain from iliopsoas inflammation and an anterior labral tear caused

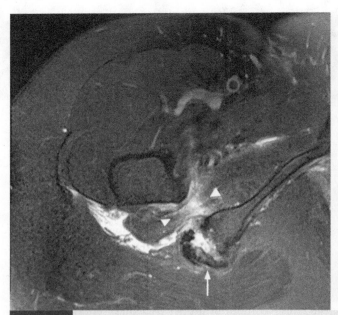 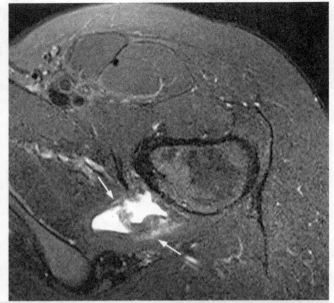

Figure 1 Axial T2-weighted fat-suppressed MRIs demonstrate findings of ischiofemoral impingement. **A,** Muscle edema in the quadratus femoris with a narrow ischiofemoral interval (arrowheads) and associated ischial tuberosity bursitis with partial tearing of the hamstring tendon complex (arrow) are shown. **B,** Development of an obturator externus bursa with mild muscle edema in the quadratus femoris (arrows) is shown.

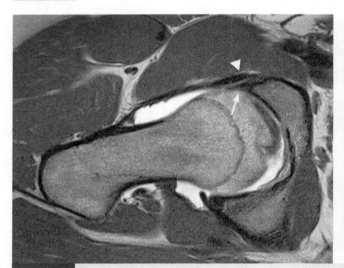 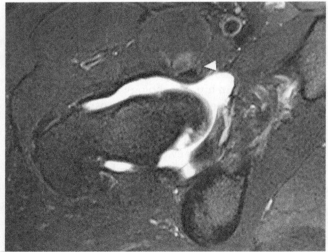

Figure 2 Images show iliopsoas impingement. **A,** Oblique axial T1-weighted magnetic resonance arthrogram shows an anterior labral tear (arrow) directly subjacent to the iliopsoas tendon (arrowhead). **B,** Axial T2-weighted fat-suppressed MRI at a position inferior to the image in **A** shows increased signal surrounding the iliopsoas tendon (arrowhead), which represents edema and bursitis.

by abnormal iliopsoas tendon traction. The labral tear is present in a specific, focal anterior location in the hip labrum at the iliopsoas notch and directly subjacent to the iliopsoas tendon (3 o'clock position).[7] This location is distinctly lower than that of labral injuries associated with femoroacetabular impingement (FAI), hip dysplasia, or trauma, which were described as occurring at the anterosuperior quadrant (1–2 o'clock position).[8] A tight,

inflamed, adherent, and thickened iliopsoas tendon can lead to iliopsoas impingement or produce a traction injury to the labrum and capsule[7] (Figure 2). A relatively narrow width and lateral dip or oblique orientation of the iliopsoas tendon, which are common in women, also can be associated with iliopsoas impingement.[8]

The symptoms of iliopsoas impingement include hip or groin pain, snapping hip (coxa saltans interna), and focal tenderness over the iliopsoas tendon at the anterior joint line. The diagnosis can be confirmed with an ultrasound-guided injection into the iliopsoas bursa, which also can provide long-term relief of symptoms.[7,8] Pain relief after the injection predicts a favorable outcome after surgical release of the iliopsoas tendon.[5]

Hip Labrum Abnormality

The diagnosis of FAI is increasingly common, and hip arthroscopy techniques are advancing. As a result, imaging of the hip has become more accurate and detailed.[9]

The acetabular labrum provides hip joint stability by deepening the acetabular cup, increasing the joint surface area, absorbing pressure or shock, distributing pressure, and sealing the joint to keep synovial fluid within the articular cartilaginous surface. In the absence of the labrum, the articular cartilage is subjected to an increase in contact stress of up to 92%, which leads to early degeneration.[10]

Labral tissue is composed of type I collagen and fibrocartilage. A triangular labral shape is common, but rounded, flattened, and other shapes are normal and are most likely to occur as patients age.[11] A labral tear can form through the substance of the labrum, at the cartilage junction, or at the osseous attachment. Most tears occur as a detachment of the labrum from the labral chondral junction or bony acetabulum.[1] The anterosuperior labrum is the typical location of a tear, especially as related to FAI (**Figure 3**). In FAI, the morphologic osseous changes of a cam deformity, acetabular retroversion, or acetabular overcoverage increase the forces across the anterosuperior hip joint.

Routine MRI of the hip is less accurate than magnetic resonance arthrography (MRA) for detecting labral tears. In comparison with arthroscopy as the gold standard, MRA was found to have sensitivity of 92% to 100% and accuracy of 93% to 96% for detecting labral tears.[12] A 2011 meta-analysis reported that comparisons of MRA and noncontrast MRI found varied sensitivity and specificity values for the detection of labral pathology.[13] Receiver operating characteristic analyses proved that the diagnostic accuracy of MRA was superior to that of noncontrast MRI of the hip. Likewise, CT arthrography with multiplanar reconstruction also can be used to detect labral tears; it offers excellent spatial resolution when iodinated contrast undermines or penetrates the labrum, indicating tear.[1,14] However, CT is inferior to MRI for the evaluation of intrasubstance labral changes, periarticular soft tissues, and edema-like marrow changes. At most institutions, CT arthrography is used to evaluate the labrum if the patient has a contraindication to the use of MRI or if a preoperative assessment of an osseous abnormality,

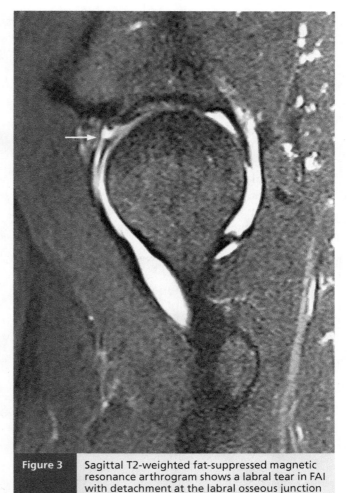

Figure 3 Sagittal T2-weighted fat-suppressed magnetic resonance arthrogram shows a labral tear in FAI with detachment at the labral osseous junction in the anterosuperior quadrant (arrow).

such as a cam or pincer deformity, is necessary. Because of the invasiveness, cost, and time requirement of MRA, improvements in the quality of noncontrast or conventional hip MRI are the subject of ongoing study. Early data suggested that 3-Tesla (T) noncontrast MRI is more effective than 1.5-T MRA for the early detection of chondral and labral pathology and that its use is cost-effective and improves patients' experience.[15]

Although there are well-known normal variants in shoulder labral anatomy, sublabral sulci or recesses in the hip labrum have only been widely reported beginning in 2004.[16-18] A labroligamentous sulcus is created when fluid distends the junction of the labrum and the transverse ligament, especially anteriorly. Therefore, this normal variant can be seen with fluid distension of MRA and should not be mistaken for a tear.

Sublabral sulci are found to be present in approximately 20% to 24% of hips.[17,18] Although a posteroinferior sublabral sulcus (**Figure 4**) initially was described as a potential pitfall in the diagnosis of labral tears,[16] sulci were found at all locations and quadrants of the acetabular labrum. Sulci were most common in the anteroinferior and posterior quadrants.[17] Distinguishing labral tears from sublabral sulci requires a detailed evaluation of the depth and morphology of labral detachment from bone, the subjacent osseous changes, and paralabral cysts. On MRA, sublabral sulci have incomplete labral undermining by contrast or fluid at the labral base–bone junction, have linear morphology, and are less than 2 mm thick. In addition, sublabral sulci lack subjacent osseous changes such as osteophytes, subchondral cysts, sclerosis, and marrow edema (Figure 5). In contrast, labral tears typically are located in the anterosuperior quadrant, have complete to near-complete depth of contrast or fluid undermining of the torn labrum, have a nonlinear appearance, and can be associated with a paralabral cyst or osseous abnormality[17,18] (Figure 6).

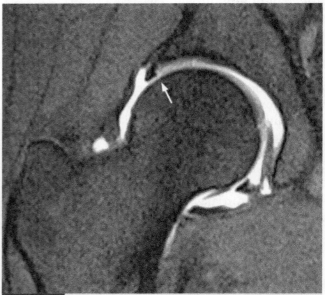

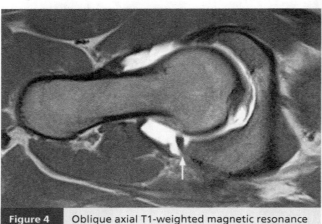

Figure 4 — Oblique axial T1-weighted magnetic resonance arthrogram shows a focal, smooth-margined normal-variant posterior sulcus (arrow) and normal subjacent bone.

Figure 5 — Coronal T1-weighted fat-suppressed magnetic resonance arthrogram shows linear partial undermining by high-signal gadolinium at the labral-chondral junction (arrow). The subjacent bone, surrounding pericapsular structures, and cartilage are normal.

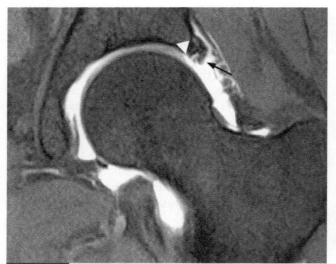

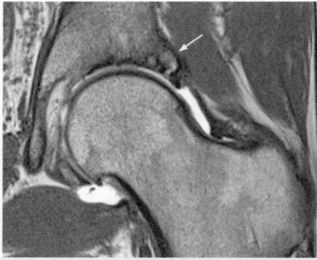

Figure 6 — A, Coronal T1-weighted fat-suppressed magnetic resonance arthrogram shows a chondral defect (arrowhead) and irregular labral undermining by gadolinium (arrow). B, Coronal T1-weighted magnetic resonance arthrogram shows subchondral cysts (arrow) and deficient cartilage at the labral-chondral interface. These findings suggest the presence of a labral tear rather than a sublabral sulcus.

© 2016 American Academy of Orthopaedic Surgeons

Hip Cartilage Abnormality

Imaging and cadaver studies revealed that the greatest hip cartilage thickness is along the superolateral acetabulum and the anterosuperior femoral head.[19,20] Appropriately, these areas must absorb the greatest force during weight bearing and walking. Chondral damage was found in 73% of patients with a labral tear.[21] Therefore, the detection of chondral abnormality should lead to careful evaluation of the labrum, and vice versa. Ninety-four percent of chondral damage was found to occur at the labral-chondral junction, especially in the anterosuperior acetabular labrum, and the presence of labral tears doubled the risk of chondral damage. Relatively young patients were found to have an isolated labral tear, but older patients had both labral and chondral lesions; therefore, it was postulated that labral tears can precede and lead to chondral damage.[21]

Early detection of cartilage disease is preferable, and imaging can be used to provide a noninvasive assessment of chondral areas at risk before irreversible degenerative joint disease occurs. Radiography, CT, and MRI for evaluating articular cartilage traditionally depicted only morphologic defects.[22] However, new MRI cartilage-mapping techniques make it possible to assess the biochemical ultrastructure and health of cartilage before the development of distinct macroscopic defects.[20] The new techniques include T2 mapping, delayed gadolinium-enhanced MRI of cartilage (dGEMRIC), T1-rho MRI, sodium imaging, and diffusion tensor imaging.[20]

Proton-density fast spin-echo and T2-weighted sequences are commonly used in the evaluation of cartilage. Both of these fluid-sensitive sequences show excellent contrast between the osseous, chondral, and fluid interfaces. The associated subchondral cysts and bone marrow edema pattern are most accurately seen in these sequences[22] (Figure 7). MRA is widely used for evaluating articular cartilage in the hip. The distention of the joint with fluid and gadolinium contrast improves the evaluation of the thin and tightly congruent chondral surfaces of the femoral head and acetabulum. Additional joint distraction can be accomplished by applying traction to the hip or lower leg during MRI by using MRI-compatible weights.[23,24] When 6 kg of traction was used in MRA, an average 1.7 mm of separation along the femoral and acetabular surfaces improved detection of chondral defects such as delamination.[24] Noncontrast MRI can be used for the evaluation of cartilage, but relatively few studies have been published.[20] Nonarthrographic MRI of the hip was found to be 88% to 93% sensitive and 78% to 87% specific for the detection of arthroscopy-proved cartilage defects.[25]

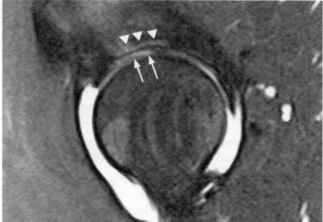

| Figure 7 | Sagittal T2-weighted fat-suppressed magnetic resonance arthrogram shows chondral delamination with subjacent bone marrow edema. This fluid-sensitive sequence shows fluid undermining a flap of acetabular cartilage (arrows) and abnormal reactive edemalike signal in the subchondral bone subjacent to the cartilage defect (arrowheads). |

T2 mapping is sensitive for the collagen and extracellular matrix components of cartilage. Degraded cartilage has a disruption of collagen fiber architecture, decreased concentration of collagen, and increased free water content.[26] Therefore, degenerating cartilage typically produces higher T2 values than normal, healthy cartilage. The use of dGEMRIC sequences provides information on the proteoglycan-glycosaminoglycan (GAG) content of cartilage. The large, negatively charged GAG molecule draws in positively charged sodium ions and binds water into the extracellular matrix of cartilage. Like GAG, gadopentetate dimeglumine has a negative charge, and increased concentrations of gadolinium are distributed into areas with a low GAG density and, therefore, into cartilage that is abnormal and unhealthy.[20] On T1-weighted sequences, this increased or concentrated uptake of gadolinium has shorter T1 values and can be distinguished from the remainder of the chondral surface.[20] Before dGEMRIC sequences are obtained, an intravenous dose of gadolinium is administered. The patient exercises for 15 minutes to aid gadolinium delivery to the hip joint, and a subsequent 30-minute delay allows uptake and concentration of gadolinium in the cartilage. Intravenous gadolinium enters the cartilage from blood perfusion at both the synovium-cartilage and bone-cartilage interfaces.[27]

Summary

Imaging of the hip, especially using MRI, can help distinguish intra-articular and extra-articular etiologies of pain. The diagnosis and treatment of FAI is becoming more prevalent; therefore, understanding hip labral normal variants and pitfalls are crucial for accurate diagnosis. Also, new MRI sequences and technology appear promising for early detection of cartilage degeneration. Ischiofemoral and iliopsoas impingement syndromes need to be distinguished from FAI, and imaging with MRI allows for direct visualization of the regions of interest.

Key Study Points

- The ischiofemoral interval measurement varies with internal and external rotation of the leg. The diagnosis is made when there is impingement type pain and abnormal edema/fluid in the muscle traversing the ischiofemoral space.
- MRI findings of iliopsoas impingement are edema/fluid surrounding the iliopsoas tendon and lower anterior labral tears. Fluoroscopic or ultrasound-guided injection of the iliopsoas bursa is an important diagnostic test and treatment option.
- Hip labral normal variants and sublabral sulci and clefts have been described throughout the labrum. These normal variants will not have complete deattachment of the labrum, adjacent chondral defects, or osseous changes.

Annotated References

1. Sutter R, Zanetti M, Pfirrmann CW: New developments in hip imaging. *Radiology* 2012;264(3):651-667.

   Technical advances in hip imaging and recent anatomic and pathologic insights were reviewed as related to hip diagnoses.

2. Torriani M, Souto SC, Thomas BJ, Ouellette H, Bredella MA: Ischiofemoral impingement syndrome: An entity with hip pain and abnormalities of the quadratus femoris muscle. *AJR Am J Roentgenol* 2009;193(1):186-190.

   The author reviewed the anatomy of the ischiofemoral interval, along with results of internal or external position of the leg.

3. Ali AM, Whitwell D, Ostlere SJ: Imaging and surgical treatment of a snapping hip due to ischiofemoral impingement. *Skeletal Radiol* 2011;40(5):653-656.

   The clinical, anatomic, and imaging aspects of ischiofemoral impingement were discussed in this case report.

4. Tosun O, Algin O, Yalcin N, Cay N, Ocakoglu G, Karaoglanoglu M: Ischiofemoral impingement: Evaluation

with new MRI parameters and assessment of their reliability. *Skeletal Radiol* 2012;41(5):575-587.

   Substantial narrowing of the ischiofemoral space was reported in patients with hip pain and muscle changes to the quadratus femoris, compared with asymptomatic control subjects. MRI with the hip in neutral position detected differences in ischiofemoral space intervals compared with studies with the hip in internal rotation.

5. Blankenbaker DG, Tuite MJ: Non-femoroacetabular impingement. *Semin Musculoskelet Radiol* 2013;17(3):279-285.

   Hip pain caused by ischiofemoral, anteroinferior iliac spine or subspine, or iliopsoas impingement was reviewed, with a focus on MRI findings and pathophysiology.

6. Taneja AK, Bredella MA, Torriani M: Ischiofemoral impingement. *Magn Reson Imaging Clin N Am* 2013;21(1):65-73.

   The anatomic and clinical background of ischiofemoral impingement was reviewed. Ischiofemoral impingement is difficult to diagnosis on radiographs and CT. MRI is the preferred modality for seeing a narrowed ischiofemoral space and quadratus femoris muscle edema changes.

7. Domb BG, Shindle MK, McArthur B, Voos JE, Magennis EM, Kelly BT: Iliopsoas impingement: A newly identified cause of labral pathology in the hip. *HSS J* 2011;7(2):145-150.

   Iliopsoas impingement causes labral tearing directly subjacent to the iliopsoas tendon at the level of the iliopsoas notch. An inflamed, adherent iliopsoas tendon can cause impingement or traction injury to the labrum and capsule.

8. Blankenbaker DG, Tuite MJ, Keene JS, del Rio AM: Labral injuries due to iliopsoas impingement: Can they be diagnosed on MR arthrography? *AJR Am J Roentgenol* 2012;199(4):894-900.

   A review of arthroscopically proved iliopsoas impingement found that related labral tears were focally present at the 3 o'clock position. This position is lower than the typical 1 to 2 o'clock labral tears in FAI or osteoarthritis. Especially in women, a narrow width and oblique orientation of the iliopsoas tendon may be associated with iliopsoas impingement.

9. Thomas JD, Li Z, Agur AM, Robinson P: Imaging of the acetabular labrum. *Semin Musculoskelet Radiol* 2013;17(3):248-257.

   Imaging of labral tears was reviewed with a focus on MRI. Labral tears resulting from FAI, hip hypermobility, degeneration, dysplasia, and trauma were discussed, with pitfalls in labral imaging, such as sublabral sulci. The effectiveness of noncontrast 3-T MRI was compared with that of 1.5-T MRA. Early data suggest that 3-T noncontrast MRI is preferable to 1.5-T MRA.

10. Ferguson SJ, Bryant JT, Ganz R, Ito K: The influence of the acetabular labrum on hip joint cartilage

© 2016 American Academy of Orthopaedic Surgeons

consolidation: A poroelastic finite element model. *J Biomech* 2000;33(8):953-960.

11. Lecouvet FE, Vande Berg BC, Malghem J, et al: MR imaging of the acetabular labrum: Variations in 200 asymptomatic hips. *AJR Am J Roentgenol* 1996;167(4):1025-1028.

12. Beaulé PE, O'Neill M, Rakhra K: Acetabular labral tears. *J Bone Joint Surg Am* 2009;91(3):701-710.

    This study compared the accuracy of MRA to arthroscopy as the gold standard for labral tears.

13. Smith TO, Hilton G, Toms AP, Donell ST, Hing CB: The diagnostic accuracy of acetabular labral tears using magnetic resonance imaging and magnetic resonance arthrography: A meta-analysis. *Eur Radiol* 2011;21(4):863-874.

    This meta-analysis included 19 articles and a total of 881 hips. Although there was a wide range of sensitivities and specificities for the use of noncontrast MRI and MRA, the diagnostic accuracy of MRA was found to be superior.

14. Llopis E, Fernandez E, Cerezal L: MR and CT arthrography of the hip. *Semin Musculoskelet Radiol* 2012;16(1):42-56.

    MRI and CT arthrography of the hip were reviewed, with imaging findings related to several intra-articular hip pathologies, especially labral tears and chondral defects.

15. Robinson P: Conventional 3-T MRI and 1.5-T MR arthrography of femoroacetabular impingement. *AJR Am J Roentgenol* 2012;199(3):509-515.

    The concept of FAI and the MRI findings associated with FAI were reviewed. The current status of 1.5-T MRA was described and compared with noncontrast 3-T MRI. With its increasing availability, powerful new sequences, and noninvasive nature, noncontrast 3-T MRI has the potential to be superior to 1.5-T MRA.

16. Dinauer PA, Murphy KP, Carroll JF: Sublabral sulcus at the posteroinferior acetabulum: A potential pitfall in MR arthrography diagnosis of acetabular labral tears. *AJR Am J Roentgenol* 2004;183(6):1745-1753.

17. Saddik D, Troupis J, Tirman P, O'Donnell J, Howells R: Prevalence and location of acetabular sublabral sulci at hip arthroscopy with retrospective MRI review. *AJR Am J Roentgenol* 2006;187(5):W507-11.

18. Studler U, Kalberer F, Leunig M, et al: MR arthrography of the hip: Differentiation between an anterior sublabral recess as a normal variant and a labral tear. *Radiology* 2008;249(3):947-954.

19. Kurrat HJ, Oberländer W: The thickness of the cartilage in the hip joint. *J Anat* 1978;126(Pt 1):145-155.

20. Petchprapa CN, Recht MP: Imaging of chondral lesions including femoroacetabular impingement. *Semin Musculoskelet Radiol* 2013;17(3):258-271.

    The function and structure of cartilage were emphasized to improve understanding of traditional MRI of the physical, morphologic defects of cartilage and new, biochemically based MRI sequences for evaluating the ultrastructure of cartilage.

21. McCarthy JC, Noble PC, Schuck MR, Wright J, Lee J: The role of labral lesions to development of early degenerative hip disease. *Clin Orthop Relat Res* 2001;393:25-37.

22. Strickland CD, Kijowski R: Morphologic imaging of articular cartilage. *Magn Reson Imaging Clin N Am* 2011;19(2):229-248.

    MRI sequences and their ability to show hip cartilage were discussed.

23. Nishii T, Nakanishi K, Sugano N, Masuhara K, Ohzono K, Ochi T: Articular cartilage evaluation in osteoarthritis of the hip with MR imaging under continuous leg traction. *Magn Reson Imaging* 1998;16(8):871-875.

24. Llopis E, Cerezal L, Kassarjian A, Higueras V, Fernandez E: Direct MR arthrography of the hip with leg traction: Feasibility for assessing articular cartilage. *AJR Am J Roentgenol* 2008;190(4):1124-1128.

    Continuous traction provided with 6-kg MRI-compatible weights achieved 1.6 mm of separation between the acetabular and femoral chondral surfaces. The increased separation may improve detection of chondral defects such as delamination.

25. Mintz DN, Hooper T, Connell D, Buly R, Padgett DE, Potter HG: Magnetic resonance imaging of the hip: Detection of labral and chondral abnormalities using noncontrast imaging. *Arthroscopy* 2005;21(4):385-393.

26. Mosher TJ, Dardzinski BJ: Cartilage MRI T2 relaxation time mapping: Overview and applications. *Semin Musculoskelet Radiol* 2004;8(4):355-368.

27. Burstein D, Gray M, Mosher T, Dardzinski B: Measures of molecular composition and structure in osteoarthritis. *Radiol Clin North Am* 2009;47(4):675-686.

    This article reviews new specialized magnetic resonance sequences to evaluate the ultrastructure of cartilage to detect early cartilage degeneration and change.

Chapter 56

Imaging of the Knee

Meredith C. Northam, MD

Abstract

The knee is one of the most commonly injured joints in the body and is also a common source of chronic pain. The menisci, articular cartilage, and major ligaments of the knee may be injured and require surgical exploration and/or intervention. These structures are well evaluated with MRI so this can be a useful tool for preoperative planning or when diagnosis is uncertain. Familiarity with the appearance of these key structures and their injuries on MRI can be beneficial to the clinical practice of the orthopaedic surgeon.

Keywords: anterior cruciate ligament; cartilage; knee imaging; MRI; meniscus; posterior cruciate ligament

Introduction

The knee is one of the most important joints in the human body and knee pain is a common complaint among patients. Although an orthopaedic surgeon gathers a great deal of clinical information from the patient and by performing a physical examination, a basic understanding of the appearance of the knee on MRI can be extremely beneficial. In addition, it is important for the orthopaedic surgeon to review the appearance of the major structures of the knee and the appearance of common injuries on MRI.

The Anterior Cruciate Ligament

The anterior cruciate ligament (ACL) is the most commonly injured major ligament of the knee. The ACL stabilizes the knee primarily by resisting anterior translation

Neither Dr. Northam nor any immediate family member has received anything of value from or has stock or stock options held in a commercial company or institution related directly or indirectly to the subject of this chapter.

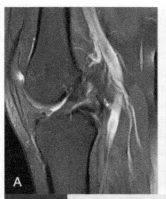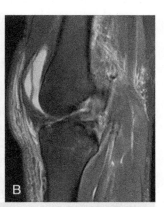

Figure 1 Sagittal T2-weighted fat-suppressed MRI of the anterior cruciate ligament (ACL). **A,** A normal ACL with homogenous low signal intensity and intact fibers paralleling the intercondylar roof. **B,** An intrasubstance tear of the ACL.

and secondarily by resisting varus and valgus forces.[1] Approximately 90% of ACL tears can be diagnosed based on the patient's clinical history and a thorough physical examination. MRI is the imaging study of choice for diagnosing pathology and tears in the ACL as well as associated injuries. The accuracy of MRI for ACL tears was found to be 95% to 100%.[2] To avoid magic angle artifact, which can mimic a tear, T2-weighted sequences are recommended for evaluation of the ACL rather than T1-weighted sequences. An intact ACL usually is seen as taut fibers paralleling the intercondylar roof on sagittal MRI studies, but confirmation on axial and coronal views is recommended (Figure 1, A). ACL tears most commonly involve the intrasubstance fibers (approximately 70%), but 7% to 20% occur proximally at the femoral attachment of the ACL and 3% to 10% occur distally at the tibial insertion.[3,4]

On MRI, the primary sign of a complete tear of the ACL is complete disruption of the fibers (Figure 1, B). Occasionally the ACL is completely torn, although the fibers initially appear to be intact on MRI. The fibers are wavy in appearance and have a relatively horizontal or flat angle with respect to the intercondylar roof, and this subtle appearance is consistent with a tear. Secondary MRI signs of an ACL tear also have been reported. Pivot-shift bone contusions often are seen as bone marrow edema in the lateral femoral condyle and posterolateral tibial plateau. The contusion occurs when the tibia is displaced anteriorly and impacts onto the lateral femoral condyle. This mechanism also can produce an impaction fracture (the so-called deep femoral notch sign).[5,6] A contrecoup bone contusion in the posteromedial tibial plateau, a Segond fracture (a small avulsion fracture of the lateral tibial plateau related to the meniscotibial ligament and/or slips from the iliotibial band or lateral collateral ligament), and anterior translation of the tibia also have been described.[3,5,7] Patients with an ACL tear with a cortical depression fracture were reported to have an increased incidence of meniscal tears in the same knee as well as a relatively poor clinical outcome 1 year after ACL reconstruction.[8] In the same study, an increased volume of bone marrow edema without fracture was not associated with a poor postoperative clinical outcome.

A partial ACL tear usually is treated nonsurgically. There are relatively few published studies on this type of tear because it is not common and can be difficult to diagnose clinically or radiographically. MRI findings suggesting a partial tear include an increased T2 signal along the course of the ligament, with predominantly intact fibers; unexpected focal angulation of intact fibers; and, in a chronic tear, attenuation of the fibers.[2] Narrowing of the transverse dimension with a normal anterior-posterior dimension on axial imaging has been described in a stable partial tear; the absence of the anteromedial or posterolateral bundle suggests an unstable partial tear.[9] New imaging planes have been suggested for use in the diagnosis of partial ACL tears. A recent study reported that 32% of suspected ACL injuries were selective bundle tears, and there were three times as many anteromedial bundle tears as posterolateral bundle tears.[10] The study also found that 3-Tesla (3-T) imaging in the oblique coronal plane yielded significantly greater specificity (92% to 96%) for selective bundle tears than imaging in conventional orthogonal (sagittal and coronal) planes (67%). The use of this imaging approach can be beneficial in selective ACL bundle reconstructions.

Pitfalls in the diagnosis of ACL tears are related to increased T2-weighted signal abnormality along the course of the ligament that results from mucoid degeneration or an ACL ganglion. These patients usually have no instability, may have no symptoms, and occasionally have a history of swelling or fullness in the knee. An ACL ganglion is best identified on MRI as a globular mass-like cyst within the ACL, although with intact fibers (Figure 2). An ACL ganglion is difficult to diagnose through an arthroscopic anterior portal because it is difficult to see superficially or anteriorly. Probing or aspirating from a posterior portal usually is required.[11-13]

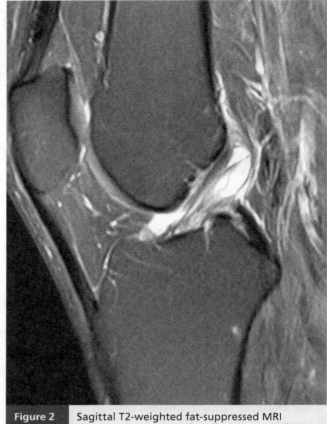

Figure 2 Sagittal T2-weighted fat-suppressed MRI shows an anterior cruciate ligament ganglion with a globular, masslike hyperintense signal abnormality within the ligament, with intact fibers.

The Posterior Cruciate Ligament

The posterior cruciate ligament (PCL) is not often torn. The PCL also is infrequently repaired or reconstructed, although surgical correction is becoming more common. On MRI, the normal PCL is seen curving into the intercondylar notch, is usually less than 6 mm thick in the anterior-posterior dimension (as measured on T2-weighted sagittal images), and has a low signal intensity on all sequences.[14] The PCL is unusual in that the fibers most often do not frankly disrupt with tearing, although complete intrasubstance tears and avulsions are possible (Figure 3). Instead, the ligament stretches significantly and subsequently becomes structurally incompetent.[14] On MRI, a torn PCL ligament appears as thickened to more than 7 mm, with a sensitivity of 94% and specificity of 92%, and usually the T1- and proton density–weighted intrasubstance signal abnormality is greater than the T2-weighted signal abnormality.[14] Unlike other ligament tears, for unknown reasons PCL tears only rarely have a significantly increased T2-weighted intrasubstance signal

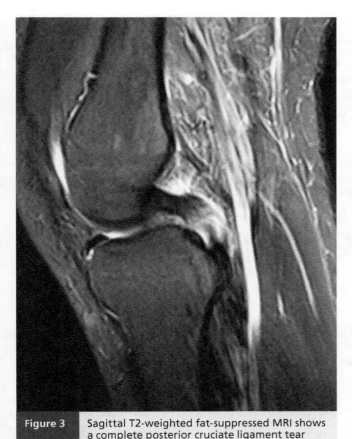

Figure 3 Sagittal T2-weighted fat-suppressed MRI shows a complete posterior cruciate ligament tear with disruption of the fibers.

abnormality. Because of these features, radiologists sometimes miss the diagnosis of PCL tear.

MRI can suggest mucoid degeneration of the PCL, as in the ACL.[15] With mucoid degeneration, the PCL usually is thickened and has increased T2- and proton density–weighted signal abnormality (although the intensity of the signal abnormality is less than in a tear). The similarity of these findings to those for a PCL tear can lead to confusion. A so-called tram-track appearance of the PCL on MRI helps to distinguish mucoid degeneration from a PCL tear. The tram-track appearance is associated with a functionally intact ligament and is described as a homogeneous longitudinal T2- and proton density–weighted intrasubstance signal abnormality that usually extends along the course of the entire ligament, with intact fibers coursing through the signal abnormality on all three planes and an adjacent peripheral rim of intact hypointense ligament fibers.[15]

The Menisci and Hyaline Cartilage

MRI is the most accurate imaging modality for diagnosing a meniscal tear. The menisci are C- shaped and thicker at the periphery than at the center. The posterior horn of the medial meniscus is larger than the anterior horn, and the horns are roughly equal in size to those of the lateral meniscus. A meniscus should be seen as having a homogeneously low signal intensity on all imaging sequences, although some mildly increased intrasubstance signal in the posterior horn of the medial meniscus is normal in children and young adults and is related to normal vascularity. Older adults may have a predominantly intrasubstance signal abnormality that does not extend to the articular surface. This finding represents mucoid degeneration, which is not always a source of pain and does not always lead to a meniscal tear but is mentioned in imaging reports to acknowledge signal abnormality that does not represent a tear.[2,16]

Several variants should be noted when evaluating the menisci. Meniscal flounce usually occurs along the free edge of the medial meniscus and typically is secondary to flexion and redundancy of the free edge. A meniscal ossicle is of uncertain etiology and can be congenital, posttraumatic, or degenerative. The ossicle most often is seen in the posterior horn of the medial meniscus and should not be called a loose body. A discoid meniscus is most common in the lateral meniscus and is a central extension of the meniscal fibrocartilage to cover the central tibial plateau. A discoid extension can be diagnosed if the body of the meniscus measures 15 mm or more on a relevant central coronal image or if three or more bowtie shapes are identified on contiguous (4-mm-thick) sagittal images (**Figure 4**). Chondrocalcinosis also can been seen on MRI, and it is important to correlate the images with corresponding radiographs.[16]

A meniscal tear has been defined as a "distortion in the absence of prior surgery or increased intrasubstance signal intensity unequivocally contacting the articular surface."[16]

If the signal is seen on two contiguous slices, the positive predictive value for a tear is 94% in the medial meniscus and 96% in the lateral meniscus.[16] Meniscal tears are best diagnosed on MRI sequences with a low echo time, such as T1- and proton density–weighted sequences. Oblique, horizontal, longitudinal, radial, complex, and root meniscal tears can occur. A horizontal tear runs parallel to the tibial articular surface and divides the meniscus into superior and inferior halves (**Figure 5**). These tears most often are degenerative and often are associated with a parameniscal cyst. A longitudinal tear runs perpendicular to the tibial articular surface and divides the meniscus into peripheral and central halves. These tears usually occur in relatively young patients after a traumatic event, and they are strongly associated with ACL tears. A radial tear is both perpendicular and parallel to the tibial articular

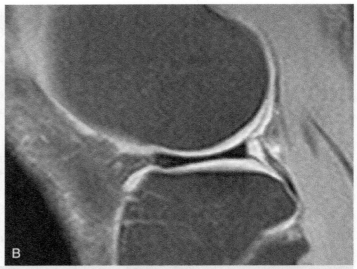

Figure 4 MRI shows a discoid lateral meniscus. **A,** Coronal T2-weighted fat-suppressed sequence. **B,** Sagittal proton density–weighted fat-suppressed sequence.

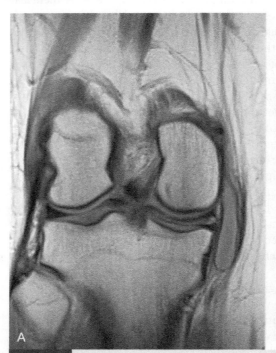

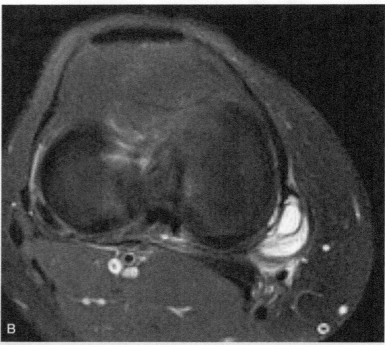

Figure 5 MRI shows a horizontal tear of the medial meniscus with an adjacent parameniscal cyst. **A,** Coronal proton density–weighted sequence. **B,** Axial T2-weighted fat-suppressed sequence.

surface; it disrupts the hoop strength of the meniscus, causing significant loss of meniscal function. A root tear typically is a type of radial tear, and it can result in meniscal extrusion of more than 3 mm beyond the tibial plateau (**Figure 6**). These tears are well known for being missed on MRI and during arthroscopy. The coronal plane is best for diagnosing a root tear. A complex tear is a combination of horizontal, vertical, and radial tears.[2,16]

The indirect signs of a meniscal tear include a parameniscal cyst, a meniscal extrusion, and subchondral bone marrow edema. Parameniscal cysts are strongly associated with an underlying meniscal tear, and the likelihood of an underlying meniscal tear varies with the location of the parameniscal cyst.[17] Specifically, 100% of patients with a lateral parameniscal cyst adjacent to the body and posterior horn of the lateral meniscus had an underlying

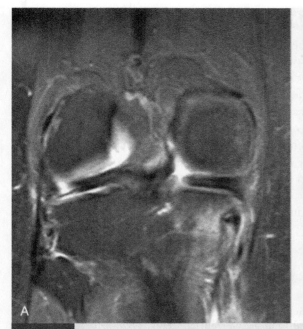
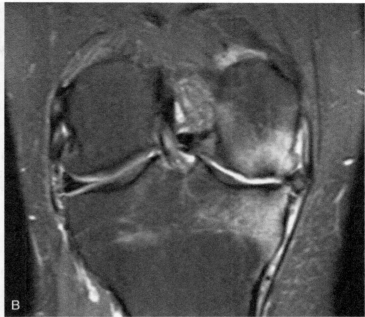

Figure 6 MRI shows a posterior root tear. **A,** Coronal T2-weighted fat-suppressed sequence showing a complete tear of the posterior root of the medial meniscus. **B,** A more anterior sequence shows associated meniscal extrusion and severe osteoarthrosis.

meniscal tear, but an underlying meniscal tear was not present in 36% of the patients with a parameniscal cyst adjacent to the anterior horn-body region of the lateral meniscus.[17] It is necessary to be aware that a parameniscal cyst within the region of the anterior horn of the lateral meniscus is less likely to have underlying tear than a parameniscal cyst elsewhere in the knee.

Meniscal root tears reportedly are difficult to diagnose on MRI or during arthroscopy. These tears were described using 3-T MRI correlated with dissection photographs of cadaver knee specimens.[18] Posterior root tears of the lateral meniscus were found to be associated with meniscal extrusion and ACL tears.[19] The posterior root of the lateral meniscus does not have the isosceles triangular configuration seen elsewhere in the menisci. The usefulness of MRI in diagnosing a tear of the posterior root of the lateral meniscus was evaluated, with the question of whether an associated ACL tear alters diagnostic accuracy.[20] The standard criteria for diagnosing meniscal tears were found to be adequate to diagnose a posterior root tear of the lateral meniscus, and the presence or absence of an ACL tear did not affect the ability to diagnose a meniscal root tear.

An association between medial meniscal root tears and medial tibiofemoral cartilage loss has primarily been described in small studies. An association between medial meniscal root tears and the development or worsening of medial tibiofemoral chondrosis was found in a study that

used a longitudinal design.[21] The significantly greater prevalence of severe chondral loss in patients with a root tear than in those without a meniscal root tear supported the theory that meniscal root tears have a pseudomeniscectomy-like effect.[21]

Hyaline cartilage is an extremely important intra-articular tissue that supports joints and often is injured by trauma or degenerative change in the knee. Damaged cartilage rarely heals spontaneously, and its subsequent degeneration leads to osteoarthrosis of the knee. Surgical and pharmacologic advancements have become extremely important in the treatment of damaged cartilage. MRI is the most important and widely used imaging modality for evaluating cartilage because of its superior contrast resolution. Multiple grading systems can be used for cartilage abnormalities, but for clinical purposes it is best to describe the abnormality in terms of focal abnormal signal, surface fibrillation, partial- or full-thickness chondral loss, and underlying bone marrow signal abnormality. It is also important to note any delamination, which appears as high-signal abnormality at the bone-cartilage interface.[2]

Many sequences can be used for cartilage evaluation, but the most common are the two dimensional fast spin-echo proton density–weighted and T2-weighted imaging sequences, with or without fat suppression. Many institutions prefer an intermediate-weighted sequence that combines the contrast advantage of proton density weighting with that of T2 weighting by using an echo time of 33 to 60 msec. T1-weighted sequences do not provide adequate contrast between the joint fluid and the cartilage and should not be the primary type of sequence.

The field strength of the imaging magnet has important implications for the assessment of hyaline cartilage. In patients with symptoms, 3-T MRI offered better diagnostic performance than 1.5-T MRI for assessing articular cartilage.[22] The specificity and accuracy of 3-T MRI was greater for detecting cartilage lesions, but it did not have greater sensitivity than 1.5-T imaging. In addition, 3-T imaging had greater accuracy than 1.5-T imaging for grading articular surfaces and cartilage lesions.[22] Additional sequences also are being studied for the evaluation of cartilage; with 3-T MRI, T2 mapping was shown to improve sensitivity in the detection of cartilage lesions within the knee from 74.6% to 88.9%.[23] The greatest improvement in sensitivity was noted in patients with early cartilage degeneration, and this sequence can have a significant effect on early detection and possibly prevention of further cartilage degeneration.[23]

Summary

The knee joint is a common source of pain in patients presenting to an orthopaedic clinic. The ACL and PCL are two of the major ligaments of the knee; the former being commonly injured and the latter being infrequently torn. The ACL may be completely or partially torn, or may have a bulbous appearance suggestive of mucoid degeneration. The PCL may be torn with seemingly intact thickened fibers on MRI or be disrupted and/or avulsed. The appearance of mucoid degeneration of the PCL has recently been described as a tram-track appearance with increased proton density and T2 signal abnormality diffusely along its course. Signal abnormality within the meniscus that extends to the articular surface on at least two images is suggestive of tear. Many types of meniscal tears have been described and include oblique/horizontal, vertical, radial and complex tears. Parameniscal cysts are a secondary sign of meniscal tear, but may not always be when located along the anterior horn of the lateral meniscus. Hyaline cartilage is best evaluated on proton density– and T2-weighted images with or without fat saturation, and diagnostic accuracy is increased when imaging on a 3-T magnet.

Key Study Points

- The ACL may be completely or partially torn, or may have a bulbous appearance suggestive of mucoid degeneration.
- The PCL may be torn with seemingly intact thickened fibers on MRI or be disrupted and/or avulsed.
- Parameniscal cysts are often a secondary sign of meniscal tear.
- Hyaline cartilage is best evaluated on proton density– and T2-weighted images with or without fat saturation; imaging on a 3-T magnet increases diagnostic accuracy.

Annotated References

1. Swenson TM, Harner CD: Knee ligament and meniscal injuries: Current concepts. *Orthop Clin North Am* 1995;26(3):529-546.

2. Helms C, Major N, Anderson M, Kaplan P, Dussault R: *Musculoskeletal MRI*.Philadelphia, PA, Saunders, 2009.

3. Resnick D, Kransdorf M: *Bone and Joint Imaging*.Philadelphia, PA, Saunders, 2004.

4. Remer EM, Fitzgerald SW, Friedman H, Rogers LF, Hendrix RW, Schafer MF: Anterior cruciate ligament injury: MR imaging diagnosis and patterns of injury. *Radiographics* 1992;12(5):901-915.

5. Kaplan PA, Walker CW, Kilcoyne RF, Brown DE, Tusek D, Dussault RG: Occult fracture patterns of the knee associated with anterior cruciate ligament tears: Assessment with MR imaging. *Radiology* 1992;183(3):835-838.

6. Garth WP Jr, Greco J, House MA: The lateral notch sign associated with acute anterior cruciate ligament disruption. *Am J Sports Med* 2000;28(1):68-73.

7. Campos JC, Chung CB, Lektrakul N, et al: Pathogenesis of the Segond fracture: Anatomic and MR imaging evidence of an iliotibial tract or anterior oblique band avulsion. *Radiology* 2001;219(2):381-386.

8. Kijowski R, Sanogo ML, Lee KS, et al: Short-term clinical importance of osseous injuries diagnosed at MR imaging in patients with anterior cruciate ligament tear. *Radiology* 2012;264(2):531-541.

   This retrospective study evaluated patients with an ACL tear and a depression fracture. Clinical outcome scores were decreased 1 year after ACL reconstruction surgery. Bone marrow edema volume was not associated with the decrease in clinical outcome scores.

© 2016 American Academy of Orthopaedic Surgeons

9. Roychowdhury S, Fitzgerald SW, Sonin AH, Peduto AJ, Miller FH, Hoff FL: Using MR imaging to diagnose partial tears of the anterior cruciate ligament: Value of axial images. *AJR Am J Roentgenol* 1997;168(6):1487-1491.

10. Park HJ, Kim SS, Lee SY, et al: Comparison between arthroscopic findings and 1.5-T and 3-T MRI of oblique coronal and sagittal planes of the knee for evaluation of selective bundle injury of the anterior cruciate ligament. *AJR Am J Roentgenol* 2014;203(2):W199-206.

   In this study, the oblique coronal plane and the combination of the orthogonal planes and both sagittal oblique and coronal oblique planes provide better diagnostic information with increased specificity on 3-T MRI compared with orthogonal views alone for the diagnosis of selective bundle tears. The results were not similar for 1.5-T MRI.

11. McIntyre J, Moelleken S, Tirman P: Mucoid degeneration of the anterior cruciate ligament mistaken for ligamentous tears. *Skeletal Radiol* 2001;30(6):312-315.

12. Fealy S, Kenter K, Dines JS, Warren RF: Mucoid degeneration of the anterior cruciate ligament. *Arthroscopy* 2001;17(9):E37.

13. Bergin D, Morrison WB, Carrino JA, Nallamshetty SN, Bartolozzi AR: Anterior cruciate ligament ganglia and mucoid degeneration: Coexistence and clinical correlation. *AJR Am J Roentgenol* 2004;182(5):1283-1287.

14. Rodriguez W Jr, Vinson EN, Helms CA, Toth AP: MRI appearance of posterior cruciate ligament tears. *AJR Am J Roentgenol* 2008;191(4):1031.

15. McMonagle JS, Helms CA, Garrett WE Jr, Vinson EN: Tram-track appearance of the posterior cruciate ligament (PCL): Correlations with mucoid degeneration, ligamentous stability, and differentiation from PCL tears. *AJR Am J Roentgenol* 2013;201(2):394-399.

   On MRI, PCL tears and findings suggestive of mucoid degeneration show intrasubstance signal abnormality and ligament thickening. Tram-track appearance with peripheral rim of hypointense signal is seen with mucoid degeneration. Patients with mucoid degeneration usually are asymptomatic and have no instability.

16. Nguyen JC, De Smet AA, Graf BK, Rosas HG: MR imaging-based diagnosis and classification of meniscal tears. *Radiographics* 2014;34(4):981-999.

   The MRI findings of meniscal tearing of the knee were reviewed in this study.

17. De Smet AA, Graf BK, del Rio AM: Association of parameniscal cysts with underlying meniscal tears as identified on MRI and arthroscopy. *AJR Am J Roentgenol* 2011;196(2):W180-6.

   Compared with parameniscal cysts associated with the medial meniscus or other locations in the lateral meniscus, parameniscal cysts adjacent to the anterior horn or root of the lateral meniscus are less likely to have an underlying meniscal tear.

18. Brody JM, Hulstyn MJ, Fleming BC, Tung GA: The meniscal roots: Gross anatomic correlation with 3-T MRI findings. *AJR Am J Roentgenol* 2007;188(5):W446-50.

19. Brody JM, Lin HM, Hulstyn MJ, Tung GA: Lateral meniscus root tear and meniscus extrusion with anterior cruciate ligament tear. *Radiology* 2006;239(3):805-810.

20. De Smet AA, Blankenbaker DG, Kijowski R, Graf BK, Shinki K: MR diagnosis of posterior root tears of the lateral meniscus using arthroscopy as the reference standard. *AJR Am J Roentgenol* 2009;192(2):480-486.

   Standard imaging findings suggesting a meniscal tear can be used to diagnose root tears of the lateral meniscus. The concurrent presence of an ACL tear did not decrease diagnostic accuracy for a lateral root tear.

21. Guermazi A, Hayashi D, Jarraya M, et al: Medial posterior meniscal root tears are associated with development or worsening of medial tibiofemoral cartilage damage: The multicenter osteoarthritis study. *Radiology* 2013;268(3):814-821.

   Isolated medial meniscal root tears are associated with the development and progression of medial tibiofemoral cartilage loss.

22. Kijowski R, Blankenbaker DG, Davis KW, Shinki K, Kaplan LD, De Smet AA: Comparison of 1.5- and 3.0-T MR imaging for evaluating the articular cartilage of the knee joint. *Radiology* 2009;250(3):839-848.

   The use of 3-T MRI has improved the diagnostic performance of MRI (in specificity and accuracy but not sensitivity) in evaluation of the articular cartilage compared with 1.5-T MRI.

23. Kijowski R, Blankenbaker DG, Munoz Del Rio A, Baer GS, Graf BK: Evaluation of the articular cartilage of the knee joint: Value of adding a T2 mapping sequence to a routine MR imaging protocol. *Radiology* 2013;267(2):503-513.

   The addition of a T2 mapping sequence to routine 3-T MRI protocols improved sensitivity for cartilage lesions of the knee, with the greatest effect in the detection of early cartilage deterioration, from 74.6% to 88.9%. There was a small reduction in specificity.

Chapter 57

Diagnostic Ultrasound and Ultrasound-Guided Procedures

Jennifer L. Pierce, MD   Nicholas C. Nacey, MD

Abstract

Ultrasound can provide valuable information in many musculoskeletal disorders. Its low cost, nonionizing multiplanar imaging, easy accessibility, and dynamic real-time imaging make ultrasound attractive for use in patients with a sports injury or another joint-related condition. With knowledge of musculoskeletal anatomy, pathophysiology, and specific ultrasound techniques, diagnosis and effective therapeutic intervention can be performed.

Keywords: calcific tendinitis; foreign bodies; joint aspiration; musculoskeletal ultrasound; tendinosis; tendon tears; ultrasound; ultrasound-guided interventions

Introduction

Musculoskeletal ultrasound increasingly is used in both diagnostic and interventional applications. Ultrasound offers several advantages for musculoskeletal evaluation, including the absence of exposure to ionizing radiation, good soft-tissue resolution, potential for dynamic imaging, easy comparison with the contralateral side, safety for patients who cannot undergo MRI (such as those with a pacemaker), and low cost.[1,2] Ultrasound also has several disadvantages, however. Ultrasound provides a more limited field-of-view examination than other cross-sectional techniques, it has limited ability to show some structures (particularly bones and cartilage) that are easily observable on MRI, the examination is time

Neither of the following authors nor any immediate family member has received anything of value from or has stock or stock options held in a commercial company or institution related directly or indirectly to the subject of this chapter: Dr. Pierce and Dr. Nacey.

consuming, and the examination quality depends on the skill of the technician.[1] Although ultrasound can be used to complete a systematic examination of an entire joint, it is most effective when used to answer a particular clinical question or to examine a focal area.

Choosing the appropriate ultrasound transducer is critical (**Figure 1**). A high-frequency probe produces a higher resolution image of superficial structures, but a lower frequency probe is necessary to penetrate into deep tissues, as in the hip. A small-footprint, high-frequency transducer (a so-called hockey stick transducer) is used to obtain high-resolution images of superficial structures in the hands and feet or ankles. A linear high-frequency probe can be used to obtain high-resolution images of superficial structures and yields a larger field of view than the small-footprint transducer. A curved, lower frequency transducer is used to produce images of deep tissues with an even larger field of view.[1]

Modern ultrasound machines incorporate a wide array of parameters that can be used to obtain an optimal imaging examination.[1] After the appropriate transducer is chosen, a presetting is selected for the body part to be examined. The appropriate imaging depth allows the chosen structure to be studied but does not include unnecessary deeper tissues. The focal zone should be adjusted so that it lies at the targeted structure. The gain setting can be adjusted to obtain the appropriate image brightness, and time gain compensation can be adjusted so that the image brightness is homogenous throughout the superficial and deep aspects of the image. The color and power Doppler settings show an increase in blood flow and may be beneficial in detecting areas of hyperemia within inflamed tissues.[3] Many units offer extended field-of-view imaging in which the probe can be moved and multiple images can be stitched together to produce an image that is much larger than the intrinsic field of view of the transducer. A structure can be described as being hyperechoic (bright), hypoechoic (dark), or anechoic (black and typical of simple fluid). Assessment of the echogenicity, or brightness, of a structure is a critical component of the examination

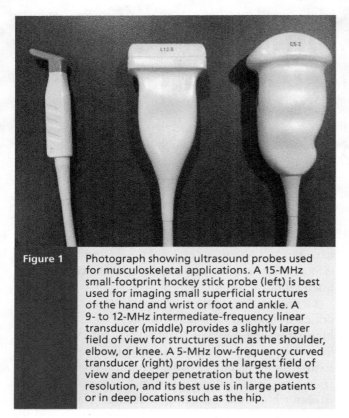

Figure 1 Photograph showing ultrasound probes used for musculoskeletal applications. A 15-MHz small-footprint hockey stick probe (left) is best used for imaging small superficial structures of the hand and wrist or foot and ankle. A 9- to 12-MHz intermediate-frequency linear transducer (middle) provides a slightly larger field of view for structures such as the shoulder, elbow, or knee. A 5-MHz low-frequency curved transducer (right) provides the largest field of view and deeper penetration but the lowest resolution, and its best use is in large patients or in deep locations such as the hip.

that can be adversely affected by inappropriate settings.

Many potential ultrasound artifacts must be considered. Anisotropy, which is most commonly seen in tendons, is an artifact unique to musculoskeletal ultrasound.[1,3] Tendon imaging must be done with the ultrasound beam aimed perpendicular to the course of the tendon to show the normal echogenic, fibrillar pattern of the tendon. If the probe is not perpendicular to the tendon, the tendon will appear to be hypoechoic, and tendinosis could mistakenly be diagnosed.

The presence of air reduces the ability of ultrasound to obtain images, and therefore it is critical to use a sufficient quantity of ultrasound gel and to maintain skin contact with the entire ultrasound transducer. The hand holding the transducer can be kept in contact with the patient's skin to improve stability. Images should be obtained in orthogonal planes to confirm an abnormality in any targeted structure. Most interventions are done using a freehand technique in which one hand holds the probe and the other holds the needle. The needle is in the plane along the long axis of the transducer so that its entire course can be seen until it reaches the target.[4] It is critical to observe the needle tip to avoid advancing more deeply than expected. Some small joints can be reached with a needle using an out-of-plane approach in which only a small cross-section of the needle is observed.[1]

Shoulder Ultrasound

One of the primary uses of musculoskeletal ultrasound is to evaluate the shoulder and in particular the rotator cuff. Ultrasound is particularly beneficial in patients who cannot undergo MRI because of claustrophobia or an implanted medical device. MRI and ultrasound by an experienced technician both have approximately 95% sensitivity and specificity for detecting a rotator cuff tear, in comparison with arthroscopy.[5] Shoulder ultrasound is limited by its dependence on the skill of the technician because of the difficulty of appropriately scanning the complicated shoulder anatomy. MRI remains the test of choice for evaluating the bones, cartilage, labrum, and intra-articular portion of the biceps because these structures cannot be well seen using ultrasound.

The supraspinatus is the most commonly torn rotator cuff tendon. Positioning the patient's hand with an anterior-facing palm along the ipsilateral lower back (the modified Crass position) moves the tendon out from under the acromion and aids visualization[6] (Figure 2). The criteria for diagnosing a rotator cuff tear include nonvisualization of the tendon, partial- or full-thickness tendon interruption with or without a hypoechoic defect, focal tendon thinning, and loss of the normal bursal surface tendon convexity.[7] Tendinosis appears as hypoechoic enlargement of the tendon with loss of its normal fibrillar echotexture, although care must be taken to distinguish this appearance from anisotropy artifact.[5] The infraspinatus and teres minor tendons are best seen from the posterior aspect of the shoulder, with the hand crossing the chest and touching the contralateral shoulder.[6] The criteria for diagnosing tears of these tendons are similar to those for diagnosing a supraspinatus tear. The nondistended subacromial-subdeltoid bursa can be seen as a thin echogenic line representing the potential space between the deltoid and supraspinatus; in bursitis, anechoic fluid is present in this space.[5]

The subscapularis tendon and extra-articular portion of the biceps tendon can be seen on ultrasound by placing the transducer along the anterior aspect of the shoulder (Figure 3). The anatomy in this area is most easily identified with the patient's shoulder externally rotated and the transducer in a horizontal position to produce a short-axis image of the biceps tendon and a long-axis image of the subscapularis tendon, similar to an axial MRI image.[6] Abnormal findings in the biceps tendon include surrounding fluid from tenosynovitis, focal anechoic slits or tendon splitting in a partial tear, and nonvisualization of the tendon in a complete disruption.[5] Subscapularis tendon tearing can be diagnosed using the criteria for a supraspinatus tear, except that the subscapularis tendon

© 2016 American Academy of Orthopaedic Surgeons

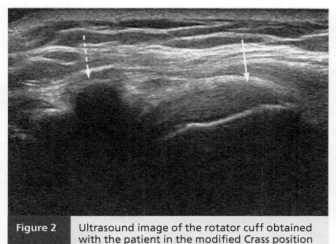

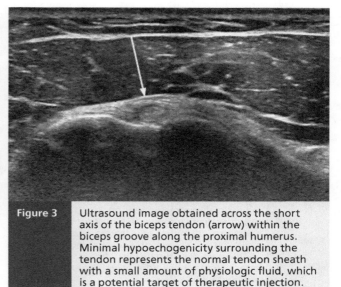

Figure 2   Ultrasound image of the rotator cuff obtained with the patient in the modified Crass position and the transducer along the long axis of the supraspinatus tendon, showing the normal fibrillar appearance of the tendon (solid arrow) and its attachment on the greater tuberosity. Posterior shadowing from the acromion (dashed arrow) can increase the difficulty of imaging the medial portion of the tendon.

Figure 3   Ultrasound image obtained across the short axis of the biceps tendon (arrow) within the biceps groove along the proximal humerus. Minimal hypoechogenicity surrounding the tendon represents the normal tendon sheath with a small amount of physiologic fluid, which is a potential target of therapeutic injection.

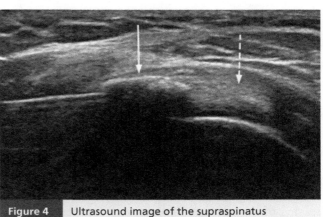

Figure 4   Ultrasound image of the supraspinatus tendon, (dashed arrow), showing a markedly hyperechoic focus (solid arrow) with posterior acoustic shadowing representing calcium hydroxyapatite deposition. A hyperechoic needle can be seen entering the calcium from the left side of the image for therapeutic calcium fenestration and aspiration.

has a multipennate appearance on short-axis images from its multiple tendon slips, which should not be misinterpreted as a tear.[8]

Ultrasound of the shoulder has multiple interventional applications. Ultrasound can be used as an alternative to fluoroscopy to guide injections into the glenohumeral or acromioclavicular joint. Subacromial-subdeltoid bursa injection can be done under ultrasound guidance as an alternative to fluoroscopy- or palpation-guided injection. The biceps tendon sheath can be quickly located with ultrasound for a peritendinous injection. Calcific tendinitis can be treated using a unique interventional application of ultrasound in the shoulder (**Figure 4**). Ultrasound can exquisitely reveal hyperechoic foci from calcium deposits. Both single- and double-needle techniques have been described.[9,10] A needle is inserted into the calcific deposit, and saline and/or anesthetic are introduced to break up the calcium, which is aspirated. After the procedure, steroids should be injected into the subacromial bursa to decrease reactive inflammation.[11] Usually it is not possible to remove all of the calcium, but at 1-year follow-up 90% of patients had improvement in symptoms and calcifications even if no calcium was removed.[12]

Elbow Ultrasound

Because of the superficial location of the distal biceps tendon, ultrasound is able to accurately diagnose a tear and determine the extent of proximal retraction of the tendon stump (**Figure 5**). Specific techniques may be necessary to

observe the distal aspect of the tendon as it courses deep to its insertion at an oblique angle and is predisposed to anisotropy.[13] During imaging in the long axis of the tendon, the application of additional pressure to the distal aspect of the transducer (the so-called heel-toe maneuver) can help keep the transducer parallel to the tendon. The long axis of the distal biceps also can be observed by flexing the elbow and positioning the transducer in the coronal plane from a lateral or medial approach.[14] Complete tears are seen as tendon discontinuity with a gap between the tendon stump and radial tuberosity. Fluid and/or hemorrhage can be seen in the tendon gap. A partial tear may be more challenging to diagnose than

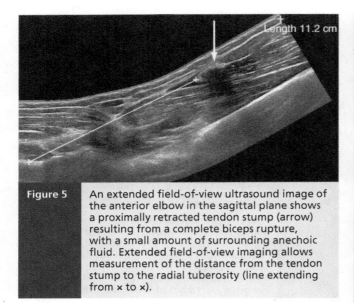

Figure 5 An extended field-of-view ultrasound image of the anterior elbow in the sagittal plane shows a proximally retracted tendon stump (arrow) resulting from a complete biceps rupture, with a small amount of surrounding anechoic fluid. Extended field-of-view imaging allows measurement of the distance from the tendon stump to the radial tuberosity (line extending from × to ×).

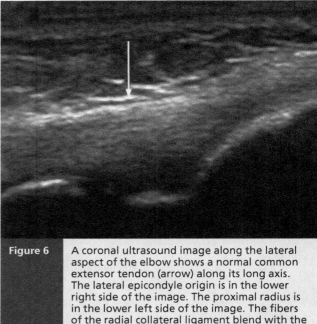

Figure 6 A coronal ultrasound image along the lateral aspect of the elbow shows a normal common extensor tendon (arrow) along its long axis. The lateral epicondyle origin is in the lower right side of the image. The proximal radius is in the lower left side of the image. The fibers of the radial collateral ligament blend with the undersurface fibers of the common extensor tendon and can be difficult to distinguish.

a complete tear, but tendon thinning, irregularity, or hypoechogenicity may be observable, sometimes with fluid in the bicipitoradial bursa.[14]

Long-axis images of the common flexor or extensor tendon can be obtained by placing the probe in the coronal plane of the flexed elbow along the medial or lateral epicondyle, respectively[13] (**Figure 6**). Tendinosis in either tendon appears as hypoechoic swelling without fiber disruption, cortical irregularity of adjacent bone, increased Doppler blood flow, or intratendinous calcifications.[15] Focal anechoic areas with fiber disruption are seen with tearing of the common flexor or extensor tendon.[13] Imaging in the same plane can be used during peritendinous steroid injection, dry tenotomy, or platelet-rich plasma injection. The collateral ligaments can be seen underlying the common extensor and flexor tendons. Ultrasound is not commonly used specifically to evaluate these ligaments, but they should be evaluated concurrently with the overlying tendons because their disruption can cause persistent symptoms after the tendinopathy is treated.[13]

Elbow neuropathy can be observed under ultrasound as enlargement of the nerve cross-sectional area and loss of the normal fascicular pattern. The ulnar nerve is easily seen in its short axis by placing the transducer transversely across the cubital tunnel.[13] As the elbow flexes, dynamic subluxation of the ulnar nerve can be seen across the apex of the medial epicondyle. If the medial head of the triceps moves along with the ulnar nerve, snapping triceps syndrome can be diagnosed.[16,17] The median and radial nerves also can be observed more anteriorly in the elbow if neuropathy is suspected, although an underlying etiology usually is difficult to identify in these sites.[13]

Wrist and Hand Ultrasound

High-resolution images of wrist and hand tendons are easy to obtain because of their superficial location. Peritendinous injection can be effectively done under ultrasound guidance.[18] Tendon rupture can occur as a result of trauma, chronic irritation caused by adjacent hardware, or an underlying inflammatory condition such as rheumatoid arthritis.[19] The torn tendon stump and extent of retraction are readily identifiable with ultrasound, which may aid in presurgical planning (**Figure 7**). In chronic tendon rupture, scar tissue along the path of the torn tendon can form a pseudotendon, which is a pitfall in ultrasound interpretation. However, the structured fibrillar-appearing collagen fibers of normal tendon usually are absent if scar tissue has replaced the normal tendon.[20]

Supporting soft-tissue structures in the fingers can be evaluated with ultrasound. Direct observation of a disrupted sagittal band can be difficult, but dynamic imaging with the hand in a clenched-fist position can show subluxation of the tendon away from the side of the ruptured sagittal band.[21] A flexor tendon pulley injury can produce tendon bowstringing, particularly in the flexed position. A distance of 1 mm between the phalanx and flexor tendon at the location of a pulley was suggested as the maximal normal distance in the flexed position, with a higher value suggesting a pulley injury.[22] Patients with trigger finger may have a thickened, hypervascular A1 pulley with associated tendinosis or tenosynovitis of

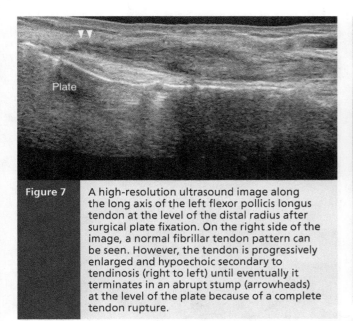

Figure 7 A high-resolution ultrasound image along the long axis of the left flexor pollicis longus tendon at the level of the distal radius after surgical plate fixation. On the right side of the image, a normal fibrillar tendon pattern can be seen. However, the tendon is progressively enlarged and hypoechoic secondary to tendinosis (right to left) until eventually it terminates in an abrupt stump (arrowheads) at the level of the plate because of a complete tendon rupture.

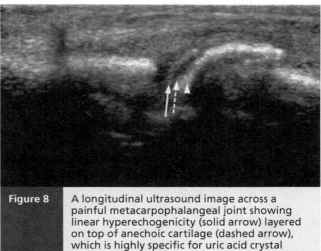

Figure 8 A longitudinal ultrasound image across a painful metacarpophalangeal joint showing linear hyperechogenicity (solid arrow) layered on top of anechoic cartilage (dashed arrow), which is highly specific for uric acid crystal deposition in gout. The underlying cortex and subchondral bone plate of the metacarpal (arrowhead) appear hyperechoic, as expected.

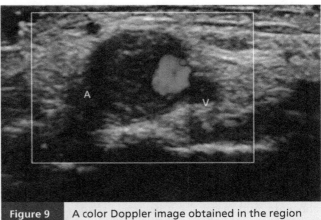

Figure 9 A color Doppler image obtained in the region of a palpable abnormality clinically suspected to be a ganglion cyst. Color flow in a rounded lesion is compatible with blood flow in a radial artery pseudoaneurysm. The echogenic material in the remainder of the mass probably represents thrombus. A ganglion cyst would be expected to be anechoic (black) and not show any internal Doppler color flow. A = artery, V = vein.

the underlying flexor tendon and possibly thickening of the volar plate.[19,23] Dynamic imaging done longitudinally along the affected tendon may show loss of normal smooth tendon gliding at the level of the A1 pulley with catching of the tendon adjacent to the pulley.[17] Collateral ligaments of the fingers, particularly the ulnar collateral ligament of the thumb, can be examined with ultrasound. Ultrasound accurately shows proximal retraction of a ruptured ulnar collateral ligament in patients with a Stener lesion.[24] Flexing the thumb at the interphalangeal joint produces motion of the adductor aponeurosis and is useful for distinguishing the adductor aponeurosis from the underlying ulnar collateral ligament.[25]

Rheumatologic evaluation can be done with ultrasound. Joint effusion appears as anechoic compressible fluid signal; in comparison, synovitis has a more heterogeneous appearance and is noncompressible.[26] Synovitis also can be distinguished from effusion on Doppler imaging by the demonstration of internal vascularity within areas of synovitis, whereas vascularity is not present in an effusion. Erosions can be identified as focal areas of cortical disruption that appear in two planes.[26] A survey of multiple joints can be done to assess for disease severity or progression. A patient with a crystal deposition disease such as gout may have effusion and synovitis as well as small hyperechoic foci within the area of synovitis or along the cartilage surface secondary to uric acid crystal deposition[27] (Figure 8).

Ultrasound can be used to confirm a suspected diagnosis of ganglion cyst in the hand or wrist. Ganglia appear as rounded, sometimes multilocular, anechoic foci, sometimes with a small neck extending toward a joint or tendon sheath. Color Doppler imaging is mandatory to exclude the possibility of an arterial aneurysm or pseudoaneurysm mimicking a ganglion cyst, particularly if aspiration is being considered (Figure 9). The presence of blood flow or echogenic signal within the lesion suggests the presence of a solid mass rather than a ganglion. Ganglion cyst fenestration and aspiration, with or without steroid injection, is effective in 89% of patients, although the lesion may reccur.[18]

Ultrasound is promising for the evaluation of carpal tunnel syndrome when used in combination with clinical examination and nerve conduction velocity studies. The

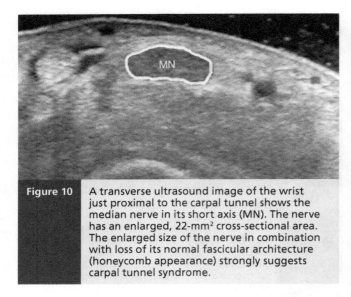

Figure 10 A transverse ultrasound image of the wrist just proximal to the carpal tunnel shows the median nerve in its short axis (MN). The nerve has an enlarged, 22-mm² cross-sectional area. The enlarged size of the nerve in combination with loss of its normal fascicular architecture (honeycomb appearance) strongly suggests carpal tunnel syndrome.

median nerve can be distinguished from the tendons of the carpal tunnel because of its honeycomb appearance and because it does not show as much loss in echogenicity with anisotropy as do the adjacent flexor tendons. A nerve cross-sectional area of less than 8 mm² can be considered normal, and a cross-sectional area of more than 12 mm² can be considered abnormal[28] (Figure 10).

Although radiography is the first-line imaging modality for the detection of foreign bodies, some foreign bodies (such as those made of glass or wood) are radiographically occult. Ultrasound is effective in screening for radiolucent foreign bodies. Most foreign bodies are echogenic, and many show posterior shadowing[29] (Figure 11). Hypoechoic tissue from a reactive inflammatory or granulomatous reaction can be seen surrounding the foreign body. Complications such as abscess formation or tendon rupture also can be detected.

Hip Ultrasound

The evaluation of patients with hip pain is elusive and challenging because of the many structures in the area and many potential pain sources. The pain may arise in superficial or deep structures, and therefore finding the optimal ultrasound transducer is important. High-frequency transducers (> 10 MHz) are ideal for examining superficial structures, but lower frequency and curvilinear transducers should be considered for the deep structures of the hip.

Placing the transducer along the anterior hip parallel to the long axis of the femoral neck allows a relative sagittal-plane image of the acetabulum, femoral head, and femoral neck to be obtained, and this location is best for

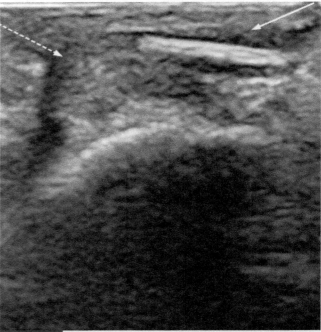

Figure 11 A high-resolution ultrasound image of a finger in its short axis showing a linear hyperechoic focus just beneath the skin surface, as is compatible with the presence of a glass foreign body (solid arrow). The foreign body was not visible on radiographs. Minimal hypoechogenicity surrounding the foreign body is compatible with inflammatory change. The foreign body is in contact with the adjacent flexor tendon (dashed arrow), but the tendon appears intact.

the evaluation of fluid or synovitis in the hip joint. Normally the anterior joint capsule of the hip is concave and will bow with convexity when distended with fluid. With this location and transducer orientation, the hip may be accessed for joint aspiration or synovial biopsy to detect infection, inflammatory arthritis, or a metal hardware complication (Figure 12). Superficial to the anterior hip capsule is the thin tendon and bulky muscle of the iliopsoas. By turning the transducer 90° and moving superiorly, an axial- or transverse-plane image of the femoral head is produced, and the oval echogenic iliopsoas tendon can be seen directly anterior to the femoral head (Figure 13). The iliopsoas tendon can be dynamically assessed for snapping or internal coxa saltans in the transverse plane with flexion, abduction, and internal rotation. Iliopsoas tendinosis and, rarely, bursitis can be detected.[30,31] Although surgical release is the definitive treatment, an initial successful response from steroid injection may be a predictor of favorable surgical outcome.[32]

Evaluation of the lateral hip over the greater trochanter is essential, particularly if gluteal tendon pathology

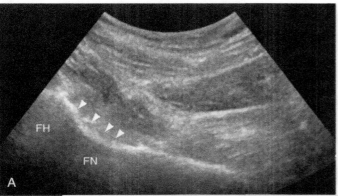

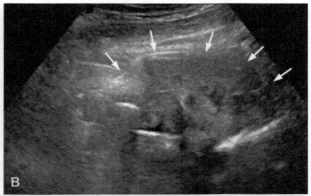

Figure 12 Ultrasound images in the longitudinal plane of the anterior hip with the transducer parallel to the femoral neck. **A,** Normal hip joint without effusion, showing the concave anterior joint capsule (arrowheads), femoral head (FH), and femoral neck (FN). **B,** A so-called bowed-out anterior capsule (arrows) with convex contours caused by a large joint effusion and synovitis secondary to an adverse reaction to metal-on-metal hip arthroplasty.

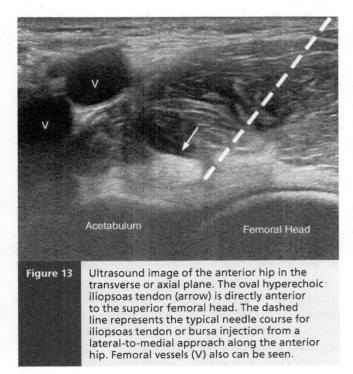

Figure 13 Ultrasound image of the anterior hip in the transverse or axial plane. The oval hyperechoic iliopsoas tendon (arrow) is directly anterior to the superior femoral head. The dashed line represents the typical needle course for iliopsoas tendon or bursa injection from a lateral-to-medial approach along the anterior hip. Femoral vessels (V) also can be seen.

is suspected. The patient is placed in the lateral decubitus position on the opposite hip, and the transducer is placed in the transverse plane over the lateral hip and bony protuberance of the greater trochanter. With movement slightly anterior to posterolateral on the greater trochanter, it is possible to see the gluteal tendons and their corresponding bursae: the gluteus minimus attachment at the anterior facet with the subjacent subgluteus minimus bursa, the gluteus medius attachment onto the lateral and superoposterior facets with the subgluteus medius bursa below it, and the large gluteus maximus attachment on the posterior facet with the interposed trochanteric or

subgluteus maximus bursa.[33] Areas of thickening and hypoechogenicity represent tendinosis or tearing. At these attachment sites on the greater trochanter, calcific tendinitis and osseous spurring with enthesopathic changes are common pain generators that can be treated with ultrasound-guided aspiration or lavage or with steroid injection, respectively.[32,33]

With the patient prone, the piriformis and the hamstring complex can be seen using a curvilinear probe that is less than 10 MHz. To locate the piriformis, the transducer is placed in the transverse plane along the inferior sacroiliac joint. As the transducer is moved caudally and laterally toward the greater trochanter, the region of the greater sciatic notch with the piriformis is seen. Passive internal and external rotation of the hip dynamically moves the piriformis muscle and confirms its location on the ultrasound image. The sciatic nerve is a large oval hypoechoic multifasciculated structure seen deep to the gluteus maximus. An ultrasound-guided piriformis injection can be done in this transverse plane with the needle coursing medial to lateral (Figure 14). A cadaver study found that ultrasound-guided piriformis injections had a 95% accuracy rate (19 of 20 injections were correctly placed into the piriformis muscle belly), compared with a 30% rate for fluoroscopy-guided injections (6 of 20 were correctly placed). Many of the fluoroscopic injections were erroneously placed into the gluteus maximus, and in one patient the placement was within the sciatic nerve.[34]

The hamstring complex, composed of the semimembranosus, semitendinosus, and biceps femoris, can be evaluated by ultrasound starting in the transverse plane at the level of the ischial tuberosity near the lower buttock or gluteal fold region. At the ischial tuberosity, the conjoined tendon of the semitendinosus and the biceps femoris inserts medially; the semimembranosus tendon

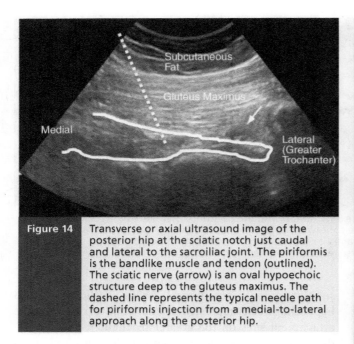

Figure 14 Transverse or axial ultrasound image of the posterior hip at the sciatic notch just caudal and lateral to the sacroiliac joint. The piriformis is the bandlike muscle and tendon (outlined). The sciatic nerve (arrow) is an oval hypoechoic structure deep to the gluteus maximus. The dashed line represents the typical needle path for piriformis injection from a medial-to-lateral approach along the posterior hip.

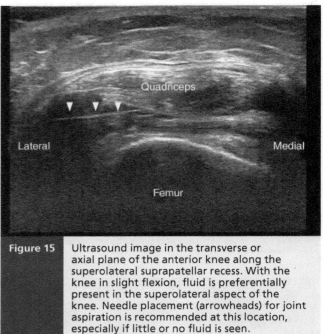

Figure 15 Ultrasound image in the transverse or axial plane of the anterior knee along the superolateral suprapatellar recess. With the knee in slight flexion, fluid is preferentially present in the superolateral aspect of the knee. Needle placement (arrowheads) for joint aspiration is recommended at this location, especially if little or no fluid is seen.

is lateral and slightly deeper. The sciatic nerve is lateral to the hamstring tendons in a region of surrounding fat at the level of the ischial tuberosity. Hypoechoic enlargement of tendon represents tendinosis and degeneration, and anechoic fluid filling a gap between disrupted, frayed tendons is diagnostic of a tendon tear.

Knee Ultrasound

Although the intra-articular and osseous structures of the knee are best evaluated using MRI, the superficial tendons and soft tissues are ideal for ultrasound examination. The normal hyperechoic and fibrillar appearance of the quadriceps and patellar tendons can be evaluated using a linear transducer of approximately 10 MHz in the sagittal plane, parallel to the extensor mechanism. The ability to dynamically evaluate the quadriceps and patellar tendons in flexion-extension motion is a unique advantage of ultrasound. Tendinosis of the quadriceps or patellar tendon is seen as hypoechoic thickening or swelling of the tendon with observable continuous fibers. Well-defined anechoic defects suggest tearing of the tendon fibers; occasionally, neovascularity and hyperemia are seen and are best depicted with power Doppler ultrasound imaging.

Just deep to the quadriceps tendon is the suprapatellar recess, which is preferentially distended by fluid in the knee. This location can be used to obtain joint aspirations in both native and postarthroplasty knee joints. With the knee in slight flexion and the transducer placed transverse to the knee, the superolateral aspect of the knee adjacent to the patella is the ideal location for joint aspiration, even

when little or no joint effusion has been seen (**Figure 15**). This location also can be used for knee injections if ultrasound guidance is necessary.

A joint effusion can communicate posteromedially into a Baker cyst (a semimembranosus–medial gastrocnemius bursa). A Baker cyst is diagnosed by location and has a small neck arising between the tendons of the semimembranosus and the medial head of the gastrocnemius. Identification of this anatomic position and relationship is critical to confirming the diagnosis of a Baker cyst and differentiating it from a heterogeneous, cystic soft-tissue neoplasm. Aspiration and injection of steroids and local anesthetic can be done if a Baker cyst is symptomatic, although fluid may reaccumulate. Ultrasound guidance of Baker cyst aspiration and injection is ideal because it provides real-time visualization of needle placement and vessel location (Figure 16).

Foot and Ankle Ultrasound

The Achilles tendon is best evaluated from a posterior approach with the patient prone. A high-frequency transducer (> 10 MHz) can be used because of the superficial location of the tendon. In the sagittal plane or parallel to the long axis of the tendon fibers, the Achilles tendon is a large uniformly hyperechoic, fibrillar tendon approximately 6 mm thick. The tendon should be scanned proximally from the gastrocnemius-soleus musculotendinous junction and distally to the calcaneal

© 2016 American Academy of Orthopaedic Surgeons

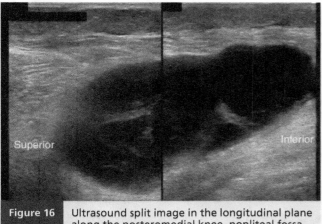

Figure 16 Ultrasound split image in the longitudinal plane along the posteromedial knee–popliteal fossa showing a predominately anechoic Baker cyst between the tendons of the semimembranosus and the medial head of the gastrocnemius. Internal debris, septations, and synovial thickening often are present in a Baker cyst.

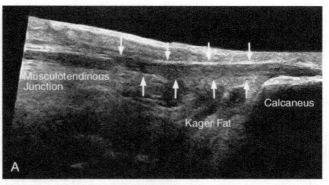

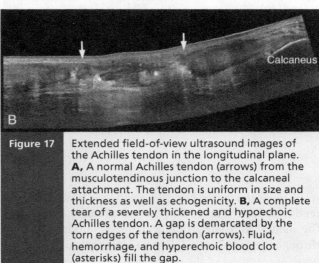

Figure 17 Extended field-of-view ultrasound images of the Achilles tendon in the longitudinal plane. **A,** A normal Achilles tendon (arrows) from the musculotendinous junction to the calcaneal attachment. The tendon is uniform in size and thickness as well as echogenicity. **B,** A complete tear of a severely thickened and hypoechoic Achilles tendon. A gap is demarcated by the torn edges of the tendon (arrows). Fluid, hemorrhage, and hyperechoic blood clot (asterisks) fill the gap.

insertion. Hypoechogenicity and fusiform thickening indicate chronic tendinosis and degeneration, which typically occur 5 to 6 cm proximal to the calcaneal insertion. The dynamic capabilities of ultrasound allow the Achilles tendon to be evaluated with dorsiflexion or plantar flexion of the foot, which can assist in the evaluation of tendon disruption or gliding dysfunction within the paratenon (Figure 17). Turning the transducer 90° produces an axial-plane image of the Achilles tendon, in which the tendon should maintain a flat to concave anterior border and not be diffusely convex. Like other ultrasound examinations of tendons, the Achilles tendon evaluation requires care to reduce anisotropy artifact and should be implemented with a back-and-forth toggle of the transducer in the transverse plane and a heel-toe maneuver in the longitudinal plane.[8]

The plantar fascia or aponeurosis is seen by placing a linear-frequency transducer along the plantarmedial aspect of the heel in the longitudinal plane. The normal fascia is uniformly hyperechoic and less than 4 mm in thickness.[35] Thickening and hypoechoic regions near the calcaneal attachment are a common finding in patients with plantar fasciitis. Comparison with an asymptomatic contralateral plantar fascia can be helpful. The transducer is turned 90° perpendicular to the long axis of the foot. An evaluation in the transverse-axial plane also should be done. Corticosteroid injection or needle tenotomy of the plantar fascia can be done in the transverse plane, with the needle entrance along the medial or lateral aspect of the heel to avoid penetrating the more sensitive plantar surface of the foot.

The superficial nature of the foot and ankle tendons and ligaments makes them well suited to ultrasound evaluation, especially with the addition of dynamic testing with motion or stressing of ligaments. Unlike postoperative MRI or CT of the foot, ultrasound of tendons and soft tissues around hardware is not degraded by metal artifact. Fluid collections and nerve or tendon impingement by adjacent plates and screws can be detected with ultrasound.

High-resolution ultrasound transducers are excellent for the evaluation of most peripheral nerves.[36] Ultrasound can reveal nerve abnormalities caused by entrapment syndromes. Dynamic testing depicts nerve impingment, abnormal motion, and nerve enlargement indicating neuritis. Ultrasound-guided local injection with corticosteroids and local anesthetic around the nerve can be beneficial for both the diagnosis and treatment of nerve entrapment or neuritis.

At the posteromedial ankle, abnormalities in the fibro-osseous tarsal tunnel can cause tarsal tunnel syndrome from impingement on the tibial nerve. The tibial nerve is large (similar in caliber to a small tendon), and it is recognized by multiple tiny hypoechoic nerve fascicles as well as its location superficial to the flexor hallucis longus. The distal phalanx of the great toe can be flexed

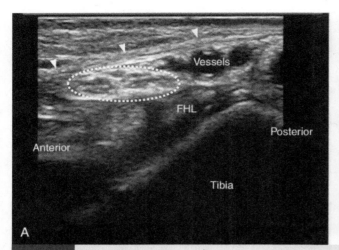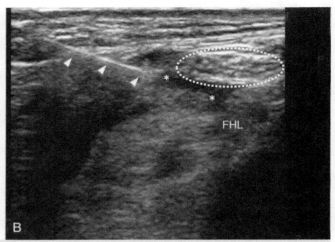

Figure 18 Ultrasound images in the transverse or axial plane of the posteromedial ankle at the tarsal tunnel. **A,** The flexor retinaculum (arrowheads) outlines the tarsal tunnel. Within the tarsal tunnel, the oval, echogenic, and multifasciculated tibial nerve (dashed circle) courses adjacent to vessels. The flexor hallucis longus (FHL) is subjacent to the tibial nerve. **B,** Combined perineural injection of corticosteroid and bupivacaine, which is hypoechoic (asterisks). The needle (arrowheads) courses anterior to posterior near the tibial nerve.

to observe the contraction of the flexor hallucis longus tendon-muscle (**Figure 18**). The tibial nerve divides into the medial and lateral plantar nerves along its course through the tarsal tunnel. If there is clinical concern about nerve entrapment of the branches of the tibial nerve, such as the first branch of the lateral plantar nerve (the Baxter nerve), ultrasound-guided injections are more effective than injections done without guidance or with fluoroscopic guidance.[37]

Summary

Ultrasound has advantages that allow it to play an important role in the diagnosis and management of many musculoskeletal disorders. Its low cost, nonionizing multiplanar imaging, easy accessibility, and dynamic real-time imaging make ultrasound attractive for use in patients with a sports injury or another joint-related condition. However, ultrasound can be significantly time consuming, is heavily technician dependent, and requires a steep initial learning curve. Knowledge of musculoskeletal anatomy, pathophysiology, and specific techniques are required for accurate diagnosis and effective therapeutic intervention in all musculoskeletal ultrasound examinations.

Key Study Points

- Higher frequency probes (> 9 MHz) are ideal for the evaluation of superficial musculoskeletal structures. A lower frequency curvilinear probe (5-6 MHz) aids in the evaluation of deeper structures and is recommended for hip ultrasound examinations.

- The normal tendons exhibit a well-defined very linear fibrillar pattern of fibers. Tendinosis is diagnosed when there is fusiform enlargement, hypochogenicity, and loss of the fibrillar pattern. If there is an anechoic gap in the tendon with separation of tendon fibers, tendon tear is highly likely.

- Anistropy is an important artifact in musculoskeletal ultrasound that can mimic pathology, such as tendon tear or tendinosis. Subtle movements of the transducer can eliminate anisotropy, such as "toggling" back and forth in the transverse plane and "heel-toeing" in the longitudinal plane. Ultrasound by an experienced technician has approximately 95% sensitivity and specificity for detecting a rotator cuff tear in comparison with arthroscopy, similar to the sensitivity and specificity of MRI.

- Ultrasound can be used as real-time guidance for musculoskeletal percutaneous interventions and injections with significant improvement in accurate needle placement as compared to the "blind approach" and fluoroscopy.

Annotated References

1. Smith J, Finnoff JT: Diagnostic and interventional musculoskeletal ultrasound: Part 1. Fundamentals. *PM R* 2009;1(1):64-75.

   This review article provides information on the physics of ultrasound, a description of basic techniques of imaging the musculoskeletal system with ultrasound, and describes the normal appearance of structures such as tendons, muscles, and nerves.

2. Nazarian LN: The top 10 reasons musculoskeletal sonography is an important complementary or alternative technique to MRI. *AJR Am J Roentgenol* 2008;190(6):1621-1626.

3. Lin J, Fessell DP, Jacobson JA, Weadock WJ, Hayes CW: An illustrated tutorial of musculoskeletal sonography: Part I. Introduction and general principles. *AJR Am J Roentgenol* 2000;175(3):637-645.

4. Louis LJ: Musculoskeletal ultrasound intervention: Principles and advances. *Radiol Clin North Am* 2008;46(3):515-533, vi.

5. Yablon CM, Bedi A, Morag Y, Jacobson JA: Ultrasonography of the shoulder with arthroscopic correlation. *Clin Sports Med* 2013;32(3):391-408.

   This review for orthopaedic surgeons describes normal rotator cuff anatomy, common pathologic findings, and common pitfalls in shoulder ultrasonography.

6. Jacobson JA: Shoulder US: Anatomy, technique, and scanning pitfalls. *Radiology* 2011;260(1):6-16.

   The author discusses technique and positioning for a thorough shoulder ultrasound examination.

7. Rutten MJ, Jager GJ, Blickman JG: US of the rotator cuff: Pitfalls, limitations, and artifacts. *Radiographics* 2006;26(2):589-604.

8. Jamadar DA, Robertson BL, Jacobson JA, et al: Musculoskeletal sonography: Important imaging pitfalls. *AJR Am J Roentgenol* 2010;194(1):216-225.

   A review of common ultrasound pitfalls for an inexperienced musculoskeletal sonographer is presented, with an emphasis on anisotropy.

9. Lee KS, Rosas HG: Musculoskeletal ultrasound: How to treat calcific tendinitis of the rotator cuff by ultrasound-guided single-needle lavage technique. *AJR Am J Roentgenol* 2010;195(3):638.

   The technique for single-needle injection or aspiration of rotator cuff calcific tendinitis is described.

10. Serafini G, Sconfienza LM, Lacelli F, Silvestri E, Aliprandi A, Sardanelli F: Rotator cuff calcific tendonitis: Short-term and 10-year outcomes after two-needle US-guided percutaneous treatment. Nonrandomized controlled trial. *Radiology* 2009;252(1):157-164.

    This 10-year study on patients treated for rotator cuff calcific tendinitis demonstrated that treated patients had improve outcomes compared to nontreated patients at 1 year; however, outcomes were similar at 5 and 10 years whether or not rotator cuff calcific tendinitis aspiration was performed.

11. Bureau NJ: Calcific tendinopathy of the shoulder. *Semin Musculoskelet Radiol* 2013;17(1):80-84.

    The imaging manifestations of shoulder calcific tendinosis are discussed, including its stages of development and interventional injection or aspiration using a single-needle technique.

12. del Cura JL, Torre I, Zabala R, Legórburu A: Sonographically guided percutaneous needle lavage in calcific tendinitis of the shoulder: Short- and long-term results. *AJR Am J Roentgenol* 2007;189(3):W128-34.

13. Konin GP, Nazarian LN, Walz DM: US of the elbow: Indications, technique, normal anatomy, and pathologic conditions. *Radiographics* 2013;33(4):E125-E147.

    Normal anatomy and the technique for an elbow ultrasound examination are described, as well as pathologic findings with an emphasis on distal biceps, common forearm flexor-extensor, and nerve pathology.

14. Brigido MK, De Maeseneer M, Morag Y: Distal biceps brachii. *Semin Musculoskelet Radiol* 2013;17(1):20-27.

    Ultrasound of the distal biceps tendon is described, with an emphasis on techniques used to identify the distal aspect of the tendon. Common pathologic entities including tendinosis and tears are discussed.

15. Radunovic G, Vlad V, Micu MC, et al: Ultrasound assessment of the elbow. *Med Ultrason* 2012;14(2):141-146.

    The elbow anterior, posterior, medial, and lateral regions are described, with a discussion of anatomy and pathology in each region.

16. Zbojniewicz AM: US for diagnosis of musculoskeletal conditions in the young athlete: Emphasis on dynamic assessment. *Radiographics* 2014;34(5):1145-1162.

    This review articles describes multiple scenarios in which dynamic maneuvers can be performed when performing musculoskeletal ultrasound. Most of these maneuvers are not possible with cross-sectional imaging, thus providing a potential advantage of ultrasound compared to cross-sectional modalities.

17. Khoury V, Cardinal E, Bureau NJ: Musculoskeletal sonography: A dynamic tool for usual and unusual disorders. *AJR Am J Roentgenol* 2007;188(1):W63-73.

18. Orlandi D, Corazza A, Silvestri E, et al: Ultrasound-guided procedures around the wrist and hand: How to do. *Eur J Radiol* 2014;83(7):1231-1238.

Techniques for common ultrasound-guided procedures are described, with an emphasis on injection of small joints, DeQuervain tenosynovitis, and trigger finger.

19. Bodor M, Fullerton B: Ultrasonography of the hand, wrist, and elbow. *Phys Med Rehabil Clin N Am* 2010;21(3):509-531.

This review intended for physiatrists describes diagnostic imaging and interventions in the hand, wrist, and elbow.

20. Pappas N, Gay AN, Major N, Bozentka D: Case report: Pseudotendon formation after a type III flexor digitorum profundus avulsion. *Clin Orthop Relat Res* 2011;469(8):2385-2388.

This case report describes the MRI appearance of a pseudotendon that formed after a complete finger tendon disruption.

21. Lopez-Ben R, Lee DH, Nicolodi DJ: Boxer knuckle (injury of the extensor hood with extensor tendon subluxation): Diagnosis with dynamic US. Report of three cases. *Radiology* 2003;228(3):642-646.

22. Klauser A, Frauscher F, Bodner G, et al: Finger pulley injuries in extreme rock climbers: Depiction with dynamic US. *Radiology* 2002;222(3):755-761.

23. Guerini H, Pessis E, Theumann N, et al: Sonographic appearance of trigger fingers. *J Ultrasound Med* 2008;27(10):1407-1413.

24. Ebrahim FS, De Maeseneer M, Jager T, Marcelis S, Jamadar DA, Jacobson JA: US diagnosis of UCL tears of the thumb and Stener lesions: Technique, pattern-based approach, and differential diagnosis. *Radiographics* 2006;26(4):1007-1020.

25. Martinoli C, Perez MM, Bignotti B, et al: Imaging finger joint instability with ultrasound. *Semin Musculoskelet Radiol* 2013;17(5):466-476.

The use of ultrasound is described for the evaluation of finger instability, with an emphasis on collateral ligament and palmar plate injuries.

26. Grainger AJ, Rowbotham EL: Rheumatoid arthritis. *Semin Musculoskelet Radiol* 2013;17(1):69-73.

Common ultrasound findings in patients with rheumatoid arthritis are described, with discussion of potential advancements in ultrasound and comparison with other modalities.

27. O'Connor PJ: Crystal deposition disease and psoriatic arthritis. *Semin Musculoskelet Radiol* 2013;17(1):74-79.

Ultrasound findings pertaining to crystal deposition disease are described, with emphasis on gout and psoriatic arthritis.

28. Peetrons PA, Derbali W: Carpal tunnel syndrome. *Semin Musculoskelet Radiol* 2013;17(1):28-33.

The use of ultrasound in evaluation of carpal tunnel syndrome is described, and multiple studies were synthesized to suggest a median nerve cross-sectional area below 8 mm^2 as normal and above 12 mm^2 as abnormal.

29. Jarraya M, Hayashi D, de Villiers RV, et al: Multimodality imaging of foreign bodies of the musculoskeletal system. *AJR Am J Roentgenol* 2014;203(1):W92-102.

The use of radiography, ultrasound, and MRI is described for the evaluation of foreign bodies, with the clinical implications of metal, glass, and wood foreign bodies.

30. Deslandes M, Guillin R, Cardinal E, Hobden R, Bureau NJ: The snapping iliopsoas tendon: New mechanisms using dynamic sonography. *AJR Am J Roentgenol* 2008;190(3):576-581.

31. Blankenbaker DG, De Smet AA, Keene JS: Sonography of the iliopsoas tendon and injection of the iliopsoas bursa for diagnosis and management of the painful snapping hip. *Skeletal Radiol* 2006;35(8):565-571.

32. Pfirrmann CW, Chung CB, Theumann NH, Trudell DJ, Resnick D: Greater trochanter of the hip: Attachment of the abductor mechanism and a complex of three bursae. MR imaging and MR bursography in cadavers and MR imaging in asymptomatic volunteers. *Radiology* 2001;221(2):469-477.

33. Labrosse JM, Cardinal E, Leduc BE, et al: Effectiveness of ultrasound-guided corticosteroid injection for the treatment of gluteus medius tendinopathy. *AJR Am J Roentgenol* 2010;194(1):202-206.

In a prospective study, 54 patients with a clinical diagnosis of gluteus medius tendinosis were evaluated after ultrasound-guided peritendinous injection with triamcinolone and bupivacaine. An average 55% reduction in pain was reported, and 70% of patients were satisfied with the results of the injection. Peritendinous ultrasound-guided corticosteroid injections may be an effective treatment of gluteus medius tendinopathy.

34. Finnoff JT, Hurdle MF, Smith J: Accuracy of ultrasound-guided versus fluoroscopically guided contrast-controlled piriformis injections: A cadaveric study. *J Ultrasound Med* 2008;27(8):1157-1163.

35. Cardinal E, Chhem RK, Beauregard CG, Aubin B, Pelletier M: Plantar fasciitis: Sonographic evaluation. *Radiology* 1996;201(1):257-259.

36. Chiou HJ, Chou YH, Chiou SY, Liu JB, Chang CY: Peripheral nerve lesions: Role of high-resolution US. *Radiographics* 2003;23(6):e15.

37. Presley JC, Maida E, Pawlina W, Murthy N, Ryssman DB, Smith J: Sonographic visualization of the first branch of the lateral plantar nerve (Baxter nerve): Technique and validation using perineural injections in a cadaveric model. *J Ultrasound Med* 2013;32(9):1643-1652.

Twelve ankle-foot cadaver specimens underwent ultrasound-guided Baxter nerve perineural injections with diluted colored latex. An optimal location for the perineural injection was found to be at the abductor hallucis–quadratus plantae interval. Surgical dissection was performed to assess injection location, and all 12 injections were found to have accurately placed the injectate around the Baxter nerve.

Index

©2016 American Academy of Orthopaedic Surgeons
Orthopaedic Knowledge Update: Sports Medicine 5

©2016 American Academy of Orthopaedic Surgeons

©2016 American Academy of Orthopaedic Surgeons

Radial nerve
    abnormal, 736f
    causes of neuropathy, 735–736
    course of, 735–736
Radiation, heat dissipation, 632f
Radiation exposure, eye injuries, 610
Radiocapitellar compartment, 734f
Radiocapitellar joint overload, 74–75
Randomization, clinical studies, 482–483
Range of motion (ROM) exercises
    after ACL injuries, 361
    circumduction, 353, 354f
    early *versus* delayed
        in rotator cuff rehabilitation, 322–323
RC Allograft, 528, 529
Realignment osteotomy, 243, 243f
Rectal sheath hematoma, 618
Rectus abdominis muscle
    abdominal wall, 163–164
    activity of, 396
Rectus femoris muscle
    activity of, 396
    anatomy, 156, 157f
    bulls-eye lesions, 157f
    injuries
        classification, 157
        treatment, 157–158, 158f
Registries
    research based on, 485–487
    sports medicine, 479–491
Rehabilitation
    before ACL reconstruction, 360
    after ACL reconstruction, 359–370
    early
        after ACL reconstruction, 360–362
    elbow injuries
        overhead athletes, 329–349
        phase I, 330–333
        phase II, 333–334
        phase III, 334–336
        phase IV, 336–338
        postoperative, 331t
    late, after ACL reconstruction, 362–366
    patellofemoral pain syndrome, 371–382
    rotator cuff, 311–328, 320t
    in skeletally immature athletes, 659
Relative risk (RR), 482
Relocation test, 4
Remplissage, Hill-Sachs lesions, 8
Renal injuries
    adult, 622
    management of, 623t
    pediatric, 621–622
Research studies
    hypotheses, 480
    knee registries, 486
    protocols, 481t
    in sports medicine, 479–491

statistics, 483–485
study design, 479–480
study types, 480–483
Resistance exercises, 322
Resistance training, 711–712
Resisted clam shell exercises, 352f
Resisted sidestep exercise, 352f
Rest, ice, compression and elevation (RICE), 152
Resting metabolic rate (RMR) testing, 578
Restore Orthobiologic soft-tissue implant, 528
Retinal injuries, 610
Retrobulbar hemorrhage, 609–610
Return to activity, elbow injuries, 336–338
Return to learn, after head injury, 689–690
Return to sport
    adolescents after head injury, 690
    after ACL injury, 366t
    after ACL reconstruction, 359–370
    after ACL repair, 179
    after concussions, 418, 419t
    after spinal injury, 428
    athletes with hip injuries, 355
    graduated protocol, 474t
    protocols, 151–152
    proximal thigh injuries, 151–152
    team physicians and, 470, 471
Reverse total shoulder arthroplasty, 38
Revo knots, 534
Rheumatologic inflammation, ultrasound of, 759
Rhinorrhea, clear, 606
Rhinovirus, 594–595
Ringworm, 591
Robbery exercise, 315f
Robinson classification, 24f
Roman numeral X reconstruction, 27f
Romberg sign, 436, 436t
Romberg test, positive, 453
Rotational osteotomy, 8
Rotator cuff, 33–41
    anatomy, 33–34
    biomechanics, 33–34
    etiology of disease, 34
    genetics, 33–34
    glenohumeral MRI, 723–730
    imaging of, 35, 37f
    interval, 726–728, 728f
    muscle degeneration, 34t
    natural history of disease, 33
    pathology of
        nonsurgical treatment, 35–36
        surgical considerations, 36–37
    physical examination of, 34–35
    postoperative concerns, 37
    rehabilitation, 311–328, 320t–321t
    repair
        implants in, 527–529

platelet-rich plasma in, 506–508, 508t
    stem cells in, 511
    ROM, early *versus* delayed, 322–323
    societal effect of disease, 33
    tears, 34, 35f, 724f
        MRA, 723
        MRI, 723
        prevalence by age, 34f
    tendon transfers, 37–38
    ultrasound evaluation of, 756, 757f
Rotavirus, 595–596
RotorloC, 532
Roux-Goldthwait procedure, 669
Rowing motion exercises, 313–314
Royal London Hospital Test, 386
Running athletes, rehabilitation, 354
Ruptured globe, 609

S

S100B protein, 416
Sacroiliac joint laxity, 394
Saddle-nose deformities, 606
Sagittal band injury, 104
Salicylic acid, for verruca, 588
Salmonella
    etiology, 597t
    GI infections, 596
Salter-Harris physeal fractures, 655
San Diego knots, 534
Scaffolds, tissue therapies, 512–513
Scapholunate interval, 108f
Scapholunate ligament injuries, 107
Scapular plane elevation
    early stabilization exercises, 320
    musculature, 333t
    for rotator cuff pathology, 312–313, 313f
Scapular retraction exercises, 313–314
Scapulothoracic dyskinesia, 47
Sciatic nerve
    anatomy of, 144f
    ultrasound evaluation of, 761
Sciatic notch, ultrasound of, 762f
Scleraxis gene, 499
Sclerotherapy, in tendinopathy, 498
Scoliosis Research Society questionnaire, 460
Scranton-McDermott classification, 285
Seated knee extension, 361
Seattle Criteria, 562, 563t
Second-impact syndrome
    in adolescents, 691–692
    concussions, 419–420
Selective serotonin reuptake inhibitors (sSRIs), 419
Sensory Organization Test (SOT), 415
Sequent device, 535
Sertaconazole, 590
Sesamoid disorders, 291
Sexually transmitted infections, 596, 597

©2016 American Academy of Orthopaedic Surgeons

©2016 American Academy of Orthopaedic Surgeons

©2016 American Academy of Orthopaedic Surgeons